CASE STUDY

☞ Case Studies illustrate key points.

CASE STUDY

☞ See examples on pages 239, 251, 495, and 780.

"Contents in Brief" located on page x.

TEST YOUR CRITICAL THINKING SKILLS

Boxes reinforce problem-solving skills.

☞ See examples on pages 333, 351, 529, 554, 699 and 847.

RESEARCH NOTE

Offer additional background material.

☞ See examples on pages 352, 530, 705, 733, and 783.

INTERNET REFERENCES

- Internet Reference boxes list websites for additional information.
- For examples, see pages 334, 498, 530, 705 and 733.

PSYCHIATRIC MENTAL HEALTH NURSING

CONCEPTS OF CARE

PSYCHIATRIC MENTAL HEALTH NURSING
CONCEPTS OF CARE

THIRD EDITION

MARY C. TOWNSEND, RN, MN, CS

Clinical Nurse Specialist
Adult Psychiatric/Mental Health Nursing
Private Practice
Oklahoma City, Oklahoma

Former Assistant Professor and
Coordinator, Mental Health Nursing
Kramer School of Nursing
Oklahoma City University
Oklahoma City, Oklahoma

F.A. DAVIS COMPANY / PUBLISHERS • PHILADELPHIA

F. A. Davis Company
1915 Arch Street
Philadelphia, PA 19103

Printed in the United States of America

List digit indicates print number: 10 9 8 7 6 5 4 3 2

Publisher, Nursing: Robert G. Martone
Production Editor: Michael Schnee
Cover Designer: Louis J. Forgione

As new scientific information becomes available through basic and clinical research, recommended treatments and drug therapies undergo changes. The author and publisher have done everything possible to make this book accurate, up to date, and in accord with accepted standards at the time of publication. The author, editors, and publisher are not responsible for errors or omissions or for consequences from application of the book, and make no warranty, expressed or implied, with regard to the contents of the book. Any practice described in this book should be applied by the reader in accordance with professional standards of care used with regard to the unique circumstances that may apply in each situation. The reader is advised always to check product information (package inserts) for changes and new information regarding dose and contraindications before administering any drug. Caution is especially urged when using new or infrequently ordered drugs.

Library of Congress Cataloging-in-Publication Data

Townsend, Mary C., 1941–
    Psychiatric mental health nursing : concepts of care / Mary C.
  Townsend.—3rd ed.
      p. cm.
    Includes bibliographic references and index.
    ISBN 0-8036-0483-1 (alk. paper)
    1. Psychiatric nursing. I. Title.
    [DNLM: 1. Psychiatric Nursing—methods. 2. Mental Disorders—
nursing. 3. Psychotherapy Nurses' Instruction. WY 160 T749p
2000]
  RC440.T693   2000
  610.73′68—dc21
  DNLM/DLC
  for Library of Congress   99-37381
                                          CIP

THIS BOOK IS DEDICATED

To Francie:

God made sisters for sharing laughter

and wiping tears.

PREFACE

TO THE THIRD EDITION

As we arrive at the door to the 21st century, psychiatric nursing finds itself in the midst of numerous complex challenges. The movement toward the use of sophisticated technology has required that psychiatric nurses be knowledgeable about computerized scans and imaging techniques in this major shift toward the "medicalization" of psychiatry. This biological shift in psychiatry has also made it necessary for psychiatric nurses to be familiar with the concepts of psychoimmunology, neuroendocrinology, and genetics, and the role these may play in mental illness. The *Statement on Psychiatric–Mental Health Clinical Nursing Practice and Standards of Psychiatric–Mental Health Clinical Nursing Practice* (American Nurses Association, 1994) states:

> "Some fear that the pendulum may swing too far in the direction of relying on medical treatments for all psychiatric and mental health problems, to the exclusion of psychotherapeutic interventions. This is unlikely since research to date substantiates the superiority of the combined treatment of psychopharmacology and psychotherapy in severe mental illness to any one treatment by itself." (p. 3)

Another challenge is the continuation of the shift of psychiatric nursing to the community setting and away from the acute care setting. There is little doubt that today health care is driven by cost rather than by need. Only the very severely ill clients are hospitalized. Pressure is then placed on health care providers to ensure stabilization as quickly as possible—usually with pharmacological intervention—and to release the client to the community, often while he or she is still acutely ill. This generally means that intensive case management or psychiatric home care is required.

The trend of caring for these individuals in the community parallels the U.S. Department of Health and Human Services' goals outlined in the 1990 report, *Healthy People 2000: National Health Promotion and Disease Prevention.* The overall objective of this effort was to work toward an increase in a healthy life span for all Americans, which was to be accomplished through health promotion and disease prevention strategies. In light of this perspective, the focus of psychiatric nursing is changing. Greater emphasis is being placed on primary prevention (e.g., education about stress management, healthy coping, and the effects of substances) and tertiary prevention (e.g., psychiatric rehabilitation to prevent reinstitutionalization) than in the past, when the emphasis was on secondary prevention (e.g., care of individuals after they became mentally ill).

Features That Have Been Retained

This textbook has attempted since the first edition to include aspects of the three levels of prevention as they apply to individuals with emotional illness, or to those who are at risk for such illness. The concept of pyschobiology was strengthened in the second edition with the addition of a chapter devoted entirely to this topic. Changes in the theories behind some psychiatric disorders—from the implication of purely psychological predisposing factors to purely biological ones—have been discussed. The major conceptual framework of stress/adaptation has been retained for its ease of comprehensibility and workability in the realm of psychiatric nursing. This framework continues to emphasize the multiple causes of mental illness while accepting the increasing biological implications in the etiology of certain disorders.

The concept of holistic nursing is retained in the third edition. I have attempted to ensure that the physical aspects of psychiatric/mental health nursing are not overlooked. Both physical and psychosocial nursing diagnoses are included for physiological disorders (such as asthma, migraine headache, and HIV disease) and for psychological disorders (such as depression and anxiety). In all relevant situations, the mind-body connection is addressed.

Nursing process is retained in the third edition, as the tool for delivery of care to the individual with a psychiatric disorder, or to assist in the primary prevention or the mitigation of mental illness symptoms. The six steps of the nursing process, as described in the *Standards of Clinical Nursing Practice, 2nd Ed.* (ANA, 1998), are used to provide guidelines for the nurse. These standards of care are included for the *DSM-IV* diagnoses and as they relate to the aging individual, the individual with HIV disease, and as examples in several of the therapeutic approaches. The six steps include:

Assessment: Data collection, under the format of *Background Assessment Data: Symptomatology*, which provides extensive assessment data for the nurse to draw upon when performing an assessment. Several assessment tools are also included.

Diagnosis: Analysis of the data is included, from which nursing diagnoses common to specific psychiatric disorders are derived.

Outcome Identification: Outcomes are derived from the nursing diagnoses and stated as measurable goals.

Planning: A plan of care is presented with selected nursing diagnoses for all *DSM-IV* diagnoses, as well as for the elderly client, the client with HIV disease, the elderly homebound client, and the primary caregiver of the client with a chronic mental illness. *Critical Pathways of Care* are included for clients in alcohol withdrawal, schizophrenic psychosis, depression, mania, PTSD, and anorexia nervosa. The planning standard now also includes tables that list topics for educating clients and families about mental illness.

Implementation: The interventions that have been identified in the plan of care are included along with a rationale for each. Case studies at the end of each *DSM-IV* chapter assist the student in the practical application of theoretical material. Also included as a part of this particular standard is Unit II of the textbook: *Therapeutic Approaches in Psychiatric Nursing Care.* This section of the book addresses psychiatric nursing intervention in depth, and frequently speaks to the differentiation in scope of practice between the basic-level psychiatric nurse and the advanced practice–level psychiatric nurse. Advanced-practice nurses with prescriptive authority will find the extensive chapter on psychopharmacology particularly helpful.

Evaluation: The evaluation standard includes a set of questions that the nurse may use to assess whether the nursing actions have been successful in achieving the objectives of care.

New to the Third Edition

Several new chapters, as well as new features, are included in this third edition. Two new chapters are included in Unit II: *Therapeutic Approaches in Psychiatric Nursing Care.* One new chapter, "Cognitive Therapy," was chosen because of the continued expansion of its use. Cognitive therapy was originally developed for use with depression. Today it is used for a broad range of emotional disorders, both alone or in combination with behavior therapy. An example of how cognitive therapy is used with a client is included in this chapter.

The second new chapter in Unit II is titled "Complementary Therapies." Complementary therapies include methods that deviate from the traditional methods of treating illness. This is a growing practice in the United States, where more than $15 billion is currently spent each year on these alternative methodologies. The enormity of this behavioral pattern emphasizes the importance for nurses to have knowledge about these alternative methods so that they may communicate them to and educate their clients about them.

Two additional new chapters have been included in Unit IV: *Special Topics in Psychiatric/Mental Health Nursing.* These chapters are "Psychiatric Home Nursing Care" and "Forensic Nursing." Both of these topics are emerging and expanding in the realm of psychiatric nursing and providing challenges that must be addressed. All chapters throughout the text have been updated and revised to reflect today's health care reformation and to provide information based on the current state of the discipline of nursing.

Additional features new to the third edition include:

- Abstracts describing research studies conducted on *DSM-IV* diagnoses
- Tables with guidelines for client education related to specific psychiatric illnesses
- An appendix with a list of common psychiatric behaviors and associated NANDA nursing diagnoses
- Internet references for each *DSM-IV* diagnosis, with website listing for information related to the disorder

It is my hope that the revisions and additions to this third edition continue to satisfy a need within psychiatric/mental health nursing practice. Many of the changes reflect feedback that I have received from users of the first and second editions. To those individuals I express a heartfelt thanks. I welcome comments, in an effort to retain what some have called the "user friendliness" of the text. I hope that this third edition continues to promote and advance the commitment to psychiatric/mental health nursing.

MARY C. TOWNSEND

Acknowledgments

I owe a great deal of thanks to many people who supported me with their time and encouragement throughout this second revision. To name a few, I thank:

Ruth DeGeorge, Editorial Assistant, F. A. Davis Company, for your bright and cheerful voice on the other end of the phone, and for your never-ending willingness to provide assistance. It seems I only needed to ask.

Robert G. Martone, Publisher, Nursing, F. A. Davis Company, for your sense of humor and continuous optimistic outlook.

Robert C. Butler, Director of Production, and Michael Schnee, Production Editor, F. A. Davis Company, for their sincere and diligent efforts to ensure a timely publication of the text.

The nursing educators and clinicians who provide input and help keep me informed about current clinical and state-of-the-discipline issues.

My mother, Camalla Welsh, who continues to be a bright spot in the lives of all who know her.

My daughters, Kerry and Tina, for all the joy you have provided me and all the hope that you instill in me. You keep me young at heart.

My constant companions, Affie and Bucky, for the pure pleasure you bring into my life every day that you live.

My husband, Jim, who gives meaning to my life in so many ways. You are the one whose encouragement keeps me motivated, whose support gives me strength, and whose gentleness gives me comfort.

Contents in Brief

CONTENTS

CHAPTER **4**

Concepts of Psychobiology 49

UNIT TWO

THERAPEUTIC APPROACHES IN PSYCHIATRIC NURSING CARE 77

CHAPTER **5**

Relationship Development 79

CHAPTER **6**

Therapeutic Communication 89

CHAPTER 11

Crisis Intervention 167

CHAPTER 12

Relaxation Therapy 177

CHAPTER 13

Assertiveness Training 187

CHAPTER 14

Promoting Self-Esteem 199

CHAPTER 15
Anger/Aggression Management   213

CHAPTER 16
The Suicidal Client   225

CHAPTER 17
Behavior Therapy   235

CHAPTER **23**

**Delirium, Dementia,
and Amnestic Disorders** 339

CHAPTER **24**

Substance-Related Disorders 357

CHAPTER **27**

Anxiety Disorders 469

CHAPTER **28**

Somatoform and Sleep Disorders 504

CHAPTER **29**

Dissociative Disorders 535

CHAPTER **30**

Sexual and Gender Identity Disorders 559

UNIT ONE

BASIC CONCEPTS IN PSYCHIATRIC/MENTAL HEALTH NURSING

AN INTRODUCTION TO THE CONCEPT OF STRESS

CHAPTER OUTLINE

OBJECTIVES

INTRODUCTION

STRESS AS A BIOLOGICAL RESPONSE

STRESS AS AN ENVIRONMENTAL EVENT

STRESS AS A TRANSACTION BETWEEN THE INDIVIDUAL AND THE ENVIRONMENT

STRESS MANAGEMENT

SUMMARY

REVIEW QUESTIONS

KEY TERMS

stress
adaption
maladaptation

"fight or flight syndrome"
general adaptation
  syndrome

precipitating event
predisposing factors

OBJECTIVES

After reading this chapter, the student will be able to:

1. Define *adaptation* and *maladaptation*
2. Identify physiological responses to stress.
3. Explain the relationship between stress and "diseases of adaptation."
4. Describe the concept of stress as an environmental event.
5. Explain the concept of stress as a transaction between the individual and the environment.
6. Discuss adaptive coping strategies in the management of stress.

sychologists and others have struggled for many years to establish an effective definition of the term **stress**. This term is used loosely today and still lacks definitive explanation. As one researcher said, "Stress, in addition to being itself, and the result of itself, is also the cause of itself" (Wallis, 1983). Responses directed at stabilizing internal biological processes and the preserving of self-esteem can be viewed as healthy **adaptation** to stress.

Roy (1976) defined adaptive response as behavior that maintains the integrity of the individual. Adaptation is viewed as positive and is correlated with a healthy response. When behavior disrupts the integrity of the individual, it is perceived as **maladaptive** (Roy, 1976). Maladaptive responses by the individual are considered to be negative or unhealthy.

Various researchers of this century have contributed to several different concepts of stress. Three of these concepts include stress as a biological response, stress as an environmental event, and stress as a transaction between the individual and the environment.

STRESS AS A BIOLOGICAL RESPONSE

In 1956, Hans Selye published the results of his research concerning the physiological response of a biological system to a change imposed on it. Since his initial publication, he has revised his definition of stress to " . . . the state manifested by a specific syndrome which consists of all the nonspecifically-induced changes within a biologic system" (Selye, 1976). This syndrome of symptoms has come to be known as the **"fight or flight syndrome."** Schematics of these biological responses, both initially and with sustained stress, are presented in Figures 1.1 and 1.2. Selye called this general reaction of the body to stress the **general adaptation syndrome.** He described the reaction in three distinct stages:

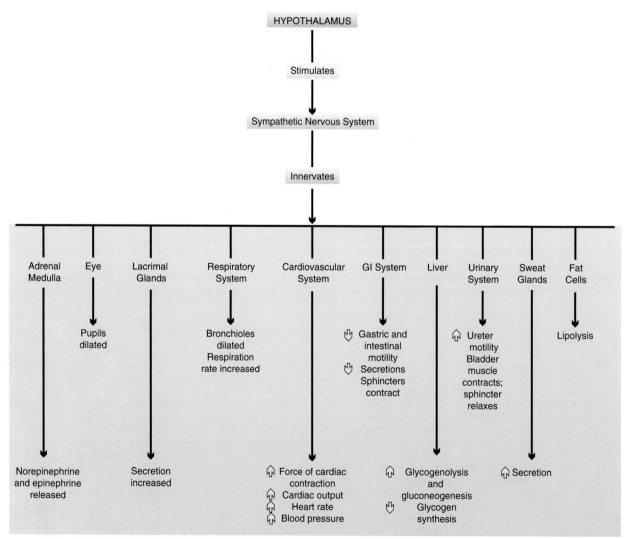

Figure 1.1   The "fight or flight syndrome": the initial stress response.

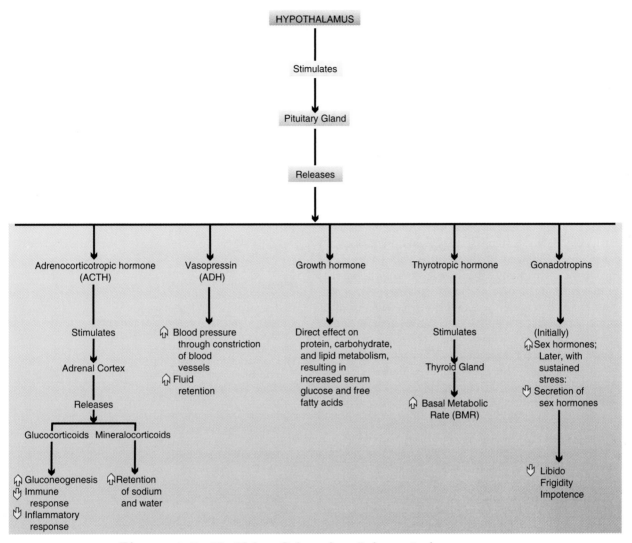

Figure 1.2 The "fight or flight syndrome": the sustained stress response.

1. **Alarm Reaction Stage.** During this stage, the physiological responses of the "fight or flight syndrome" are initiated.

2. **Stage of Resistance.** The individual uses the physiological responses of the first stage as a defense in the attempt to adapt to the stressor. If adaptation occurs, the third stage is prevented or delayed. Physiological symptoms may disappear.

3. **Stage of Exhaustion.** This stage occurs when there is a prolonged exposure to the stressor to which the body has become adjusted. The adaptive energy is depleted, and the individual can no longer draw from the resources for adaptation described in the first two stages. Diseases of adaptation (e.g., headaches, mental disorders, coronary artery disease, ulcers, colitis) may occur. Without intervention for reversal, exhaustion and even death ensue (Selye, 1956, 1974).

This "fight or flight" response undoubtedly served our ancestors well. Those *Homo sapiens* who had to face the giant grizzly bear or the saber-toothed tiger as a facet of their struggle for survival must have used these adaptive resources to their advantage. The response was elicited in the emergency situation, used in the preservation of life, and followed by restoration of the compensatory mechanisms to the preemergent condition (homeostasis).

Selye performed his extensive research in a controlled setting with laboratory animals as subjects. He elicited the physiological responses with physical stimuli, such as exposure to heat or frigid temperatures, electric shock, injection of toxic agents, restraint, and surgical injury. Since the publication of his original research, it has become apparent that the "fight or flight" syndrome of symptoms occurs in response to psychological or emotional stimuli, just as it does to physical stimuli. The psychological or emotional stressors are often not resolved as rapidly as some physical stressors, and therefore the body may be depleted of its adaptive energy more readily than it is from physical stressors. The "fight or flight" response may be inappropriate, even dangerous, to the lifestyle of today, in which stress has been described as "a pervasive, chronic and relentless psychosocial situation" (Wallis, 1983). It is this chronic response that maintains the body in the aroused condition for extended periods of time that promotes susceptibility to diseases of adaptation (Hafen, Karren, Frandsen, & Smith, 1996).

STRESS AS AN ENVIRONMENTAL EVENT

A second concept defines stress as the "thing" or "event" that triggers the adaptive physiological and psychological responses in an individual. The event is one that creates change in the life pattern of the individual, requires significant adjustment in lifestyle, and taxes available personal resources. The change can be either positive, such as outstanding personal achievement, or negative, such as being fired from a job. The emphasis here is on *change* from the existing steady state of the individual's life pattern.

Holmes and Rahe (1967) developed a method of correlating the effects of life change with illness. They tested their hypotheses with more than 5000 people. From their research, they devised the Social Readjustment Rating Scale (Table 1.1). Numerical values were assigned to various events, or changes, that are common in people's lives. Holmes and Rahe concluded from the results of their research that the higher the score on the Social Readjustment Rating Scale, the greater the susceptibility of that individual to physical or psychological illness. The score can be interpreted in the following manner:

0–150	No significant possibility of stress-related illness
150–199	Mild life crisis level—35 percent chance of illness
200–299	Moderate life crisis level—50 percent chance of illness
300 or more	Major life crisis level—80 percent chance of illness

It is unknown whether stress overload merely predisposes a person to illness or actually precipitates it, but there does appear to be a causal link (Pelletier, 1992). The Holmes and Rahe Social Readjustment Rating Scale has been criticized because it does not consider the individual's perception of the event. Individuals differ in their reactions to life events, and these variations are related to the degree to which the change is perceived as stressful. The Social Readjustment Rating Scale also fails to consider the individual's coping strategies and available support systems at the time of the life change. Positive coping mechanisms and strong social or familial support can reduce the intensity of the stressful life change and promote a more adaptive response.

TABLE 1.1 SOCIAL READJUSTMENT RATING SCALE

LIFE EVENT	MEAN VALUE
Death of spouse	100
Divorce	73
Marital separation	65
Jail term	63
Death of close family member	63
Personal illness or injury	53
Marriage	50
Fired from work	47
Marital reconciliation	45
Retirement	45
Change in family member's health	44
Pregnancy	40
Sex difficulties	39
Addition to family	39
Business readjustment	39
Change in financial status	38
Death of close friend	37
Change to different line of work	36
Change in number of marital arguments	35
Mortgage or loan greater than $10,000	31
Foreclosure of mortgage or loan	30
Change in work responsibilities	29
Son or daughter leaving home	29
Trouble with in-laws	29
Outstanding personal achievement	28
Spouse begins or stops work	26
Starting or finishing school	26
Change in living conditions	25
Revision of personal habits	24
Trouble with boss	23
Change in work hours, conditions	20
Change in residence	20
Change in schools	20
Change in recreational habits	19
Change in church activities	19
Change in social activities	18
Mortgage or loan less than $10,000	17
Change in sleeping habits	16
Change in number of family gatherings	15
Change in eating habits	15
Vacation	13
Christmas season	12
Minor violation of the law	11

SOURCE: Reprinted with permission from Journal of Psychosomatic Research, Vol 11, Holmes, T & Rahe, R, The Social Readjustment Rating Scale. Copyright © 1967, Pergamon Press, plc.

STRESS AS A TRANSACTION BETWEEN THE INDIVIDUAL AND THE ENVIRONMENT

This definition of stress emphasizes the *relationship* between the individual and the environment. Personal characteristics as well as the nature of the environmental event are considered (Lazarus & Folkman, 1984). This illustration parallels the modern concept of the etiology of disease. No longer is causation viewed solely as an external organism; whether or not illness occurs depends also on the receiving organism's susceptibility. Similarly, to predict psychological stress as a reaction, the properties of the person in relation to the environment must be considered.

Precipitating Event

Lazarus and Folkman (1984) define *stress* as a relationship between the person and the environment that is appraised by the person as taxing or exceeding his or her resources and endangering his or her well-being. A **precipitating event** is a stimulus arising from the internal or external environment and is perceived by the individual in a specific manner. Determination that a particular person/environment relationship is stressful depends on the individual's cognitive appraisal of the situation. *Cognitive appraisal* is an individual's evaluation of the personal significance of the event or occurrence. The event "precipitates" a response on the part of the individual, and the response is influenced by the individual's perception of the event. The *cognitive response* consists of a primary appraisal and a secondary appraisal.

Individual's Perception of the Event

Primary Appraisal

Lazarus and Folkman (1984) identify three types of primary appraisal: irrelevant, benign-positive, and stressful. An event is judged *irrelevant* when the outcome holds no significance for the individual. A *benign-positive* outcome is one that is perceived as producing pleasure for the individual. *Stress* appraisals include harm/loss, threat, and challenge. *Harm/loss* appraisals refer to damage or loss already experienced by the individual. Appraisals of a *threatening* nature are perceived as anticipated harms or losses. When an event is appraised as *challenging*, the individual focuses on potential for gain or growth, rather than on risks associated with the event. Challenge produces stress even though the emotions associated with it (eagerness and excitement) are viewed as positive, and coping mechanisms must be called upon to face the new encounter. Challenge and threat may occur together when an individual experiences these positive emotions along with fear or anxiety over possible risks associated with the challenging event.

When stress is produced in response to harm/loss, threat, or challenge, a secondary appraisal is made by the individual.

Secondary Appraisal

This secondary appraisal is an assessment of skills, resources, and knowledge that the person possesses to deal with the situation. The individual evaluates:

- What coping strategies are available to me?
- Will the option I choose be effective in this situation?
- Do I have the ability to use that strategy in an effective manner?

The interaction between the primary appraisal of the event that has occurred and the secondary appraisal of available coping strategies determines the individual's quality of adaptation response to stress.

Predisposing Factors

A variety of elements influence how an individual perceives and responds to a stressful event. These **predisposing factors** strongly influence whether the response is adaptive or maladaptive. Types of predisposing factors include genetic influences, past experiences, and existing conditions.

Genetic influences are those circumstances of an individual's life that are acquired by heredity. Examples include family history of physical and psychological conditions (strengths and weaknesses) and temperament (behavioral characteristics present at birth that evolve with development).

Past experiences are occurrences that result in learned patterns that can influence an individual's adaptation response. They include previous exposure to the stressor or other stressors, learned coping responses, and degree of adaptation to previous stressors.

Existing conditions incorporate vulnerabilities that influence the adequacy of the individual's physical, psychological, and social resources for dealing with adaptive demands (Murphy & Moriarty, 1976). Examples include current health status, motivation, developmental maturity, severity and duration of the stressor, financial and educational resources, age, existing coping strategies, and a support system of caring others.

This transactional model of stress/adaptation will serve as a framework for the process of nursing in this text. A graphic display of the model is presented in Figure 1.3.

STRESS MANAGEMENT*

Stress management has become a multimillion-dollar-a-year business. Stress management involves the use of coping strategies in response to stressful situations. Coping strategies are adaptive when they protect the individual from harm (or additional harm) or strengthen the individual's ability to meet challenging situations. Adaptive responses help restore homeostasis to the body and impede the development of diseases of adaptation.

---

*Techniques of stress management are discussed at greater length in Unit Two of this text.

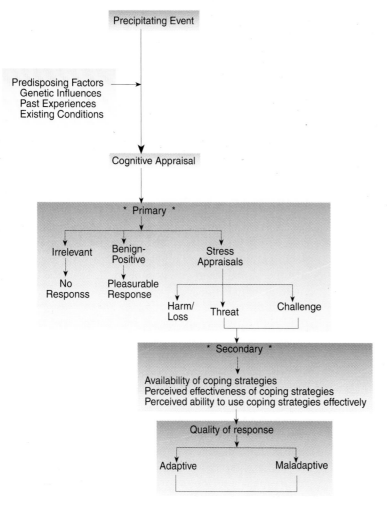

Figure 1.3 Transactional model of stress/adaptation.

Coping strategies are considered maladaptive when the conflict being experienced goes unresolved or intensifies. Energy resources become depleted as the body struggles to compensate for the chronic physiological and psychological arousal being experienced. The effect is a significant vulnerability to physical or psychological illness. (A detailed discussion of the types of diseases of adaptation can be found in Chapter 33.)

Adaptive Coping Strategies

Awareness

The initial step in managing stress is awareness—to become aware of the factors that create stress and the feelings associated with a stressful response. Stress can be controlled only when one recognizes that it is being experienced. As one becomes aware of stressors, they can be either omitted, avoided, or accepted.

Relaxation

Individuals experience relaxation in different ways. Some individuals relax by engaging in large motor activities, such as sports, jogging, and physical exercise. Still others use techniques such as breathing exercises and progressive relaxation to relieve stress. (A discussion of relaxation therapy can be found in Chapter 12.)

Meditation

Practiced 20 minutes once or twice daily, meditation has been shown to produce a lasting reduction in blood pressure and other stress-related symptoms (Wallis, 1983). Meditation involves assuming a comfortable position, closing the eyes, casting off all other thoughts, and concentrating on a single word, sound, or phrase that has positive meaning to the individual. The technique is described in detail in Chapter 12.

Interpersonal Communication With Caring Other

As previously mentioned, the strength of one's available support systems is an existing condition that significantly influences the adaptiveness of coping with stress. Sometimes just "talking the problem out" with an individual who is empathetic is sufficient to interrupt escalation of the stress response. Writing about one's feelings in a journal or diary can also be very therapeutic.

Problem Solving

An extremely adaptive coping strategy is to view the situation objectively (or to seek assistance from another individual to accomplish this if the anxiety level is too high to concentrate). After an objective assessment of the situation, the problem-solving/decision-making model can be instituted:

1. Assess the facts of the situation.
2. Formulate goals for resolution of the stressful situation.
3. Study the alternatives for dealing with the situation.
4. Determine the risks and benefits of each alternative.
5. Select an alternative.
6. Implement the alternative selected.
7. Evaluate the outcome of the alternative implemented.
8. If the first choice is ineffective, select and implement a second alternative.

Pets

Recent psychological studies have begun to uncover evidence that those who care for pets, especially dogs and cats, are better able to cope with the stressors of life (Leepson, 1984). The physical act of stroking or petting a dog or cat can be therapeutic. It gives the animal the intuitive knowledge that it is being cared for and also gives the individual the calming feeling of warmth, affection, and interdependence with a reliable, trusting being. One study showed that among people who had had heart attacks, pet owners had one-fifth the death rate of those who did not have pets (Ornstein & Sobel, 1989).

Music

It is true that music can "soothe the savage beast." Creating and listening to music both stimulate motivation, enjoyment, and relaxation. Music reduces depression and brings about measurable changes in mood and general activity (Feder & Feder, 1981).

Individuals must determine what coping strategies are adaptive for them. A few examples have been presented here. Various therapies for assisting individuals to cope adaptively are presented in Unit Two of this text.

SUMMARY

Stress has become a chronic and pervasive condition in the United States today. We live in a world of uncertain-

ties, with a sophisticated media that keeps us informed and knowledgeable about the upheavals occurring around the world. In our own country, "life in the fast lane," a continuous drive for advancement, competitiveness, and the search for "the good life" have created a stress epidemic that has individuals, corporations, and health professionals searching for ways to calm the collective masses.

The term *stress* has only recently come into vogue, partly because of the persistent lack of an adequate definition for the concept. Selye, who has become known as the founding father of stress research, defined stress as ". . . the state manifested by a specific syndrome which consists of all the nonspecifically-induced changes within a biologic system." He determined that physical beings respond to stressful stimuli with a predictable set of physiological changes. He described the response in three distinct stages: (1) the alarm reaction stage, (2) the stage of resistance, and (3) the stage of exhaustion. Many illnesses, or diseases of adaptation, have their origin in this aroused state, this preparation for "fight or flight."

Holmes and Rahe viewed stress not as the physiological response but as the environmental event that produced the physiological response. Their research centered around the study of life changes, or "events," that trigger the adapative physiological and psychological responses in an individual. From their research, they devised the Social Readjustment Rating Scale, which is used to determine an individual's vulnerability to stress-related illness. This concept of stress has received criticism based on its lack of consideration of the individual's personal perception of the event, potential for coping, and available support systems at the time of the life change.

Lazarus and others have expanded the concept of stress to encompass more than just change in an individual's existing steady state or the physiological response it produces. They define stress as a relationship between the person and the environment that is appraised by the person as taxing or exceeding his or her resources and endangering his or her well-being. Response to stimuli from the internal or external environment is determined by the individual's perception of the event through cognitive appraisal. A primary appraisal is made, during which the individual determines the personal significance of the event. If the event is perceived as threatening, the individual then makes a secondary appraisal to determine the availability and effectiveness of coping strategies to manage the stressful situation. Another consideration is the predisposing factors that influence how an individual perceives and responds to a stressful event. Genetic influences, past experiences, and existing conditions strongly influence whether the response is adaptive or maladaptive.

Adaptive responses protect the individual from harm (or additional harm) and help restore homeostasis to the body. They impede the development of diseases of adaptation. With maladaptive responses conflict goes unresolved, energy resources become depleted, and the individual becomes vulnerable to physical or psychological illness.

Adaptive coping strategies for management of stress are varied and individual. Becoming aware of situations that create stress and the feelings associated with the stress response is an essential foundation in successful stress management.

Relaxation can be achieved by practicing breathing exercises or progressive relaxation techniques. Some individuals relax by exercising, playing sports, or doing other large motor activities. *Meditation* for 20 minutes once or twice daily has been shown to be an effective stress-reduction technique for some people. *Interpersonal communication with a caring other* or writing one's feelings in a journal or diary often interrupts escalation of the stress response. Using the *problem-solving/decision-making model* in an objective manner (or seeking assistance in doing so during a crisis situation) is adaptive and gives the individual a feeling of control over his or her life situation. *Pet ownership* has been shown to help individuals better cope with the stressors of life. The reliability and loyalty experienced, along with the giving and receiving of warmth and affection, produce a feeling of security as well as a unique and therapeutic coping strategy for an individual. *Music* is an adaptive coping strategy that has the capacity for stimulating motivation, enjoyment, and relaxation in some people.

Individual requirements for stress reduction vary widely. Nurses are in a unique position to assist individuals in identifying adaptive coping strategies. Stress has reached epidemic proportions in today's society, and efforts aimed at control are essential.

REVIEW QUESTIONS

SELF-EXAMINATION/LEARNING EXERCISE

Select the answer that is most appropriate for questions 1 through 4.

1. Sondra, who lives in Maine, hears on the evening news that 25 people were killed in a tornado in south Texas. Sondra experiences no anxiety upon hearing of this stressful situation. This is most likely because Sondra:
   a. Is selfish and does not care what happens to other people.
   b. Appraises the event as irrelevant to her own situation.
   c. Assesses that she has the skills to cope with the stressful situation.
   d. Uses suppression as her primary defense mechanism.

2. Cindy regularly develops nausea and vomiting when she is faced a stressful situation. Which of the following is *most* likely a predisposing factor to this maladaptive response by Cindy?
   a. Cindy inherited her mother's "nervous" stomach.
   b. Cindy is fixed in a lower level of development.
   c. Cindy has never been motivated to achieve success.
   d. Cindy's mother pampered her and kept her home from school when she was ill as a child.

3. When an individual's stress response is sustained over a long period of time, the endocrine system involvement results in:
   a. Decreased resistance to disease.
   b. Increased libido.
   c. Decreased blood pressure.
   d. Increased inflammatory response.

4. Management of stress is extremely important in today's society because:
   a. Evolution has diminished human capability for "fight or flight."
   b. The stressors of today tend to be ongoing, resulting in a sustained response.
   c. We have stress disorders that did not exist in the time of our ancestors.
   d. One never knows when one will have to face a grizzly bear or saber-toothed tiger in today's society.

5. Match each of the following situations to its correct component of the transactional model of stress/adaptation.
   _____ 1. Mr. T is fixed in a lower level of development.   a. Precipitating stressor
   _____ 2. Mr. T's father had diabetes mellitus.   b. Past experiences
   _____ 3. Mr. T has been fired from his last five jobs.   c. Existing conditions
   _____ 4. Mr. T's baby was stillborn last month.   d. Genetic influences

6. Match the following types of primary appraisals to their correct definition of the event as perceived by the individual.
   _____ 1. Irrelevant   a. Perceived as producing pleasure
   _____ 2. Benign-positive   b. Perceived as anticipated harms or losses
   _____ 3. Harm/loss   c. Perceived as potential for gain or growth
   _____ 4. Threat   d. Perceived as having no significance to the individual
   _____ 5. Challenge   e. Perceived as damage or loss already experienced

REFERENCES

Feder, E., & Feder, B. (1981). *The expressive arts therapies.* Englewood Cliffs, NJ: Prentice-Hall.

Hafen, B.Q., Karren, K.J., Frandsen, K.J., & Smith, N.L. (1996). *Mind/body health: The effects of attitudes, emotions, and relationships.* Boston: Allyn & Bacon.

Holmes, T., & Rahe, R. (1967). The Social Readjustment Rating Scale. *Journal of Psychosomatic Research, 11,* 213–218.

Lazarus, R.S., & Folkman, S. (1984). *Stress, appraisal and coping.* New York: Springer Publishing.

Leepson, M. (1984). *The alive and well stress book.* New York: Bantam Books.

Murphy, L.B., & Moriarty, A.E. (1976). *Vulnerability, coping, and growth.* New Haven, CT: Yale University Press.

Ornstein, R., & Sobel, D. (1989). *Healthy pleasures.* Reading, MA: Addison-Wesley.

Pelletier, K.R. (1992). *Mind as healer, mind as slayer.* New York: Dell.

Roy, C. (1976). *Introduction to nursing: An adaptation model.* Englewood Cliffs, NJ: Prentice-Hall.

Selye, H. (1956). *The stress of life.* New York: McGraw-Hill.

Selye, H. (1974). *Stress without distress.* New York: Signet Books.

Selye, H. (1976). *The stress of life* (rev. ed.). New York: McGraw-Hill.

Wallis, C. (1983, June 6). Stress: Can we cope? *Time,* pp. 48–54.

Bibliography

Axelrod, J., & Reisine, T.E. (1984). Stress hormones: Their interaction and regulation. *Science, 224,* 452–459.

Horowitz, M.J. (1986). *Stress response syndromes* (2nd ed.). Northvale, NJ: Jason Aronson.

Krames Communications. (1985). *A guide to managing stress.* Daly City, CA: Krames Communications.

McCance, K.L., & Huether, S.E. (1990). *Pathophysiology—The biologic basis for disease in adults and children.* St. Louis, MO: CV Mosby.

Rachman, S.J., & Philips, C. (1980). *Psychology and behavioral medicine.* Cambridge, England: Cambridge University Press.

Sobel, D.S., & Orstein, R. (1996). *The healthy mind, healthy body handbook.* Los Altos, CA: DRx.

MENTAL HEALTH AND MENTAL ILLNESS

CHAPTER OUTLINE

OBJECTIVES

INTRODUCTION

HISTORICAL OVERVIEW OF PSYCHIATRIC CARE

MENTAL HEALTH

MENTAL ILLNESS

PSYCHOLOGICAL ADAPTATION TO STRESS

MENTAL HEALTH/MENTAL ILLNESS CONTINUUM

THE *DMS-IV* MULTIAXIAL EVALUATION SYSTEM

SUMMARY

REVIEW QUESTIONS

KEY TERMS

mental health
mental illness
anxiety
grief
humors
"ship of fools"
defense mechanisms
    compensation
    denial

displacement
identification
intellectualization
introjection
isolation
projection
rationalization
reaction formation
regression

repression
sublimation
suppression
undoing
neurosis
psychosis
anticipatory grieving
bereavement overload

OBJECTIVES

After reading this chapter, the student will be able to:

1. Discuss the history of psychiatric care.
2. Define *mental health* and *mental illness.*
3. Discuss cultural elements that influence attitudes toward mental health and mental illness.
4. Describe psychological adaptation responses to stress.
5. Identify correlation of adaptive/maladaptive behaviors to the mental health/mental illness continuum.

he consideration of mental health and mental illness has its basis in the cultural beliefs of the society in which the behavior takes place. Some cultures are quite liberal in the range of behaviors that are considered acceptable, whereas others have very little tolerance for behaviors that deviate from the cultural norms.

A study of the history of psychiatric care reveals some shocking truths about past treatment of mentally ill individuals. Many were kept in control by means that could be considered less than humane.

This chapter deals with the evolution of psychiatric care from ancient times to the present. **Mental health** and **mental illness** are defined, and the psychological adaptation to stress is explained in terms of the two major responses: **anxiety** and **grief**. A mental health/mental illness continuum and the *Diagnostic and Statistical Manual of Mental Disorders*, 4th edition, (*DSM-IV*), multiaxial evaluation system are presented.

HISTORICAL OVERVIEW OF PSYCHIATRIC CARE

Primitive beliefs regarding mental disturbances took several views. Some thought that an individual with mental illness had been dispossessed of his or her soul and that the only way wellness could be achieved was if the soul returned. Others believed that evil spirits or supernatural or magical powers had entered the body. The "cure" for these individuals involved a ritualistic exorcism to purge the body of these unwanted forces. This often consisted of brutal beatings, starvation, or other torturous means. Still others considered that the mentally ill individual may have broken a taboo or sinned against another individual or God, for which ritualistic purification was required or various types of retribution were demanded. The correlation of mental illness to demonology or witchcraft led to some mentally ill individuals being burned at the stake.

The position of these ancient beliefs evolved with increasing knowledge about mental illness, as well as changes in cultural, religious, and sociopolitical attitudes. The work of Hippocrates, about 400 BC, began the movement away from belief in the supernatural. Hippocrates associated insanity and mental illness with an irregularity in the interaction of the four body fluids—blood, black bile, yellow bile, and phlegm. He called these body fluids **humors,** and associated each with a particular disposition. Disequilibrium among these four humors was thought to cause mental illness, and it was often treated by inducing vomiting and diarrhea with potent cathartic drugs.

During the Middle Ages (AD 500 to 1500), the association of mental illness with witchcraft and the supernatural continued to prevail in the European community. During this period, many severely mentally ill people were sent out to sea on sailing boats with little guidance and in search of their lost rationality. This operation is credited with engendering the expression **"ship of fools."**

In the same period in the Middle Eastern Islamic countries, however, a change in attitude began to occur, from one of mental illness as the result of witchcraft or the supernatural to the idea that these individuals were actually ill. This notion gave rise to the establishment of special units for the mentally ill within general hospitals, as well as institutions specifically designed to house the insane. They can likely be considered the first asylums for the mentally ill.

Colonial Americans tended to reflect the attitudes of the European communities from which they had emigrated. Particularly in the New England area, individuals were punished for behavior attributed to witchcraft. In the 16th and 17th centuries, institutions for the mentally ill were not available in America and care of these individuals became a family responsibility. Those without family or other resources became the responsibility of the communities in which they lived and were incarcerated in places where they could do no harm to themselves or others.

The first hospital in America to admit mentally ill clients was established in Philadelphia in the middle of the 18th century. Benjamin Rush, often called the father of American psychiatry, was a physician at the hospital. He initiated the provision of humanistic treatment and care for the mentally ill. Although he included kindness, exercise, and socialization, he also employed harsher methods such as bloodletting, purging, various types of physical restraints, and extremes of temperatures, reflecting the medical therapies of that era.

The 19th century brought the establishment of a system of state asylums, largely the result of the work of Dorothea Dix, a former New England school teacher, who lobbied tirelessly on behalf of the mentally ill population. She was unfaltering in her belief that mental illness was curable and that state hospitals should provide humanistic therapeutic care. This system of hospital care for the mentally ill grew, but the mentally ill population grew faster. The institutions became overcrowded and understaffed, and conditions deteriorated. Therapeutic care reverted to custodial care. These state hospitals provided the largest resource for the mentally ill until the initiation of the community health movement of the 1960s (see Chapter 38).

The emergence of psychiatric nursing began in 1873 with the graduation of Linda Richards from the nursing program at the New England Hospital for Women and Children in Boston. She has come to be known as the first American psychiatric nurse. Richards was instrumental in the establishment of a number of psychiatric hospitals during her career, as well as the first school of psychiatric nursing at the McLean Asylum in Waverly, Massachusetts, in 1882. The focus in this school, and those that followed, was "training" in how to provide custodial care for clients in psychiatric asylums—training that did not include the study of psychological concepts. Significant change did not occur until 1955, when incorporation of psychiatric nursing into their curricula became a requirement for all undergraduate schools of nursing (Sills, 1973).

Nursing curricula emphasized the importance of the nurse-patient relationship and therapeutic communication techniques. Nursing intervention in the somatic therapies (e.g., insulin and electroconvulsive therapy) provided impetus for the incorporation of these concepts into nursing's body of knowledge.

With the apparently increasing need for psychiatric care in the aftermath of World War II, the government passed the National Mental Health Act of 1946. This legislation provided funds for the education of psychiatrists, psychologists, social workers, and psychiatric nurses. Graduate-level education in psychiatric nursing was established during this period. Also of significance during this period was the discovery of antipsychotic medications, which made it possible for psychotic clients to more readily participate in therapeutic care, including nursing therapies.

Knowledge of the history of psychiatric/mental health care contributes to the understanding of the concepts presented in this chapter, as well as those in Chapter 3, which describe the theories of personality development according to various 19th-century and 20th-century leaders in the psychiatric/mental health movement. Modern American psychiatric care has its roots in ancient times. A great deal of opportunity exists for continued advancement of this specialty within the practice of nursing.

MENTAL HEALTH

A number of theorists have attempted to define the concept of mental health. Many of these concepts deal with various aspects of individual functioning. Maslow (1970) emphasized an individual's motivation in the continuous quest for self-actualization. He identified a "hierarchy of needs," the lower ones requiring fulfillment before those at higher levels can be achieved, with self-actualization being fulfillment of one's highest potential. Individuals may reverse their position in the hierarchy from a higher level to a lower level based on life circumstances. For example, an individual facing major surgery who has been working on tasks to achieve self-actualization may become preoccupied, if only temporarily, with the need for physiological safety. A representation of this needs hierarchy is presented in Figure 2.1.

Maslow described self-actualization as being "psychologically healthy, fully human, highly evolved, and fully mature." He believed that "healthy," or "self-actualized," individuals possessed the following characteristics:

1. An appropriate perception of reality
2. The ability to accept oneself, others, and human nature
3. The ability to manifest spontaneity

4. The capacity for focusing concentration on problem solving
5. A need for detachment and desire for privacy
6. Independence, autonomy, and a resistance to enculturation
7. An intensity of emotional reaction
8. A frequency of "peak" experiences that validate the worthwhileness, richness, and beauty of life
9. An identification with humankind
10. The ability to achieve satisfactory interpersonal relationships
11. A democratic character structure and strong sense of ethics
12. Creativeness
13. A degree of nonconformance

Jahoda (1958) has identified a list of six indicators that she suggests are a reflection of mental health:

1. **A Positive Attitude Toward Self.** This includes an objective view of self, including knowledge and acceptance of strengths and limitations. The individual feels a strong sense of personal identity and a security within the environment.

2. **Growth, Development, and the Ability to Achieve Self-Actualization.** This indicator correlates with whether the individual successfully achieves the tasks associated with each level of development (see Erikson, Chapter 3). With successful achievement in each level the individual gains motivation for advancement to his or her highest potential.

3. **Integration.** The focus here is on maintaining an equilibrium or balance among various life processes. Integration includes the ability to adaptively respond to the environment and the development of a philosophy of life, both of which help the individual maintain anxiety at a manageable level in response to stressful situations.

4. **Autonomy.** This refers to the individual's ability to perform in an independent, self-directed manner. The individual makes choices and accepts responsibility for the outcomes.

5. **Perception of Reality.** Accurate reality perception is a positive indicator of mental health. This includes perception of the environment without distortion, as well as the capacity for empathy and social sensitivity—a respect and concern for the wants and needs of others.

6. **Environmental Mastery.** This indicator suggests that the individual has achieved a satisfactory role within the group, society, or environment. It suggests that he or she is able to love and accept the love of others. When faced with life situations, the individual is able to strategize, make decisions, change, adjust, and adapt. Life offers satisfaction to the individual who has achieved environmental mastery.

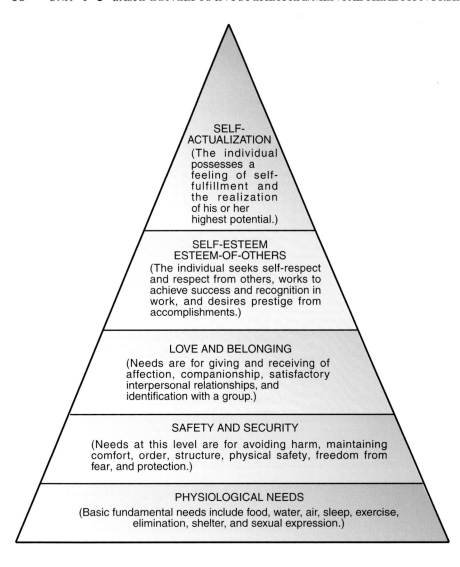

Figure 2.1 Maslow's hierarchy of needs.

The American Psychiatric Association (APA) (1980) defines mental health as:

> ". . . simultaneous success at working, loving, and creating with the capacity for mature and flexible resolution of conflicts between instincts, conscience, important other people and reality."

Robinson (1983) has offered the following definition of mental health:

> ". . . a dynamic state in which thought, feeling, and behavior that is age-appropriate and congruent with the local and cultural norms is demonstrated."

For purposes of this text, and in keeping with the framework of stress/adaptation, a modification of Robinson's definition of mental health will be considered. Thus, *mental health* will be viewed as the successful adaptation to stressors from the internal or external environment, evidenced by thoughts, feelings, and behaviors that are age-appropriate and congruent with local and cultural norms.

MENTAL ILLNESS

A universal concept of mental illness is difficult, owing to the cultural factors that influence such a definition. However, certain elements are associated with individuals' perceptions of mental illness, regardless of cultural origin. Horwitz (1982) identifies two of these elements as (1) incomprehensibility and (2) cultural relativity.

Incomprehensibility relates to the inability of the general population to understand the motivation behind the behavior. When observers are unable to find meaning or comprehensibility in behavior, they are likely to label that behavior as mental illness. Horwitz states, "Observers attribute labels of mental illness when the rules, conventions, and understandings they use to interpret behavior fail to find any intelligible motivation behind an action." The element of *cultural relativity* considers that these rules, conventions, and understandings are conceived within an individual's own particular culture. Behavior that is considered "normal" and "abnormal" is defined by one's cultural or societal norms. Therefore, a behavior that is recognized as mentally ill in one society may be viewed as "normal" in another society, and vice versa. Horwitz identified a number of cultural aspects of mental illness, which are presented in Table 2.1.

In the *DSM-IV* (American Psychiatric Association [APA], 1994), the APA defined mental illness or a mental disorder as

"... a clinically significant behavioral or psychological syndrome or pattern that occurs in a person and that is associated with present distress (a painful symptom) or disability (impairment in one or more important areas of functioning), a significantly increased risk of suffering death, pain, disability, or an important loss of freedom ... and is not merely an expectable response to a particular event."

For purposes of this text, and in keeping with the framework of stress/adaptation, *mental illness* will be characterized as maladaptive responses to stressors from the internal or external environment, evidenced by thoughts, feelings, and behaviors that are incongruent with the local and cultural norms, and interfere with the individual's social, occupational, and/or physical functioning.

PSYCHOLOGICAL ADAPTATION TO STRESS

All individuals exhibit some characteristics associated with both mental health and mental illness at any given point in time. Chapter 1 described how an individual's response to stressful situations was influenced by his or her personal perception of the event, as well as a variety of predisposing factors, such as heredity, temperament, learned response patterns, developmental maturity, existing coping strategies, and support systems of caring others.

Anxiety and grief have been described as two major, primary psychological response patterns to stress. A variety of thoughts, feelings, and behaviors are associated with each of these response patterns. Adaptation is determined by the degree to which the thoughts, feelings, and behaviors interfere with an individual's functioning.

Anxiety

Anxiety has been defined as a diffuse apprehension that is vague in nature and is associated with feelings of uncertainty and helplessness (May, 1950). Feelings of anxiety are so common as to almost be considered universal in our society. Low levels of anxiety are adaptive and can provide the motivation required for survival. Anxiety becomes problematic when the individual is unable to prevent the anxiety from escalating to a level that interferes with the ability to meet basic needs.

Peplau (1963) described four levels of anxiety: mild, moderate, severe, and panic. It is important for nurses to be able to recognize the symptoms associated with each level in order to plan for appropriate intervention with anxious individuals.

1. **Mild Anxiety.** This level of anxiety is seldom a problem for the individual. It is associated with the

---

TABLE 2.1 CULTURAL ASPECTS OF MENTAL ILLNESS

1. The initial recognition that an individual's behavior deviates from the societal norms usually is by members of the lay community rather than by a psychiatric professional.
2. People who are related to an individual or who are of the same cultural or social group are less likely to label an individual's behavior as mentally ill than someone who is relationally or culturally distant. Relatives (or people of the same cultural or social group) try to "normalize" the behavior, try to find an explanation for the behavior.
3. Psychiatrists see a mentally ill person most often when the family members can no longer deny the illness, often when the behavior is at its worst. The local or cultural norms define pathological behavior.
4. The lowest social class usually displays the highest amount of mental illness symptoms. However, they tend to tolerate a wider range of behaviors that deviate from societal norms and are less likely to consider these behaviors as indicative of mental illness. Mental illness labels are most often applied by psychiatric professionals.
5. The higher the social class, the greater the recognition of mental illness behaviors. Members of the higher social classes are likely to be self-labeled or labeled by family members or friends. Psychiatric assistance is sought near the first signs of emotional disturbance.
6. The more highly educated a person is, the greater the recognition of mental illness behaviors. However, even more relevant than *amount* of education is *type* of education. Individuals in the more humanistic types of professions (lawyers, social workers, artists, teachers, nurses) are more likely to seek psychiatric assistance than professionals such as business executives, computer specialists, accountants, and engineers.
7. In terms of religion, Jewish people are more likely to seek psychiatric assistance than are Catholics or Protestants.
8. Women are more likely than men to recognize the symptoms of mental illness and seek assistance.
9. The greater the cultural distance from the *mainstream* of society (i.e., the fewer the ties with *conventional* society), the greater the likelihood of negative response by society to their illness. For example, immigrants have a greater distance from the mainstream than the native born, blacks more than whites, and "bohemians" more than bourgeoisie. They are more likely to be subjected to coercive treatment, and involuntary psychiatric commitments are more common.

SOURCE: Adapted from Horwitz (1982).

tension experienced in response to the events of day-to-day living. Mild anxiety prepares people for action. It sharpens the senses, increases motivation for productivity, increases the perceptual field, and results in a heightened awareness of the environment. Learning is enhanced and the individual is able to function at his or her optimal level.

2. **Moderate Anxiety.** As the level of anxiety increases, the extent of the perceptual field diminishes. The moderately anxious individual is less alert to events occurring within the environment. The individual's attention span and ability to concentrate decrease, although he or she may still attend to needs with direction. Assistance with problem solving may be required. Increased muscular tension and restlessness are evident.

3. **Severe Anxiety.** The perceptual field of the severely anxious individual is so greatly diminished that concentration centers on one particular detail only or on many extraneous details. Attention span is extremely limited, and the individual has much difficulty completing even the most simple task. Physical symptoms (e.g., headaches, palpitations, insomnia) and emotional symptoms (e.g., confusion, dread, horror) may be evident. Discomfort is experienced to the degree that virtually all overt behavior is aimed at relieving the anxiety.

4. **Panic Anxiety.** In this most intense state of anxiety, the individual is unable to focus on even one detail within the environment. Misperceptions are common, and a loss of contact with reality may occur. The individual may experience hallucinations or delusions. Behavior may be characterized by wild and desperate actions or extreme withdrawal. Human functioning and communication with others is ineffective. Panic anxiety is associated with a feeling of terror, and individuals may be convinced that they have a life-threatening illness or fear that they are "going crazy," losing control, or are emotionally weak (APA, 1994). Prolonged panic anxiety can lead to physical and emotional exhaustion and can be a life-threatening situation.

A synopsis of the characteristics associated with each of the four levels of anxiety is presented in Table 2.2.

Behavioral Adaptation Responses to Anxiety

A variety of behavioral adaptation responses occur at each level of anxiety. Figure 2.2 depicts these behavioral responses on a continuum of anxiety ranging from mild to panic.

Mild Anxiety. At the mild level, individuals employ any of a number of coping behaviors that satisfy their needs for comfort. Menninger (1963) described the following types of coping mechanisms that individuals use to relieve anxiety in stressful situations:

- Sleeping
- Eating
- Physical exercise
- Smoking
- Crying
- Pacing
- Foot swinging
- Fidgeting
- Yawning
- Drinking
- Daydreaming
- Laughing
- Cursing
- Nail biting
- Finger tapping
- Talking to someone with whom one feels comfortable

Undoubtedly there are many more responses too numerous to mention here, considering that each individual develops his or her own unique ways to relieve anxiety at the mild level. Some of these behaviors are much more adaptive than others.

Mild-to-Moderate Anxiety. Sigmund Freud (1961) identified the ego as the reality component of the personality that governs problem solving and rational thinking. As the level of anxiety increases, the strength of the ego is tested, and energy is mobilized to confront the threat. Anna Freud (1953) identified a number of **defense mechanisms** employed by the ego in the face of threat to biological or psychological integrity. Some of these ego defense mechanisms are more adaptive than others, but all are used either consciously or unconsciously as a protective device for the ego in an effort to relieve mild-to-moderate anxiety. They become maladaptive when they are "used to such an extreme degree that they distort reality, interfere with interpersonal relationships, limit one's ability to work productively, and promote ego disintegration instead of self-integrity" (Stuart & Sundeen, 1987). The major ego defense mechanisms identified by Anna Freud are discussed here and summarized in Table 2.3.

1. **Compensation** is the covering up of a real or perceived weakness by emphasizing a trait one considers more desirable.

EXAMPLES

(a) A handicapped boy who is unable to participate in sports compensates by becoming a great scholar. (b) A young man who is the shortest among members of his peer group views this as a deficiency and compensates by being overly aggressive and daring.

2. **Denial** is the refusal to acknowledge the existence of a real situation or the feelings associated with it.

TABLE 2.2   LEVELS OF ANXIETY

LEVEL	PERCEPTUAL FIELD	ABILITY TO LEARN	PHYSICAL CHARACTERISTICS	EMOTIONAL/BEHAVIORAL CHARACTERISTICS
Mild	Heightened perception (e.g., noises may seem louder; details within the environment are clearer) Increased awareness Increased alertness	Enhanced learning	Restlessness Irritability	May remain superficial with others Rarely experienced as distressful Increased motivation
Moderate	Reduction in perceptual field Reduced alertness to environmental events (e.g., someone talking may not be heard; part of the room may not be noticed)	Ability to learn but not optimally Decreased attention span Decreased ability to concentrate	Increased restlessness Increased heart and respiration rate Increased perspiration Gastric discomfort Increased muscular tension Increase in speech rate, volume, and pitch	Feeling of discontent May lead to a degree of impairment in interpersonal relationships as individual begins to focus on self and the need to relieve personal discomfort
Severe	Greatly diminished perceptual field (e.g., only extraneous details are perceived, or fixation on a single detail may occur; may not take notice of an event even when attention is directed by another)	Extremely limited attention span Inability to concentrate or problem solve Inability to learn effectively	Headaches Dizziness Nausea Trembling Insomnia Palpitations Tachycardia Hyperventilation Urinary frequency Diarrhea	Feelings of dread, loathing, horror Total focus on self and intense desire to relieve the anxiety
Panic	Inability to focus on even one detail within the environment Misperceptions of the environment common (e.g., a perceived detail may be elaborated and out of proportion)	Inability to learn Inability to concentrate Inability to comprehend even simple directions	Dilated pupils Labored breathing Severe trembling Sleeplessness Palpitations Diaphoresis and pallor Muscular incoordination Immobility or purposeless hyperactivity Incoherence or inability to verbalize	Sense of impending doom Terror Bizarre behavior, including shouting, screaming, running about wildly, clinging to anyone or anything from which a sense of safety and security is derived Hallucinations; delusions Extreme withdrawal into self

EXAMPLES

(a) A woman has been told by her family doctor that she has a lump in her breast. An appointment is made for her with a surgeon; however, she does not keep the appointment and goes about her activities of daily living with no evidence of concern. (b) Individuals continue to smoke cigarettes even though they have been told of the health risk involved.

3. **Displacement** is the transferring of feelings from one target to another that is considered less threatening or neutral.

EXAMPLES

(a) A man who is passed over for promotion on his job says nothing to his boss but later belittles his son for not making the basketball team. (b) A

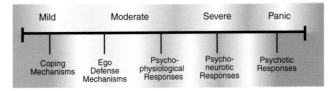

Figure 2.2 Adaptation responses on a continuum of anxiety.

◤ TABLE 2.3 EGO DEFENSE MECHANISMS

DEFENSE MECHANISM	EXAMPLE	DEFENSE MECHANISM	EXAMPLE
Compensation Covering up a real or perceived weakness by emphasizing a trait one considers more desirable	A physically handicapped boy is unable to participate in football, so he compensates by becoming a great scholar.	**Rationalization** Attempting to make excuses or formulate logical reasons to justify unacceptable feelings or behaviors	John tells the rehab nurse, "I drink because it's the only way I can deal with my bad marriage and my worse job."
Denial Refusing to acknowledge the existence of a real situation or the feelings associated with it	A woman drinks alcohol every day and cannot stop, failing to acknowledge that she has a problem.	**Reaction formation** Preventing unacceptable or undesirable thoughts or behaviors from being expressed by exaggerating opposite thoughts or types of behaviors	Jane hates nursing. She attended nursing school to please her parents. During career day, she speaks to prospective students about the excellence of nursing as a career.
Displacement The transfer of feelings from one target to another that is considered less threatening or that is neutral	A client is angry at his physician, does not express it, but becomes verbally abusive with the nurse.	**Regression** Retreating in response to stress to an earlier level of development and the comfort measures associated with that level of functioning	When 2-year-old Jay is hospitalized for tonsillitis he will drink only from a bottle, even though his mom states he has been drinking from a cup for 6 months.
Identification An attempt to increase self-worth by acquiring certain attributes and characteristics of an individual one admires	A teenager who required lengthy rehabilitation after an accident decides to become a physical therapist as a result of his experiences.	**Repression** Involuntarily blocking unpleasant feelings and experiences from one's awareness	An accident victim can remember nothing about his accident.
Intellectualization An attempt to avoid expressing actual emotions associated with a stressful situation by using the intellectual processes of logic, reasoning, and analysis	S's husband is being transferred with his job to a city far away from her parents. She hides anxiety by explaining to her parents the advantages associated with the move.	**Sublimation** Rechanneling of drives or impulses that are personally or socially unacceptable into activities that are constructive	A mother whose son was killed by a drunk driver channels her anger and energy into being the president of the local chapter of Mothers Against Drunk Drivers.
Introjection Integrating the beliefs and values of another individual into one's own ego structure	Children integrate their parents' value system into the process of conscience formation. A child says to friend, "Don't cheat. It's wrong."	**Suppression** The voluntary blocking of unpleasant feelings and experiences from one's awareness	Scarlett O'Hara says, "I don't want to think about that now. I'll think about that tomorrow."
Isolation Separating a thought or memory from the feeling, tone, or emotion associated with it	A young woman describes being attacked and raped, without showing any emotion.	**Undoing** Symbolically negating or canceling out an experience that one finds intolerable	Joe is nervous about his new job and yells at his wife. On his way home he stops and buys her some flowers and himself a new video game.
Projection Attributing feelings or impulses unacceptable to one's self to another person	Sue feels a strong sexual attraction to her track coach and tells her friend, "He's coming on to me!"		

boy who is teased and hit by the class bully on the playground comes home after school and kicks his dog.

4. **Identification** is an attempt to increase self-worth by acquiring certain attributes and characteristics of an individual one admires.

EXAMPLES

(a) A teenage girl emulates the mannerisms and style of dress of a popular female rock star. (b) The young son of a famous civil rights worker adopts his father's attitudes and behaviors with the intent of pursuing similar aspirations.

5. **Intellectualization** is an attempt to avoid expressing actual emotions associated with a stressful situation by using the intellectual processes of logic, reasoning, and analysis.

EXAMPLES

(a) A man whose brother is in a cardiac intensive care unit following a severe myocardial infarction (MI) spends his allotted visiting time in discussion with the nurse analyzing test results and making a reasonable determination about the pathophysiology that may have occurred to induce the MI. (b) A young psychology professor receives a letter from his fiancée breaking off their engagement. He shows no emotion when discussing this with his best friend. Instead he analyzes his fiancée's behavior and tries to reason why the relationship failed.

6. **Introjection** is the internalization of the beliefs and values of another individual such that they symbolically become a part of the self to the extent that the feeling of separateness or distinctness is lost.

EXAMPLES

(a) A small child develops her conscience by internalizing what the parents believe is right and wrong. The parents literally become a part of the child. The child says to a friend while playing, "Don't hit people. It's not nice!" (b) A psychiatric client claims to be the son of God, drapes himself in sheet and blanket, "performs miracles" on other clients, and refuses to respond unless addressed as Jesus Christ.

7. **Isolation** is the separation of a thought or a memory from the feeling tone or emotions associated with it (sometimes called *emotional isolation*).

EXAMPLES

(a) A young woman describes being attacked and raped by a street gang. She displays an apathetic expression and no emotional tone. (b) A physician is able to isolate her feelings about the eventual death of a terminally ill cancer client by focusing her attention instead on the chemotherapy that will be given.

8. **Projection** is the attribution of feelings or impulses unacceptable to one's self to another person. The individual "passes the blame" for these undesirable feelings or impulses to another, thereby providing relief from the anxiety associated with them.

EXAMPLES

(a) A young soldier who has an extreme fear of participating in military combat tells his sergeant that the others in his unit are "a bunch of cowards." (b) A businessperson who values punctuality is late for a meeting and states, "Sorry I'm late. My assistant forgot to remind me of the time. It's so hard to find good help these days."

9. **Rationalization** is the attempt to make excuses or formulate logical reasons to justify unacceptable feelings or behaviors.

EXAMPLES

(a) A young woman is turned down for a secretarial job after a poor performance on a typing test. She claims, "I'm sure I could have done a better job on a word processor. Hardly anyone uses an electric typewriter anymore!" (b) A young man is unable to afford the sports car he wants so desperately. He tells the salesperson, "I'd buy this car but I'll be getting married soon. This is really not the car for a family man."

10. **Reaction formation** is the prevention of unacceptable or undesirable thoughts or behaviors from being expressed by exaggerating opposite thoughts or types of behaviors.

EXAMPLES

(a) The young soldier who has an extreme fear of participating in military combat volunteers for dangerous front-line duty. (b) A secretary is sexually attracted to her boss and feels an intense dislike toward his wife. She treats her boss with detachment and aloofness while performing her secretarial duties and is overly courteous, polite, and flattering to his wife when she comes to the office.

11. **Regression** is the retreating to an earlier level of development and the comfort measures associated with that level of functioning.

EXAMPLES

(a) When his mother brings his new baby sister home from the hospital, 4-year-old Tommy, who had been toilet trained for more than a year, begins to wet his pants, cry to be held, and suck his thumb. (b) A person who is depressed may withdraw to his or her room, curl up in a fetal position on the bed, and sleep for long periods of time.

12. **Repression** is the involuntary blocking of unpleasant feelings and experiences from one's awareness.

EXAMPLES

(a) A woman cannot remember being sexually assaulted when she was 15 years old. (b) A teenage boy cannot remember driving the car that was involved in an accident in which his best friend was killed.

13. **Sublimation** is the rechanneling of drives or impulses that are personally or socially unacceptable (e.g., aggressiveness, anger, sexual drives) into activities that are more tolerable and constructive.

EXAMPLES

(a) A teenage boy with strong competitive and aggressive drives becomes the star football player on his high school team. (b) A young unmarried woman with a strong desire for marriage and a family achieves satisfaction and success in establishing and operating a day-care center for preschool children.

14. **Suppression** is the voluntarily blocking of unpleasant feelings and experiences from one's awareness.

EXAMPLES

(a) Scarlett O'Hara says, "I'll think about that tomorrow." (b) A young woman who is depressed about a pending divorce proceeding tells the nurse, "I just don't want to talk about the divorce. There's nothing I can do about it anyway."

15. **Undoing** is the act of symbolically negating or canceling out a previous action or experience that one finds intolerable.

EXAMPLES

(a) A man spills some salt on the table, then sprinkles some over his left shoulder to "prevent bad luck." (b) A man who is anxious about giving a presentation at work yells at his wife during breakfast. He stops on his way home from work that evening to buy her a dozen red roses.

Moderate-to-Severe Anxiety. Anxiety at the moderate-to-severe level that remains unresolved over an extended period of time can contribute to a number of physiological disorders. The *DSM-IV* (APA, 1994) describes these disorders as ". . . the presence of one or more specific psychological or behavioral factors that adversely affect a general medical condition." The psychological factors may exacerbate symptoms of, delay recovery from, or interfere with treatment of the medical condition. The condition may be initiated or exacerbated by an environmental situation that the individual perceives as stressful. Measurable pathophysiology can be demonstrated.

Common examples of psychophysiological conditions include but are not limited to tension and migraine headaches, angina pectoris, obesity, anorexia nervosa, bulimia nervosa, rheumatoid arthritis, ulcerative colitis, gastric and duodenal ulcers, asthma, irritable bowel syndrome, nausea and vomiting, gastritis, cardiac arrhythmias, myocardial infarction, diabetes, premenstrual syndrome, muscle spasms and pain, sexual dysfunction, and cancer (APA, 1994; Halmi, 1982; Kaplan & Sadock, 1985; LeShan, 1977; Mims & Swensen, 1980). A more comprehensive discussion of specific psychophysiological disorders is presented in Chapter 33.

Severe Anxiety. Extended periods of repressed severe anxiety can result in psychoneurotic patterns of behaving. **Neurosis** is no longer a separate category of disorders in the *DSM-IV* (APA, 1994). However, the term is still used in the literature to further describe the symptomatology of certain disorders. Neuroses are psychiatric disturbances characterized by excessive anxiety or depression, disrupted bodily functions, unsatisfying interpersonal relationships, and behaviors that interfere with routine functioning (Kirkham, 1980). People with neuroses:

1. Are aware that they are experiencing distress.
2. Are aware that their behaviors are maladaptive.
3. Are unaware of any possible psychological causes of the distress.
4. Feel helpless to change their situation.
5. Experience no loss of contact with reality.

The following disorders are examples of psychoneurotic responses to anxiety as they appear in the *DSM-IV*. They are discussed in this text in Chapters 27, 28, and 29.

1. **Anxiety Disorders.** Disorders in which the characteristic features are symptoms of anxiety and avoidance behavior (e.g., phobias, obsessive-compulsive disorder, panic disorder, generalized anxiety disorder, and posttraumatic stress disorder).
2. **Somatoform Disorders.** Disorders in which the characteristic features are physical symptoms for which there is no demonstrable organic pathology. Psychological factors are judged to play a significant role in the onset, severity, exacerbation, or maintenance of the symptoms (e.g., hypochondriasis, conversion disorder, somatization disorder, pain disorder).
3. **Dissociative Disorders.** Disorders in which the characteristic feature is a disruption in the usually integrated functions of consciousness, memory, identity, or perception of the environment (e.g., dissociative amnesia, dissociative fugue, dissociative identity disorder, and depersonalization disorder).

Panic Anxiety. At this extreme level of anxiety, an individual is not capable of processing what is happening in the environment, and may lose contact with reality. **Psychosis** is defined as a loss of ego boundaries or a gross impairment in reality testing (APA, 1994). Psychoses are serious psychiatric disturbances characterized by the presence of delusions or hallucinations and the impairment of interpersonal functioning and relationship to the external world. People with psychoses:

1. Experience minimal distress (emotional tone is flat, bland, or inappropriate).
2. Are unaware that their behavior is maladaptive.
3. Are unaware of any psychological problems.
4. Are exhibiting a flight from reality into a less stressful world or into one in which they are attempting to adapt.

Examples of psychotic responses to anxiety include the schizophrenic, schizoaffective, and delusional disorders. They are discussed at length in Chapter 25.

Grief

Grief is a subjective state of emotional, physical, and social responses to the loss of a valued entity. The loss may be real, in which case it can be substantiated by others (e.g., death of a loved one, loss of personal possessions), or it may be *perceived* by the individual alone, unable to be shared or identified by others (e.g., loss of the feeling of femininity following mastectomy). Any situation that creates *change* for an individual can be identified as a loss. *Failure* (either real or perceived) can be viewed as a loss.

The loss, or anticipated loss, of anything of value to an individual can trigger the grief response. This period of characteristic emotions and behaviors is called *mourning*. The "normal" mourning process is adaptive and is characterized by feelings of sadness, guilt, anger, helplessness, hopelessness, and despair. Indeed, an absence of mourning may be considered maladaptive.

Stages of Grief

Kübler-Ross (1969), in extensive research with terminally ill patients, identified five stages of feelings and behaviors that individuals experience in response to a real, perceived, or anticipated loss:

Stage 1—Denial. This is a stage of shock and disbelief. The response may be one of "No, it can't be true!" The reality of the loss is not acknowledged. Denial is a protective mechanism that allows the individual to cope within an immediate time frame while organizing more effective defense strategies.
Stage 2—Anger. "Why me?" and "It's not fair!" are comments often expressed during the anger stage. Envy and resentment toward individuals not affected by the loss are common. Anger may be di-

rected at the self or displaced on loved ones, caregivers, and even God. There may be a preoccupation with an idealized image of the lost entity.
Stage 3—Bargaining. "If God will help me through this, I promise I will go to church every Sunday and volunteer my time to help others." During this stage, which is usually not visible or evident to others, a "bargain" is made with God in an attempt to reverse or postpone the loss. Sometimes the promise is associated with feelings of guilt for not having performed satisfactorily, appropriately, or sufficiently.
Stage 4—Depression. During this stage, the full impact of the loss is experienced. The sense of loss is intense, and feelings of sadness and depression prevail. This is a time of quiet desperation and disengagement from all association with the lost entity. This stage differs from pathological depression in that this is a stage of advancement toward resolution rather than the fixation in an earlier stage of the grief process.
Stage 5—Acceptance. The final stage brings a feeling of peace regarding the loss that has occurred. It is a time of quiet expectation and resignation. The focus is on the reality of the loss and its meaning for the individuals affected by it.

All individuals do not experience each of these stages in response to a loss, nor do they necessarily experience them in this order. Some individuals' grieving behaviors may fluctuate, and even overlap, between stages.

Anticipatory Grief

When a loss is anticipated, individuals often begin the work of grieving before the actual loss occurs. Most people reexperience the grieving behaviors once the loss occurs, but having this time to prepare for the loss can facilitate the process of mourning, actually decreasing the length and intensity of the response. Problems arise, particularly in anticipating the death of a loved one, when family members experience **anticipatory grieving** and the mourning process is completed prematurely. They disengage emotionally from the dying person, who may then experience feelings of being rejected by loved ones at a time when this psychological support is so necessary.

Resolution

The grief response can last from weeks to years. It cannot be hurried, and individuals must be allowed to progress at their own pace. In the loss of a loved one, grief work usually lasts for at least a year, during which the grieving person experiences each significant "anniversary" date for the first time without the loved one present.

Length of the grief process may be prolonged by a number of factors. If the relationship with the lost entity had been marked by ambivalence or if there had been an enduring "love-hate" association, reaction to the loss may be burdened with guilt. Guilt lengthens the grief reaction by promoting feelings of anger toward the self for having committed a wrongdoing or behaved in an unacceptable manner toward that which is now lost, even perhaps to feeling that one's behavior has contributed to the loss.

Anticipatory grieving is thought to shorten the grief response in some individuals who are able to work through some of the feelings before the loss occurs. If the loss is sudden and unexpected, mourning may take longer than it would if individuals were able to grieve in anticipation of the loss.

Length of the grieving process is also affected by the number of recent losses experienced by an individual and whether he or she is able to complete one grieving process before another loss occurs. This is particularly true for elderly individuals who may be experiencing numerous losses, such as spouse, friends, other relatives, independent functioning, home, personal possessions, and pets, in a relatively short period of time. Grief accumulates, and this represents a type of **bereavement overload,** which for some individuals presents an impossible task of grief work.

Resolution of the process of mourning is thought to have occurred when an individual can look back on the relationship with the lost entity and accept both the pleasures and the disappointments (both the positive and the negative aspects) of the association (Bowlby and Parkes, 1970). Disorganization and emotional pain have been experienced and tolerated. Preoccupation with the lost entity has been replaced with energy and the desire to pursue new situations and relationships.

Maladaptive Grief Responses

Maladaptive responses to loss occur when an individual is not able to satisfactorily progress through the stages of grieving to achieve resolution. Maladaptive responses generally occur when an individual becomes fixed in the denial or anger stage of the grief process. Several types of grief responses have been identified as pathological (Jackson, 1957; Lindemann, 1944; Parkes, 1972). They include responses that are prolonged, delayed or inhibited, or distorted. The *prolonged* response is characterized by an intense preoccupation with memories of the lost entity for *many years after the loss has occurred.* Behaviors associated with the stages of denial or anger are manifested, and disorganization of functioning and intense emotional pain related to the lost entity are evidenced.

In the *delayed or inhibited* response, the individual becomes fixed in the denial stage of the grieving process. The emotional pain associated with the loss is not experienced, but anxiety disorders (e.g., phobias, hypochondriasis) or sleeping and eating disorders (e.g., insomnia, anorexia) may be evident. The individual may remain in denial for many years until the grief response is triggered by a reminder of the loss or even by another, unrelated loss.

The individual who experiences a *distorted* response is fixed in the anger stage of grieving. In the distorted response, all the normal behaviors associated with grieving, such as helplessness, hopelessness, sadness, anger, and guilt, are exaggerated out of proportion to the situation. The individual turns the anger inward on the self, is consumed with overwhelming despair, and is unable to function in normal activities of daily living. Pathological depression is a distorted grief response (see Chapter 26).

MENTAL HEALTH/MENTAL ILLNESS CONTINUUM

Anxiety and grief have been described as two major, primary responses to stress. In Figure 2.3, both of these responses are presented on a continuum according to degree of symptom severity. Disorders as they appear in the *DSM-IV* are identified at their appropriate placement along the continuum.

THE *DSM-IV* MULTIAXIAL EVALUATION SYSTEM

The APA endorses case evaluation on a multiaxial system, "to facilitate comprehensive and systematic evaluation with attention to the various mental disorders and general medical conditions, psychosocial and environmental problems, and level of functioning that might be overlooked if the focus were on assessing a single presenting problem." Each individual is evaluated on five axes. They are defined by the *DSM-IV* in the following manner:

Axis I—Clinical Disorders and Other Conditions That May Be a Focus of Clinical Attention. This includes all mental disorders (except personality disorders and mental retardation).

Axis II—Personality Disorders and Mental Retardation. These disorders usually begin in childhood or adolescence and persist in a stable form into adult life.

Axis III—General Medical Conditions. These include any current general medical condition that is potentially relevant to the understanding or management of the individual's mental disorder.

Axis IV—Psychosocial and Environmental Problems. These are problems that may affect the diagnosis, treatment, and prognosis of mental disorders named on axes I and II. These include problems re-

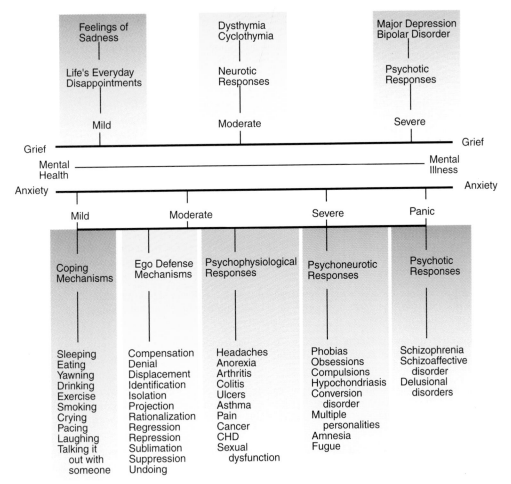

Figure 2.3 Conceptualization of anxiety and grief responses along the mental health/mental illness continuum.

lated to primary support group, social environment, education, occupation, housing, economics, access to health care services, interaction with the legal system or crime, and other types of psychosocial and environmental problems.

Axis V—Global Assessment of Functioning. This allows the clinician to rate the individual's overall functioning on the Global Assessment of Functioning (GAF) Scale. This scale represents in global terms a single measure of the individual's psychological, social, and occupational functioning. A copy of GAF Scale appears in Table 2.4. The *DSM-IV* outline of axes I and II categories and codes is presented in Appendix C.

SUMMARY

The history of psychiatric care has an unquestionable influence on the manner in which treatment of the mentally ill is provided today. Psychiatric care has its roots in ancient times, when etiology was based in superstition and ideas related to the supernatural. Treatment was inhu-

mane, and accounts of torturous methods abound in the literature. Conditions have improved, largely because of the influence of leaders such as Benjamin Rush, Dorothea Dix, and Linda Richards, whose endeavors provided a model for humanistic treatment of the mentally ill.

Various definitions of mental health and mental illness from the literature were presented. For purposes of this text, *mental health* is defined as "the successful adaptation to stressors from the internal or external environment, evidenced by thoughts, feelings, and behaviors that are age-appropriate and congruent with local and cultural norms." *Mental illness* is defined as "maladaptive responses to stressors from the internal or external environment, evidenced by thoughts, feelings, and behaviors that are incongruent with the local and cultural norms, and interfere with the individual's social, occupational, and/or physical functioning."

Most cultures label behavior as mental illness on the basis of *incomprehensibility* and *cultural relativity*. When observers are unable to find meaning or comprehensibility in behavior, they are likely to label that behavior as mental illness. The meaning of behaviors is determined within individual cultures.

TABLE 2.4 GLOBAL ASSESSMENT OF FUNCTIONING (GAF) SCALE

Consider psychological, social, and occupational functioning on a hypothetical continuum of mental health–illness. Do not include impairment in functioning due to physical (or environmental) limitations.

Code	(Note: Use intermediate codes when appropriate, e.g., 45, 68, 72)
100 91	**Superior functioning in a wide range of activities, life's problems never seem to get out of hand, is sought out by others because of his or her many positive qualities. No symptoms.**
90 81	**Absent or minimal symptoms** (e.g., mild anxiety before an exam), **good functioning in all areas, interested and involved in a wide range of activities, socially effective, generally satisfied with life, no more than everyday problems or concerns** (e.g., an occasional argument with family members).
80 71	**If symptoms are present, they are transient and expectable reactions to psychosocial stressors** (e.g., difficulty concentrating after family argument); **no more than slight impairment in social, occupational, or school functioning** (e.g., temporarily falling behind in schoolwork).
70 61	**Some mild symptoms** (e.g., depressed mood and mild insomnia) **OR some difficulty in social, occupational, or school functioning** (e.g., occasional truancy, or theft within the household), **but generally functioning pretty well, has some meaningful interpersonal relationships.**
60 51	**Moderate symptoms** (e.g., flat affect and circumstantial speech, occasional panic attacks) **OR moderate difficulty in social, occupational, or school functioning** (e.g., few friends, conflicts with peers or coworkers).
50 41	**Serious symptoms** (e.g., suicidal ideation, severe obsessional rituals, frequent shoplifting) **OR any serious impairment in social, occupational, or school functioning** (e.g., no friends, unable to keep a job).
40 31	**Some impairment in reality testing or communication** (e.g., speech is at times illogical, obscure, or irrelevant) **OR major impairment in several areas, such as work or school, family relations, judgment, thinking, or mood** (e.g., depressed man avoids friends, neglects family, and is unable to work; child frequently beats up younger children, is defiant at home, and is failing at school).
30 21	**Behavior is considerably influenced by delusions or hallucinations OR serious impairment in communication or judgment** (e.g., sometimes incoherent, acts grossly inappropriately, suicidal preoccupation) **OR inability to function in almost all areas** (e.g., stays in bed all day; no job, home, or friends).
20 11	**Some degree of hurting self or others** (e.g., suicide attempts without clear expectation of death; frequently violent; manic excitement) **OR occasionally fails to maintain minimal personal hygiene** (e.g., smears feces) **OR gross impairment in communication** (e.g., largely incoherent or mute).
10 1	**Persistent danger of severely hurting self or others** (e.g., recurrent violence) **OR persistent inability to maintain minimal personal hygiene OR serious suicidal act with clear expectation of death.**
0	**Inadequate information.**

SOURCE: APA (1994), with permission.

Anxiety and *grief* have been identified as the two major, primary responses to stress. Peplau (1963) defined anxiety by levels of symptom severity: mild, moderate, severe, and panic. Behaviors associated with levels of anxiety include coping mechanisms, ego defense mechanisms, psychophysiological responses, psychoneurotic responses, and psychotic responses.

Grief is described as a response to loss of a valued entity. Stages of normal mourning as identified by Kübler-Ross (1969) are denial, anger, bargaining, depression, and acceptance. Anticipatory grief is grief work that is begun, and sometimes completed, before the loss occurs. Resolu-tion is thought to occur when an individual is able to re-member and accept both the positive and negative aspects associated with the lost entity. Grieving is thought to be maladaptive when the mourning process is prolonged, de-layed or inhibited, or becomes distorted and exaggerated out of proportion to the situation. Pathological depres-sion is considered to be a distorted reaction. The behav-iors and associated disorders of anxiety and grief were pre-sented on the mental health/mental illness continuum.

The *DSM-IV* multiaxial system of diagnostic classifi-cation was explained and an outline of axes I and II cate-gories and codes presented.

REVIEW QUESTIONS

SELF-EXAMINATION/LEARNING EXERCISE

Situation: Anna is 72 years old. She has been a widow for 20 years. When her husband had been dead for a year, her daughter gave Anna a puppy, whom she named Lucky. Lucky was a happy, lively mutt of unknown origin, and he and Anna soon became inseparable. Lucky lived to a ripe old age of 16, dying in Anna's arms 3 years ago. Anna's daughter has consulted the community mental health nurse practitioner about her mother, stating, "She doesn't do a thing for herself anymore, and all she wants to talk about is Lucky. She visits his grave every day! She still cries when she talks about him. I don't know what to do!"

Select the answer that is most appropriate for this situation.

1. Anna's behavior would be considered maladaptive because:
   a. It has been over three years since Lucky died.
   b. Her grief is too intense to be just over the loss of a dog.
   c. She continues to be preoccupied with Lucky's loss after a prolonged period.
   d. People in our culture do not comprehend such behavior over loss of a pet.

2. Anna's grieving behavior would most likely be considered to be:
   a. Delayed
   b. Inhibited
   c. Prolonged
   d. Distorted

3. Anna is most likely fixed in which stage of the grief process?
   a. Denial
   b. Anger
   c. Depression
   d. Acceptance

4. Anna is of the age when she may have experienced many losses coming close together. What is this called?
   a. Bereavement overload
   b. Normal mourning
   c. Isolation
   d. Cultural relativity

5. Anna's daughter has likely put off seeking help for Anna because:
   a. Women are less likely to seek help for emotional problems than men.
   b. Relatives often try to "normalize" the behavior, rather than label it mental illness.
   c. She knows that all old people are expected to be a little depressed.
   d. She is afraid that the neighbors "will think her mother is crazy."

6. Lucky got away from Anna while they were taking a walk. He ran into the street and was hit by a car. Anna cannot remember any of these circumstances of his death. This is an example of what defense mechanism?
   a. Rationalization
   b. Suppression
   c. Denial
   d. Repression

7. Lucky sometimes refused to obey Anna, and indeed he did not come back to her when she called to him on the day he was killed. But Anna continues to insist, "He was the very best dog. He always minded me. He always did everything I told him to do." This represents the defense mechanism of:

   a. Sublimation

   b. Compensation

   c. Reaction formation

   d. Undoing

8. Anna's maladaptive grief response may be attributed to:

   a. Unresolved grief over loss of her husband.

   b. Loss of several relatives and friends over the last few years.

   c. Repressed feelings of guilt over the way in which Lucky died.

   d. Any or all of the above.

9. For what reason would Anna's illness be considered a neurosis rather than a psychosis?

   a. She is unaware that her behavior is maladaptive.

   b. She exhibits inappropriate affect (emotional tone).

   c. She experiences no loss of contact with reality.

   d. She tells the nurse, "There is nothing wrong with me!"

10. Which of the following statements by Anna might suggest that she is achieving resolution of her grief over Lucky's death?

   a. "I don't cry anymore when I think about Lucky."

   b. "It's true. Lucky didn't always mind me. Sometimes he ignored my commands."

   c. "I remember how it happened now. I should have held tighter to his leash!"

   d. "I won't ever have another dog. It's just too painful to lose them."

Match the following defense mechanisms to the appropriate situation:

_____ 11. Compensation

_____ 12. Denial

_____ 13. Displacement

_____ 14. Identification

_____ 15. Intellectualization

_____ 16. Introjection

_____ 17. Isolation

_____ 18. Projection

_____ 19. Rationalization

_____ 20. Reaction formation

_____ 21. Regression

_____ 22. Repression

_____ 23. Sublimation

_____ 24. Suppression

_____ 25. Undoing

a. Tommy, who is small for his age, is teased at school by the older boys. When he gets home from school, he yells at and hits his little sister.

b. Johnny is in a wheelchair as a result of paralysis of the lower limbs. Before his accident, he was the star athlete on the football team. Now he obsessively strives to maintain a 4.0 grade point average in his courses.

c. Nancy and Sally are 4 years old. While playing with their dolls, Nancy says to Sally, "Don't hit your dolly. It's not nice to hit people!"

d. Jackie is 4 years old. He has wanted a baby brother very badly, yet when his mother brings the new sibling home from the hospital, Jackie cries to be held when the baby is being fed and even starts to soil his clothing, although he has been toilet trained for 2 years.

e. A young man is late for class. He tells the professor, "Sorry I'm late, but my stupid wife forgot to set the alarm last night!"

f. Nancy was emotionally abused as a child and hates her mother. However, when she talks to others about her mother, she tells them how wonderful she is and how much she loves her.

g. Pete grew up in a rough neighborhood where fighting was a way of coping. He is tough and aggressive and is noticed by the football coach, who makes him a member of the team. Within the year he becomes the star player.

h. Fred stops at the bar every night after work and has several drinks. During the last 6 months he has been charged twice with driving under the influence, both times while driving recklessly after leaving the bar. Last night, he was stopped again. The judge ordered rehabilitation services. Fred responded, "I don't need rehab. I can stop drinking anytime I want to!"

   i. Mary tries on a beautiful dress she saw in the store window. She discovers that it costs more than she can afford. She says to the salesperson, "I'm not going to buy it. I really don't look good in this color."

   j. Janice is extremely upset when her boyfriend of 2 years breaks up with her. Her best friend tries to encourage her to talk about the breakup, but Janice says, "No need to talk about him anymore. He's history!"

   k. While jogging in the park, Linda was kidnapped and taken as a hostage by two men who had just robbed a bank. She was held at gunpoint for 2 days until she was able to escape from the robbers. In her account to the police, she speaks of the encounter with no display of emotion whatsoever.

   l. While Mark is on his way to work a black cat runs across the road in front of his car. Mark turns the car around, drives back in the direction from which he had come, and takes another route to work.

   m. Fifteen-year-old Zelda has always wanted to be a teacher. Ms. Fry is Zelda's history teacher. Zelda admires everything about Ms. Fry and wants to be just like her. She changes her hair and dress style to match that of Ms. Fry.

   n. Bart is turned down for a job he desperately wanted. He shows no disappointment when relating the situation to his girlfriend. Instead he reviews the interview and begins to analyze systematically why the interaction was ineffective for him.

   o. Eighteen-year-old Jennifer can recall nothing related to an automobile accident in which she was involved 8 years ago and in which both of her parents were killed.

REFERENCES

American Psychiatric Association. (1980). *A psychiatric glossary* (5th ed.). Washington, DC: American Psychiatric Press.

American Psychiatric Association. (1994). *Diagnostic and statistical manual of mental disorders* (4th ed.). Washington, DC: American Psychiatric Association.

Bowlby, J., & Parkes, C.M. (1970). Separation and loss. In E.J. Anthony & C. Koupernik (Eds.), *International yearbook for child psychiatry and allied disciplines: The child and his family* (Vol. 1). New York: John Wiley & Sons.

Freud, A. (1953). *The ego and mechanisms of defense.* New York: International Universities Press.

Freud, S. (1961). The ego and the id. In *Standard edition of the complete psychological works of Freud,* Vol. XIX. London: Hogarth Press.

Halmi, K.A. (1982). Pragmatic information on eating disorders. *Psychiatric Clinics of North America, 5*(2):371–377.

Horwitz, A.V. (1982). *The social control of mental illness.* New York: Academic Press.

Jackson, E.N. (1957). *Understanding grief: Its roots, dynamics and treatment.* Nashville: Abingdon.

Jahoda, M. (1958). *Current concepts of positive mental health.* New York: Basic Books.

Kaplan, H.I., & Sadock, B.J. (1985). *Comprehensive textbook of psychiatry* (4th ed.). Baltimore: Williams & Wilkins.

Kirkham, A.K. (1980). Neuroses. In J. Lancaster (Ed.), *Adult psychiatric nursing.* Garden City, NY: Medical Examination Publishing.

Kübler-Ross, E. (1969). *On death and dying.* New York: Macmillan.

LeShan, R. (1977). *You can fight for your life.* New York: M. Evans & Co.

Lindemann, E. (1944). Symptomatology and management of acute grief. *American Journal of Psychiatry, 101*:141.

Maslow, A. (1970). *Motivation and personality* (2nd ed.). New York: Harper & Row.

May, R. (1950). *The meaning of anxiety.* New York: Ronald Press.

Menninger, K. (1963). *The vital balance.* New York: Viking Press.

Mims, F.H., & Swensen, M. (1980). *Sexuality: A nursing perspective.* New York: McGraw-Hill.

Parkes, C.M. (1972). *Bereavement: Studies of grief in adult life.* New York: International Universities Press.

Peplau, H. (1963). A working definition of anxiety. In S. Burd & M. Marshall (Eds.), *Some clinical approaches to psychiatric nursing.* New York: Macmillan.

Robinson, L. (1983). *Psychiatric nursing as a human experience* (3rd ed.). Philadelphia: W.B. Saunders.

Sills, G. (1973). Historical developments and issues in psychiatric mental health nursing. In M. Leininger (Ed.), *Contemporary issues in mental health nursing.* Boston: Little, Brown.

Stuart, G., and Sundeen, S. (1987). *Principles and practice of psychiatric nursing* (3rd ed.). St. Louis, MO: C.V. Mosby.

Bibliography

Alexander, F., and Selesnick, S. (1966). *The history of psychiatry.* New York: Harper & Row.

Carter, F.M. (1981). *Psychosocial nursing* (3rd ed.). New York: Macmillan.

Ellenberger, F. (1970). *The discovery of the unconscious.* New York: Basic Books.

Maslow, A. (1968). *Towards a psychology of being* (2nd ed.). New York: D. Van Nostrand.

THEORIES OF PERSONALITY DEVELOPMENT

CHAPTER OUTLINE

OBJECTIVES

INTRODUCTION

PSYCHOANALYTIC THEORY

INTERPERSONAL THEORY

THEORY OF PSYCHOSOCIAL DEVELOPMENT

THEORY OF OBJECT RELATIONS

COGNITIVE DEVELOPMENT THEORY

THEORY OF MORAL DEVELOPMENT

A NURSING MODEL—HILDEGARD E. PEPLAU

SUMMARY

REVIEW QUESTIONS

KEY TERMS

personality
temperament
id
ego
superego

libido
symbiosis
cognitive
    development
cognitive maturity

psychodynamic
    nursing
counselor
technical expert
surrogate

OBJECTIVES

After reading this chapter, the student will be able to:

1. Define *personality*.
2. Identify the relevance of knowledge associated with personality development to nursing in the psychiatric/mental health setting.
3. Discuss the major components of the following developmental theories:
   a. Psychoanalytic theory—Freud
   b. Interpersonal theory—Sullivan
   c. Theory of psychosocial development—Erikson
   d. Theory of object relations development—Mahler
   e. Cognitive development theory—Piaget
   f. Theory of moral development—Kohlberg
   g. A nursing model of interpersonal development—Peplau

he *DSM-IV* (American Psychiatric Association [APA], 1994) defines **personality** as "enduring patterns of perceiving, relating to, and thinking about the environment and oneself."

Nurses must have a basic knowledge of human personality development to understand maladaptive behavioral responses commonly seen in psychiatric clients. Developmental theories identify behaviors associated with various *stages* through which individuals pass, thereby specifying what is appropriate or inappropriate at each developmental level.

Specialists in child development have historically believed that infancy and early childhood are the major life periods for the origin and occurrence of developmental change (Clunn, 1991). Specialists in life-cycle development believe that people continue to develop and change throughout life, thereby suggesting the possibility for renewal and growth in adults (Schaie, 1984).

Developmental stages are identified by age. Behaviors can then be evaluated by whether or not they are recognized as age-appropriate. Ideally, an individual successfully fulfills all the tasks associated with one stage before moving on to the next stage (at the appropriate age). Realistically, however, this seldom happens. One reason is related to temperament. **Temperament** refers to inborn personality characteristics that influence an individual's manner of reacting to the environment, and ultimately their developmental progression (Chess & Thomas, 1986). The environment may also influence one's developmental pattern. Individuals who are reared in a dysfunctional family system often have retarded ego development. According to specialists in life-cycle development, behaviors from an unsuccessfully completed stage can be modified and corrected in a later stage.

Stages overlap, and an individual may be working on tasks associated with several stages at one time. When an individual becomes fixed in a lower level of development, with age-inappropriate behaviors focused on fulfillment of those tasks, psychopathology may become evident. Only when personality traits are inflexible and maladaptive and cause either significant functional impairment or subjective distress do they constitute "personality disorders" (APA, 1994). These disorders are discussed in Chapter 34.

PSYCHOANALYTIC THEORY

Freud (1961), who has been called the father of psychiatry, is credited as the first to identify development by stages. He considered the first 5 years of a child's life to be the most important, as he believed that an individual's basic character had been formed by the age of 5.

Freud's personality theory can be conceptualized according to structure and dynamics of the personality, topography of the mind, and stages of personality development.

Structure of the Personality

Freud organized the structure of the personality into three major components: the **id, ego,** and **superego.** They are distinguished by their unique functions and different characteristics.

Id

The *id* is the locus of instinctual drives—the "pleasure principle." Present at birth, it endows the infant with instinctual drives that seek to satisfy needs and achieve immediate gratification. Id-driven behaviors are impulsive and may be irrational.

Ego

The *ego,* also called the *rational self* or the "reality principle," begins to develop between the ages of 4 and 6 months. The ego experiences the reality of the external world, adapts to it, and responds to it. As the ego develops and gains strength, it seeks to bring the influences of the external world to bear upon the id, to substitute the reality principle for the pleasure principle (Kaplan & Sadock, 1989). A primary function of the ego is one of mediator; that is, to maintain harmony among the external world, the id, and the superego.

Superego

If the id is identified as the pleasure principle, and the ego the reality principle, the *superego* might be referred to as the "perfection principle." The superego, which develops between ages 3 and 6 years, internalizes the values and morals set forth by primary caregivers. Derived out of a system of rewards and punishments, the superego is composed of two major components: the *ego-ideal* and the *conscience.* When a child is consistently rewarded for "good" behavior, the self-esteem is enhanced, and the behavior becomes part of the ego-ideal; that is, it is internalized as part of his or her value system. The conscience is formed when the child is consistently punished for "bad" behavior. The child learns from feedback received from parental figures and from society or culture what is considered morally right or wrong. When moral and ethical principles or even internalized ideals and values are disregarded, the conscience generates a feeling of guilt within the individual. The superego is important in the socialization of the individual as it assists the ego in the control of id impulses. When the superego becomes rigid and punitive, problems with low self-confidence and low self-esteem arise.

Topography of the Mind

Freud classified all mental contents and operations into three categories: the conscious, the preconscious, and the unconscious.

* The *conscious* includes all memories that remain within an individual's awareness. It is the smallest of the three categories. Events and experiences that are easily remembered or retrieved are considered to be within one's conscious awareness. Examples include telephone numbers, birthdays of self and significant others, the dates of special holidays, and what one had for lunch this noon. The conscious mind is thought to be under the control of the ego, the rational and logical structure of the personality.
* The *preconscious* includes all memories that may have been forgotten or are not in present awareness but with attention can be readily recalled into consciousness. Examples include telephone numbers or addresses once known but little used and feelings associated with significant life events that may have occurred at sometime in the past. The preconscious enhances awareness by helping to *suppress* unpleasant or nonessential memories from consciousness. It is thought to be partially under the control of the superego, which helps to suppress unacceptable thoughts and behaviors.
* The *unconscious* includes all memories that one is unable to bring to conscious awareness. It is the largest of the three topographical levels. Unconscious material consists of unpleasant or nonessential memories that have been *repressed* and can only be retrieved through therapy, hypnosis, and with certain substances that alter the awareness and have the capacity to restructure repressed memories. Unconscious material may also emerge in dreams and in seemingly incomprehensible behavior.

Dynamics of the Personality

Freud believed that *psychic energy* is the force or impetus required for mental functioning. Originating in the id, it instinctually fulfills basic physiological needs. Freud called this psychic energy (or the drive to fulfill basic physiological needs such as hunger, thirst, and sex) the **libido.** As the child matures, psychic energy is diverted from the id to form the ego and then from the ego to form the superego. Psychic energy is distributed within these three components, with the ego retaining the largest share to maintain a balance between id impulsive behavior and the idealistic behaviors of the superego. If an excessive amount of psychic energy is stored in one of these personality components, behavior will reflect that part of the personality. For instance, impulsive behavior will prevail when excessive psychic energy is stored in the id. Overinvestment in the ego will be reflected in self-absorbed, or narcissistic, behaviors, and an excess within the superego will result in rigid, self-deprecating behaviors.

Freud used the terms *cathexis* and *anticathexis* to describe the forces within the id, ego, and superego that are used to invest psychic energy in external sources in order to satisfy needs. Cathexis is the process by which the id invests energy into an object in an attempt to achieve gratification. An example is the individual who instinctively turns to alcohol to relieve stress. Anticathexis is the use of psychic energy by the ego and the superego to control id impulses. In the example cited, the ego would attempt to control the use of alcohol with rational thinking, such as, "I already have ulcers from drinking too much. I will call my AA counselor for support. I will not drink." The superego would exert control with, "I shouldn't drink. If I drink, my family will be hurt and angry. I should think of how it affects them. I'm such a weak person." Freud believed that an imbalance between cathexis and anticathexis resulted in internal conflicts, producing tension and anxiety within the individual. Freud's daughter Anna devised a comprehensive list of defense mechanisms believed to be used by the ego as a protective device against anxiety in mediating between the excessive demands of the id and the excessive restrictions of the superego (see Chapter 2).

Freud's Stages of Personality Development

Freud described formation of the personality through five stages of *psychosexual* development. He placed much emphasis on the first 5 years of life and believed that characteristics developed during these early years bore heavily on one's adaptation patterns and personality traits in adulthood. Fixation in an early stage of development will almost certainly result in psychopathology. An outline of these five stages is presented in Table 3.1.

Oral Stage: Birth to 18 Months

During this stage, behavior is directed by the id, and the goal is immediate gratification of needs. The focus of energy is the mouth, with behaviors that include sucking, chewing, and biting. The infant feels a sense of attachment and is unable to differentiate the self from the person who is providing the mothering. This includes feelings such as anxiety, so that a pervasive feeling of anxiety on the part of the mother may be passed on to her infant, leaving the child vulnerable to similar feelings of insecurity. With the beginning of development of the ego at age 4 to 6 months, the infant starts to view the self as separate from the mothering figure. A sense of security and the ability to trust others is derived out of gratification from fulfillment of basic needs during this stage.

Anal Stage: 18 Months to 3 Years

The major tasks in this stage are gaining independence and control, with particular focus on the excretory func-

TABLE 3.1 FREUD'S STAGES OF PSYCHOSEXUAL DEVELOPMENT

AGE	STAGE	MAJOR DEVELOPMENTAL TASKS
Birth–18 months	Oral	Relief from anxiety through oral gratification of needs
18 months–3 years	Anal	Learning independence and control, with focus on the excretory function
3–6 years	Phallic	Identification with parent of same sex; development of sexual identity; focus on genital organs
6–12 years	Latency	Sexuality repressed; focus on relationships with same-sex peers
13–20 years	Genital	Libido reawakened as genital organs mature; focus on relationships with members of the opposite sex

tion. Freud believed that the manner in which the parents and other primary caregivers approach the task of toilet training may have long-term effects on the child in terms of values and personality characteristics. When toilet training is strict and rigid, the child may choose to retain the feces, becoming constipated. Adult retentive personality traits influenced by this type of training include stubbornness, stinginess, and miserliness. An alternate reaction to strict toilet training is for the child to expel feces in an unacceptable manner or at inappropriate times. Far-reaching effects of this behavior pattern include malevolence, cruelty to others, destructiveness, disorganization, and untidiness.

Toilet training that is more permissive and accepting attaches the feeling of importance and desirability to feces production. The child becomes extroverted, productive, and altruistic.

Phallic Stage: 3 to 6 Years

In this stage, the focus of energy shifts to the genital area. Discovery of differences between genders results in a heightened interest in the sexuality of self and others. This interest may be manifested in sexual self-exploratory or group-exploratory play. Freud proposed that the development of the *Oedipus complex* occurred during this stage of development. He described this as the child's unconscious desire to eliminate the parent of the same sex and to possess the parent of the opposite sex for himself or herself. Guilt feelings result with the emergence of the superego during these years. Resolution of this internal conflict occurs when the child develops a strong identification with the parent of the same sex and that parent's attitudes, beliefs, and value system are subsumed by the child.

Latency Stage: 6 to 12 Years

During the elementary school years, the focus changes from egocentrism to one in which there is more interest in group activities, learning, and socialization with peers. Sexuality is not absent during this period but remains obscure and imperceptible to others. The preference is ho-

mosexual; children of this age show a distinct preference for same-sex relationships, even rejecting members of the opposite sex.

Genital Stage: 13 to 20 Years

In the genital stage, there is a reawakening of the libidinal drive with the maturing of the genital organs. The focus is on relationships with members of the opposite sex and preparations for selecting a mate. The development of sexual maturity evolves from self-gratification to behaviors that have been deemed acceptable by societal norms. Interpersonal relationships are based on genuine pleasure derived from the interaction rather than the more self-serving implications of childhood associations.

Relevance of Psychoanalytic Theory to Nursing Practice

Knowledge about the structure of the personality can assist nurses who work in the mental health setting. Being able to recognize behaviors associated with the id, the ego, and the superego will assist in the assessment of developmental level. Understanding the use of ego defense mechanisms is important in making determinations about maladaptive behaviors, in planning care for clients to assist in creating change, if desired, or in helping clients accept themselves as unique individuals.

INTERPERSONAL THEORY

Sullivan (1953) believed that individual behavior and personality development are the direct result of interpersonal relationships. Prior to the development of his own theoretical framework, Sullivan embraced the concepts of Freud. Later, he changed the focus of his work from the *intrapersonal* view of Freud to one with more *interpersonal* flavor in which human behavior could be observed in social interactions with others. His ideas, which were not universally accepted at the time, have been integrated into the practice of psychiatry through publication only since his death in 1949. Sullivan's major concepts include:

Anxiety is a feeling of emotional discomfort, toward the relief or prevention of which all behavior is aimed. Sullivan believed that anxiety is the "chief disruptive force in interpersonal relations and the main factor in the development of serious difficulties in living." It arises out of one's inability to satisfy needs or achieve interpersonal security.

Satisfaction of needs is the fulfillment of all requirements associated with an individual's physicochemical environment. Sullivan identified examples of these requirements as oxygen, food, water, warmth, tenderness, rest, activity, sexual expression—virtually anything that, when absent, produces discomfort in the individual.

Interpersonal security is the feeling associated with relief from anxiety. When all needs have been met, one experiences a sense of total well-being, which Sullivan termed *interpersonal security*. He believed individuals have an innate need for interpersonal security.

Self-system is a collection of experiences, or security measures, adopted by the individual to protect against anxiety. Sullivan identified three components of the self-system, which are based on interpersonal experiences early in life:

* The "*good me*" is the part of the personality that develops in response to positive feedback from the primary caregiver. Feelings of pleasure, contentment, and gratification are experienced. The child learns which behaviors elicit this positive response as it becomes incorporated into the self-system.

* The "*bad me*" is the part of the personality that develops in response to negative feedback from the primary caregiver. Anxiety is experienced, eliciting feelings of discomfort, displeasure, and distress. The child learns to avoid these negative feelings by altering certain behaviors.

* The "*not me*" is the part of the personality that develops in response to situations that produce intense anxiety in the child. Feelings of horror, awe, dread, and loathing are experienced in response to these situations, leading the child to deny these feelings in an effort to relieve anxiety. These feelings, having then been denied, become "not me," but someone else. This withdrawal from emotions has serious implications for mental disorders in adult life.

Sullivan's Stages of Personality Development

Infancy: Birth to 18 Months

During this beginning stage, the major developmental task for the child is the gratification of needs. This is accomplished around activity associated with the mouth, such as crying, nursing, and thumb sucking.

Childhood: 18 Months to 6 Years

At this age, the child learns that interference with fulfillment of personal wishes and desires may result in delayed gratification. He or she learns to accept this and feel comfortable with it, recognizing that delayed gratification often results in parental approval, a more lasting type of reward. Tools of this stage include the mouth, language, the anus, experimentation, manipulation, and identification.

Juvenile: 6 to 9 Years

The major task of this stage is formation of satisfactory relationships within peer groups. This is accomplished through the use of competition, cooperation, and compromise.

Preadolescence: 9 to 12 Years

The tasks at this level focus on developing relationships with persons of the same sex. One's ability to collaborate with and show love and affection for another person begins at this stage.

Early Adolescence: 12 to 14 Years

During early adolescence, the child is struggling with developing a sense of identity, separate and independent from the parents. The major task is formation of satisfactory relationships with members of the opposite sex. Sullivan saw the emergence of lust in response to biological changes as a major force occurring during this period.

Late Adolescence: 14 to 21 Years

The late adolescent period is characterized by tasks associated with the attempt to achieve interdependence within the society and the formation of a lasting, intimate relationship with a selected member of the opposite sex. The genital organs are the major developmental focus of this stage.

An outline of the stages of personality development according to Sullivan's interpersonal theory is presented in Table 3.2.

Relevance of Interpersonal Theory to Nursing Practice

The interpersonal theory has significant relevance to nursing practice. Relationship development is a major concept of this theory, and relationship development is a major psychiatric nursing intervention. Nurses develop therapeutic relationships with clients in an effort to help them generalize this ability to interact successfully with others.

TABLE 3.2 STAGES OF DEVELOPMENT IN SULLIVAN'S INTERPERSONAL THEORY

AGE	STAGE	MAJOR DEVELOPMENTAL TASKS
Birth–18 months	Infancy	Relief from anxiety through oral gratification of needs
18 months–6 years	Childhood	Learning to experience a delay in personal gratification without undo anxiety
6–9 years	Juvenile	Learning to form satisfactory peer relationships
9–12 years	Preadolescence	Learning to form satisfactory relationships with persons of same sex; initiating feelings of affection for another person
12–14 years	Early adolescence	Learning to form satisfactory relationships with persons of the opposite sex; developing a sense of identity
14–21 years	Late adolescence	Establishing self-identity; experiencing satisfying relationships; working to develop a lasting, intimate opposite-sex relationship

Knowledge about the behaviors associated with all levels of anxiety and methods for alleviating anxiety helps nurses to assist clients achieve interpersonal security and a sense of well-being. Nurses use the concepts of Sullivan's theory to help clients achieve a higher degree of independent and interpersonal functioning.

THEORY OF PSYCHOSOCIAL DEVELOPMENT

Erikson (1963) studied the influence of social processes on the development of the personality. He described eight stages of the life cycle during which individuals struggle with developmental "crises." Specific tasks associated with each stage must be completed for resolution of the crisis and for emotional growth to occur. An outline of Erikson's stages of psychosocial development is presented in Table 3.3.

Erikson's Stages of Personality Development

Trust versus Mistrust: Birth to 18 Months

Major Developmental Task. In this stage, the major task is to develop a basic trust in the mothering figure and be able to generalize it to others.

* Achievement of the task results in self-confidence, optimism, faith in the gratification of needs and desires, and hope for the future. The infant learns to trust when basic needs are consistently met.
* Nonachievement results in emotional dissatisfaction with the self and others, suspiciousness, and difficulty with interpersonal relationships. The task remains unresolved when primary caregivers fail to respond to the infant's distress signal promptly and consistently.

TABLE 3.3 STAGES OF DEVELOPMENT IN ERIKSON'S PSYCHOSOCIAL THEORY

AGE	STAGE	MAJOR DEVELOPMENTAL TASKS
Infancy (Birth–18 months)	Trust vs. mistrust	To develop a basic trust in the mothering figure and be able to generalize it to others
Early childhood (18 months–3 years)	Autonomy vs. shame and doubt	To gain some self-control and independence within the environment
Late childhood (3–6 years)	Initiative vs. guilt	To develop a sense of purpose and the ability to initiate and direct own activities
School age (6–12 years)	Industry vs. inferiority	To achieve a sense of self-confidence by learning, competing, performing successfully, and receiving recognition from significant others, peers, and acquaintances
Adolescence (12–20 years)	Identity vs. role confusion	To integrate the tasks mastered in the previous stages into a secure sense of self
Young adulthood (20–30 years)	Intimacy vs. isolation	To form an intense, lasting relationship or a commitment to another person, cause, institution, or creative effort
Adulthood (30–65 years)	Generativity vs. stagnation	To achieve the life goals established for oneself, while also considering the welfare of future generations
Old age (65 years–death)	Ego integrity vs. despair	To review one's life and derive meaning from both positive and negative events, while achieving a positive sense of self-worth

Autonomy versus Shame and Doubt: 18 Months to 3 Years

Major Developmental Task. The major task in this stage is to gain some self-control and independence within the environment.

* Achievement of the task results in a sense of self-control and the ability to delay gratification, and a feeling of self-confidence in one's ability to perform. Autonomy is achieved when parents encourage and provide opportunities for independent activities.
* Nonachievement results in a lack of self-confidence, a lack of pride in the ability to perform, a sense of being controlled by others, and a rage against the self. The task remains unresolved when primary caregivers restrict independent behaviors, both physically and verbally, or set the child up for failure with unrealistic expectations.

Initiative versus Guilt: 3 to 6 Years

Major Developmental Task. During this stage the goal is to develop a sense of purpose and the ability to initiate and direct one's own activities.

* Achievement of the task results in the ability to exercise restraint and self-control of inappropriate social behaviors. Assertiveness and dependability increase, and the child enjoys learning and personal achievement. The conscience develops, thereby controlling the impulsive behaviors of the id. Initiative is achieved when creativity is encouraged and performance is recognized and positively reinforced.
* Nonachievement results in feelings of inadequacy and a sense of defeat. Guilt is experienced to an excessive degree, even to the point of accepting liability in situations for which one is not responsible. The child may view himself or herself as evil and deserving of punishment. The task remains unresolved when creativity is stifled and parents continually expect a higher level of achievement than the child produces.

Industry versus Inferiority: 6 to 12 Years

Major Developmental Task. The major task here is to achieve a sense of self-confidence by learning, competing, performing successfully, and receiving recognition from significant others, peers, and acquaintances.

* Achievement of the task results in a sense of satisfaction and pleasure in the interaction and involvement with others. The individual masters reliable work habits and develops attitudes of trustworthiness. He or she is conscientious, feels pride in achievement, and enjoys play but desires a balance between fantasy and "real world" activities. Industry is achieved when encouragement is given to activities and responsibilities in the school and community, as well as those within the home, and recognition is given for accomplishments.
* Nonachievement results in difficulty in interpersonal relationships owing to feelings of personal inadequacy. The individual can neither cooperate and compromise with others in group activities nor problem solve or complete tasks successfully. He or she may become either passive and meek or overly aggressive to cover up for feelings of inadequacy. If this occurs, the individual may manipulate or violate the rights of others to satisfy his or her own needs or desires; he or she may become a workaholic with unrealistic expectations for personal achievement. This task remains unresolved when parents set unrealistic expectations for the child, when discipline is harsh and tends to impair self-esteem, and when accomplishments are consistently met with negative feedback.

Identity versus Role Confusion: 12 to 20 Years

Major Developmental Task. At this stage, the goal is to integrate the tasks mastered in the previous stages into a secure sense of self.

* Achievement of the task results in a sense of confidence, emotional stability, and a view of the self as a unique individual. Commitments are made to a value system, to the choice of a career, and to relationships with members of both genders. Identity is achieved when adolescents are allowed to experience independence by making decisions that influence their lives. Parents should be available to offer support when needed but should gradually relinquish control to the maturing individual in an effort to encourage the development of an independent sense of self.
* Nonachievement results in a sense of self-consciousness, doubt, and confusion about one's role in life. Personal values or goals for one's life are absent. Commitments to relationships with others are nonexistent, but instead are superficial and brief. A lack of self-confidence is often expressed by delinquent and rebellious behavior. Entering adulthood, with its accompanying responsibilities, may be an underlying fear. This task can remain unresolved for many reasons. Examples include: when independence is discouraged by the parents, and the adolescent is nurtured in the dependent position; when discipline within the home has been overly harsh, inconsistent, or absent; and when there has been

parental rejection or frequent shifting of parental figures.

Intimacy versus Isolation: 20 to 30 Years

Major Developmental Task. The objective during this phase is to form an intense, lasting relationship or a commitment to another person, a cause, an institution, or a creative effort (Murray & Zentner, 1997).

* Achievement of the task results in the capacity for mutual love and respect between two people and the ability of an individual to pledge a total commitment to another. The intimacy goes far beyond the sexual contact between two people. It describes a commitment in which personal sacrifices are made for another, whether it be another person or, if one chooses, a career or other type of cause or endeavor to which an individual elects to devote his or her life. Intimacy is achieved when an individual has developed the capacity for giving of oneself to another. This is learned when one has been the recipient of this type of giving within the family unit.
* Nonachievement results in withdrawal, social isolation, aloneness. The individual is unable to form lasting, intimate relationships, often seeking intimacy through numerous superficial sexual contacts. No career is established; he or she may have a history of occupational changes (or may fear change and thus remain in an undesirable job situation). The task remains unresolved when love in the home has been deprived or distorted through the younger years (Murray & Zentner, 1997). One fails to achieve the ability to give of the self without having been the recipient early on from primary caregivers.

Generativity versus Stagnation or Self-Absorption: 30 to 65 Years

Major Developmental Tasks. The major task here is to achieve the life goals established for oneself while also considering the welfare of future generations.

* Achievement of the task results in a sense of gratification from personal and professional achievements, and from meaningful contributions to others. The individual is active in the service of and to society. Generativity is achieved when the individual expresses satisfaction with this stage in life and demonstrates responsibility for leaving the world a better place in which to live.
* Nonachievement results in lack of concern for the welfare of others and total preoccupation with the self. He or she becomes withdrawn, isolated, and highly self-indulgent, with no capacity for giving of the self to others. The task remains unresolved when earlier developmental tasks are not fulfilled and the individual does not achieve the degree of maturity required to derive gratification out of a personal concern for the welfare of others.

Ego Integrity versus Despair: 65 Years to Death

Major Developmental Task. During this phase, the goal is to review one's life and derive meaning from both positive and negative events, while achieving a positive sense of self at this stage in life.

* Achievement of the task results in a sense of self-worth and self-acceptance as one reviews life goals, accepting that some were achieved and some were not. The individual derives a sense of dignity from his or her life experiences and does not fear death, rather viewing it as another phase of development. Ego integrity is achieved when individuals have successfully completed the developmental tasks of the other stages and would have little desire to make major changes in how their lives have progressed.
* Nonachievement results in a sense of self-contempt and disgust with how life has progressed. The individual would like to start over and have a second chance at life. He or she feels worthless and helpless to change. Anger, depression, and loneliness are evident. The focus may be on past failures or perceived failures. Impending death is feared or denied, or ideas of suicide may prevail. The task remains unresolved when earlier tasks are not fulfilled: self-confidence, a concern for others, and a strong sense of self-identity were never achieved.

Relevance of Psychosocial Development Theory to Nursing Practice

Erikson's theory is particularly relevant to nursing practice in that it incorporates sociocultural concepts into the development of personality. He provides a systematic, stepwise approach and outlines specific tasks that should be completed during each stage. This information can be used quite readily in psychiatric/mental health nursing. Many individuals with mental health problems are still struggling to achieve tasks from a number of developmental stages. Nurses can plan care to assist these individuals to fulfill these tasks and move on to a higher developmental level.

THEORY OF OBJECT RELATIONS

Mahler (Mahler, Pine, & Bergman, 1975) has formulated a theory that describes the separation-individuation process of the infant from the maternal figure (primary caregiver). She describes this process as progressing through three major phases. She further delineates phase 3, the separation-individuation phase, into four subphases. Mahler's developmental theory is outlined in Table 3.4.

Phase I: The Autistic Phase (Birth to 1 Month)

In this phase, also called *normal autism*, the infant exists in a half-sleeping, half-waking state and does not perceive the existence of other people or an external environment. The fulfillment of basic needs for survival and comfort is the focus and is merely accepted as it occurs. Fixation in this phase predisposes the child to autistic disorder.

Phase II: The Symbiotic Phase (1 to 5 Months)

Symbiosis is a type of "psychic fusion" of mother and child. The child views the self as an extension of the mother, but with a developing awareness that it is she who fulfills his or her every need. Mahler suggests that absence of, or rejection by, the maternal figure at this phase can lead to symbiotic psychosis. Fixation in the symbiotic phase of development predisposes the child to adolescent- or adult-onset schizophrenia.

Phase III: Separation-Individuation (5 to 36 Months)

This third phase represents what Mahler calls the "psychological birth" of the child. *Separation* is defined as the physical and psychological attainment of a sense of personal distinction from the mothering figure. *Individuation* occurs with a strengthening of the ego and an acceptance of a sense of "self," with independent ego boundaries.

Four subphases through which the child evolves in his or her progression from a symbiotic extension of the mothering figure to a distinct and separate being are described.

Subphase 1—Differentiation (5 to 10 Months). This phase begins with the child's initial physical movements away from the mothering figure. A primary recognition of separateness commences.

Subphase 2—Practicing (10 to 16 Months). With advanced locomotor functioning, the child experiences feelings of exhilaration from increased independence. He or she is now able to move away from, and return to, the mothering figure. A sense of omnipotence is manifested.

Subphase 3—Rapprochement (16 to 24 Months). This third subphase is extremely critical to the child's healthy ego development. During this time, the child becomes increasingly aware of his or her separateness from the mothering figure, while the sense of fearlessness and omnipotence diminishes. The child, now recognizing the mother as a separate individual, wishes to reestablish closeness with her but shuns the total reengulfment of the symbiotic stage. The need is for the mothering figure to be available to provide "emotional refueling" on demand.

Critical to this subphase is the mothering figure's response to the child. If she is available to fulfill emotional needs as they are required, the child develops a sense of security in the knowledge that he or she is loved and will not be abandoned. However, if emotional needs are inconsistently met or if the mother rewards clinging, dependent behaviors and withholds nurturing when the child demonstrates independence, feelings of rage and a fear of abandonment develop and often persist into adulthood.

Subphase 4—Consolidation (24 to 36 Months). With achievement of this subphase, a definite individuality and sense of separateness of self are

---

TABLE 3.4   STAGES OF DEVELOPMENT IN MAHLER'S THEORY OF OBJECT RELATIONS

AGE	PHASE/SUBPHASE		MAJOR DEVELOPMENTAL TASKS
Birth–1 month	I.	Normal autism	Fulfillment of basic needs for survival and comfort
1–5 months	II.	Symbiosis	Development of awareness of external source of need fulfillment
	III.	Separation-Individuation	
5–10 months		a. Differentiation	Commencement of a primary recognition of separateness from the mothering figure
10–16 months		b. Practicing	Increased independence through locomotor functioning; increased sense of separateness of self
16–24 months		c. Rapprochement	Acute awareness of separateness of self; learning to seek "emotional refueling" from mothering figure to maintain feeling of security
24–36 months		d. Consolidation	Sense of separateness established; on the way to object constancy (i.e., able to internalize a sustained image of loved object/person when it is out of sight); resolution of separation anxiety

established. Objects are represented as whole, with the child having the ability to integrate both "good" and "bad." A degree of object constancy is established as the child is able to internalize a sustained image of the mothering figure as enduring and loving, while maintaining the perception of her as a separate person in the outside world.

Relevance of Object Relations Theory to Nursing Practice

Understanding of the concepts of Mahler's theory of object relations assists the nurse to assess the client's level of individuation from primary caregivers. The emotional problems of many individuals can be traced to lack of fulfillment of the tasks of separation/individuation. Examples include problems related to dependency and excessive anxiety. The individual with borderline personality disorder is thought to be fixed in the rapprochement phase of development, harboring fears of abandonment and underlying rage. This knowledge is important in the provision of nursing care to these individuals.

COGNITIVE DEVELOPMENT THEORY

Piaget (Piaget & Inhelder, 1969) has been called the father of child psychology. His work concerning **cognitive development** in children is based on the premise that human intelligence is an extension of biological adaptation—or one's ability to adapt psychologically to the environment. He believed that human intelligence progresses through a series of stages that are related to age, demonstrating at each successive stage a higher level of logical organization than at the previous stages.

From his extensive studies of cognitive development in children, Piaget discovered four major stages, each of which he believed to be a necessary prerequisite for the one that follows. An outline is presented in Table 3.5.

Stage 1: Sensorimotor (Birth to 2 Years)

From the beginning, the child is concerned only with satisfying basic needs and comforts. The self is not differentiated from the external environment. As the sense of differentiation occurs, with increasing mobility and awareness, the mental system is expanded. The child develops a greater understanding regarding objects within the external environment and their effects upon him or her. Knowledge is gained regarding the ability to manipulate objects and experiences within the environment. The sense of *object permanence*, the notion that an object will continue to exist when it is no longer present to the senses, is initiated.

Stage 2: Preoperational (2 to 6 years)

Piaget believed that preoperational thought is characterized by egocentrism. Personal experiences are thought to be universal, and the child is unable to accept the differing viewpoints of others. Language development progresses, as does the ability to attribute special meaning to symbolic gestures (e.g., bringing a story book to mother is a symbolic invitation to have a story read). Reality is often given to inanimate objects. Object permanence culminates in the ability to conjure up mental representations of objects or people.

Stage 3: Concrete Operations (6 to 12 Years)

The ability to apply logic to thinking begins in this stage; however, "concreteness" still predominates. An understanding of the concepts of reversibility and spatiality is developed. For example, the child recognizes that changing the shape of objects does not necessarily change the amount, weight, volume, or the ability of the object to return to its original form. Another achievement of this stage is the ability to classify objects by any of their several characteristics. For example, he or she can classify all poodles as dogs but recognizes that all dogs are not poodles.

TABLE 3.5 PIAGET'S STAGES OF COGNITIVE DEVELOPMENT

AGE	STAGE	MAJOR DEVELOPMENTAL TASKS
Birth–2 years	Sensorimotor	With increased mobility and awareness, development of a sense of self as separate from the external environment; the concept of object permanence emerges as the ability to form mental images evolves
2–6 years	Preoperational	Learning to express self with language; development of understanding of symbolic gestures; achievement of object permanence
6–12 years	Concrete operations	Learning to apply logic to thinking; development of understanding of reversibility and spatiality; learning to differentiate and classify; increased socialization and application of rules
12–15+ years	Formal operations	Learning to think and reason in abstract terms; making and testing hypotheses; capability of logical thinking and reasoning expand and are refined; cognitive maturity achieved

The concept of a lawful self is developed at this stage as the child becomes more socialized and rule conscious. Egocentrism decreases, the ability to cooperate in interactions with other children increases, and understanding and acceptance of established rules grow.

Stage 4: Formal Operations (12 to 15+ Years)

At this stage, the individual is able to think and reason in abstract terms. He or she can make and test hypotheses using logical and orderly problem solving. Current situations and reflections of the future are idealized, and a degree of egocentrism returns during this stage. There may be some difficulty reconciling idealistic hopes with more rational prospects. Formal operations, however, enable individuals to distinguish between the ideal and the real. Piaget's theory suggests that most individuals achieve **cognitive maturity,** the capability to perform all mental operations needed for adulthood, in middle to late adolescence.

Relevance of Cognitive Development Theory to Nursing Practice

Nurses who work in psychiatry are likely to be involved in helping clients, particularly depressed clients, with techniques of cognitive therapy. In cognitive therapy, the individual is taught to control thought distortions that are considered to be a factor in the development and maintenance of mood disorders. In the cognitive model, depression is characterized by a triad of negative distortions related to expectations of the environment, self, and the future. In this model, depression is viewed as a distortion in cognitive development, the self is unrealistically devalued, and the future is perceived as hopeless. Therapy focuses on changing "automatic thoughts" that occur spontaneously and contribute to the distorted affect. Nurses who assist with this type of therapy must have knowledge of how cognition develops in order to help clients identify the distorted thought patterns and make the changes required for improvement in affective functioning.

THEORY OF MORAL DEVELOPMENT

Kohlberg's (1968) stages of moral development are not closely tied to specific age groups. Research was conducted with males ranging in age from 10 to 28 years. Kohlberg believes that each stage is necessary and basic to the next stage and that all individuals must progress through each stage sequentially. He defined three major levels of moral development, each of which is further subdivided into two stages each. Most people do not progress through all six stages. An outline of Kohlberg's developmental stages is presented in Table 3.6.

Level I: Preconventional Level (Prominent from Ages 4 to 10 Years)

Stage 1—Punishment and Obedience Orientation. At this stage the individual is responsive to cultural guidelines of good and bad, right and wrong, but primarily in terms of the known related consequences. Fear of punishment is likely to be the incentive for conformity (e.g., "I'll do it, because if I don't I can't watch TV for a week.")

Stage 2—Instrumental Relativist Orientation. Behaviors of this stage are guided by egocentrism and concern for self. There is an intense desire to satisfy one's own needs, but occasionally the needs of others are considered. For the most part, decisions are based on personal benefits derived (e.g., "I'll do it if I get something in return," or occasionally, ". . . because you asked me to").

TABLE 3.6 KOHLBERG'S STAGES OF MORAL DEVELOPMENT

LEVEL/AGE*	STAGE	DEVELOPMENTAL FOCUS
I. Preconventional (common from age 4 to 10 years)	1. Punishment and obedience orientation	Behavior motivated by fear of punishment
	2. Instrumental relativist orientation	Behavior motivated by egocentrism and concern for self
II. Conventional (common from age 10 to 13 years, and into adulthood)	3. Interpersonal concordance orientation	Behavior motivated by expectations of others; strong desire for approval and acceptance
	4. Law and order orientation	Behavior motivated by respect for authority
III. Postconventional (can occur from adolescence on)	5. Social contract legalistic orientation	Behavior motivated by respect for universal laws and moral principles; guided by internal set of values
	6. Universal ethical principle orientation	Behavior motivated by internalized principles of honor, justice, and respect for human dignity; guided by the conscience

*Ages in Kohlberg's theory are not well defined. The stage of development is determined by the motivation behind the individual's behavior.

Level II: Conventional Level (Prominent from Ages 10 to 13 Years and into Adulthood)*

Stage 3—Interpersonal Concordance Orientation. Behavior at this stage is guided by the expectations of others. Approval and acceptance within one's societal group provide the incentive to conform (e.g., "I'll do it because you asked me to," ". . . because it will help you," or ". . . because it will please you").

Stage 4—Law and Order Orientation. There is a personal respect for authority. Rules and laws are required and override personal principles and group mores. The belief is that all individuals and groups are subject to the same code of order, and no one is exempt (e.g., "I'll do it because it is the law").

Level III. Postconventional Level (Can Occur from Adolescence on)

Stage 5—Social Contract Legalistic Orientation. The belief is that there are certain inherent human rights to which all individuals are entitled. Individuals who reach stage 5 have developed a system of values and principles that determine for them what is right or wrong; behaviors are acceptably guided by this value system, provided they do not violate the human rights of others. The individual at stage 5 lives according to universal laws and principles; however, he or she holds the idea that the laws are subject to scrutiny and change as needs within society evolve and change (e.g., "I'll do it because it is the moral and legal thing to do, even though it is not my personal choice").

Stage 6—Universal Ethical Principle Orientation. Behavior at this stage is directed by internalized principles of honor, justice, and respect for human dignity. Laws are abstract and unwritten, such as the "Golden Rule," "equality of human rights," and "justice for all," not the concrete rules established by society. The conscience is the guide, and when one fails to meet the self-expected behaviors, intense guilt is the personal consequence. The allegiance to these ethical principles is so strong that the individual will stand by them even knowing that negative consequences will result (e.g., "I'll do it because I believe it is the right thing to do, even though it is illegal and I will be imprisoned for doing it").

*Eighty percent of adults are fixed in level II, with a majority of women in stage 3 and a majority of men in stage 4.

Relevance of Moral Development Theory to Nursing Practice

Moral development has relevance to psychiatric nursing in that it affects critical thinking about how individuals ought to behave and treat others. Moral behavior reflects the way a person interprets basic respect for other persons, such as the respect for human life, freedom, justice, or confidentiality (Davis, 1981). Psychiatric nurses must be able to assess the level of moral development of their clients in order to be able to help them in their effort to advance in their progression toward a higher level of developmental maturity.

A NURSING MODEL— HILDEGARD E. PEPLAU

Peplau (1991) applied interpersonal theory to nursing practice and, most specifically, to nurse-client relationship development. She provides a framework for "psychodynamic nursing," the interpersonal involvement of the nurse with a client in a given nursing situation. Peplau states, "Nursing is helpful when both the patient and the nurse grow as a result of the learning that occurs in the nursing situation."

Peplau correlates the stages of personality development in childhood to stages through which clients advance during the progression of an illness. She also views these interpersonal experiences as learning situations for nurses to facilitate forward movement in the development of personality. She believes that when there is fulfillment of psychological tasks associated with the nurse-client relationship, the personalities of both can be strengthened. Key concepts include the following:

Nursing is a human relationship between an individual who is sick, or in need of health services, and a nurse especially educated to recognize and to respond to the need for help.

Psychodynamic nursing is being able to understand one's own behavior, to help others identify felt difficulties, and to apply principles of human relations to the problems that arise at all levels of experience.

Roles are sets of values and behaviors that are specific to functional positions within social structures. Peplau identifies the following *nursing roles*:

* *Resource person* is one who provides specific, needed information that aids the client to understand his or her problem and the new situation.

* **Counselor** is one who listens as the client reviews feelings related to difficulties he or she is experiencing in any aspect of life. "Interpersonal techniques" have been identified to facilitate the nurse's interaction in the process of helping the client solve problems and make decisions concerning these difficulties.

* *Teacher* is one who identifies learning needs and provides information to the client or family that may aid in improvement of the life situation.
* *Leader* is one who directs the nurse-client interaction and ensures that appropriate actions are undertaken to facilitate achievement of the designated goals.
* **Technical expert** is one who understands various professional devices and possesses the clinical skills necessary to perform the interventions that are in the best interest of the client.
* **Surrogate** is one who serves as a substitute figure for another.

Phases of nurse-client relationship are stages of overlapping roles or functions in relation to health problems, during which the nurse and client learn to work cooperatively to resolve difficulties. Peplau identifies four phases:
* *Orientation* is the phase during which the client, nurse, and family work together to recognize, clarify, and define the existing problem (Belcher & Fish, 1980).
* *Identification* is the phase after which the client's initial impression has been clarified and when he or she begins to respond selectively to persons who seem to offer the help that is needed. Clients may respond in one of three ways: (1) on the basis of participation or interdependent relations with the nurse; (2) on the basis of independence or isolation from the nurse; or (3) on the basis of helplessness or dependence on the nurse (Peplau, 1991).
* *Exploitation* is the phase during which the client proceeds to take full advantage of the services offered to him or her. Having learned which services are available, feeling comfortable within the setting, and serving as an active participant in his or her own health care, the client exploits the services available and explores all possibilities of the changing situation.
* *Resolution* occurs when the client is freed from identification with helping persons and gathers strength to assume independence. Resolution is the direct result of successful completion of the other three phases.

Psychological tasks are developmental lessons that must be learned on the way to achieving maturity of the personality.

Peplau's Stages of Personality Development

Peplau identifies four psychological tasks that she associates with the stages of infancy and childhood described by Freud and Sullivan. She states,

"When psychological tasks are successfully learned at each era of development, biological capacities are used productively and relations with people lead to productive living. When they are not successfully learned they carry over into adulthood and attempts at learning continue in devious ways, more or less impeded by conventional adaptations that provide a superstructure over the baseline of actual learning" (Peplau, 1991, p. 166).

In the context of nursing, Peplau (1991) relates these four psychological tasks to the demands made on nurses in their relations with clients. She maintains that

"...nursing can function as a maturing force in society. Since illness is an event that is experienced along with feelings that derive from older experiences but are reenacted in the relationship of nurse to patient, the nurse-patient relationship is seen as an opportunity for nurses to help patients to complete the unfinished psychological tasks of childhood in some degree" (p. 159).

Peplau's psychological tasks of personality development include the following four stages.

Learning to Count on Others

Nurses and clients first come together as strangers. Both bring to the relationship certain "raw materials," such as inherited biological components, personality characteristics (*temperament*), individual intellectual capacity, and specific cultural or environmental influences. Peplau relates these to the same "raw materials" with which an infant comes into this world. The newborn is capable of experiencing *comfort* and *discomfort*. He or she soon learns to communicate feelings in a way that results in the fulfillment of comfort needs by the mothering figure who provides love and care unconditionally. However, fulfillment of these dependency needs is inhibited when goals of the mothering figure become the focus, and love and care are contingent upon meeting the needs of the caregiver rather than the infant.

Clients with unmet dependency needs will regress during illness and demonstrate behaviors that relate to this stage of development. Other clients will regress to this level because of physical disabilities associated with their illness. Peplau believes that when nurses provide unconditional care, they help these clients progress toward more mature levels of functioning. This may involve the role of "surrogate mother," in which the nurse fulfills needs for the client with the intent of helping him or her grow, mature, and become more independent.

Learning to Delay Satisfaction

Peplau relates this stage to that of toddlerhood, or the first step in the development of interdependent social relations. Psychosexually, it is compared to the anal stage of development, when a child learns that, because of cultural mores, he or she cannot empty the bowels for relief of discomfort at will, but must delay to use the toilet, which is considered more culturally acceptable. Toilet training that occurs too early, is very rigid and renders the child powerless, is presented as a dirty and disgusting behavior, or is set forth as a condition for love and caring results in a child's unfulfillment of the tasks associated with this stage. The child fails to learn the satisfaction of pleasing others by delaying self-gratification in small ways. He or she may also exhibit rebellious behavior by failing to comply with demands of the mothering figure in an effort to counter feelings of powerlessness. The child may accomplish this by withholding the fecal product or failing to deposit it in the culturally acceptable manner.

Peplau cites Fromm (1949) in describing the following potential behaviors of individuals who have failed to complete the tasks of the second stage of development:

* Exploitation and manipulation of others to satisfy their own desires because they are unable to do so independently
* Suspiciousness and envy of others, directing hostility toward others in an effort to enhance their own self-image
* Hoarding and withholding possessions from others; miserliness
* Inordinate neatness and punctuality
* Inability to relate to others through sharing of feelings, ideas, or experiences
* Ability to vary the personality characteristics to those required to satisfy personal desires at any given time

When nurses observe these types of behaviors in clients, it is important to encourage full expression and to convey unconditional acceptance. When the client learns to feel safe and unconditionally accepted, he or she is more likely to let go of the oppositional behavior and advance in the developmental progression. Peplau states:

> "Nurses who aid patients to feel safe and secure, so that wants can be expressed and satisfaction eventually achieved, also help them to strengthen personal power that is needed for productive social activities."

Identifying Oneself

"A concept of self develops as a product of interaction with adults" (Peplau, 1991, p. 211). A child learns to structure self-concept by observing how others interact with him or her as a person. Roles and behaviors are established out of the child's perception of the expectations of others. When children perceive that adults expect them to maintain more-or-less permanent roles as infants, they perceive themselves as helpless and dependent. When the perceived expectation is that the child must behave in a manner beyond his or her maturational level, the child is deprived of the fulfillment of emotional and growth needs at the lower levels of development. Children who are given freedom to respond to situations and experiences unconditionally (i.e., with behaviors that are appropriate to their feelings) learn to improve on and reconstruct behavioral responses at their own individual pace. Peplau states, "The ways in which adults appraise the child and the way he functions in relation to his experiences and perceptions are taken in or introjected and become the child's view of himself" (Peplau, 1991, p. 213).

In nursing, it is important for the nurse to recognize cues that communicate how the client feels about himself or herself, and about the presenting medical problem. In the initial interaction, it is difficult for the nurse to perceive the "wholeness" of the client, for the focus is on the condition that has caused him or her to seek help. Likewise, it is difficult for the client to perceive the nurse as a "mother (or father)" or "somebody's wife (or husband)" or as having a life aside from being there to offer assistance with the immediate presenting problem. As the relationship develops, nurses must be able to recognize client behaviors that indicate unfulfilled needs and provide experiences that promote growth. For example, the client who very proudly announces that she has completed activities of daily living (ADLs) independently and wants the nurse to come and inspect her room may still be craving the positive reinforcement that is so necessary at lower levels of development.

Nurses must also be aware of the predisposing factors that they bring to the relationship. Attitudes and beliefs about certain issues can have a deleterious effect on the client and interfere not only with the therapeutic relationship but also with the client's ability for growth and development. For example, a nurse who has strong beliefs against abortion may treat a client who has just undergone an abortion with disapproval and disrespect. The nurse may respond in this manner without even realizing he or she is doing so. Attitudes and values are introjected during early development and can be integrated so completely as to become a part of the self-system. Nurses must have knowledge and appreciation of their own concept of self in order to develop the flexibility required to accept all clients as they are, unconditionally. Effective resolution of problems that arise in the interdependent relationship can be the means for both client and nurse to reinforce positive personality traits and modify those more negative views of self.

Developing Skills in Participation

Peplau cites Sullivan's (1953) description of the "juvenile" stage of personality development (ages 6 through 9). During this stage, the child develops the capacity to "compromise, compete, and cooperate" with others. These skills are considered to be basic to one's ability to

▰ TABLE 3.7   STAGES OF DEVELOPMENT IN PEPLAU'S INTERPERSONAL THEORY

AGE	STAGE	MAJOR DEVELOPMENTAL TASKS
Infancy	Learning to count on others	Learning to communicate in various ways with the primary caregiver in order to have comfort needs fulfilled
Toddlerhood	Learning to delay satisfaction	Learning the satisfaction of pleasing others by delaying self-gratification in small ways
Early childhood	Identifying oneself	Learning appropriate roles and behaviors by acquiring the ability to perceive the expectations of others
Late childhood	Developing skills in participation	Learning the skills of compromise, competition, and cooperation with others; establishment of a more realistic view of the world and a feeling of one's place in it.

participate collaboratively with others. If a child tries to use the skills of an earlier level of development, e.g., crying, whining, or demanding, he or she may be rejected by peers of this juvenile stage. As this stage progresses, children begin to view themselves through the eyes of their peers. Sullivan (1953) called this "consensual validation." Preadolescents take on a more realistic view of the world and a feeling of their place in it. The capacity to love others (besides the mother figure) develops at this time and is expressed in relation to one's self-acceptance.

Failure to develop appropriate skills at any point along the developmental progression results in an individual's difficulty with participation in confronting the recurring problems of life. It is not the responsibility of the nurse to teach solutions to problems, but rather to help clients improve their problem-solving skills so that they may achieve their own resolution. This is accomplished through development of the skills of competition, compromise, cooperation, consensual validation, and love of self and others. Nurses can assist clients to develop or refine these skills by helping them to identify the problem, define a goal, and take the responsibility for performing the actions necessary to reach that goal. Peplau (1991) states:

> "Participation is required by a democratic society. When it has not been learned in earlier experiences, nurses have an opportunity to facilitate learning in the present and thus to aid in the promotion of a democratic society" (p. 259).

An outline of the stages of personality development according to Peplau's theory is presented in Table 3.7.

Relevance of Peplau's Model to Nursing Practice

Peplau's model provides nurses with a framework to interact with clients, many of whom are fixed in, or because of illness have regressed to, an earlier level of development. She suggests roles that nurses may assume in order to assist clients to progress and to achieve or resume their appropriate developmental level. Appropriate developmental progression arms the individual with the ability to confront the recurring problems of life. Nurses serve to facilitate learning of that which has not been learned in earlier experiences.

SUMMARY

Growth and development are unique with each individual and continue throughout the life span. With each stage, there evolves an increasing complexity in the growth of the personality. This chapter has provided a description of the theories of Freud, Sullivan, Erikson, Mahler, Piaget, and Kohlberg. In addition, the theoretical concepts of Peplau, and their application to interpersonal relations in nursing, were presented. These theorists together provide a multifaceted approach to personality development, encompassing cognitive, psychosocial, and moral aspects.

Nurses must have a basic knowledge of human personality development to understand maladaptive behavioral responses commonly seen in psychiatric clients. Knowledge of the appropriateness of behaviors at each developmental level is vital to the planning and implementation of quality nursing care.

REVIEW QUESTIONS

SELF-EXAMINATION/LEARNING EXERCISE

Situation: Mr. J. is 35 years old. He has been admitted to the psychiatric unit for observation and evaluation following his arrest on charges that he robbed a convenience store and sexually assaulted the store clerk. Mr. J. was the illegitimate child of a teenage mother who deserted him when he was 6 months old. He was shuffled from one relative to another until it was clear that no one wanted him. Social services placed him in foster homes, from which he continuously ran away. During his teenage years he was arrested a number of times for stealing, vandalism, arson, and various other infractions of the law. He was shunned by his peers and to this day has little interaction with others. On the unit, he appears very anxious, paces back and forth, and darts his head from side to side in a continuous scanning of the area. He is unkempt and unclean. He has refused to eat, making some barely audible comment related to "being poisoned." He has shown no remorse for his misdeeds.

Select the answer that is most appropriate for this situation.

1. Theoretically, in which level of psychosocial development (according to Erikson) would you place Mr. J.?
   a. Intimacy versus isolation
   b. Generativity versus self-absorption
   c. Trust versus mistrust
   d. Autonomy versus shame and doubt

2. According to Erikson's theory, where would you place Mr. J. based on his behavior?
   a. Intimacy versus isolation
   b. Generativity versus self-absorption
   c. Trust versus mistrust
   d. Autonomy versus shame and doubt

3. According to Mahler's theory, Mr. J. did not receive the critical "emotional refueling" required during the rapprochement phase of development. What are the consequences of this deficiency?
   a. He has not yet learned to delay gratification.
   b. He does not feel guilt about wrongdoings to others.
   c. He is unable to trust others.
   d. He has internalized rage and fears of abandonment.

4. In what stage of development is Mr. J. fixed according to Sullivan's interpersonal theory?
   a. Infancy. He relieves anxiety through oral gratification.
   b. Childhood. He has not learned to delay gratification.
   c. Early adolescence. He is struggling to form an identity.
   d. Late adolescence. He is working to develop a lasting relationship.

5. Which of the following describes the psychoanalytical structure of Mr. J.'s personality?
   a. Weak id, strong ego, weak superego
   b. Strong id, weak ego, weak superego
   c. Weak id, weak ego, punitive superego
   d. Strong id, weak ego, punitive superego

6. In which of Peplau's stages of development would you assess Mr. J.?
   a. Learning to count on others
   b. Learning to delay satisfaction
   c. Identifying oneself
   d. Developing skills in participation

7. In planning care for Mr. J., which of the following would be the primary focus for nursing?
   a. To decrease anxiety and develop trust
   b. To set limits on his behavior
   c. To ensure that he gets to group therapy
   d. To attend to his hygiene needs

Match the nursing role as described by Peplau with the nursing care behaviors listed on the right.

_____ 8. Surrogate

_____ 9. Counselor

_____ 10. Resource person

a. "Mr. J., please tell me what it was like when you were growing up."
b. "What questions do you have about being here on this unit?"
c. "Some changes will have to be made in in your behavior. I care about what happens to you."

REFERENCES

American Psychiatric Association (1994). *Diagnostic and statistical manual of mental disorders* (4th ed.). Washington, DC: American Psychiatric Association.

Belcher, J.R., & Fish, L.J.B. (1980). Hildegard E. Peplau. In The Nursing Theories Conference Group, J.B. George (Chairperson), *Nursing theories: The base for professional nursing practice.* Englewood Cliffs, NJ: Prentice-Hall.

Chess, S., & Thomas, A. (1986). *Temperament in clinical practice.* New York: The Guilford Press.

Clunn, P. (1991). *Child psychiatric nursing.* St. Louis: Mosby Year Book.

Davis, C.M. (1981). Affective education for the health professions. *Physical Therapy 61* (11): 1587–1593.

Erikson, E. (1963). *Childhood and society* (2nd ed.). New York: WW Norton.

Freud, S. (1961). The ego and the id. *Standard edition of the complete psychological works of Freud,* Vol XIX. London: Hogarth Press.

Fromm, E. (1949). *Man for himself.* New York: Farrar & Rinehart.

Kaplan, H.I., & Sadock, B.J. (1989). *Comprehensive textbook of psychiatry,* (5th ed.). Baltimore: Williams & Wilkins.

Kohlberg, L. (1968). Moral development. In *International encyclopedia of social science.* New York: Macmillan.

Mahler, M., Pine, F., & Bergman, A. (1975). *The psychological birth of the human infant.* New York: Basic Books.

Murray, R., & Zentner, J. (1997). *Health assessment and promotion strategies through the life span.* Stanford, CT: Appleton & Lange.

Peplau, H.E. (1991). *Interpersonal relations in nursing.* New York: Springer.

Piaget, J., & Inhelder, B. (1969). *The psychology of the child.* New York: Basic Books.

Schaie, K. (1984). Historical time and cohort effects. In K. McClusky & H. Reese (Eds.), *Life-span developmental psychology.* New York: Academic Press.

Sullivan, H.S. (1953). *The interpersonal theory of psychiatry.* New York: WW Norton.

Bibliography

Chapman, A.H. (1976). *Harry Stack Sullivan, his life and his work.* New York: GP Putnam's Sons.

Chess, S., Thomas, A., & Birch, H. (1970). The origins of personality. *Scientific American 223*:102.

Kernberg, O. (1976). *Object relations theory and clinical psychoanalysis.* New York: Jason Aronson.

Kohlberg, L. (1975, November). The cognitive-developmental approach to moral judgment. *Phi Delta Kappan,* 56:571–577.

Kohlberg, L. (1977). *Recent research in moral development.* New York: Holt, Rinehart & Winston.

Mahler, M. (1968). *On human symbiosis and the vicissitudes of individuation.* New York: International Universities Press.

Piaget, J. (1952). *The origin of intelligence in children.* New York: International Universities Press.

Piaget, J. (1963). *The psychology of intelligence.* Paterson, NJ: Littlefield Adams.

CONCEPTS OF PSYCHOBIOLOGY

CHAPTER OUTLINE

OBJECTIVES

INTRODUCTION

THE NERVOUS SYSTEM: AN ANATOMICAL REVIEW

NEUROENDOCRINOLOGY

GENETICS

PSYCHOIMMUNOLOGY

IMPLICATIONS FOR NURSING

SUMMARY

REVIEW QUESTIONS

KEY TERMS

neuron
limbic system
cell body
dendrites

axon
synapse
neurotransmitter
receptor sites

circadian rhythms
genotype
phenotype

OBJECTIVES

After reading this chapter, the student will be able to:

1. Identify gross anatomical structures of the brain and describe their functions.
2. Discuss the physiology of neurotransmission within the central nervous system.
3. Describe the role of neurotransmitters in human behavior.
4. Discuss the association of endocrine functioning to the development of psychiatric disorders.
5. Describe the role of genetics in the development of psychiatric disorders.
6. Discuss the correlation of alteration in brain functioning to various psychiatric disorders.
7. Identify various diagnostic procedures used to detect alteration in biological functioning that may be contributing to psychiatric disorders.
8. Discuss the influence of psychological factors on the immune system.
9. Discuss the implications of psychobiological concepts to the practice of psychiatric/mental health nursing.

he 101st legislature of the United States designated the 1990s as the "decade of the brain." With this legislation came the challenge for studying the biological basis of behavior. Peschel and Peschel (1991) have stated:

"The revolution occurring in neurobiology and molecular biology has documented that serious mental illnesses are, in fact, physical illnesses characterized by, or resulting from, malfunctions and/or malformations of the brain. Among these physical illnesses are schizophrenia, schizo-affective disorder, bipolar and major depressive disorders, autism, pervasive developmental disorders, obsessive compulsive disorder, Tourette's disorder, anxiety and panic disorders, and attention deficit hyperactivity disorder." (p. 4.)

This is not to imply that psychosocial and sociocultural influences are totally discounted. Such a notion would negate the transactional model of stress/adaptation on which the framework of this textbook is conceptualized. In keeping with the "neuroscientific revolution," however, greater emphasis is placed on the study of the organic basis for psychiatric illness.

Grebb (1989) has stated, "There is no contest: nature is nurtured and nurture has a nature." He believes that nature and nurture are not mutually exclusive, but are interacting systems clearly indicated by the fact that individuals experience biological changes in response to various environmental events. He also suggests that the dichotomous thinking of biology versus psychology, which has been prevalent in our society, is misleading, and that each of *several* disciplines (e.g., biology, psychology, and sociology) may at various times be most appropriate for explaining behavioral phenomena.

This chapter focuses on the role of neurophysiological, neurochemical, genetic, and endocrine influences on psychiatric illness. Various diagnostic procedures used to detect alteration in biological function that may contribute to psychiatric illness are identified, and the implications to psychiatric/mental health nursing are discussed.

THE NERVOUS SYSTEM: AN ANATOMICAL REVIEW

The Brain

The brain has three major divisions, subdivided into six major parts:

1. Forebrain
   a. Cerebrum
   b. Diencephalon
2. Midbrain
   a. Mesencephalon
3. Hindbrain
   a. Pons
   b. Medulla
   c. Cerebellum

Each of these structures will be discussed individually. A summary is presented in Table 4.1.

Cerebrum

The cerebrum consists of a right and left hemisphere and constitutes the largest part of the human brain. The right and left hemispheres are connected by a deep groove, which houses a band of 200 million **neurons** (nerve cells) called the corpus callosum. Because each hemisphere controls different functions, information is processed through the corpus callosum so that each hemisphere is aware of the activity of the other.

The surface of the cerebrum consists of gray matter and is called the cerebral cortex. The gray matter is so called because the neuron cell bodies of which it is composed look gray to the eye (Haroutunian, 1991). These gray matter cell bodies are thought to be the actual thinking structures of the brain. Another pair of masses of gray matter called *basal ganglia* are found deep within the cerebral hemispheres. They are responsible for certain subconscious aspects of voluntary movement, such as swinging the arms when walking, gesturing while speaking, and regulating muscle tone (Scanlon & Sanders, 1995).

The cerebral cortex is identified by numerous folds, called gyri, and deep grooves between the folds, called sulci. This extensive folding extends the surface area of the cerebral cortex, and thus permits the presence of millions more neurons than would be possible without it (as is the case in the brains of some animals, such as dogs and cats). Each hemisphere of the cerebral cortex is divided into the frontal lobe, parietal lobe, temporal lobe, and occipital lobe. These lobes, which are named for the overlying bones in the cranium, are identified in Figure 4.1.

The Frontal Lobes. Voluntary body movement is controlled by the impulses through the frontal lobes. The right frontal lobe controls motor activity on the left side of the body and the left frontal lobe controls motor activity on the right side of the body. Movements that permit speaking are also controlled by the frontal lobe, usually only on the left side (Scanlon & Sanders, 1995). The frontal lobe may also play a role in the emotional experience, as evidenced by changes in mood and character after damage to this area. The alterations include fear, aggressiveness, depression, rage, euphoria, irritability, and apathy and are likely related to a frontal lobe connection to the **limbic system** (Vander, Sherman, & Luciano, 1975). The frontal lobe may also be involved (indirectly through association fibers linked to primary sensory areas) in thinking and perceptual interpretation of information (Vander, Sherman, & Luciano, 1975).

The Parietal Lobes. Somatosensory input occurs in the parietal lobe area of the brain. These include touch, pain and pressure, taste, temperature, perception of joint and body position, and visceral sensations. The parietal

◢ TABLE 4.1 STRUCTURE AND FUNCTION OF THE BRAIN

STRUCTURE	PRIMARY FUNCTION
I. The Forebrain 　A. Cerebrum	Composed of two hemispheres separated by a deep groove that houses a band of 200 million neurons called the corpus callosum. The outer shell is called the cortex. It is extensively folded and consists of billions of neurons. The left hemsphere appears to be dominant in most people. It controls speech, comprehension, rationality, and logic. The right hemisphere is nondominant in most people. It may be called the "creative" brain and is associated with affect, behavior, and spacial-perceptual functions. Each hemisphere is divided into four lobes.
1. Frontal lobes	Voluntary body movement, including movements that permit speaking; thinking and judgment formation; expression of feelings.
2. Parietal lobes	Perception and interpretation of most sensory information (including touch, pain, taste, and body position).
3. Temporal lobes	Hearing, short-term memory, and sense of smell; expression of emotions through connection with limbic system.
4. Occipital lobes	Visual reception and interpretation.
B. Diencephalon	Connects cerebrum with lower brain structures.
1. Thalamus	Integrates all sensory input (except smell) on way to cortex; some involvement with emotions and mood.
2. Hypothalamus	Regulates anterior and posterior lobes of pituitary gland; exerts control over actions of the autonomic nervous system; regulates appetite and temperature.
3. Limbic system	Consists of medially placed cortical and subcortical structures and the fiber tracts connecting them with one another and with the hypothalamus. It is sometimes called the "emotional brain"—associated with feelings of fear and anxiety; anger and aggression; love, joy, and hope; and with sexuality and social behavior.
II. The Midbrain 　A. Mesencephalon	Responsible for visual, auditory, and balance ("righting") reflexes.
III. The Hindbrain 　A. Pons	Regulation of respiration and skeletal muscle tone; ascending and descending tracts connect brainstem with cerebellum and cortex.
B. Medulla	Pathway for all ascending and descending fiber tracts; contains vital centers that regulate heart rate, blood pressure, and respiration; reflex centers for swallowing, sneezing, coughing, and vomiting.
C. Cerebellum	Regulates muscle tone and coordination and maintains posture and equilibrium.

lobes also contain association fibers linked to the primary sensory areas through which interpretation of sensory-perceptual information is made. Language interpretation is associated with the left hemisphere of the parietal lobe.

The Temporal Lobes. The upper anterior temporal lobe is concerned with auditory functions, while the lower part is dedicated to short-term memory. The sense of smell has a connection to the temporal lobes, as the impulses carried by the olfactory nerves end in this area of the brain (Scanlon & Sanders, 1995). The temporal lobes also play a role in the expression of emotions through an interconnection with the limbic system. The left temporal lobe, along with the left parietal lobe, is involved in language interpretation.

The Occipital Lobes. The occipital lobes are the primary area of visual reception and interpretation. Visual perception, which gives individuals the ability to judge spacial relationships such as distance and to see in three dimensions, is also processed in this area (Scanlon & Sanders, 1995). Language interpretation is influenced by the occipital lobes through an association with the visual experience.

Diencephalon

The second part of the forebrain is the diencephalon, which connects the cerebrum with lower structures of the brain. The major components of the diencephalon include the thalamus, the hypothalamus, and the limbic system. These structures may be identified in Figures 4.2 and 4.3.

Thalamus. The thalamus integrates all sensory input (except smell) on its way to the cortex. This helps the cerebral cortex interpret the whole picture very rapidly, rather than experiencing each sensation individually. The thalamus is also involved in temporarily blocking minor sensations, so that an individual can concentrate on one important event when necessary. For example, an individual who is studying for an examination may be unaware of the clock ticking in the room, or even of another person walking into the room, because the thalamus has temporarily blocked these incoming sensations from the cortex (Scanlon & Sanders, 1995).

Hypothalamus. The hypothalamus is located just below the thalamus and just above the pituitary gland and has a number of diverse functions.

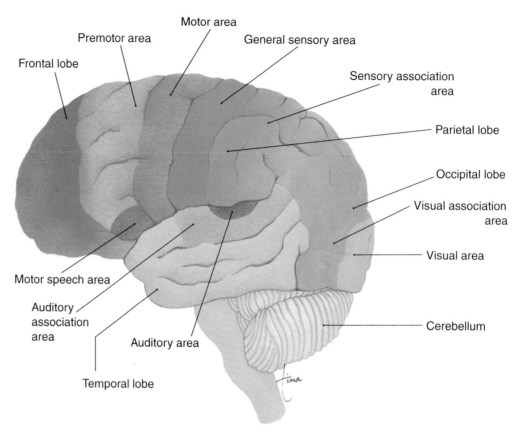

Figure 4.1   Left cerebral hemisphere showing some of the functional areas that have been mapped. (Reprinted with permission from Scanlon & Sanders: Essentials of Anatomy and Physiology 3/E, 1999 F.A. Davis Company.)

1. **Regulation of the Pituitary Gland.** The pituitary gland consists of two lobes: the posterior lobe and the anterior lobe.
   a. *The posterior lobe* of the pituitary gland is actually extended tissue from the hypothalamus. The posterior lobe stores antidiuretic hormone (which helps to maintain blood pressure through regulation of water retention) and oxytocin (the hormone responsible for stimulation of the uterus during labor and the release of milk from the mammary glands). Both of these hormones are produced in the hypothalamus. When the hypothalamus detects the body's need for these hormones, it sends nerve impulses to the posterior pituitary for their release.
   b. *The anterior lobe* of the pituitary gland consists of glandular tissue that produces a number of hormones used by the body. These hormones are regulated by "releasing factors" from the hypothalamus. When the hormones are required by the body, the releasing factors stimulate the release of the hormone from the anterior pituitary and the hormone in turn stimulates its target organ to carry out its specific functions.
2. **Direct Neural Control Over the Actions of the Autonomic Nervous System.** The hypothalamus regulates the appropriate visceral responses during various emotional states. The actions of the autonomic nervous system are described later in this chapter.
3. **Regulation of Appetite.** Appetite is regulated through response to blood nutrient levels.
4. **Regulation of Temperature.** The hypothalamus senses internal temperature changes in the blood that flows through the brain. It receives information through sensory input from the skin about external temperature changes. The hypothalamus then uses this information to promote certain types of responses (e.g., sweating or shivering) that help to maintain body temperature within the normal range (Scanlon & Sanders, 1995).

Limbic System. The part of the brain known as the limbic system consists of portions of the cerebrum and the diencephalon. The major components include the medially placed cortical and subcortical structures and the fiber tracts connecting them with one another and with the hypothalamus (Landau, 1976). The system is composed of the amygdala, mammillary body, olfactory tract, hypothalamus, cingulate gyrus, septum pellucidum, thalamus, hippocampus, and neuronal connecting pathways, such as the fornix and others. This system has been called "the emotional brain" and is associated with feelings of fear and anxiety; anger, rage, and aggression; and love, joy, and hope; and with sexuality and social behavior.

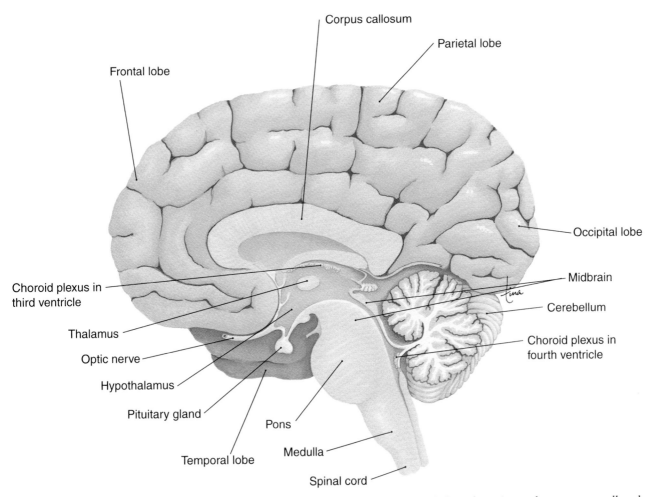

Figure 4.2 Midsagittal section of the brain as seen from the left side. This medial plane shows internal anatomy as well as the lobes of the cerebrum. (Reprinted with permission from Scanlon & Sanders: Essentials of Anatomy and Physiology 3/E, 1999 F.A. Davis Company.)

Mesencephalon

Structures of major importance in the mesencephalon, or midbrain, include nuclei and fiber tracts. The mesencephalon extends from the pons to the hypothalamus and is responsible for integration of various reflexes, including visual reflexes (e.g., automatically turning away from a dangerous object when it comes into view), auditory reflexes (e.g., automatically turning toward a sound that is heard), and righting reflexes (e.g., automatically keeping the head upright and maintaining balance) (Scanlon & Sanders, 1995). The mesencephalon may be identified in Figure 4.2.

Pons

The pons is a bulbous structure that lies between the midbrain and the medulla (see Fig. 4.2). It is composed of large bundles of fibers and forms a major connection between the cerebellum and the brainstem. It also contains the central connections of cranial nerves V through VIII and centers for respiration and skeletal muscle tone (Landau, 1976).

Medulla

The medulla is the connecting structure between the spinal cord and the pons, and all of the ascending and descending fiber tracts pass through it. The vital centers are contained within the medulla, and it is responsible for regulation of heart rate, blood pressure, and respiration. Also in the medulla are reflex centers for swallowing, sneezing, coughing, and vomiting (Scanlon & Sanders, 1995). It also contains nuclei for cranial nerves IX through XII. The medulla, pons, and midbrain form the structure known as the brainstem. These structures may be identified in Figure 4.2.

Cerebellum

The cerebellum is separated from the brainstem by the fourth ventricle but has connections to the brainstem through bundles of fiber tracts. It is situated just below the occipital lobes of the cerebrum (see Figs. 4.1 and 4.2). The functions of the cerebellum are concerned with involuntary movement, such as muscular tone and coordination and the maintenance of posture and equilibrium.

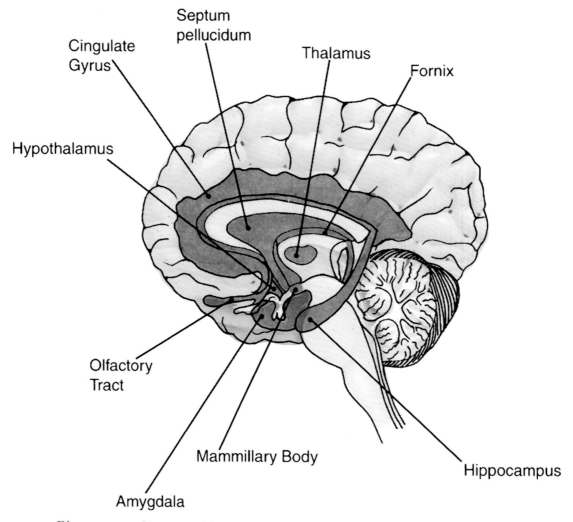

Figure 4.3 Structures of the limbic system. *Source:* Adapted from Scanlon and Sanders (1995).

Nerve Tissue

The tissue of the central nervous system (CNS) consists of nerve cells called *neurons* that generate and transmit electrochemical impulses. The structure of a neuron is composed of a cell body, an axon, and dendrites. The **cell body** contains the nucleus and is essential for the continued life of the neuron. The **dendrites** are processes that transmit impulses toward the cell body, and the **axon** transmits impulses away from the cell body. The axons and dendrites are covered by layers of cells called *neuroglia* that form a coating, or "sheath," of myelin. *Myelin* is a phospholipid that provides insulation against short-circuiting of the neurons during their electrical activity and increases the velocity of the impulse. The white matter of the brain and spinal cord is so called because of the whitish appearance of the myelin sheath over the axons and dendrites. The gray matter is composed of cell bodies that contain no myelin.

The three classes of neurons include afferent (sensory), efferent (motor), and interneurons. The *afferent neurons* carry impulses from receptors in the internal and external periphery to the central nervous system, where they are then interpreted into various sensations. The *efferent neurons* carry impulses from the CNS to *effectors* in the periphery, such as muscles (that respond by contracting) and glands (that respond by secreting). A schematic of afferent and efferent neurons is presented in Figure 4.4.

Interneurons exist entirely within the CNS, and 99 percent of all nerve cells belong to this group (Vander, Sherman, & Luciano, 1975). They may carry only sensory or motor impulses, or they may serve as integrators in the pathways between afferent and efferent neurons. They account in large part for thinking, feelings, learning, language, and memory. The directional pathways of afferent, efferent, and interneurons are presented in Figure 4.5.

Synapses

Information is transmitted through the body from one neuron to another. Some messages may be processed

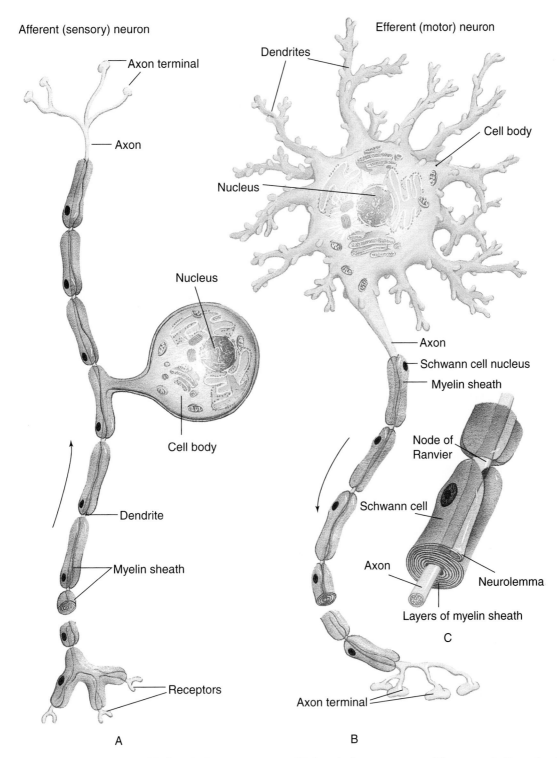

Afferent (sensory) neuron

Axon terminal

Axon

Nucleus

Cell body

Dendrite

Myelin sheath

Receptors

A

Efferent (motor) neuron

Dendrites

Cell body

Nucleus

Axon

Schwann cell nucleus

Myelin sheath

Node of Ranvier

Schwann cell

Axon

Neurolemma

Layers of myelin sheath

C

Axon terminal

B

Figure 4.4 Neuron structure. (A) A typical sensory neuron. (B) A typical motor neuron. The arrows indicate the direction of impulse transmission. (C) Details of the myelin sheath and neurolemma formed by Schwann cells. (Reprinted with permission from Scalon & Sanders: Essentials of Anatomy and Physiology 3/E, 1999 F.A. Davis Company.)

through only a few neurons, while others may require thousands of neuronal connections. The neurons that transmit the impulses do not actually touch each other. The junction between two neurons is called a **synapse.** The small space between the axon terminals of one neu-

ron and the cell body or dendrites of another is called the *synaptic cleft.* Neurons conducting impulses toward the synapse are called *presynaptic neurons* and those conducting impulses away are called *postsynaptic neurons.*

A chemical, called a **neurotransmitter,** is stored in the

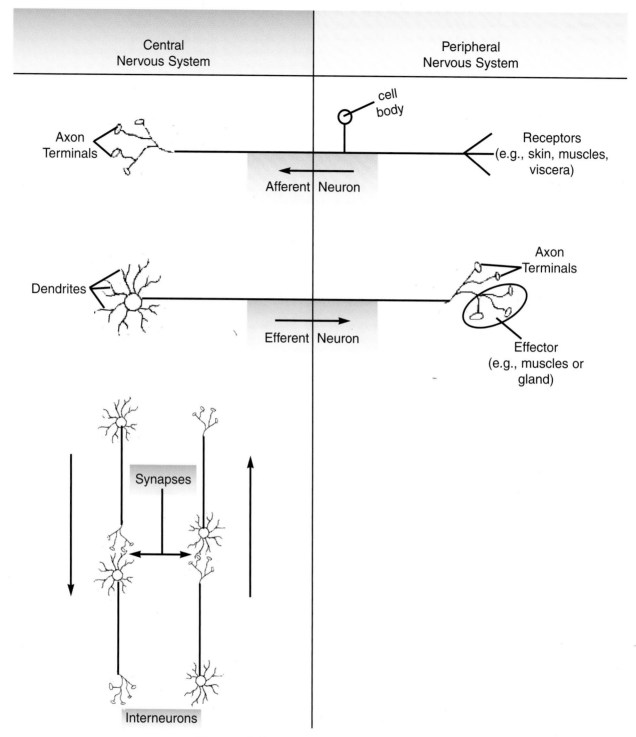

Figure 4.5 Directional pathways of neurons.

axon terminals of the presynaptic neuron. An electrical impulse through the neuron will cause the release of this neurotransmitter into the synaptic cleft. The neurotransmitter then diffuses across the synaptic cleft and combines with **receptor sites** that are situated on the cell membrane of the postsynaptic neuron. The result of the combination of neurotransmitter–receptor site is the determi-

nation of whether or not another electrical impulse is generated. If one is generated, the result is called an *excitatory response* and the electrical impulse moves on to the next synapse, where the same process reoccurs. If another electrical impulse is not generated by the neurotransmitter–receptor site combination, the result is called an *inhibitory response*, and synaptic transmission is terminated.

The cell body or dendrite of the postsynaptic neuron also contains a chemical *inactivator* that is specific to the neurotransmitter that has been released by the presynaptic neuron. When the synaptic transmission has been completed, the chemical inactivator quickly inactivates the neurotransmitter to prevent unwanted, continuous impulses, until a new impulse from the presynaptic neuron releases more neurotransmitter. A schematic representation of a synapse is presented in Figure 4.6.

Autonomic Nervous System

The autonomic nervous system (ANS) is actually considered part of the peripheral nervous system. However, its regulation is integrated by the hypothalamus and therefore the emotions exert a great deal of influence over its functioning. It is for this reason that the ANS has been implicated in the etiology of a number of psychophysiological disorders. These diseases of adaptation are discussed in detail in Chapter 33.

The ANS has two divisions: the sympathetic and the parasympathetic. The sympathetic division is dominant in stressful situations, and prepares the body for the "fight or flight" response that was discussed in Chapter 1. The neuronal cell bodies of the sympathetic division originate in the thoracolumbar region of the spinal cord. Their axons extend to the chains of sympathetic ganglia where they synapse with other neurons that subsequently innervate the visceral effectors. This results in an increase in heart rate and respirations and a decrease in digestive secretions and peristalsis. Blood is shunted to the vital organs and to skeletal muscles to ensure adequate oxygenation.

The neuronal cell bodies of the parasympathetic division originate in the brainstem and the sacral segments of the spinal cord, and extend to the parasympathetic ganglia where the synapse takes place either very close to or actually in the visceral organ being innervated. In this way, a very localized response is possible. The parasympathetic division dominates when an individual is in a relaxed, nonstressful condition. The heart and respirations are maintained at a normal rate, and secretions and peristalsis increase for normal digestion. Elimination functions are promoted. A schematic representation of the autonomic nervous system is presented in Figure 4.7.

Neurotransmitters

Neurotransmitters were described during the explanation of synaptic activity. They are being discussed separately and in detail because of the essential function they play in

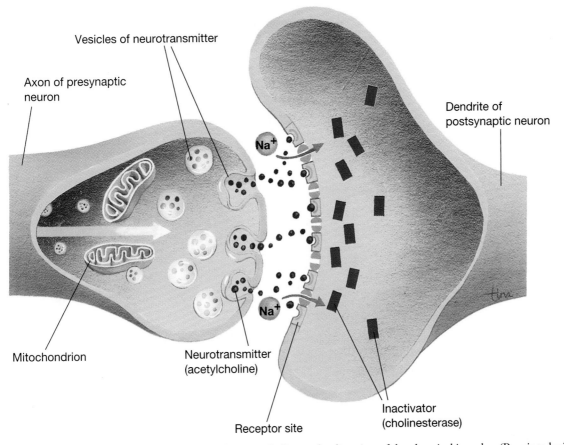

Figure 4.6 Impulse transmission at a synapse. The arrow indicates the direction of the electrical impulse. (Reprinted with permission from Scanlon & Sanders: Essentials of Anatomy and Physiology 3/E, 1999 F.A. Davis Company.)

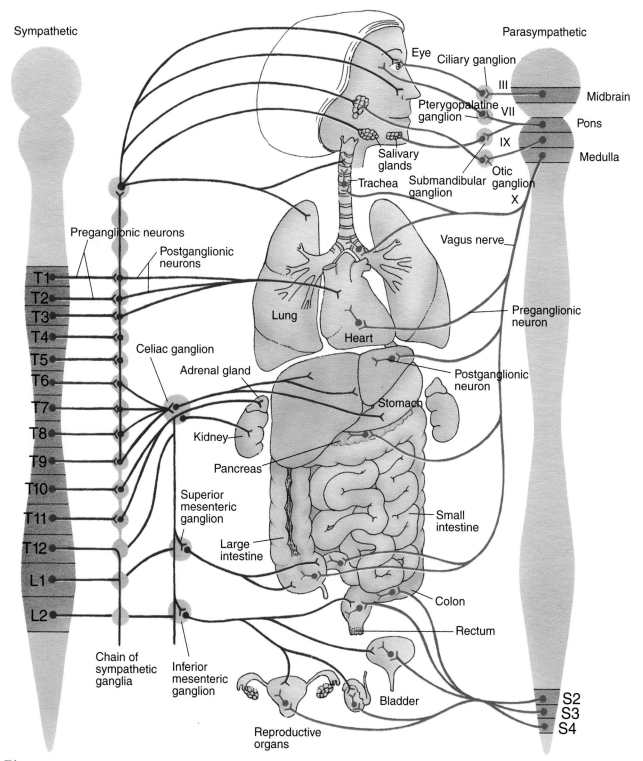

Figure 4.7   The autonomic nervous system. The sympathetic division is shown on the left, and the parasympathetic division is shown on the right (both divisions are bilateral). (Reprinted with permission from Scanlon & Sanders: Essentials of Anatomy and Physiology 3/E, 1999 F.A. Davis Company.)

the role of human emotion and behavior, and because they are the target for mechanism of action of many of the psychotropic medications.

Neurotransmitters are chemicals that convey informa-

tion, contained within action potentials, across synaptic clefts to neighboring target cells (Murphy & Deutsch, 1991). They are stored in small vesicles in the axon terminals of neurons. When the action potential, or electrical impulse, reaches this point, the neurotransmitters are released from the vesicles. They cross the synaptic cleft and bind with receptor sites on the cell body or dendrites of the adjacent neuron to allow the impulse to continue its course, or to prevent the impulse from continuing. After the neurotransmitter has performed its function in the synapse, it either returns to the vesicles to be stored and used again, or it is inactivated and dissolved by enzymes. The process of being stored for reuse is called *reuptake*, a function that holds significance for understanding the mechanism of action of certain psychotropic medications.

Many neurotransmitters exist within the central and peripheral nervous systems, but only a limited number have implications for psychiatry. Major categories include cholinergics, monoamines, amino acids, and neuropeptides. Each of these is discussed separately and summarized in Table 4.2.

Cholinergics

Acetylcholine. Acetylcholine was the first chemical to be identified and proven as a neurotransmitter (Kruk & Pycock, 1983). It is a major effector chemical within the ANS, producing activity at all sympathetic and parasympathetic presynaptic nerve terminals and all parasympathetic postsynaptic nerve terminals. It is highly significant in the neurotransmission that occurs at the junctions of nerves and muscles. Acetylcholinesterase is the enzyme that destroys acetylcholine or inhibits its activity.

In the CNS, acetylcholine neurons innervate the cerebral cortex, hippocampus, and limbic structures. The pathways are especially dense through the area of the basal ganglia in the brain.

Functions of acetylcholine are manifold and include sleep, arousal, pain perception, the modulation and coordination of movement, and memory acquisition and retention (Murphy & Deutsch, 1991). Cholinergic mechanisms may have some role in certain disorders of motor behavior and memory, such as Parkinson's disease, Huntington's chorea, and Alzheimer's disease (Chafetz, 1990).

Monoamines

Norepinephrine. Norepinephrine is the neurotransmitter that produces activity at the sympathetic postsynaptic nerve terminals in the ANS resulting in the "fight or flight" responses in the effector organs. In the central nervous system, norepinephrine pathways originate in the pons and medulla and innervate the thalamus, dorsal hypothalamus, limbic system, hippocampus, cerebellum, and cerebral cortex. When norepinephrine is not returned for storage in the vesicles of the axon terminals, it is metabolized and inactivated by the enzymes monoamine oxidase (MAO) and catechol-*O*-methyltransferase (COMT).

The functions of norepinephrine include the regulation of mood, cognition, perception, locomotion, cardiovascular functioning, and sleep and arousal (Murphy & Deutsch, 1991). The mechanism of norepinephrine transmission has been implicated in certain mood disorders such as depression and mania (Kaplan & Sadock, 1985), in anxiety states (Murphy & Handelsman, 1991), and in schizophrenia (Davis & Greenwald, 1991).

Dopamine. Dopamine pathways arise from the midbrain and hypothalamus and terminate in the frontal cortex, limbic system, basal ganglia, and thalamus. Dopamine neurons in the hypothalamus innervate the posterior pituitary, and those from the posterior hypothalamus project to the spinal cord. As with norepinephrine, the inactivating enzymes for dopamine are MAO and COMT.

Dopamine functions include regulation of movements and coordination, emotions, voluntary decision-making ability, and because of its influence on the pituitary gland, it inhibits the release of prolactin (Halperin, 1991). Dopamine transmission has been implicated in the etiology of certain mental disorders, such as depression and mania (Siever, Davis, & Gorman, 1991), schizophrenia (Davis & Greenwald, 1991), and Parkinson's disease (Horvath, 1991).

Serotonin. Serotonin pathways originate from cell bodies located in the pons and medulla and project to areas including the hypothalamus, thalamus, limbic system, cerebral cortex, cerebellum, and spinal cord. Serotonin that is not returned to be stored in the axon terminal vesicles is catabolized by the enzyme monoamine oxidase.

Serotonin may play a role in sleep and arousal, libido, appetite, mood, aggression, pain perception, coordination, and the ability to pursue goal-directed behavior (Chafetz, 1990; Murphy & Deutsch, 1991). The serotoninergic system has been implicated in the etiology of certain psychopathological conditions including anxiety states (Murphy & Handelsman, 1991) and mood disorders (Siever, Davis, & Gorman, 1991).

Histamine. The role of histamine in mediating allergic and inflammatory reactions has been well documented. Its role in the CNS as a neurotransmitter has only recently been confirmed, and the availability of information is limited. The highest concentrations of histamine are found within various regions of the hypothalamus. The enzyme that catabolizes histamine is monoamine oxidase. Although the exact processes mediated by histamine with the central nervous system are uncertain, data suggest that histamine may play a role in depressive illness (Murphy & Deutsch, 1991).

Amino Acids

Inhibitory Amino Acids

Gamma-Aminobutyric Acid. Gamma-aminobutyric acid (GABA) has a widespread distribution in the central

TABLE 4.2 NEUROTRANSMITTERS IN THE CENTRAL NERVOUS SYSTEM

NEUROTRANSMITTER	LOCATION/FUNCTION	POSSIBLE IMPLICATIONS FOR MENTAL ILLNESS
I. Cholinergics A. Acetylcholine	ANS: Sympathetic and parasympathetic presynaptic nerve terminals; parasympathetic postsynaptic nerve terminals. CNS: Cerebral cortex, hippocampus, limbic structures, and basal ganglia. Functions: Sleep, arousal, pain perception, movement, memory.	Increased levels: Depression. Decreased levels: Alzheimer's disease, Huntington's chorea, Parkinson's disease.
II. Monoamines A. Norepinephrine	ANS: Sympathetic postsynaptic nerve terminals. CNS: Thalamus, hypothalamus, limbic system, hippocampus, cerebellum, cerebral cortex. Functions: Mood, cognition, perception, locomotion, cardiovascular functioning, and sleep and arousal.	Decreased levels: Depression. Increased levels: Mania, anxiety states, schizophrenia.
B. Dopamine	Frontal cortex, limbic system, basal ganglia, thalamus, posterior pituitary, and spinal cord. Functions: Movement and coordination, emotions, voluntary judgment, release of prolactin.	Decreased levels: Parkinson's disease and depression. Increased levels: Mania and schizophrenia.
C. Serotonin	Hypothalamus, thalamus, limbic system, cerebral cortex, cerebellum, spinal cord. Functions: Sleep and arousal, libido, appetite, mood, aggression, pain perception, coordination, judgment.	Decreased levels: Depression. Increased levels: Anxiety states.
D. Histamine	Hypothalamus	Decreased levels: Depression.
III. Amino Acids A. Gamma-amino-butyric acid (GABA)	Hypothalamus, hippocampus, cortex, cerebellum, basal ganglia, spinal cord, retina. Functions: Slowdown of body activity.	Decreased levels: Huntington's chorea, anxiety disorders, schizophrenia, and various forms of epilepsy.
B. Glycine	Spinal cord and brainstem Functions: Recurrent inhibition of motor neurons.	Toxic levels: "glycine encephalopathy," decreased levels are correlated with spastic motor movements.
C. Glutamate and aspartate	Pyramidal cells of the cortex, cerebellum, and the primary sensory afferent systems; hippocampus, thalamus, hypothalamus, spinal cord. Functions: Relay of sensory information and in the regulation of various motor and spinal reflexes.	Increased levels: Huntington's chorea, temporal lobe epilepsy, spinal cerebellar degeneration.
IV. Neuropeptides A. Endorphins and enkephalins	Hypothalamus, thalamus, limbic structures, midbrain, and brainstem. Enkephalins are also found in the gastrointestinal tract. Functions: Modulation of pain and reduced peristalsis (enkephalins).	Modulation of dopamine activity by opioid peptides may indicate some link to the symptoms of schizophrenia.
B. Substance P	Hypothalamus, limbic structures, midbrain, brainstem, thalamus, basal ganglia, and spinal cord; also found in gastrointestinal tract and salivary glands. Function: Regulation of pain.	Decreased levels: Huntington's chorea.
C. Somatostatin	Cerebral cortex, hippocampus, thalamus, basal ganglia, brainstem, and spinal cord. Function: Inhibits release of norepinephrine; stimulates release of serotonin, dopamine, and acetylcholine.	Decreased levels: Alzheimer's disease. Increased levels: Huntington's chorea

nervous system, with high concentrations in the hypothalamus, hippocampus, cortex, cerebellum, and basal ganglia of the brain, in the gray matter of the dorsal horn of the spinal cord, and in the retina. Most GABA is associated with short inhibitory interneurons, although some long-axon pathways within the brain have also been indentified (Kruk & Pycock, 1983). GABA is catabolized by the enzyme GABA transaminase (Baraban & Coyle, 1989).

Inhibitory neurotransmitters, such as GABA, prevent postsynaptic excitation, interrupting the progression of the electrical impulse at the synaptic junction. This function is significant when slowdown of body activity is advantageous. Enhancement of the GABA system is the mechanism of action by which the benzodiazepines produce their calming effect.

Alterations in the GABA system have been implicated in the etiology of anxiety disorders, movement disorders (e.g., Huntington's chorea), and various forms of epilepsy.

Glycine. The highest concentrations of glycine in the CNS are found in the spinal cord and brainstem. Little is known about the possible enzymatic metabolism of glycine (Kruk & Pycock, 1983).

Glycine appears to be the neurotransmitter of recurrent inhibition of motor neurons within the spinal cord, and is possibly involved in the regulation of spinal and brainstem reflexes. It has been implicated in the pathogenesis of certain types of spastic disorders and in "glycine encephalopathy," which is known to occur with toxic accumulation of the neurotransmitter in the brain and cerebrospinal fluid (Murphy & Deutsch, 1991).

Excitatory Amino Acids

Glutamate and Aspartate. Glutamate and aspartate have largely descending pathways that interconnect functional regions of the CNS (Chafetz, 1990). They appear to be primary excitatory neurotransmitters in the pyramidal cells of the cortex, the cerebellum, and the primary sensory afferent systems. They are also found in the hippocamus, thalamus, hypothalamus, and spinal cord. Glutamate seems to be the primary neurotransmitter of the auditory nerve (Chafetz, 1990). Glutamate and aspartate are inactivated by uptake into the tissues and through assimilation in various metabolic pathways.

Glutamate and aspartate function in the relay of sensory information and in the regulation of various motor and spinal reflexes (Kruk & Pycock, 1983). Alteration in these systems has been implicated in the etiology of certain neurodegenerative disorders, such as Huntington's chorea, temporal lobe epilepsy, and spinal cerebellar degeneration (Schwarcz & Meldrum, 1985).

Neuropeptides

Numerous neuropeptides have been identified and studied. They are classified by the area of the body in which they are located or by their pharmacological or functional properties. Although their role as neurotransmitters has not been clearly established, it is known that they often coexist with the classic neurotransmitters within a neuron; however, the functional significance of this coexistence still requires further study. Hormonal neuropeptides are discussed in the section of this chapter on psychoendocrinology.

Opioid Peptides. Opioid peptides, which include the endorphins and enkephalins, have been widely studied. Opioid peptides are found in various concentrations in the hypothalamus, thalamus, limbic structures, midbrain, and brainstem. Enkephalins are also found in the gastrointestinal (GI) tract. Opioid peptides are thought to have a role in pain modulation, with their natural morphine-like properties. They are released in response to painful stimuli and may be responsible for producing the analgesic effect following acupuncture (Kruk & Pycock, 1983). Opioid peptides alter the release of dopamine and affect the spontaneous activity of the dopaminergic neurons (Davidson, 1991). These findings may have some implication for opioid peptide–dopamine interaction in the etiology of schizophrenia.

Substance P. Substance P was the first neuropeptide to be discovered. It is present in high concentrations in the hypothalamus, limbic structures, midbrain, and brainstem, and is also found in the thalamus, basal ganglia, and spinal cord. Substance P has been found to be highly concentrated in sensory fibers, and for this reason is thought to play a role in sensory transmission, and particularly in the regulation of pain. Decreased concentrations have been found in the substantia nigra of the basal ganglia of clients with Huntington's chorea (Davidson, 1991).

Somatostatin. Somatostatin (also called growth hormone–inhibiting hormone) is found in the cerebral cortex, hippocampus, thalamus, basal ganglia, brainstem, and spinal cord, and has multiple effects on the CNS. It exerts inhibitory effects on the release of norepinephrine and stimulatory effects on serotonin. It stimulates the turnover and release of dopamine in the basal ganglia and acetylcholine in the brainstem and hippocampus (Davidson, 1991). High concentrations of somatostatin have been reported in brain specimens of clients with Huntington's chorea, and low concentrations in those with Alzheimer's disease.

NEUROENDOCRINOLOGY

Human endocrine functioning has a strong foundation in the CNS, under the direction of the hypothalamus, which has direct control over the pituitary gland. The pituitary gland has two major lobes—the anterior lobe (also called the *adenohypophysis*) and the posterior lobe (also called the *neurohypophysis*). The pituitary gland is only about the size of a pea, but despite its size and because of the powerful control it exerts over endocrine functioning in humans, it is sometimes called the "master gland." (Figure 4.8 shows

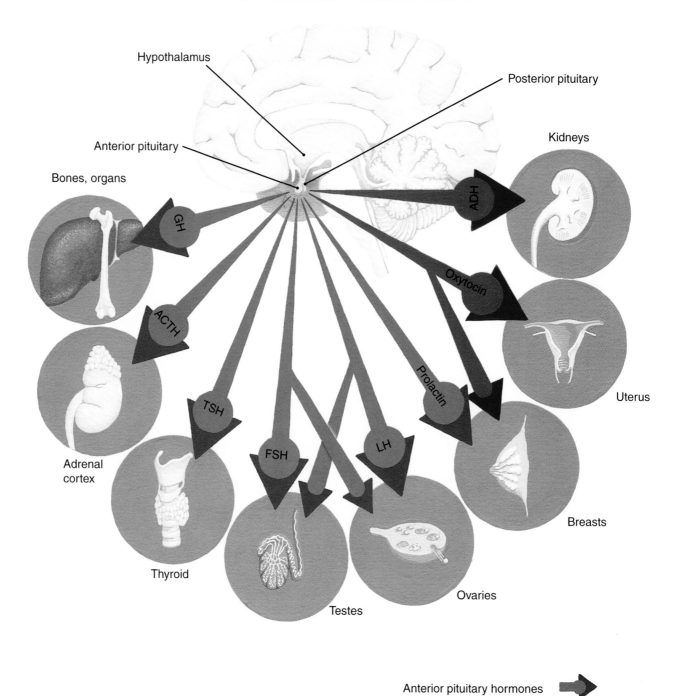

Figure 4.8 Hormones of the pituitary gland and their target organs. (Reprinted with permission from Scanlon & Sanders: Essentials of Anatomy and Physiology 3/E, 1999 F.A. Davis Company.)

the hormones of the pituitary gland and their target organs.) Many of the hormones subject to hypothalamus-pituitary regulation may have implications for behavioral functioning. Discussion of these hormones is summarized in Table 4.3.

Pituitary Gland

The Posterior Pituitary (Neurohypophysis)

The hypothalamus has direct control over the posterior pituitary through efferent neural pathways. Two hor-

◀ TABLE 4.3   **HORMONES OF THE NEUROENDOCRINE SYSTEM**

HORMONE	LOCATION AND STIMULATION OF RELEASE	TARGET ORGAN	FUNCTION	POSSIBLE BEHAVIORAL CORRELATION TO ALTERED SECRETION
Antidiuretic hormone (ADH)	Posterior pituitary; release stimulated by dehydration, pain, stress	Kidney (causes increased reabsorption)	Conservation of body water and maintenance of blood pressure	Polydipsia; altered pain response; modified sleep pattern
Oxytocin	Posterior pituitary; release stimulated by end of pregnancy; stress; during sexual arousal	Uterus; breasts	Contraction of the uterus for labor; release of breast milk	May play role in stress response by stimulation of ACIH
Growth hormone (GH)	Anterior pituitary; release stimulated by growth hormone–releasing hormone from hypothalamus	Bones and tissues	Growth in children; protein synthesis in adults	Anorexia nervosa
Thyroid-stimulating hormone (TSH)	Anterior pituitary; release stimulated by thyrotropin-releasing hormone from hypothalamus	Thyroid gland	Stimulation of secretion of needed thyroid hormones for metabolism of food and regulation of temperature	Increased levels: insomnia, anxiety, emotional lability Decreased levels: fatigue, depression
Adrenocorticotropic hormone (ACTH)	Anterior pituitary; release stimulated by corticotropin-releasing hormone from hypothalamus	Adrenal cortex	Stimulation of secretion of cortisol, which plays a role in response to stress	Increased levels: mood disorders, psychosis Decreased levels: depression, apathy, fatigue
Prolactin	Anterior pituitary; release stimulated by prolactin-releasing hormone from hypothalamus	Breasts	Stimulation of milk production	Increased levels: depression, anxiety decreased libido, irritability
Gonadotropic hormones	Anterior pituitary; release stimulated by gonadotropin-releasing hormone from hypothalamus	Ovaries and testes	Stimulation of secretion of estrogen, progesterone, and testosterone; role in ovulation and sperm production	Decreased levels: depression and anorexia nervosa Increased testosterone: increased sexual behavior and aggressiveness
Melanocyte-stimulating hormone (MSH)	Anterior pituitary; release stimulated by onset of darkness	Pineal gland	Stimulation of secretion of melatonin	Increased levels: depression

mones are found in the posterior pituitary: vasopressin, or antidiuretic hormone, and oxytocin. They are actually produced by the hypothalamus and stored in the posterior pituitary. Their release is mediated by neural impulses from the hypothalamus (Fig. 4.9).

Antidiuretic Hormone. The main function of antidiuretic hormone (ADH) is to conserve body water and maintain normal blood pressure. The release of ADH is stimulated by pain, emotional stress, dehydration, increased plasma concentration, and decreases in blood volume (Reus, 1989). An alteration in the secretion of this hormone may be a factor in the polydipsia observed in about 10 to 15 percent of hospitalized psychiatric patients. Other factors correlated with this behavior include adverse effects of psychotropic medications and features of the behavioral disorder itself. Some studies have indicated that ADH may also play a role in learning and memory, in alteration of the pain response, and in the modification of sleep patterns (Kruk & Pycock, 1983).

Ocytocin. Oxytocin stimulates contraction of the uterus at the end of pregnancy and stimulates release of milk from the mammary glands (Scanlon & Sanders, 1995). It is also released in response to stress and during sexual arousal (Halperin, 1991). Its role in behavioral functioning is unclear, although it is possible that oxytocin may act in certain situations to stimulate the release of adrenocorticotropic hormone (ACTH), thereby playing a key role in the overall hormonal response to stress (Reus, 1989).

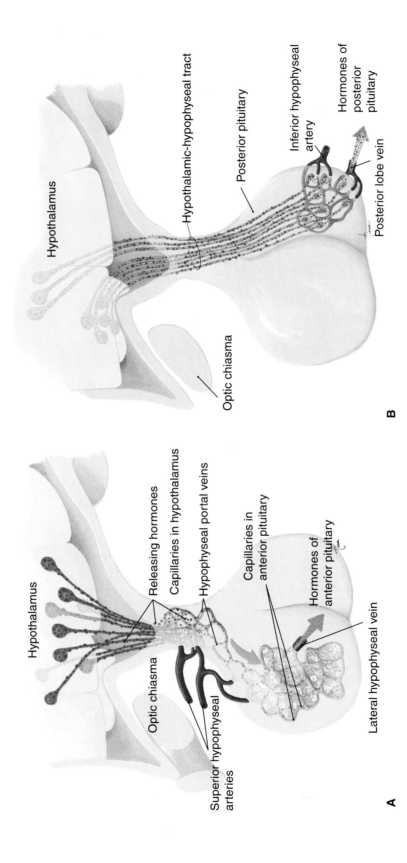

Figure 4.9 Structural relationships of hypothalamus and pituitary gland. (A) Releasing hormones of the hypothalamus circulate directly to the anterior pituitary and influence its secretions. Notice the two networks of capillaries. (B) Posterior pituitary stores hormones produced in the hypothalamus. (Reprinted with permission from Scanlon & Sanders: Essentials of Anatomy and Physiology 3/E, 1999 F.A. Davis Company)

The Anterior Pituitary (Adenohypophysis)

The hypothalamus produces *releasing hormones* that pass through capillaries and veins of the hypophyseal portal system to capillaries in the anterior pituitary, where they stimulate secretion of specialized hormones. This pathway is presented in Figure 4.9. The hormones of the anterior pituitary gland regulate multiple body functions and include growth hormone, thyroid-stimulating hormone, ACTH, prolactin, gonadotropin-stimulating hormone, and melanocyte-stimulating hormone. Most of these hormones are regulated by a *negative feedback mechanism*. Once the hormone has exerted its effects, the information is "fed back" to the anterior pituitary, which inhibits the release, and ultimately decreases the effects, of the stimulating hormones.

Growth Hormone. The release of growth hormone (GH), also called somatotropin, is stimulated by growth hormone–releasing hormone (GHRH) from the hypothalamus. Its release is inhibited by growth hormone–inhibiting hormone (GHIH), or somatostatin, also from the hypothalamus. It is responsible for growth in children, as well as continued protein synthesis throughout life. During periods of fasting, it stimulates the release of fat from the adipose tissue to be used for increased energy. The release of GHIH is stimulated in response to periods of hyperglycemia. GHRH is stimulated in response to hypoglycemia and to stressful situations. During prolonged stress, GH has a direct effect on protein, carbohydrate, and lipid metabolism, resulting in increased serum glucose and free fatty acids to be used for increased energy. There has been some indication of a possible correlation between abnormal secretion of growth hormone and anorexia nervosa (Halperin, 1991).

Thyroid-Stimulating Hormone. Thyrotropin-releasing hormone (TRH) from the hypothalamus stimulates the release of thyroid-stimulating hormone (TSH), or thyrotropin, from the anterior pituitary. TSH stimulates the thyroid gland to secrete triiodothyronine (T_3) and thyroxine (T_4). Thyroid hormones are integral to the metabolism of food and the regulation of temperature.

A correlation between thyroid dysfunction and altered behavioral functioning has been studied. Early reports in the medical literature associated hyperthyroidism with irritability, insomnia, anxiety, restlessness, weight loss, and emotional lability, and in some instances with progressing to delirium or psychosis (Reus, 1989). Symptoms of fatigue, decreased libido, memory impairment, depression, and suicidal ideations have been associated with chronic hypothyroidism. Studies have correlated various forms of thyroid dysfunction with mood disorders, anxiety, eating disorders, schizophrenia, and dementia (Reus, 1989).

Adrenocorticotropic Hormone. Corticotropin-releasing hormone (CRH) from the hypothalamus stimulates the release of ACTH from the anterior pituitary. ACTH stimulates the adrenal cortex to secrete cortisol.

The role of cortisol in human behaviors is not well understood, although it seems to be secreted under stressful situations (Siever, 1991). Disorders of the adrenal cortex can result in hyposecretion or hypersecretion of cortisol.

Addison's disease is the result of hyposecretion of the hormones of the adrenal cortex. Behavioral symptoms of hyposecretion include mood changes with apathy, social withdrawal, impaired sleep, decreased concentration, and fatigue. Hypersecretion of cortisol results in Cushing's disease and is associated with behaviors that include depression, mania, psychosis, and suicidal ideation. Cognitive impairments are also commonly observed (Reus, 1989).

Prolactin. Serum prolactin levels are regulated by prolactin-releasing hormone (PRH) and prolactin-inhibiting hormone (PIH) from the hypothalamus. Prolactin stimulates milk production by the mammary glands in the presence of high levels of estrogen and progesterone during pregnancy. Behavioral symptoms associated with hypersecretion of prolactin include depression, decreased libido, stress intolerance, anxiety, and increased irritability (Reus, 1989).

Gonadotropic Hormones. The gonadotropic hormones are so called because they produce an effect on the gonads—the ovaries and the testes. The gonadotropins include follicle-stimulating hormone (FSH) and luteinizing hormone (LH), and their release from the anterior pituitary is stimulated by gonadotropin-releasing hormone (GnRH) from the hypothalamus. In women, FSH initiates maturation of ovarian follicles into the ova and stimulates their secretion of estrogen. LH is responsible for ovulation and the secretion of progesterone from the corpus luteum. In men, FSH initiates sperm production in the testes and LH increases secretion of testosterone by the interstitial cells of the testes (Scanlon & Sanders, 1995). The gonadotropins are regulated by a negative feedback of gonadal hormones at the hypothalamic or pituitary level.

Limited evidence exists to correlate gonadotropins to behavioral functioning, although some observations have been made to warrant hypothetical consideration. Studies have indicated decreased levels of testosterone, LH, and FSH in depressed men. Increased sexual behavior and aggressiveness have been linked to elevated testosterone levels in both men and women. Decreased plasma levels of LH and FSH commonly occur in patients with anorexia nervosa. Supplemental estrogen therapy has resulted in improved mentation and mood in some depressed women.

Melanocyte-Stimulating Hormone. Melanocyte-stimulating hormone (MSH) from the hypothalamus stimulates the pineal gland to secrete melatonin. The release of melatonin appears to depend on the onset of darkness and is suppressed by light. Studies of this hormone have indicated that environmental light can affect neuronal activity and influence *circadian rhythms*. Correlation between abnormal secretion of melatonin and symptoms of depression has led to the recent implication of mela-tonin in the etiology of seasonal affective disorder (SAD), in which individuals become depressed only during the fall and winter months when the amount of daylight decreases.

Circadian Rhythms

Human biological rhythms are largely determined by genetic coding, with input from the external environment influencing the cyclic effects. **Circadian rhythms** in humans follow a near–24-hour cycle and may influence a variety of regulatory functions, including the sleep-wake cycle, body temperature regulation, patterns of activity such as eating and drinking, and hormone secretion (Jarrett, 1989). The 24-hour rhythm in humans is affected to a large degree by the cycles of lightness and darkness. This occurs because of a "pacemaker" in the brain that sends messages to other systems in the body and maintains the 24-hour rhythm. This endogenous pacemaker appears to be the suprachiasmatic nuclei of the hypothalamus. These nuclei receive projections of light through the retina, and in turn stimulate electrical impulses to various other systems in the body, mediating the release of neurotransmitters or hormones that regulate bodily functioning.

Most of the biological rhythms of the body operate over a period of about 24 hours, but cycles of longer lengths have been studied. For example, women of menstruating age show monthly cycles of progesterone levels in the saliva, of skin temperature over the breasts, and of prolactin levels in the plasma of the blood (Hughes, 1989).

The concentration of red blood cells in plasma has been measured in weekly cycles, with the peak occurring between Sunday evenings and Monday mornings in one study (Hughes, 1989). Some rhythms may even last as long as a year. These circannual rhythms are particularly relevant to certain medications, such as cyclosporine, that appear to be more effective at some times than others during the period of about a year (Hughes, 1989).

The Role of Circadian Rhythms in Psychopathology

Circadian rhythms may play a role in psychopathology. Because many hormones have been implicated in behavioral functioning, it is reasonable to believe that peak secretion times could be influential in predicting certain behaviors. The association of depression to increased secretion of melatonin during darkness hours has already been discussed. External manipulation of the light-dark cycle and removal of external time cues often have beneficial effects on mood disorders (Siever, 1991).

Symptoms that occur in the premenstrual cycle have also been linked to disruptions in biological rhythms. A number of the symptoms associated with this syndrome strongly resemble those attributed to depression, and hormonal changes have been implicated in the etiology. Some of these changes include progesterone-estrogen imbalance, increase in prolactin and mineralocorticoids, high level of prostaglandins, decrease in endogenous opiates, changes in metabolism of biogenic amines (serotonin, dopamine, norepinephrine, acetylcholine), and variations in secretion of glucocorticoids or melatonin (Sack et al., 1987).

Sleep disturbances are common in both depression and premenstrual dysphoric disorder. Because the sleep-wake cycle is probably the most fundamental of biological rhythms, it will be discussed in greater detail. A representation of bodily functions affected by 24-hour biological rhythms is presented in Figure 4.10.

Sleep

The sleep-wake cycle is genetically determined rather than learned and is established some time after birth (Moore, Karacan, & Williams, 1989). Even when environmental cues such as the ability to detect light and darkness are removed, the human sleep-wake cycle generally develops about a 25-hour periodicity, which is close to the 24-hour normal circadian rhythm.

Sleep can be measured by the types of brain waves that occur during various stages of sleep activity. Dreaming episodes are characterized by rapid eye movement and are called REM sleep. Non-REM sleep is represented by four distinct stages.

1. **Stage 0—Alpha Rhythm.** This stage of the sleep-wake cycle is characterized by a relaxed, waking state with eyes closed. The alpha brain wave rhythm has a frequency of 8 to 12 cycles per second.
2. **Stage 1—Beta Rhythm.** Stage 1 characterizes the "transition" into sleep, or a period of dozing. Thoughts wander, and there is a drifting in and out of sleep. Beta brain wave rhythm has a frequency of 18 to 25 cycles per second.
3. **Stage 2—Theta Rhythm.** This stage characterizes the manner in which about half of sleep time is spent. Eye movement and muscular activity are minimal. Theta brain wave rhythm has a frequency of 4 to 7 cycles per second.
4. **Stage 3—Delta Rhythm.** This is a period of deep and restful sleep. Muscles are relaxed, heart rate and blood pressure fall, and breathing slows. No eye movement occurs. Delta brain wave rhythm has a frequency of 1.5 to 3 cycles per second.
5. **Stage 4—Delta Rhythm.** The stage of deepest sleep. Individuals who suffer from insomnia or other sleep disorders often do not experience this stage of sleep. Eye movement and muscular activity are minimal. Delta waves predominate.
6. **REM Sleep—Beta Rhythm.** The dream cycle. Eyes dart about beneath closed eyelids, moving

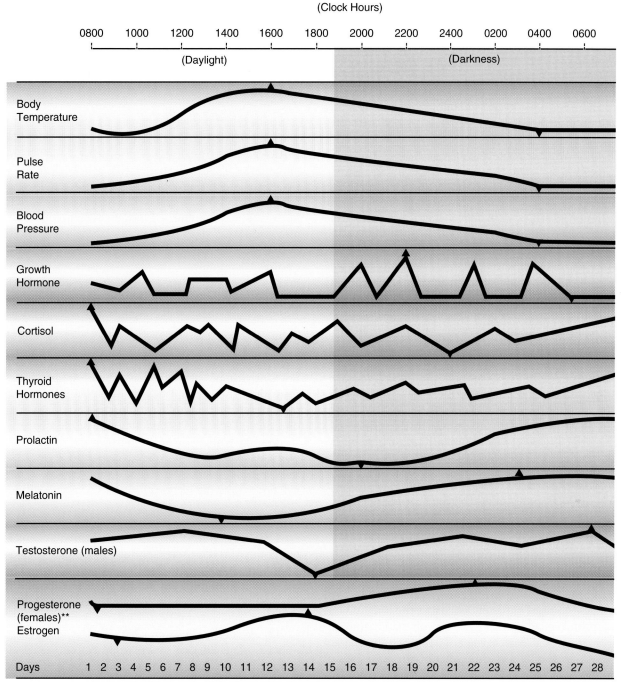

Figure 4.10 Circadian biological rhythms.*

*The female hormones are presented on a monthly rhythm because of their influence on the reproductive cycle. Daily rhythms of female gonadotropins are difficult to assay and are probably less significant than monthly.

more rapidly than when awake. The brain wave pattern is similar to that of stage 1 sleep. Heart and respiration rates increase and blood pressure may increase or decrease. Muscles are hypotonic during REM sleep.

Stage 2 through REM repeat themselves throughout the cycle of sleep. One is more likely to experience longer periods of stages 3 and 4 sleep early in the cycle and longer periods of REM sleep later in the sleep cycle. Most people experience REM sleep about four to five times during the night. The amount of REM sleep and deep sleep decreases with age, while the time spent in drowsy wakefulness and dozing increases.

Neurochemical Influences. A number of neurochemicals have been shown to influence the sleep-wake cycle. Several studies have revealed information about the sleep-inducing characteristics of serotonin. Applying serotonin directly to areas of the brain induces electroencephalographic (EEG) sleep (Moore, Karacan, & Williams, 1989). L-tryptophan, the amino acid precursor to serotonin, has been used for many years as an effective sedative-hypnotic to induce sleep in individuals with sleep-onset disorder. Some researchers speculate that the occurrence of REM sleep may require norepinephrine neurotransmission, while dopamine may be involved in maintaining arousal and in decreasing stage 4 and REM sleep (Moore, Karacan, & Williams, 1989). The exact role of GABA in sleep facilitation is unclear, although the sedative effects of drugs that enhance GABA transmission, such as the benzodiazepines, suggest that this neurotransmitter plays an important role in regulation of sleep and arousal. Some studies have suggested that acetylcholine induces and prolongs REM sleep, whereas histamine appears to have an inhibitive effect. Neuroendocrine mechanisms seem to be more closely tied to circadian rhythms than to the sleep-wake cycle. One exception is growth hormone secretion, which exhibits increases during the early sleep period and may be associated with slow-wave sleep (Siever, 1991).

GENETICS

Kendler and Silverman (1991) describe *behavior genetics* as a "science that combines aspects of psychology, psychiatry, physiology, and genetics," the goal of which "is to clarify the role that genetic factors play in the determination of behavior." The term **genotype** refers to the total set of genes present in an individual at the time of conception, and coded in the DNA. The physical manifestations of a particular genotype are designated by characteristics that specify a specific **phenotype.** Examples of phenotypes include eye color, height, blood type, language, and hair type. As evident by the examples presented, phenotypes are not *only* genetic, but may also be acquired (i.e., influenced by the environment) or a combination of both. It is likely that most psychiatric disorders are the result of a combination of genetics and environmental influences (Kendler & Silverman, 1991).

Investigators who study the etiological implications for psychiatric illness may explore several risk factors. Studies to determine if an illness is *familial* compare the percentages of family members with the illness to those in the general population or within a control group of unrelated individuals. These studies estimate the prevalence of psychopathology among relatives and make predictions about the predisposition to an illness based on familial risk factors. Schizophrenia, bipolar disorder, major depression, anorexia nervosa, panic disorder, somatization disorder, antisocial personality disorder, and alcoholism are examples of psychiatric illness in which familial tendencies have been indicated (Rieder & Kaufmann, 1988).

Studies that are purely genetic in nature search for a specific gene that is responsible for an individual having a particular illness. A number of disorders exist in which the mutation of a specific gene or change in the number or structure of a chromosome has been associated with the etiology. Examples include Huntington's chorea, cystic fibrosis, phenylketonuria, Duchenne's muscular dystrophy, and Down's syndrome.

The search for genetic links to certain psychiatric disorders continues. An investigation of early-onset Alzheimer's disease has reported a possible linkage to markers on chromosome 21 (Kendler & Silverman, 1991). Other studies have refuted this evidence. A great deal of additional research is required before definitive confirmation can be made.

In addition to familial and purely genetic investigations, other types of studies have been conducted to estimate the existence and degree of genetic and environmental contributions to the etiology of certain psychiatric disorders. Twin studies and adoption studies have been successfully employed for this purpose.

Twin studies examine the frequency of a disorder in monozygotic (genetically identical) and dizygotic (fraternal; not genetically identical) twins. Twins are called *concordant* when both members suffer from the same disorder in question. Concordance in monozygotic twins is considered stronger evidence of genetic involvement than it is in dizygotic twins. Disorders in which twin studies have suggested a possible genetic link include alcoholism, schizophrenia, major depression, bipolar disorder, anorexia nervosa, panic disorder, and obsessive-compulsive disorder (Kendler & Silverman, 1991; Rieder & Kaufmann, 1988).

Adoption studies allow comparisons to be made of the influences of genetics versus environment on the development of a psychiatric disorder. Rieder & Kaufmann (1988) describe four types of adoption studies that have been conducted:

1. The study of adopted children whose biological parent(s) had a psychiatric disorder but whose adoptive parent(s) did not.
2. The study of adopted children whose adoptive parent(s) had a psychiatric disorder but whose biological parent(s) did not.
3. The study of adoptive and biological relatives of adopted children who developed a psychiatric disorder.
4. The study of monozygotic twins reared apart by different adoptive parents.

▰ TABLE 4.4 BIOLOGICAL IMPLICATIONS OF PSYCHIATRIC DISORDERS

ANATOMICAL BRAIN STRUCTURES INVOLVED	NEUROTRANSMITTER HYPOTHESIS	POSSIBLE ENDOCRINE CORRELATION	IMPLICATIONS OF CIRCADIAN RHYTHMS	POSSIBLE GENETIC LINK
Schizophrenia Frontal cortex, temporal lobes, limbic system	Dopamine hyperactivity	Decreased prolactin levels	May correlate antipsychotic medication administration to times of lowest level	Twin, familial, and adoption studies suggest genetic link
Depressive Disorders Frontal lobes, limbic system, temporal lobes	Decreased levels of norepinephrine, dopamine, and serotonin	Increased coltisol levels; thyroid hormone hyposecretion; increased melatonin	DST* used to predict effectiveness of antidepressants; melatonin linked to depression during periods of darkness	Twin, familial, and adoption studies suggest a genetic link
Bipolar Disorder Frontal lobes, limbic system, temporal lobes	Increased levels of norepinephrine, dopamine, and serotonin in acute mania	Some indication of elevated thyroid hormones in acute mania		Twin, familial, and adoption studies suggest genetic link
Panic Disorder Limbic system, midbrain	Increased levels of norepinephrine; decreased GABA activity	Elevated levels of thyroid hormones	May have some application for times of medication administration	Twin and familial studies suggest a genetic link
Anorexia nervosa Limbic system, particularly the hypothalamus	Decreased levels of norepinephrine, serotonin, and dopamine	Decreased levels of gonadotropins and growth hormone; increased cortisol levels	DST* often shows same results as in depression	Twin and familial studies suggest a genetic link
Obsessive-Compulsive Disorder Limbic system, basal ganglia (specifically caudate nucleus)	Decreased levels of serotonin	Increased cortisol levels	DST* often shows same results as in depression	Twin studies suggest a possible genetic link
Alzheimer's Disease Temporal, parietal, and occipital regions of cerebral cortex; hippocampus	Decreased levels of acetylcholine, norepinephrine, serotonin, and somatostatin	Decreased corticotropin-releasing hormone	Decreased levels of acetylcholine and serotonin may inhibit hypothalamic-pituitary axis and interfere with hormonal releasing factors	Familial studies suggest a genetic predisposition; early-onset disorder linked to marker on chromosome 21

*DST = dexamethasone suppression test. Dexamethasone is a synthetic glucocorticoid that suppresses cortisol secretion via the feedback mechanism. In this test, 1 mg of dexamethasone is administered at 11:30 PM and blood samples are drawn at 8:00 AM, 4:00 PM, and 11:00 PM on the following day. A plasma value greater than 5 μg/dl suggests that the individual is not suppressing cortisol in response to the dose of dexamethasone. This is a positive result for depression and may have implications for other disorders as well.

Disorders in which adoption studies have suggested a possible genetic link include alcoholism, schizophrenia, major depression, bipolar disorder, somatization disorder, and antisocial personality disorder (Kendler & Silverman, 1991; Rieder & Kaufmann, 1988).

A summary of various psychiatric disorders and the possible biological influences discussed in this chapter is presented in Table 4.4. Various diagnostic procedures used to detect alteration in biological functioning that may contribute to psychiatric disorders are presented in Table 4.5.

▰ TABLE 4.5 DIAGNOSTIC PROCEDURES USED TO DETECT ALTERED BRAIN FUNCTIONING

EXAM	TECHNIQUE USED	PURPOSE OF THE EXAM AND POSSIBLE FINDINGS
Electroencephalography (EEG)	Electrodes are place on the scalp in a standardized position. Amplitude and frequency of beta, alpha, theta, and delta brain waves are graphically recorded on paper by ink markers for multiple areas of the brain surface.	Measures brain electrical activity; identifies dysrhythmias, asymmetries, or suppression of brain rhythms; used in the diagnosis of epilepsy, neoplasm, stroke, metabolic or degenerative disease.
Computerized EEG mapping	EEG tracings are summarized by computer-assisted systems in which various regions of the brain are identified and functioning is interpreted by color coding or gray shading.	Measures brain electrical activity; used largely in research to represent statistical relationships between individuals and groups or between two populations of subjects (e.g., patients with schizophrenia vs. control subjects).
Computed tomographic (CT) scan	May be used with or without contrast medium. X rays are taken of various transverse planes of the brain while a computerized analysis produces a precise reconstructed image of each segment.	Measures accuracy of brain structure to detect possible lesions, abscesses, areas of infarction, or aneurysm. CT has also identified various anatomical differences in patients with schizophrenia, organic mental disorders, and bipolar disorder.
Magnetic resonance imaging (MRI)	Within a strong magnetic field, the nuclei of hydrogen atoms absorb and reemit electromagnetic energy that is computerized and transformed into image information. No radiation or contrast medium is used.	Measures anatomical and biochemical status of various segments of the brain; detects brain edema, ischemia, infection, neoplasm, trauma, and other changes such as demyelination. Morphological differences have been noted in brains of patients with schizophrenia as compared with control subjects.
Positron emission tomography (PET)	The patient receives an intravenous (IV) injection of a radioactive substance (type dependent upon brain activity to be visualized). The head is surrounded by detectors that relay data to a computer that interprets the signals and produces the image.	Measures specific brain functioning, such as glucose metabolism, oxygen utilization, blood flow, and, of particular interest in psychiatry, neurotransmitter-receptor interaction.
Single photon emission computed tomography (SPECT)	The technique is similar to PET, but longer-acting radioactive substance must be used to allow time for a gamma-camera to rotate about the head and gather the data, which are then computer assembled into a brain image.	Measures various aspects of brain functioning, as with PET; has also been used to image activity or cerebrospinal fluid circulation.

PSYCHOIMMUNOLOGY

Normal Immune Response

Cells responsible for *nonspecific* immune reactions include neutrophils, monocytes, and macrophages. They work to destroy the invasive organism and initiate and facilitate damaged tissue. If these cells are not effective in accomplishing a satisfactory healing response, *specific* immune mechanisms take over.

Specific immune mechanisms are divided into two major types: the cellular response and the humoral response. The controlling elements of the cellular response are the T lymphocytes (T cells); those of the humoral response are called B lymphocytes (B cells). When the body is invaded by a specific antigen, the T cells, and particularly the T4 lymphocytes (also called *T helper cells*), become sensitized to and specific for the foreign antigen. These antigen-specific T4 cells divide many times, producing antigen-specific T4 cells with other functions. One of these, the *T killer cell*, destroys viruses that reproduce inside other cells by punctur-

ing the cell membrane of the host cell and allowing the contents of the cell, including viruses, to spill out into the bloodstream, where they can be engulfed by macrophages (Perdew, 1990). Another cell produced through division of the T4 cells is the suppressor T cell, which serves to stop the immune response once the foreign antigen has been destroyed (Scanlon & Sanders, 1995).

The humoral response is activated when antigen-specific T4 cells communicate with the B cells in the spleen and lymph nodes. The B cells in turn produce the antibodies specific to the foreign antigen. Antibodies attach themselves to foreign antigens so that they are unable to invade body cells. These invader cells are then destroyed without being able to multiply.

Implications for Psychiatric Illness

In studies of the biological response to stress, it has been hypothesized that individuals become more susceptible to physical illness following exposure to a stressful stimulus or life event (see Chapter 1). This response is thought to be due to the effect of increased glucocorticoid release from the adrenal cortex following stimulation from the hypothalamic-pituitary-adrenal axis during stressful situations. The result is a suppression in lymphocyte proliferation and function.

Studies have shown that nerve endings exist in tissues of the immune system. The CNS has connections in both bone marrow and the thymus, where immune system cells are produced, and in the spleen and lymph nodes, where those cells are stored (Ader, Cohen, & Felton, 1987).

Growth hormone, which may be released in response to certain stressors, may enhance immune functioning, while testosterone is thought to inhibit immune functioning. Increased production of epinephrine and norepinephrine occurs in response to stress and may decrease immunity (Stein, Schleifer, & Keller, 1985). Serotonin has demonstrated both enhancing and inhibitory effects on immunity (Stein, Schleifer, & Keller, 1991).

Studies have correlated a decrease in lymphocyte functioning with periods of grief, bereavement, and depression, associating the degree of altered immunity with severity of the depression (Schleifer, Keller, & Siris, 1985). A number of research studies have been conducted attempting to correlate the onset of schizophrenia to abnormalities of the immune system. These studies have considered autoimmune responses, viral infections, and immunogenetics (Kaplan, Sadock, & Grebb, 1994). The role of these factors in the onset and course of schizophrenia remains unclear. Immunological abnormalities have also been investigated in a number of other psychiatric illnesses, including alcoholism, autism, and dementia.

Evidence exists to support a correlation between psychosocial stress and the onset of illness. Research is still required to determine the specific processes involved in stress-induced modulation of the immune system.

IMPLICATIONS FOR NURSING

The discipline of psychiatric/mental health nursing has always spoken of its role in holistic health care, but historical review reveals that emphasis has been placed on treatment approaches that focus on psychological and social factors (Abraham, Fox, & Cohen, 1992). Psychiatric nurses must integrate knowledge of the biological sciences into their practices if they are to ensure safe and effective care to people with mental illness. Lowery (1992) states:

> "The 'medicalization' of psychiatry seems to be well underway. It is psychiatry's turn to reap the benefits of technology and science. Perhaps more than any other specialty, psychiatric nursing will change as the result of these developments that are revolutionizing the way in which we think about our patients and ourselves." (p. 13.)

To ensure a smooth transition from a psychosocial focus to one of biopsychosocial emphasis, nurses must have a clear understanding of the following:

Neuroanatomy and neurophysiology: the structure and functioning of the various parts of the brain and their correlation to human behavior and psychopathology.

Neuronal processes: the various functions of the nerve cells, including the role of neurotransmitters, receptors, synaptic activity, and informational pathways.

Neuroendocrinology: the interaction of the endocrine and nervous systems, and the role that the endocrine glands and their respective hormones play in behavioral functioning.

Circadian rhythms: regulation of biochemical functioning over periods of rhythmic cycles and their influence in predicting certain behaviors.

Genetic influences: hereditary factors that predispose individuals to certain psychiatric disorders.

Psychoimmunology: the influence of stress on the immune system and its role in the susceptibility to illness.

Psychopharmacology: the increasing use of psychotropics in the treatment of mental illness, demanding greater knowledge of psychopharmacological principles and nursing interventions necessary for safe and effective management.

Diagnostic technology: the importance of keeping informed about the latest in technological procedures for diagnosing alterations in brain structure and function.

Why are these concepts important to the practice of psychiatric/mental health nursing? The interrelationship between psychosocial adaptation and physical functioning has been established. The "bio" must remain an integral part of biopsychosocial nursing. As Lowery (1992) proclaims:

> "Nursing's near future is full of challenges: we have a major advocacy task to reduce the continuing stigma of mental illness and the implications for delivery of care; we must begin to rationalize the evolving specialty system and our roles in it; and we must begin to incorporate new science and technology into our practice, education, and research." (pp. 9–10).

SUMMARY

The "medicalization" of psychiatry is upon us. Nurses must be cognizant of the interaction between physical and mental factors in the development and management of psychiatric illness. These current trends have made it essential for nurses to increase their knowledge about the structure and functioning of the brain. This includes the processes of neurotransmission and the function of various neurotransmitters. This is especially important in light of the increasing role of psychotropic medication in the treatment of psychiatric illness. Because the mechanism of action of many of these drugs occurs at synaptic transmission, nurses must understand this process so that they may predict outcomes and safely manage the administration of psychotropic medications.

The endocrine system plays an important role in human behavior through the hypothalamic-pituitary axis. Hormones and their circadian rhythm of regulation significantly influence a number of physiological and psychological life-cycle phenomena, such as moods, sleep-arousal, stress response, appetite, libido, and fertility.

Research continues to validate the role of genetics in psychiatric illness. Familial, twin, and adoption studies suggest that genetics may be implicated in the etiology of schizophrenia, bipolar disorder, depression, panic disorder, anorexia nervosa, and alcoholism. Investigations to substantiate current data are ongoing and may reveal evidence of genetic influence in other psychiatric illnesses as well.

Psychoimmunology is a relatively new area of study that examines the impact of psychological factors on the immune system. Evidence exists to support a link between psychosocial stressors and suppression of the immune response. This is especially important knowledge for nurses, as they serve to assist clients in the primary prevention of mental illness.

It is also important for nurses to keep abreast of the expanding diagnostic technologies available for detecting alterations in physical functioning. Technologies such as magnetic resonance imagery (MRI) and positron emission tomography (PET) are facilitating the growth of knowledge linking mental illness to disorders of the brain. Trygstad (1994) states, "Psychiatric nursing in the 1990s requires integrating an expanding biological focus into nursing practice to accommodate both the growing biological knowledge base and changing patients' needs."

REVIEW QUESTIONS

SELF-EXAMINATION/LEARNING EXERCISE

Match the following parts of the brain to their functions described in the right-hand column:

_____ 1. Frontal lobe

_____ 2. Parietal lobe

_____ 3. Temporal lobe

_____ 4. Occipital lobe

_____ 5. Thalamus

_____ 6. Hypothalamus

_____ 7. Limbic system

a. Sometimes called the "emotional brain"; associated with multiple feelings and behaviors.

b. Concerned with visual reception and interpretation.

c. Voluntary body movement; thinking and judgment; expression of feeling.

d. Integrates all sensory input (except smell) on way to cortex.

e. Part of the cortex that deals with sensory perception and interpretation.

f. Hearing, short-term memory, and sense of smell.

g. Control over pituitary gland and autonomic nervous system. Regulates appetite and temperature.

Select the answer that is most appropriate for each of the following questions.

8. At a synapse, the determination of further impulse transmission is accomplished by means of

    a. Potassium ions
    b. Interneurons
    c. Neurotransmitters
    d. The myelin sheath

9. A decrease in which of the following neurotransmitters has been implicated in depression?

    a. GABA, acetylcholine, and aspartate
    b. Norepinephrine, serotonin, and dopamine
    c. Somatostatin, substance P, and glycine
    d. Glutamate, histamine, and opioid peptides

10. Which of the following hormones has been implicated in the etiology of seasonal affective disorder (SAD)?

    a. Increased levels of melatonin
    b. Decreased levels of oxytocin
    c. Decreased levels of prolactin
    d. Increased levels of thyrotropin

11. In which of the following psychiatric disorders do genetic tendencies appear to exist?

    a. Schizophrenia
    b. Dissociative disorder
    c. Conversion disorder
    d. Narcissistic personality disorder

12. With which of the following diagnostic imaging technologies can neurotransmitter-receptor interaction be visualized?

    a. Magnetic resonance imaging (MRI)
    b. Positron emission tomography (PET)
    c. Electroencephalography (EEG)
    d. Computerized EEG mapping

13. During stressful situations, stimulation of the hypothalamic-pituitary-adrenal axis results in suppression of the immune system because of the effect of
    a. Antidiuretic hormone from the posterior pituitary
    b. Increased secretion of gonadotropins from the gonads
    c. Decreased release of growth hormone from the anterior pituitary
    d. Increased glucocorticoid release from the adrenal cortex

REFERENCES

Abraham, I.L., Fox, J.C., & Cohen, B.T. (1992). Integrating the bio into the biopsychosocial: Understanding and treating biological phenomena in psychiatric-mental health nursing. *Archives of Psychiatric Nursing, 6*(5), 296–305.

Ader, R., Cohen, N., & Felton,. D. (1987). Brain, behavior, and immunity. *Brain Behavior and Immunity, 1*, 1.

Baraban, J.M., & Coyle, J.T. (1989). Receptors, monoamines, and amino acids. In H.I. Kaplan & B.J. Sadock (Eds.)., *Comprehensive textbook of psychiatry* (Vol. 1) (5th ed.). Baltimore: Williams & Wilkins.

Chafetz, M.D. (1990). *Nutrition and neurotransmitters: The nutrient bases of behavior.* Englewood Cliffs, NJ: Prentice Hall.

Davidson, M. (1991). Neuropeptides. In K. Davis, H. Klar, & J.T. Coyle (Eds.), *Foundations of psychiatry.* Philadelphia: W.B. Saunders.

Davis, K.L., & Greenwald, B. (1991). Biology of schizophrenia. In K. Davis, H. Klar, & J.T. Coyle (Eds.), *Foundations of psychiatry.* Philadelphia: W.B. Saunders.

Grebb, J.A. (1989). Introduction and overview of neural science. In H.I. Kaplan & B.J. Sadock (Eds.), *Comprehensive textbook of psychiatry* (Vol. 1) (5th ed.). Baltimore: Williams & Wilkins.

Halperin, R. (1991). Hypothalamic control. In K. Davis, H. Klar, & J.T. Coyle (Eds.), *Foundations of psychiatry.* Philadelphia: W.B. Saunders.

Horvath, T.B. (1991). Integrative brain mechanisms. In K. Davis, H. Klar, & J.T. Coyle (Eds.), *Foundations of psychiatry.* Philadelphia: W.B. Saunders.

Hughes, M. (1989). *Body clock: The effects of time on human health.* New York: Andromeda Oxford Ltd.

Jarrett, D.B. (1989). Chronobiology. In H.I. Kaplan & B.J. Sadock (Eds.), *Comprehensive textbook of psychiatry* (Vol. 1) (5th ed.). Baltimore: Williams & Wilkins.

Kaplan, H.I., & Sadock, B.J. (1985). *Modern synopsis of comprehensive textbook of psychiatry* (4th ed.). Baltimore: Williams & Wilkins.

Kaplan, H.I., Sadock, B.J., & Grebb, J. A. (1994). *Synopsis of psychiatry* (7th ed.). Baltimore: Williams & Wilkins.

Kendler, K.S., & Silverman, J.M. (1991). Behavior genetics. In K. Davis, H. Klar, & J.T. Coyle (Eds.), *Foundations of psychiatry.* Philadelphia: W.B. Saunders.

Kruk, Z.L., & Pycock, C.J. (1983). *Neurotransmitters and drugs.* Baltimore: University Park Press.

Landau, B.R. (1976). *Essential human anatomy and physiology.* Glenview, IL: Scott, Foresman & Co.

Lowery, B.J. (1992). Psychiatric nursing in the 1990's and beyond. *Journal of Psychosocial Nursing, 30*(1), 7–13.

Moore, C.A., Karacan, I., & Williams, R.L. (1989). Basic science of sleep. In H.I. Kaplan & B.J. Sadock (Eds.), *Comprehensive textbook of psychiatry* (Vol. 1) (5th ed.). Baltimore: Williams & Wilkins.

Murphy, M., & Deutsch, S.I. (1991). Neurophysiological and neurochemical basis of behavior. In K. Davis, H. Klar, & J.T. Coyle (Eds.), *Foundations of psychiatry.* Philadelphia: W.B. Saunders.

Murphy, M., & Handelsman, L. (1991). Anxiety. In K. Davis, H. Klar, & J.T. Coyle (Eds.), *Foundations of psychiatry.* Philadelphia: W.B. Saunders.

Perdew, S. (1990). *Facts About AIDS: A guide for health care providers.* Philadelphia: J.B. Lippincott.

Peschel, E., & Peschel, R. (1991). Neurobiological disorders. *Journal of the California Alliance for the Mentally Ill, 2*(4), 4.

Reus, V.I. (1989). Psychoneuroendocrinology. In H.I. Kaplan & B.J. Sadock (Eds.), *Comprehensive textbook of psychiatry* (Vol. 1) (5th ed.). Baltimore: Williams & Wilkins.

Rieder, R.O., & Kaufmann, C.A. (1988). Genetics. In J.A. Talbott, R.E. Hales, & S.C. Yudofsky (Eds.), *Textbook of psychiatry.* Washington, DC: The American Psychiatric Press.

Sack, D., Rosenthal, N., Parry, B., & Wehr, T. (1987). Biological rhythms in psychiatry. In H. Meltzer (Ed.), *Psychopharmacology.* New York: Raven Press.

Scanlon, V.C., & Sanders, T. (1995). *Essentials of anatomy and physiology* (2nd ed.). Philadelphia: F.A. Davis.

Scanlon, V.C., & Sanders, T. (1999). *Essentials of anatomy and physiology* (3rd ed.). Philadelphia: F.A. Davis.

Schleifer, S.J., Keller, S.E., & Siris, S.G. (1985). Depression and immunity. *Archives of General Psychiatry, 42*, 129–133.

Schwarcz, R., & Meldrum, B. (1985). Excitatory amino acid antagonists provide a therapeutic approach to neurologic disorders. *Lancet, 2:*140–143.

Siever, L.J. (1991). Biological rhythms and the neuroendocrine system. In K. Davis, H. Klar, & J.T. Coyle (Eds.), *Foundations of psychiatry.* Philadelphia: W.B. Saunders.

Siever, L.J., Davis, K.L., & Gorman, L.K. (1991). Pathogenesis of mood disorders. In K. Davis, H. Klar, & J.T. Coyle (Eds.), *Foundations of psychiatry.* Philadelphia: W.B. Saunders.

Stein, M., Schleifer, S.J., & Keller, S.E. (1985). Immune disorders. In H.I. Kaplan & B.J. Sadock (Eds.), *Comprehensive textbook of psychiatry* (4th ed.). Baltimore: Williams & Wilkins.

Stein, M., Schleifer, S.J., & Keller, S.E. (1991). Stress and the immune system. In K. Davis, H. Klar, & J.T. Coyle (Eds.), *Foundations of psychiatry.* Philadelphia: W.B. Saunders.

Trygstad, L.N. (1994). The need to know: Biological learning needs identified by practicing psychiatric nurses. *Journal of Psychosocial Nursing, 32*(2), 13–18.

Vander, A.J., Sherman, J.H., & Luciano, D.S. (1975). *Human physiology: The mechanisms of body function* (2nd ed.). New York: McGraw-Hill.

Bibliography

Altshuler, L. (1991). Neuroanatomy in schizophrenia and affective disorder. *Journal of the California Alliance for the Mentally Ill, 2*(4), 27–30.

American Nurses Association. (1994). *Psychiatric mental health nursing psychopharmacology project.* Washington, DC: American Nurses Publishing.

Barondes, S.H. (1991). Genetics of mental illness: Problems and promise. *Journal of the California Alliance for the Mentally Ill, 2*(4), 19–20.

Binkley, S. (1990). *The clockwork sparrow: Time, clocks, and calendars in biological organisms.* Englewood Cliffs, NJ: Prentice Hall.

Crow, T.J. (1995). The meaning of the morphological changes in the brain in schizophrenia. *Current Approaches to Psychoses: Diagnosis and Management, 4*(1), 8–9.

Gillin, J.C. (1991). A PET study: Sleeping . . . dreaming . . . hallucinating. *Journal of the California Alliance for the Mentally Ill, 2*(4), 11–13.

Gilman, S., & Newman, S.W. (1992). *Essentials of clinical neuroanatomy and neurophysiology.* Philadelphia: F.A. Davis.

Glod, C.A., & Cawley, D. (1997). The neurobiology of obsessive-compulsive disorder. *Journal of the American Psychiatric Nurses Association, 3*(4): 120–122.

Mauron, J. (1986). *Nutrition: Neurotransmitter function and behavior.* Toronto: Hans Huber Publishers.

Mazziotta, J.C., & Gilman, S. (1992). *Clinical brain imaging: Principles and applications.* Philadelphia: F.A. Davis.

Mesulam, M. (1985). *Principles of behavioral neurology.* Philadelphia: F.A. Davis.

Minors, D.S., & Waterhouse, J.M. (1981). *Circadian rhythms and the human.* Bristol, England: John Wright & Sons.

National Institute of Mental Health. (1991). Caring for people with severe mental disorders: A national plan of research to improve services. DHHS Pub. No. (ADM)91–1762. Washington, DC: U.S. Government Printing Office.

Sedvall, G. (1995). PET studies on the neuroreceptor effects of antipsychotic drugs. *Current Approaches to Psychoses: Diagnosis and Management, 4*(1), 1–3.

VanRee, J.M., & Matthysse, S. (1986). *Psychiatric disorders: Neurotransmitters and neuropeptides.* Amsterdam, The Netherlands: Elsevier Science Publishers.

Walker, E., & Neumann, C. (Spring 1994). Neurodevelopmental origins of schizophrenia. *NARSAD Research Newsletter,* 14–16.

Wirshing, W.C. (1991). Searching the brain: Trying to see neuro-biological disorders. *Journal of the California Alliance for the Mentally Ill, 2*(4), 2–3.

UNIT TWO

THERAPEUTIC APPROACHES IN PSYCHIATRIC NURSING CARE

RELATIONSHIP DEVELOPMENT

KEY TERMS

beliefs
attitudes
values
rapport

concrete thinking
confidentiality
unconditional positive
    regard

genuineness
empathy
sympathy

OBJECTIVES

After reading this chapter, the student will be able to:

1. Describe the relevance of a therapeutic nurse-client relationship.
2. Discuss the dynamics of a therapeutic nurse-client relationship.
3. Discuss the importance of self-awareness in the nurse-client relationship.
4. Identify goals of the nurse-client relationship.
5. Identify and discuss essential conditions for a therapeutic relationship to occur.
6. Describe the phases of relationship development and the tasks associated with each phase.

he nurse-client relationship is the foundation upon which psychiatric nursing is established. It is a relationship in which both participants must recognize each other as unique and important human beings. It is also a relationship in which mutual learning occurs. Peplau (1991) states:

> "Shall a nurse do things *for* a patient or can participant relationships be emphasized so that a nurse comes to do things *with* a patient as her share of an agenda of work to be accomplished in reaching a goal—health. It is likely that the nursing process is educative and therapeutic when nurse and patient can come to know and to respect each other, as persons who are alike, and yet, different, as persons who share in the solution of problems." (p. 9.)

This chapter examines the role of the psychiatric nurse and the use of self as the therapeutic tool in the nursing of clients with emotional illness. Phases of the therapeutic relationship are explored and conditions essential to the development of a therapeutic relationship are discussed. The importance of values clarification in the development of self-awareness is emphasized.

ROLE OF THE PSYCHIATRIC NURSE

What is a nurse? Undoubtedly, this question would elicit as many different answers as the number of people to whom it was presented. Nursing as a *concept* has probably existed since the beginning of the civilized world, with the provision of "care" to the ill or infirm by anyone in the environment who took the time to administer to those in need. The emergence of nursing as a *profession* only began in the late 1800s, however, with the graduation of Linda Richards from the New England Hospital for Women and Children in Boston, upon achievement of the diploma in nursing. Since that time, the nurse's role has evolved from that of custodial caregiver and physician's handmaiden to being recognized as a unique, independent member of the professional health care team.

Peplau (1957) has identified several subroles within the role of the nurse:

1. **The Mother-Surrogate.** In this subrole, the nurse fulfills basic needs associated with mothering, such as bathing, feeding, dressing, toileting, warning, disciplining, and approving.
2. **The Technician.** The focus of this subrole is on the competent, efficient, and correct performance of technical procedures.
3. **The Manager.** In this subrole the nurse manages and manipulates the environment to improve conditions for the client's recovery.
4. **The Socializing Agent.** The major function here is participating in social activities with the client.
5. **The Health Teacher.** In this subrole the nurse identifies learning needs and provides information

required by the client or family to improve the health situation.
6. **The Counselor or Psychotherapist.** The nurse uses "interpersonal techniques" to assist clients to learn to adapt to difficulties or changes in life experiences.

Peplau (1962) believes that the emphasis in psychiatric nursing is on the counseling or psychotherapeutic subrole. How then does this emphasis influence the role of the nurse in the psychiatric setting? Many sources define the *nurse therapist* as having graduate preparation in psychiatric/mental health nursing. He or she has developed skills through intensive supervised educational experiences to provide helpful individual, group, or family therapy.

Peplau suggests that it is essential for the *staff nurse working in psychiatry* to have a general knowledge of basic counseling techniques. A therapeutic or "helping" relationship is established through use of these interpersonal techniques and is based on a knowledge of theories of personality development and human behavior.

Sullivan (1953) believed that emotional problems stem from difficulties with interpersonal relationships. Interpersonal theorists, such as Peplau and Sullivan, emphasize the importance of relationship development in the provision of emotional care. Through establishment of a satisfactory nurse-client relationship, individuals learn to generalize the ability to achieve satisfactory interpersonal relationships to other aspects of their lives.

DYNAMICS OF A THERAPEUTIC NURSE-CLIENT RELATIONSHIP

Travelbee (1971), who expanded on Peplau's theory of interpersonal relations in nursing, has stated that it is only when each individual in the interaction perceives the other as a human being that a relationship is possible. She refers not to a nurse-client relationship, but rather to a human-to-human relationship, which she describes as a "mutually significant experience." That is, both the nurse and the recipient of care have needs met when each views the other as a unique human being, not as "an illness," as "a room number, " or as "all nurses" in general.

Therapeutic relationships are goal oriented. Ideally, the nurse and client decide together what the goal of the relationship will be. Most often the goal is directed at learning and growth promotion, in an effort to bring about some type of change in the client's life. In general, the goal of a therapeutic relationship may be based on a problem-solving model.

EXAMPLE

Goal

The client will demonstrate more adaptive coping strategies for dealing with (specific life situation).

Interventions

1. Identify what is troubling the client at this time.
2. Encourage the client to discuss changes he or she would like to make.
3. Discuss with the client which changes are possible and which are not possible.
4. Have the client explore feelings about aspects that cannot be changed and alternative ways of coping more adaptively.
5. Discuss alternative strategies for creating changes the client desires to make.
6. Weigh the benefits and consequences of each alternative.
7. Assist the client to select an alternative.
8. Encourage the client to implement the change.
9. Provide positive feedback for the client's attempts to create change.
10. Assist the client to evaluate outcomes of the change and make modifications as required.

Therapeutic Use of Self

Travelbee (1971) described the instrument for delivery of the process of interpersonal nursing as the *therapeutic use of self*, which she defined as "the ability to use one's personality consciously and in full awareness in an attempt to establish relatedness and to structure nursing interventions."

Use of the self in a therapeutic manner requires that the nurse have a greater deal of self-awareness and self-understanding; that he or she has arrived at a philosophical belief about life, death, and the overall human condition. The nurse must understand that the ability and extent to which one can effectively help others in time of need is strongly influenced by this internal value system—a combination of intellect and emotions.

Gaining Self-Awareness

Values Clarification

Knowing and understanding oneself enhances the ability to form satisfactory interpersonal relationships. Self-awareness requires that an individual recognize and accept what he or she values and learn to accept the uniqueness and differences in others. This concept is important in everyday life and in the nursing profession in general; but it is *essential* in psychiatric nursing.

An individual's value system is established very early in life and has its foundations in the value system held by the primary caregivers. It is culturally oriented; it may change many times over the course of a lifetime; and it consists of beliefs, attitudes, and values. Values clarification is one process by which an individual may gain self-awareness.

Beliefs. A **belief** is an idea that one holds to be true, and it can take any of several forms:

1. **Rational Beliefs.** Ideas for which objective evidence exists to substantiate its truth.

EXAMPLE

Alcoholism is a disease.

2. **Irrational Beliefs.** Ideas that an individual holds as true despite the existence of objective contradictory evidence. Delusions can be a form of irrational beliefs.

EXAMPLE

Once an alcoholic has been through detox and rehab, he or she can drink socially if desired.

3. **Faith (Sometimes Called "Blind Beliefs").** Ideals that an individual holds as true for which no objective evidence exists.

EXAMPLE

Belief in a higher power can help an alcoholic stop drinking.

4. **Stereotype.** A socially shared belief that describes a concept in an oversimplified or undifferentiated manner.

EXAMPLE

All alcoholics are skid-row bums.

Attitudes. An **attitude** is a frame of reference around which an individual organizes knowledge about his or her world. An attitude also has an emotional component. It can be a prejudgment and may be selective and biased. Attitudes fulfill the need to find meaning in life and to provide clarity and consistency for the individual. The prevailing stigma attached to mental illness is an example of a negative attitude. An associated belief might be that "all people with mental illness are dangerous."

Values. **Values** are abstract standards, positive or negative, that represent an individual's ideal mode of conduct and ideal goals. Some examples of ideal mode of conduct include seeking truth and beauty; being clean and orderly; and behaving with sincerity, justice, reason, compassion, humility, respect, honor, and loyalty. Examples of ideal goals are security, happiness, freedom, equality, ecstasy, fame, and power.

Values differ from attitudes and beliefs in that they are action-oriented or action-producing. One may hold many attitudes and beliefs without behaving in a way that shows one holds those attitudes and beliefs. For example, a nurse may believe that all clients have the right to be told the truth about their diagnosis; however, he or she may not always act on the belief and tell all clients the complete truth about their condition. It is only when the belief is acted on that it becomes a value.

Attitudes and beliefs flow out of one's set of values. An individual may have thousands of beliefs, hundreds of attitudes, but his or her values probably only number in the dozens. Values may be viewed as a kind of core concept or basic standards that determine one's attitudes and beliefs, and ultimately, one's behavior. Raths, Merril, and Simon (1966) identified a seven-step process of valuing that can be used to help clarify personal values. This process is presented in Table 5.1. The process can be used by applying these seven steps to an attitude or belief that one holds. When an attitude or belief has met each of the seven criteria, it can be considered a value.

The Johari Window

The self arises out of self-appraisal and the appraisal of others and represents each individual's unique pattern of values, attitudes, beliefs, behaviors, emotions, and needs (Ujhely, 1968). Self-awareness is the recognition of these aspects and understanding about their impact on the self and others. The Johari window is a representation of the self and a tool that can be used to increase self-awareness (Luft, 1970). The Johari window is presented in Figure 5.1 and is divided into four quadrants.

The Open or Public Self. The upper left quadrant of the window represents the part of the self that is public; that is, aspects of the self about which both the individual and others are aware.

EXAMPLE

Susan, a nurse who is the adult child of an alcoholic, has strong feelings about helping alcoholics to achieve sobri-ety. She volunteers her time to be a support person on call to help recovering alcoholics. She is aware of her feelings and her desire to help others. Members of the Alcoholics Anonymous group in which she volunteers her time are also aware of Susan's feelings, and they feel comfortable calling her when they need help refraining from drinking.

The Unknowing Self. The upper right (blind) quadrant of the window represents the part of the self that is known to others but remains hidden from the awareness of the individual.

EXAMPLE

When Susan takes care of patients in detox, she does so without emotion, tending to the technical aspects of the task in a way that the clients perceive as cold and judgmental. She is unaware that she comes across to the clients in this way.

The Private Self. The lower left quadrant of the window represents the part of the self that is known to the individual but which the individual deliberately and consciously conceals from others.

EXAMPLE

Susan would prefer not to take care of the clients in detox because doing so provokes painful memories from her childhood. However, because she does not want the other staff members to know about these feelings, she volunteers to take care of the detox clients whenever they are assigned to her unit.

The Unknown Self. The lower right quadrant of the window represents the part of the self that is unknown to both the individual and to others.

TABLE 5.1 THE PROCESS OF VALUES CLARIFICATION

LEVEL OF OPERATIONS	CATEGORY	CRITERIA	EXPLANATION
Cognitive	Choosing	1. Freely 2. From alternatives 3. After careful consideration of the consequences	"This value is mine. No one forced me to choose it. I understand and accept the consequences of holding this value."
Emotional	Prizing	4. Satisfied; pleased with the choice 5. Making public affirmation of the choice, if necessary	"I am proud that I hold this value, and I am willing to tell others about it."
Behavioral	Acting	6. Taking action to demonstrate the value behaviorally 7. Demonstrating this pattern of behavior consistently and repeatedly	The value is reflected in the individual's behavior for as long as he or she holds it.

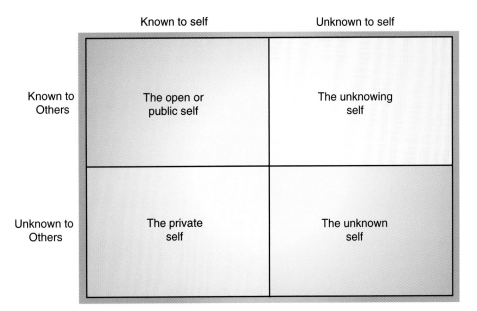

Known to self   Unknown to self

Known to Others — The open or public self | The unknowing self

Unknown to Others — The private self | The unknown self

Figure 5.1 The Johari window. *Source:* Luft (1970).

EXAMPLE

Susan felt very powerless as a child growing up with an alcoholic father. She seldom knew in what condition she would find her father or what his behavior would be. She learned over the years to find small ways to maintain control over her life situation, and left home as soon as she graduated from high school. Needing to stay in control has always been very important to Susan, and she is unaware that working with recovering alcoholics helps to fulfill this need in her. The people whom she is helping are also unaware that Susan is satisfying an unfulfilled personal need as she provides them with assistance.

The goal of increasing self-awareness by using the Johari window is to increase the size of the quadrant that represents the open or public self. The individual who is open to self and others has the ability to be spontaneous and to share emotions and experiences with others. This individual also has a greater understanding of personal behavior and of others' responses to him or her. Increased self-awareness allows an individual to interact with others comfortably, to accept the differences in others, and to observe each person's right to respect and dignity.

CONDITIONS ESSENTIAL TO DEVELOPMENT OF A THERAPEUTIC RELATIONSHIP

Several theorists have identified characteristics that enhance the achievement of a therapeutic relationship (Rogers et al., 1967; Travelbee, 1971; Peplau, 1969; Carkhuff, 1968). These concepts are highly significant to the use of self as the therapeutic tool in interpersonal relationship development.

Rapport

Getting acquainted and establishing **rapport** is the primary task in relationship development. Rapport implies special feelings on the part of both the client and the nurse based on acceptance, warmth, friendliness, common interest, a sense of trust, and a nonjudgmental attitude. Establishing rapport may be accomplished by discussing non-health-related topics. Travelbee (1971) states:

> "[To establish rapport] is to create a sense of harmony based on knowledge and appreciation of each individual's uniqueness. It is the ability to be still and experience the other as a human being—to appreciate the unfolding of each personality one to the other. The ability to truly care for and about others is the core of rapport."

Trust

To trust another, one must feel confidence in that person's presence, reliability, integrity, veracity, and sincere desire to provide assistance when requested. As previously discussed, trust is the initial developmental task described by Erikson. When this task has not been achieved, this component of relationship development becomes more difficult. That is not to say that trust cannot be established, but only that additional time and patience may be required on the part of the nurse.

It is imperative for the nurse to convey an aura of trustworthiness which requires that he or she possess a sense of self-confidence. Confidence in the self is derived out of knowledge gained through achievement of personal and professional goals, as well as the ability to integrate these roles and to function as a unified whole.

Trust cannot be presumed; it must be earned. Trustworthiness is demonstrated through nursing interventions that convey a sense of warmth and caring to the client. These interventions are initiated simply and concretely, and directed toward activities that address the client's basic needs for physiological and psychological safety and security. Many psychiatric clients experience **concrete thinking** which focuses their thought processes on specifics rather than generalities and immediate issues rather than eventual outcomes. Examples of nursing interventions that would promote trust in an individual who is thinking concretely include the following:

- Providing a blanket when the client is cold.
- Providing food when the client is hungry.
- Keeping promises.
- Being honest (e.g., saying "I don't know the answer to your question, but I'll try to find out") and then following through.
- Simply and clearly providing reasons for certain policies, procedures, and rules.
- Providing a written, structured schedule of activities.
- Attending activities with the client if he or she is reluctant to go alone.
- Being consistent in adhering to unit guidelines.
- Taking the client's preferences, requests, and opinions into consideration when possible in decisions concerning his or her care.
- Ensuring **confidentiality;** providing reassurance that what is discussed will not be repeated outside the boundaries of the health care team.

Trust is the basis of a therapeutic relationship. The nurse working in psychiatry must perfect the skills that foster the development of trust. Without the establishment of trust, the helping relationship will not progress beyond the level of mechanical provision for tending to superficial needs (Sundeen et al., 1985).

Respect

To show respect is to believe in the dignity and worth of an individual regardless of his or her unacceptable behavior. Rogers (1951) called this **unconditional positive regard.** The attitude is nonjudgmental, and the respect is unconditional in that it does not depend on the behavior of the client to meet certain standards. The nurse, in fact, may not approve of the client's lifestyle or pattern of behaving. However, with unconditional positive regard, the client is accepted and respected for no other reason than that he or she is considered to be a worthwhile and unique human being.

Many psychiatric clients have very little self-respect owing to the fact that, because of their behavior, they have been rejected by others in the past. Recognition that they are being accepted and respected as unique individuals on an unconditional basis can serve to elevate feelings of self-worth and self-respect. The nurse can convey an attitude of respect by:

- Calling the client by name (and title, if the client prefers).
- Spending time with the client.
- Allowing for sufficient time to answer the client's questions and concerns.
- Promoting an atmosphere of privacy during therapeutic interactions with the client or when the client may be undergoing physical examination or therapy.
- Always being open and honest with the client, even when the truth may be difficult to discuss.
- Taking the client's ideas, preferences, and opinions into considerations when planning care.
- Striving to understand the motivation behind the client's behavior, regardless of how unacceptable it may seem.

Genuineness

The concept of **genuineness** refers to the nurse's ability to be open, honest, and "real" in interactions with the client. To be "real" is to be aware of what one is experiencing internally and to allow the quality of this inner experiencing to be apparent in the therapeutic relationship (Meador & Rogers, 1979). When one is genuine, there is *congruence* between what is felt and what is being expressed. The nurse who possesses the quality of genuineness responds to the client with truth and honesty, rather than with responses he or she may consider more "professional" or ones that merely reflect the "nursing role."

Genuineness may call for a degree of *self-disclosure* on the part of the nurse. This is not to say that the nurse must disclose to the client *everything* he or she is feeling or *all* personal experiences that may relate to what the client is going through. Indeed, care must be taken when using self-disclosure to avoid transposing the roles of nurse and client.

When the nurse uses self-disclosure, a quality of "humanness" is revealed to the client, creating a role for the client to model in similar situations. The client may then feel more comfortable revealing personal information to the nurse.

Most individuals have an uncanny ability to detect other people's artificiality. When the nurse does not bring the quality of genuineness to the relationship, a reality base for trust cannot be established. These qualities are essential if the actualizing potential of the client is to be released and for change and growth to occur (Meador & Rogers, 1979).

Empathy

Empathy is a process wherein an individual is able to see beyond outward behavior and sense accurately another's inner experience at a given point in time (Travelbee, 1971). With empathy, the nurse can accurately perceive and understand the meaning and relevance of the client's thoughts and feelings. The nurse must also be able to communicate this perception to the client. This is done by attempting to translate words and behaviors into feelings.

It is not uncommon for the concept of empathy to be confused with that of **sympathy.** The major difference is that with *empathy* the nurse "accurately perceives or understands" what the client is feeling and encourages the client to explore these feelings. With *sympathy* the nurse actually "shares" what the client is feeling and experiences a need to alleviate distress.

Empathy is considered to be one of the most important characteristics of a therapeutic relationship. Accurate empathetic perceptions on the part of the nurse assist the client to identify feelings that may have been suppressed or denied. Positive emotions are generated as the client realizes that he or she is truly understood by another. As the feelings surface and are explored, the client learns aspects about self of which he or she may have been unaware. This contributes to the process of personal identification and the promotion of positive self-concept.

With empathy, while understanding the client's thoughts and feelings, the nurse is able to maintain sufficient objectivity to allow the client to achieve problem resolution with minimal assistance. With sympathy, the nurse actually feels what the client is feeling, objectivity is lost, and the nurse may become focused on relief of personal distress rather than on helping the client resolve the problem at hand. The following is an example of an empathetic and sympathetic response to the same situation.

> *Situation:* BJ is a client on the psychiatric unit with a diagnosis of dysthymic disorder. She is 5′5″ tall and weights 295 lb. BJ has been overweight all her life. She is single, has no close friends, and has never had an intimate relationship with another person. It is her first day on the unit, and she is refusing to come out of her room. When she appeared for lunch in the dining room following admission, she was embarrassed when several of the other clients laughed out loud and called her "fatso."
>
> *Sympathetic response:* Nurse: "I can certainly identify with what you are feeling. I've been overweight most of my life, too. I just get so angry when people act like that. They are so insensitive! It's just so typical of skinny people to act that way. You have a right to want to stay away from them. We'll just see how loud they laugh when *you* get to choose what movie is shown on the unit after dinner tonight."
>
> *Empathetic response:* Nurse: "You feel angry and embarrassed by what happened at lunch today." As tears fill BJ's eyes, the nurse encourages her to cry if she feels like it and to express her anger at the situation. She stays with BJ but does not dwell on her *own* feelings about what happened. Instead she focuses on BJ and what the client perceives are her most immediate needs at this time.

PHASES OF A THERAPEUTIC NURSE-CLIENT RELATIONSHIP

Psychiatric nurses use interpersonal relationship development as the primary intervention with clients in various psychiatric/mental health settings. This is congruent with Peplau's (1962) identification of *counseling* as the major subrole of nursing in psychiatry. If what Sullivan (1953) believed is true (i.e., that all emotional problems stem from difficulties with interpersonal relationships), then this role of the nurse in psychiatry becomes especially meaningful and purposeful. It becomes an integral part of the total therapeutic regimen.

The therapeutic interpersonal relationship is the means by which the nursing process is implemented. Through the relationship, problems are identified and resolution is sought. Tasks of the relationship have been categorized into four phases: the preinteraction phase, the orientation (introductory) phase, the working phase, and the termination phase. Although each phase is presented as specific and distinct from the others, there may be some overlapping of tasks, particularly when the interaction is limited.

The Preinteraction Phase

The preinteraction phase involves preparation for the first encounter with the client. Tasks include:

1. Obtaining available information about the client from his or her chart, significant others, or other health team members. From this information, the initial assessment is begun. This initial information may also allow the nurse to become aware of personal responses to knowledge about the client.
2. Examining one's feelings, fears, and anxieties about working with a particular client. For example, the nurse may have been reared in an alcoholic family and have ambivalent feelings about caring for a client who is alcohol dependent. All individuals bring attitudes and feelings from prior experiences to the clinical setting. The nurse needs to be aware of how these preconceptions may affect his or her ability to care for individual clients.

The Orientation (Introductory) Phase

During the orientation phase, the nurse and client become acquainted. Tasks include:

1. Creating an environment for the establishment of trust and rapport.
2. Establishing a contract for intervention that details the expectations and responsibilities of both nurse and client.
3. Gathering assessment information to build a strong client data base.
4. Identifying the client's strengths and limitations.
5. Formulating nursing diagnoses.

6. Setting goals that are mutually agreeable to the nurse and client.
7. Developing a plan of action that is realistic for meeting the established goals.
8. Exploring feelings of both the client and nurse in terms of the introductory phase. Introductions are often uncomfortable, and the participants may experience some anxiety until a degree of rapport has been established. Interactions may remain on a superficial level until anxiety subsides. Several interactions may be required to fulfill the tasks associated with this phase.

The Working Phase

The therapeutic work of the relationship is accomplished during this phase. Tasks include:

1. Maintaining the trust and rapport that was established during the orientation phase.
2. Promoting the client's insight and perception of reality.
3. Problem solving using the model presented earlier in this chapter.
4. Overcoming resistance behaviors on the part of the client as the level of anxiety rises in response to discussion of painful issues.
5. Continuously evaluating progress toward goal attainment.

The Termination Phase

Termination of the relationship may occur for a variety of reasons: the mutually agreed-on goals may have been reached, the client may be discharged from the hospital, or in the case of a student nurse, it may be the end of a clinical rotation. Termination can be a difficult phase for both the client and nurse. Tasks include:

1. Bringing a therapeutic conclusion to the relationship. This occurs when:
   a. Progress has been made toward attainment of mutually set goals.
   b. A plan for continuing care or for assistance during stressful life experiences is mutually established by the nurse and client.
   c. Feelings about termination of the relationship are recognized and explored. Both the nurse and client may experience feelings of sadness and loss. The nurse should share his or her feelings with the client. Through these interactions, the client learns that it is acceptable to undergo these feelings at a time of separation. Through this knowledge, the client experiences growth during the process of termination.

TABLE 5.2 PHASES OF RELATIONSHIP DEVELOPMENT AND MAJOR NURSING GOALS

PHASE	GOALS
1. Preinteraction	Explore self-perceptions
2. Orientation (introductory)	Establish trust
	Formulate contract for intervention
3. Working	Promote client change
4. Termination	Evaluate goal attainment
	Ensure therapeutic closure

NOTE: When the client feels sadness and loss, behaviors to delay termination may become evident. If the nurse experiences the same feelings, he or she may allow the client's behaviors to delay termination. For therapeutic closure, the nurse must establish the reality of the separation and resist being manipulated into repeated delays by the client.

The major nursing goals during each phase of the nurse-client relationship are listed in Table 5.2.

SUMMARY

Nurses who work in the psychiatric/mental health field use special skills, or "interpersonal techniques," to assist clients in adapting to difficulties or changes in life experiences. A therapeutic or "helping" relationship is established through use of these interpersonal techniques and is based on a knowledge of theories of personality development and human behavior.

Therapeutic nurse-client relationships are goal oriented. Ideally, the goal is mutually agreed on by the nurse and client, and is directed at learning and growth promotion. The problem-solving model is used in an attempt to bring about some type of change in the client's life. The instrument for delivery of the process of interpersonal nursing is the therapeutic use of self, which requires that the nurse possess a strong sense of self-awareness and self-understanding.

A number of characteristics that enhance the achievement of a therapeutic relationship have been identified. They include rapport, trust, respect, genuineness, and empathy.

The tasks associated with the development of a therapeutic interpersonal relationship have been categorized into four phases: the preinteraction phase, the orientation (introductory) phase, the working phase, and the termination phase.

The concepts and tasks presented herein can facilitate the promotion of a helping relationship and effective nursing care for clients requiring psychosocial intervention.

REVIEW QUESTIONS

SELF-EXAMINATION/LEARNING EXERCISE

Test your knowledge of therapeutic nurse-client relationships by answering the following questions:

1. Name the six subroles of nursing identified by Peplau.

2. Which subrole is emphasized in psychiatric nursing?

3. Why is relationship development so important in the provision of emotional care?

4. In general, what is the goal of a therapeutic relationship? What method is recommended for intervention?

5. What is the instrument for delivery of the process of interpersonal nursing?

6. Several characteristics that enhance the achievement of a therapeutic relationship have been identified. Match the therapeutic concept with the corresponding definition.

   _____ 1. Rapport

   _____ 2. Trust

   _____ 3. Respect

   _____ 4. Genuineness

   _____ 5. Empathy

   a. The feeling of confidence in another person's presence, reliability, integrity, and desire to provide assistance.
   b. Congruence between what is felt and what is being expressed.
   c. The ability to accurately sense what another person is feeling at a given point in time.
   d. Special feelings between two people based on acceptance, warmth, friendliness, and a shared common interest.
   e. Unconditional acceptance of an individual as a worthwhile and unique human being.

7. Match the actions listed on the right to the appropriate phase of nurse-client relationship development on the left.

   _____ 1. Preinteraction phase

   _____ 2. Orientation (introductory) phase

   _____ 3. Working phase

   _____ 4. Termination phase

   a. Kim tells Nurse Jones she wants to learn more adaptive ways to handle her anger. Together, they set some goals.
   b. The goals of therapy have been met, but Kim cries and says she has to keep coming to therapy in order to be able to handle her anger appropriately.
   c. Nurse Jones reads Kim's previous medical records. She explores her feelings about working with a woman who has abused her child.
   d. Nurse Jones helps Kim practice various techniques to control her angry outbursts. She gives Kim positive feedback for attempting to improve maladaptive behaviors.

REFERENCES

Carkhuff, R. (1968). *Helping and human relations* (Vols. 1 & 2). New York: Holt, Rinehart & Winston.

Luft, J. (1970). *Group processes: An introduction to group dynamics.* Palo Alto, CA: National Press Books.

Meador, B.D., & Rogers, C. R. (1979) Person-centered therapy. In R. J. Corsini (Ed.), *Current psychotherapies* (2nd ed.). Itasca, IL: F.E. Peacock Publishers.

Peplau, H.E. (1957). Therapeutic concepts. In *National league for nursing, aspects of psychiatric nursing.* New York: National League for Nursing.

Peplau, H.E. (1962). Interpersonal techniques: The crux of psychiatric nursing. *American Journal of Nursing*, 62(6):50–54.

Peplau, H.E. (1969). *Basic principles of patient counseling* (2nd ed.). Philadelphia: Smith, Kline, & French Laboratories.

Peplalu, H.E. (1991). *Interpersonal relations in nursing*. New York: Springer.

Raths, L., Merril, H., & Simon, S. (1966). *Values and teaching*. Columbus, OH: Merrill.

Rogers, C.R. (1951). *Client Centered Therapy*. Boston: Houghton Mifflin.

Rogers, C.R., Gendlin, E.T., Kiesler, D.J., & Louax, C. (1967). *The therapeutic relationship and its impact*. Madison, WI: University of Wisconsin Press.

Sullivan, H.S. (1953). *The interpersonal theory of psychiatry*. New York: W.W. Norton.

Sundeen, S.J., Stuart, G.W., Rankin, E.D., & Cohen, S.A. (1985). *Nurse-client interaction—Implementing the nursing process*. St. Louis, MO: C.V. Mosby.

Travelbee, J. (1971). *Interpersonal aspects of nursing* (2nd ed.). Philadelphia: F.A. Davis.

Ujhely, G. (1968). *Determinants of the nurse-patient relationship*. New York: Springer.

Bibliography

Cormier, L.S., Cormier, W.H., & Weisser, R.J., Jr. (1984). *Interviewing and helping skills for health professionals*. Monterey, CA: Wadsworth Health Sciences Division.

Duldt, B.W., Griffin, K., & Patton, B.R. (1984). *Interpersonal communication in nursing*. Philadelphia: F.A. Davis.

Maloney, E. (1962, June). Does the psychiatric nurse have independent functions? *American Journal of Nursing*, 62(6):61–63.

Northouse, P.G., & Northouse, L.L. (1985). *Health communication, A handbook for health professionals*. Englewood Cliffs, NJ: Prentice-Hall.

Rogers, C.R. (1961). *On becoming a person*. Boston: Houghton Mifflin.

Rogers, C.R. (1957). The necessary and sufficient conditions of therapeutic personality change. *Journal of Consulting Psychology*, 21:95–103.

THERAPEUTIC COMMUNICATION

CHAPTER OUTLINE

OBJECTIVES

INTRODUCTION

WHAT IS COMMUNICATION?

THE IMPACT OF PREEXISTING CONDITIONS

NONVERBAL COMMUNICATION

THERAPEUTIC COMMUNICATION TECHNIQUES

NONTHERAPEUTIC COMMUNICATION TECHNIQUES

ACTIVE LISTENING

PROCESS RECORDINGS

FEEDBACK

SUMMARY

REVIEW QUESTIONS

KEY TERMS

territoriality
density
distance

intimate distance
personal
   distance

social distance
public distance
paralanguage

OBJECTIVES

After reading this chapter, the student will be able to:

1. Discuss the transactional model of communication.
2. Identify types of preexisting conditions that influence the outcome of the communication process.
3. Define *territoriality*, *density*, and *distance* as components of the environment.
4. Identify components of nonverbal expression.
5. Describe therapeutic and nontherapeutic verbal communication techniques.
6. Describe active listening.
7. Discuss therapeutic feedback.

evelopment of the *therapeutic interpersonal relationship* was described in Chapter 5 as the process by which nurses provide care for clients in need of psychosocial intervention. *Therapeutic use of self* was identified as the instrument for delivery of care. The focus of this chapter is on techniques, or more specifically, *interpersonal communication techniques*, to facilitate the delivery of that care.

Hays and Larson (1963) have stated, "To relate therapeutically with a patient it is necessary for the nurse to understand his or her role and its relationship to the patient's illness." They describe the role of the nurse as providing the client with the opportunity to:

1. Identify and explore problems in relating to others.
2. Discover healthy ways of meeting emotional needs.
3. Experience a satisfying interpersonal relationship.

This is accomplished through use of interpersonal communication techniques (both verbal and nonverbal). The nurse must be aware of the therapeutic or nontherapeutic value of the communication techniques used with the client, as they are the "tools" of psychosocial intervention.

WHAT IS COMMUNICATION?

It has been said, "You cannot not communicate." Every word that is spoken and every movement that is made gives a message to someone. Interpersonal communication is a *transaction* between the sender and the receiver. In the transactional model of communication, both persons are participating simultaneously. They are mutually perceiving each other, simultaneously listening to each other, and simultaneously and mutually engaged in the process of creating meaning in a relationship (Smith & Williamson, 1981). The transactional model is illustrated in Figure 6.1.

THE IMPACT OF PREEXISTING CONDITIONS

In all interpersonal transactions, both the sender and receiver bring certain preexisting conditions to the exchange that influence both the intended message and the way in which it is interpreted. Examples of these conditions include one's value system, internalized attitudes and beliefs, culture or religion, social status, gender, background knowledge and experience, and age or developmental level. The type of environment in which the communication takes place may also influence the outcome of the transaction. Figure 6.2 shows how these influencing factors are positioned on the transactional model.

Values, Attitudes, and Beliefs

Values, attitudes, and beliefs are learned ways of thinking. Children generally adopt the value systems and internalize the attitudes and beliefs of their parents. Children may retain this way of thinking into adulthood or develop a different set of attitudes and values as they mature.

Values, attitudes, and beliefs can influence communication in numerous ways. For example, prejudice is expressed verbally through negative stereotyping.

One's value system may be communicated with behaviors that are more symbolic in nature. For example, an individual who values youth may dress and behave in a manner that is characteristic of one who is much younger. A person who values freedom and the American way of life may fly the U.S. flag in front of his or her home each day. In each of these situations, a message is being communicated.

Culture or Religion

Communication has its roots in culture. Cultural mores, norms, ideas, and customs provide the basis for our way of thinking. Cultural values are learned and differ from society to society. For example, in some European countries (e.g., Italy, Spain, and France), men may greet each other with hugs and kisses. These behaviors are appropriate in those cultures but would communicate a different message in America or Great Britain.

Religion can influence communication as well. Priests and ministers who wear clerical collars publicly communicate their mission in life. The collar may also influence the way in which others relate to them, either positively or negatively. Other symbolic gestures, such as wearing a cross around the neck or hanging a crucifix on the wall, also communicate an individual's religious beliefs.

Social Status

Mehrabian (1972) conducted studies of nonverbal indicators of social status or power. He reports that high-status

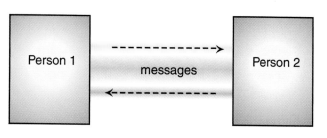

Figure 6.1 The transactional model of communication.

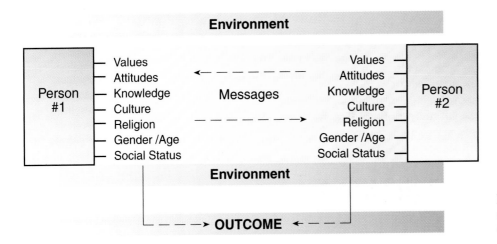

Figure 6.2 Factors influencing the transactional model of communication.

persons are associated with gestures that communicate their higher-power position. For example, they use less eye contact, a more relaxed posture, louder voice pitch, more frequent use of hands on hips, "power dressing," greater height, and more distance when communicating with individuals considered to be of lower social status.

Gender

Gender influences the manner in which individuals communicate. Each culture has *gender signals* that are recognized as either masculine or feminine and provide a basis for distinguishing between members of each sex (Smith & Williamson, 1981). Examples include differences in posture, both standing and sitting, between American men and women. Men stand with thighs 10 to 15 degrees apart, the pelvis rolled back, and the arms slightly away from the body. Women are seen with legs close together, the pelvis tipped forward, and the arms close to the body. When sitting, men may lean back in the chair with legs apart or may rest the ankle of one leg over the knee of the other. Women tend to sit more upright in the chair with legs together, perhaps crossed at the ankles, or one leg crossed over the other at thigh level.

Roles have traditionally been identified as either male or female. For example, in America masculinity has been traditionally communicated through such roles as husband, father, breadwinner, doctor, lawyer, or engineer. Traditional female roles have included wife, mother, homemaker, nurse, teacher, or secretary.

Gender signals are changing in American society as sexual roles become less distinct. Behaviors that have been considered typically masculine or feminine in the past may now be generally acceptable in both sexes. Words such as "unisex" communicate a desire by some individuals to diminish the distinction between the sexes and minimize the discrimination of either. Gender roles are changing as both women and men enter professions that were once dominated by members of the opposite sex.

Age or Developmental Level

Age influences communication and it is never more evident than during adolescence. In their struggle to separate from parental confines and establish their own identity, adolescents generate a pattern of communication that is unique and changes from generation to generation. Words such as "awesome," "groovy," and "cool" have had special meaning for certain generations of adolescents.

Developmental influences on communication may relate to physiological alterations. One example is American Sign Language, the system of unique gestures used by many people who are deaf or hearing impaired. Individuals who are blind at birth never learn the subtle nonverbal gesticulations that accompany language and can totally change the meaning of the spoken word.

Environment in Which the Transaction Takes Place

The place where the communication occurs influences the outcome of the interaction. Some individuals who feel uncomfortable and refuse to speak during a group therapy session may be open and willing to discuss problems privately on a one-to-one basis with the nurse.

Territoriality, density, and **distance** are aspects of environment that communicate messages. *Territoriality* is the innate tendency to own space. Individuals lay claim to areas around them as their own. This influences communication when an interaction takes place in the territory "owned" by one or the other. Interpersonal communication can be more successful if the interaction takes place in a "neutral" area. For example, with the concept of territoriality in mind, the nurse may choose to conduct the psychosocial assessment in an interview room rather than in his or her office or in the client's room.

Density refers to the number of people within a given environmental space and has been shown to influence interpersonal interaction. Some studies indicate that a correlation exists between prolonged high-density situations and certain behaviors, such as aggression, stress, criminal activity, hostility toward others, and a deterioration of mental and physical health (Knapp, 1980).

Distance is the means by which various cultures use space to communicate. Hall (1966) identified four kinds of spatial interaction, or distances, that people maintain from each other in their interpersonal interactions and the kinds of activities in which people engage at these various distances. **Intimate distance** is the closest distance that individuals will allow between themselves and others. In America, this distance, which is restricted to interactions of an intimate nature, is 0 to 18 inches. **Personal distance** is approximately 18 to 40 inches and reserved for interactions that are personal in nature, such as close conversations with friends or colleagues. Our **social distance** is about 4 to 12 feet away from the body. Interactions at this distance include conversations with strangers or acquaintances, such as at a cocktail party or in a public building. **Public distances** are those that exceed 12 feet. Examples include speaking in public or yelling to someone some distance away. This distance is considered public space, and communicants are free to move about in it during the interaction.

NONVERBAL COMMUNICATION

Some aspects of nonverbal expression have been discussed in the previous section on preexisting conditions that influence communication. Other components of nonverbal communication include physical appearance and dress, body movement and posture, touch, facial expressions, eye behavior, and vocal cues or paralanguage. These nonverbal messages vary from culture to culture.

Physical Appearance and Dress

Physical appearance and dress are part of the total nonverbal stimuli that influence interpersonal responses and, under some conditions, they are the primary determiners of such responses (Knapp, 1980). Body coverings—both dress and hair—are manipulated by the wearer in a manner that conveys a distinct message to the receiver. Dress can be formal or casual, stylish or sloppy. Hair can be long or short, and even the presence or absence of hair conveys a message about the person. Other body adornments that are also considered potential communicative stimuli include tattoos, masks, cosmetics, badges, jewelry, and eyeglasses. Some jewelry worn in specific ways can give special messages (e.g., a gold band or diamond ring worn on the fourth finger of the left hand, a boy's class ring worn on a chain around a girl's neck, or a pin bearing Greek letters worn on the lapel). Some individuals convey a specific message with the total absence of any type of body adornment.

Body Movement and Posture

The way in which an individual positions his or her body communicates messages regarding self-esteem, gender identity, status, and interpersonal warmth or coldness. The individual whose posture is slumped, with head and eyes pointed downward, conveys a message of low self-esteem. Specific ways of standing or sitting are considered to be either feminine or masculine within a defined culture. To stand straight and tall with head high and hands on hips indicates a superior status over the person being addressed. Reece and Whitman (1962) identified response behaviors that were used to designate individuals as either "warm" or "cold" persons. Individuals who were perceived as warm responded to others with a shift of posture toward the other person, a smile, direct eye contact, and hands that remained still. Individuals who responded to others with a slumped posture, by looking around the room, drumming fingers on the desk, and not smiling were perceived as cold.

Touch

Touch is a powerful communication tool. It can elicit both negative and positive reactions, depending on the people involved and the circumstances of the interaction. It is a very basic and primitive form of communication, and the appropriateness of its use is culturally determined.

Touch can be categorized according to the message communicated (Knapp, 1980):

1. **Functional-Professional.** This type of touch is impersonal and businesslike. It is used to accomplish a task.

   EXAMPLE

   A tailor measuring a customer for a suit or a physician examining a client.

2. **Social-Polite.** This type of touch is still rather impersonal, but it conveys an affirmation or acceptance of the other person.

   EXAMPLE

   A handshake.

3. **Friendship-Warmth.** Touch at this level indicates a strong liking for the other person, a feeling that he or she is a friend.

   EXAMPLE

   Laying one's hand on the shoulder of another.

4. **Love-Intimacy.** This type of touch conveys an emotional attachment or attraction for another person.

EXAMPLE

Engaging in a strong, mutual embrace.

5. **Sexual Arousal.** Touch at this level is an expression of physical attraction only.

EXAMPLE

Touching another in the genital region.

Some cultures encourage more touching of various types than others. The nurse should understand the cultural meaning of touch before using this method of communication in specific situations.

Facial Expressions

Next to human speech, facial expression is the primary source of communication. Facial expressions primarily reveal an individual's emotional states, such as happiness, sadness, anger, surprise, and fear. The face is a complex multimessage system. Facial expressions serve to complement and qualify other communication behaviors, and at times even take the place of verbal messages.

Eye Behavior

Smith and Williamson (1981) identified behaviors by which individuals communicate with their eyes: eye contact and gazing or staring. Eyes have been called the "windows of the soul." It is through eye contact that individuals view and are viewed by others in a revealing way. An interpersonal connectedness occurs through eye contact. In American culture, eye contact conveys a personal interest in the other person. Eye contact indicates that the communication channel is open, and it is often the initiating factor in verbal interaction between two people.

Patterns of gazing or staring are regulated by social rules. These rules dictate where we can look, when we can look, for how long we can look, and at whom we can look (Smith & Williamson, 1981). Staring is often used to register disapproval of the behavior of another. People are extremely sensitive to being looked at, and if the gazing or staring behavior violates social rules, they often assign meaning to it, such as the following statement implies: "He kept staring at me, and I began to wonder if I was dressed inappropriately or had mustard on my face!"

Vocal Cues, or Paralanguage

Paralanguage is the gestural component of the spoken word. It consists of pitch, tone, and loudness of spoken messages, the rate of speaking, expressively placed pauses, and emphasis assigned to certain words. These vocal cues greatly influence the way individuals interpret verbal messages. A normally soft-spoken individual whose pitch and rate of speaking increases may be perceived as being anxious or tense.

Different vocal emphases can alter interpretation of the message.

Three examples follow:

1. "I felt SURE you would notice the change." *Interpretation:* I was SURE you would, but you didn't.
2. "I felt sure YOU would notice the change." *Interpretation:* I thought YOU would, even if nobody else did.
3. "I felt sure you would notice the CHANGE." *Interpretation:* Even if you didn't notice anything else, I thought you would notice the CHANGE.

Verbal cues play a major role in determining responses in human communication situations. *How* a message is verbalized can be as important as *what* is verbalized.

THERAPEUTIC COMMUNICATION TECHNIQUES

Hays and Larson (1963) identified a number of techniques to assist the nurse in interacting more therapeutically with clients. These are the "technical procedures" carried out by the nurse working in psychiatry, and they should serve to enhance development of a therapeutic nurse-client relationship. Table 6.1 includes a list of these techniques, a short explanation of their usefulness, and examples of each.

NONTHERAPEUTIC COMMUNICATION TECHNIQUES

Several approaches are considered to be barriers to open communication between the nurse and client. Hays and Larson (1963) identified a number of these techniques, which are presented in Table 6.2. The nurse should recognize and eliminate the use of these patterns in his or her relationships with clients. Avoiding these communication barriers will maximize the effectiveness of communication and enhance the nurse-client relationship.

ACTIVE LISTENING

To listen actively is to be attentive to what the client is saying, both verbally and nonverbally. Attentive listening creates a climate in which the client can communicate (Bernstein & Bernstein, 1980). With active listening the nurse communicates acceptance and respect for the client, and trust is enhanced. A climate is established within the relationship that promotes openness and honest expression.

▬ TABLE 6.1 THERAPEUTIC COMMUNICATION TECHNIQUES

TECHNIQUE	EXPLANATION/RATIONALE	EXAMPLES
Using silence	Gives the client the opportunity to collect and organize thoughts, to think through a point, or to consider introducing a topic of greater concern than the one being discussed.	
Accepting	Conveys an attitude of reception and regard	"Yes, I understand what you said." Eye contact; nodding.
Giving recognition	Acknowledging; indicating awareness; better than complimenting, which reflects the nurse's judgment.	"Hello, Mr. J. I noticed that you made a ceramic ash tray in OT." "I see you made your bed."
Offering self	Making oneself available on an unconditional basis, increasing client's feelings of self-worth.	"I'll stay with you awhile." "We can eat our lunch together." "I'm interested in you."
Giving broad openings	Allows the client to take the initiative in introducing the topic; emphasizes the importance of the client's role in the interaction.	"What would you like to talk about today?" "Tell me what you are thinking."
Offering general leads	Offers the client encouragement to continue.	"Yes, I see." "Go on." "And after that?"
Placing the event in time or sequence	Clarifies the relationship of events in time so that the nurse and client can view them in perspective.	"What seemed to lead up to . . .?" "Was this before or after . . .?" "When did this happen.?"
Making observations	Verbalizing what is observed or perceived. This encourages the client to recognize specific behaviors and compare perceptions with the nurse.	"You seem tense." "I notice you are pacing a lot." "You seem uncomfortable when you . . ."
Encouraging description of perceptions	Asking the client to verbalize what is being perceived; often used with clients experiencing hallucinations.	"Tell me what is happening now." "Are you hearing the voices again?" "What do the voices seem to be saying?"
Encouraging comparison	Asking the client to compare similarities and differences in ideas, experiences, or interpersonal relationships. This helps the client recognize life experiences that tend to recur as well as those aspects of life that are changeable.	"Was this something like . . .?" "How does this compare with the time when . . .?" "What was your response the last time this situation occurred?"
Restating	The main idea of what the client has said is repeated; lets the client know whether or not an expressed statement has been understood and gives him or her the chance to continue, or to clarify if necessary.	Cl: "I can't study. My mind keeps wandering." Ns: "You have difficulty concentrating." Cl: "I can't take that new job. What if I can't do it?" Ns: "You're afraid you will fail in this new position."
Reflecting	Questions and feelings are referred back to the client so that they may be recognized and accepted, and so that the client may recognize that his or her point of view has value—a good technique to use when the client asks the nurse for advice.	Cl: "What do you think I should do about my wife's drinking problem?" Ns: "What do *you* think you should do?" Cl: "My sister won't help a bit toward my mother's care. I have to do it all!" Ns: "You feel angry when she doesn't help."
Focusing	Taking notice of a single idea or even a single word; works especially well with a client who is moving rapidly from one thought to another. This technique is *not* therapeutic, however, with the client who is very anxious. Focusing should not be pursued until the anxiety level has subsided.	"This point seems worth looking at more closely. Perhaps you and I can discuss it together."
Exploring	Delving further into a subject, idea, experience, or relationship; especially helpful with clients who tend to remain on a superficial level of communication. However, if the client chooses not to disclose further information, the nurse should refrain from pushing or probing in an area that obviously creates discomfort.	"Please explain that situation in more detail." "Tell me more about that particular situation."
Seeking clarification and validation	Striving to explain that which is vague or incomprehensible and searching for mutual	"I'm not sure that I understand. Would you please explain?"

TABLE 6.1   THERAPEUTIC COMMUNICATION TECHNIQUES

TECHNIQUE	EXPLANATION/RATIONALE	EXAMPLES
	understanding; clarifying the meaning of what has been said facilitates and increases understanding for both client and nurse.	"Tell me if my understanding agrees with yours." "Do I understand correctly that you said . . .?"
Presenting reality	When the client has a misperception of the environment, the nurse defines reality or indicates his or her perception of the situation for the client.	"I understand that the voices seem real to you, but I do not hear any voices." "There is no one else in the room but you and me."
Voicing doubt	Expressing uncertainty as to the reality of the client's perceptions; often used with clients experiencing delusional thinking.	"I find that hard to believe." "That seems rather doubtful to me."
Verbalizing the implied	Putting into words what the client has only implied or said indirectly; can also be used with the client who is mute or is otherwise experiencing impaired verbal communication. This clarifies that which is *implicit* rather than *explicit*.	Cl: "It's a waste of time to be here. I can't talk to you or anyone." Ns: "Are you feeling that no one understands?" Cl: (Mute) Ns: "It must have been very difficult for you when your husband died in the fire."
Attempting to translate words into feelings	When feelings are expressed indirectly, the nurse tries to "desymbolize" what has been said and to find clues to the underlying true feelings.	Cl: "I'm way out in the ocean." Ns: "You must be feeling very lonely now."
Formulating a plan of action	When a client has a plan in mind for dealing with what is considered to be a stressful situation, it may serve to prevent anger or anxiety from escalating to an unmanageable level.	"What could you do to let your anger out harmlessly?" "Next time this comes up, what might you do to handle it more appropriately?

SOURCE: Adapted from Hays & Larson (1963).

Several nonverbal behaviors have been designated as facilitative skills for attentive listening. Those listed here can be identified by the acronym SOLER.

S—Sit squarely facing the client. This gives the message that the nurse is there to listen and is interested in what the client has to say.

O—Observe an open posture. Posture is considered "open" when arms and legs remain uncrossed. This suggests that the nurse is "open" to what the client has to say. With a "closed" position, the nurse can convey a somewhat defensive stance, possibly invoking a similar response in the client.

L—Lean forward toward the client. This conveys to the client that you are involved in the interaction, interested in what is being said, and making a sincere effort to be attentive.

E—Establish eye contact. Direct eye contact is another behavior that conveys the nurse's involvement and willingness to listen to what the client has to say. The absence of eye contact, or the constant shifting of eye contact, gives the message that the nurse is not really interested in what is being said.

NOTE: Ensure that eye contact conveys warmth and is accompanied by smiling and intermittent nodding of the head, and that it does not come across as staring or glaring, which can create intense discomfort in the client.

R—Relax. Whether sitting or standing during the interaction, the nurse should communicate a sense of being relaxed and comfortable with the client. Restlessness and fidgetiness communicate a lack of interest and a feeling of discomfort that are likely to be transferred to the client.

PROCESS RECORDINGS

Process recordings are written reports of verbal interactions with clients. They are verbatim (to the extent that this is possible) accounts, written by the nurse or student as a tool for improving interpersonal communication techniques. Although the process recording can take many forms, it usually includes the verbal and nonverbal communication of both nurse and client. It provides a means for the nurse to analyze both the content and the pattern of the interaction. The process recording, which is not documentation in and of itself, should be used as a learning tool for professional development. An example of one type of process recording is presented in Table 6.3.

FEEDBACK

Feedback is a method of communication for helping the client consider a modification of behavior. Feedback gives information to clients about how they are being perceived by others. It should be presented in a manner that discourages defensiveness on the part of the client. Feedback can be useful to the client if presented with objectivity by a trusted individual.

TABLE 6.2 NONTHERAPEUTIC COMMUNICATION TECHNIQUES

TECHNIQUE	EXPLANATION/RATIONALE	EXAMPLES
Giving reassurance	Indicates to the client that there is no cause for anxiety, thereby devaluing the client's feelings; may discourage the client from further expression of feelings if he or she believes they will only be downplayed or ridiculed.	"I wouldn't worry about that if I were you." "Everything will be all right." **Better to say:** "We will work on that together."
Rejecting	Refusing to consider or showing contempt for the client's ideas or behavior. This may cause the client to discontinue interaction with the nurse for fear of further rejection.	"Let's not discuss . . ." "I don't want to hear about . . ." **Better to say:** "Let's look at that a little closer."
Giving approval or disapproval	Sanctioning or denouncing the client's ideas or behavior; implies that the nurse has the right to pass judgment on whether the client's ideas or behaviors are "good" or "bad" and that the client is expected to please the nurse. The nurse's acceptance of the client is then seen as conditional, depending on the client's behavior.	"That's good. I'm glad that you . . ." "That's bad. I'd rather you wouldn't . . ." **Better to say:** "Let's talk about how your behavior invoked anger in the other clients at dinner."
Agreeing/disagreeing	Indicating accord with or opposition to the client's ideas or opinions; implies that the nurse has the right to pass judgment on whether the client's ideas or opinions are "right" or "wrong." Agreement prevents the client from later modifying his or her point of view without admitting error. Disagreement implies inaccuracy, provoking the need for defensiveness on the part of the client.	"That's right. I agree." "That's wrong. I disagree." "I don't believe that." **Better to say:** "Let's discuss what you feel is unfair about the new community rules."
Giving advice	Telling the client what to do or how to behave implies that the nurse knows what is best and that the client is incapable of any self-direction. It nurtures the client in the dependent role by discouraging independent thinking.	"I think you should . . ." "Why don't you . . ." **Better to say:** "What do you think you should do?"
Probing	Persistent questioning of the client; pushing for answers to issues the client does not wish to discuss. This causes the client to feel used and valued only for what is shared with the nurse and places the client on the defensive.	"Tell me how your mother abused you when you were a child." "Tell me how you feel toward your mother now that she is dead." "Now tell me about . . ." **Better technique:** The nurse should be aware of the client's response and discontinue the interaction at the first sign of discomfort.
Defending	Attempting to protect someone or something from verbal attack. To defend what the client has criticized is to imply that he or she has no right to express ideas, opinions, or feelings. Defending does not change the client's feelings and may cause the client to think the nurse is taking sides with those being criticized and against the client.	"No one here would lie to you." "You have a very capable physician. I'm sure he only has your best interests in mind." **Better to say:** "I will try to answer your questions and clarify some issues regarding your treatment."
Requesting an explanation	Asking the client to provide the reasons for thoughts, feelings, behavior, and events. Asking "why" a client did something or feels a certain way can be very intimidating and implies that the client must defend his or her behavior or feelings.	"Why do you think that?" "Why do you feel this way?" "Why did you do that?" **Better to say:** "Describe what you were feeling just before that happened."
Indicating the existence of an external source of power	Attributing the source of thoughts, feelings, and behavior to others or to outside influences. This encourages the client to project blame for his or her thoughts or behaviors upon others rather than accepting the responsibility personally.	"What makes you say that?" "What made you do that?" "What made you so angry last night?" **Better to say:** "You became angry when your brother insulted your wife."

TABLE 6.2 NONTHERAPEUTIC COMMUNICATION TECHNIQUES

TECHNIQUE	EXPLANATION/RATIONALE	EXAMPLES
Belittling feelings expressed	When the nurse misjudges the degree of the client's discomfort, a lack of empathy and understanding may be conveyed. The nurse may tell the client to "perk up" or "snap out of it." This causes the client to feel insignificant or unimportant. When one is experiencing discomfort, it is no relief to hear that others are or have been in similar situations.	Cl: "I have nothing to live for. I wish I were dead." Ns: "Everybody gets down in the dumps at times. I feel that way myself sometimes." **Better to say:** "You must be very upset. Tell me what you are feeling right now."
Making stereotyped comments	Cliches and trite expressions are meaningless in a nurse-client relationship. For the nurse to make empty conversation is to encourage a like response from the client.	"I'm fine, and how are you?" "Hang in there. It's for your own good." "Keep your chin up." **Better to say:** "The therapy must be difficult for you at times. How do you feel about your progress at this point?"
Using denial	When the nurse denies that a problem exists, he or she blocks discussion with the client and avoids helping the client identify and explore areas of difficulty.	Cl: "I'm nothing." Ns: "Of course you're something. Everybody is somebody." **Better to say:** "You're feeling like no one cares about you right now"
Interpreting	With this technique the therapist seeks to make conscious that which is unconscious, to tell the client the meaning of his experience.	"What you really mean is . . ." "Unconsciously you're saying . . ." **Better technique:** The nurse must leave interpretation of the client's behavior to the psychiatrist. The nurse has not been prepared to perform this technique, and in attempting to do so, may endanger other nursing roles with the client.
Introducing an unrelated topic	Changing the subject causes the nurse to take over the direction of the discussion. This may occur in order to get to something that the nurse wants to discuss with the client or to get away from a topic that he or she would prefer not to discuss.	Cl: "I don't have anything to live for." Ns: "Did you have visitors this weekend?" **Better technique:** The nurse must remain open and free to hear the client, to take in all that is being conveyed, both verbally and nonverbally.

SOURCE: Adapted from Hays & Larson (1963), with permission.

Some criteria about useful feedback include

1. Feedback is descriptive rather than evaluative and focuses on the behavior rather than on the client. Avoiding evaluative language reduces the need for the client to react defensively. An objective description allows the client to take the information and use it in whatever way he or she chooses. When the focus is on the client, the nurse makes judgments about the client.

EXAMPLES

Descriptive and focused on behavior	"Jane was very upset in group today when you called her 'fatty' and laughed at her in front of the others."
Evaluative	"You were very rude and inconsiderate to Jane in group today."
Focus on client	"You are a very insensitive person."

2. Feedback should be specific rather than general. Information that gives details about the client's behavior can be used more easily than a generalized description for modifying the behavior.

EXAMPLES

General	"You just don't pay attention."
Specific	"You were talking to Joe when we were deciding on the issue. Now you want to argue about the outcome."

TABLE 6.3   SAMPLE PROCESS RECORDING

NURSE VERBAL (NONVERBAL)	CLIENT VERBAL (NONVERBAL)	NURSE'S THOUGHTS AND FEELINGS CONCERNING THE INTERACTION	ANALYSIS OF THE INTERACTION
Do you still have thoughts about harming yourself? (Sitting facing the client; looking directly at client)	Not really. I still feel sad, but I don't want to die. (Looking at hands in lap.)	Felt a little uncomfortable. Always a hard question to ask.	**Therapeutic.** Asking a direct question about suicidal intent.
Tell me what you were feeling before you took all the pills the other night. (Still using SOLER techniques of active listening.)	I was just so angry! To think that my husband wants a divorce now that he has a good job. I worked hard to put him through college. (Fists clenched. Face and neck reddened.)	Beginning to feel more comfortable. Client seems willing to talk and I think she trusts me.	**Therapeutic.** Exploring. Delving further into the experience.
You wanted to hurt him because you felt betrayed. (SOLER)	Yes! If I died, maybe he'd realize that he loved me more than that other woman. (Tears starting to well up in her eyes.)	Starting to feel sorry for her.	**Therapeutic.** Attempting to translate words into feelings.
Seems like a pretty drastic way to get your point across. (Small frown.)	I know. It was a stupid thing to do. (Wiping eyes.)	Trying hard to remain objective.	**Nontherapeutic.** Sounds disapproving. Better to have pursued her feelings.
How are you feeling about the situation now? (SOLER)	I don't know. I still love him. I want him to come home. I don't want him to marry her. (Starting to cry again.)	Wishing there was an easy way to help relieve some of her pain.	**Therapeutic.** Focusing on her feelings.
Yes, I can understand that you would like things to be the way they were before. (Offer client a tissue.)	(Silence. Continues to cry softly.)	I'm starting to feel some anger toward her husband. Sometimes it's so hard to remain objective!	**Therapeutic.** Conveying empathy.
What do you think are the chances of your getting back together? (SOLER)	None. He's refused marriage counseling. He's already moved in with her. He says it's over. (Wipes tears. Looks directly at nurse.)	Relieved to know that she isn't using denial about the reality of the situation.	**Therapeutic.** Reflecting. Seeking client's perception of the situation.
So how are you preparing to deal with this inevitable outcome? (SOLER)	I'm going to do the things we talked about: join a divorced women's support group; increase my job hours to full-time; do some volunteer work; and call you or the suicide hot line if I feel like taking pills again. (Looks directly at nurse. Smiles.)	Positive feeling to know that she remembers what we discussed earlier and plans to follow through.	**Therapeutic.** Formulating a plan of action.
It won't be easy. But you have come a long way, and I feel you have gained strength in your ability to cope. (Standing. Looking at client. Smiling.)	Yes, I know I will have hard times. But I also know I have support, and I want to go on with my life and be happy again. (Standing, smiling at nurse.)	Feeling confident that the session has gone well; hopeful that the client will succeed in what she wants to do with her life.	**Therapeutic.** Presenting reality.

3. Feedback should be directed toward behavior that the client has the capacity to modify. To provide feedback about a characteristic or situation that the client cannot change will only provoke frustration.

EXAMPLES

| Can modify | "I noticed that you did not want to hold your baby when the nurse brought her to you." |
| Cannot modify | "Your baby daughter is mentally retarded because you took drugs when you were pregnant." |

4. Feedback should impart information rather than offering advice. Giving advice fosters dependence and may convey the message to the client that he or she is not capable of making decisions and solving problems independently. It is the client's right and privilege to be as self-sufficient as possible.

EXAMPLES

| Imparting information | "There are various methods of assistance for people who want to lose weight, such as Overeaters Anonymous, Weight Watchers, regular visits to a dietitian, the Physician's Weight Loss Program. You can decide what is best for you." |
| Giving advice | "You obviously need to lose a great deal of weight. I think the Physician's Weight Loss Program would be best for you." |

5. Feedback should be well-timed. Feedback is most useful when given at the earliest appropriate opportunity following the specific behavior.

EXAMPLES

| Prompt response | "I saw you hit the wall with your fist just now when you hung up the phone from talking to your mother." |
| Delayed response | "You need to learn some more appropriate ways of dealing with your anger. Last week after group I saw you pounding your fist against the wall." |

SUMMARY

Interpersonal communication is a transaction between the sender and the receiver. In all interpersonal transactions, both the sender and receiver bring certain preexisting conditions to the exchange that influence both the intended message and the way in which it is interpreted. Examples of these conditions include one's value system, internalized attitudes and beliefs, culture or religion, social status, gender, background knowledge and experience, age or developmental level, and the type of environment in which the communication takes place.

Nonverbal expression is a primary communication system in which meaning is assigned to various gestures and patterns of behavior. Some components of nonverbal communication include physical appearance and dress, body movement and posture, touch, facial expressions, eye behavior, and vocal cues or paralanguage. The meaning of each of these nonverbal components is culturally determined.

Hays and Larson (1963) have described various techniques of communication that can facilitate interaction between nurse and client. They have also identified a number of barriers in communication that can interfere with a satisfactory nurse-client interaction. Examples of both were presented in this chapter.

Active listening is described as being attentive to what the client is saying, through both verbal and nonverbal cues. Facilitative skills for attentive listening include sitting squarely facing the client, observing an open posture, leaning forward toward the client, establishing eye contact, and relaxing. They can be identified by the acronym SOLER.

Feedback is a method of communication for helping the client consider a modification of behavior. It is most useful when it:

1. Is descriptive rather than evaluative.
2. Focuses on behavior rather than on the person.
3. Is specific rather than general.
4. Is directed toward behavior that the client can change.
5. Imparts information rather than gives advice.
6. Is well-timed.

The nurse must be aware of the therapeutic or nontherapeutic value of the communication techniques used with the client, as they are the "tools" of psychosocial intervention.

REVIEW QUESTIONS

SELF-EXAMINATION/LEARNING EXERCISE

Test your knowledge about the concept of communication by answering the following questions:

1. Describe the transactional model of communication.
2. List eight types of preexisting conditions that can influence the outcome of the communication process.
3. Define *territoriality*. How does it affect communication?
4. Define *density*. How does it affect communication?
5. Identify four types of spatial distance and give an example of each.
6. Identify six components of nonverbal communication that convey special messages and give an example of each.
7. Describe five facilitative skills for active, or attentive, listening that can be identified by the acronym SOLER.

Identify the correct answer in each of the following questions. Provide explanation where requested. Identify the technique used (both therapeutic and nontherapeutic) in all choices given.

8. A client states: "I refuse to shower in this room. I must be very cautious. The FBI has placed a camera in here to monitor my every move." Which of the following is the therapeutic response? What is this technique called?
   a. "That's not true."
   b. "I have a hard time believing that is true."

9. Nancy, a depressed client who has been unkept and untidy for weeks, today comes to group therapy wearing a clean dress, makeup, and having washed and combed her hair. Which of the following responses by the nurse is most appropriate? Give the rationale.
   a. "Nancy, I see you have put on a clean dress and combed your hair."
   b. "Nancy, you look wonderful today!"

10. Dorothy was involved in an automobile accident while under the influence of alcohol. She swerved her car into a tree and narrowly missed hitting a child on a bicycle. She is in the hospital with multiple abrasions and contusions. She is talking about the accident with the nurse. Which of the following statements by the nurse is most appropriate? Identify the therapeutic or nontherapeutic technique in each.
    a. "Now that you know what can happen when you drink and drive, I'm sure you won't let it happen again. I'm sure everything will be okay."
    b. "That was a terrible thing you did. You could have killed that child!"
    c. "Now I guess you'll have to buy a new car. Can you afford that?"
    d. "What made you do such a thing?"
    e. "Tell me how you are feeling about what happened."

11. Judy has been in the hospital for 3 weeks. She has used Valium "to settle my nerves" for the past 15 years. She was admitted by her psychiatrist for safe withdrawal from the drug. She has passed the physical symptoms of withdrawal at this time but states to the nurse, "I don't know if I will make it without Valium after I go home. I'm already starting to feel nervous. I have so many personal problems." Which is the most appropriate response by the nurse? Identify the technique in each.

a. "Why do you think you have to have drugs to deal with your problems?"

b. "You'll just have to pull yourself together. Everybody has problems, and everybody doesn't use drugs to deal with them. They just do the best that they can."

c. "I don't want to talk about that now. Look at that sunshine. It's beautiful outside. You and I are going to take a walk!"

d. "Starting today you and I are going to think about some alternative ways for you to deal with those problems—things that you can do to decrease your anxiety without resorting to drugs."

12. Mrs. S. asks the nurse, "Do you think I should tell my husband about my affair with my boss?" Give one therapeutic response and one nontherapeutic response, give your rationale, and identify the technique used in each response.

13. Carol, an adolescent, just returned from group therapy and is crying. She says to the nurse, "All the other kids laughed at me! I try to fit in, but I always seem to say the wrong thing. I've never had a close friend. I guess I never will." Which is the most appropriate response by the nurse? Identify each technique used.

a. "You're feeling pretty down on yourself right now."

b. "Why do you feel this way about yourself?"

c. "What makes you think you will never have any friends?"

d. "The next time they laugh at you, you should just get up and leave the room!"

e. "I'm sure they didn't mean to hurt your feelings."

f. "Keep your chin up and hang in there. Your time will come."

REFERENCES

Bernstein, L., & Bernstein, R. (1980). *Interviewing: A guide for health professionals*. New York: Appleton-Century-Crofts.

Hall, E.T. (1966). *The hidden dimension*. Garden City, NY: Doubleday.

Hays, J.S., & Larson, K.H. (1963). *Interacting with patients*. New York: Macmillan.

Knapp, M.L. (1980). *Essentials of nonverbal communication*. New York: Holt, Rinehart & Winston.

Mehrabian, A. (1972). *Nonverbal communication*. Chicago: Aldine-Atherton.

Reece, M., & Whitman, R. (1962). Expressive movements, warmth, and verbal reinforcement. *Journal of Abnormal and Social Psychology, 64*, 234–236.

Smith, D.R., & Williamson, L.K. (1981). *Interpersonal communication* (2nd ed.). Dubuque, IA: W.C. Brown Co. Publishers.

Duldt, B.W., Giffin, K., & Patton, B.R. (1984). *Interpersonal communication in nursing*. Philadelphia: F.A. Davis.

Egan, G. (1977). *You and me*. Monterey, CA: Brooks/Cole.

Fritz, P.A., Russell, C.G., Wilcox, E.M., & Shirk, F.I. (1984). *Interpersonal communication in nursing*. Norwalk, CT: Appleton-Century-Crofts.

Hein, E.C. (1980). *Communication in nursing practice* (2nd ed.). Boston: Little, Brown.

Northouse, P.G., & Northouse, L.L. (1985). *Health communication—A handbook for health professionals*. Englewood Cliffs, NJ: Prentice-Hall.

Sundeen, S.J., Stuart, G.W., Rankin, E.D., & Cohen, S.A. (1985). *Nurse-client interaction—Implementing the nursing process* (3rd ed.). St. Louis, MO: C.V. Mosby.

Watzlawick, P., Beavin, J., & Jackson, D.D. (1967). *The pragmatics of human communication*. New York: W.W. Norton.

Bibliography

Cormier, L.S., Cormier, W.H., & Weisser, R.J., Jr. (1984). *Interviewing and helping skills for health professionals*. Monterey, CA: Wadsworth Health Sciences Division.

THE NURSING PROCESS IN PSYCHIATRIC/MENTAL HEALTH NURSING

CHAPTER OUTLINE

OBJECTIVES

INTRODUCTION

THE NURSING PROCESS

WHY NURSING DIAGNOSIS?

NURSING CASE MANAGEMENT

APPLYING THE NURSING PROCESS IN THE PSYCHIATRIC SETTING

DOCUMENTATION TO THE NURSING PROCESS

SUMMARY

REVIEW QUESTIONS

KEY TERMS

nursing process
nursing diagnosis
case management
managed care

case manager
critical pathways
of care
interdisciplinary

problem-oriented recording
Focus Charting®
PIE charting

OBJECTIVES

After reading this chapter, the student will be able to:

1. Define *nursing process*.
2. Identify six steps of the nursing process and describe nursing actions associated with each.
3. Describe the benefits of using nursing diagnosis.
4. Discuss the list of nursing diagnoses approved by the North American Nursing Diagnosis Association for clinical use and testing.
5. Define and discuss the utilization of case management and critical pathways of care in the clinical setting.
6. Apply the six steps of the nursing process in the care of a client within the psychiatric setting.
7. Document client care that validates use of the nursing process.

he **nursing process** has for many years provided a systematic framework for the delivery of nursing care. It is nursing's means of fulfilling the requirement for a *scientific methodology* in order to be considered a profession.

This chapter examines the steps of the nursing process as they are set forth by the American Nurses' Association in the *Standards of Clinical Nursing Practice* (ANA, 1991). A list of the nursing diagnoses approved for clinical use and testing through the 13th conference of the North American Nursing Diagnosis Association (NANDA) is presented. An explanation is provided for the implementation of case management and the tool used in the delivery of care with this methodology, critical pathways of care. Documentation that validates the use of the nursing process is discussed.

THE NURSING PROCESS

Definition

The nursing process consists of six steps and uses a problem-solving approach that has come to be accepted as nursing's scientific methodology. It is goal-directed, with the objective being delivery of quality client care.

Nursing process is dynamic, not static. It is an ongoing process that continues for as long as the nurse and client have interactions directed toward change in the client's physical or behavioral responses. Figure 7.1 presents a schematic of the ongoing nursing process.

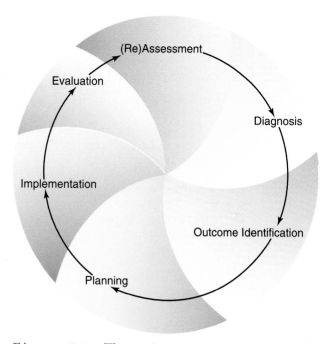

Figure 7.1 The ongoing nursing process.

Standards of Care

The Coalition of Psychiatric Nursing Organizations of the American Nurses' Association (ANA) has delineated a set of standards that psychiatric nurses are expected to follow as they provide care for their clients. The ANA (1994) states:

> "Standards of care pertain to professional nursing activities that are demonstrated by the nurse through the nursing process. These involve assessment, diagnosis, outcome identification, planning, implementation, and evaluation. The nursing process is the foundation of clinical decision making and encompasses all significant action taken by nurses in providing psychiatric–mental health care to all clients."

The standards are presented by the Coalition as follows:

Standard I. Assessment

The Psychiatric/Mental Health Nurse Collects Client Health Data

Rationale. The assessment interview—which requires linguistically and culturally effective communications skills, interviewing, behavioral observation, database record review, and comprehensive assessment of the client and relevant systems—enables the psychiatric/mental health nurse to make sound clinical judgments and plan appropriate interventions with the client (ANA, 1994).

In this first step, information is gathered from which to establish a database for determining the best possible care for the client. Information for this database is gathered from a variety of sources including interviewing the client or family, observing the client and his or her environment, consulting other health team members, reviewing the client's records, and conducting a nursing physical examination. A biopsychosocial assessment tool based on the stress-adaptation framework is included in Table 7.1.

Standard II. Diagnosis

The Psychiatric/Mental Health Nurse Analyzes the Assessment Data in Determining Diagnoses

Rationale. The basis for providing psychiatric/mental health nursing care is the recognition and identification of patterns of response to actual or potential psychiatric illnesses and mental health problems (ANA, 1994).

In the second step, data gathered during the assessment are analyzed. Diagnoses and potential problem statements are formulated and prioritized. Diagnoses conform to accepted classification systems, such as the North American Nursing Diagnosis Association (NANDA) Nursing Diagnosis Classification (see Table 7.3); *International*

◢ TABLE 7.1 NURSING HISTORY AND ASSESSMENT TOOL

I. General Information

Client name: _____   Allergies: _____

Room number: _____   Diet: _____

Doctor: _____   Height/weight: _____

Age: _____   Vital signs: TPR/BP _____

Sex:_____   Name and phone no. of

Race: _____   significant other: _____

Dominant language:_____   _____

Marital status: _____   City of residence: _____

Chief complaint:_____   Diagnosis (admitting & current): _____

_____   _____

_____   _____

Conditions of admission:

Date: _____   Time: _____

Accompanied by: _____

Route of admission (wheelchair; ambulatory; cart): _____

Admitted from:_____

II. Predisposing Factors

A. *Genetic Influences*

1. Family configuration (use genograms):

Family of origin: Present family:

Family dynamics (describe significant relationships between family members): _____

_____

_____

_____

2. Medical/psychiatric history:
   a. Client: _____

   _____

   _____

   b. Family members: _____

   _____

   _____

3. Other genetic influences affecting present adaptation. This might include effects specific to gender, race, appearance, such as genetic physical defects, or any other factor related to genetics that is affecting the client's adaptation that has not been mentioned elsewhere in this assessment.

_____

_____

B. *Past Experiences*

1. Cultural and social history:
   a. Environmental factors (family living arrangements, type of neighborhood, special working conditions): _____

   _____

   _____

Continued on following page

TABLE 7.1 NURSING HISTORY AND ASSESSMENT TOOL *Continued*

b. Health beliefs and practices (personal responsibility for health; special self-care practices): _____
_____
_____

c. Religious beliefs and practices: _____
_____
_____

d. Educational background: _____
_____
_____

e. Significant losses/changes (include dates): _____
_____
_____

f. Peer/friendship relationships: _____
_____
_____

g. Occupational history: _____
_____
_____

h. Previous pattern of coping with stress: _____
_____
_____

i. Other lifestyle factors contributing to present adaptation: _____
_____
_____

C. *Existing Conditions*
  1. Stage of development (Erikson): _____
    a. Theoretically: _____
    b. Behaviorally: _____
    c. Rationale:_____
    _____
    _____

  2. Support systems: _____
    _____

  3. Economic security: _____
    _____

  4. Avenues of productivity/contribution:
    a. Current job status: _____
    _____

    b. Role contributions and responsibility for others: _____
    _____

III. Precipitating Event
  Describe the situation or events that precipitated this illness/hospitalization:_____
  _____
  _____

IV. Client's Perception of the Stressor
  Client's or family member's understanding or description of stressor/illness and expectations of hospitalization: _____
  _____
  _____

TABLE 7.1   NURSING HISTORY AND ASSESSMENT TOOL

V. Adaptation Responses
  A. *Psychosocial*
    1. Anxiety level (circle level, and check the behaviors that apply):   mild   moderate   severe   panic
       calm _____   friendly _____   passive _____   alert _____   perceives environment correctly _____
       cooperative _____   impaired attention _____   "jittery" _____   unable to concentrate _____
       hypervigilant _____   tremors _____   rapid speech _____   withdrawn _____   confused _____
       disoriented _____   fearful _____   hyperventilating _____   misinterpreting the environment (hallucinations
       or delusions) _____   depersonalization _____   obsessions _____   compulsions _____
       somatic complaints _____   excessive hyperactivity _____   other _____

    2. Mood/affect (circle as many as apply):   happiness   sadness   dejection   despair   elation   euphoria   suspiciousness
       apathy (little emotional tone)   anger/hostility
    3. Ego defense mechanisms (describe how used by client):
       Projection _____
       Suppression _____
       Undoing _____
       Displacement _____
       Intellectualization _____
       Rationalization _____
       Denial _____
       Repression _____
       Isolation _____
       Regression _____
       Reaction Formation _____
       Splitting _____
       Religiosity _____
       Sublimation _____
       Compensation _____
    4. Level of self-esteem (circle one):   low   moderate   high
       Things client likes about self _____

       Things client would like to change about self _____
       Objective assessment of self-esteem:
       Eye contact_____
       General appearance_____

       Personal hygiene _____
       Participation in group activities and interactions with others _____

    5. Stage and manifestations of grief (circle one):
       denial   anger   bargaining   depression   acceptance
       Describe the client's behaviors that are associated with this stage of grieving in response to loss or change.
       _____
       _____
       _____

    6. Thought processes (circle as many as apply):   clear   logical   easy to follow   relevant   confused   blocking
       delusional   rapid flow of thoughts   slowness in thought association   suspicious
       recent memory: loss   intact   remote memory: loss   intact
       other _____

Continued on following page

TABLE 7.1 NURSING HISTORY AND ASSESSMENT TOOL *Continued*

7. Communication patterns (circle as many as apply):   clear   coherent   slurred speech   incoherent   neologisms   loose associations   flight of ideas   aphasic   perseveration   rumination   tangential speech   loquaciousness   slow, impoverished speech   speech impediment (describe) _____

   other _____

   _____

8. Interaction patterns (describe client's pattern of interpersonal interactions with staff and peers on the unit, e.g., manipulative, withdrawn, isolated, verbally or physically hostile, argumentative, passive, assertive, aggressive, passive-aggressive, other): _____

   _____

   _____

   _____

9. Reality orientation (check those that apply):

   Oriented to: time _____   person _____

               place _____   situation _____

10. Ideas of destruction to self/others?   Yes   No

   If yes, consider plan; available means _____

   _____

   _____

   _____

B. *Physiological*

   1. Psychosomatic manifestations (describe any somatic complaints that may be stress-related):

   _____

   _____

   _____

   2. Drug history and assessment:

   Use of prescribed drugs:

NAME	DOSAGE	PRESCRIBED FOR	RESULTS

   Use of over-the-counter drugs:

NAME	DOSAGE	USED FOR	RESULTS

   Use of street drugs or alcohol:

NAME	AMOUNT USED	HOW OFTEN USED	WHEN LAST USED	EFFECTS PRODUCED

   3. Pertinent physical assessments:

   a. Respirations: normal _____   labored _____

        Rate _____   Rhythm _____

TABLE 7.1   NURSING HISTORY AND ASSESSMENT TOOL

b. Skin: warm _____   dry _____   moist _____   cool _____

clammy _____   pink _____   cyanotic _____

poor turgor _____   edematous _____

Evidence of: rash ——— bruising _____

needle tracks _____   hirsutism _____

loss of hair _____   other _____

c. Musculoskeletal status: weakness _____   tremors _____

Degree of range of motion (describe limitations) _____

_____

Pain (describe)_____

Skeletal deformities (describe)_____

Coordination (describe limitations) _____

d. Neurologic status:

History of (check all that apply): seizures _____

(describe method of control) _____

headaches (describe location and frequency) _____

fainting spells _____   dizziness _____

tingling/numbness (describe location) _____

e. Cardiovascular: B/P _____   Pulse _____

History of (check all that apply):

hypertension _____   palpitations _____

heart murmur _____   chest pain _____

shortness of breath _____   pain in legs _____

phlebitis _____   ankle/leg edema _____

numbness/tingling in extremities _____

varicose veins_____

f. Gastrointestinal:

Usual diet pattern: _____

Food allergies:_____

Dentures? _____   Upper _____   Lower _____

Any problems with chewing or swallowing? _____

Any recent change in weight? _____

Any problems with:

indigestion/heartburn?_____

relieved by_____

nausea/vomiting? _____

relieved by_____

loss of appetite? _____

History of ulcers? _____

Usual bowel pattern _____

Constipation? _____   Diarrhea? _____

Type of self-care assistance provided for either of the above problems _____

g. Genitourinary/Reproductive:

Usual voiding pattern_____

Urinary hesitancy? _____   Frequency _____

Nocturia? _____   Pain/burning? _____

Incontinence? _____

Any genital lesions? _____

Continued on following page

TABLE 7.1   NURSING HISTORY AND ASSESSMENT TOOL *Continued*

Discharge? _____ Odor? _____

History of sexually transmitted disease? _____

If yes, please explain: _____

_____

Any concerns about sexuality/sexual activity?

_____

_____

Method of birth control used _____

Females:

Date of last menstrual cycle _____

Length of cycle _____

Problems associated with menstruation? _____

_____

Breasts: Pain/tenderness?_____

Swelling? _____ Discharge? _____

Lumps? _____ Dimpling? _____

Practice self-breast examination?

Frequency? _____

Males:

Penile discharge? _____

Prostate problems? _____

h. Eyes: YES   NO   EXPLAIN

Glasses?   _____   _____   _____

Contacts?   _____   _____   _____

Swelling?   _____   _____   _____

Discharge?   _____   _____   _____

Itching?   _____   _____   _____

Blurring?   _____   _____   _____

Double vision?   _____   _____   _____

i. Ears: YES   NO   EXPLAIN

Pain?   _____   _____   _____

Drainage?   _____   _____   _____

Difficulty hearing? _____   _____   _____

Hearing aid?   _____   _____   _____

Tinnitus?   _____   _____   _____

j. Medication side effects:

What symptoms is the client experiencing that may be attributed to current medication usage? _____

_____

_____

k. Altered lab values and possible significance: _____

_____

_____

l. Activity/rest patterns:

Exercise (amount, type, frequency) _____

_____

Leisure time activities: _____

_____

◢ TABLE 7.1 NURSING HISTORY AND ASSESSMENT TOOL

Patterns of sleep: Number of hours per night _____

   Use of sleep aids? _____

   Pattern of awakening during the night? _____

_____

   Feel rested upon awakening? _____

m. Personal hygiene/activities of daily living:

   Patterns of self-care: independent _____

   Requires assistance with: mobility _____

                  hygiene _____

                  toileting _____

                  feeding _____

                  dressing _____

                  other _____

   Statement describing personal hygiene and general appearance _____

_____

_____

n. Other pertinent physical assessments: _____

_____

_____

VI: Summary of Initial Psychosocial/Physical Assessment

KNOWLEDGE DEFICITS IDENTIFIED:

NURSING DIAGNOSES INDICATED:

SOURCE: From Townsend (1997), with permission.

Classification of Diseases (WHO, 1993); and *DSM-IV* (APA, 1994) (see Appendix C).

Standard III. Outcome Identification

The Psychiatric/Mental Health Nurse Identifies Expected Outcomes Individualized to the Client

Rationale. Within the context of providing nursing care, the ultimate goal is to influence health outcomes and improve the client's health status (ANA, 1994).

Expected outcomes are derived from the diagnosis. They must be measurable and estimate a time for attainment. They must be realistic for the client's capabilities, and are most effective when formulated by the interdisciplinary team members, the client, and significant others together.

Standard IV. Planning

The Psychiatric/Mental Health Nurse Develops a Plan of Care That Prescribes Interventions to Attain Expected Outcomes

Rationale. A plan of care is used to guide therapeutic intervention systematically and achieve the expected client outcomes (ANA, 1994).

The care plan is individualized to the client's mental health problems, condition, or needs and is developed in collaboration with the client, significant others, and interdisciplinary team members, if possible. For each diagnosis identified, the most appropriate interventions, based on current psychiatric/mental health nursing practice and research, are selected. Client education and necessary referrals are included. Priorities for delivery of nursing care are determined.

Standard V. Implementation

The Psychiatric/Mental Health Nurse Implements the Interventions Identified in the Plan of Care

Rationale. In implementing the plan of care, psychiatric/mental health nurses use a wide range of interventions designed to prevent mental and physical illness, and promote, maintain, and restore mental and physical health. Psychiatric/mental health nurses select interventions according to their level of practice. At the basic level, the nurse may select counseling, milieu therapy, self-care activities, psychobiological interventions, health teaching, case management, health promotion and health maintenance, and a variety of other approaches to meet the mental health needs of clients. In addition to the intervention options available to the basic-level psychiatric/mental health nurse, at the advanced level the certified specialist may provide consultation, engage in psychotherapy, and prescribe pharmacological agents where permitted by state statutes or regulations (ANA, 1994).

Interventions selected during the planning stage are executed, taking into consideration the nurse's level of practice, education, and certification. The care plan serves as a blueprint for delivery of safe, ethical, and appropriate interventions. Documentation of interventions also occurs at this step in the nursing process.

Several specific interventions are included among the standards of psychiatric/mental health clinical nursing practice (ANA, 1994):

Standard Va. Counseling. The psychiatric/mental health nurse uses counseling interventions to assist clients in improving or regaining their previous coping abilities, fostering mental health, and preventing mental illness and disability.

Standard Vb. Milieu Therapy. The psychiatric/mental health nurse provides, structures, and maintains a therapeutic environment in collaboration with the client and other health care providers.

Standard Vc. Self-Care Activities. The psychiatric/mental health nurse structures interventions around the client's activities of daily living to foster self-care and mental and physical well-being.

Standard Vd. Psychobiological Interventions. The psychiatric/mental health nurse uses knowledge of psychobiological interventions and applies clinical skills to restore the client's health and prevent further disability.

Standard Ve. Health Teaching. The psychiatric/mental health nurse, through health teaching, assists clients in achieving satisfying, productive, and healthy patterns of living.

Standard Vf. Case Management. The psychiatric/mental health nurse provides case management to coordinate comprehensive health services and ensure continuity of care.

Standard Vg. Health Promotion and Health Maintenance. The psychiatric/mental health nurse employs strategies and interventions to promote and maintain mental health and prevent mental illness.

Advanced Practice Interventions

Standard Vh. Psychotherapy. The certified specialist in psychiatric/mental health nursing uses individual, group, and family psychotherapy, child psychotherapy, and other therapeutic treatments to assist clients in fostering mental health, preventing mental illness and disability, and improving or regaining previous health status and functional abilities.

Standard Vi. Prescription of Pharmacological Agents. The certified specialist uses prescription of pharmacological agents, in accordance with the state nursing practice act, to treat symptoms of psychiatric illness and improve functional health status.

Standard Vj. Consultation. The certified specialist provides consultation to health care providers and others to influence the plans of care for clients and to enhance the abilities of others to provide psychiatric and mental health care and effect change in systems.

Standard VI. Evaluation

The Psychiatric/Mental Health Nurse Evaluates the Client's Progress in Attaining Expected Outcomes

Rationale. Nursing care is a dynamic process involving change in the client's health status over time, giving rise to the need for new data, different diagnoses, and modifications in the plan of care. Therefore, evaluation is a continuous process of appraising the effect of nursing interventions and the treatment regimen on the client's health status and expected health outcomes (ANA, 1994).

During the evaluation step, the nurse measures the success of the interventions in meeting the outcome criteria. The client's response to treatment is documented, validating use of the nursing process in the delivery of care. The diagnoses, outcomes, and plan of care are reviewed and revised as need is determined by the evaluation.

WHY NURSING DIAGNOSIS?

The concept of **nursing diagnosis** is not new. For centuries, nurses have identified specific client responses for which nursing interventions were employed in an effort to improve quality of life. Therefore, it is not surprising that some nurses who have been in practice for many years have been heard to ask: "What is this thing called nursing diagnosis? Why must changes be made if what we are doing works?" Historically lacking in the provision of nursing care was the autonomy of practice to which nurses were entitled by virtue of their licensure. Nursing was described as a set of tasks, and nurses were valued as "hand-maidens" for the physician (Gordon, 1987).

The term *diagnosis* in relation to nursing first began to appear in the literature in the early 1950s. The formalized organization of the concept, however, was only initiated in 1973 with the convening of the First National Conference on Nursing Diagnosis. The National Task Force for Classification of Nursing Diagnoses was developed during this conference. These individuals were charged with the task of identifying and classifying nursing diagnoses.

Also in the 1970s, the ANA began to write standards of practice around the steps of the nursing process, of which nursing diagnosis is an inherent part (ANA, 1973). This format encompassed both the general and specialty standards outlined by the ANA. The standards of psychiatric/mental health nursing practice are summarized in Table 7.2.

From this progression a statement of policy was published in 1980 and included a definition of nursing. The ANA defined nursing as ". . . the diagnosis and treatment of human responses to actual or potential health problems" (ANA, 1980).

Decisions regarding professional negligence are made based on the standards of practice defined by the ANA and the individual state nursing practice acts. A number of states have incorporated the steps of the nursing process, including nursing diagnosis, into the scope of nursing practice described in their nursing practice acts. When this is the case, it is the legal duty of the nurse to show that nursing process and nursing diagnosis were accurately implemented in the delivery of nursing care.

NANDA evolved from the National Task Force for Classification of Nursing Diagnoses. The major purpose of NANDA is to provide a forum for discussion about the development, refinement, and promotion of a taxonomy of nursing diagnostic terminology (Lancour, 1990). As of the 13th national conference held in 1998, 145 nursing diagnoses have been approved by NANDA for use and for testing (Table 7.3). This list is by no means exhaustive or all-inclusive. For purposes of this text, however, the existing list will be used in an effort to maintain a common language within nursing and to encourage clinical testing of what is available.

An official definition of *nursing diagnosis* has been formulated through the work of NANDA and was presented to the membership in 1990. The definition is as follows:

TABLE 7.2 STANDARDS OF PSYCHIATRIC/MENTAL HEALTH CLINICAL NURSING PRACTICE

Standard I. Assessment
The psychiatric/mental health nurse collects client health data.

Standard II. Diagnosis
The psychiatric/mental health nurse analyzes the assessment data in determining diagnoses.

Standard III. Outcome Identification
The psychiatric/mental health nurse identifies expected outcomes individualized to the client.

Standard IV. Planning
The psychiatric/mental health nurse develops a plan of care that prescribes interventions to attain expected outcomes.

Standard V. Implementation
The psychiatric/mental health nurse implements the interventions identified in the plan of care.

Standard Va. Counseling
The psychiatric/mental health nurse uses counseling interventions to assist clients in improving or regaining their previous coping abilities, fostering mental health, and preventing mental illness and disability.

Standard Vb. Milieu Therapy
The psychiatric/mental health nurse provides, structures, and maintains a therapeutic environment in collaboration with the client and other health care providers.

Standard Vc. Self-Care Activities
The psychiatric/mental health nurse structures interventions around the client's activities of daily living to foster self-care and mental and physical well-being.

Standard Vd. Psychobiological Interventions
The psychiatric/mental health nurse uses knowledge of psychobiological interventions and applies clinical skills to restore the client's health and prevent further disability.

Standard Ve. Health Teaching
The psychiatric/mental health nurse, through health teaching, assists clients in achieving satisfying, productive, and healthy patterns of living.

Standard Vf. Case Management
The psychiatric/mental health nurse provides case management to coordinate comprehensive health services and ensure continuity of care.

Standard Vg. Health Promotion and Health Maintenance
The psychiatric/mental health nurse employs strategies and interventions to promote and maintain mental health and prevent mental illness.

Advanced Practice Interventions

Standard Vh. Psychotherapy
The certified specialist in psychiatric/mental health nursing uses individual, group, and family psychotherapy, child psychotherapy, and other therapeutic treatments to assist clients in fostering mental health, preventing mental illness and disability, and improving or regaining previous health status and functional abilities.

Standard Vi. Prescription of Pharmacologic Agents
The certified specialist uses prescription of pharmacological agents, in accordance with the state nursing practice act, to treat symptoms of psychiatric illness and improve functional health status.

Standard Vj. Consultation
The certified specialist provides consultation to health care providers and others to influence the plans of care for clients, and to enhance the abilities of others to provide psychiatric and mental health care and effect change in systems.

Standard VI. Evaluation
The psychiatric/mental health nurse evaluates the client's progress in attaining expected outcomes.

SOURCE: Adapted from ANA (1994).

TABLE 7.3 NURSING DIAGNOSES APPROVED BY NANDA (For Use and Testing)

Activity Intolerance (specify level)
Activity Intolerance, risk for
Adaptive Capacity: Intracranial, decreased
*Adult Failure to Thrive
Adjustment, impaired
Airway Clearance, ineffective
*Altered Dentition
*Altered Development, risk for
*Altered Growth, risk for
Anxiety (specify level)
Aspiration, risk for
*Autonomic Dysreflexia, risk for

*Bed Mobility, impaired
Body Image disturbance
Body Temperature, risk for altered
Bowel Incontinence
Breastfeeding, effective
Breastfeeding, ineffective
Breastfeeding, interrupted
Breathing Pattern, ineffective

Cardiac Output, decreased
Caregiver Role Strain
Caregiver Role Strain, risk for
*Chronic Sorrow
Communication, impaired verbal
Community Coping, potential for enhanced
Community Coping, ineffective
Confusion, acute
Confusion, chronic
Constipation
Constipation, perceived
*Constipation, risk for
Coping, defensive
Coping, Individual, ineffective

*Death Anxiety
Decisional Conflict (specify)
*Delayed Surgical Recovery
Denial, ineffective
Diarrhea
Disuse Syndrome, risk for
Diversional Activity deficit
Dysreflexia

Energy Field disturbance
Environmental Interpretation Syndrome, impaired

Family Coping: ineffective, compromised
Family Coping: ineffective, disabling
Family Coping: potential for growth
Family Process, altered: alcoholism
Family Processes, altered
Fatigue
Fear
Fluid Volume deficit
Fluid Volume risk for deficit
Fluid Volume excess
*Fluid Volume Imbalance, risk for

Gas Exchange, impaired
Grieving, anticipatory
Grieving, dysfunctional
Growth & Development, altered

Health Maintenance, altered
Health-Seeking Behaviors (specify)

Home Maintenance Management, impaired
Hopelessness
Hyperthermia
Hypothermia

Incontinence, functional
Incontinence, reflex
Incontinence, stress
Incontinence, total
Incontinence, urge
Infant Behavior, disorganized
Infant Behavior, risk for disorganized
Infant Behavior, organized, potential for enhanced
Infant Feeding Pattern, ineffective
Infection, risk for
Injury, risk for
Knowledge deficit (specify)

*Latex Allergy
*Latex Allergy, risk for
Loneliness, risk for

Memory, impaired

*Nausea
Noncompliance (specify)
Nutrition, altered, less than body requirements
Nutrition: altered, more than body requirements
Nutrition: altered, risk for more than body requirements

Oral Mucous Membrane, altered

Pain
Pain, chronic
Parental Role conflict
Parent/Infant/Child Attachment, risk for altered
Parenting, altered
Parenting, risk for altered
Perioperative Positioning Injury, risk for
Peripheral Neurovascular dysfunction, risk for
Personal Identity disturbance
Physical Mobility, impaired
Poisoning, risk for
Post-Trauma Response
*Post-Trauma Syndrome
Powerlessness
Protection, altered

Rape-Trauma Syndrome
Rape-Trauma Syndrome: compound reaction
Rape-Trauma Syndrome: silent reaction
Relocation Stress Syndrome
Role Performance, altered

Self-Care deficit: feeding, bathing/hygiene,
   dressing/grooming, toileting
Self Esteem, chronic low
Self Esteem disturbance
Self Esteem, situational low
Self Mutilation, risk for
Sensory/Perceptual alterations (specify): visual, auditory,
   kinesthetic, gustatory, tactile, olfactory
Sexual dysfunction
Sexuality Patterns, altered
Skin Integrity, impaired
Skin Integrity, risk for impaired
Sleep Pattern disturbance
Social Interaction, impaired

TABLE 7.3   NURSING DIAGNOSES APPROVED BY NANDA (For Use and Testing)

Social Isolation	Thought Processes, altered
Spiritual Distress (distress of the human spirit)	Tissue Integrity, impaired
Spiritual Well-Being, potential for enhanced	Tissue Perfusion, altered (specify): cerebral,
Spontaneous Ventilation, inability to sustain	cardiopulmonary, renal, gastrointestinal, peripheral
Suffocation, risk for	Trauma, risk for
Swallowing, impaired	Unilateral Neglect
	Urinary Elimination, altered
Therapeutic Regimen: Community, ineffective management	Urinary Retention
Therapeutic Regimen: Families, ineffective management	Ventilatory Weaning Response, dysfunctional
Therapeutic Regimen: Individual, effective management	(DVWR)
Therapeutic Regimen: (Individuals) ineffective	Violence risk for, directed at self
management	Violence risk for, directed at others
Thermoregulation, ineffective	

SOURCE: Adapted from NANDA, 1999–2000. *New diagnoses accepted in 1998.

"Nursing diagnoses are clinical judgments about individual, family, or community responses to actual and potential health problems/life processes. Nursing diagnoses provide the basis for selection of nursing interventions to achieve outcomes for which the nurse is accountable." (Carroll-Johnson, 1990, p. 50)

The use of nursing diagnosis affords a degree of autonomy that historically has been lacking in the practice of nursing. Nursing diagnosis describes the client's condition, facilitating the prescription of interventions and establishment of parameters for outcome criteria based upon what is uniquely nursing. The ultimate benefit is to the client, who receives effective and consistent nursing care based on knowledge of the problems that the client is experiencing and of the most beneficial nursing interventions for resolution (Miller, 1989).

NURSING CASE MANAGEMENT

With the advent of diagnosis-related groups (DRGs) and shorter hospital stays, the concept of **case management** has evolved. Case management is an innovative model of care delivery that can result in improved client care. The ANA (1988) describes nursing case management as

"... a health care delivery process whose goals are to provide quality health care, decrease fragmentation, enhance the client's quality of life and contain costs."

Case management in the acute care setting strives to organize client care through an episode of illness so that specific clinical and financial outcomes are achieved within an allotted time frame (Zander, 1988). Commonly, the allotted time frame is determined by the established protocols for length of stay as defined by the DRGs.

Case management is becoming a recommended method of treatment for individuals with a chronic mental illness (Forchuk et al., 1989). This type of care strives to improve functioning by assisting the individual to solve problems

and improve work and socialization skills, to promote leisure-time activities, and to enhance overall independence.

Ideally, case management incorporates concepts of care at the primary, secondary, and tertiary levels of prevention. Various definitions have emerged and should be clarified, as follows.

Managed care is a concept purposefully designed to control the balance between cost and quality of care (Zander, 1988). In a managed care program, individuals receive health care based on need, as assessed by coordinators of the providership. Managed care exists in many settings, including (but not limited to)

- Insurance-based programs
- Employer-based medical providerships
- Social service programs
- The public health sector

Managed care may exist in virtually any setting in which medical providership is a part of the service; that is, in any setting in which an organization (whether private or government-based) is responsible for payment of health care services for a group of people. Examples of managed care are the health maintenance organizations (HMOs) and preferred provider organizations (PPOs).

Case management is the method used to achieve managed care. It is the actual coordination of services required to meet the needs of the client. Goals of case management are to

"facilitate access to needed services and coordinate care for clients within the fragmented health care delivery system, prevent avoidable episodes of illness among at-risk clients, and control or reduce the cost of care borne by the client or third-party payers." (Bower, 1992, p. 8)

Types of clients who benefit from case management include (but are not limited to)

- The frail elderly
- The developmentally disabled
- The physically handicapped
- The mentally handicapped

- Individuals with long-term medically complex problems that require multifaceted, costly care (e.g., high-risk infants, those with human immunodeficiency virus [HIV] or acquired immunodeficiency syndrome [AIDS], and transplant clients)
- Individuals who are severely compromised by an acute episode of illness or an acute exacerbation of a chronic illness (e.g., schizophrenia)

The **case manager** is responsible for negotiating with multiple health care providers to obtain a variety of services for the client. Bower (1992) states, "Nurses are particularly suited to provide case management for clients with multiple health problems that have a health-related component." The very nature of nursing, which incorporates knowledge about the biological, psychological, and sociocultural aspects related to human functioning, makes nurses highly appropriate as case managers. The ANA recommends that the minimum preparation for a nurse case manager is a baccalaureate degree in nursing with 3 years of appropriate clinical experience (Bower, 1992). Some case management programs prefer master's-prepared clinical nurse specialists who have experience working with the specific populations for whom the case management service will be rendered.

Critical Pathways of Care

Critical pathways of care (CPCs) have emerged as the tools for provision of care in a case management system. A critical pathway is a type of abbreviated plan of care that provides outcome-based guidelines for goal achievement within a designated length of stay. CPCs have been included in this text for selected psychiatric diagnoses. A sample CPC is presented in Table 7.4. Only one nursing diagnosis is used in this sample. A CPC may have nursing diagnoses for several individual problems.

Critical pathways of care are meant to be used by the entire interdisciplinary team, which may include nurse case manager, clinical nurse specialist, social worker, psychiatrist, psychologist, dietitian, occupational therapist, recreational therapist, chaplain, and others. The team decides what categories of care are to be performed, by what date, and by whom. Each member of the team is then expected to carry out his or her functions according to the time line designated on the CPC. The nurse, as case manager, is ultimately responsible to ensure that each of the assignments is carried out. If variations occur at any time in any of the categories of care, the rationale must be documented in the progress notes.

For example, with the sample CPC presented, the nurse case manager may admit the client into the detoxification center. The nurse contacts the psychiatrist to inform him or her of the admission. The psychiatrist performs additional assessments to determine if other consults are required. The psychiatrist also writes the orders for the initial diagnostic work-up and medication regimen. Within 24 hours, the interdisciplinary team meets to decide on other categories of care, to complete the CPC, and to make individual care assignments from the CPC. This particular sample CPC relies heavily on nursing care of the client through the critical withdrawal period. However, other problems for the same client, such as altered nutrition, impaired physical mobility, or spiritual distress, may utilize other members of the team to a greater degree. Each member of the team stays in contact with the nurse case manager regarding individual assignments. Ideally, team meetings are held daily or every other day to review progress and modify as required.

Critical pathways of care can be standardized, as they are intended to be used with uncomplicated cases. A CPC can be viewed as protocol for various clients with problems for which a designated outcome can be predicted.

APPLYING THE NURSING PROCESS IN THE PSYCHIATRIC SETTING

Based on the definition of mental health set forth in Chapter 2, the role of the nurse in psychiatry focuses on assisting the client to successfully adapt to stressors within the environment. Goals are directed toward change in thoughts, feelings, and behaviors that are age-appropriate and congruent with local and cultural norms.

Therapy within the psychiatric setting is very often team, or **interdisciplinary,** oriented. Therefore, it is important to delineate nursing's involvement in the treatment regimen. Nurses are indeed valuable members of the team. Having progressed beyond the role of custodial caregiver in the psychiatric setting, nurses now provide services that are defined within the scope of nursing practice. Nursing diagnosis is helping to define these nursing boundaries, providing the degree of autonomy and professionalism that has for so long been unrealized.

For example, a newly admitted client with the medical diagnosis of schizophrenia may be demonstrating the following behaviors:

- Inability to trust others
- Verbalizing hearing voices
- Refusing to interact with staff and peers
- Expressing a fear of failure
- Poor personal hygiene

From these assessments, the treatment team may determine that the client has the following problems:

- Paranoid delusions
- Auditory hallucinations
- Social withdrawal
- Developmental regression

Team goals would be directed toward

- Reducing suspiciousness
- Terminating auditory hallucinations
- Increasing feelings of self-worth

TABLE 7.4   SAMPLE CRITICAL PATHWAY OF CARE FOR CLIENT IN ALCOHOL WITHDRAWAL

Estimated Length of Stay: 7 days. Variations from designated pathway should be documented in progress notes.

Nursing Diagnosis: Risk for Injury related to CNS agitation
Outcome objective: Client shows no evidence of injury obtained during ETOH withdrawal.

Day	1	2	3	4	5	6	7
Categories of care: Referrals	Psychiatrist Assess need for: Neurologist Cardiologist Internist	Dietitian					Discharge with follow-up appointments as required
Diagnostic studies	Blood alcohol level Drug screen SMAC 27 Urinalysis	Chest x-ray ECG		Repeat of selected diagnostic studies as necessary			
Additional assessments	VS q4h I&O Restraints prn Assess withdrawal symptoms: tremors, n/v, tachycardia, sweating, high blood pressure, seizures, insomnia, hallucinations	VS q8h if stable I&O Restraints prn Assess withdrawal symptoms (see day 1)	VS q8h I&O Restraints prn Assess withdrawal symptoms	VS bid I&O Restraints prn Assess withdrawal symptoms	VS bid I&O Restraints prn Assess withdrawal symptoms	VS bid DC I&O	Discharge VS stable Absence of objective withdrawal symptoms
Medications	Librium 200 mg (in divided doses) Librium 25–50 mg prn Maalox ac & hs	Librium 160 mg (in divided doses) Librium 25 mg prn Maalox ac & hs	Librium 120 mg (in divided doses) Librium 15 mg prn Maalox ac & hs	Librium 80 mg (divided doses) Librium 10 mg prn Maalox ac & hs	Librium 40 mg (divided doses) Librium 5 mg prn Maalox ac & hs	DC scheduled Librium Librium 5 mg prn bid Maalox ac & hs	Discharge; no withdrawal symptoms; no meds
Client education					Discuss goals of AA and need for rehab therapy		Discharge with info on AA and rehab or other outpatient therapy

From this team treatment plan, nursing may identify the following nursing diagnoses:

1. Altered thought processes
2. Sensory-perceptual alteration (auditory)
3. Self-esteem disturbance
4. Self-care deficit (hygiene)

Nursing in psychiatry, regardless of the setting—hospital (inpatient or outpatient), office, home, community—is goal-directed care. The goals (or expected outcomes) are client oriented, are measurable, and focus on resolution of the problem if this is realistic or on a more short-term outcome if resolution is unrealistic. For example, in the previous situation, expected outcomes for the identified nursing diagnoses might be as follows:

1. The client will demonstrate trust in one staff member within 5 days.
2. The client will verbalize understanding that the voices are not real (not heard by others) within 10 days.
3. The client will complete one simple craft project within 7 days.
4. The client will take responsibility for own self-care and perform activities of daily living independently by discharge.

Nursing's contribution to the interdisciplinary treatment regimen will focus on establishing trust on a one-to-one basis, reducing the level of anxiety that is promoting hallucinations, giving positive feedback for small day-to-day accomplishments in an effort to build self-esteem, and assisting with and encouraging independent self-care. These interventions describe *independent nursing* actions and goals that are evaluated apart from, while also being directed toward achievement of, the *team's* treatment goals.

In this manner of collaboration with other team members, nursing provides a service that is unique and based on sound knowledge of psychopathology, scope of practice, and legal implications of the role. Although there is no dispute that "following doctor's orders" continues to be accepted in the priority of care, nursing intervention that enhances achievement of the overall goals of treatment is being recognized for its important contribution. The nurse who administers a medication prescribed by the physician to decrease anxiety may also choose to stay with the anxious client and offer reassurance of safety and security, thereby providing an independent nursing action that is distinct from, yet complementary to, the medical treatment.

DOCUMENTATION TO THE NURSING PROCESS

Equally as important as using the nursing process in the delivery of care is the written documentation that it has been used. Some contemporary nursing leaders are advocating that with solid standards of practice and procedures in place within the institution, nurses need only chart when there has been a deviation in the care as outlined by that standard. However, many legal decisions are still based on the precept that "if it was not charted, it was not done."

Because nursing process and nursing diagnosis are mandated by some nursing practice acts, documentation of their use is being considered in those states as evidence in determining certain cases of negligence by nurses. Some health care organization accrediting agencies also require that the nursing process be reflected in the delivery of care. Therefore, documentation must bear written testament to the use of the nursing process.

A variety of documentation methods can be used to reflect use of the nursing process in the delivery of nursing care. Three examples are presented here: problem-oriented recording (POR), Focus Charting®, and the problem, intervention, evaluation (PIE) system of documentation.

Problem-Oriented Recording

Problem-oriented recording follows the subjective, objective, assessment, plan, implementation, and evaluation (SOAPIE) format. It has as its basis a list of problems. When it is used by nursing, the problems (nursing diagnoses) are identified on a written plan of care with appropriate nursing interventions described for each. Documentation written in the SOAPIE format includes:

S = Subjective data: Information gathered from what the client, family, or other source has said or reported.

O = Objective data: Information gathered by direct observation of the person doing the assessment; may include a physiological measurement such as blood pressure or a behavioral response such as affect.

A = Assessment: The nurse's interpretation of the subjective and objective data.

P = Plan: The actions or treatments to be carried out (may be omitted in daily charting if the plan is clearly explained in the written nursing care plan and no changes are expected).

I = Intervention: Those nursing actions that were actually carried out.

E = Evaluation of the problem following nursing intervention (some nursing interventions cannot be evaluated immediately, so this section may be optional).

TABLE 7.5 VALIDATION OF THE NURSING PROCESS WITH PROBLEM-ORIENTED RECORDING

PROBLEM-ORIENTED RECORDING	WHAT IS RECORDED	NURSING PROCESS
S and O (Subjective and Objective data)	Verbal reports to, and direct observation and examination by, the nurse	Assessment
A (Assessment)	Nurse's interpretation of S and O	Diagnosis and outcome identification
P (Plan) Omitted in charting if written plan describes care to be given	Description of appropriate nursing actions to resolve the identified problem	Planning
I (Intervention)	Description of nursing actions actually carried out	Implementation
E (Evaluation)	A reassessment of the situation to determine results of nursing actions implemented	Evaluation

Table 7.5 shows how POR corresponds to the steps of the nursing process. Following is an example of a three-column documentation in the POR format.

EXAMPLE:

Date/Time	Problem	Progress Notes
6-22-99 1000	Social isolation	S: States he does not want to sit with or talk to others; "they frighten me" O: Stays in room alone unless strongly encouraged to come out; no group involvement; at times listens to group conversations from a distance but does not interact; some hypervigilance and scanning noted A: Inability to trust; panic level of anxiety; delusional thinking I: Initiated trusting relationship by spending time alone with the client; discussed his feelings regarding interactions with others; accompanied client to group activities; provided positive feedback for voluntarily participating in assertiveness training

Focus Charting

Another type of documentation that reflects use of the nursing process is **Focus Charting®**. Focus Charting® differs from POR in that the main perspective has been changed from "problem" to "focus," and data, action, and response (DAR) has replaced SOAPIE.

Lampe (1985) suggests that a focus for documentation can be any of the following:

1. Nursing diagnosis
2. Current client concern or behavior
3. Significant change in the client status or behavior
4. Significant event in the client's therapy

The focus cannot be a medical diagnosis. The documentation is organized in the format of DAR. These categories are defined as follows:

D = Data: Information that supports the stated focus or describes pertinent observations about the client

A = Action: Immediate or future nursing actions that address the focus, and evaluation of the present care plan along with any changes required

R = Response: Description of client's responses to any part of the medical or nursing care.

Table 7.6 shows how Focus Charting® corresponds to the steps of the nursing process. Following is an example of a three-column documentation in the DAR format.

EXAMPLE:

Date/Time	Focus	Progress Notes
6-22-99 1000	Social isolation related to mistrust, panic anxiety, delusions	D: States he does not want to sit with or talk to others; they "frighten" him; stays in room alone unless strongly encouraged to come

TABLE 7.6 VALIDATION OF THE NURSING PROCESS WITH FOCUS CHARTING

FOCUS CHARTING	WHAT IS RECORDED	NURSING PROCESS
D (Data)	Information that supports the stated focus or describes pertinent observations about the client.	Assessment
Focus	A nursing diagnosis; current client concern or behavior; significant change in client status; significant event in the client's therapy. **NOTE:** If outcome appears on written care plan, it need not be repeated in daily documentation unless a change occurs.	Diagnosis and outcome identification
A (Action)	Immediate or future nursing actions that address the focus; appraisal of the care plan along with any changes required.	Plan and implementation
R (Response)	Description of client responses to any part of the medical or nursing care.	Evaluation

out; no group involvement; at times listens to group conversations from a distance, but does not interact; some hypervigilance and scanning noted

A: Initiated trusting relationship by spending time alone with client; discussed his feelings regarding interactions with others; accompanied client to group activities; provided positive feedback for voluntarily participating in assertiveness training

R: Cooperative with therapy; still acts uncomfortable in the presence of a group of people; accepted positive feedback from nurse

The PIE Method

PIE, or more specifically "APIE" (assessment, problem, intervention, evaluation), is a systematic method of documenting to nursing process and nursing diagnosis. A problem-oriented system, **PIE charting** uses accompanying flow sheets that are individualized by each institution. Criteria for documentation are organized in the following manner:

A = Assessment: A complete client assessment is conducted at the beginning of each shift. Results are documented under this section in the progress notes. Some institutions elect instead to use a daily client assessment sheet designed to meet specific needs of the unit. Explanation of any deviation from the norm is included in the progress notes.

P = Problem: A problem list, or list of nursing diagnoses, is an important part of the APIE method of charting. The name or number of the problem being addressed is documented in this section.

I = Intervention: Nursing actions are performed, directed at resolution of the problem.

E = Evaluation: Outcomes of the implemented inverventions are documented, including an evaluation of client responses to determine the effectiveness of nursing interventions and the presence or absence of progress toward resolution of a problem.

Table 7.7 shows how APIE charting corresponds to the steps of the nursing process. Following is an example of a three-column documentation in the APIE format.

EXAMPLE:

Date/Time	Problem	Progress Notes
6-22-99 1000	Social isolation	A: States he does not want to sit with or talk to others; they "frighten" him; stays in room alone unless strongly encouraged to come out; no group involvement; at times listens to group conversations from a distance but does not interact; some hypervigilance and scanning noted

TABLE 7.7 VALIDATION OF THE NURSING PROCESS WITH APIE METHOD

APIE CHARTING	WHAT IS RECORDED	NURSING PROCESS
A (Assessment)	Subjective and objective data about the client that is gathered at the beginning of each shift	Assessment
P (Problem)	Name (or number) of nursing diagnosis being addressed from written problem list, and identified outcome for that problem. **NOTE:** If outcome appears on written care plan, it need not be repeated in daily documentation unless a change occurs.	Diagnosis and outcome identification
I (Intervention)	Nursing actions performed, directed at problem resolution	Plan and implementation
E (Evaluation)	Appraisal of client responses to determine effectiveness of nursing interventions	Evaluation

P: Social isolation related to inability to trust, panic level of anxiety, and delusional thinking

I: Initiated trusting relationship by spending time alone with client; discussed his feelings regarding interactions with others; accompanied client to group activities; provided positive feedback for voluntarily participating in assertiveness training

E: Cooperative with therapy; still uncomfortable in the presence of a group of people; accepted positive feedback from nurse

SUMMARY

The nursing process provides a methodology by which nurses may deliver care using a systematic, scientific approach. The focus is goal directed and based on a decision-making or problem-solving model, consisting of six steps: assessment, diagnosis, outcome identification, planning, implementation, and evaluation.

Nursing diagnosis is inherent within the nursing process. The concept of nursing diagnosis is not new, but has only become formalized with the organization of NANDA in the 1970s. Nursing diagnosis defines the scope and boundaries for nursing, thereby offering a degree of autonomy and independence so long restricted within the practice of nursing. Nursing diagnosis also provides a common language for nursing and assists nurses to provide consistent, quality care for their clients based on an increase in the body of nursing knowledge through research. As of the 13th National NANDA Conference held in 1998, 145 nursing diagnoses have been approved for use and testing.

The psychiatric nurse uses the nursing process to assist clients to adapt successfully to stressors within the environment. Goals are directed toward change in thoughts, feelings, and behaviors that are age- appropriate and congruent with local and cultural norms. The nurse serves as a valuable member of the interdisciplinary treatment team, working both independently and cooperatively with other team members. Nursing diagnosis, in its ability to define the scope of nursing practice, is facilitating nursing's role in the psychiatric setting by differentiating that which is specifically nursing from interventions associated with other disciplines.

Nursing in psychiatry is goal-directed care. These goals are evaluated apart from, while also being directed toward achievement of, the team's treatment goals. The role of case management in psychiatric nursing is being expanded, and some institutions that employ this concept are using CPCs as the tool for treatment planning. The concept of case management was explored in this chapter and a sample CPC was included with an explanation for its use.

Nurses must document that the nursing process has been used in the delivery of care. Its use is mandated in some states by the nurse practice act and also required by some health care organization accrediting agencies. Three methods of documentation, POR, Focus Charting®, and the PIE system, were presented with examples to demonstrate how they reflect use of the nursing process.

REVIEW QUESTIONS

SELF-EXAMINATION/LEARNING EXERCISE

Test your knowledge of nursing process by supplying the information requested.

1. Name the six steps of the nursing process.

2. Identify the step of the nursing process to which each of the following nursing actions applies:
   a. Obtains a short-term contract from the client to seek out staff if feeling suicidal
   b. Identifies nursing diagnosis: Potential for self-directed violence
   c. Determines if nursing interventions have been appropriate to achieve desired results
   d. Client's family reports recent suicide attempt
   e. Prioritizes the necessity for maintaining a safe environment for the client
   f. Establishes goal of care: Client will not harm self during hospitalization

3. S.T. is a 15-year-old girl who has just been admitted to the adolescent psychiatric unit with a diagnosis of anorexia nervosa. She is 5'5" tall and weighs 82 lb. She was elected to the cheerleading squad for the fall but states that she is not as good as the others on the squad. The treatment team has identified the following problems: refusal to eat, occasional purging, refusing to interact with staff and peers, and fear of failure.

   Formulate three nursing diagnoses and identify outcomes for each that, as a part of the treatment team, nursing could use to contribute both independently and cooperatively to the team treatment plan.

4. Review various methods of documentation that reflect delivery of nursing care via the nursing process. Practice making entries for the case described in question 3 using the various methods.

REFERENCES

American Nurses' Association (ANA). (1994). *Statement on psychiatric–mental health clinical nursing practice and standards of psychiatric–mental health clinical nursing practice.* Washington, DC: American Nurses' Association.

ANA. (1991). *Standards of clinical nursing practice.* Kansas City, MO: American Nurses' Association.

ANA. (1980). *Nursing—A social policy statement.* Kansas City, MO: American Nurses' Association.

ANA. (1988). *Nursing case management.* Publication No. NS-32. Kansas City, MO: American Nurses' Association.

ANA. (1973). *Standards of nursing practice.* Kansas City, MO: American Nurses' Association.

American Psychiatric Association (APA). (1994). *Diagnosis and statistical manual of mental disorders* (4th ed.). Washington, DC: American Psychiatric Association.

Bower, K. A. (1992). *Case management by nurses.* Washington, DC: American Nurses Publishing.

Carroll-Johnson, R. M. (1990). Reflections on the Ninth Biennial Conference. *Nursing Diagnosis, 1*(2), 49–50.

Faherty, B. (1990, July). Case management: The latest buzzword—What it is, and what it isn't. *CARING,* 20–22.

Forchuk, C., Beaton, S., Crawford, L., Ide, L., Voorberg, N., & Bethune, J. (1989). Incorporating Peplau's theory and case management. *Journal of Psychosocial Nursing, 27*(2), 35–38.

Gordon, M. (1987). *Nursing diagnosis—Process and application* (2nd ed.). New York: McGraw-Hill.

Lampe, S.S. (1985). Focus charting: Streamlining documentation. *Nursing Management, 16*(7), 43–46.

Lancour, J. (1990). President's message. *Nursing diagnosis, 1*(1):4.

McHugh, M.K. (1987, August). Has nursing outgrown the nursing process? *Nursing 87,* 50–51.

Miller, E. (1989). *How to make nursing diagnosis work.* Norwalk, CT: Appleton & Lange.

North American Nursing Diagnosis Association (NANDA). (1998). *Nursing diagnoses: Definitions and classification, 1999–2000.* Philadelphia: NANDA.

World Health Organization (WHO). (1993). *International classification of diseases* (10th ed.). Geneva: World Health Organization.

Zander, K. (1988). Managed care within acute care settings: Design and implementation via nursing case management. *Health Care Supervisor, 6*(2), 27–43.

Bibliography

Alfaro, R. (1990). *Applying nursing diagnosis and nursing process* (2nd ed.). Philadelphia: J.B. Lippincott.

Atkinson, L.D., & Murray, M.E. (1983). *Understanding the nursing process* (2nd ed.). New York: Macmillan.

Buckley-Womack, C., & Gidney, S. (1987, October). A new dimension in documentation: The PIE method. *Journal of Neuroscience Nursing,* 256–260.

Doenges, M.E., & Moorhouse, M.F. (1998). *Nurse's pocket guide: Nursing diagnoses with interventions* (6th ed.). Philadelphia: F.A. Davis.

Doenges, M.E., Townsend, M.C., & Moorhouse, M.F. (1998). *Psychiatric care plans: Guidelines for client care* (3rd ed.). Philadelphia: F.A. Davis.

Eggland, E.T. (1988, November). Charting: How and why to document your care daily—and fully. *Nursing88,* 76–84.

Hickey, P.W. (1990). *Nursing process handbook.* St. Louis: C.V. Mosby.

Iyer, P.W., Taptich, B.J., & Bernocchi-Losey, D. (1986). *Nursing process and nursing diagnosis.* Philadelphia: W.B. Saunders.

Iyer, P.W. (1991, January). New trends in charting. *Nursing 91,* 48–50.

LaMonica, E.L. (1979). *The nursing process—A humanistic approach.* Menlo Park, CA: Addison-Wesley.

Pinnell, N.N., & deMeneses, M. (1986). *The nursing process—Theory, application, and related processes.* Norwalk, CT: Appleton-Century-Crofts.

Siegrist, L., Dettor, R.E., & Stocks, B. (1985, June). The PIE system: Complete planning and documentation of nursing care. *Quality Review Bulletin,* 186–189.

Townsend, M.C. (1997). *Nursing diagnoses in psychiatric nursing: A pocket guide for care plan construction* (4th ed.). Philadelphia: F.A. Davis.

Yura, H., and Walsh, M.B. (1988). *The nursing process* (5th ed.). Norwalk, CT: Appleton & Lange.

THERAPEUTIC GROUPS

CHAPTER OUTLINE

OBJECTIVES

INTRODUCTION

THE GROUP, DEFINED

FUNCTIONS OF A GROUP

TYPES OF GROUPS

PHYSICAL CONDITIONS

CURATIVE FACTORS

PHASES OF GROUP DEVELOPMENT

LEADERSHIP STYLES

MEMBER ROLES

PSYCHODRAMA

THE ROLE OF THE NURSE IN GROUP THERAPY

SUMMARY

REVIEW QUESTIONS

KEY TERMS

group therapy
universality
altruism

catharsis
autocratic
democratic

laissez-faire
psychodrama

OBJECTIVES

After reading this chapter, the student will be able to:

1. Define a *group*.
2. Discuss eight functions of a group.
3. Identify various types of groups.
4. Describe physical conditions that influence groups.
5. Discuss "curative factors" that occur in groups.
6. Describe the phases of group development.
7. Identify various leadership styles in groups.
8. Identify various roles that members assume within a group.
9. Discuss psychodrama as a specialized form of group therapy.
10. Describe the role of the nurse in group therapy.

uman beings are complex creatures who share their activities of daily living with various *groups* of people. Sampson and Marthas (1990) state:

"We are *biological* organisms possessing qualities shared with all living systems and with others of our species. We are *psychological* beings with distinctly human capabilities for thought, feeling, and action. We are also social beings, who function as part of the complex webs that link us with other people." (p. 3)

Health care professionals not only share their personal lives with groups of people but also encounter multiple group situations in their professional operations. Team conferences, committee meetings, grand rounds, and inservice sessions are to name but a few. In psychiatry, work with clients and families often takes the form of groups. With group work, not only does the nurse have the opportunity to reach out to a greater number of people at one time, but those individuals also assist each other by bringing to the group and sharing their feelings, opinions, ideas, and behaviors. Clients learn from each other in a group setting.

This chapter explores various types and methods of therapeutic groups that can be used with psychiatric clients, and the role of the nurse in group intervention.

THE GROUP, DEFINED

A *group* is defined as "a collection of individuals whose association is founded upon shared commonalities of interest, values, norms, or purpose." Membership in a group is generally by chance (born into the group), by choice (voluntary affiliation), or by circumstance (the result of life-cycle events over which an individual may or may not have control).

FUNCTIONS OF A GROUP

Sampson and Marthas (1990) have outlined eight functions that groups serve for their members. They contend that groups may serve more than one function and usually serve different functions for different members of the group. The eight functions are

1. **Socialization.** The cultural group into which we are born begins the process of teaching social norms. This is continued throughout our lives by members of other groups with which we become affiliated.
2. **Support.** One's fellow group members are available in time of need. Individuals derive a feeling of security from group involvement.
3. **Task completion.** Group members provide assistance in endeavors that are beyond the capacity of one individual alone or when results can be achieved more effectively as a team.
4. **Camaraderie.** Members of a group provide the joy and pleasure that individuals seek from interactions with significant others.
5. **Informational.** Learning takes place within groups. Explanations regarding world events occur in groups. Knowledge is gained when individual members learn how others in the group have resolved situations similar to those with which they are currently struggling.
6. **Normative.** This function relates to the ways in which groups enforce the established norms.
7. **Empowerment.** Groups help to bring about improvement in existing conditions by providing support to individual members who seek to bring about change. Groups have power that individuals alone do not.
8. **Governance.** An example of the governing function is that of rules being made by committees within a larger organization.

TYPES OF GROUPS

The functions of a group vary depending on the reason the group was formed. Clark (1987) identifies three types of groups in which nurses most often participate: task groups, teaching groups, and supportive/therapeutic groups.

Task Groups

The function of a task group is to accomplish a specific outcome or task. The focus is on solving problems and making decisions to achieve this outcome. Often a deadline is placed on completion of the task, and such importance is placed on a satisfactory outcome that conflict within the group may be smoothed over or ignored in order to focus on the priority at hand.

Teaching Groups

Teaching, or educational, groups exist to convey knowledge and information to a number of individuals. Nurses can be involved in teaching groups of many varieties, such as medication education, childbirth education, breast self-examination, and effective parenting classes. These groups usually have a set time frame or a set number of meetings. Members learn from each other as well as from the designated instructor. The objective of teaching groups is verbalization or demonstration by the learner of the material presented by the end of the designated period.

Supportive/Therapeutic Groups

The primary concern of support groups is to prevent future upsets by teaching participants effective ways of dealing with emotional stress arising from situational or developmental crises (Clark, 1987).

For the purposes of this text, it is important to differentiate between "therapeutic groups" and "**group therapy.**" Leaders of group therapy generally have advanced degrees in psychology, social work, nursing, or medicine. They often have additional training or experience under the supervision of an accomplished professional in conducting group psychotherapy based on various theoretical frameworks such as psychoanalytic, psychodynamic, interpersonal, or family dynamics. Approaches based on these theories are used by the group therapy leaders to encourage improvement in the ability of group members to function on an interpersonal level.

Therapeutic groups, on the other hand, are based to a lesser degree in theory. Focus is more on group relations, interactions among group members, and the consideration of a selected issue. Like group therapists, individuals who lead therapeutic groups must be knowledgeable in *group process*; that is, the *way* in which group members interact with each other. Interruptions, silences, judgments, glares, and scapegoating are examples of group processes (Clark, 1987). They must also have thorough knowledge of *group content*, the topic or issue being discussed within the group, and the ability to present the topic in language that can be understood by all group members. Many nurses who work in psychiatry lead supportive/therapeutic groups.

Self-Help Groups

An additional type of group, in which nurses may or may not be involved, is the self-help group. Self-help groups have grown in numbers and in credibility in recent years and serve to reduce the possibilities of further emotional distress leading to pathology and necessary treatment (Newton, 1984). Examples of self-help groups are Alzheimer's Disease and Related Disorders, Anorexia Nervosa and Associated Disorders, Weight Watchers, Alcoholics Anonymous, Reach to Recovery, Parents Without Partners, Overeaters Anonymous, Adult Children of Alcoholics, and many others related to specific needs or illnesses. These groups may or may not have a professional leader or consultant. They are run by the members, and leadership often rotates from member to member.

Nurses may become involved with self-help groups either voluntarily, or because their advice or participation has been requested by the members. The nurse may function as a referral agent, resource person, member of an advisory board, or leader of the group. Self-help groups are a valuable source of referral for clients with specific problems. However, nurses must be knowledgeable about the purposes of the group, membership, leadership, benefits, and problems that might threaten the suc-

cess of the group before making referrals to their clients for a specific self-help group. The nurse may find it necessary to attend several meetings of a particular group, if possible, to assess its effectiveness of purpose and appropriateness for client referral.

PHYSICAL CONDITIONS

Seating

The physical conditions for the group should be set up so that there is no barrier between the members. For example, a circle of chairs is better than chairs set around a table. Members should be encouraged to sit in different chairs each meeting. This openness and change creates an uncomfortableness that encourages anxious and unsettled behaviors that can then be explored within the group.

Size

Various authors have suggested different ranges of size as ideal for group interaction: 5 to 10 (Lego, 1987), 2 to 15 (Sampson & Marthas, 1990), and 4 to 12 (Clark, 1987). Group size does make a difference in the interaction among members. The larger the group, the less time there is available to devote to each member. In fact, in larger groups, those more aggressive individuals are most likely to be heard, while quieter members may be left out of the discussions altogether. On the other hand, larger groups provide more opportunities for individuals to learn from other members. The wider range of life experiences and knowledge provides a greater potential for effective group problem solving. Studies have indicated that 7 or 8 members provides a favorable climate for optimal group interaction and relationship development.

Membership

Whether the group is open- or closed-ended is another condition that influences the dynamics of group process. Open-ended groups are those in which members leave and others join at any time during the existence of the group. The continuous movement of members in and out of the group creates the type of uncomfortableness described previously that encourages unsettled behaviors in individual members and fosters the exploration of feelings. These are the most common types of groups held on short-term inpatient units, although they are used in outpatient and long-term care facilities as well. Closed-ended groups usually have a predetermined, fixed time frame. All members join at the time the group is organized and terminate at the end of the designated time period. Closed-ended groups are often composed of individuals with common issues or problems they wish to address.

CURATIVE FACTORS

Why are therapeutic groups helpful? Yalom (1985) identified 11 curative factors that individuals can achieve through interpersonal interactions within the group. Some of the factors are present in most groups in varying degrees. These curative factors identified by Yalom include:

1. **The Instillation of Hope.** By observing the progress of others in the group with similar problems, a group member garners hope that his or her problems can also be resolved.

2. **Universality.** Individuals come to realize that they are not alone in the problems, thoughts, and feelings they are experiencing. Anxiety is relieved by the support and understanding of others in the group who share similar (**universal**) experiences.

3. **The Imparting of Information.** Knowledge is gained through formal instruction as well as the sharing of advice and suggestions among group members.

4. **Altruism.** Altruism is assimilated by group members through mutual sharing and concern for each other. Providing assistance and support to others creates a positive self-image and promotes self-growth.

5. **The Corrective Recapitulation of the Primary Family Group.** Group members are able to re-experience early family conflicts that remain unresolved. Attempts at resolution are promoted through feedback and exploration.

6. **The Development of Socializing Techniques.** Through interaction with and feedback from other members within the group, individuals are able to correct maladaptive social behaviors and learn and develop new social skills.

7. **Imitative Behavior.** In this setting, one who has mastered a particular psychosocial skill or developmental task can be a valuable role model for others. Individuals may imitate selected behaviors that they wish to develop in themselves.

8. **Interpersonal Learning.** The group offers many and varied opportunities for interacting with other people. Insight is gained regarding how one perceives and is being perceived by others.

9. **Group Cohesiveness.** Members develop a sense of belonging that separates the individual ("I am") from the group ("we are"). Out of this alliance emerges a common feeling that both individual members and the total group are of value to each other.

10. **Catharsis.** Within the group, members are able to express both positive and negative feelings—perhaps feelings that have never been expressed before—in a nonthreatening atmosphere. This **catharsis,** or open expression of feelings, is beneficial for the individual within the group.

11. **Existential Factors.** The group is able to help individual members take direction of their own lives and to accept responsibility for the quality of their existence.

It may be helpful for a group leader to explain these curative factors to members of the group. Boyer (1982) stated that positive responses were experienced by group members who understood and were able to recognize curative factors as they occurred within the group.

PHASES OF GROUP DEVELOPMENT

Groups, like individuals, move through phases of life-cycle development. Ideally, groups will progress from the phase of infancy to advanced maturity in an effort to fulfill the objectives set forth by the membership. Unfortunately, as with individuals, some groups become fixed in early developmental levels and never progress, or experience periods of regression in the developmental process. Three phases of group development are discussed here.

Phase I. Initial or Orientation Phase

Group Activities

Leader and members work together to establish the rules that will govern the group (when and where meetings will occur, the importance of confidentiality, how meetings will be structured). Goals of the group are established. Members are introduced to each other.

Leader Expectations

The leader is expected to orient members to specific group processes, encourage members to participate without disclosing too much too soon, promote an environment of trust, and ensure that rules established by the group do not interfere with fulfillment of the goals.

Member Behaviors

In phase I, members have not yet established trust and will respond to this lack of trust by being overly polite. There is a fear of not being accepted by the group. They may try to "get on the good side" of the leader with compliments and conforming behaviors. A power struggle may ensue as members compete for their position in the "pecking order" of the group.

Phase II. Middle or Working Phase

Group Activities

Ideally, during the working phase, cohesiveness has been established within the group. This is when the productive work toward completion of the task is undertaken. Problem solving and decision making occur within the group. In the mature group, cooperation prevails, and differences and disagreements are confronted and resolved.

Leader Expectations

The role of leader diminishes and becomes more one of facilitator during the working phase. Some leadership functions are shared by certain members of the group as they progress toward resolution. The leader helps to resolve conflict and continues to foster cohesiveness among the members, while ensuring that they do not deviate from the intended task or purpose for which the group was organized.

Member Behaviors

At this point trust has been established among the members. They turn more often to each other and less often to the leader for guidance. They accept criticism from each other, using it in a constructive manner to create change. Occasionally, subgroups will form in which two or more members conspire with each other to the exclusion of the rest of the group. To maintain group cohesion, these subgroups must be confronted and discussed by the entire membership. Conflict is managed by the group with minimal assistance from the leader.

Phase III. Final or Termination Phase

Group Activities

The longer a group has been in existence, the more difficult termination is likely to be for the members. Termination should be mentioned from the outset of group formation. It should be discussed in depth for several meetings prior to the final session. A sense of loss that precipitates the grief process may be in evidence, particularly in groups that have been successful in their stated purpose.

Leader Expectations

In the termination phase, the leader encourages the group members to reminisce about what has occurred within the group, to review the goals and discuss the actual outcomes, and to encourage members to provide feedback to each other about individual progress within the group.

The leader encourages members to discuss feelings of loss associated with termination of the group.

Member Behaviors

Members may express surprise over the actual materialization of the end. This represents the grief response of denial, which may then progress to anger. Anger toward other group members or toward the leader may reflect feelings of abandonment (Sampson & Marthas, 1990). These feelings may lead to individual members' discussions of previous losses for which similar emotions were experienced. Successful termination of the group may help members develop the skills needed when losses occur in other dimensions of their lives.

LEADERSHIP STYLES

Three of the most common group leadership styles have been described by Lippitt and White (1958). They include autocratic, democratic, and laissez-faire.

Autocratic

Autocratic leaders have personal goals for the group. They withhold information from group members, particularly issues that may interfere with achievement of their own objectives. The message that is conveyed to the group is: "We will do it my way. My way is best." The focus in this style of leadership is on the leader. Members are dependent on the leader for problem solving, decision making, and permission to perform. The approach of the autocratic leader is one of persuasion, striving to persuade others in the group that his or her ideas and methods are superior. Productivity is high with this type of leadership, but often morale within the group is low owing to lack of member input and creativity.

Democratic

The **democratic** leadership style focuses on the members of the group. Information is shared with members in an effort to allow them to make decisions regarding achieving the goals for the group. Members are encouraged to participate fully in problem solving of issues that relate to the group, including taking action to effect change. The message that is conveyed to the group is: "Decide what must be done, consider the alternatives, make a selection, and proceed with the actions required to complete the task." The leader provides guidance and expertise as needed. Productivity is lower than it is with autocratic leadership, but morale is much higher because of the extent of input allowed all members of the group and the potential for individual creativity.

Laissez-Faire

This leadership style allows people to do as they please. There is no direction from the leader. In fact, the **laissez-faire** leader's approach is noninvolvement. Goals for the group are undefined. No decisions are made, no problems are solved, and no action is taken. Members become frustrated and confused, and productivity and morale are low.

Table 8.1 shows an outline of various similarities and differences among the three leadership styles.

MEMBER ROLES

Benne and Sheats (1948) identified three major types of roles that individuals play within the membership of the group. These are roles that serve to:

1. Complete the task of the group.
2. Maintain or enhance group processes.
3. Fulfill personal or individual needs.

Task roles and maintenance roles contribute to the success or effectiveness of the group. Personal roles satisfy needs of the individual members, sometimes to the extent of interfering with the effectiveness of the group.

Table 8.2 presents an outline of specific roles within these three major types and the behaviors associated with each.

PSYCHODRAMA

A specialized type of therapeutic group, called **psychodrama**, was introduced by J. L. Moreno, a Viennese psychiatrist. Moreno's method employs a dramatic approach in which clients become "actors" in life-situation scenarios.

The group leader is called the *director*, group members are the *audience*, and the *set*, or *stage*, may be specially designed or may just be any room or part of a room selected for this purpose. Actors are members from the audience who agree to take part in the "drama" by role playing a situation about which they have been informed by the director. Usually the situation is an issue with which one individual client has been struggling. The client plays the role of himself or herself and is called the *protagonist*. In this role, the client is able to express true feelings toward individuals (represented by group members) with whom he or she has unresolved conflicts.

In some instances, the group leader may ask for a client to volunteer to be the protagonist for that session. The client may chose a situation he or she wishes to enact and select the audience members to portray the roles of others in the life situation.

The psychodrama setting provides the client with a safer and less threatening atmosphere than the real situation in which to express true feelings. Resolution of interpersonal conflicts is facilitated.

When the drama has been completed, group members from the audience discuss the situation they have observed, offer feedback, express their feelings, and relate their own similar experiences. In this way, all group members benefit from the session, either directly or indirectly.

Nurses often serve as actors, or role players, in psychodrama sessions. Leaders of psychodrama have graduate degrees in psychology, social work, nursing, or medicine, with additional training in group therapy and specialty preparation to become a psychodramatist.

THE ROLE OF THE NURSE IN GROUP THERAPY

Nurses participate in group situations on a daily basis. Within health care settings, nurses serve on or lead task groups that create policy, describe procedures, plan client care, as well as a variety of other groups aimed at the in-

TABLE 8.1 LEADERSHIP STYLES—SIMILARITIES AND DIFFERENCES

CHARACTERISTICS	AUTOCRATIC	DEMOCRATIC	LAISSEZ-FAIRE
1. Focus	Leader	Members	Undetermined
2. Task strategy	Members are persuaded to adopt leader ideas	Members engage in group problem solving	No defined strategy exists
3. Member participation	Limited	Unlimited	Inconsistent
4. Individual creativity	Stifled	Encouraged	Not addressed
5. Member enthusiasm and morale	Low	High	Low
6. Group cohesiveness	Low	High	Low
7. Productivity	High	High (may not be as high as autocratic)	Low
8. Individual motivation and commitment	Low (tending to work only when leader is present to urge them to do so)	High (satisfaction derived from personal input and participation)	Low (feelings of frustration from lack of direction or guidance)

TABLE 8.2   MEMBER ROLES WITHIN GROUPS

ROLE	BEHAVIORS
Task Roles	
Coordinator	Clarifies ideas and suggestions that have been made within the group; brings relationships together to pursue common goals
Evaluator	Examines group plans and performance, measuring against group standards and goals
Elaborator	Explains and expands upon group plans and ideas
Energizer	Encourages and motivates group to perform at its maximum potential
Initiator	Outlines the task at hand for the group and proposes methods for solution
Orienter	Maintains direction within the group
Maintenance Roles	
Compromiser	Relieves conflict within the group by assisting members to reach a compromise agreeable to all
Encourager	Offers recognition and acceptance of others' ideas and contributions
Follower	Listens attentively to group interaction; is passive participant
Gatekeeper	Encourages acceptance of, and participation by, all members of the group
Harmonizer	Minimizes tension within the group by intervening when disagreements produce conflict
Individual (Personal) Roles	
Aggressor	Expresses negativism and hostility toward other members; may use sarcasm in effort to degrade the status of others
Blocker	Resists group efforts; demonstrates rigid and sometimes irrational behaviors that impede group progress
Dominator	Manipulates others to gain control; behaves in authoritarian manner
Help-seeker	Uses the group to gain sympathy from others; seeks to increase self-confidence from group feedback; lacks concern for others or for the group as a whole
Monopolizer	Maintains control of the group by dominating the conversation
Mute or silent member	Does not participate verbally; remains silent for a variety of reasons—may feel uncomfortable with self-disclosure or may be seeking attention through silence
Recognition-seeker	Talks about personal accomplishments in an effort to gain attention for self
Seducer	Shares intimate details about self with group; is the least reluctant of the group to do so; may frighten others in the group and inhibit group progress with excessive premature self-disclosure

SOURCE: Adapted from Benne & Sheats (1948).

stitutional effort of serving the consumer. Nurses are encouraged to use the steps of the nursing process as a framework for task group leadership.

In psychiatry, nurses may lead various types of therapeutic groups, such as client education, assertiveness training, support, parent, and transition to discharge groups, among others. To function effectively in the leadership capacity for these groups, nurses need to be able to recognize various processes that occur in groups (such as the phases of group development, the various roles that people play within group situations, and the motivation behind the behavior) and to be able to select the most appropriate leadership style for the type of group being led. Generalist nurses may develop these skills as part of their undergraduate education, or they may pursue additional study while serving and learning as the coleader of a group with a more experienced nurse leader.

Generalist nurses in psychiatry rarely serve as leaders of psychotherapy groups. ANA guidelines specify that nurses who serve as group psychotherapists should have a minimum of a master's degree in psychiatric nursing.

Other criteria that have been suggested are educational preparation in group theory, extended practice as a group coleader or leader under the supervision of an experienced psychotherapist, and participation in group therapy on an experiential level. Additional specialist training is required beyond the master's level to prepare nurses to become family therapists or psychodramatists.

Leading therapeutic groups is within the realm of nursing practice. Because group work is such a common therapeutic approach in the discipline of psychiatry, nurses working in this field must continually strive to expand their knowledge and use of group process as a significant psychiatric nursing intervention.

SUMMARY

A *group* has been defined as "a collection of individuals whose association is founded upon shared commonalities of interest, values, norms, or purpose." Groups serve various functions for their members. Eight group functions were defined by Sampson and Marthas (1990). They include *socialization, support, task completion, camaraderie, informational, normative, empowerment,* and *governance.*

Three types of groups were identified: (1) task groups, whose function it is to solve problems, make decisions, and achieve a specific outcome; (2) teaching groups, in which knowledge and information are conveyed to a number of individuals; and (3) supportive/therapeutic groups, whose function it is to educate people to deal effectively with emotional stress in their lives. Self-help groups can be beneficial to clients with specific problems. In self-help groups, members share the same problem and help each other to prevent decompensation related to that problem. Professionals may or may not be a part of self-help groups.

Group therapy is differentiated from *therapeutic groups* by degree of educational preparation of the leader. Group psychotherapists have advanced degrees in psychology, social work, medicine, or nursing. The focus of group psychotherapy is more theoretically based than it is in therapeutic groups.

Certain physical conditions, such as placement of the seating and size of the group, influence group interaction. Whether the group is open-ended or closed-ended can also affect group performance. In an *open-ended* group members leave and others join at any time during the existence of the group. *Closed-ended* groups have a predetermined, fixed time frame. All members join the group at the same time and leave at the end of the designated time period.

Yalom (1985) identified a number of benefits that individuals derive from participation in therapeutic groups. He called these benefits *curative factors.* They include the instillation of hope, universality, the imparting of information, altruism, the corrective recapitulation of the primary family group, the development of socializing techniques, imitative behavior, interpersonal learning, group cohesiveness, catharsis, and existential factors.

Groups progress through three major phases of development. In the initial (orientation) phase, members are introduced to each other, rules and goals of the group are established, and a trusting relationship is initiated. In the second phase, called the middle or working phase, the actual work of the group takes place. As the group matures, trust is established and members cooperate in decision making and problem solving, with the leader then serving more as a facilitator. The final or termination phase can be difficult, particularly if the group has been together for a long time. A sense of loss can trigger the grief response, and it is essential that members confront these feelings and work through them before the final session.

Group leadership styles may vary. The *autocratic* leader concentrates on fulfillment of his or her own objectives for the group. This is achieved through persuasive selling of personal ideas to the group. Productivity is high with this type of leader, but morale and motivation are low. With a *democratic* leader, group members are encouraged to participate fully in the decision-making process. The leader provides guidance and expertise as needed. Productivity is lower than with autocratic leadership, but morale and motivation are much higher. In a group with *laissez-faire* leadership, the members essentially receive no direction at all. Goals are not established, decisions are not made, everyone does as he or she pleases, and confusion prevails. Productivity, morale, and motivation are low.

Members play various roles within groups. These roles are categorized according to *task roles, maintenance roles,* and *personal roles.* Task roles and maintenance roles contribute to the success or effectiveness of the group. Personal roles satisfy needs of the individual members, sometimes to the extent of interfering with the effectiveness of the group.

Psychodrama is a specialized type of group therapy that uses a dramatic approach in which clients become "actors" in life-situation scenarios. The psychodrama setting provides the client with a safer and less threatening atmosphere than the real situation in which to express and work through unresolved conflicts. Specialized training, in addition to a master's degree, is required for nurses to serve as psychodramatists.

Nurses lead various types of therapeutic groups in the psychiatric setting. Knowledge of human behavior in general and the group process in particular is essential to effective group leadership.

REVIEW QUESTIONS

SELF-EXAMINATION/LEARNING EXERCISE

Test your knowledge of group process by supplying the information requested.

1. Define a *group*.

2. Identify the type of group and leadership style in each of the following situations:

   a. NJ is the nurse leader of a childbirth preparation group. Each week she shows various films and sets out various reading materials. She expects the participants to utilize their time on a topic of their choice or practice skills they have observed in the films. Two couples have dropped out of the group, stating, "This is a big waste of time."

   Type of group _____

   Style of leadership _____

   b. MK is a psychiatric nurse who has been selected to lead a group for women who desire to lose weight. The criteria for membership is that they must be at least 20 lb overweight. All have tried to lose weight on their own many times in the past without success. At their first meeting, MK provides suggestions as the members determine what their goals will be and how they plan to go about achieving those goals. They decided how often they wanted to meet and what they plan to do at each meeting.

   Type of group _____

   Style of leadership _____

   c. JJ is a staff nurse on a surgical unit. He has been selected as leader of a newly established group of staff nurses organized to determine ways to decrease the number of medication errors occurring on the unit. JJ has definite ideas about how to bring this about. He has also applied for the position of Head Nurse on the unit and believes that if he is successful in leading the group toward achievement of its goals, he can also facilitate his chances for promotion. At each meeting he addresses the group in an effort to convince the members to adopt his ideas.

   Type of group _____

   Style of leadership _____

3. Match the situation on the right to the curative factor or benefit it describes on the left.

   _____ 1. Instillation of hope

   _____ 2. Universality

   _____ 3. Imparting of information

   _____ 4. Altruism

   _____ 5. Corrective recapitulation of the primary family group

   _____ 6. Development of socializing techniques

   _____ 7. Imitative behavior

   _____ 8. Interpersonal learning

   a. Sam admires the way Jack stands up for what he believes. He decides to practice this himself.

   b. Nancy sees that Jane has been a widow for 5 years now and has adjusted well. She thinks maybe she can too.

   c. Susan has come to realize that she has the power to shape the direction of her life.

   d. John is able to have a discussion with another person for the first time in his life.

   e. Linda now understands that her mother really did love her, although she was not able to show it.

   f. Alice has come to feel as though the other group members are like a family to her. She looks forward to the meetings each week.

   g. Tony talks in the group about the abuse he experienced as a child. He has never told anyone about this before.

   h. Sandra felt so good about herself when she left group tonight. She had provided both physical and emotional support to Judy, who shared for the first time about being raped.

   i. Judy appreciated Sandra's support as she expressed her feelings related to the rape. She had come to believe that no one else felt as she did.

_____ 9. Group cohesiveness

_____ 10. Catharsis

_____ 11. Existential factors

j. Paul knew that people did not want to be his friend because of his violent temper. In the group he has learned to control his temper and form satisfactory interpersonal relationships with others.

k. Henry learned about the effects of alcohol on the body when a nurse from the chemical dependency unit spoke to the group.

4. Match the individual on the right to the role he or she is playing within the group.

_____ 1. Aggressor

_____ 2. Blocker

_____ 3. Dominator

_____ 4. Help-seeker

_____ 5. Monopolizer

_____ 6. Mute or silent member

_____ 7. Recognition-seeker

_____ 8. Seducer

a. Nancy talks incessantly in group. When someone else tries to make a comment, she refuses to allow them to speak.

b. On the first day the group meets, Valarie shares the intimate details of her incestual relationship with her father.

c. Colleen listens with interest to everything the other members say, but she does not say anything herself in group.

d. Violet is obsessed with her physical appearance. Although she is beautiful, she has little self-confidence and needs continuous positive feedback. She states, "Maybe if I became a blonde my boyfriend would love me more."

e. Larry states to Violet, "Listen, dummy, you need more than blonde hair to keep the guy around. A bit more in the brains department would help!"

f. At the beginning of the group meeting Dan says, "All right now, I have a date tonight. I want this meeting over on time! I'll keep track of the time and let everyone know when their time is up. When I say you're done, you're done, understand?"

g. Joyce says, "I won my first beauty contest when I was 6 months old. Can you imagine? And I've been winning them ever since. I was prom queen when I was 16, Miss Rose Petal when I was 19, Miss Silver City at 21. And next I go to the state contest. It's just all so exciting!"

h. Joe, an RN on the care-planning committee, says, "What a stupid suggestion. Nursing Diagnosis!?! I won't even discuss the matter. We have been doing our care plans this way for 20 years. I refuse to even consider changing."

REFERENCES

Benne, K.B., & Sheats, P. (1948, Spring). Functional roles of group members. *Journal of Social Issues, 4*(2), 42–49.

Boyer, V.B. (1982). Process and content: Distinctions and implications. In E.H. Janosik & L.B. Phipps (Eds.), *Life cycle group work in nursing.* Monterey, CA: Wadsworth Health Sciences.

Clark, C.C. (1987). *The nurse as group leader* (2nd ed.). New York: Springer.

Lego, S. (1987). Group psychotherapy. In J. Haber, P.P. Hoskins, A.M. Leach, & B.F. Sidelau (Eds.), *Comprehensive psychiatric nursing* (3rd ed.). New York: McGraw-Hill.

Lippitt, R., & White, R.K. (1958). An experimental study of leadership and group life. In E.E. Maccoby, T.M. Newcomb, & E.L. Hartley (Eds.), *Readings in social psychology* (3rd ed.). New York: Holt, Rinehart & Winston.

Newton, G. (1984). Self-help groups. *Journal of Psychosocial Nursing and Mental Health Services, 22*(7), 27–31.

Sampson, E.E., & Marthas, M. (1990). *Group process for the health professions* (3rd ed.). Albany, NY: Delmar Publishers.

Yalom, I. (1985). *The theory and practice of group psychotherapy* (3rd ed.). New York: Basic Books.

Bibliography

Blatner, A. (1995). Psychodrama. In R.J. Corsini & D. Wedding (Eds.), *Current Psychotherapies* (5th ed.). Itasca, IL: F.E. Peacock.

Clarke, D.E., Adomoski, E., & Joyce, B. (1998). Inpatient group psychotherapy: The role of the staff nurse. *Journal of Psychosocial Nursing, 36*(5): 22–26.

Friedman, W.H. (1994). *How to do groups* (2nd ed.). Northvale, NJ: Jason Aronson Inc.

Hare, A.P. (1952). A study of interaction and consensus in different sized groups. *American Sociological Review, 17,* 261–267.

Larson, M.L., & Williams, R.A. (1978, August). How to become a better group leader? *Nursing78,* 65–72.

Pollack, L. (1995). Treatment of inpatients with bipolar disorder: A role for self-management groups. *Journal of Psychosocial Nursing, 33*(1): 11–16.

Staples, N., & Schwartz M. (1990). Anorexia nervosa support group: Providing transitional support. *Journal of Psychosocial Nursing, 28*(2): 6.

Yalom, I.E., & Vinogradov, S. (1989). *Group psychotherapy.* Washington, DC: American Psychiatric Press.

INTERVENTION WITH FAMILIES

CHAPTER OUTLINE

OBJECTIVES

INTRODUCTION

STAGES OF FAMILY DEVELOPMENT

MAJOR VARIATIONS

FAMILY FUNCTIONING

THERAPEUTIC MODALITIES WITH FAMILIES

THE NURSING PROCESS—A CASE STUDY

SUMMARY

REVIEW QUESTIONS

KEY TERMS

double-bind communication
family system
triangles
scapegoating
genogram
subsystems

boundaries
disengagement
enmeshment
family structure
pseudomutuality
pseudohostility

marital schism
marital skew
paradoxical intervention
reframing

OBJECTIVES

After reading this chapter, the student will be able to:

1. Define the term *family*.
2. Identify stages of family development.
3. Describe major variations to the American middle-class family life cycle.
4. Discuss characteristics of adaptive family functioning.
5. Describe behaviors that interfere with adaptive family functioning.
6. Discuss the essential components of family systems, structural, and strategic therapies.
7. Construct a family genogram.
8. Apply the steps of the nursing process in therapeutic intervention with families.

hat is a family? Wright and Leahey (1994) propose the following definition: a family is who they say they are. Many family forms exist within society today, such as the biological family of procreation, the nuclear family that incorporates one or more members of the extended family (family of origin), the sole-parent family, the stepfamily, the communal family, and the homosexual couple or family. However, labeling individuals as "families" based on their group composition may not be the best way. Instead, family consideration may be more appropriately determined based on attributes of affection, strong emotional ties, a sense of belonging, and durability of membership (Wright & Leahey, 1994).

Many nurses have interactions with family members on a daily basis. A client's illness or hospitalization affects all members of the family, and nurses must understand how to work with the family as a unit, knowing that family members can have a profound effect on the client's healing process.

Nurse generalists should be familiar with the tasks associated with adaptive family functioning. With this knowledge, they are able to assess family interaction and recognize when problems arise. They can provide support to families with an ill member and make referrals to other professionals when assistance is required to restore adaptive functioning.

Nurse specialists usually possess an advanced degree in nursing. Some nurse specialists have education or experience that qualifies them to perform family therapy. Family therapy is broadly defined as "the attempt to modify the relationships in a family to achieve harmony" (Foley, 1979). Family therapy has a strong theoretical focus, and a number of conceptual approaches have been introduced and suggested as frameworks for this intervention.

This chapter explores the stages of family development and compares the "typical" family within various subcultures. Characteristics of adaptive family functioning, as well as behaviors that interfere with this adaptation, are discussed. Theoretical components of selected therapeutic approaches are described. Instructions for construction of a family genogram are included. Nursing process provides the framework for nursing intervention with families.

STAGES OF FAMILY DEVELOPMENT

Carter and McGoldrick (1989) have identified six stages that describe the life cycle of the North American middle-class family. It is acknowledged that these tasks would vary greatly among cultural groups, as well as the various forms of families previously described. However, these stages provide a valuable framework from which the nurse may study families, emphasizing expansion (the addition of members), contraction (the loss of members), and realignment of relationships as members experience devel-

opmental changes. These stages of family development are summarized in Table 9.1.

Stage I. The Single Young Adult

This model begins with the launching of the young adult from the family of origin. This is a difficult stage, as the young adult must decide what social standards from the family of origin will be preserved and what they will change for themselves to be incorporated into a new family. Tasks of this stage include forming an identity separate from the parents, establishing intimate peer relationships, and advancing toward financial independence. Problems can arise when either the young adults or the parents encounter difficulty terminating the interdependent relationship that has existed in the family of origin.

Stage II. The Newly Married Couple

Marriage is a difficult transition because renegotiation must include the integration of contrasting issues that each partner brings to the relationship, as well as issues they may have redefined for themselves as a couple. In addition, the new couple must renegotiate relationships with parents, siblings, and other relatives in view of the new marriage (L'Abate, Ganahl, & Hansen, 1986). Tasks of this stage include establishing a new identity as a couple, realigning relationships with members of extended family, and making decisions about having children. Problems can arise if either partner remains too enmeshed with their family of origin or when the couple chooses to cut themselves off completely from extended family (L'Abate, Ganahl, & Hansen, 1986).

Stage III. The Family With Young Children

Adjustments in relationships must occur with the arrival of children. The entire family system is affected and role realignments are necessary for both new parents and new grandparents. Tasks of this stage include making adjustments within the marital system to meet the responsibilities associated with parenthood while maintaining the integrity of the couple relationship, sharing equally in the tasks of childrearing, and integrating the roles of extended family members into the newly expanded family organization. Problems can arise when parents lack knowledge about normal childhood development and adequate patience to allow children to express themselves through behavior.

Stage IV. The Family With Adolescents

This stage of family development is characterized by a great deal of turmoil and transition. Both parents, who are

TABLE 9.1 STAGES OF THE NORTH AMERICAN MIDDLE-CLASS FAMILY LIFE CYCLE

FAMILY LIFE CYCLE STAGES	EMOTIONAL PROCESS OF TRANSITION: KEY PRINCIPLES	CHANGES REQUIRED IN FAMILY STATUS TO PROCEED DEVELOPMENTALLY
I. The Single Young Adult	Accepting separation from parents and responsibility for self	Differentiation of self in relation to family of origin Development of intimate peer relationships Establishment of self in work
II. The Newly Married Couple	Commitment to new system	Formation of marital system Realignment of relationships with extended families and friends to include spouse
III. The Family With Young Children	Accepting new generation of members into the system	Adjusting marital system to make space for child(ren) Taking on parenting roles Realignment of relationships with extended family to include parenting and grandparenting roles
IV. The Family With Adolescents	Increasing flexibility of family boundaries to include children's independence and grandparents' increasing dependence	Shifting of parent-child relationships to permit adolescents to move in and out of system Refocus on midlife marital and career issues Beginning shift toward concerns for older generation
V. The Family Launching Grown Children	Accepting a multitude of exits from and entries into the family system	Renegotiation of marital system as a dyad Development of adult-to-adult relationships between grown children and their parents Realignment of relationships to include in-laws and grandchildren Dealing with disabilities and death of parents (grandparents)
VI. The Family in Later Life	Accepting the shifting of generational roles	Maintaining own and/or couple functioning and interests in face of physiological decline; exploration of new familial and social role options Support for a more central role for middle generation Making room in the system for the wisdom and experience of the elderly; supporting the older generation without overfunctioning for them Dealing with loss of spouse, siblings, and other peers, and preparation for own death; life review and integration

SOURCE: From Carter, B & McGoldrick, M (eds): The changing family life cycle: A framework for family therapy (2nd ed.). Copyright © 1989 by Allyn and Bacon. Reprinted by permission.

approaching a midlife stage, and adolescents are undergoing biological, emotional, and sociocultural changes that place demands on each individual, as well as on the family unit. Grandparents, too, may require assistance with the tasks of later life. These developments can create a "sandwich" effect for the parents, who must deal with issues confronting three generations. Tasks of this stage include redefining the level of dependence so that adolescents are provided with greater autonomy while parents remain responsive to the teenager's dependency needs. Midlife issues related to marriage, career, and aging parents must also be resolved during this period. Problems can arise when parents are unable to relinquish control and allow the adolescent greater autonomy and freedom to make independent decisions, or when parents are unable to agree and support each other in this effort.

Stage V. The Family Launching Grown Children

A great deal of realignment of family roles occurs during this stage. This stage is characterized by the intermittent exiting and entering of various family members. Children leave home for further education and careers; marriages occur, and new spouses, in-laws, and children enter the system; and new grandparent roles are established. Adult-to-adult relationships are renegotiated between grown children and their parents. Tasks associated with this stage include reestablishing the bond of the dyadic marital relationship; realigning relationships to include grown children, in-laws, and new grandchildren; and accepting the additional caretaking responsibilities and eventual death of elderly parents. Problems can arise when feelings of loss and depression become overwhelming in response to the departure of children from the home, when parents are unable to accept their children as adults or cope with the disability or death of their own parents, and when the marital bond has deteriorated.

Stage VI. The Family in Later Life

This stage begins with retirement and lasts until the death of both spouses (Wright & Leahey, 1994). Most adults in their later years are still a prominent part of the family system, and many are able to offer support to their grown children in the middle generation. Tasks associated with this stage include exploring new social roles related to retirement and possible change in socioeconomic status; accepting some decline in physiological functioning; dealing with the deaths of spouse, siblings, and friends; and confronting and preparing for one's own death. Problems may arise when older adults have failed to fulfill the tasks associated with earlier levels of development and are dissatisfied with the way their lives have gone. They are unable to find happiness in retirement or emotional satisfaction with children and grandchildren, and they are unable to accept the deaths of loved ones or to prepare for their own impending death.

MAJOR VARIATIONS

Divorce

Carter and McGoldrick (1989) also discuss stages and tasks of families experiencing divorce and remarriage. In 1982, nearly half of all American marriages ended in divorce (Messinger, 1982). Some statistics indicate that the divorce rate may be on the decline since the 1970s. However, in 1988, 11 percent of all families in the United States were headed by solo parents (Glick, 1989). Stages in the family life cycle of divorce include deciding to divorce, planning the break-up of the system, separation, and divorce. Tasks include accepting one's own part in the failure of the marriage, working cooperatively on problems related to custody and visitation of children and finances, realigning relationships with extended family, and mourning the loss of the marriage relationship and the intact family.

After the divorce, the custodial parent must adjust to functioning as the single leader of an ongoing family, while working to rebuild a new social network. The noncustodial parent must find ways to continue to be an effective parent while remaining outside the normal parenting role (L'Abate, Ganahl, & Hansen, 1986).

Remarriage

Studies suggest that between two thirds and three fourths of those who divorce will eventually remarry (Glick,

1989). In 1987, an estimated 11 million remarried families and 4.3 million stepfamilies were living in the United States (Glick, 1989). The challenges that face the joining of two established families are immense, and statistics reveal that the rate of redivorce for remarried couples is even higher than the divorce rate following first marriages (Pill, 1990). Stages in the remarried family life cycle include entering the new relationship, planning the new marriage and family, and remarriage and reestablishment of family. Tasks include making a firm commitment to confronting the complexities of combining two families, maintaining open communication, facing fears, realigning relationships with extended family to include new spouse and children, and encouraging healthy relationships with biological (noncustodial) parents and grandparents.

Problems can arise when there is a blurring of boundaries between the custodial and noncustodial families. Children may contemplate, "Who is the boss now? Who is most important, the child or the new spouse? Mom loves her new husband more than she loves me. Dad lets me do more than my new stepdad. I don't have to mind him; he's not my real dad." Confusion and distress for both the children and the parents can be avoided with the establishment of clear boundaries (Ahrons & Perlmutter, 1982).

L'Abate, Ganahl, and Hansen (1986) state:

"The most common problem in a remarriage family is the development of an adversarial relationship between the new stepparent and the biological parent. Both individuals may feel some conflict and role strain, and if the children are caught in between, it will be a negative factor in the children's development and the restructuring of the new family."

Cultural Variations

It is difficult to generalize about variations in family life-cycle development according to culture. Most families have become acculturated to the American society and conform to the life-cycle stages previously described. However, cultural diversity does exist and nurses must be aware of possible differences in family expectations related to sociocultural beliefs. They must also be aware of a great deal of variation within ethnic groups as well as among them. Some variations that may be considered follow.

Marriage

A number of American subcultures maintain traditional values in terms of marriage. Traditional views about family life and Roman Catholicism exert important influences upon attitudes toward marriage in many Italian American and Latino American families. Although the tradition of arranged marriages is disappearing in Asian American families, there is still frequently a much stronger influence by the family on mate selection than there is for other cultures in the United States (Shon & Ja, 1982). In these subcultures, the father is considered the authority figure and head of the household and the mother assumes the role of homemaker and caretaker. Family loyalty is intense and a breach of this loyalty brings considerable shame to the family.

Herz and Rosen (1982) make the following statement about Jewish families:

"The importance of the family is commonly expressed in the images of the Jewish man as a good father, husband, and provider and the Jewish woman as devoted wife and mother of intelligent children. Pressure is exerted upon men and women to marry. Intermarriage has always been perceived as the most flagrant breach of family togetherness, and total emotional cutoffs are not uncommon in such instances."

Children

In traditional Latino American and Italian American cultures, children are central to the family system. Many of these individuals have strong ties to Roman Catholicism, which historically has promoted marital relations for procreation only and encouraged families to have large numbers of children. Regarding birth control, the Catechism of the Catholic Church (1995) states, "Periodic continence, that is, the methods of birth regulation based on self-observation and the use of infertile periods, is in conformity with the objective criteria of morality." In the traditional Jewish community, having children is seen as a scriptural and social obligation. "You shall be fruitful and multiply" is the first commandment in the Torah (Herz & Rosen, 1982).

In traditional Asian American cultures, sons are clearly more highly valued than are daughters, and the most important child is the oldest son (Shon & Ja, 1982). Younger siblings are expected to follow the guidance of the oldest son throughout their lives, and when the father dies, the oldest son takes over the leadership of the family.

In all of these cultures, children are expected to be respectful of their parents and not bring shame to the family. Especially in Asian cultures, children learn a sense of obligation to their parents for bringing them into this world and caring for them when they were helpless. This is viewed as a debt that can never be truly repaid, and no matter what the parents may do the child is still obligated to give respect and obedience (Shon & Ja, 1982).

Extended Family

Extended family plays a central role in all aspects of Italian family life, including decision making (Rotunno & McGoldrick, 1982). Respect for and responsibility toward older family members is a strong norm, and families strongly resist admitting elderly relatives to nursing homes.

In some American subcultures, such as Asian, Latino, Italian, and Iranian, it is not uncommon to find several generations living together. Older family members are valued for their experience and wisdom. Because extended families often share living quarters, or at least live nearby, tasks of childrearing may be shared by several generations.

Divorce

In the Jewish community, divorce is often seen as a violation of family togetherness (Herz & Rosen, 1982). Some Jewish parents take their child's divorce personally, with the response, "How could you possibly do this to me?"

Because Roman Catholicism has traditionally opposed divorce, those cultures that are largely Catholic have followed this dictate. Historically, a low divorce rate has existed among Italian Americans, Irish Americans, and Latino Americans. However, the number of divorces among these subcultures is on the rise, particularly in successive generations that have become more acculturated into a society where divorce is more acceptable.

FAMILY FUNCTIONING

Boyer and Jeffrey (1984) describe six elements on which families are assessed to be either functional or dysfunctional. Each can be viewed on a continuum, although families rarely fall at extreme ends of the continuum. Rather, they tend to be dynamic and fluctuate from one point to another within the different areas. These six elements of assessment are described below and summarized in Table 9.2.

Communication

Functional communication patterns are those in which verbal and nonverbal messages are clear, direct, and congruent between sender and intended receiver. Family members are encouraged to express honest feelings and opinions, and all members participate in decisions that affect the family system. Each member is an active listener to the other members of the family.

Behaviors that interfere with functional communication include the following.

Making Assumptions

With this behavior, one assumes that others will know what is meant by an action or an expression (or sometimes even what one is thinking); or, on the other hand, assumes

TABLE 9.2   FAMILY FUNCTIONING: ELEMENTS OF ASSESSMENT

| ELEMENTS OF ASSESSMENT | CONTINUUM | |
	FUNCTIONAL	DYSFUNCTIONAL
Communication	Clear, direct, open, and honest, with congruence between verbal and nonverbal	Indirect, vague, controlled, with many double-bind messages
Self-concept reinforcement	Supportive, loving, praising, approving, with behaviors that instill confidence	Unsupportive, blaming, "put-downs," refusing to allow self-responsibility
Family members' expectations	Flexible, realistic, individualized	Judgmental, rigid, controlling, ignoring individuality
Handling differences	Tolerant, dynamic, negotiating	Attacking, avoiding, surrendering
Family interactional patterns	Workable, constructive, flexible, and promoting the needs of all members	Contradictory, rigid, self-defeating, and destructive
Family climate	Trusting, growth-promoting, caring, general feeling of well-being	Distrusting, emotionally painful, with absence of hope for improvement

SOURCE: Adapted from Boyer & Jeffrey (1984).

to know what another member is thinking or feeling without checking to make certain.

Example. A mother says to her teenage daughter, "You should have known that I expected you to clean up the kitchen while I was gone!"

Belittling Feelings

This action involves ignoring or minimizing another's feelings when they are expressed. This encourages the individual to withhold honest feelings to avoid being hurt by the negative response.

Example. When the young woman confides to her mother that she is angry because the grandfather has touched her breast, the mother responds, "Oh, don't be angry. He doesn't mean anything by that."

Failing to Listen

With this behavior, one does not hear what the other individual is saying. This can mean not hearing the words by "tuning out" what is being said, or it can be "selective" listening, in which a person hears only a selective part of the message or interprets it in a selective manner.

Example. The father explains to Johnny, "If the contract comes through and I get this new job, we'll have a little extra money and we will consider sending you to State U." Johnny relays the message to his friend, "Dad says I can go to State U!"

Communicating Indirectly

This usually means that an individual does not or cannot present a message to a receiver directly, so seeks to communicate through a third person.

Example. A father does not want his teenage daughter

to see a certain boyfriend, but wants to avoid the angry response he expects from his daughter if he tells her so. He expresses his feelings to his wife, hoping she will share them with their daughter.

Presenting Double-Bind Messages

Double-bind communication conveys a "damned if I do and damned if I don't" message. A family member may respond to a direct request by another family member, only to be rebuked when the request is fulfilled.

Example. The father tells his son he is spending too much time playing football and falling down in his grades. He is expected to bring his grades up over the next 9 weeks or he gets his car taken away. When the son tells the father he has quit the football team so he can study more, Dad responds angrily, "I won't allow any son of mine to be a quitter!"

Self-Concept Reinforcement

Functional families strive to reinforce and strengthen each member's self-concept, with the positive results being that family members feel loved and valued. Boyer and Jeffrey (1984) state:

> "The manner in which children see and value themselves is influenced most significantly by the messages they receive concerning their value to other members of the family. Messages that convey praise, approval, appreciation, trust, and confidence in decisions and that allow family members to pursue individual needs and ultimately to become independent are the foundation blocks of a child's feelings of self-worth. Adults also need and depend heavily on this kind of reinforcement for their own emotional well-being." (p. 27)

Behaviors that interfere with self-concept reinforcement follow.

Expressing Denigrating Remarks

These remarks are commonly called "put downs." Individuals receive messages that they are worthless or unloved.

Example. A child spills a glass of milk at the table. The mother responds, "You are hopeless! How could anybody be so clumsy?!"

Withholding Supportive Messages

Some family members find it very difficult to provide others with reinforcing and supportive messages. This may be because they themselves have not been the recipients of reinforcement from significant others and have not learned how to provide support to others.

Example. A 10-year-old boy playing Little League baseball retrieves the ball and throws it to second base for an out. After the game he says to his Dad, "Did you see my play on second base?" Dad responds, "Yes, I did, son, but if you had been paying better attention, you could have caught the ball for a direct and immediate out."

Taking Over

This occurs when one family member fails to permit another member to develop a sense of responsibility and self-worth, by doing things for the individual instead of allowing him or her to manage the situation independently.

Example. Twelve-year-old Eric has a job delivering the evening paper, which he usually begins right after school. Today he must serve a 1-hour detention after school for being late to class yesterday. He tells his Mom, "Tommy said he would throw my papers for me today if I help him wash his Dad's car on Saturday." Mom responds, "Never mind. Tell Tommy to forget it. I'll take care of your paper route today."

Family Members' Expectations

All individuals have some expectations about the outcomes of the life situations they experience. These expectations are related to and significantly influenced by earlier life experiences. In functional families, expectations are realistic, thereby avoiding setting family members up for failure. In functional families, expectations are also flexible. Life situations are full of extraneous and unexpected interferences. Flexibility allows for changes and interruptions to occur without creating conflict. Finally, in functional families, expectations are individualized. Each family member is different, with different strengths and limitations. The outcome of a life situation for one family member may not be realistic for another. Each member must be valued independently, and comparison among members avoided.

Behaviors that interfere with adaptive functioning in terms of member expectations include the following.

Ignoring Individuality

This occurs when family members expect others to do things or behave in ways that do not fit with the latter's individuality or current life situation (Boyer & Jeffrey, 1984). This sometimes happens when parents expect their children to fulfill the hopes and dreams the parents have failed to achieve, when the children have their own, different hopes and dreams.

Example. Bob, an only child, leaves for college next year. Bob's father, Robert, inherited a hardware store that was founded by Bob's great-grandfather and has been in the family for three generations. Robert expects Bob to major in business, work in the store after college, and take over the business when Robert retires. Bob, however, has a talent for writing; he wants to major in journalism and work on a big-city newspaper when he graduates. Robert sees this as a betrayal of the family.

Demanding Proof of Love

Boyer and Jeffrey (1984) state, "Family members place expectations on others' behavior that are used as standards by which the expecting member determines how much the other members care for him or her. The message attached to these expectations is: 'If you will not be as I wish you to be, you don't love me.' "

Example. This is the message that Bob receives from his father in the example cited in the previous paragraph.

Handling Differences

It is difficult to conceive of two or more individuals living together who agree on everything all of the time. Serious problems in a family's functioning appear when differences become equated with "badness" or when disagreement is seen as "not caring" (Boyer & Jeffrey, 1984). Members of a functional family understand that it is acceptable to disagree and deal with differences in an open, nonattacking manner. Members are willing to hear the other person's position, respect the other person's right to hold an opposing position, and work to modify the expectations on both sides of the issue in order to negotiate a workable solution.

Behaviors that interfere with successful family negotiations are as follows.

Attacking

A difference of opinion can deteriorate into a direct personal attack and may be manifested by blaming another person, bringing up the past, making destructive comparisons, or lashing out with other expressions of anger and hurt (Boyer & Jeffrey, 1984).

Example. When Nancy's husband, John, buys an expensive set of golf clubs, Nancy responds, "How could you do such a thing? You know we can't afford those! No wonder we don't have a nice house like all our friends. You spend all our money before we can save for a down payment. You're so selfish! We'll never have anything nice and it's all your fault!"

Avoiding

With this tactic, differences are never acknowledged openly. The individual who disagrees avoids discussing it for fear that the other person will withdraw love or approval or become angry in response to the disagreement. Avoidance also occurs when an individual fears loss of control of his or her temper if the disagreement is brought out into the open.

Example. Vicki and Clint have been married 6 months. This is Vicki's second marriage and she has a 4-year-old son from her first marriage, Derek, who lives with her and Clint. Both Vicki and Clint work, and Derek goes to day care. Since the marriage 6 months ago, Derek cries every night continuously unless Vicki spends all her time with him, which she does in order to keep him quiet. Clint resents this but says nothing for fear he will come across as interfering; however, he has started going back to work in his office in the evenings to avoid the family situation.

Surrendering

The person who surrenders in the face of disagreement does so at the expense of denying his or her own needs or rights. The individual avoids expressing a difference of opinion for fear of angering another person or of losing approval and support.

Example. Elaine is the only child of wealthy parents. She attends an exclusive private college in a small New England town, where she met Andrew, the son of a farming couple from the area. Andrew attended the local community college for 2 years but chose to work on his parents' farm rather than continue college. Elaine and Andrew love each other and want to be married, but Elaine's parents say they will disown her if she marries Andrew, who they believe is below her social status. Elaine breaks off her relationship with Andrew rather than challenge her parents' wishes.

Family Interactional Patterns

Interactional patterns have to do with the ways in which families "behave." All families develop recurring, predictable patterns of interaction over time. These are often thought of as "family rules." The mentality conveys "this is the way we have always done it" and provides a sense of security and stability for family members that comes from predictability. These interactions may have to do with communication, self-concept reinforcement, expressing expectations, and handling differences (all of the behaviors that were discussed previously), but because they are repetitive, and recur over time, they become the "rules" that govern patterns of interaction among family members.

Family rules are functional when they are workable, are constructive, and promote the needs of all family members. They are dysfunctional when they become contradictory, self-defeating, and destructive. Family therapists often find that individuals are unaware that dysfunctional family rules exist and may vehemently deny their existence even when confronted with a specific behavioral interaction. The development of dysfunctional interactional patterns occurs through a habituation process and out of fear of change or reprisal or a lack of knowledge as to how a given situation might be handled differently (Boyer & Jeffrey, 1984). Many are derived out of the parents' own growing-up experiences.

Patterns of interaction that interfere with adaptive family functioning include the following.

Patterns That Cause Emotional Discomfort

Interactions can promote hurt and anger in family members. This is particularly true of emotions that individuals feel uncomfortable expressing or are not permitted (according to "family rules") to express openly. These interactional patterns include behaviors such as never apologizing or never admitting that one has made a mistake, forbidding flexibility in life situations ("you must do it my way, or you will not do it at all"), making statements that devalue the worth of others, or withholding statements that promote increased self-worth.

Example. Priscilla and Bill had been discussing buying a new car but could not agree on the make or model to buy. One day, Bill appeared at Priscilla's office over the lunch hour and said, "Come outside and see our new car." In front of the building, Bill had parked a brand-new sports car that he explained he had purchased with their combined savings. Priscilla was furious, but kept quiet and proceeded to finish her workday. At home she expressed her anger to Bill for making the purchase without consulting her. Bill refused to apologize or admit to making a mistake. They both remained cool and hardly spoke to each other for weeks.

Patterns That Perpetuate or Intensify Problems Rather Than Solve Them

When problems go unresolved over a long period of time, it sometimes appears to be easier just to ignore them. If problems of the same nature occur, the tendency to ignore them then becomes the safe and predictable pattern of interaction for dealing with this type of situation. This may occur until the problem intensifies to a point when it can no longer be ignored.

Example. Dan works hard in the automobile factory and demands peace and quiet from his family when he comes home from work. His children have learned over the years not to share their problems with him because they fear his explosive temper. Their mother attempts to handle unpleasant situations alone as best she can. When son Ron was expelled from school for being caught the third time smoking pot, Dan yelled, "Why wasn't I told about this before?"

Patterns That Are in Conflict With Each Other

Some family rules may appear to be functional—very workable and constructive—on the surface but in practice may serve to destroy healthy interactional patterns. Boyer and Jeffrey (1984) describe the following scenario as an example.

Example. Dad insists that all members of the family eat dinner together every evening. No one may leave the table until everyone is finished because dinnertime is one of the few times left when the family can be together. Yet Dad frequently uses the time to reprimand Bobby about his poor grades in math, to scold Ann for her sloppy room, or to make not-so-subtle gibes at Mom for "spending all day on the telephone and never getting anything accomplished."

Family Climate

The atmosphere or climate of a family is composed of a blend of the feelings and experiences that are the result of family members' verbal and nonverbal sharing and interacting. Boyer and Jeffrey (1984) suggest that a positive family climate is founded on trust and is reflected in openness, appropriate humor and laughter, expressions of caring, mutual respect, a valuing of the quality of each individual, and a general feeling of well-being. A dysfunctional family climate is evidenced by tension, pain, physical disabilities, frustration, guilt, persistent anger, and feelings of hopelessness.

THERAPEUTIC MODALITIES WITH FAMILIES

The Family as a System

General systems theory is a way of organizing thought according to the holistic perspective. A system is considered greater than the sum of its parts. A system is considered dynamic and ever-changing. A change in one part of the system causes a change in the other parts of the system and in the system as a whole. When studying families, it is helpful to conceptualize a hierarchy of systems.

The family can be viewed as a system composed of various subsystems, such as the marital subsystem, parent-child subsystems, and sibling subsystems. Each of these subsystems is further divided into subsystems of individuals. The **family system** is also a subsystem of a larger suprasystem, such as the neighborhood or community. A schematic of a hierarchy of systems is presented in Figure 9.1.

Major Concepts

Bowen (1978) has done a great deal of work with families using a systems approach. Bowen's theoretical approach to family therapy is composed of eight major concepts: (1) differentiation of self, (2) triangles, (3) nuclear family emotional process, (4) family projection process, (5) multigenerational transmission process, (6) sibling position profiles, (7) emotional cutoff, and (8) societal regression.

Differentiation of Self. Differentiation of self is the ability to define oneself as a separate being. Freeman (1981) characterizes emotionally differentiated individuals as those who are "able to define who they are, what they want, what they think, what their goals are, and what they are prepared to work on, in a way that is minimally influenced by others."

The degree of differentiation of self can be viewed on a continuum from high levels, in which an individual manifests a clearly defined sense of self, to low levels, or undifferentiated, in which emotional fusion exists and the individual is unable to function separately from a relationship system. Healthy families encourage differentiation, and the process of separation from the family ego mass is most pronounced during the ages of 2 to 5 and again between the ages of 13 and 15 (Freeman, 1981). Families that do not understand the child's need to be different during these times may perceive their behavior as objectionable.

Bowen (1971) uses the term *stuck-togetherness* to describe the family with the fused ego mass. When family fusion occurs, none of the members has a true sense of self as an independent individual. Boundaries between members are blurred, and the family becomes enmeshed without individual distinguishing characteristics. In this situation, family members can neither gain true intimacy nor separate and become individuals. They have a quality of *stuck-togetherness* that gives them no freedom or option to move closer or to get away (Foley, 1979).

Triangles. The concept of **triangle** refers to a three-person emotional configuration which is considered the basic building block of the family system. Bowen (1978) offers the following description of triangles:

> "The basic building block of any emotional system is the triangle. When emotional tension in a two-person system exceeds a certain level, it triangles in a third person, permitting the tension to shift about within the triangle. Any two in the original triangle can add a new triangle. An emotional system is composed of a series of interlocking triangles." (p. 306)

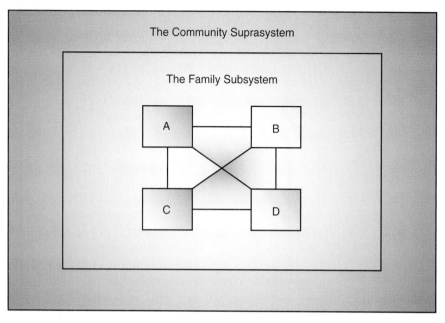

The Community Suprasystem

The Family Subsystem

Key: A = Father Subsystem
      B = Mother Subsystem
      C = Child Subsystem
      D = Child Subsystem
      AB = Marital Subsystem

      CD = Sibling Subsystem
      AD = Parent-child Subsystem
      BC = Parent-child Subsystem
      AC = Parent-child Subsystem
      BD = Parent-child Subsystem

Figure 9.1   A hierarchy of systems.

Triangles are dysfunctional in that they offer relief from anxiety through diversion rather than through resolution of the issue. For example, when stress develops in a marital relationship, the couple may redirect their attention to a child, whose misbehavior gives them something aside from the tension in their relationship on which to focus. When the dynamics within a triangle stabilize, a fourth person may be brought in to form additional triangles, in an effort to reduce tension. This triangulation can continue almost indefinitely as extended family and people outside the family, including the family therapist, can become entangled in the process. The therapist working with families must strive to remain de-triangled from this emotional system.

Nuclear Family Emotional Process. The nuclear family emotional process describes the patterns of emotional functioning in a single generation. The nuclear family begins with a relationship between two people who form a couple. The most open relationship usually occurs during courtship, when most individuals choose partners with similar levels of differentiation. The lower the level of differentiation, the greater the possibility of problems in the future. A degree of fusion occurs with permanent commitment. This fusion results in anxiety and must be dealt with by each partner in an effort to maintain a healthy degree of differentiation.

Family Projection Process. Spouses who are unable to work through the undifferentiation or fusion that occurs with permanent commitment may, when they become parents, project the resulting anxiety onto the children. This

occurrence is manifested as a father-mother-child triangle. These triangles are common and exist, in various gradations of intensity, in most families with children.

The child who becomes the target of the projection may be selected for various reasons:

1. If a particular child reminds one of the parents of an unresolved childhood issue.
2. If the child is of a particular sex or position within the family.
3. If the child is born with a deformity.
4. If the parent has a negative attitude about the pregnancy.

Bell and Vogel (1968) call this behavior **scapegoating.** They contend that scapegoating is harmful to both the child's emotional stability and ability to function outside the family. Trimpey (1982) states:

> "The child slowly internalizes the scapegoat role and absorbs the hostility until it builds then in turn releases tension by punishing the parents. When this counteraggression raises family anxiety to an intolerable level, or when the child moves from the home into the school or community and is identified as disturbed, the family may seek help." (p. 192)

Multigenerational Transmission Process. Bowen (1978) describes the multigenerational transmission process as the manner in which interactional patterns are transferred from one generation to another. Attitudes, values, beliefs, behaviors, and patterns of interaction are passed along from parents to children over many lifetimes, so that it becomes possible to show in a family assessment that a certain behavior has existed within a family through multiple generations.

Genograms

A convenient way to plot a multigenerational assessment is with the use of **genograms.** Genograms offer the convenience of a great deal of information in a small amount of space. They can also be used as teaching tools with the family itself. An overall picture of the life of the family over several generations can be conveyed, including roles that various family members play as well as emotional distance between specific individuals. Areas for change can be easily identified. A sample genogram is presented in Figure 9.2.

Sibling Position Profiles. The thesis regarding sibling position profiles is that the position one holds in a family influences the development of predictable personality characteristics. For example, first-born children are thought to be perfectionistic, reliable, and conscientious; middle children are described as independent, loyal, and intolerant of conflict; and youngest children tend to be charming, precocious, and gregarious (Leman, 1985). Bowen uses this to help determine level of differentiation within a family and the possible direction of the family projection process. For example, if an oldest child exhibits characteristics more representative of a youngest child, there is evidence that this child may be the product of triangulation. Sibling position profiles are also used when studying multigenerational transmission processes and verifiable data are missing for certain family members.

Emotional Cutoff. Emotional cutoff describes differentiation of self from the perception of the child. All individuals have some degree of unresolved emotional attachment to their parents, and the lower the level of differentiation, the greater the degree of unresolved emotional attachment (Jones, 1980).

Emotional cutoff has very little to do with how far away one lives from the family of origin. Individuals who live great distances from their parents can still be undifferentiated, while some individuals are emotionally cut off from their parents who live in the same town or even the same neighborhood.

Bowen (1976) suggests that emotional cutoff is the result of dysfunction within the family of origin in which fusion has occurred, and that emotional cutoff promotes the same type of dysfunction in the new nuclear family. He contends that maintaining some emotional contact with the family of origin promotes healthy differentiation.

Societal Regression. The Bowen theory views society as an emotional system. The concept of societal regression compares society's response to stress to the same type of response seen in individuals and families in response to emotional crisis: stress creates uncomfortable levels of anxiety, which leads to hasty solutions, which add to the problems, and the cycle continues. Jones (1980) states:

> "This concept extends Bowen's notion of an emotional system composed of interlocking triangles in logical steps from the individual to the family, to larger social groups, to the total of society."

Goal and Techniques of Therapy

The goal of Bowen's systems approach to family therapy is to increase the level of differentiation of self, while

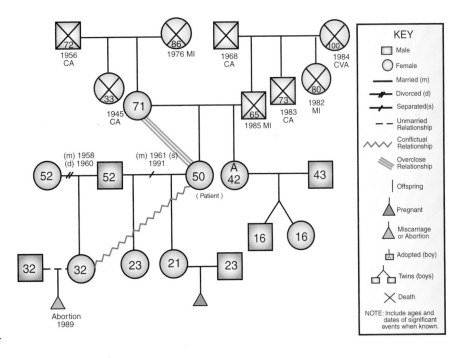

Figure 9.2 Sample genogram.

remaining in touch with the family system. The premise is that intense emotional problems within the nuclear family can be resolved only by resolving undifferentiated relationships with the family of origin. Emphasis is given to the understanding of past relationships.

The therapeutic role is that of "coach" or supervisor, and emotional involvement with the family is minimized. Therapist techniques include:

1. Defining and clarifying the relationship between the spouses.
2. Keeping the self de-triangled from the family emotional system.
3. Teaching family members about the functioning of emotional systems.
4. Demonstrating differentiation by taking "I position" stands during the course of therapy (Jones, 1980).

The Structural Model

Structural family therapy is associated with a model developed by Minuchin (1974). In this model, the family is viewed as a social system within which the individual lives and to which the individual must adapt (Jones, 1980). The individual both contributes and responds to stresses within the family.

Major Concepts

Systems. The structural model views the family as a system. The structure of the *family system* is founded on a set of invisible principles that influence the interaction among family members. These principles concern how, when, and with whom to relate, and are established over time and through repeated transactions, until they become "laws" that govern the conduct of various family members (Jones, 1980).

Transactional Patterns. Transactional patterns are the "laws" that have been established over time that organize the ways in which family members relate to one another. A hierarchy of authority is one example of a transactional pattern. Usually, parents have a higher level of authority in a family than the children, so parental behavior will reflect this role. A balance of authority may exist between husband and wife, or one may reflect a higher level than the other. These patterns of behavioral expectations differ from family to family, and may trace their origin over generations of family negotiations.

Subsystems. Minuchin (1974) describes **subsystems** as smaller elements that make up the larger family system. Subsystems can be individuals or can consist of two or more persons united by gender, relationship, generations, interest, or function (Jones, 1980). A family member may belong to several subsystems at the same time, in which he or she may experience different levels of power and re-

quire different types of skills. For example, a young man has a different level of power, as well as a different set of expectations, in his father-son subsystem than he would in a subsystem with his younger brother.

Boundaries. **Boundaries** define the level of participation and interaction among subsystems. Boundaries are appropriate when they permit appropriate contact with others while preventing excessive interference (Nygaard, 1982). Clearly defined boundaries promote adaptive functioning. Maladaptive functioning can occur when boundaries are *rigid* or *diffuse*.

A rigid boundary is characterized by decreased communication and lack of support and responsiveness. Rigid boundaries prevent a subsystem (family member or subgroup) from achieving appropriate closeness or interaction with others in the system. Rigid boundaries promote **disengagement,** or extreme separateness, among family members.

A diffuse boundary is characterized by dependency and overinvolvement. Diffuse boundaries interfere with adaptive functioning because of the overinvestment, overinvolvement, and lack of differentiation between certain subsystems. Diffuse boundaries promote **enmeshment,** or exaggerated connectedness, among family members.

EXAMPLE:

Sally and Jim have been married for 12 years, during which time they have tried without success to have children. Six months ago they were thrilled to have the opportunity to adopt a 5-year-old girl, Annie. Since both Sally and Jim have full-time teaching jobs, Annie stays with her maternal grandmother, Krista, during the day after she gets home from half-day kindergarten.

At first, Annie was a polite and obedient child. However, in the last few months, she has become insolent and oppositional, and has temper tantrums when she cannot have her way. Sally and Krista agree that Annie should have whatever she desires and should not be punished for her behavior. Jim believes that discipline is necessary, but Sally and Krista refuse to enforce any guidelines he tries to establish. Annie is aware of this discordance and manipulates it to her full advantage.

In this situation, diffuse boundaries exist among the Sally/Krista/Annie subsystems. They have become enmeshed. They have also established a rigid boundary against Jim, disengaging him from the system.

Goal and Techniques of Therapy

The goal of structural family therapy is to facilitate change in the **family structure.** Family structure is changed with modification of the family "principles" or transactional patterns that are contributing to dysfunction within the family. The family is viewed as the unit of therapy, and all members are counseled together. Little, if any, time is spent exploring past experiences. The focus of structural therapy is on the present. Therapist techniques include the following:

1. **Joining the Family.** The therapist must become a part of the family if restructuring is to occur. The therapist joins the family but maintains a leadership position. He or she may at different times join various subsystems within the family, but ultimately includes the entire family system as the target of intervention.

2. **Evaluating the Family Structure.** Even though a family may come for therapy because of the behavior of one family member (the identified patient), the family as a unit is considered problematic. The family structure is evaluated by assessing transactional patterns, system flexibility and potential for change, boundaries, family developmental stage, and role of the identified patient within the system.

3. **Restructuring the Family.** An alliance or contract for therapy is established with the family. By becoming an actual part of the family, the therapist is able to manipulate the system and facilitate the circumstances and experiences that can lead to structural change.

The Strategic Model

The strategic model of family therapy uses the interactional or communications approach. Communication theory is viewed as the foundation for this model. Communication is the actual transmission of information between and among individuals. All behavior sends a message, so all behavior in the presence of two or more individuals is communication. Young (1982) describes differences between functional and dysfunctional families based on the communication model. She states that functional families are open systems where clear and precise messages, congruent with the situation, are sent and received. Healthy communication patterns promote nurturance and individual self-worth. In dysfunctional families, viewed as partially closed systems, communication is vague, and messages are often inconsistent and incongruent with the situation. Destructive patterns of communication tend to inhibit healthful nurturing and decrease individual feelings of self-worth.

Major Concepts

Double-Bind Communication. Double-bind communication occurs when a statement is made and succeeded by a contradictory statement. It also occurs when a statement is made accompanied by nonverbal expression that is inconsistent with the verbal communication. These incompatible communications can interfere with ego development in an individual and promote mistrust of all communications. Double-bind communication often results in a "damned if I do and damned if I don't" situation.

Example. A mother freely gives and receives hugs and kisses from her 6-year-old son some of the time, while at other times she pushes him away saying, "Big boys don't act like that." The little boy receives a conflicting message and is presented with an impossible dilemma: "To please my mother I must not show her that I love her, but if I do not show her that I love her, I'm afraid I will lose her."

Pseudomutuality and Pseudohostility. A healthily functioning individual is able to relate to other people while still maintaining a sense of separate identity. In a dysfunctional family, patterns of interaction may be reflected in the remoteness or closeness of relationships. These relationships may reflect erratic interaction (that is, sometimes remote and sometimes close) or inappropriate interaction (that is, excessive closeness or remoteness).

Pseudomutuality and **pseudohostility** are seen as collective defenses against recognition of the underlying meaninglessness of the relationships within a dysfunctional family system (Jones, 1980). Pseudomutuality is characterized by a facade of mutual regard. Emotional investment is directed at maintaining outward representation of reciprocal fulfillment rather than in the relationship itself. The style of relating is fixed and rigid, and pseudomutuality allows family members to deny underlying fears of separation and hostility.

Example. Janet, age 16, is the only child of State Senator J and his wife. Janet was recently involved in a joyriding experience with a group of teenagers her parents call "the wrong crowd." In family therapy, Mrs. J says, "We have always been a close family. I can't imagine why she is doing these things." Senator J states, "I don't know another colleague who has a family that is as close as mine." Janet responds, "Yes, we are close. I just don't see my parents very much. Dad has been in politics since I was a baby, and Mom is always with him. I wish I could spend more time with them. But we are a close family."

Pseudohostility is also a fixed and rigid style of relating, but the facade being maintained is that of a state of chronic conflict and alienation among family members (Jones, 1980). This relationship pattern allows family members to deny underlying fears of tenderness and intimacy.

Example. Jack, 14, and his sister Jill, 15, will have nothing to do with each other. When they are together they can agree on nothing, and the barrage of "put downs" is constant. This behavior reflects pseudohostility used by individuals who are afraid to reveal feelings of intimacy.

Schism and Skew. Lidz, Cornelison, Fleck, and Terry (1957) observed two patterns within families that relate to a dysfunctional marital dyad. A **marital schism** is defined as "a state of severe chronic disequilibrium and discord, with recurrent threats of separation." Each partner undermines the other, mutual trust is absent, and a competition exists for closeness with the children. Often a partner establishes an alliance with his or her parent against the spouse. Children lack appropriate role models.

Marital skew describes a relationship in which there is lack of equal partnership. One partner dominates the relationship and the other partner. The marriage remains intact as long as the passive partner allows the domination to continue. Children also lack role models when a marital skew exists.

Goal and Techniques of Therapy

The goal of strategic family therapy is to create change in destructive behavior and communication patterns among family members. The identified family *problem* is the unit of therapy, and all family members need not be counseled together. In fact, strategic therapists may prefer to see subgroups or individuals separately in an effort to achieve problem resolution. Therapy is oriented within the present and the therapist assumes full responsibility for devising an effective strategy for family change. Therapeutic techniques include:

1. **Paradoxical Intervention.** A paradox can be called a contradiction in therapy, or "prescribing the symptom." With **paradoxical intervention,** the therapist requests that the family continue to engage in the behavior that they are trying to change. Alternatively, specific directions may be given for continuing the defeating behavior. For example, a couple that regularly engages in insulting shouting matches is instructed to have one of these encounters on Tuesdays and Thursdays from 8:30 to 9:00 PM. Boyer and Jeffrey (1984) explain:

   "A family using its maladaptive behavior to control or punish other people loses control of the situation when it finds itself continuing the behavior under a therapist's direction and being praised for following instructions. If the family disobeys the therapist's instruction, the price it pays is sacrificing the old behavior pattern and experiencing more satisfying ways of interacting with one another. A family that maintains it has no control over its behavior, or whose members contend that others must change before they can themselves, suddenly finds itself unable to defend such statements."

2. **Reframing.** Watzlawick, Weakland, and Fisch (1974) describe **reframing** as "changing the conceptual and/or emotional setting or viewpoint in relation to which a situation is experienced and placing it in another frame that fits the 'facts' of the same concrete situation equally well or even better and thereby changing its entire meaning." Therefore, with reframing, the *behavior* may not actually change, but the *consequences* of the behavior may change, owing to a change in the meaning attached to the behavior. This technique is sometimes referred to as *positive reframing*.

EXAMPLE

Tom has a construction job and makes a comfortable living for his wife, Sue, and their two children. Tom and Sue have been arguing a lot and came to the therapist for counseling. Sue says Tom frequently drinks too much and is often late getting home from work. Tom counters, "I never used to drink on my way home from work, but Sue started complaining to me the minute I walked in the door about being so dirty and about tracking dirt and mud on 'her nice, clean floors.' It was the last straw when she made me undress before I came in the house and leave my dirty clothes and shoes in the garage. I thought a man's home was his castle. Well, I sure don't feel like a king. I need a few stiff drinks to face her nagging!" The therapist used reframing to attempt change by helping Sue to view the situation in a more positive light. He suggested to Sue that she try to change her thinking by focusing on how much her husband must love her and her children to work as hard has he does. He asked her to focus on the dirty clothes and shoes as symbols of his love for them, and to respond to his "dirty" arrivals home with greater affection. This positive reframing set the tone for healing and for increased intimacy within the marital relationship.

THE NURSING PROCESS

Assessment

Wright and Leahey (1994) have developed the Calgary Family Assessment Model (CFAM), a multidimensional model originally adapted from a framework developed by Tomm and Sanders (1983). The CFAM consists of three major categories: structural, developmental, and functional. Wright and Leahey (1994) state:

"Each category contains several subcategories. It is important for each nurse to decide which subcategories are relevant and appropriate to explore and assess with each family at each point in time. That is, not all subcategories need to be assessed at a first meeting with a family, and some subcategories need never be assessed. If nurses use too many subcategories, they may become overwhelmed by all the data. If they assess too few, they may have a distorted view of the family situation." (p. 37)

A diagram of the CFAM is presented in Figure 9.3. The three major categories are listed, along with the subcategories for assessment under each. Assessment of the Marino family will follow this diagram.

Structural Assessment. A graphic representation of the Marino family structure is presented in the genogram in Figure 9.4.

CASE STUDY

THE MARINO FAMILY

John and Nancy Marino have been married for 19 years. They have a 17-year-old son, Peter, and a 15-year-old daughter, Anna. Anna was recently hospitalized for taking an overdose of fluoxetine, her mother's prescription antidepressant. The family is attending family therapy sessions while Anna is in the hospital. Anna states, "I just couldn't take the fighting anymore! Our house is an awful place to be. Everyone hates each other, and everyone is unhappy. Dad drinks too much and Mom is always sick! Peter stays away as much as he can and I don't blame him. I would too if I had someplace to stay. I just thought I'd be better off dead."

John Marino, age 44, is the oldest of five children. His father, Paulo, age 66, is a first-generation Italian American whose parents immigrated from Italy in the early 1900s. Paulo retired last year after 32 years as a cutter in a meat-packing plant. His wife, Carla, age 64, has never worked outside the home. John and his siblings all worked at minimum-wage jobs during high school, and John and his two brothers worked their way through college. His two sisters married young, and both are housewives and mothers. John was able to go to law school with the help of loans, grants, and scholarships. He has held several positions since graduation and is currently employed as a corporate attorney for a large aircraft company.

Nancy, age 43, is the only child of Sam and Ethyl Jones. Sam, age 67, inherited a great deal of money from his family, who had been in the shipping business. He is currently the chief executive officer of this business. Ethyl, also 67, was an aspiring concert pianist when she met Sam. She chose to give up her career for marriage and family, although Nancy believes her mother always resented doing so. Nancy was reared in an affluent lifestyle. She attended private boarding schools as she was growing up, and chose an exclusive college in the East to pursue her interest in art. She studied in Paris during her junior year. Nancy states that she was never emotionally close to her parents. They traveled a great deal and she spent much of her time under the supervision of a nanny.

Nancy's parents were opposed to her marrying John. They perceived John's family to be below their social status. Nancy, on the other hand, loved John's family. She

felt them to be very warm and loving, so unlike what she was used to in her own family. Her family are Protestants, and also disapproved of her marrying in the Roman Catholic church.

Family Dynamics. As their marriage progressed, Nancy's health became very fragile. She had continued her artistic pursuits but seemed to achieve little satisfaction from it. She tried to keep in touch with her parents but often felt spurned by them. They traveled a great deal and often did not even inform her of their whereabouts. They were not present at the birth of her children. She experiences many aches and pains, and spends many days in bed. She sees several physicians, who have prescribed various pain medications, antianxiety agents, and antidepressants but can find nothing organically wrong. Five years ago she learned that John had been having an affair with his secretary. He promised to break it off and fired the secretary, but Nancy has had difficulty trusting him since that time. She brings up his infidelity whenever they have an argument, which is more and more lately. When he is home, John drinks, usually until he falls asleep. Peter frequently comes home smelling of alcohol and a number of times has been clearly intoxicated.

When Nancy called her parents to tell them that Anna was in the hospital, Ethyl replied, "I'm sorry to hear that, dear. We certainly never had any of those kinds of problems on our side of the family. But I'm sure everything will be okay now that you are getting help. Please give our love to your family. Your father and I are leaving for Europe on Saturday and will be gone for 6 weeks."

Although more supportive, John's parents view this situation as somewhat shameful for the family. John's dad responded, "We had hard times when you were growing up, but never like this. We always took care of our own problems. We never had to tell a bunch of strangers about them. It's not right to air your dirty laundry in public. Bring Anna home. Give her your love and she will be okay."

In therapy, Nancy blames John's drinking and his admitted affair for all their problems. John states that he drinks because it is the only way he can tolerate his wife's complaining about his behavior, as well as her many illnesses. Peter is very quiet most of the time but says he will be glad when he graduates in 4 months and can leave "this looney bunch of people." Anna cries as she listens to her family in therapy, "Nothing's ever going to change."

Internal Structure. This is a family that consists of a husband, wife, and their biological son and daughter who live together in the same home. They conform to the traditional gender roles. John is the eldest child from a rather large family, and Nancy has no siblings. In this family, their son, Peter, is the first-born and his sister, Anna, is 2 years younger. Neither spousal, sibling, nor spousal-sibling subsystems appear to be close in this family, and some are clearly conflictual. Problematic subsystems include John-Nancy, John-Nancy-children, and Nancy-Ethyl. The subsystem boundaries are quite rigid, and the family members appear to be emotionally disengaged from one another.

External Structure. This family has ties to extended family, although the availability of support is questionable. Nancy's parents offered little emotional support to her as a developing child. They never approved of her marriage to John and still remain distant and cold. John's family consists of a father, mother, two brothers, and two sisters. They are warm and supportive most of the time, but cultural influences interfere with their understanding of this current situation. At this time, the Marino family is probably receiving the most support from health care professionals who have intervened during Anna's hospitalization.

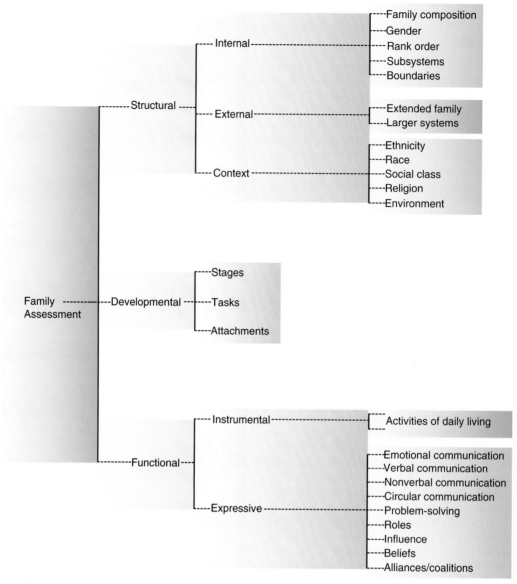

Figure 9.3   Branching diagram of the Calgary family assessment model (CFAM). *Source:* Wright and Leahey (1994), with permission.

Context. John is a second-generation Italian American. His family of origin is large, warm, and supportive. However, John's parents believe that family problems should be dealt with in the family, and disapprove of bringing "strangers" in to hear what they consider to be private information. They believe that Anna's physical condition should be stabilized, and then she should be discharged to deal with family problems at home.

John and Nancy were reared in different social classes. In John's family, money was not available to seek out professional help for every problem that arose. Italian cultural beliefs promote the provision of help within the nuclear and extended family network. If outside counseling is sought, it is often with the family priest. John and Nancy did not seek this type of counseling because they no longer attend church regularly.

In Nancy's family, money was available to obtain the very best professional help at the first sign of trouble. However, Nancy's parents refused to acknowledge, both then and now, that any difficulty ever existed in their family situation.

The Marino family lives comfortably on John's salary as a corporate attorney. They have health insurance and access to any referrals that are deemed necessary. They are well-educated but have been attempting to deny the dysfunctional dynamics that exist within their family.

Developmental Assessment. The Marino family is in stage IV of Carter and McGoldrick's family life cycle, the family with adolescents. In stage IV, parents are expected to respond to adolescents' requests for increasing independence, while being available to continue to fulfill dependency needs. They may also be required to provide

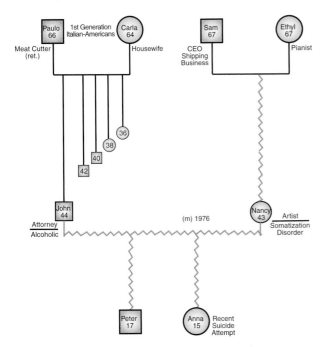

Figure 9.4 Genogram of the Marino family.

additional support to aging grandparents. This may be a time when parents may also begin to reexamine their own marital and career issues.

The Marino family is not fulfilling the dependency needs of its adolescents; in fact, they may be establishing premature independence. The parents are absorbed in their own personal problems to the exclusion of their children. Peter responds to this neglect by staying away as much as possible, drinking with his friends, and planning to leave home at the first opportunity. Anna's attempted suicide is a cry for help. She has needs that are going unfulfilled by her parents, and this crisis situation may be required in order for them to recognize that a problem exists. This may be the time when they begin to reexamine their unresolved marital issues. Extended family are still self-supporting and do not require assistance from John and Nancy at this time.

Functional Assessment. *Instrumental Functioning.* This family has managed to adjust to the maladaptive functioning in an effort to meet physical activities of daily living. They subsist on fast food, or sometimes Nancy or Anna will prepare a meal. Seldom do they sit down at table to eat together. Nancy must take pain medication or sedatives to sleep. John usually drinks himself to sleep. Anna and Peter take care of their own needs independently. Often they do not even see their parents in the evenings. Each manages to do fairly well in school. Peter says, "I don't intend to ruin my chances of getting out of this hell hole as soon as I can!"

Expressive Functioning. John and Nancy Marino argue a great deal about many topics. This family seldom shows affection to one another. Nancy and Anna express sadness with tears, while John and Peter have a tendency to with-

draw or turn to alcohol when experiencing unhappiness. Nancy somaticizes her internal pain, and numbs this pain with medication. Anna internalized her emotional pain until it became unbearable. A notable lack of constructive communication is evident.

This family is unable to solve its problems effectively. In fact, it is unlikely that it has even identified its problems, which undoubtedly have been in existence for a long while. These problems have only recently been revealed in light of Anna's suicide attempt.

Diagnosis

The following nursing diagnoses were identified for the Marino family:

1. Altered family processes
   related to: unsuccessful achievement of family developmental tasks and dysfunctional coping strategies
   evidenced by: inability of family members to relate to each other in an adaptive manner; adolescents' unmet dependency needs; inability of family members to express a wide range of feelings and to send and receive clear messages.

2. Ineffective family coping
   related to: highly ambivalent family relationships and lack of support
   evidenced by: inability to problem solve; each member copes in response to dysfunctional family processes with destructive behavior: John drinks; Nancy somaticizes; Peter drinks and withdraws; and Anna attempts suicide.

Outcome Identification

The following criteria were identified as measurement of outcomes in counseling of the Marino family:

1. Family members will demonstrate effective communication patterns.
2. Family members will express feelings openly and honestly.
3. Family members will establish more adaptive coping strategies.
4. Family members will be able to identify destructive patterns of functioning and problem-solve them effectively.
5. Boundaries between spousal subsystems and spousal-children subsystems will become more clearly defined.
6. Family members will establish stronger bonds with extended family.

Planning/Implementation

The Marino family will undoubtedly require many months of outpatient therapy. It is even likely that each member will need individual psychotherapy in addition to the family therapy. Once Anna has been stabilized physiologically and is discharged from the hospital, family/individual therapy will begin.

Several strategies for family therapy have been discussed in this chapter. As mentioned previously, family therapy has a strong theoretical framework and is performed by individuals with specialized education in family theory and process. Some clinical nurse specialists possess the credentials required to perform family therapy. It is important, however, for all nurses to have some knowledge about working with families, to be able to assess family interaction, and to recognize when problems exist.

Some interventions with the Marino family might include:

1. Create a therapeutic environment that fosters trust, and in which the family members can feel safe and comfortable. The nurse can promote this type of environment by being empathetic, listening actively (see Chapter 6), accepting feelings and attitudes, and being nonjudgmental.

2. Promote effective communication by
   a. Seeking clarification when vague and generalized statements are made (e.g., Anna states, "I just want my family to be like my friends' families." Nurse: "Anna, would you please explain to the group exactly what you mean by that?").
   b. Setting clear limits (e.g., "Peter, it is okay to state when you are angry about something that has been said. It is not okay to throw the chair against the wall.").
   c. Being consistent and fair (e.g., "I encourage each of you to contribute to the group process and to respect one another's opportunity to contribute equally.").
   d. Addressing each individual clearly and directly and encouraging family members to do the same (e.g., "Nancy, I think it would be more appropriate if you directed that statement to John instead of to me.").

3. Identify patterns of interaction that interfere with successful problem resolution. For example, John asks Nancy many "Why?" questions that keep her on the defensive. He criticizes her for "always being sick." Nancy responds by frequently reminding John of his infidelity. Peter and Anna interrupt each other and their parents when the level of conflict reaches a certain point. Provide examples of more appropriate ways to communicate that can improve interpersonal relations and lead to more effective patterns of interaction.

4. Help the Marino family to identify problems that may necessitate change. Encourage each member to discuss a family process that he or she would like to change. As a group, promote discussion of what must take place for change to occur and allow each member to explore whether he or she could realistically cooperate with the necessary requirements for change.

5. As the problem-solving process progresses, encourage all family members to express honest feelings. Address each one directly: "John (Nancy, Peter, Anna), how do you feel about what the others are suggesting?" Ensure that all participants understand that each member may express honest feelings (e.g., anger, sadness, fear, anxiety, guilt, disgust, helplessness) without criticism, judgment, or fear of personal reprisal.

6. Avoid becoming triangled within the family emotional system. Remain neutral and objective. Do not take sides in family disagreements; instead, provide alternative explanations and suggestions (e.g., "Perhaps we can look at that situation in a different light. . .).

7. Reframe vague problem descriptions into ones for which resolution is more realistic. For example, rather than defining the problem as "We don't love each other any more," the problem could be defined as, "We do not spend time together in family activities any more." This definition evolves from the family members' description of what they mean by the more general problem description (Cox et al., 1993).

8. Discuss present coping strategies. Encourage each family member to describe how he or she copes with stress and with the adversity within the family. Explore each member's possible contribution to the family's problems. Encourage family members to discuss possible solutions among themselves.

9. Identify community resources that may assist individual family members and provide support for establishing more adaptive coping mechanisms. For example, Alcoholics Anonymous for John; Al Anon for Nancy; and Al Ateen for Peter and Anna. Other groups that may be of assistance to this family include Emotions Anonymous, Parent's Support Group, Families Helping Families, Marriage Enrichment, Parents of Teenagers, and We Saved Our Marriage (WESOM). Local self-help networks often provide a directory of resources within specific communities.

10. Discuss with the family the possible need for psychotherapy for individual members. Provide names of therapists who would perform assessments to determine individual needs. Encourage follow-through with appointments.

11. Assist family members in planning fun activities together. This could include time to play together, exercise together, or engage in a shared project (Cox et al., 1993).

Evaluation

Evaluation is the final step in the nursing process. In this step, progress toward attainment of outcomes is measured.

1. Do family members demonstrate effective patterns of communication?
2. Can family members express feelings openly and honestly without fear of reprisal?
3. Can family members accept their own personal contribution to the family's problems?
4. Can individual members identify maladaptive coping methods and express a desire to improve?
5. Do family members work together to solve problems?
6. Can family members identify resources within the community from whom they can seek assistance and support?
7. Do family members express a desire to form stronger bonds with the extended family?
8. Are family members willing to seek individual psychotherapy?
9. Are family members pursuing shared activities?

SUMMARY

Nurses interact with families daily. They must have enough knowledge of family functioning to assess family interaction and recognize when problems arise. Some nurse specialists perform therapy with families.

Carter and McGoldrick (1989) identified six stages that describe the family life cycle. They include

1. The single young adult
2. The newly married couple
3. The family with young children
4. The family with adolescents
5. The family launching grown children
6. The family in later life

They also discuss tasks of families experiencing divorce and remarriage, and those that vary according to cultural norms.

Families are assessed as functional or dysfunctional based on six elements (Boyer & Jeffrey, 1984). These elements include communication, self-concept reinforcement, family members' expectations, handling differences, family interactional patterns, and family climate.

Three models for family therapy were presented: the family as a system, the structural model, and the strategic model. Major concepts, goal, and techniques of therapy were presented for each. Explanation for use of the genogram in family assessment was included.

The nursing process, as the tool for delivery of nursing care, was presented in the form of a case study. Structure, development, and functioning were assessed, nursing diagnoses and outcome criteria were identified, and strategies for intervention and evaluation were discussed.

REVIEW QUESTIONS

Self-Examination/Learning Exercise

Match the tasks in the column on the left to the family-life cycle stages listed on the right.

_____ 1. Renegotiation of the marital system as a dyad.

_____ 2. Differentiation of self in relation to family of origin.

_____ 3. Dealing with loss of spouse, siblings, and peers.

_____ 4. Adjusting marital system to make space for children.

_____ 5. Formation of the marital system.

_____ 6. Refocus on midlife marital and career issues.

a. The Single Young Adult
b. The Newly Married Couple
c. The Family With Young Children
d. The Family With Adolescents
e. The Family Launching Grown Children
f. The Family in Later Life

Select the answer that is most appropriate in each of the following questions.

7. The nurse-therapist is counseling the Smith family: Mr. and Mrs. Smith, 10-year-old Rob, and 8-year-old Lisa. When Mr. and Mrs. Smith start to argue, Rob hits Lisa and Lisa starts to cry. The Smiths then turn their attention to comforting Lisa and scolding Rob, complaining that he is "out of control and we don't know what to do about his behavior." These dynamics are an example of

a. Double-bind messages.
b. Triangulation.
c. Pseudohostility.
d. Multigenerational transmission.

8. Using Bowen's systems approach to therapy with the Smiths, the therapist would

a. Try to change family principles that may be promoting dysfunctional behavior patterns.
b. Strive to create change in destructive behavior through improvement in communication and interaction patterns.
c. Encourage increase in the differentiation of individual family members.
d. Promote change in dysfunctional behavior by encouraging the formation of more diffuse boundaries between family members.

9. Using the structural approach to therapy with the Smiths, the therapist would

a. Try to change family principles that may be promoting dysfunctional behavior patterns.
b. Strive to create change in destructive behavior through improvement in communications and interaction patterns.
c. Encourage increase in the differentiation of individual family members.
d. Promote change in dysfunctional behavior by encouraging the formation of more diffuse boundaries between family members.

10. Using the strategic approach to therapy with the Smiths, the therapist would

a. Try to change family principles that may be promoting dysfunctional behavior patterns.
b. Strive to create change in destructive behavior through improvement in communication and interaction patterns.
c. Encourage increase in the differentiation of individual family members.
d. Promote change in dysfunctional behavior by encouraging the formation of more diffuse boundaries between family members.

REFERENCES

Ahrons, C., & Perlmutter, M. (1982). The relationship between former spouses: A fundamental subsystem in the remarriage family. In L. Messinger (Ed.), *Therapy with remarriage families.* Rockville, MD: Aspen Systems Corporation.

Bell, N.W., & Vogel, E.F. (1968). *A modern introduction to the family.* New York: The Free Press.

Bowen, M. (1971). The use of family theory in clinical practice. In J. Haley (Ed.), *Changing families.* New York: Grune & Stratton.

Bowen, M. (1976). Theory in the practice of psychotherapy. In P. Guerin (Ed.), *Family therapy: Theory and practice.* New York: Gardner Press.

Bowen, M. (1978). *Family therapy in clinical practice.* New York: Jason Aronson.

Boyer, P.A., & Jeffrey, R.J. (1984). *A guide for the family therapist.* Northvale, NJ: Jason Aronson.

Carter, B., & McGoldrick, M. (Eds.). (1989). *The changing family life cycle: A framework for family therapy* (2nd ed.). New York: Gardner Press.

Catechism of the Catholic Church. (1995). New York: Doubleday.

Cox, H.C., Hinz, M.D., Lubno, M.A., Newfield, S.A., Ridenour, N.A., Slater, M.M., & Sridaromont, K.L. (1993). *Clinical applications of nursing diagnosis* (2nd ed.).Philadelphia: F.A. Davis.

Foley, V.D. (1979). Family therapy. In R.J. Corsini (Ed.), *Current psychotherapies* (2nd ed.). Itasca, IL: F.E. Peacock.

Freeman, D. (1981). *Techniques of family therapy.* New York: Jason Aronson.

Glick, P.C. (1989). The family life cycle and social change. *Family Relations, 38,* 123–129.

Herz, F.M., & Rosen, E.J. (1982). Jewish families. In M. McGoldrick, J.K. Pearce, & J. Giordano (Eds.), *Ethnicity and family therapy.* New York: The Guilford Press.

Jones, S.L. (1980). *Family therapy: A comparison of approaches.* Bowie, MD: Robert J. Brady.

L'Abate, L., Ganahl, G., & Hansen, J.C. (1986). *Methods of family therapy.* Englewood Cliffs, NJ: Prentice-Hall.

Leman, K. (1985). *The birth order book: Why you are the way you are.* New York: Dell Publishing.

Lidz, T., Cornelison, A., Fleck, S., & Terry, D. (1957). The intrafamilial environment of schizophrenic patients: II. Marital schism and marital skew. *American Journal of Psychiatry, 114:*241–248.

Messinger, L. (1982). *Therapy with remarriage families.* Rockville, MD: Aspen Systems Corporation.

Minuchin, S. (1974). *Families and family therapy.* Cambridge, MA: Harvard University Press.

Nygaard, N.L. (1982). Family ego mass and family structure. In I.W. Clements, & D.M. Buchanan (Eds.), *Family therapy: A nursing perspective.* New York: John Wiley & Sons.

Pill, C. (1990). Stepfamilies: Redefining the family. *Family relations, 39:*186–193.

Rotunno, M., & McGoldrick, M. (1982). Italian families. In M. McGoldrick, J.K. Pearce, & J. Giordano (Eds.), *Ethnicity and family therapy.* New York: The Guilford Press.

Shon, S.P., & Ja, D.Y. (1982). Asian families. In M. McGoldrick, J.K. Pearce, & J. Giordano (Eds.), *Ethnicity and family therapy.* New York: The Guilford Press.

Tomm, K., & Sanders, G. (1983). Family assessment in a problem oriented record. In J.C. Hansen & B.F. Keeney (Eds.), *Diagnosis and assessment in family therapy.* London: Aspen Systems.

Trimpey, M.M. (1982). Family projection system and scapegoating. In I.W. Clements & D.M. Buchanan (Eds.), *Family therapy: A nursing perspective.* New York: John Wiley & Sons.

Watzlawick, P., Weakland, J., & Fisch, R. (1974). *Change: Principles of problem formulation and problem resolution.* New York: W.W. Norton.

Wright, L.M. & Leahey, M. (1994). *Nurses and families: A guide to family assessment and intervention* (2nd ed.). Philadelphia: F.A. Davis.

Young, B. (1982). Family communication model. In I.W. Clements & D.M. Buchanan (Eds.), *Family therapy: A nursing perspective.* New York: John Wiley & Sons.

Bibliography

Clements, I.W. & Buchanan, D.M. (Eds.). (1982). *Family therapy: A nursing perspective.* New York: John Wiley & Sons.

Freeman, D.S. (1992). *Family therapy with couples: The family-of-origin approach.* Northvale, NJ: Jason Aronson.

Hoffman, L. (1981). *Foundations of family therapy: A conceptual framework for systems change.* New York: Basic Books.

Martin, P.A. (1994). *A marital therapy manual.* Northvale, NJ: Jason Aronson.

McGoldrick, M., & Gerson, R. (1986). *Genograms and family assessment.* New York: W.W. Norton.

Satir, V. (1972). *Peoplemaking.* Palo Alto, CA: Science and Behavior Books.

Satir, V. (1983). *Conjoint family therapy.* Palo Alto, CA: Science and Behavior Books.

MILIEU THERAPY—THE THERAPEUTIC COMMUNITY

KEY TERMS

milieu   milieu therapy   therapeutic community

OBJECTIVES

After reading this chapter, the student will be able to:

1. Define *milieu therapy*.
2. Explain the goal of therapeutic community/milieu therapy.
3. Identify seven basic assumptions of a therapeutic community.
4. Discuss conditions that characterize a therapeutic community.
5. Identify the various therapies that may be included within the program of the therapeutic community and the health care workers that make up the interdisciplinary treatment team.
6. Describe the role of the nurse on the interdisciplinary treatment team.

tandard Vb of the Standards of Psychiatric-Mental Health Clinical Nursing Practice (ANA, 1994) states that, "The psychiatric-mental health nurse provides, structures, and maintains a therapeutic environment in collaboration with the client and other health care providers."

This chapter defines and explains the goal of milieu therapy. The conditions necessary for a therapeutic environment are discussed, and the roles of the various health care workers within the interdisciplinary team are delineated. An interpretation of the nurse's role in milieu therapy is included.

MILIEU, DEFINED

The word *milieu* is French for "middle." The English translation of the word is "surroundings, or environment." In psychiatry, therapy involving the **milieu,** or environment, may be called **milieu therapy,** therapeutic community, or therapeutic environment. In this context it is defined as "a scientific structuring of the environment in order to effect behavioral changes and to improve the psychological health and functioning of the individual" (Skinner, 1979). Thus, the goal of milieu therapy is to manipulate the environment so that all aspects of the client's hospital experience are considered therapeutic. Within this therapeutic community setting the client is expected to learn adaptive coping, interaction, and relationship skills that can be generalized to other aspects of his or her life.

BASIC ASSUMPTIONS

Skinner (1979) outlined seven basic assumptions on which a therapeutic community is based:

1. **The Health in Each Individual Is to Be Realized and Encouraged to Grow.** All individuals are considered to have strengths as well as limitations. These healthy aspects of the individual are identified and serve as a foundation for growth in the personality and in the ability to function more adaptively and productively in all aspects of life.
2. **Every Interaction is an Opportunity for Therapeutic Intervention.** Within this structured setting, it is virtually impossible to avoid interpersonal interaction. The ideal situation exists for clients to improve communication and relationship development skills. Learning occurs from immediate feedback of personal perceptions.
3. **The Client Owns His or Her Own Environment.** Clients make decisions and solve problems related to government of the unit. In this way, personal needs for autonomy as well as needs that pertain to the group as a whole are fulfilled.
4. **Each Client Owns His or Her Behavior.** Each individual within the therapeutic community is expected to take responsibility for his or her own behavior.
5. **Peer Pressure Is a Useful and a Powerful Tool.** Behavioral group norms are established through peer pressure. Feedback is direct and frequent, so that behaving in a manner acceptable to the other members of the community becomes essential.
6. **Inappropriate Behaviors Are Dealt With as They Occur.** Individuals examine the significance of their behavior, look at how it affects other people, and discuss more appropriate ways of behaving in certain situations.
7. **Restrictions and Punishment Are to Be Avoided.** Destructive behaviors can usually be controlled with group discussion. However, if an individual requires external controls, temporary isolation is preferred over lengthy restriction or other harsh punishment.

CONDITIONS THAT PROMOTE A THERAPEUTIC COMMUNITY

In a **therapeutic community** setting, everything that happens to the client, or within the client's environment, is considered to be part of the treatment program. The community setting is the foundation for the program of treatment. Community factors, such as social interactions, the physical structure of the unit, and schedule of activities, may generate negative responses from some clients. These stressful experiences are used as examples to help the client learn how to manage stress more adaptively in real-life situations.

Under what conditions, then, is a hospital environment considered therapeutic? A number of criteria have been identified:

1. **Basic Physiological Needs Are Fulfilled.** As Maslow (1968) has suggested, individuals do not move to higher levels of functioning until the basic biological needs for food, water, air, sleep, exercise, elimination, shelter, and sexual expression have been met.
2. **The Physical Facilities Are Conducive to Achievement of the Goals of Therapy.** Space is provided so that each client has sufficient privacy, as well as physical space, for therapeutic interaction with others. Furnishings are arranged to present a homelike atmosphere, usually in spaces that accommodate communal living, dining, and activity areas, for facilitation of interpersonal interaction and communication.
3. **A Democratic Form of Self-Government Exists.** In the therapeutic community, clients participate in the decision making and problem solving that affect

the management of the unit. This is accomplished through regularly scheduled community meetings. These meetings are attended by staff and clients, and all individuals have equal input into the discussions. At these meetings, unit norms and rules and behavioral limits are set forth. This reinforces the democratic posture of the unit, as these are expectations that affect all clients on an equal basis. An example might be the unit rule that no client may enter a room being occupied by a client of the opposite sex. Consequences of violating the rules are explained.

Other issues that may be discussed at the community meetings include those with which certain clients have some disagreements. A decision is then made by the entire group in a democratic manner. For example, several clients may disagree with the hours that have been designated for watching television on a weekend night. They may elect to bring up this issue at a community meeting and suggest an extension in television-viewing time. After discussion by the group, a vote will be taken and clients and staff agree to abide by the expressed preference of the majority.

Meetings are usually held each morning right after breakfast. Some therapeutic communities elect officers (usually a president and a secretary) who serve for a period of a week or even for a few days. The president calls the meeting to order, conducts the business of discussing old and new unit issues, and asks for volunteers (or makes appointments, alternately, so that all clients have a turn) to accomplish the daily tasks associated with community living; for example, cleaning the tables after each meal and watering plants on the unit. New assignments are made each morning.

The secretary reads the minutes of yesterday's meeting and takes minutes of the current meeting. Minutes are important in the event that clients have a disagreement about issues that were discussed at various meetings. Minutes provide written evidence of decisions made by the group.

On units whose clients have short attention spans or disorganized thinking, meetings are brief. Business is generally limited to introductions and expectations of the here and now. Discussions also may include comments about a recent occurrence on the unit or something that has been bothering a member and about which he or she has some questions. These meetings are usually conducted by staff, although all clients have equal input into the discussions.

All clients are expected to attend the meetings each morning. Exceptions are made for times when aspects of therapy interfere (e.g., scheduled testing, X-ray examinations, electroencephalograms). An explanation is made to clients present so that false perceptions of danger are not generated by another person's absence. All staff members, except those required to manage the unit and provide necessary care for clients, are expected to attend the daily meetings.

4. **Unit Responsibilities Are Assigned According to Client Capabilities.** Increasing self-esteem is an ultimate goal of the therapeutic community. Therefore, a client should not be set up for failure by being assigned a responsibility that is beyond his or her level of ability. By assigning clients responsibilities that promote achievement, self-esteem is enhanced. Consideration must also be given to times during which the client will show some regression in the treatment regimen. Adjustments in assignments should be made in a way that preserves self-esteem and provides for progression to greater degrees of responsibility as the client returns to previous level of functioning.

5. **A Structured Program of Social and Work-Related Activities Is Scheduled as Part of the Treatment Program.** Each client's therapeutic program consists of group activities in which interpersonal interaction and communication with other individuals are emphasized. Time is also devoted to personal problems. Various group activities may be selected for clients with specific needs; for example, an exercise group for a person who expresses anger inappropriately, an assertiveness group for a person who is passive-aggressive, or a stress-management group for a person who is anxious. A structured schedule of activities is the major focus of a therapeutic community. Through these activities, change in the client's personality and behavior can be effected. New coping strategies are learned and social skills are developed. In the group situation, the client is able to practice what he or she has learned in order to prepare for transition to the general community.

6. **Community and Family Are Included in the Program of Therapy in an Effort to Facilitate Discharge From the Hospital.** An attempt is made to include family members, as well as certain aspects of the community that affect the client, in the treatment program. It is important to keep as many links to the client's life outside the hospital as possible. Family members are invited to participate in specific therapy groups and, in some instances, to share meals with the client in the communal dining room. Connection with community life may be maintained through client group activities, such as shopping, picnicking, attending movies, bowling, and visiting the zoo. Clients may also be awarded passes to visit family or may participate in work-related activities, the length of time being determined by the activity and the client's condition. These connections with family and

community facilitate the discharge process and may also help to prevent the client from becoming too dependent on hospitalization.

THE PROGRAM OF THERAPEUTIC COMMUNITY

Care for clients in the therapeutic community is directed by an interdisciplinary treatment (IDT) team. An initial assessment is made by the admitting psychiatrist, nurse, or other designated admitting agent who establishes a priority of care. The IDT team meets within 48 hours of admission to determine a comprehensive treatment plan and goals of therapy and to assign intervention responsibilities. All members sign the treatment plan and meet weekly to update the plan as needed. Depending on the size of the institution and scope of the treatment program, members representing a variety of disciplines may participate in the promotion of a therapeutic community. For example, an IDT team may include a psychiatrist, clinical psychologist, psychiatric clinical nurse specialist, psychiatric nurse, mental health technician, psychiatric social worker, occupational therapist, recreational therapist, art therapist, music therapist, psychodramatist, dietitian, and chaplain. Table 10.1 provides an explanation of responsibilities and educational preparation required for these members of the IDT team.

THE ROLE OF THE NURSE

Nurses are generally the only members of the IDT team who spend time with the clients on a 24-hour basis. They assume responsibility for management of the therapeutic milieu, and accomplish this through use of the nursing process. An ongoing assessment, diagnosis, outcome identification, planning, implementation, and evaluation of the environment is necessary for the successful management of a therapeutic milieu. Nurses are involved in all day-to-day activities that pertain to client care. Suggestions and opinions of nursing staff are given serious consideration in the planning of care for individual clients. Information from the initial nursing assessment is used to create the IDT plan. Nurses have input into the goals of therapy and participate in the weekly updates and modification of the treatment plans.

In some institutions, a separate nursing care plan is required in addition to the IDT plan. When this is the case, the nursing care plan must reflect diagnoses that are specific to nursing and include problems and interventions from the IDT plan that have been assigned specifically to the discipline of nursing.

In the therapeutic milieu, nurses are responsible for ensuring that clients' physiological needs are met. Clients must be encouraged to perform as independently as possible in fulfilling activities of daily living. However, the nurse must make ongoing assessments to provide assistance for those who require it. Assessing physical status is an important nursing responsibility that must not be overlooked on the psychiatric unit that emphasizes holistic care.

Reality orientation for clients who have disorganized thinking or who are disoriented or confused is important in the therapeutic milieu. Clocks with large hands and numbers, calendars that give the day and date in large print, and orientation boards that discuss daily activities and news happenings can help keep clients oriented to reality. Nurses ensure that clients have written schedules of activities to which they are assigned and that they arrive at those activities on schedule. Some clients may require an identification sign on their door to remind them which room is theirs. All of these determinations are made from ongoing nursing assessments.

Nurses are responsible for the management of medication administration. On some psychiatric units, clients are expected to accept the responsibility and request their medication at the appropriate time. Although ultimate responsibility lies with the nurse, he or she must encourage clients to be self-reliant. Nurses must work with the clients to determine methods that result in achievement and provide positive feedback for successes.

A major focus of nursing in the therapeutic milieu is the one-to-one relationship, which grows out of a developing trust between client and nurse. Many clients with psychiatric disorders have never achieved the ability to trust. If this can be accomplished in a relationship with the nurse, the trust may be generalized to other relationships in the client's life. Developing trust means keeping promises that have been made. It means total acceptance of the individual as a person, separate from behavior that is unacceptable. It means responding to the client with concrete behaviors that are understandable to him or her (e.g., "If you are frightened, I will stay with you"; "If you are cold, I will bring you a blanket"; "If you are thirsty, I will bring you a drink of water"). Within an atmosphere of trust, the client is encouraged to express feelings and emotions and to discuss unresolved issues that are creating problems in his or her life.

The nurse is responsible for setting limits on unacceptable behavior in the therapeutic milieu. This requires stating to the client in understandable terminology what behaviors are not acceptable and what the consequences will be should the limits be violated. These limits must be established, written, and carried out by all staff on all shifts. Consistency in carrying out the consequences of violation of the established limits is essential if the learning is to be reinforced.

The role of client teacher is important in the psychiatric area, as it is in all areas of nursing. Nurses must be able to assess learning readiness in individual clients. Do they want to learn? What is their level of anxiety? What is their level of ability to understand the information being presented? Topics for client education in psychiatry include information about medical diagnoses, side effects

TABLE 10.1 THE INTERDISCIPLINARY TREATMENT TEAM IN PSYCHIATRY

TEAM MEMBER	RESPONSIBILITIES	EDUCATION REQUIRED
Psychiatrist	Serves as the leader of the team. Responsible for diagnosis and treatment of mental disorders. Performs psychotherapy; prescribes medication and other somatic therapies.	Medical degree with residency in psychiatry and license to practice medicine.
Clinical psychologist	Conducts individual, group, and family therapy. Administers, interprets, and evaluates psychological tests that assist in the diagnostic process.	Doctorate in clinical psychology with 2–3 year internship supervised by a licensed clinical psychologist. State license is required to practice.
Psychiatric clinical nurse specialist	Conducts individual, group, and family therapy. Presents educational programs for nursing staff. Provides consultation services to nurses who require assistance in the planning and implementation of care for individual clients.	Registered nurse with minimum of a master's degree in psychiatric nursing.
Psychiatric nurse	Provides ongoing assessment of client condition, both mentally and physically. Manages the therapeutic milieu on a 24-hour basis. Administers medications. Assists clients with all therapeutic activities as required. Focus is on one-to-one relationship development.	Registered nurse with hospital diploma, associate degree, or baccalaureate degree.
Mental health technician (also called psychiatric aide or assistant or psychiatric technician)	Functions under the supervision of the psychiatric nurse. Provides assistance to clients in the fulfillment of their activities of daily living. Assists activity therapists as required in conducting their groups. May also participate in one-to-one relationship development.	Varies from state to state. Requirements include high school education, with additional vocational education or on-the-job training. Some hospitals hire individuals with bachelor of science degree in psychology in this capacity. Some states require a licensure examination to practice.
Psychiatric social worker	Conducts individual, group, and family therapy. Is concerned with client's social needs, such as placement, financial support, and community requirements. Conducts in-depth psychosocial history on which the needs assessment is based. Works with client and family to ensure that requirements for discharge are fulfilled and needs can be met by appropriate community resources.	Minimum of a master's degree in social work (MSW). Some states require additional supervision and subsequent licensure by examination (LSCSW).
Occupational therapist	Works with clients to help develop (or redevelop) independence in performance of activities of daily living. Focus is on rehabilitation and vocational training in which clients learn to be productive, thereby enhancing self-esteem. Creative activities and therapeutic relationship skills are used.	Baccalaureate or master's degree in occupational therapy.
Recreational therapist	Uses recreational activities to promote clients to redirect their thinking or to rechannel destructive energy in an appropriate manner. Clients learn skills that can he used during leisure time and during times of stress following discharge from the hospital. Examples include bowling, volleyball, exercises, and jogging. Some programs include activities such as picnics, swimming, and even group attendance at the state fair when it is in session.	Baccalaureate or master's degree in recreational therapy.
Music therapist	Encourages clients in self-expression through music. Clients listen to music, play instruments, sing, dance, even compose songs that help them get in touch with feelings and emotions that they may not be able to experience in any other way.	Graduate degree with specialty in music therapy.
Art therapist	Uses the client's creative abilities to encourage expression of emotions and feelings through artwork. Helps clients to analyze their own work in an effort to recognize and resolve underlying conflict.	Graduate degree with specialty in art therapy.

Continued on following page

TABLE 10.1 THE INTERDISCIPLINARY TREATMENT TEAM IN PSYCHIATRY *Continued*

TEAM MEMBER	RESPONSIBILITIES	EDUCATION REQUIRED
Psychodramatist	Directs clients in the creation of a "drama" that portrays real-life situations. Individuals select problems they wish to enact, and other clients play the roles of significant others in the situations. Some clients are able to "act out" problems that they are unable to work through in a more traditional manner. All members benefit through intensive discussion that follows.	Graduate degree in psychology, social work, nursing, or medicine with additional training in group therapy and specialty preparation to become a psychodramatist.
Dietitian	Plans nutritious meals for all clients. Works on consulting basis for clients with specific eating disorders, such as anorexia nervosa, bulimia nervosa, obesity, and pica.	Baccalaureate or master's degree with specialty in dietetics.
Chaplain	Assesses, identifies, and attends to the spiritual needs of clients and their family members. Provides spiritual support and comfort as requested by client or family. May provide counseling if educational background includes this type of preparation.	College degree with advanced education in theology, seminary, or rabbinical studies.

of medications, the importance of continuing to take medications, and stress management, among others. Some topics must be individualized for specific clients, whereas others may be taught in group situations. Table 10.2 outlines various topics of nursing concern for client education in psychiatry.

Devine (1981) has stated:

"It would appear that the role of the nurse is all-encompassing in a therapeutic environment. The nurse must be supportive and encourage the client to become self-reliant. Normal natural social relationships must be fostered, and a consistent, positive outlook is the primary tool with which to practice milieu therapy." (p. 23)

SUMMARY

In psychiatry, milieu therapy, or a therapeutic community, constitutes a manipulation of the environment in an effort to create behavioral changes and to improve the psychological health and functioning of the individual. The goal of therapeutic community is for the client to learn adaptive coping, interaction, and relationship skills that can be generalized to other aspects of his or her life. The community environment itself serves as the primary tool of therapy.

According to Skinner (1979), a therapeutic community is based on seven basic assumptions:

1. The health in each individual is to be realized and encouraged to grow.
2. Every interaction is an opportunity for therapeutic intervention.

TABLE 10.2 THE THERAPEUTIC MILIEU— TOPICS FOR CLIENT EDUCATION

1. Ways to increase self-esteem
2. Ways to deal with anger appropriately
3. Stress-management techniques
4. How to recognize signs of increasing anxiety and intervene to stop progression
5. Normal stages of grieving and behaviors associated with each stage
6. Assertiveness techniques
7. Relaxation techniques
   a. Progressive relaxation
   b. Tense and relax
   c. Deep breathing
   d. Autogenics
8. Medications (specify)
   a. Harmless side effects
   b. Side effects to report to physician
   c. Importance of taking regularly
   d. Importance of not stopping abruptly
9. Effects of (substance) on the body
   a. Alcohol
   b. Other depressants
   c. Stimulants
   d. Hallucinogens
   e. Narcotics
   f. Cannabinols
10. Problem-solving skills
11. Thought-stopping/thought-switching techniques
12. Sex education
    a. Structure and function of reproductive system
    b. Contraceptives
    c. Sexually transmitted diseases
13. The essentials of good nutrition
14. (For parents/guardians)
    a. Signs and symptoms of substance abuse
    b. Effective parenting techniques

3. The client owns his or her own environment.
4. Each client owns his or her behavior.
5. Peer pressure is a useful and a powerful tool.
6. Inappropriate behaviors are dealt with as they occur.
7. Restrictions and punishment are to be avoided.

Because the goals of milieu therapy relate to helping the client learn to generalize that which is learned to other aspects of his or her life, the conditions that promote a therapeutic community in the hospital setting are similar to the types of conditions that exist in real-life situations. They include the following:

1. The fulfillment of basic physiological needs.
2. Physical facilities that are conducive to achievement of the goals of therapy.
3. The existence of a democratic form of self-government.
4. The assignment of unit responsibilities according to client capabilities.
5. A structured program of social and work-related activities.
6. The inclusion of community and family in the program of therapy in an effort to facilitate discharge from the hospital.

The program of therapy on the milieu unit is conducted by the IDT team. The team includes some, or all, of the following disciplines, and may include others that are not specified here: psychiatrist, clinical psychologist, psychiatric clinical nurse specialist, psychiatric nurse, mental health technician, psychiatric social worker, occupational therapist, recreational therapist, art therapist, music therapist, psychodramatist, dietitian, and chaplain.

Nurses play a crucial role in the management of a therapeutic milieu. They are involved in the assessment, diagnosis, outcome identification, planning, implementation, and evaluation of all treatment programs. They have significant input into the IDT plans that are developed for all clients. They are responsible for ensuring that clients' basic needs are fulfilled, for continual assessment of physical and psychosocial status, for medication administration, for the development of trusting relationships, for setting limits on unacceptable behaviors, for client education, and ultimately, for helping clients, within the limits of their capability, become productive members of society.

REVIEW QUESTIONS

SELF-EXAMINATION/LEARNING EXERCISE

Test your knowledge of milieu therapy by supplying the information requested.

1. Define *milieu therapy*.

2. What is the goal of milieu therapy/therapeutic community?

Select the best response in each of the following questions:

3. In prioritizing care within the therapeutic environment, which of the following nursing interventions would receive the highest priority?

   a. Ensuring that the physical facilities are conducive to achievement of the goals of therapy.
   b. Scheduling a community meeting for 8:30 each morning.
   c. Attending to the nutritional and comfort needs of all clients.
   d. Establishing contacts with community resources.

4. In the community meeting, which of the following actions is most important for reinforcing the democratic posture of the unit?

   a. Allowing each person a specific equal amount of time to talk.
   b. Reviewing unit rules and behavioral limits that apply to all clients.
   c. Reading the minutes from yesterday's meeting.
   d. Waiting until all clients are present before initiating the meeting.

5. One of the goals of therapeutic community is for clients to become more independent and accept self-responsibility. Which of the following approaches by staff best encourages fulfillment of this goal?

   a. Including client input and decisions into the treatment plan.
   b. Insisting that each client take a turn as "president" of the community meeting.
   c. Making decisions for the client regarding plans for treatment.
   d. Requiring that the client be bathed, dressed, and attend breakfast on time each morning.

6. Client teaching is an important nursing function on the milieu unit. Which of the following statements by the client indicates the need for knowledge and a readiness to learn?

   a. "Get away from me with that medicine! I'm not sick!"
   b. "I don't belong on the psych unit. It's my migraine headaches that I need help with."
   c. "I've taken Valium every day of my life for the last 20 years. I'll stop when I'm good and ready!"
   d. "The doctor says I have bipolar disorder. What does that really mean?"

7. Match the following activities with the responsible therapist from the IDT team.

   _____ 1. Psychiatrist

   _____ 2. Clinical psychologist

   _____ 3. Psychiatric social worker

   _____ 4. Psychiatric clinical nurse specialist

   _____ 5. Psychiatric nurse

   _____ 6. Mental health technician

   a. Helps clients plan, shop for, and cook a meal.
   b. Locates halfway house and arranges living conditions for client being discharged from the hospital.
   c. Helps clients get to know themselves better by having them describe what they feel when they hear a certain song.
   d. Helps clients to recognize their own beliefs so that they may draw comfort from those beliefs in time of spiritual need.
   e. Accompanies clients on community trip to the zoo.
   f. Diagnoses mental disorders, conducts psychotherapy, and prescribes somatic therapies.
   g. Manages the therapeutic milieu on a 24-hour basis.
   h. Conducts group and family therapies and administers and evaluates psychological tests that assist in the diagnostic process.

_____ 7. Occupational therapist

_____ 8. Recreational therapist

_____ 9. Music therapist

_____ 10. Art therapist

_____ 11. Psychodramatist

_____ 12. Dietitian

_____ 13. Chaplain

i. Conducts group therapies and provides consultation and education to staff nurses.

j. Assists staff nurses in the management of the milieu.

k. Encourages clients to express painful emotions by drawing pictures on paper.

l. Assesses needs, establishes, monitors, and evaluates a nutritional program for a client with anorexia nervosa.

m. Directs a group of clients in acting out a situation that is otherwise too painful for a client to discuss openly.

REFERENCES

American Nurses' Association. (1994). *Statement on psychiatric-mental health clinical nursing practice and standards of psychiatric-mental health clinical nursing practice.* Washington, DC: American Nurses' Association.

Devine, B.A. (1981, March). Therapeutic milieu/milieu therapy: An overview. *Journal of Psychiatric Nursing and Mental Health Services,* 20–24.

Maslow, A. (1968). *Towards a psychology of being* (2nd ed.). New York: D. Van Nostrand.

Skinner, K. (1979, August). The therapeutic milieu: Making it work. *Journal of Psychiatric Nursing and Mental Health Services,* 38–44.

Bibliography

Canter, D., & Canter, S. (Eds.). (1979). *Designing for therapeutic environments, a review of research.* Chichester, England: John Wiley & Sons.

Carser, D.L. (1981, February). Primary nursing in the milieu. *Journal of Psychiatric Nursing and Mental Health Services,* 35–41.

Hinds, P.S. (1980, June). Music: A milieu factor with implications for the nurse therapist. *Journal of Psychiatric Nursing and Mental Health Services,* 28–33.

Hinshelwood, R.D., & Manning, N. (Eds.). (1979). *Therapeutic communities: Reflections and progress.* London: Routledge & Kegan Paul.

Jansen, E. (1980). *The therapeutic community.* London: Croom Helm.

Jones, M. (1953). *The therapeutic community.* New York: Basic Books.

Sharp, V. (1975). *Social control in the therapeutic community.* Westmead, England: Saxon House, D.C. Heath.

CRISIS INTERVENTION

CHAPTER OUTLINE

OBJECTIVES

INTRODUCTION

CRISIS, DEFINED

PHASES IN THE DEVELOPMENT
OF A CRISIS

TYPES OF CRISES

CRISIS INTERVENTION

PHASES OF CRISIS INTERVENTION:
THE ROLE OF THE NURSE

SUMMARY

REVIEW QUESTIONS

KEY TERMS

crisis   crisis intervention

OBJECTIVES

After reading this chapter, the student will be able to:

1. Define *crisis*.
2. Describe four phases in the development of a crisis.
3. Identify types of crises that occur in people's lives.
4. Discuss the goal of crisis intervention.
5. Describe the steps in crisis intervention.
6. Identify the role of the nurse in crisis intervention.

tressful situations are a part of everyday life. Any stressful situation can precipitate a crisis. Crises result in a disequilibrium from which many individuals require assistance to recover. Crisis intervention requires problem-solving skills that are often diminished by the level of anxiety accompanying disequilibrium. Assistance with problem-solving during the crisis period preserves self-esteem and promotes growth with resolution.

This chapter examines the phases in the development of a crisis and the types of crises that occur in people's lives. The methodology of crisis intervention, including the role of the nurse, is explored.

CRISIS, DEFINED

The term **crisis** was defined by Caplan (1964) as the

"... psychological disequilibrium in a person who confronts a hazardous circumstance that for him constitutes an important problem which he can for the time being neither escape nor solve with his customary problem-solving resources."

Certain characteristics have been identified by various individuals who have studied crisis theory (Caplan, 1964; France, 1982; Geissler, 1984) that can be viewed as assumptions upon which the concept of crisis is based. They include the following:

1. Crisis occurs in all individuals at one time or another and is not necessarily equated with psychopathology.
2. Crises are precipitated by specific identifiable events.
3. Crises are personal by nature. What may be considered a crisis situation by one individual may not be so for another.
4. Crises are acute, not chronic, and will be resolved in one way or another within a brief period.
5. A crisis situation contains the potential for psychological growth or deterioration.

Individuals who are in crisis feel helpless to change. They do not believe they have the resources to deal with the precipitating stressor. Levels of anxiety rise to the point that the individual becomes nonfunctional, thoughts become obsessional, and all behavior is aimed at relief of the anxiety being experienced. The feeling is overwhelming and may affect the individual physically, as well as psychosocially.

PHASES IN THE DEVELOPMENT OF A CRISIS

The development of a crisis situation follows a relatively predictable course. Caplan (1964) has outlined four specific phases through which individuals progress in response to a precipitating stressor and which culminate in the state of acute crisis.

Phase 1. The individual is exposed to a precipitating stressor. Anxiety increases; previous problem-solving techniques are employed.

Phase 2. When previous problem-solving techniques do not relieve the stressor, anxiety increases further. The individual begins to feel a great deal of discomfort at this point. Coping techniques that have worked in the past are attempted, only to create feelings of helplessness when they are not successful. Feelings of confusion and disorganization prevail.

Phase 3. All possible resources, both internal and external, are called on to resolve the problem and relieve the discomfort. The individual may try to view the problem from a different perspective, or even to overlook certain aspects of it. New problem-solving techniques may be used, and, if effectual, resolution may occur at this phase, with the individual returning to a higher, a lower, or the previous level of premorbid functioning.

Phase 4. If resolution does not occur in previous phases, Caplan states, "... the tension mounts beyond a further threshold or its burden increases over time to a breaking point. Major disorganization of the individual with drastic results often occurs." Anxiety may reach panic levels. Cognitive functions are disordered, emotions are labile, and behavior may reflect the presence of psychotic thinking.

These phases are congruent with the transactional model of stress/adaptation outlined in Chapter 1. The relationship between the two perspectives is presented in Figure 11.1. Similarly, Aguilera (1998) spoke of "balancing factors" that affect the way in which an individual perceives and responds to a precipitating stressor. A schematic of these balancing factors is illustrated in Figure 11.2.

The paradigm set forth by Aguilera suggests that whether or not an individual experiences a crisis in response to a stressful situation depends upon the following three factors:

1. **The individual's perception of the event.** If the event is perceived realistically, the individual is more likely to draw upon adequate resources to restore equilibrium. If the perception of the event is distorted, attempts at problem solving are likely to be ineffective, and restoration of equilibrium goes unresolved.
2. **The availability of situational supports.** Aguilera states, "Situational supports are those persons who are available in the environment and who can be depended on to help solve the problem" (p. 37). Without adequate situational supports during a stressful situation, an individual is most likely to feel overwhelmed and alone.

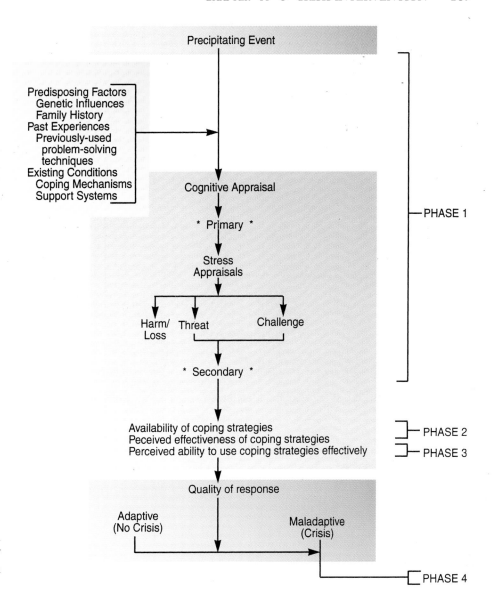

Figure 11.1 Relationship between transactional model of stress/adaptation and Caplan's phases in the development of a crisis.

3. **The availability of adequate coping mechanisms.** When a stressful situation occurs, individuals draw upon behavioral strategies that have been successful for them in the past. If these coping strategies work, a crisis may be diverted. If not, disequilibrium may continue and tension and anxiety increase.

As previously set forth, it is assumed that crises are acute, not chronic, situations that will be resolved in one way or another within a brief period. Barrell (1974) states, "Crises are by definition self-limiting and generally last from 4 to 6 weeks. During this brief period the person is psychologically vulnerable and is, consequently, *ready* for the learning and growth opportunity." Crises can become growth opportunities when individuals learn new methods of coping that can be preserved and used when similar stressors recur.

TYPES OF CRISES

Baldwin (1978) has identified six classes of emotional crises, which progress by degree of severity. As the measure of psychopathology increases, the source of the stressor changes from external to internal. The type of crisis determines the method of intervention selected.

Class 1: Dispositional Crises

Definition: An acute response to an external situational stressor.

EXAMPLE

Nancy and Ted have been married for 3 years and have a 1-year-old daughter. Ted has been hav-

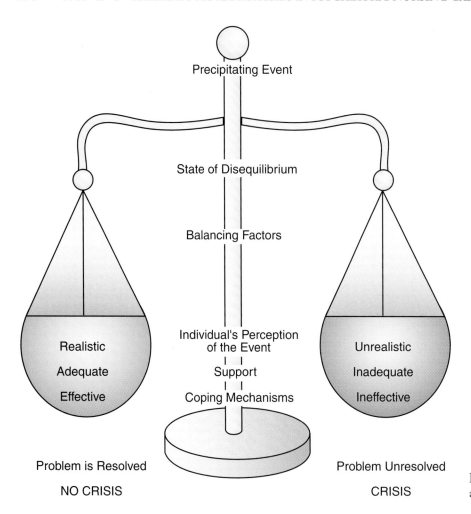

Figure 11.2 The effects of balancing factors in a stressful event.

ing difficulty with his boss at work. Twice during the past 6 months he has exploded in anger at home and become abusive with Nancy. Last night he became angry that dinner was not ready when he expected. He grabbed the baby from Nancy and tossed her, screaming, into her crib. He hit and punched Nancy until she feared for her life. This morning when he left for work, she took the baby and went to the emergency department of the city hospital, not having anywhere else to go.

Intervention: Nancy's physical wounds were cared for in the emergency department. The mental health counselor provided support and guidance in terms of presenting alternatives to her. Needs and issues were clarified, and referrals for agency assistance were made.

Class 2: Crises of Anticipated Life Transitions

Definition: Normal life-cycle transitions that may be anticipated but over which the individual may feel a lack of control.

EXAMPLE

College student JT is placed on probationary status because of low grades this semester. His wife had a baby and had to quit her job. He increased his working hours from part time to full time to compensate, and therefore had little time for studies. He presents himself to the student-health nurse clinician complaining of numerous vague physical complaints.

Intervention: Physical examination should be performed (physical symptoms could be caused by depression) and ventilation of feelings encouraged. Reassurance and support should be provided as needed. The client should be referred to services that can provide financial and other types of needed assistance. Problematic areas should be identified and approaches to change discussed.

Class 3: Crises Resulting From Traumatic Stress

Definition: Crises precipitated by unexpected external stresses over which the individual has little or no control and from which he or she feels emotionally overwhelmed and defeated.

EXAMPLE

Sally was a waitress whose shift ended at midnight. Two weeks ago, while walking to her car in the deserted parking lot, she was abducted by two men with guns, taken to an abandoned building, raped, and beaten. Since that time, her physical wounds have nearly healed. However, Sally cannot be alone, she is constantly fearful, she relives the experience in flashbacks and dreams and is unable to eat, sleep, or work on her job at the restaurant. Her friend offers to accompany her to the mental health clinic.

Intervention: The nurse should encourage Sally to talk about the experience and to ventilate feelings associated with it. The nurse should offer reassurance and support; discuss stages of grief and how rape causes a loss of self-worth, triggering the grief response; identify support systems that can help Sally to resume her normal activities; and explore new methods of coping with emotions arising from a situation with which she has had no previous experience.

Class 4: Maturational/ Developmental Crises

Definition: Crises that occur in response to situations that trigger emotions related to unresolved conflicts in one's life. These crises are of internal origin and reflect underlying developmental issues that involve dependency, value conflicts, sexual identity, control, and capacity for emotional intimacy.

EXAMPLE

Bob is 40 years old. He has just been passed over for a job promotion for the third time. He has moved many times within the large company for which he works, usually after angering and alienating himself from the supervisor. His father was domineering and became abusive when Bob did not comply with his every command. Over the years, Bob's behavioral response became one of passive-aggressiveness, first with his father, then with his supervisors. This third rejection has created feelings of depression and intense anxiety in Bob. At his wife's insistence, he has sought help at the mental health clinic.

Intervention: The primary intervention is to help the individual identify the unresolved developmental issue that is creating the conflict. Support and guidance are offered during the initial crisis period, then assistance is given to help the individual work through the underlying conflict in an effort to change response patterns that are creating problems in his current life situation.

Class 5: Crises Reflecting Psychopathology

Definition: Emotional crises in which preexisting psychopathology has been instrumental in precipitating the crisis or in which psychopathology significantly impairs or complicates adaptive resolution. Examples of psychopathology that may precipitate crises include borderline personality, severe neuroses, characterological disorders, or schizophrenia (Baldwin, 1978).

EXAMPLE

Sonja, age 29, was diagnosed with borderline personality at age 18. She has been in therapy on a weekly basis for 10 years, with several hospitalizations for suicide attempts during that time. She has had the same therapist for the past 6 years. This therapist told Sonja today that she is to be married in 1 month and will be moving across the country with her new husband. Sonja is distraught and experiencing intense feelings of abandonment. She is found wandering in and out of traffic on a busy expressway, oblivious to her surroundings. Police bring her to the emergency department of the hospital.

Intervention: The initial intervention is to help bring down the level of anxiety in Sonja that has created feelings of unreality in her. She requires that someone stay with her and reassure her of her safety and security. After the feelings of panic have subsided, she should be encouraged to verbalize her feelings of abandonment. Regressive behaviors should be discouraged. Positive reinforcement should be given for independent activities and accomplishments. The primary therapist will need to pursue this issue of termination with Sonja at length. Referral to a long-term care facility may be required.

Class 6: Psychiatric Emergencies

Definition: Crisis situations in which general functioning has been severely impaired and the individual rendered incompetent or unable to assume personal responsibility. Examples include acutely suicidal individuals, drug overdoses, reactions to hallucinogenic drugs, acute psychoses, uncontrollable anger, and alcohol intoxication (Baldwin, 1978).

EXAMPLE

Jennifer, age 16, had been dating Joe, the star high school football player, for 6 months. After the game on Friday night, Jennifer and Joe went to Jackie's house, where a number of high school students had gathered for an after-game party. No adults were present. About midnight, Joe told Jennifer that he did not want to date her anymore. Jennifer became hysterical, and Jackie was frightened by her behavior. She took Jennifer to her parents' bedroom and gave her a Valium from a bottle in her mother's medicine cabinet. She left Jennifer lying on her parents' bed and returned to the party downstairs. About an hour later, she returned to her parents' bedroom and found that Jennifer had removed the bottle of Valium from the cabinet and swallowed all of them. Jennifer was unconscious and Jackie could not awaken her. An ambulance was called and Jennifer was transported to the local hospital.

Intervention: The crisis team monitored vital signs, ensured maintenance of adequate airway, initiated gastric lavage, and administered activated charcoal to minimize absorption. Jennifer's parents were notified and rushed to the hospital. The situation was explained to them, and they were encouraged to stay by her side. When the physical crisis was resolved, Jennifer was transferred to the psychiatric unit. In therapy, she was encouraged to ventilate her feelings regarding the rejection and subsequent overdose. Family therapy sessions were conducted in an effort to clarify interpersonal issues and to identify areas for change. On an individual level, Jennifer's therapist worked with her to establish more adaptive methods of coping with stressful situations.

CRISIS INTERVENTION

Individuals experiencing crises have an urgent need for assistance. In **crisis intervention** the therapist, or other intervener, becomes a part of the individual's life situation. Because of the individual's emotional state, he or she is unable to problem solve, so requires guidance and support from another to help mobilize the resources needed to resolve the crisis.

Lengthy psychological interpretations are obviously not appropriate for crisis intervention. It is a time for doing what is needed to help the individual get relief. It is a time for calling into action all the people and other resources required to do so. Aguilera (1998) states:

"The goal of crisis intervention is the resolution of an immediate crisis. Its focus is on the supportive, with the restoration of the individual to his precrisis level of functioning or possibly to a higher level of functioning. The therapist's role is direct, supportive, and that of an active participant." (p. 24)

Crisis intervention takes place in both inpatient and outpatient settings. The basic methodology relies heavily on orderly problem-solving techniques and structured activities that are focused on change. Through adaptive change, crises are resolved and growth occurs. Because of the time limitation of crisis intervention, the individual must experience some degree of relief almost from the first interaction. Crisis intervention, then, is not aimed at major personality change or reconstruction (as may be the case in long-term psychotherapy), but rather at using a given crisis situation to, at the very least, restore functioning and also, at most, to enhance personal growth.

PHASES OF CRISIS INTERVENTION: THE ROLE OF THE NURSE

Nurses respond to crisis situations on a daily basis. Crises can occur on every unit in the general hospital, in the home setting, in the community health care setting, in schools, in offices, and in private practice. Indeed, nurses may be called upon to function as crisis helpers in virtually any setting committed to the practice of nursing.

Aguilera (1998) describes four specific phases in the technique of crisis intervention. These phases are clearly comparable to the steps of the nursing process.

Phase 1. Assessment

In this phase, the crisis helper gathers information regarding the precipitating stressor and the resulting crisis that prompted the individual to seek professional help. A nurse in crisis intervention might perform some of the following assessments:

1. Ask the individual to describe the event that precipitated this crisis.
2. Determine when it occurred.
3. Assess the individual's physical and mental status.
4. Determine if the individual has experienced this stressor before. If so, what method of coping was used? Have these methods been tried this time?
5. If previous coping methods were tried, what was the result?
6. If new coping methods were tried, what was the result?
7. Assess suicide or homicide potential, plan, and means.
8. Assess the adequacy of support systems.
9. Determine level of precrisis functioning. Assess the usual coping methods, available support systems, and ability to problem solve.
10. Assess the individual's perception of personal strengths and limitations.
11. Assess the individual's use of substances.

Information from the comprehensive assessment is then analyzed, and appropriate nursing diagnoses reflecting the immediacy of the crisis situation are identified. Some nursing diagnoses that may be relevant include:

1. Ineffective individual coping
2. Anxiety (severe to panic)
3. Altered thought processes
4. Potential for violence, self-directed or directed at others
5. Rape-trauma syndrome
6. Posttrauma response
7. Fear

Phase 2. Planning of Therapeutic Intervention

In the planning phase of the nursing process, the nurse selects the appropriate nursing actions for the identified nursing diagnoses. In planning the interventions, the type of crisis, as well as the individual's strengths and available resources for support, are taken into consideration. Goals are established for crisis resolution and a return to, or increase in, the precrisis level of functioning.

Phase 3. Intervention

During phase 3, the actions that were identified in phase 2 are implemented. Smith, Karasik, and Meyer (1984) have outlined the following interventions as the focus of nursing in crisis intervention:

1. Use a reality-oriented approach. The focus of the problem is on the here and now.
2. Remain with the individual who is experiencing panic anxiety.
3. Establish a rapid working relationship by showing unconditional acceptance, by active listening, and by attending to immediate needs.
4. Discourage lengthy explanations or rationalizations of the situation; promote an atmosphere for verbalization of true feelings.
5. Set firm limits on aggressive, destructive behaviors. At high levels of anxiety, behavior is likely to be impulsive and regressive. Establish at the outset what is acceptable and what is not, and maintain consistency.
6. Clarify the problem that the individual is facing. The nurse does this by describing his or her perception of the problem and comparing it with the individual's perception of the problem.
7. Help the individual determine what he or she believes precipitated the crisis.
8. Acknowledge feelings of anger, guilt, helplessness, and powerlessness, while taking care not to provide positive feedback for these feelings.
9. Guide the individual through a problem-solving process by which he or she may move in the direction of positive life change:
    a. Help the individual confront the source of the problem that is creating the crisis response.
    b. Encourage the individual to discuss changes he or she would like to make. Jointly determine whether or not desired changes are realistic.
    c. Encourage exploration of feelings about aspects that cannot be changed, and explore alternative ways of coping more adaptively in these situations.
    d. Discuss alternative strategies for creating changes that are realistically possible.
    e. Weigh benefits and consequences of each alternative.
    f. Assist the individual to select alternative coping strategies that will help alleviate future crisis situations.
10. Identify external support systems and new social networks from whom the individual may seek assistance in times of stress.

Phase 4. Evaluation of Crisis Resolution and Anticipatory Planning

To evaluate the outcome of crisis intervention, a reassessment is made to determine if the stated objective was achieved:

1. Have positive behavioral changes occurred?
2. Has the individual developed more adaptive coping strategies? Have they been effective?
3. Has the individual grown from the experience by gaining insight into his or her responses to crisis situations?
4. Does the individual believe that he or she could respond with healthy adaptation in future stressful situations to prevent crisis development?
5. Can the individual describe a plan of action for dealing with stressors similar to the one that precipitated this crisis?

During the evaluation period, the nurse and client summarize what has occurred during the intervention. They review what the individual has learned and "anticipate" how he or she will respond in the future. A determination is made regarding follow-up therapy; if needed, the nurse provides referral information.

SUMMARY

A *crisis* is a situation that produces

"psychological disequilibrium in a person who confronts a hazardous circumstance that for him constitutes an important problem, which he can for the time being neither escape nor solve with his customary problem-solving resources." (Caplan, 1964.)

All individuals experience crises at one time or another. This does not necessarily indicate psychopathology.

Crises are precipitated by specific identifiable events and are determined by an individual's personal perception of the situation. They are acute, not chronic, and generally last no more than 4 to 6 weeks.

Crises occur when an individual is exposed to a stressor and previous problem-solving techniques are ineffective. This causes the level of anxiety to rise. Panic may ensue when new techniques are employed and resolution fails to occur.

Baldwin (1978) identified six types of crises. They include dispositional crises, crises of anticipated life transitions, crises resulting from traumatic stress, maturation/developmental crises, crises reflecting psychopathology, and psychiatric emergencies. The type of crisis determines the method of intervention selected.

Crisis intervention is designed to provide rapid assistance for individuals who have an urgent need. Aguilera (1998) identifies the minimum therapeutic goal of crisis intervention as psychological resolution of the individual's immediate crisis and restoration to at least the level of functioning that existed before the crisis period. A maximum goal is improvement in functioning above the precrisis level.

Nurses regularly respond to individuals in crisis in all types of settings. Nursing process is the vehicle by which nurses assist individuals in crisis with a short-term problem-solving approach to change. A four-phase technique was outlined: assessment/analysis, planning of therapeutic intervention, intervention, and evaluation of crisis resolution and anticipatory planning. Through this structured method of assistance, nurses assist individuals in crisis to develop more adaptive coping strategies for dealing with stressful situations in the future.

REVIEW QUESTIONS

SELF-EXAMINATION/LEARNING EXERCISE

Select the *best* response to each of the following questions.

1. Which of the following is a correct assumption regarding the concept of crisis?

   a. Crises occur only in individuals with psychopathology.
   b. The stressful event that precipitates crisis is seldom identifiable.
   c. A crisis situation contains the potential for psychological growth or deterioration.
   d. Crises are chronic situations that recur many times during an individual's life.

2. Crises occur when an individual:

   a. Is exposed to a precipitating stressor.
   b. Perceives a stressor to be threatening.
   c. Has no support systems.
   d. Experiences a stressor and perceives coping strategies to be ineffective.

3. Amanda's mobile home was destroyed by a tornado. Amanda received only minor injuries, but is experiencing disabling anxiety in the aftermath of the event. This type of crisis is called:

   a. Crisis resulting from traumatic stress.
   b. Maturational/developmental crisis.
   c. Dispositional crisis.
   d. Crisis of anticipated life transitions.

4. The most appropriate crisis intervention with Amanda would be to:

   a. Encourage her to recognize how lucky she is to be alive.
   b. Discuss stages of grief and feelings associated with each.
   c. Identify community resources that can help Amanda.
   d. Suggest that she find a place to live that provides a storm shelter.

5. Jenny reported to the high school nurse that her mother drinks too much. She is drunk every afternoon when Jenny gets home from school. Jenny is afraid to invite friends over because of her mothers's behavior. This type of crisis is called:

   a. Crisis resulting from traumatic stress.
   b. Maturational/developmental crisis.
   c. Dispositional crisis.
   d. Crisis reflecting psychopathology.

6. The most appropriate nursing intervention with Jenny would be to:

   a. Make arrangements for her to start attending Al-Ateen meetings.
   b. Help her identify the positive things in her life and recognize that her situation could be a lot worse than it is.
   c. Teach her about the effects of alcohol on the body and that alcoholism can be hereditary.
   d. Refer her to a psychiatrist for private therapy to learn to deal with her home situation.

7. Ginger, age 19 and an only child, left 3 months ago to attend a college of her choice 500 miles away from her parents. It is Ginger's first time away from home. She has difficulty making decisions and will not undertake anything new without first consulting her mother. They talk on the phone almost every day. Ginger has recently started having anxiety attacks. She consults the nurse clinician in the student health center. This type of crisis is called:

   a. Crisis resulting from traumatic stress.
   b. Dispositional crisis.
   c. Psychiatric emergency.
   d. Maturational/developmental crisis.

8. The most appropriate nursing intervention with Ginger would be to:

   a. Suggest she move to a college closer to home.
   b. Work with Ginger on unresolved dependency issues.
   c. Help her find someone in the college town from whom she could seek assistance rather than calling her mother regularly.
   d. Recommend that the college physician prescribe an antianxiety medication for Ginger.

9. Marie, age 56, is the mother of five children. Her youngest child, who had been living at home and attending the local college, recently graduated and accepted a job in another state. Marie has never worked outside the home and has devoted her life to satisfying the needs of her husband and children. Since the departure of her last child from home, Marie has become more and more despondent. Her husband has become very concerned, and takes her to the local mental health center. This type of crisis is called:

   a. Dispositional crisis.
   b. Crisis of anticipated life transitions.
   c. Psychiatric emergency.
   d. Crisis resulting from traumatic stress.

10. The most appropriate nursing intervention with Marie would be to:

   a. Refer her to her family physician for a complete physical examination.
   b. Suggest she seek outside employment now that her children have left home.
   c. Identify convenient support systems for times when she is feeling particularly despondent.
   d. Begin grief work and assist her to recognize areas of self-worth separate and apart from her children.

REFERENCES

Aguilera, D.C. (1998). *Crisis intervention: Theory and methodology* (8th ed.). St. Louis: C.V. Mosby.

Baldwin, B.A. (1978, July). A paradigm for the classification of emotional crises: Implications for crisis intervention. *American Journal of Orthopsychiatry, 48*(3), 538–551.

Barrell, L.M. (1974, March). Crisis intervention: Partnership in problem-solving. *Nursing Clinics of North America, 9*(1), 5–16.

Caplan, G. (1964). Principles of preventive psychiatry. New York: Basic Books.

France, K. (1982). *Crisis intervention: A handbook of immediate person-to-person help.* Springfield, IL: Charles C. Thomas.

Geissler, E.M. (1984, July). Crisis: What it is and is not. Advances in Nursing Science, 6(4), 1–9.

Smith, S.F., Karasik, D.A., & Meyer, B.J. (1984). *Psychiatric and psychosocial nursing.* Los Altos, CA: National Nursing Review.

Bibliography

Brownell, M.J. (1984, July). The concept of crisis: Its utility for nursing. *Advances in Nursing Science, 6*(4), 10–21.

Duggan, H.A. (1984). *Crisis intervention: Helping individuals at risk.* Lexington, MA: Lexington Books.

Goldstein, D. (1978, December). Crisis intervention: A brief therapy model. *Nursing Clinics of North America, 13*(4), 657–663.

Hatch, C., & Schut, L. (1980, April). Description of a crisis-oriented psychiatric home visiting service. *Journal of Psychosocial Nursing and Mental Health Services, 18*(4), 31–35.

Hoff, L.A. (1989). *People in crisis: Understanding and helping* (3rd ed.). Redwood City, CA: Addison-Wesley.

Johnson, R. (1981). Applying crisis intervention techniques. In J. Robinson (Ed.), *Using crisis intervention wisely.* Nursing Skillbook Series. Horsham, PA: Intermed Communications.

RELAXATION THERAPY

KEY TERMS

stress management
progressive relaxation

meditation
mental imagery

biofeedback

OBJECTIVES

After reading this chapter, the student will be able to:

1. Identify conditions for which relaxation is appropriate therapy.
2. Describe physiological and behavioral manifestations of relaxation.
3. Discuss various methods of achieving relaxation.
4. Describe the role of the nurse in relaxation therapy.

esearchers now know that stress has a definite effect on the body. They know that stress on the body can be caused by positive events as well as negative ones, and they know that prolonged stress can result in many physiological illnesses. Many times we hear "Relax, take it easy, don't work so hard, don't worry so much; you'll live longer that way." This is good advice no doubt, but it is easier to say than to do.

Nurses are in an ideal position to assist individuals in the management of stress in their lives. This chapter discusses the therapeutic benefits to the individual of regular participation in relaxation exercises. Various methods of achieving relaxation are described, and the nurse's role in helping individuals learn how to use relaxation techniques adaptively is explored.

THE STRESS EPIDEMIC

Individuals experience stress as a daily fact of life; it cannot be avoided. It is generated by both positive and negative experiences that require adjustment to various changes in one's current routine. Whether or not there is more stress today than in the past is unknown, but some experts have suggested that it has become more pervasive. Perhaps this is due to the many uncertainties and salient risks that challenge our most basic value systems on a day-to-day basis.

In Chapter 1, a lengthy discussion was presented regarding the "fight or flight" response of the human body to stressful situations. This response served our ancestors well. The extra burst of adrenaline primed their muscles and focused their attention on the danger at hand. Indeed, the response provided early *Homo sapiens* with the essentials to deal with life-and-death situations, such as an imminent attack by a saber-toothed tiger or grizzly bear.

Today, with stress rapidly permeating our society, large segments of the population experience the "fight or flight" response on a regular basis. However, the physical reinforcements are not used in a manner by which the individual is returned to the homeostatic condition within a short period. The "fight or flight" emergency response is inappropriate to today's psychosocial stresses that persist over long periods. In fact, in today's society, rather than assisting with life-and-death situations, the response may actually be a contributing factor in some life-and-death situations. Dr. Joel Elkes, director of the behavioral medicine program at the University of Louisville (Kentucky), has said, "Our mode of life itself, the way we live, is emerging as today's principal cause of illness." Stress is now known to be a major contributor, either directly or indirectly, to coronary heart disease, cancer, lung ailments, accidental injuries, cirrhosis of the liver, and suicide—six of the leading causes of death in the United States (Hafen, Karren, Frandsen, & Smith, 1996).

Stress management has become a multimillion dollar business in this country. Corporation managers have realized increases in productivity by providing employees with stress-reduction programs. Hospitals and clinics have responded to the need for services that offer stress-management information to individuals and groups.

When, then, is relaxation therapy required? The answer to this question depends largely on *predisposing factors*, the genetic influences, past experiences, and existing conditions that influence how an individual perceives and responds to stress. For example, temperament (i.e., behavioral characteristics that are present at birth) often plays a determining role in the individual's manner of responding to stressful situations. Some individuals, by temperament, naturally respond with a greater degree of anxiety than others.

TABLE 12.1 HOW VULNERABLE ARE YOU TO STRESS?

Score each item from 1 (almost always) to 5 (never), according to how much of the time each statement applies to you.

_____ 1. I eat at least one hot, balanced meal a day.
_____ 2. I get 7 to 8 hours sleep at least four nights a week.
_____ 3. I give and receive affection regularly.
_____ 4. I have at least one relative within 50 miles on whom I can rely.
_____ 5. I exercise to the point of perspiration at least twice a week.
_____ 6. I smoke less than half a pack of cigarettes a day.
_____ 7. I take fewer than five alcoholic drinks a week.
_____ 8. I am the appropriate weight for my height.
_____ 9. I have an income adequate to meet basic expenses.
_____ 10. I get strength from my religious beliefs.
_____ 11. I regularly attend club or social activities.
_____ 12. I have a network of friends and acquaintances.
_____ 13. I have one or more friends to confide in about personal matters.
_____ 14. I am in good health (including eyesight, hearing, and teeth).
_____ 15. I am able to speak openly about my feelings when angry or worried.
_____ 16. I have regular conversations with the people I live with about domestic problems (e.g., chores, money, and daily living issues).
_____ 17. I do something for fun at least once a week.
_____ 18. I am able to organize my time effectively.
_____ 19. I drink fewer than three cups of coffee (or tea or colas) a day.
_____ 20. I take quiet time for myself during the day.
_____ TOTAL

To get your score, add up the figures and subtract 20. Any number over 30 indicates a vulnerability to stress. You are seriously vulnerable if your score is between 50 and 75, and extremely vulnerable if it is over 75.

SOURCE: From Miller & Smith (1983), p. 54, with permission.

Past experiences are occurrences that result in learned patterns that can influence an individual's adaptation response. They include previous exposure to the stressor or other stressors, learned coping responses, and degree of adaptation to previous stressors.

Existing conditions are the individual vulnerabilities that can influence the adequacy of the physical, psychological, and social resources for dealing with stressful situations. Examples include current health status, motivation, developmental maturity, severity and duration of the stressor, financial and educational resources, age, existing coping strategies, and a support system of caring others.

All individuals react to stress with predictable physiological and psychosocial responses. These predisposing factors determine the degree of severity of the response. Undoubtedly, there are very few people who would not benefit from some form of relaxation therapy. Holmes and Rahe (1967) developed the Social Readjustment Rating Scale, which correlated an individual's susceptibility to physical or psychological illness with his or her level of stress (see Chapter 1). The lay literature now provides various self-tests that individuals may perform to determine their vulnerability to stress. Two of these are presented in Tables 12.1 and 12.2.

PHYSIOLOGICAL, COGNITIVE, AND BEHAVIORAL MANIFESTATIONS OF RELAXATION

The physiological and behavioral manifestations of stress are well documented (see Chapters 1 and 2). A review of these symptoms is presented in Table 12.3. The persistence of these symptoms over long periods can contribute to the development of numerous stress-related illnesses.

The achievement of relaxation can counteract many of these symptoms. In a state of deep relaxation, the respiration rate may slow to as few as four to six breaths per minute and the heart rate to as low as 24 beats per minute (Pelletier, 1992). Blood pressure decreases and the metabolic rate slows downs. Muscle tension diminishes, pupils constrict, and blood vessels in the periphery dilate, leading to increased temperature and feeling of warmth in the extremities.

One's level of consciousness moves from beta activity, which occurs when one is mentally alert and actively thinking, to alpha activity, a state of altered consciousness (DiMotto, 1984). Benefits associated with achievement of alpha consciousness include an increase in creativity, memory, and the ability to concentrate. Ultimately, an improvement in adaptive functioning may be realized.

When deeply relaxed, individuals are less attentive to distracting stimuli in the external environment. They will

---

■ TABLE 12.2 ARE YOU "STRESSED OUT?"

Check yes or no for each of the following questions.

	Yes	No
1. Do you have recurrent headaches, neck tension, or back pain?	—	—
2. Do you often have indigestion, nausea, or diarrhea?	—	—
3. Have you unintentionally gained or lost 5–10 lb in the last month?	—	—
4. Do you have difficulty falling or staying asleep?	—	—
5. Do you often feel restless?	—	—
6. Do you have difficulty concentrating?	—	—
7. Do you drink alcohol, smoke, or take drugs to relax?	—	—
8. Have you had a major illness, surgery, or an accident in the past year?	—	—
9. Have you lost five or more days of work due to illness in the past 6 months?	—	—
10. Have you had a change in job status (been fired, laid off, promoted, demoted, and so on) in the past 6 months?	—	—
11. Do you work more than 48 hr a week?	—	—
12. Do you have serious financial problems?	—	—
13. Have you recently experienced family or marital problems?	—	—
14. Has a person of significance in your life died in the past year?	—	—
15. Have you been divorced or separated in the past year?	—	—
16. Do you find you've lost interest in hobbies, physical activity, and leisure time?	—	—
17. Have you lost interest in your relationship with your spouse, relative, or friend?	—	—
18. Do you find yourself watching more TV than you should?	—	—
19. Are you emotionally or easily irritated lately?	—	—
20. Do you seem to experience more distress and discomfort than most people?	—	—

Scoring:

Each yes is worth 1 point; each no is worth 0.   Total your points: _____

  0–3 = mildly stressed

  4–6 = moderately stressed

  7 or more = extremely vulnerable. You may be at risk for stress-related illness.

SOURCE: From The Department of Psychiatry, St. Joseph Medical Center, Wichita, KS. Printed in The *Wichita Eagle*, November 10, 1990, with permission.

TABLE 12.3 PHYSIOLOGICAL, COGNITIVE, AND BEHAVIORAL MANIFESTATIONS OF STRESS

PHYSIOLOGICAL	COGNITIVE	BEHAVIORAL
Epinephrine and norepinephrine are released into the bloodstream.	Anxiety increases.	Restlessness
Pupils dilate.	Confusion and disorientation may be evident.	Irritability
Respiration rate increases.	The person is unable to problem solve.	Use or misuse of defense mechanisms
Heart rate increases.	The person is unable to concentrate.	Disorganized routine functioning
Blood pressure increases.	Cognitive processes focus on achieving relief from anxiety	Insomnia and anorexia
Digestion subsides.	Learning is inhibited.	Compulsive or bizarre behaviors (depending on level of anxiety being experienced)
Blood sugar increases.	Thoughts may reflect obsessions and ruminations.	
Metabolism increases.		
Serum free fatty acids, cholesterol, and triglycerides increase.		

respond to questions directed at them but do not initiate verbal interaction. Physical demeanor is very composed. Virtually no muscle activity is observed. Eyes are closed, jaws may be slightly parted, palms are open with fingers curled but not clenched. Head may be slightly tilted to the side.

A summary of the physiological, cognitive, and behavioral manifestations of relaxation is presented in Table 12.4.

METHODS OF ACHIEVING RELAXATION

Deep-Breathing Exercises

Deep breathing is a simple technique that is basic to most other relaxation skills. Tension is released when the lungs are allowed to breathe in as much oxygen as possible (Sobel & Ornstein, 1996). Breathing exercises have been found to be effective in reducing anxiety, depression, irritability, muscular tension, and fatigue

(Davis, Eshelman, & McKay, 1995; Sobel & Ornstein, 1996). An advantage of this exercise is that it may be accomplished anywhere and at any time. A good guideline is to practice deep breathing for a few minutes three or four times a day or whenever a feeling of tenseness occurs.

Technique

1. Sit, stand, or lie in a comfortable position, ensuring that the spine is straight.
2. Place one hand on your abdomen and the other on your chest.
3. Inhale slowly and deeply through your nose. The abdomen should be expanding and pushing up on your hand. The chest should be moving only slightly.
4. When you have breathed in as much as possible, hold your breath for a few seconds before exhaling.
5. Begin exhaling slowly through the mouth, pursing

TABLE 12.4 PHYSIOLOGICAL, COGNITIVE, AND BEHAVIORAL MANIFESTATIONS OF RELAXATION

PHYSIOLOGICAL	COGNITIVE	BEHAVIORAL
Lower levels of epinephrine and norepinephrine in the blood	Change from beta consciousness to alpha consciousness	Distractability to environmental stimuli is decreased
Respiration rate decreases (sometimes as low as 4–6 breaths per minute)	Creativity and memory are enhanced	Will respond to questions but does not initiate verbal interaction
Heart rate decreases (sometimes as low as 24 beats per minute)	Increased ability to concentrate	Calm, tranquil demeanor; no evidence of restlessness
Blood pressure decreases		Common mannerisms include eyes closed, jaws parted, palms open, fingers curled, and head slightly tilted to the side
Metabolic rate slows down		
Muscle tension diminishes		
Pupils constrict		
Vasodilation and increased temperature in the extremities		

your lips as if you were going to whistle. Pursing the lips helps to control how fast you exhale and keeps airways open as long as possible.

6. Feel the abdomen deflate as the lungs are emptied of air.

7. Begin the inhale-exhale cycle again. Focus on the sound and feeling of your breathing as you become more and more relaxed.

8. Continue the deep-breathing exercises for 5 to 10 minutes at a time. Once mastered, the technique may be used as often as required to relieve tension.

Progressive Relaxation

Progressive relaxation, a method of deep-muscle relaxation, was developed in 1929 by Chicago physician Edmond Jacobson. His technique is based on the premise that the body responds to anxiety-provoking thoughts and events with muscle tension. Excellent results have been observed with this method in the treatment of muscular tension, anxiety, insomnia, depression, fatigue, irritable bowel, muscle spasms, neck and back pain, high blood pressure, mild phobias, and stuttering (Davis, Eshelman, & McKay, 1995).

Technique

Each muscle group is tensed for 5 to 7 seconds and then relaxed for 20 to 30 seconds, during which time the individual concentrates on the difference in sensations between the two conditions. Soft, slow background music may facilitate relaxation.

1. Sit in a comfortable chair with your hands in your lap and feet flat on the floor, your eyes closed.

2. Begin by taking three deep, slow breaths, inhaling through the nose and releasing the air slowly through the mouth.

3. Now starting with the feet, pull the toes forward toward the knees, stiffen your calves, and hold for a count of five.

4. Now release the hold. Let go of the tension. Feel the sensation of relaxation and warmth as the tension flows out of the muscles.

5. Next, tense the muscles of the thighs and buttocks, and hold for a count of five.

6. Now release the hold. Feel the tension drain away, and be aware of the difference in sensation—perhaps a heavyness or feeling of warmth that you did not feel when the muscles were tensed. Concentrate on this feeling for a few seconds.

7. Next, tense the abdominal muscles. Hold for a count of five.

8. Now release the hold. Concentrate on the feeling of relaxation in the muscles. You may feel a warm-

ing sensation. Hold on to that feeling for 15 to 20 seconds.

9. Next, tense the muscles in the back and hold for a count of five.

10. Now release the hold. Feel the sensation of relaxation and warmth as the tension flows out of the muscles.

11. Next, tense the muscles of your hands, biceps, and forearms. Clench your hands into a tight fist. Hold for a count of five.

12. Now release the hold. Notice the sensations. You may feel tingling, warmth, or a light, airy feeling. Recognize these sensations as tension leaves the muscles.

13. Next, tense the muscles of the shoulders and neck. Shrug the shoulders tightly and hold for a count of five.

14. Now release the hold. Sense the tension as it leaves the muscles and experience the feeling of relaxation.

15. Next, tense the muscles of the face. Wrinkle the forehead, frown, squint the eyes, and purse the lips. Hold for a count of five.

16. Now release the hold. Recognize a light, warm feeling flowing into the muscles.

17. Now feel the relaxation in your whole body. As the tension leaves your entire being, you feel completely relaxed.

18. Open your eyes and enjoy renewed energy.

Modified (or Passive) Progressive Relaxation

Technique

In this version of total-body relaxation the muscles are not tensed. The individual learns to relax muscles by concentrating on the feeling of relaxation within the muscle. These instructions may be presented by one person for another or they may be self-administered. Relaxation may be facilitated by playing soft, slow background music during the activity.

1. Assume a comfortable position. Some suggestions include the following:
   a. Sitting straight up in a chair with hands in the lap or at sides and feet flat on floor.
   b. Sitting in a reclining chair with hands in the lap or at sides and legs up on elevated foot of chair.
   c. Lying flat with head slightly elevated on pillow, arms at sides.

2. Close your eyes and take three deep breaths through your nose, slowly releasing the air through your mouth.

3. Allow a feeling of peacefulness to descend over you—a pleasant, enjoyable sensation of being comfortable and at ease.

4. Remain in this state for several minutes.

5. It is now time to turn your attention to various parts of your body.

6. We will begin with the muscles of the head, face, throat, and shoulders. Concentrate on these muscles, paying particular attention to those in the forehead and jaws. Feel the tension leave the area. The muscles start to feel relaxed, heavy, and warm. Concentrate on this feeling for a few minutes.

7. Now let the feeling of relaxation continue to spread downward to the muscles of your biceps, forearms, and hands. Concentrate on these muscles. Feel the tension dissolve, the muscles starting to feel relaxed and heavy. A feeling of warmth spreads through these muscles all the way to the fingertips. They are feeling very warm and very heavy. Concentrate on this feeling for a few minutes.

8. The tension is continuing to dissolve now, and you are feeling very relaxed. Turn your attention to the muscles in your chest, abdomen, and lower back. Feel the tension leave these areas. Allow these muscles to become very relaxed. They start to feel very warm, very heavy. Concentrate on this feeling for a few minutes.

9. The feeling of relaxation continues to move downward now as we move to the muscles of the thighs, buttocks, calves, and feet. Feel the tension moving down and out of your body. These muscles feel very relaxed now. Your legs are feeling very heavy, very limp. A feeling of warmth spreads over the area, all the way to the toes. You can feel that all the tension has been released.

10. Your whole body feels relaxed and warm. Listen to the music for a few moments and concentrate on this relaxed, warm feeling. Take several deep, slow breaths through your nose, releasing the air through your mouth. Continue to concentrate on how relaxed and warm you feel.

11. It is now time to refocus your concentration on the present and wake up your body to resume activity. Open your eyes and stretch or massage your muscles. Wiggle your fingers and toes. Take another deep breath, arise, and enjoy the feeling of renewed energy.

Meditation

Records and phenomenological accounts of meditative practices date back more than 2000 years, but only recently have empirical studies revealed the psychophysiological benefits of regular use (Pelletier, 1992). The goal of **meditation** is to gain "mastery over attention." It brings on a special state of consciousness as attention is concentrated solely on one thought or object.

Historically, meditation has been associated with religious doctrines and disciplines by which individuals sought enlightenment with God or another higher power. However, meditation can be practiced independently from any religious philosophy and purely as a means of achieving inner harmony and increasing self-awareness.

During meditation, the respiration rate, heart rate, and blood pressure decrease. The overall metabolism declines, and the need for oxygen consumption is reduced. Alpha brain waves, those associated with brain activity during periods of relaxation, predominate (Pelletier, 1992).

Meditation has been used successfully in the prevention and treatment of various cardiovascular diseases. It has proved helpful in curtailing obsessive thinking, anxiety, depression, and hostility. Meditation improves concentration and attention (Davis, Eshelman, & McKay, 1995).

Technique

1. Select a quiet place and a comfortable position. Various sitting positions are appropriate for meditation. Examples include:
   a. Sitting in a chair with your feet flat on the floor approximately 6 inches apart, arms resting comfortably in your lap.
   b. Cross-legged on the floor or on a cushion.
   c. In the Japanese fashion with knees on floor, great toes together, pointed backward, and buttocks resting comfortably on bottom of feet.
   d. In the lotus yoga position, sitting on the floor with the legs flexed at the knees. The ankles are crossed and each foot rests on top of the opposite thigh.

2. Select an object, word, or thought on which to dwell. During meditation the individual becomes preoccupied with the selected focus. This total preoccupation serves to prevent distractions from interrupting attention. Examples of foci include:
   a. **Counting One's Breaths.** All attention is focused on breathing in and out.
   b. **Mantras.** A *mantra* is a syllable, word, or name that is repeated many times as you free your mind of thoughts. Any mantra is appropriate if it works to focus attention and prevent distracting thoughts.
   c. **Objects for Contemplation.** Select an object, such as a rock, a marble, or anything that does not hold a symbolic meaning that might cause distraction. Contemplate the object both visually and tactilely. Focus total attention on the object.
   d. **A Thought That Has Special Meaning to You.** With eyes closed, focus total attention on a specific thought or idea.

3. Practice directing attention on your selected focus for 10 to 15 minutes a day for several weeks. It is essential that the individual does not become upset if intrusive thoughts find their way into the meditation practice. They should merely be dealt with and dismissed as the individual returns to the selected focus of attention. Worrying about one's progress in the ability to meditate is a self-inhibiting behavior.

Mental Imagery

Mental imagery uses the imagination in an effort to reduce the body's response to stress. The frame of reference is very personal, based on what each individual considers to be a relaxing environment. Some might select a scene at the seashore, some might choose a mountain atmosphere, and some might choose floating through the air on a fluffy white cloud. The choices are as limitless as one's imagination. Following is an example of how one individual uses imagery for relaxation. The information is most useful when taped and played back at a time when the individual wishes to achieve relaxation.

Technique

Sit or lie down in a comfortable position. Close your eyes. Imagine that you and someone you love are walking along the seashore. No other people are in sight in any direction. The sun is shining, the sky is blue, and a gentle breeze is blowing. You select a spot to stop and rest. You lie on the sand and close your eyes. You hear the sound of the waves as they splash against the shore. The sun feels warm on your face and body. The sand feels soft and warm against your back. An occasional wave splashes you with a cool mist that dries rapidly in the warm sun. The coconut fragrance of your suntan lotion wafts gently and pleasantly in the air. You lie in this quiet place for what seems like a very long time, taking in the sounds of the waves, the warmth of the sun, and the cooling sensations of the mist and ocean breeze. It is very quiet. It is very warm. You feel very relaxed, very contented. This is your special place. You may come to this special place whenever you want to relax.

Biofeedback

Biofeedback is the use of instrumentation to become aware of processes in your body that you usually do not notice and to help bring them under voluntary control. Biofeedback machines give immediate information about an individual's own biological conditions, such as muscle tension, skin surface temperature, brain-wave activity, skin conductivity, blood pressure, and heart rate (Davis, Eshelman, & McKay, 1995). Some conditions that can be treated successfully with biofeedback include spastic colon, hypertension, tension and migraine headaches, muscle spasms/pain, anxiety, phobias, stuttering, and teeth grinding.

Technique

Biological conditions are monitored by the biofeedback equipment. Sensors relate muscle spasticity, body temperature, brain-wave activity, heart rate, and blood pressure. Each of these conditions will elicit a signal from the equipment, such as a blinking light, a measure on a meter, or an audible tone. The individual practices using relaxation and voluntary control to modify the signal, in turn indicating a modification of the autonomic function it represents.

Various types of biofeedback equipment have been developed recently for home use. However, they have not proved very effective, as they usually measure only one autonomic function, when, in fact, modification of several functions may be required to achieve the benefits of total relaxation.

Biofeedback can help monitor the progress an individual is making toward learning to relax. It is often used together with other relaxation techniques such as deep breathing, progressive relaxation, and mental imagery.

Special training is required to become a biofeedback practitioner. Nurses can support and encourage individuals learning to use this method of stress management. Nurses can also teach other techniques of relaxation that enhance the results of biofeedback training.

Physical Exercise

Regular exercise is viewed by many as one of the most effective methods for relieving stress. Physical exertion provides a natural outlet for the tension produced by the body in its state of arousal for "fight or flight." Following exercise, physiological equilibrium is restored, resulting in a feeling of relaxation and revitalization. A sedentary lifestyle and physical inactivity are thought to be major contributors to coronary heart disease, obesity, joint and spinal disk disease, fatigue, muscular tension, and depression (Davis, Eshelman, & McKay, 1995).

Aerobic exercises strengthen the cardiovascular system and increase the body's ability to use oxygen more efficiently. Aerobic exercises include brisk walking, jogging, running, cycling, swimming, and dancing, among other activities. To achieve the benefits of aerobic exercises, they must be performed regularly—for at least 30 minutes, three times per week.

Individuals can also benefit from low-intensity physical exercise. Although there is little benefit to the cardiovascular system, low-intensity exercise can help prevent obesity, relieve muscular tension, prevent muscle spasms, and increase flexibility. Examples of low-intensity exercise include slow walking, house cleaning, shopping, light gardening, calisthenics, and weight lifting.

Studies indicate that physical exercise can be effective in reducing general anxiety and depression. Fifteen to twenty minutes of vigorous exercise has been shown to stimulate the secretion of both norepinephrine and serotonin into the brain and the release of endorphins into the blood (Davis, Eshelman, & McKay, 1994). Depressed people are often deficient in norepinephrine and serotonin. Endorphins act as natural narcotics and mood elevators.

THE ROLE OF THE NURSE IN RELAXATION THERAPY

Nurses work with anxious clients in all departments of the hospital and in community and home health services. Individuals experience stress daily; it cannot be eliminated. Management of stress must be considered a lifelong function. Nurses can help individuals recognize the sources of stress in their lives and identify methods of adaptive coping.

Assessment

Stress management requires a holistic approach. Physical and psychosocial dimensions are considered in determining the individual's adaptation to stress. Following are some examples of assessment data for collection. Other assessments may need to be made, depending on specific circumstances of each individual.

1. Genetic influences
   a. Identify medical/psychiatric history of client and biological family members.
2. Past experiences
   a. Describe your living/working conditions.
   b. When did you last have a physical examination?
   c. Do you have a spiritual or religious position from which you derive support?
   d. Do you have a job? Have you experienced any recent employment changes or other difficulties on your job?
   e. What significant changes have occurred in your life in the last year?
   f. What is your usual way of coping with stress?
   g. Do you have someone to whom you can go for support when you feel stressed?
3. Client's perception of the stressor
   a. What do you feel is the major source of stress in your life right now?
4. Adaptation responses
   a. Do you ever feel anxious? Confused? Unable to concentrate? Fearful?
   b. Do you have tremors? Stutter or stammer? Sweat profusely?
   c. Do you often feel angry? Irritable? Moody?
   d. Do you ever feel depressed? Do you ever feel like harming yourself or others?
   e. Do you have difficulty communicating with others?
   f. Do you experience pain? What part of your body? When do you experience it? When does it worsen?
   g. Do you every experience stomach upset? Constipation? Diarrhea? Nausea and vomiting?
   h. Do you ever feel your heart pounding in your chest?
   i. Do you take any drugs (prescription, over-the-counter, or street)?
   j. Do you drink alcohol? Smoke cigarettes? How much?
   k. Are you eating more/less than usual?
   l. Do you have difficulty sleeping?
   m. Do you have a significant other? Describe the relationship.
   n. Describe your relationship with other family members.
   o. Do you perceive any problems in your sexual lifestyle or behavior?

Diagnosis

Possible nursing diagnoses for individuals requiring assistance with stress management are listed here. Others may be appropriate for individuals with particular problems.

1. Adjustment, impaired
2. Anxiety (specify level)
3. Body image disturbance
4. Coping, defensive
5. Coping, ineffective, individual
6. Decisional conflict (specify)
7. Denial, ineffective
8. Fear
9. Grieving, anticipatory
10. Grieving, dysfunctional
11. Hopelessness
12. Knowledge deficit (specify)
13. Pain (acute or chronic)
14. Parental role conflict
15. Posttrauma response
16. Powerlessness
17. Rape-trauma syndrome
18. Role performance, altered
19. Self-esteem disturbance
20. Sexual dysfunction
21. Sexuality patterns, altered
22. Sleep pattern disturbance
23. Social interaction, impaired
24. Social isolation
25. Spiritual distress
26. Violence, risk for, directed at self/others

Outcome Identification/ Implementation

The immediate goal for nurses working with individuals needing assistance with stress management is to help minimize current maladaptive symptoms. The long-term goal is to assist individuals toward achievement of their highest potential for wellness. Examples of outcome criteria may include:

1. Client will verbalize a reduction in pain following progressive relaxation techniques.
2. Client will be able to voluntarily control a decrease in blood pressure following 3 weeks of biofeedback training.
3. Client will be able to maintain stress at a manageable level by performing deep breathing exercises when feeling anxious.

Implementation of nursing actions has a strong focus on the role of client teacher. Relaxation therapy, as described in this chapter, is one way to help individuals manage stress. These techniques are well within the scope of nursing practice.

Evaluation

Evaluation requires that the nurse and client assess whether or not these techniques are achieving the desired outcomes. Various alternatives may be attempted and reevaluated.

Relaxation therapy provides alternatives to old, maladaptive methods of coping with stress. Lifestyle changes may be required and change does not come easily. Nurses must help individuals analyze the usefulness of these techniques in the management of stress in their daily lives.

SUMMARY

Stress is a part of our everyday lives. It can be positive or negative, but it cannot be eliminated. Keeping stress at a manageable level is a lifelong process.

Individuals under stress respond with a physiological arousal that can be dangerous over long periods. Indeed, the stress response has been shown to be a major contributor, either directly or indirectly, to coronary heart disease, cancer, lung ailments, accidental injuries, cirrhosis of the liver, and suicide—six of the leading causes of death in the United States.

Relaxation therapy is an effective means of reducing the stress response in some individuals. The degree of anxiety that an individual experiences in response to stress is related to certain predisposing factors, such as characteristics of temperament with which he or she was born, past experiences resulting in learned patterns of responding, and existing conditions, such as health status, coping strategies, and adequate support systems.

Deep relaxation can counteract the physiological and behavioral manifestations of stress. Various methods of relaxation therapy were presented: deep-breathing exercises, progressive relaxation, passive progressive relaxation, meditation, mental imagery, biofeedback, and physical exercise.

Nurses use the nursing process in assisting individuals in the management of stress. Assessment data are collected from which nursing diagnoses are derived. Outcome criteria that help individuals reduce current maladaptive symptoms and ultimately achieve their highest potential for wellness are identified. Implementation includes instructing clients and their families in the various techniques for achieving relaxation. Behavioral changes provide objective measurements for evaluation.

REVIEW QUESTIONS

Self-Examination/Learning Exercise

1. **Learning exercise:** Practice some of the relaxation exercises presented in this chapter. It may be helpful to tape some of the exercises with soft music in the background. These tapes may be used with anxious clients or when you are feeling anxious yourself.

2. **Clinical activity:** Teach a relaxation exercise to a client. Practice it together. Evaluate the client's ability to achieve relaxation by performing the exercise.

3. **Case study:** Linda has just been admitted to the psychiatric unit. She was experiencing attacks of severe anxiety. Linda has worked in the typing pool of a large corporation for 10 years. She was recently promoted to private secretary for one of the executives. Some of her new duties include attending the board meetings and taking minutes, screening all calls and visitors for her boss, keeping track of his schedule, reminding him of important appointments, and making decisions for him in his absence. Linda felt comfortable in her old position, but has become increasingly fearful of making errors and incorrect decisions in her new job. Even though she is proud to have been selected for this position, she is constantly "nervous," has lost 10 pounds in 3 weeks, is having difficulty sleeping, and is having a recurrence of the severe migraine headaches she experienced as a teenager. She is often irritable with her husband and children for no apparent reason.

   a. Discuss some possible nursing diagnoses for Linda.
   b. Identify outcome criteria for Linda.
   c. Describe some relaxation techniques that may be helpful for her.

REFERENCES

Davis, M.D., Eshelman, E.R., & McKay, M. (1995). *The relaxation and stress reduction workbook* (4th ed.) Oakland, CA: New Harbinger Publications.

DiMotto, J.W. (1984, June). Relaxation. *American Journal of Nursing*, 754–758.

Hafen, B.Q., Karren, K.J., Frandsen, K.J., & Smith, N.L. (1996). *Mind/body health: The effects of attitudes, emotions, and relationships.* Boston: Allyn and Bacon.

Holmes, T., & Rahe, R. (1967). The social readjustment scale. *Journal of Psychosomatic Research, 11,* 213–218.

Miller, L.H., & Smith, A.D. (1983, June 6). How vulnerable are you to stress? *Time,* 54.

Pelletier, K.R. (1992). *Mind as healer, mind as slayer.* New York: Dell Publishing Co.

Sobel, D.S., & Ornstein, R. (1996). *The healthy mind, healthy body handbook.* Los Altos, CA: DRx.

Bibliography

Everly, G.S., Jr. (1989). *A clinical guide to the treatment of the human stress response.* New York: Plenum Press.

Goleman, D., & Gurin, J. (1993). *Mind body medicine: How to use your mind for better health.* New York: Consumer Reports Books.

Leepson, M. (1984). *The alive and well stress book.* New York: Bantam Books.

McGuigan, F.J., Sime, W.E., & Wallace, J.M. (1989). *Stress and tension control.* New York: Plenum Press.

Rosenbaum, L. (1989). *Biofeedback frontiers.* New York: AMS Press.

Selye, H. (1974). *Stress without distress.* New York: New American Library.

Sethi, A.S. (1989). *Meditation as an intervention in stress reactivity.* New York: AMS Press.

Smith, J.C. (1990). *Cognitive-behavioral relaxation training.* New York: Springer Publishing.

Sutherland, V.J., & Cooper, C.L. (1990). *Understanding stress: A psychological perspective for health professionals.* London: Chapman & Hall.

ASSERTIVENESS TRAINING

CHAPTER OUTLINE

KEY TERMS

nonassertiveness
assertiveness

aggressiveness
passive-aggressiveness

thought stopping

OBJECTIVES

After reading this chapter, the student will be able to:

1. Define *assertive behavior*.
2. Discuss basic human rights.
3. Differentiate between nonassertive, assertive, aggressive, and passive-aggressive behaviors.
4. Describe techniques that promote assertive behavior.
5. Demonstrate thought-stopping techniques.
6. Discuss the role of the nurse in assertiveness training.

lberti and Emmons (1990) ask:

"Do you ever feel helpless, powerless, ineffective? Do you sometimes get pushy in an effort to make yourself heard? Is it difficult for you to make your wishes known to others? Do you often find yourself 'low person on the totem pole'? Are you sometimes pushed around by others because of your own inability to stand up for yourself? Or do you push others around in order to get your way?" (p. 5)

Assertive behavior promotes a feeling of personal power and self-confidence. These two components are commonly lacking in clients with emotional disorders. Becoming more assertive empowers individuals by promoting self-esteem, without diminishing the esteem of others.

This chapter describes a number of rights that are considered basic to human beings. Various kinds of behaviors are explored, including assertive, nonassertive, aggressive, and passive-aggressive. Techniques that promote assertive behavior, as well as the nurse's role in assertiveness training, are presented.

ASSERTIVE COMMUNICATION

Alberti and Emmons (1990) have defined assertive behavior as:

"behavior that enables individuals to act in their own best interests, to stand up for themselves without undue anxiety, to express their honest feelings comfortably, or to exercise their own rights without denying the rights of others." (p. 7)

Assertive behavior helps us feel good about ourselves and increases our self-esteem. It helps us feel good about other people and increases our ability to develop satisfying relationships with others. This is accomplished out of honesty, directness, appropriateness, and respecting one's own basic rights as well as the rights of others.

Honesty is basic to assertive behavior. Assertive honesty is not an outspoken declaration of everything that is on one's mind. It is instead an accurate representation of feelings, opinions, or preferences expressed in a manner that promotes self-respect and respect for others.

Direct communication is stating what one wants to convey with clarity and candor. Hinting and "beating around the bush" are indirect forms of communication.

Communication must occur in an appropriate context in order to be considered assertive. The location and timing, as well as the manner (tone of voice, nonverbal gestures) in which the communication is presented, must be correct for the situation.

BASIC HUMAN RIGHTS

A number of authors have identified a variety of "assertive rights" (Baer, 1976; Bloom, Coburn, & Pearlman, 1975; Davis, McKay, & Eshelman, 1995; Jakubowski & Lange, 1978; Kelly, 1979; Powell & Enright, 1990; Smith, 1975). Many of these rights have been identified by participants in assertiveness training groups. Following is a composite of 10 basic assertive human rights adapted from the aggregation of sources.

1. The right to be treated with respect.
2. The right to express feelings, opinions, and beliefs.
3. The right to say "no" without feeling guilty.
4. The right to make mistakes and accept the responsibility for them.
5. The right to be listened to and taken seriously.
6. The right to change your mind.
7. The right to ask for what you want.
8. The right to put yourself first, sometimes.
9. The right to set your own priorities.
10. The right to refuse justification for your feelings or behavior.

In accepting these rights, an individual also accepts the responsibilities that accompany them. Rights and responsibilities are reciprocal entities. To experience one without the other is inherently destructive to an individual. Some responsibilities associated with basic assertive human rights are presented in Table 13.1.

RESPONSE PATTERNS

Kelly (1979) identified six ways individuals develop patterns of responding to others:

1. By watching other people (role modeling).
2. By being positively reinforced or punished for a certain response.
3. By inventing a response.
4. By not thinking of a better way to respond.
5. By not developing the proper skills for a better response.
6. By consciously choosing a response style.

The nurse should be able to recognize his or her own pattern of responding, as well as that of others. Four response patterns will be discussed here: nonassertive, assertive, aggressive, and passive-aggressive.

Nonassertive Behavior

Individuals who are **nonassertive** (sometimes called *passive*) seek to please others at the expense of denying their own basic human rights. They seldom let their true feelings show and often feel hurt and anxious because they allow others to choose for them. They seldom achieve their own desired goals (Alberti & Emmons, 1990). They come across as being very apologetic and tend to be self-deprecating. They use actions instead of words and hope some-

TABLE 13.1 ASSERTIVE RIGHTS AND RESPONSIBILITIES

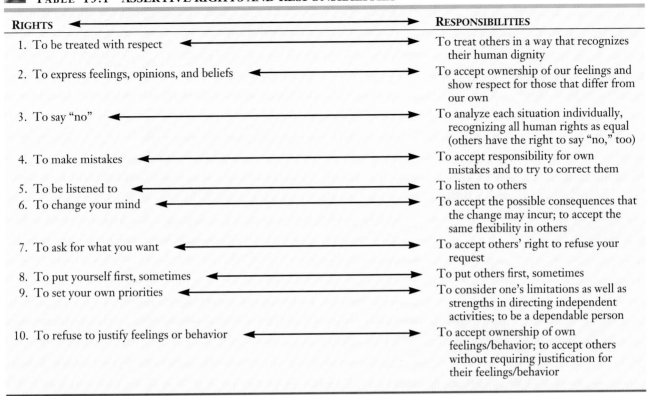

RIGHTS	RESPONSIBILITIES
1. To be treated with respect	To treat others in a way that recognizes their human dignity
2. To express feelings, opinions, and beliefs	To accept ownership of our feelings and show respect for those that differ from our own
3. To say "no"	To analyze each situation individually, recognizing all human rights as equal (others have the right to say "no," too)
4. To make mistakes	To accept responsibility for own mistakes and to try to correct them
5. To be listened to	To listen to others
6. To change your mind	To accept the possible consequences that the change may incur; to accept the same flexibility in others
7. To ask for what you want	To accept others' right to refuse your request
8. To put yourself first, sometimes	To put others first, sometimes
9. To set your own priorities	To consider one's limitations as well as strengths in directing independent activities; to be a dependable person
10. To refuse to justify feelings or behavior	To accept ownership of own feelings/behavior; to accept others without requiring justification for their feelings/behavior

one will "guess" what they want. Their voices are hesitant, weak, and expressed in a monotone. Their eyes are usually downcast. They feel uncomfortable in interpersonal interactions. All they want is to please and to be liked by others. Their behavior helps them avoid unpleasant situations and confrontations with others; however, they often harbor anger and resentment.

Assertive Behavior

Assertive individuals stand up for their own rights while protecting the rights of others. Feelings are expressed openly and honestly. They assume responsibility for their own choices and allow others to choose for themselves. They maintain self-respect and respect for others by treating everyone equally and with human dignity. They communicate tactfully, using lots of "I" statements. Their voices are warm and expressive, and eye contact is intermittent but direct. These individuals desire to communicate effectively with, and be respected by, others. They are self-confident and experience satisfactory and pleasurable relationships with others.

Aggressive Behavior

Individuals who are **aggressive** defend their own basic rights by violating the basic rights of others. Feelings are often expressed dishonestly and inappropriately. They say

what is on their mind, often at the expense of others. Aggressive behavior commonly results in a *put down* of the receiver. Rights denied, the receiver feels hurt, defensive, and humiliated (Alberti & Emmons, 1990). Aggressive individuals devalue the self-worth of others on whom they impose their choices. They express an air of superiority, and their voices are often loud, demanding, angry, or cold, without emotion. Eye contact may be "to intimidate others by staring them down." They want to increase their feeling of power by dominating or humiliating others. Aggressive behavior hinders interpersonal relationships.

Passive-Aggressive Behavior

Passive-aggressive individuals defend their own rights by expressing resistance to social and occupational demands (APA, 1994). Sometimes called *indirect aggression*, this behavior takes the form of passive, nonconfrontive action (Alberti & Emmons, 1990). These individuals are devious, manipulative, and sly, and they undermine others with behavior that expresses the opposite of what they are feeling. They are highly critical and sarcastic. They allow others to make choices for them, then resist by using passive behaviors, such as procrastination, dawdling, stubbornness, and "forgetfulness." They use actions instead of words to convey their message, and the actions express covert aggression. They become sulky, irritable, or argumentative when asked to do something they do not want to do. They may protest to others about the demands but will not confront the person who is making the demands. Instead, they may deal with the demand by "forgetting" to do it. The goal is domination through retaliation. This behavior offers a feeling of control and power, although they actually feel resentment and that they are being taken advantage of. They possess extremely low self-confidence.

A comparison of these four behavior patterns is presented in Table 13.2.

BEHAVIORAL COMPONENTS OF ASSERTIVE BEHAVIOR

Alberti and Emmons (1990) have identified several defining characteristics of assertive behavior:

1. **Eye Contact.** Eye contact is considered appropriate when it is intermittent (i.e., looking directly at the person to whom one is speaking but looking away now and then). Individuals feel uncomfortable when someone stares at them continuously and in-

tently. Intermittent eye contact conveys the message that one is interested in what is being said.

2. **Body Posture.** Sitting and leaning slightly toward the other person in a conversation suggests an active interest in what is being said. Emphasis on an assertive stance can be achieved by standing with an erect posture, squarely facing the other person. A slumped posture conveys passivity or nonassertiveness.

3. **Distance/Physical Contact.** The distance between two individuals in an interaction or the physical contact between them has a strong cultural influence. For example, in the United States, intimate distance is considered approximately 18 inches from the body. We are very careful about whom we allow to enter this intimate space. Invasion of this space may be interpreted by some individuals as very aggressive.

4. **Gestures.** Nonverbal gestures may also be culturally related. Gesturing can add emphasis, warmth, depth, or power to the spoken word.

5. **Facial Expression.** Various facial expressions convey different messages (e.g., frown, smile, surprise, anger, fear). It is difficult to "fake" these messages.

TABLE 13.2   COMPARISON OF BEHAVIORAL RESPONSE PATTERNS

	NONASSERTIVE	ASSERTIVE	AGGRESSIVE	PASSIVE-AGGRESSIVE
Behavioral characteristics	Passive, does not express true feelings, self-deprecating, denies own rights	Stands up for own rights, protects rights of others, honest, direct, appropriate	Violates rights of others, expresses feelings dishonestly and inappropriately	Defends own rights with passive resistance, is critical and sarcastic; often expresses opposite of true feelings
Examples	"Uh, Well, uh, sure, I'll be glad to stay and work an extra shift."	"I don't want to stay and work an extra shift today. I stayed over yesterday. It's someone else's turn today."	"You've got to be kidding!"	"Okay, I'll stay and work an extra shift." (Then to peer: "How dare she ask me to work over again! Well, we'll just see how much work she gets out of me!")
Goals	To please others; to be liked by others	To communicate effectively; to be respected by others	To dominate or humiliate others	To dominate through retaliation
Feelings	Anxious, hurt, disappointed with self, angry, resentful	Confident, successful, proud, self-respecting	Self-righteous, controlling, superior	Anger, resentment, manipulated, controlled
Compensation	Is able to avoid unpleasant situations and confrontations with others	Increased self-confidence, self-respect, respect for others, satisfying interpersonal relationships	Anger is released, increasing feeling of power and superiority	Feels self-righteous and in control
Outcomes	Goals not met; others meet *their* goals at nonassertive person's expense; anger and resentment grow; feels violated and manipulated	Goals met; desires most often fulfilled while defending own rights as well as rights of others	Goals may be met but at the expense of others; they feel hurt and vengeful	Goals not met, nor are the goals of others met due to retaliatory nature of the interaction

SOURCE: Adapted from Jakubowski & Lange (1978), pp. 42–43.

In assertive communication, the facial expression is congruent with the verbal message.

6. **Voice.** The voice conveys a message by its loudness, softness, degree and placement of emphasis, and evidence of emotional tone.

7. **Fluency.** Being able to discuss a subject with ease and with obvious knowledge conveys assertiveness and self-confidence. This message is impeded by numerous pauses or filler words such as "and, uh . . ." or "you know . . ."

8. **Timing.** Assertive responses are most effective when they are spontaneous and immediate. However, most people have experienced times when it was not appropriate to respond (e.g., in front of a group of people) or times when an appropriate response is generated only after the fact ("If only I had said . . . "). Alberti and Emmons (1990) state that ". . . it is never too late to be assertive!" It is correct and worthwhile to seek out the individual at a later time and express the assertive response.

9. **Listening.** Assertive listening means giving the other individual full attention, with eye contact, nodding to indicate acceptance of what is being said, and taking time to understand what is being said before giving a response.

10. **Thoughts.** Cognitive processes affect one's assertive behavior. Two such processes are (1) an individual's attitudes about the appropriateness of assertive behavior in general and (2) the appropriateness of assertive behavior for himself or herself specifically.

11. **Content.** Many times individuals do not respond to an unpleasant situation because ". . . I just didn't know what to say." Perhaps *what* is being said is not as important as how it is said. Emotions should be expressed when they are experienced. It is also important to accept ownership of those emotions and not devalue the worth of another individual in asserting oneself.

EXAMPLES:

Assertive: "I'm really angry about what you said!"

Aggressive: "You're a real jerk for saying that!"

TECHNIQUES THAT PROMOTE ASSERTIVE BEHAVIOR

Various guidelines have been established as beneficial in the process of becoming an assertive person (Bakdash, 1978; Davis, McKay, & Eshelman, 1995; Smith, 1975). The following techniques have been shown to be effective in responding to criticism and avoiding manipulation by others.

1. **Standing up for one's basic human rights.**

EXAMPLE:

"I have the right to express my opinion."

2. **Assuming responsibility for one's own statements.**

EXAMPLE:

"*I don't want* to go out with you tonight," instead of " I *can't* go out with you tonight." The latter implies a lack of power or ability.

3. **Responding as a "broken record."** Persistently repeating in a calm voice what is wanted.

EXAMPLE:

Telephone salesperson: "I want to help you save money by changing long-distance services."

Assertive response: "I don't want to change my long-distance service."

Telephone salesperson: "I can't believe you don't want to save money!"

Assertive response: "I don't want to change my long-distance service."

4. **Agreeing assertively.** Assertively accepting negative aspects about oneself; admitting when an error has been made.

EXAMPLE:

Ms. Jones: "You sure let that meeting get out of hand. What a waste of time."

Ms. Smith: "Yes, I didn't do a very good job of conducting the meeting today."

5. **Inquiring assertively.** Seeking additional information about critical statements.

EXAMPLE:

Male board member: "You made a real fool of yourself at the board meeting last night."

Female board member: "Oh, really? Just what about my behavior offended you?

Male board member: "You were so damned pushy!"

Female board member: "Were you offended that I spoke up for my beliefs, or was it because my beliefs are in direct opposition to yours?"

6. **Shifting from content to process.** Changing the focus of the communication from discussing the

topic at hand to analyzing what is actually going on in the interaction.

EXAMPLE:

Wife: "Would you please call me if you will be late for dinner?"

Husband: "Why don't you just get off my back! I always have to account for every minute of my time with you!"

Wife: "Sounds to me like we need to discuss some other things here. What are you really angry about?"

7. **Clouding/fogging.** Concurring with the critic's argument without becoming defensive and without agreeing to change.

EXAMPLE:

Nurse #1: "You make so many mistakes. I don't know how you ever got this job!"

Nurse #2: "You're right. I have made some mistakes since I started this job."

8. **Defusing.** Putting off further discussion with an angry individual until he or she is calmer.

EXAMPLE:

"You are very angry right now. I don't want to discuss this matter with you while you are so upset. I will discuss it with you in my office at 3 o'clock this afternoon."

9. **Delaying assertively.** Putting off further discussion with another individual until one is calmer.

EXAMPLE:

"That's a very challenging position you have taken, Mr. Brown. I'll need time to give it some thought. I'll call you later this afternoon."

10. **Responding assertively with irony.**

EXAMPLE:

Man: "I bet you're one of them so-called 'women's libbers,' aren't you?"

Woman: "Yes, thank you for noticing."

THOUGHT-STOPPING TECHNIQUES

Assertive thinking is sometimes inhibited by repetitive, negative thoughts of which the mind refuses to let go. In-dividuals with low self-worth may be obsessed with thoughts such as, "I know he'd never want to go out with me. I'm too ugly (or plain, or fat, or dumb)" or "I just know I'll never be able to do this job well" or "I just can't seem to do anything right." This type of thinking fosters the belief that one's individual rights do not deserve the same consideration as those of others, and reflect nonassertive communication and behavioral response patterns.

Thought-stopping techniques, as described here, were developed by psychiatrist Joseph Wolpe (1991) and are intended to eliminate intrusive, unwanted thoughts.

Method

In a practice setting, with eyes closed, the individual concentrates on an unwanted recurring thought. Once the thought is clearly established in the mind, he or she shouts aloud: "STOP!" This action will interrupt the thought, and it is actually removed from one's awareness. The individual then immediately shifts his or her thoughts to one that is considered pleasant and desirable.

It is possible that the unwanted thought may soon recur, but with practice, the length of time between recurrences will increase until the unwanted thought is no longer intrusive.

Obviously, one cannot go about one's daily life shouting "STOP!" in public places. After a number of practice sessions, the technique is equally effective if the word "stop!" is just used silently in the mind.

ROLE OF THE NURSE

It is important for nurses to become aware of and recognize their own behavioral responses. Are they mostly nonassertive? Assertive? Aggressive? Passive-aggressive? Do they consider their behavioral responses effective? Do they wish to change? Remember, all individuals have the right to choose whether or not they want to be assertive.

The ability to respond assertively is especially important to nurses who are committed to further development of the profession. Assertive skills facilitate the implementation of change—change that is required if the image of nursing is to be upgraded to the level of professionalism that most nurses desire. Assertive communication is useful in the political arena for nurses who choose to become involved at both state and national levels in striving to influence legislation and, ultimately, to improve the system of health care provision in our country.

Nurses who understand and use assertiveness skills themselves can in turn assist clients who wish to effect behavioral change in an effort to increase self-esteem and improve interpersonal relationships. The nursing process is a useful tool for nurses who are involved in helping clients increase their assertiveness.

Assessment

Nurses can help clients become more aware of their behavioral responses. Many tools for assessing the level of assertiveness have been attempted over the years. None have been terribly effective. Perhaps this is because it is so difficult to *generalize* when attempting to measure assertive behaviors. Table 13.3 and Figure 13.1 represent examples of assertiveness inventories that could be personalized to describe life situations of individual clients more specifically. Obviously, "everyday situations that may require assertiveness" are not the same for all individuals.

Diagnosis

Possible nursing diagnoses for individuals needing assistance with assertiveness include:

1. Coping, defensive
2. Coping, ineffective, individual
3. Decisional conflict (specify)
4. Denial, ineffective
5. Personal identity disturbance
6. Powerlessness
7. Rape-trauma syndrome
8. Self-esteem disturbance
9. Social interaction, impaired
10. Social isolation

Outcome Identification/Implementation

The goal for nurses working with individuals needing assistance with assertiveness is to help them develop more satisfying interpersonal relationships. Individuals who do not feel good about themselves either allow others to violate their rights or cover up their low self-esteem by being overtly or covertly aggressive. Individuals should be given information regarding their individual human rights. They must know what these rights are before they can stand up for them.

Outcome criteria would be derived from specific nursing diagnoses. Some examples might include:

1. The client verbalizes and accepts responsibility for his or her own behavior.
2. The client is able to express opinions and disagree with the opinions of others in a socially acceptable manner and without feeling guilty.
3. The client is able to verbalize positive aspects about self.
4. The client verbalizes choices made in a plan to maintain control over his or her life situation.
5. The client approaches others in an appropriate manner for one-to-one interaction.

In a clinical setting, nurses can teach clients the techniques to use in order to increase their assertive responses. This can be done on a one-to-one basis or in group situations. Once these techniques have been discussed, nurses can assist clients to practice them through role playing. Each client should compose a list of specific personal examples of situations that create difficulties for him or her. These situations will then be simulated in the therapy setting so that the client may practice assertive responses in a nonthreatening environment. In a group situation, feedback from peers can provide valuable insight about the effectiveness of the response.

An important part of this type of intervention is to ensure that clients are aware of the differences among assertive, nonassertive, aggressive, and passive-aggressive behaviors in the same situation. When discussion is held about what the best (assertive) response would be, it is also important to discuss the other types of responses as well,

---

▰ TABLE 13.3 EVERYDAY SITUATIONS THAT MAY REQUIRE ASSERTIVENESS

At Work

How do you respond when:
1. You receive a compliment on your appearance or someone praises your work?
2. You are criticized unfairly?
3. You are criticized legitimately by a superior?
4. You have to confront a subordinate for continual lateness or sloppy work?
5. Your boss makes a sexual innuendo or makes a pass at you?

In Public

How do you respond when:
1. In a restaurant, the food you ordered arrives cold or overcooked?
2. A fellow passenger in a no-smoking compartment lights a cigarette?
3. You are faced with an unhelpful shop assistant?
4. Somebody barges in front of you in a waiting line?
5. You take an inferior article back to a shop?

Among Friends

How do you respond when:
1. You feel angry with the way a friend has treated you?
2. A friend makes what you consider to be an unreasonable request?
3. You want to ask a friend for a favor?
4. You ask a friend for repayment of a loan of money?
5. You have to negotiate with a friend on which film to see or where to meet?

At Home

How do you respond when:
1. One of your parents criticizes you?
2. You are irritated by a persistent habit in someone you love?
3. Everybody leaves the cleaning-up chores to you?
4. You want to say "no" to a proposed visit to a relative?
5. Your partner feels amorous but you are not in the mood?

SOURCE: From Powell & Enright (1990), with permission.

DIRECTIONS: Fill in each block with a rating of your assertiveness on a 5-point scale. A rating of 0 means you have no difficulty asserting yourself. A rating of 5 means that you are completely unable to assert yourself. Evaluation can be made by analyzing the scores:

1. totally by activity, including all of the different people categories
2. totally by people, including all of the different activity categories
3. on an individual basis, considering specific people and specific activities

PEOPLE \ ACTIVITY	Friends of the same sex	Friends of the opposite sex	Intimate relations or spouse	Authority figures	Relatives/ family members	Colleagues and sub-ordinates	Strangers	Service workers; waiters; shop assistants, etc.
Giving and receiving compliments								
Asking for favors/help								
Initiating and maintaining conversation								
Refusing requests								
Expressing personal opinions								
Expressing anger/dis-pleasure								
Expressing liking, love, affection								
Stating your rights and needs								

Figure 13.1   Rating your assertiveness.

so that clients can begin to recognize their pattern of response and make changes accordingly.

EXAMPLE:

Linda comes to day hospital once a week to attend group therapy and assertiveness training. She has had problems with depression and low self-esteem. She is married to a man who is verbally abusive. He is highly critical, is seldom satisfied with anything Linda does, and blames her for negative consequences that occur in their lives, whether or not she was even involved.

Since the group began, the nurse who leads the assertiveness training group has taught the participants about basic human rights and the various types of response patterns. When the nurse asks for client situations to be presented in group, Linda volunteers to discuss an incident that occurred in her home this week. She related that she had just put some chicken on the stove to cook for supper when her 7-year-old son came running in the house yelling that he had been hurt. Linda went to him and observed that he had blood dripping down the side of his head from his forehead. He said he and some friends

had been playing on the jungle gym in the school yard down the street, and he had fallen and hit his head. Linda went with him to the bathroom to clean the wound and apply some medication. Her husband, Raul, was reading the newspaper in the living room. By the time she got back to the chicken on the stove, it was burned and inedible. Her husband shouted, "You stupid woman! You can't do anything right!" Linda did not respond but burst into tears.

The nurse asked the other members in the group to present some ideas about how Linda could have responded to Raul's criticism. After some discussion, they agreed that Linda might have stated, "I made a mistake. I am not stupid and I do lots of things right." They also discussed other types of responses and why they were less acceptable. They recognized that Linda's lack of verbal response and bursting into tears was a nonassertive response. They also agreed on other examples, such as:

1. An aggressive response might be, "Cook your own supper!" and toss the skillet out the back door.
2. A passive-aggressive response might be to fix sandwiches for supper and not speak to Raul for 3 days.

Practice on the assertive response began, with the nurse and various members of the group playing the role of Raul so that Linda could practice until she felt comfortable with the response. She participated in the group for 6 months, regularly submitting situations with which she needed help. She also learned from the situations presented by other members of the group. These weekly sessions gave Linda the self-confidence that she needed to stand up to Raul's criticism. She was aware of her basic human rights and, with practice, was able to stand up for them in an assertive manner. She was happy to report to the group after a few months that Raul seemed to be less critical and that their relationship was improving.

Evaluation

Evaluation requires that the nurse and client assess whether or not these techniques are achieving the desired outcomes. Reassessment might include the following questions:

Is the client able to accept criticism without becoming defensive?

Can the client express true feelings to (spouse, friend, boss, and so on) when his or her basic human rights are violated?

Is the client able to decline a request without feeling guilty?

Can the client verbalize positive qualities about himself or herself?

Does the client verbalize improvement in interpersonal relationships?

Assertiveness training serves to extend and create more flexibility in an individual's communication style so that he or she has a greater choice of responses in various situations. Although change does not come easily, assertiveness training can be an effective way of changing behavior. Nurses can assist individuals to become more assertive, thereby encouraging them to become what they want to be, promoting an improvement in self-esteem, and fostering a respect for their own rights as well as the rights of others.

SUMMARY

Assertive behavior helps individuals feel better about themselves by encouraging them to stand up for their own basic human rights. These rights have equal representation for all individuals. Along with rights comes an equal number of responsibilities. Part of being assertive includes living up to these responsibilities.

Assertive behavior increases self-esteem and the ability to develop satisfying interpersonal relationships. This is accomplished through honesty, directness, appropriateness, and respecting one's own rights as well as the rights of others.

Individuals develop patterns of responding in various ways, such as role modeling, by receiving positive or negative reinforcement, or by conscious choice. These patterns can take the form of nonassertiveness, assertiveness, aggressiveness, or passive-aggressiveness.

Nonassertive individuals seek to please others at the expense of denying their own basic human rights. *Assertive* individuals stand up for their own rights while protecting the rights of others. Those who respond *aggressively* defend their own rights by violating the basic rights of others. Individuals who respond in a *passive-aggressive* manner defend their own rights by expressing resistance to social and occupational demands.

Some important behavioral considerations of assertive behavior include eye contact, body posture, distance/physical contact, gestures, facial expression, voice, fluency, timing, listening, thoughts, and content. Various techniques have been developed to assist individuals in the process of becoming more assertive.

Negative thinking can sometimes interfere with one's ability to respond assertively. Thought-stopping techniques help individuals remove negative, unwanted thoughts from awareness and promote the development of a more assertive attitude.

Nurses can assist individuals to learn and practice assertiveness techniques. The nursing process is an effective vehicle for providing the information and support to clients as they strive to create positive change in their lives.

REVIEW QUESTIONS

SELF-EXAMINATION/LEARNING EXERCISE

Beside each response, identify it as nonassertive (NA), assertive (AS), aggressive (AG), or passive-aggressive (PA).

1. Your husband says, "You're crazy to think about going to college! You're not smart enough to handle the studies and the housework, too." You respond:

    _____ a. "I will do what I can, and the best that I can."

    _____ b. (Thinking to yourself): "We'll see how HE likes cooking dinner for a change."

    _____ c. "You're probably right. Maybe I should reconsider."

    _____ d. "I'm going to do what I want to do, when I want to do it, and you can't stop me!"

2. You are having company for dinner and they are due to arrive in 20 minutes. You are about to finish cooking and still have to shower and dress. The doorbell rings and it is a man selling a new product for cleaning windows. You respond:

    _____ a. "I don't do windows!" and slam the door in his face.

    _____ b. "I'll take a case," and write him a check.

    _____ c. "Sure, I'll take three bottles." Then to yourself you think: "I'm calling this company tomorrow and complaining to the manager about their salespeople coming around at dinnertime!"

    _____ d. "I'm very busy at the moment. I don't wish to purchase any of your product. Thank you."

3. You are in a movie theater that prohibits smoking. The person in the seat next to you just lit a cigarette and the smoke is very irritating. Your response is:

    _____ a. You say nothing.

    _____ b. "Please put your cigarette out. Smoking is prohibited."

    _____ c. You say nothing but begin to frantically fan the air in front of you and cough loudly and convulsively.

    _____ d. "Put your cigarette out, you slob! Can't you read the 'no smoking' sign?"

4. You have been studying for a nursing exam all afternoon and lost track of time. Your husband expects dinner on the table when he gets home from work. You have not started cooking yet when he walks in the door and shouts, "Why the heck isn't dinner ready?" You respond:

    _____ a. "I'm sorry. I'll have it done in no time, honey." But then you move very slowly and take a long time to cook the meal.

    _____ b. "I'm tired from studying all afternoon. Make your own dinner, you bum! I'm tired of being your slave!"

    _____ c. "I haven't started dinner yet. I'd like some help from you."

    _____ d. "I'm so sorry. I know you're tired and hungry. It's all my fault. I'm such a terrible wife!"

5. You and your best friend, Jill, have had plans for 6 months to go on vacation together to Hawaii. You have saved your money and have plane tickets to leave in 3 weeks. She has just called you and reported that she is not going. She has a new boyfriend, they are moving in together, and she does not want to leave him. You respond:

_____ a. "I'm very disappointed and very angry. I'd like to talk to you about this later. I'll call you."

_____ b. "I'm very happy for you, Jill. I think it's wonderful that you and Jack are moving in together."

_____ c. You tell Jill that you are very happy for her, but then say to another friend, "Well, that's the end of my friendship with Jill!"

_____ d. "What? You can't do that to me! We've had plans! You're acting like a real slut!"

6. A typewritten report for your psychiatric nursing class is due tomorrow at 8:00 AM. The assignment was made 4 weeks ago and you have yours ready to turn in. Your roommate says, "I finally finished writing my report, but now I have to go to work and I don't have time to type it. Please be a dear and type it for me, otherwise I'll fail!" You have a date with your boyfriend. You respond:

_____ a. "Okay, I'll call Ken and cancel our date."

_____ b. "I don't want to stay here and type your report. I'm going out with Ken."

_____ c. "You've got to be kidding! What kind of a fool do you take me for, anyway?"

_____ d. "Okay, I'll do it." However, when your roommate returns from work at midnight, you are asleep and the report has not been typed.

7. You are asked to serve on a committee on which you do not wish to serve. You respond:

_____ a. "Thank you, but I don't wish to be a member of that committee."

_____ b. "I'll be happy to serve." But then you don't show up for any of the meetings.

_____ c. "I'd rather have my teeth pulled!"

_____ d. "Okay, if I'm really needed, I'll serve."

8. You're on your way to the laundry room when you encounter a fellow dorm tenant who often asks you to "throw a few of my things in with yours." You view this as an imposition. He asks you where you're going. You respond:

_____ a. "I'm on my way to the Celtics game. Where do you think I'm going?"

_____ b. "I'm on my way to do some laundry. Do you have anything you want me to wash with mine?"

_____ c. "It's none of your damn business!"

_____ d. "I'm going to the laundry room. Please don't ask me to do some of yours. I resent being taken advantage of in that way."

9. At a hospital committee meeting, a fellow nurse who is the chairperson has interrupted you each time you have tried to make a statement. The next time it happens, you respond:

_____ a. "You make a lousy leader! You won't even let me finish what I'm trying to say!"

_____ b. You say nothing.

_____ c. "Excuse me. I would like to finish my statement."

_____ d. You say nothing but fail to complete your assignment and do not show up for the next meeting.

10. A fellow worker often borrows small amounts of money from you with the promise that she will pay you back "tomorrow." She currently owes you $15.00, and has not yet paid back any that she has borrowed. She asks if she can borrow a couple of dollars for lunch. You respond:

_____ a. "I've decided not to loan you any more money until you pay me back what you already borrowed."

_____ b. "I'm so sorry. I only have enough to pay for my own lunch today."

_____ c. "Get a life, will you? I'm tired of you sponging off me all the time!"

_____ d. "Sure, here's two dollars." Then to the other workers in the office: "Be sure you never lend Cindy any money. She never pays her debts. I'd be sure never to go to lunch with her if I were you!"

REFERENCES

Alberti, R.E., & Emmons, M.L. (1990). *Your perfect right—A guide to assertive living* (6th ed.). San Luis Obispo, CA: Impact Publishers.

American Psychiatric Association. (1994). *Diagnostic and Statistical Manual of Mental Disorders* (4th ed.). Washington, DC: American Psychiatric Association.

Baer, J. (1976). *How to be an assertive (not aggressive) woman in life, love, and on the job.* New York: New American Library.

Bakdash, D.P. (1978, October). Becoming an assertive nurse. *American Journal of Nursing,* 1710–1712.

Bloom, L., Coburn, K., & Pearlman, J. (1975). *The new assertive woman.* New York: Dell.

Davis M., McKay, M., & Eshelman, E.R. (1995). *The relaxation and stress reduction workbook* (4th ed.). Oakland, CA: New Harbinger Publications.

Jakubowski, P., & Lange, A.J. (1978). *The assertive option—Your rights and responsibilities.* Champaign, IL: Research Press Co.

Kelley, C. (1979). *Assertion training: A facilitator's guide.* La Jolla, CA: University Associates.

Powell, T.J., & Enright, S.J. (1990). *Anxiety and stress management.* London: Routledge.

Smith, M.J. (1975). *When I say no, I feel guilty.* New York: The Dial Press.

Wolpe, J. (1991). *The practice of behavior therapy* (4th ed.). Elmsford, NY: Pergamon Press.

Bibliography

Angel, G., & Petronko, D.K. (1983). *Developing the new assertive nurse.* New York: Springer Publishing.

Burley-Allen, M. (1995). *Managing assertively: How to improve your people skills.* New York: John Wiley and Sons.

Chenevert, M. (1994). *STAT: Special techniques in assertiveness training for women in the health professions* (4th ed.). St. Louis: C.V. Mosby.

Fodor, I.G. (1992). *Adolescent assertiveness and social skills training: A clinical handbook.* New York: Springer Publishing.

Loring, H., & Birch, J. (1984). *You're on . . . : Teaching assertiveness and communication skills.* Cleveland, OH: StressPress.

Phelps, S., & Austin, N. (1997). *The assertive woman.* San Louis Obispo, CA: Impact Publishers.

Shelton, N., & Burton, S. (1993). *Assertiveness skills.* New York: McGraw-Hill.

Zappe, C., & Epstein, D. (1987). Assertive training. *Journal of Psycholsocial Nursing, 25*(8), 23–25.

PROMOTING SELF-ESTEEM

CHAPTER OUTLINE

OBJECTIVES

INTRODUCTION

COMPONENTS OF SELF-CONCEPT

THE DEVELOPMENT OF SELF-ESTEEM

THE MANIFESTATIONS OF
LOW SELF-ESTEEM

BOUNDARIES

THE NURSING PROCESS

SUMMARY

REVIEW QUESTIONS

KEY TERMS

self-esteem
boundaries
self-concept
physical self
body image
personal self

personal identity
moral-ethical self
self-consistency
self-ideal
self-expectancy
focal stimuli

contextual stimuli
residual stimuli
rigid boundaries
flexible boundaries
enmeshed boundaries

OBJECTIVES

After reading this chapter, the student will be able to:

1. Identify and define components of the self-concept.
2. Discuss influencing factors in the development of self-esteem and its progression through the life span.
3. Describe the verbal and nonverbal manifestations of low self-esteem.

4. Discuss the concept of boundaries and its relationship to self-esteem.
5. Apply the nursing process with clients who are experiencing disturbances in self-esteem.

cKay and Fanning (1987) describe **self-esteem** as an emotional *sine qua non*, a component that is essential for psychological survival. They state, "Without some measure of self-worth, life can be enormously painful, with many basic needs going unmet."

The awareness of self (i.e., the ability to form an identity and then attach a value to it) is an important differentiating factor between humans and other animals. This capacity for judgment, then, becomes a contributing factor in disturbances of self-esteem.

The promotion of self-esteem is about stopping self-judgments. It is about helping individuals change how they perceive and feel about themselves. This chapter describes the developmental progression and the verbal and behavioral manifestations of self-esteem. The concept of **boundaries** and its relationship to self-esteem is explored. Nursing care of clients with disturbances in self-esteem is described in the context of the nursing process.

COMPONENTS OF SELF-CONCEPT

Driever (1976a) defines **self-concept** as:

> "The composite of beliefs and feelings that one holds about oneself at a given time, formed from perceptions particularly of others' reactions, and directing one's behavior." (p. 169)

Self-concept consists of the **physical self,** or **body image;** the **personal self** or **personal identity;** and self-esteem.

Physical Self or Body Image

An individual's body image is a personal appraisal of his or her physical being and includes physical attributes, functioning, sexuality, wellness-illness state, and appearance (Driever, 1976a). It is an integrated collection of visual, auditory, tactile, and proprioceptive information that combines with affective and cognitive processes to form the image of one's physical self (Robertson, 1991).

An individual's body image may not necessarily coincide with his or her actual appearance. For example, individuals who have been overweight for many years and then lose weight often have difficulty perceiving of themselves as thin. They may even continue to choose clothing in the size they were before they lost weight.

A disturbance in one's body image may occur with changes in structure or function. Examples of changes in bodily structure include amputations, mastectomy, and facial disfigurements. Functional alterations are conditions such as colostomy, paralysis, and impotence. Alterations in body image are often experienced as losses.

Personal Identity

Driever (1976a) identifies this component of the self-concept as the personal self and further divides it into the moral-ethical self, the self-consistency, and the self-ideal/self-expectancy.

The **moral-ethical self** is that aspect of the personal identity that functions as observer, standard setter, dreamer, comparer, and most of all evaluator of who the individual says he or she is. This component of the personal self makes judgments that influence an individual's self-evaluation.

Self-consistency is the component of the personal identity that strives to maintain a stable self-image. Even if the self-image is negative, because of this need for stability and self-consistency, the individual resists letting go of the image from which he or she has achieved a measure of constancy.

Self-ideal/self-expectancy relates to an individual's perception of what he or she wants to be, to do, or to become. The concept of the ideal self arises out of the perception one has of the expectations of others. Disturbances in self-concept can occur when individuals are unable to achieve their ideals and expectancies.

Self-Esteem

Self-esteem refers to the degree of regard or respect that individuals have for themselves and is a measure of worth that they place on their abilities and judgments. Warren (1991) states:

> "Self-esteem breaks down into two components: (1) the ability to say that "I am important," "I matter," and (2) the ability to say "I am competent," "I have something to offer to others and the world." (p. 1)

Maslow (1970) postulates that individuals must achieve a positive self-esteem before they can achieve self-actualization (see Chapter 2). On a day-to-day basis, one's self-value is challenged by changes within the environment. With a positive self-worth, individuals are able to adapt successfully to the demands associated with situational and maturational crises that occur. The ability to adapt to these environmental changes is impaired when individuals hold themselves in low esteem (Driever, 1976b).

Self-esteem is very closely related to the other components of the self-concept. Just as with body image and personal identity, the development of self-esteem is largely influenced by the perceptions of how one is viewed by significant others. It begins in early childhood and vacillates throughout the life span.

THE DEVELOPMENT OF SELF-ESTEEM

How self-esteem is established has been the topic of investigation for a number of theorists and clinicians. From a review of personality theories, Coopersmith (1981) identified the following antecedent conditions of positive self-esteem.

1. **Power.** It is important for individuals to have a feeling of control over their own life situation and an ability to claim some measure of influence over the behaviors of others.
2. **Significance.** Self-esteem is enhanced when individuals feel loved, respected, and cared for by significant others.
3. **Virtue.** Individuals feel good about themselves when their actions reflect a set of personal, moral, and ethical values.
4. **Competence.** Positive self-esteem develops out of one's ability to perform successfully or achieve self-expectations and the expectations of others.
5. **Consistently set limits.** A structured lifestyle demonstrates acceptance and caring, and provides a feeling of security.

Warren (1991) outlines the following focus areas for parents and others who work with children to emphasize when encouraging the growth and development of positive self-esteem:

1. **A sense of Competence.** Everyone needs to feel skilled at something. Warren (1991) states, "Children do not necessarily need to be THE best at a skill in order to have positive self-esteem; what they need to feel is that they have accomplished their PERSONAL best effort."
2. **Unconditional Love.** Children need to know that they are loved and accepted by family and friends regardless of success or failure. This is demonstrated by expressive touch, realistic praise, and separation of criticism of the person from criticism of the behavior.
3. **A Sense of Survival.** Everyone fails at something from time to time. Self-esteem is enhanced when individuals learn from failure and grow in the knowledge that they are stronger for having experienced it.
4. **Realistic Goals.** Low self-esteem can be the result of not being able to achieve established goals. Individuals may "set themselves up" for failure by setting goals that are unattainable. Goals can be unrealistic when they are beyond a child's capability to achieve, require an inordinate amount of effort to accomplish, and are based on exaggerated fantasy.
5. **A Sense of Responsibility.** Children gain positive self-worth when they are assigned areas of responsibility or are expected to complete tasks that they perceive are valued by others.
6. **Reality Orientation.** Personal limitations abound within our world, and it is important for children to recognize and achieve a healthy balance between what they can possess and achieve, and what is beyond their capability or control.

Driever (1976c) cites the following factors as influential in the development of self-esteem:

1. **The Perceptions of Responses by Others, Particularly Significant Others.** The development of self-esteem can be positively or negatively influenced by the responses of others and by how individuals perceive those responses.
2. **Genetic Factors.** Factors that are genetically determined, such as physical appearance, size, or inherited infirmity can have an effect on the development of self-esteem.
3. **Environmental Factors.** The development of self-esteem can be influenced by demands from the environment. For example, intellectual prowess may be incorporated into the self-worth of an individual who is reared in an academic environment.

Developmental Progression of the Self-Esteem Through the Life Span

The development of self-esteem progresses throughout the life span. Erikson's (1963) theory of personality development provides a useful framework for illustration (see Chapter 3). Erikson describes eight transitional or maturational crises, the resolution of which can have a profound influence on the self-esteem. If a crisis is successfully resolved at one stage, the individual develops healthy coping strategies that he or she can draw on to help fulfill tasks of subsequent stages. Driever (1976c) states, "Should adaptation be less than successful, the person develops negative behaviors and views of himself which make him less healthy and less able to adapt successfully to the next maturational crisis or any situational crises that also may be encountered."

Trust Versus Mistrust

The development of trust results in a feeling of confidence in the predictability of the environment. Achievement of trust results in positive self-esteem through the instillation of self-confidence, optimism, and faith in the gratification of needs.

Unsuccessful resolution results in the individual experiencing emotional dissatisfaction with the self and suspiciousness of others, thereby promoting negative self-esteem.

Autonomy Versus Shame and Doubt

With motor and mental development come greater movement and independence within the environment.

The child begins active exploration and experimentation. Achievement of the task results in a sense of self-control and the ability to delay gratification, as well as a feeling of self-confidence in one's ability to perform.

This task remains unresolved when the child's independent behaviors are restricted or when the child fails because of unrealistic expectations. Negative self-esteem is promoted by a lack of self-confidence, a lack of pride in the ability to perform, and a sense of being controlled by others.

Initiative Versus Guilt

Positive self-esteem is gained through initiative when creativity is encouraged and performance is recognized and positively reinforced. In this stage, children strive to develop a sense of purpose and the ability to initiate and direct their own activities.

This is the stage during which the child begins to develop a conscience. He or she becomes vulnerable to the labeling of behaviors as "good" or "bad." Guidance and discipline that relies heavily on shaming the child creates guilt and results in a decrease in self-esteem.

Industry Versus Inferiority

Self-confidence is gained at this stage through learning, competing, performing successfully, and receiving recognition from significant others, peers, and acquaintances.

Negative self-esteem is the result of nonachievement, unrealistic expectations, or when accomplishments are consistently met with negative feedback. The child develops a sense of personal inadequacy.

Identity Versus Role Confusion

During adolescence, the individual is striving to redefine the sense of self. Positive self-esteem occurs when individuals are allowed to experience independence by making decisions that influence their lives.

Failure to develop a new self-definition results in a sense of self-consciousness, doubt, and confusion about one's role in life. This can occur when adolescents are encouraged to remain in the dependent position; when discipline in the home has been overly harsh, inconsistent, or absent; and when parental support has been lacking. These conditions are influential in the development of low self-esteem.

Intimacy Versus Isolation

Intimacy is achieved when one is able to form a lasting relationship or a commitment to another person, a cause, an institution, or a creative effort (Murray & Zentner, 1997).

Positive self-esteem is promoted through this capacity for giving of oneself to another.

Failure to achieve intimacy results in behaviors such as withdrawal, social isolation, aloneness, and the inability to form lasting intimate relationships. Isolation occurs when love in the home has been lacking or distorted through the younger years, causing a severe impairment in self-esteem.

Generativity Versus Stagnation

Generativity promotes positive self-esteem through gratification from personal and professional achievements, and from meaningful contributions to others.

Failure to achieve generativity occurs when earlier developmental tasks are not fulfilled and the individual does not achieve the degree of maturity required to derive gratification out of a personal concern for the welfare of others. He or she lacks self-worth and becomes withdrawn and isolated.

Ego Integrity Versus Despair

Ego integrity results in a sense of self-worth and self-acceptance as one reviews life goals, accepting that some were achieved and some were not. The individual has little desire to make major changes in how his or her life has progressed. Positive self-esteem is evident.

Individuals in despair possess a sense of self-contempt and disgust with how life has progressed. They would like to have a second chance at life and feel worthless and helpless. Earlier developmental tasks of self-confidence, self-identity, and concern for others remain unfulfilled. Negative self-esteem prevails.

THE MANIFESTATIONS OF LOW SELF-ESTEEM

Individuals with low self-esteem perceive themselves to be incompetent, unlovable, insecure, and unworthy. The number of manifestations exhibited is influenced by the degree to which an individual experiences low self-esteem. Roy (1976) categorizes behaviors according to the type of stimuli that give rise to these behaviors and affirms the importance of including this type of information in the nursing assessment. Stimulus categories are identified as *focal*, *contextual*, and *residual*. A summary of these types of influencing factors is presented in Table 14.1.

Focal Stimuli

A **focal stimulus** is the immediate concern that is causing the threat to self-esteem and the stimulus that is engendering the current behavior. Examples of focal stimuli include

▰ TABLE 14.1   FACTORS THAT INFLUENCE MANIFESTATIONS OF LOW SELF-ESTEEM

FOCAL	CONTEXTUAL	RESIDUAL
1. Any experience or situation causing the individual to question or decrease his or her value of self. Experiences of loss are particularly significant.	1. Body changes experienced because of growth or illness. 2. Maturational crises associated with developmental stages. 3. Situational crises and the individual's ability to cope. 4. The individual's perceptions of feedback from significant others. 5. Ability to meet expectations of self and others. 6. The feeling of control one has over life situation. 7. One's self-definition and the use of it to measure self-worth. 8. How one copes with feelings of guilt, shame, and powerlessness. 9. How one copes with the required changes in self-perception. 10. Awareness of what affects self-concept and the manner with which these stimuli are dealt. 11. The number of failures experienced before judging self as worthless. 12. The degree of self-esteem one possesses. 13. How one copes with limits within the environment. 14. The type of support from significant others and how one responds to it. 15. One's awareness of and ability to express feelings. 16. One's current feeling of hope and comfort with the self.	1. Age and coping mechanisms one has developed. 2. Stressful situations previously experienced and how well one coped with them. 3. Previous feedback from significant others that contributed to self-worth. 4. Coping strategies developed through experiences with previous developmental crises. 5. Previous experiences with powerlessness and hopelessness and how one coped with them. 6. Coping with previous losses. 7. Coping with previous failures. 8. Previous experiences meeting expectations of self and others. 9. Previous experiences with control of self and the environment and quality of coping response. 10. Previous experience with decision making and subsequent consequences. 11. Previous experience with childhood limits, and whether or not those limits were clear, defined, and enforced.

SOURCE: Adapted from Driever (1976b), with permission.

termination of a significant relationship, loss of employment, and failure to pass the nursing state board examination.

Contextual Stimuli

Contextual stimuli are all of the other stimuli present in the person's environment that *contribute* to the behavior being caused by the focal stimulus. Examples of contextual stimuli related to the previously mentioned focal stimuli might be a child of the relationship becoming emotionally disabled in response to the divorce, advanced age interfering with obtaining employment, or a significant other who states, "I knew you weren't smart enough to pass state boards."

Residual Stimuli

Residual stimuli are factors that *may* influence one's maladaptive behavior in response to focal and contextual stimuli. An individual conducting a self-esteem assessment might *presume* from previous knowledge that certain beliefs, attitudes, experiences, or traits have an effect on client behavior, even though it cannot be clearly substantiated. For example, being reared in an atmosphere of ridicule and deprecation may be affecting current adaptation to failure on the state board examination.

Symptoms of Low Self-Esteem

Driever (1976b) identifies a number of behaviors manifested by the individual with low self-esteem. These behaviors are presented in Table 14.2.

BOUNDARIES

The word *boundary* is used to denote the personal space, both physical and psychological, that individuals identify as their own. Boundaries are sometimes referred to as limits:

TABLE 14.2 MANIFESTATIONS OF LOW SELF-ESTEEM

1. Loss of appetite/weight loss
2. Overeating
3. Constipation or diarrhea
4. Sleep disturbances (insomnia or difficulty falling or staying asleep)
5. Hypersomnia
6. Complaints of fatigue
7. Poor posture
8. Withdrawal from activities
9. Difficulty initiating new activities
10. Decreased libido
11. Decrease in spontaneous behavior
12. Expression of sadness, anxiety, or discouragement
13. Expression of feeling of isolation, being unlovable, unable to express or defend oneself, and too weak to confront or overcome difficulties
14. Fearful of angering others
15. Avoidance of situations of self-disclosure or public exposure
16. Tendency to stay in background; be a listener rather than a participant
17. Sensitivity to criticism; self-conscious
18. Expression of feelings of helplessness
19. Various complaints of aches and pains
20. Expression of being unable to do anything "good" or productive; expression of feelings of worthlessness and inadequacy
21. Expressions of self-deprecation, self-dislike, and unhappiness with self
22. Denial of past successes/accomplishments and of possibility for success with current activities
23. Feeling that anything one does will fail or be meaningless.
24. Rumination about problems
25. Seeking reinforcement from others; making efforts to gain favors, but failing to reciprocate such behavior
26. Seeing self as a burden to others
27. Alienation from other by clinging and self-preoccupation
28. Self-accusatory
29. Demanding reassurance but not accepting it
30. Hostile behavior
31. Angry at self and others but unable to express these feelings directly
32. Decreased ability to meet responsibilities
33. Decreased interest, motivation, concentration
34. Decrease in self-care, hygiene

SOURCE: From Driever (1976b), with permission.

the limit or degree to which individuals feel comfortable in a relationship. Whitfield (1993) states, "Boundaries delineate where I and my physical and psychological space end and where you and yours begin."

Boundaries help individuals define the self and are part of the individuation process. Individuals who are aware of their boundaries have a healthy self-esteem because they must know and accept their inner selves. The inner self includes beliefs, thoughts, feelings, decisions, choices, experiences, wants, needs, sensations, and intuitions (Whitfield, 1993).

Types of physical boundaries include physical closeness, touching, sexual behavior, eye contact, privacy (e.g., mail, diary, doors, nudity, bathroom, telephone), and pollution (e.g., noise and smoke), among others. Examples of invasions of physical boundaries are reading someone else's diary, smoking in a nonsmoking public area, and touching someone who does not wish to be touched.

Types of psychological boundaries include beliefs, feelings, choices, needs, time alone, interests, confidences, individual differences, and spirituality, among others. Examples of invasions of psychological boundaries are being criticized for doing something differently than others, having personal information shared in confidence told to others, and being told one "should" believe, feel, decide, choose, or think in a certain way.

Boundary Pliancy

Boundaries can be rigid, flexible, or enmeshed. Katherine (1991) suggests that dogs and cats can be a good illustra-

tion of **rigid boundaries** and **flexible boundaries.** She quotes author Mary Bly, "Dogs come when they're called; cats take a message and get back to you." Most dogs want to be as close to people as possible. When "their people" walk into the room, the dog is likely to be all over them. They want to be where their people are and do what they are doing. Dogs have very flexible boundaries.

Cats, on the other hand, have very distinct boundaries. They do what they want, when they want. They decide how close they will be to their people, and when. Cats take notice when their people enter a room, but may not even acknowledge their presence (until the cat decides the time is right). Their boundaries are less flexible than those of dogs.

Rigid Boundaries

Katherine (1991) states:

"When boundaries are very rigid, new ideas or experiences can't get in. A person who has very rigid boundaries may be difficult to bond with. Such a person has a narrow perspective on life, sees things one way, and can't discuss matters that lie outside his field of vision." (p. 78)

EXAMPLE:

Fred and Alice were seeing a marriage counselor because they were unable to agree on many aspects of raising their children and it was beginning to interfere with their relationship. Alice runs a day-care service out of their home, and Fred is an accountant. Alice states, "He never once changed a diaper or got up at night with a child. Now that they are older, he refuses to discipline them in any way." Fred responds, "In my family, my Mom took care of the house and kids and my Dad kept us clothed and fed. That's the way it should be. It's Alice's job to raise the kids. It's my job to make the money." Fred's boundaries are considered rigid because he refuses to consider the ideas of others or to experience alternative ways of doing things.

Flexible Boundaries

Healthy boundaries are flexible. That is, individuals must be able to let go of their boundaries and limits when appropriate. In order to have flexible boundaries, one must be aware of who is considered safe and when it is safe to let others invade our personal space.

EXAMPLE:

Nancy always takes the hour from 4 to 5 PM for her own. She takes no phone calls and tells the children that she is not to be disturbed during that hour. She reads or takes a long leisurely bath and relaxes before it is time to start dinner. Today her private time was interrupted when her 15-year-old daughter came home from school crying because she had not made the cheerleading squad. Nancy used her private time to comfort her daughter, who was experiencing a traumatic response to the failure.

Sometimes boundaries can be too flexible. Individuals with boundaries that are too loose are like chameleons. They take their "colors" from whomever they happen to be with at the time. That is, they allow others to make their choices and direct their behavior. For example, at a cocktail party Diane agreed with one person that the winter had been so unbearable she had hardly been out of the house. Later at the same party, she agreed with another person that the winter had seemed milder than usual.

Enmeshed Boundaries

Enmeshed boundaries occur when two people's boundaries are so blended together that neither can be sure where one stops and the other begins, or one individual's boundaries may be blurred with another's. The individual with the enmeshed boundaries may be unable to differentiate his or her feelings, wants, and needs from the other person's.

EXAMPLES:

1. Fran's parents are in town for a visit. They say to Fran, "Dear, we want to take you and Dave out to dinner tonight. What is your favorite restaurant?" Fran automatically responds, "Villa Roma," knowing that the Italian restaurant is Dave's favorite.

2. If a mother has difficulty allowing her daughter to individuate, the mother may perceive the daughter's experiences as happening to her (Katherine, 1991). For example, Aileen got her hair cut without her mother's knowledge. It was styled with spikes across the top of her head. When her mother saw it, she said, "How dare you go around looking like that! What will people think of me?"

Establishing Boundaries

Boundaries are established in childhood. Unhealthy boundaries are the products of unhealthy, troubled, or dysfunctional families. The boundaries enclose painful feelings that have their origin in the dysfunctional family and that have not been dealt with. McKay and Fanning (1987) explain the correlation between unhealthy boundaries and self-esteem disturbances and how they can arise out of negative role models:

> "Modeling self-esteem means valuing oneself enough to take care of one's own basic needs. When parents put themselves last, or chronically sacrifice for their kids, they teach them that a person is only worthy insofar as he or she is of service to others. When parents set consistent, supportive limits and protect themselves from overbearing demands, they send a message to their children that both are important and both have legitimate needs." (p. 256)

In addition to the lack of positive role models, unhealthy boundaries may also be the result of abuse or neglect. These circumstances can cause a delay in psychosocial development. The individual must then resume the grief process as an adult in order to continue the developmental progression. They learn to recognize feelings, work through core issues, and tolerate emotional pain as their own. They complete the individuation process, go on to develop healthy boundaries, and learn to appreciate their self-worth.

THE NURSING PROCESS

Assessment

Clients with self-esteem problems may manifest any of the symptoms presented in Table 14.2. Some clients with disturbances in self-esteem will make direct statements that reflect guilt, shame, or negative self-appraisal, but often it is necessary for the nurse to ask specific questions to obtain this type of information. In particular, clients who have experienced abuse or other severe trauma will often have kept feelings and fears buried for years, and behavioral manifestations of low self-esteem may not be readily evident.

Various tools for measuring self-esteem exist. One is presented in Table 14.3. This particular tool can be used as a self-inventory by the client, or it can be adapted and used by the nurse to format questions for assessing level of self-esteem in the client.

◄ Table 14.3 SELF-ESTEEM INVENTORY

Place a check mark in the column that most closely describes your answer to each statement. Each check is worth the number of points listed above each column.

	3 Often or a Great Deal	2 Sometimes	1 Seldom or Occasionally	0 Never or Not at All
1. I become angry or hurt when criticized.				
2. I am afraid to try new things.				
3. I feel stupid when I make a mistake.				
4. I have difficulty looking people in the eye.				
5. I have difficulty making small talk.				
6. I feel uncomfortable in the presence of strangers.				
7. I am embarrassed when people compliment me.				
8. I am dissatisfied with the way I look.				
9. I am afraid to express my opinions in a group.				
10. I prefer staying home alone rather than participating in group social situations.				
11. I have trouble accepting teasing.				
12. I feel guilty when I say "no" to people.				
13. I am afraid to make a commitment to a relationship for fear of rejection.				
14. I believe that most people are more competent than I.				
15. I feel resentment toward people who are attractive and successful.				
16. I have trouble thinking of any positive aspects about my life.				
17. I feel inadequate in the presence of authority figures.				
18. I have trouble making decisions.				
19. I fear the disapproval of others.				
20. I feel tense, stressed out, or "uptight."				

Problems with low self-esteem are indicated by items scored with a "3" or by a total score >46.

Diagnosis/Outcome Identification

The North American Nursing Diagnosis Association (NANDA) has accepted, for use and testing, three nursing diagnoses that relate to self-esteem. These diagnoses are self-esteem disturbance, chronic low self-esteem, and situational low self-esteem (NANDA, 1999). Each is described here with its definitions and defining characteristics.

Self-Esteem Disturbance

Definition. Negative self-evaluation/feelings about self or self-capabilities, which may be directly or indirectly expressed.

DEFINING CHARACTERISTICS
  1. Self-negating verbalization.
  2. Expressions of shame/guilt.
  3. Evaluates self as unable to deal with events.
  4. Rationalizes away/rejects positive feedback and exaggerates negative feedback about self.
  5. Hesitant to try new things/situations.
  6. Denial of problems obvious to others.
  7. Projection of blame/responsibility for problems.
  8. Rationalizing personal failures.
  9. Hypersensitive to slight or criticism.
 10. Grandiosity.

Chronic Low Self-Esteem

Definition. Longstanding negative self-evaluation/ feelings about self or self-capabilities.

DEFINING CHARACTERISTICS
Long-standing or chronic
  1. Self-negating verbalizations.
  2. Expressions of shame/guilt.
  3. Evaluates self as unable to deal with events.
  4. Rationalizes away/rejects positive feedback and exaggerates negative feedback about self.
  5. Hesitant to try new things/situations.
  6. Frequent lack of success in work or other life events.
  7. Overly conforming, dependent on others' opinions.

8. Lack of eye contact.
9. Nonassertive/passive.
10. Indecisive.
11. Excessively seeks reassurance.

Situational Low Self-Esteem

Definition. Negative self-evaluation/feelings about self that develop in response to a loss or change in an individual who previously had a positive self-evaluation.

DEFINING CHARACTERISTICS

1. Episodic occurrence of negative self-appraisal in response to life events in a person with a previous positive self-evaluation.
2. Verbalization of negative feelings about the self (helplessness, uselessness).
3. Self-negating verbalizations.
4. Expressions of shame/guilt.
5. Evaluates self as unable to handle situations and events.
6. Difficulty making decisions.

Outcome Criteria

The following criteria may be used for measurement of outcomes in the care of the client with self-esteem disturbances.

THE CLIENT:

1. Is able to express positive aspects about self and life situation.
2. Is able to accept positive feedback from others.
3. Is able to attempt new experiences.
4. Is able to accept personal responsibility for own problems.
5. Is able to accept constructive criticism without becoming defensive.
6. Is able to make independent decisions about life situation.
7. Uses good eye contact.
8. Is able to develop positive interpersonal relationships.
9. Is able to communicate needs and wants to others assertively.

Planning/Implementation

In Table 14.4, a plan of care using the three self-esteem diagnoses accepted by NANDA is presented. Outcome criteria, appropriate nursing interventions, and rationales are included for each diagnosis.

Evaluation

Reassessment is conducted to determine if the nursing actions have been successful in achieving the objectives of care. Evaluation of the nursing actions for the client with self-esteem disturbances may be facilitated by gathering information using the following types of questions.

Is the client able to discuss past accomplishments and other positive aspects about his or her life?

Does the client accept praise and recognition from others in a gracious manner?

Is the client able to try new experiences without extreme fear of failure?

Can he or she accept constructive criticism now without becoming overly defensive and shifting the blame to others?

Does the client accept personal responsibility for problems, rather than attributing feelings and behaviors to others?

Does the client participate in decisions that affect his or her life?

Can the client make rational decisions independently?

Has he or she become more assertive in interpersonal relations?

Is improvement observed in the physical presentation of self-esteem, such as eye contact, posture, changes in eating and sleeping, fatigue, libido, elimination patterns, self-care, and complaints of aches and pains?

SUMMARY

Emotional wellness requires that an individual have some degree of self-worth—a perception that he or she possesses a measure of value to self and others. Self-concept consists of body image, personal identity, and self-esteem. Body image encompasses one's appraisal of personal attributes, functioning, sexuality, wellness-illness state, and appearance.

The personal identity component is composed of the moral-ethical self, the self-consistency, and the self-ideal. The moral-ethical self functions as observer, standard setter, dreamer, comparer, and most of all evaluator of who the individual says he or she is. Self-consistency is the component of the personal identity that strives to maintain a stable self-image. Self-ideal relates to an individual's perception of what he or she wants to be, do, or become.

Self-esteem refers to the degree of regard or respect that individuals have for themselves and is a measure of worth that they place on their abilities and judgments. It is largely influenced by the perceptions of how one is viewed by significant others. Predisposing factors to the development of positive self-esteem include a sense of competence, unconditional love, a sense of survival, realistic

TABLE 14.4 CARE PLAN FOR THE CLIENT WITH PROBLEMS RELATING TO SELF-ESTEEM

NURSING DIAGNOSIS: SELF-ESTEEM DISTURBANCE
RELATED TO: Lack of positive feedback; repeated negative feedback; dysfunctional family system
EVIDENCED BY: Blaming others for problems; grandiosity

OUTCOME CRITERIA	NURSING INTERVENTIONS	RATIONALE
Client will take personal responsibility for own problems and be able to graciously accept positive feedback from others.	1. Accept and respect client as a unique and valued human being. 2. Promote feelings of personal control by encouraging independent decision making. 3. Acknowledge client's strengths and incorporate the employment of these strengths in care planning. 4. Discuss fears, encourage involvement in new activities.	1. Respect and dignity are basic human rights. 2. Powerlessness contributes to low self-esteem. 3. Promotes feelings of self-worth. 4. Confronting concerns and engaging in new tasks promotes personal growth and new skills.

NURSING DIAGNOSIS: CHRONIC LOW SELF-ESTEEM
RELATED TO: Childhood neglect/abuse; numerous failures; negative feedback from others
EVIDENCED BY: Longstanding self-negating verbalizations and expressions of shame and guilt

OUTCOME CRITERIA	NURSING INTERVENTIONS	RATIONALE
Client will verbalize positive aspects of self and abandon judgmental self-perceptions.	1. Be supportive, accepting, and respectful without invading the client's personal space. 2. Discuss inaccuracies in self-perception with client. 3. Have client list successes and strengths. Provide positive feedback. 4. Assess content of negative self-talk.	1. Individuals who have had longstanding feelings of low self-worth may be uncomfortable with personal attentiveness. 2. Client may not see positive aspects of self that others see, and bringing it to awareness may help change perception. 3. Helps client to develop internal self-worth and new coping behaviors. 4. Self-blame, shame, and guilt promote feelings of low self-worth. Depending on chronicity and severity of the problem, this is likely to be the focus of long-term psychotherapy with this client.

NURSING DIAGNOSIS: SITUATIONAL LOW SELF-ESTEEM
RELATED TO: Failure (either real or perceived) in a situation of importance to the individual or loss (either real or perceived) of a concept of value to the individual
EVIDENCED BY: Negative self-appraisal in a person with a previous positive self-evaluation

OUTCOME CRITERIA	NURSING INTERVENTIONS	RATIONALE
Client will identify source of threat to self-esteem and work through the stages of the grief process to resolve the loss or failure.	1. Convey an accepting attitude; encourage client to express self openly. 2. Encourage client to express anger. Do not become defensive if initial expression of anger is displaced on nurse/therapist. Assist client to explore angry feelings and direct them toward the intended object/person or other loss.	1. An accepting attitude enhances trust and communicates to the client that you believe he or she is a worthwhile person, regardless of what is expressed. 2. Verbalization of feelings in a nonthreatening environment may help client come to terms with unresolved issues related to the loss.

Continued on following page

TABLE 15.2 *Continued*

3. Assist client to avoid ruminating about past failures. Withdraw attention if client persists.	3. Lack of attention to these undesirable behaviors may discourage their repetition.
4. Client needs to focus on positive attributes if self-esteem is to be enhanced. Encourage discussion of past accomplishments and offer support in undertaking new tasks. Offer recognition of successful endeavors and positive reinforcement of attempts made.	4. Recognition and positive reinforcement enhance self-esteem and encourage repetition of desirable behaviors.

goals, a sense of responsibility, and reality orientation. Genetics and environmental conditions may also be influencing factors.

The development of self-esteem progresses throughout the life span. Erikson's theory of personality development was used in this chapter as a framework for illustration of this progression.

The behaviors associated with low self-esteem are numerous. Stimuli that trigger these behaviors were presented according to focal, contextual, or residual types.

Boundaries, or personal limits, help individuals define the self and are part of the individuation process. Boundaries are physical and psychological and may be rigid, flexible, or enmeshed. Unhealthy boundaries are often the result of dysfunctional family systems.

The nursing process was presented as the vehicle for delivery of care to clients needing assistance with self-esteem disturbances. An inventory for assessing self-esteem was included. The three nursing diagnoses relating to self-esteem that have been accepted by NANDA were discussed, along with definitions and defining characteristics. Outcome criteria for clients with low self-esteem were presented. A plan of care for clients experiencing self-esteem disturbances was included, along with reassessment questions for evaluation.

REVIEW QUESTIONS

SELF-EXAMINATION/LEARNING EXERCISE

Situation: Karen is 23 years old. She has always been a good student and liked by her peers. She made As and Bs in high school, was captain of the cheerleading squad, and was chosen best-liked girl by her senior classmates at graduation. She entered nursing school at a nearby university and graduated with a 3.2/4.0 grade point average in 4 years. The summer after graduation, Karen took the state board examination and did not pass. She was disappointed but was allowed to continue working at her hospital job as a graduate nurse until she was able to take the examination again. After a few months, she retook the exam and again she did not pass. She was not able to keep her job any longer and became despondent. She has sought counseling at the local mental health clinic.

Select the answer that is most appropriate for this situation.

1. Karen says to the psychiatric nurse, "I am a complete failure. I'm so dumb, I can't do anything right." What is the most appropriate nursing diagnosis for Karen?

    a. Chronic low self-esteem.
    b. Situational low self-esteem.
    c. Defensive coping.
    d. Self-esteem disturbance.

2. Which of the following outcome criteria would be most appropriate for Karen?

    a. Karen is able to express positive aspects about herself and her life situation.
    b. Karen is able to accept constructive criticism without becoming defensive.
    c. Karen is able to develop positive interpersonal relationships.
    d. Karen is able to accept positive feedback from others.

3. Which of the following nursing interventions is *best* for Karen's specific problem?

    a. Encourage Karen to talk about her feeling of shame over the failure.
    b. Assist Karen to problem solve her reasons for failing the exam.
    c. Help Karen understand the importance of good self-care and personal hygiene in the maintenance of self-esteem.
    d. Explore with Karen her past successes and accomplishments.

4. The psychiatric nurse encourages Karen to express her anger. Why is this an appropriate nursing intervention?

    a. Anger is the basis for self-esteem problems.
    b. The nurse suspects that Karen was abused as a child.
    c. The nurse is attempting to guide Karen through the grief process.
    d. The nurse recognizes that Karen has longstanding repressed anger.

5. Karen is demonstrating a number of behaviors attributed to low self-esteem that were triggered by her failure of the examination. In Karen's case, failure of the exam can be considered a

    a. Focal stimulus.
    b. Contextual stimulus.
    c. Residual stimulus.
    d. Spatial stimulus.

Match the following words to the statements that follow:

_____ a. Rigid boundary.

_____ b. Too flexible boundary.

_____ c. Enmeshed boundary.

_____ d. A boundary violation.

_____ e. Showing respect for the boundary of another.

6. "What do you want to do tonight?" "Whatever you want to do."
7. Twins Jan and Jean still dress alike even though they are grown and married.
8. Karen's counselor asks her if she would like a hug.
9. Velma told Betty a secret that Mary had told her.
10. Tommy says to his friend, "I can't ever talk to my Daddy until after he has read his newspaper."

REFERENCES

Coopersmith, S. (1981). *The antecedents of self-esteem.* Palo Alto, CA: Consulting Psychologists Press.

Driever, M.J. (1976a). Theory of self-concept. In C. Roy (Ed.), *Introduction to nursing: An adaptation model.* Englewood Cliffs, NJ: Prentice-Hall.

Driever, M.J. (1976b). Problem of low self-esteem. In C. Roy (Ed.), *Introduction to nursing: An adaptation model.* Englewood Cliffs, NJ: Prentice-Hall.

Driever, M.J. (1976c). Development of self-concept. In C. Roy (Ed.), *Introduction to nursing: An adaptation model.* Englewood Cliffs, NJ: Prentice-Hall.

Erikson, E.H. (1963). *Childhood and society* (2nd ed.). New York: W.W. Norton.

Katherine, A. (1991). *Boundaries: Where you end and I begin.* New York: Simon & Schuster.

Maslow, A. (1970). *Motivation and personality* (2nd ed.). New York: Harper & Row.

McKay, M., & Fanning, P. (1987). *Self-esteem.* Oakland, CA: New Harbinger Publications.

Murray, R.B., & Zentner, J.P. (1997). *Health assessment and promotion strategies through the life span* (6th ed.). Stamford, CT: Appleton & Lange.

North American Nursing Diagnosis Association (NANDA). (1999). *Nursing diagnoses: Definitions and classification 1999–2000.* Philadelphia: NANDA.

Robertson, S.M. (1991). Self-concept disturbance. In G.K. McFarland, & M.D. Thomas (Eds.), *Psychiatric mental health nursing: Application of the nursing process.* Philadelphia: J.B. Lippincott.

Roy, C. (1976). *Introduction to nursing: An adaptation model.* Englewood Cliffs, NJ: Prentice-Hall.

Warren, J. (1991). Your child and self-esteem. *The Prairie View, 30*(2):1.

Whitfield, C.L. (1993). *Boundaries and relationships: Knowing, protecting, and enjoying the self.* Deerfield Beach, FL: Health Communications.

Bibliography

Burns, D.D. (1980) *Feeling good: The new mood therapy.* New York: New American Library.

Burns, D.D. (1993). *Ten days to self-esteem.* New York: William Morrow & Co.

Fanning, P. (1988). *Visualization for change.* Oakland, CA: New Harbinger Publications.

Klose, P., & Tinius, T. (1992). Confidence builders: A self-esteem group at an inpatient psychiatric hospital. *Journal of Psychosocial Nursing, 30*(7), 5–9.

LeMone, P. (1991). Analysis of a human phenomenon: Self-concept. *Nursing Diagnosis, 2*(3), 126–130.

Norris, J. (1992). Nursing intervention for self-esteem disturbances. *Nursing Diagnosis, 3*(2), 48–53.

O'Connor, R. (1981). Self-consistency as a dimension of self-concept related to birth order in families of five to seven siblings. *Issues in Mental Health Nursing, 3,* 185–193.

Reardon, J.A. (1993). A clinical ladder for milieu counselors: An opportunity to contribute to self-esteem. *Journal of Psychosocial Nursing, 31*(1), 27–29.

Tinelli, S.O. (1981). The relationship of family concept to individual self-esteem. Issues in *Mental Health Nursing, 3,* 251–270.

Waitley, D. (1983). *Seeds of greatness.* Old Tappan, NJ: Fleming H. Revell.

ANGER/AGGRESSION MANAGEMENT

CHAPTER OUTLINE

OBJECTIVES

INTRODUCTION

ANGER AND AGGRESSION, DEFINED

PREDISPOSING FACTORS TO ANGER AND AGGRESSION

THE NURSING PROCESS

SUMMARY

REVIEW QUESTIONS

KEY TERMS

anger
aggression

modeling
operant conditioning

preassaultive
   tension state

OBJECTIVES

After reading this chapter, the student will be able to:

1. Define and differentiate between anger and aggression.
2. Identify when the expression of anger becomes a problem.
3. Discuss predisposing factors to the maladaptive expression of anger.
4. Apply the nursing process to clients expressing anger or aggression.
   a. **Assessment:** Describe physical and psychological responses to anger.
   b. **Diagnosis/outcome identification:** For-

mulate nursing diagnoses and outcome criteria for clients expressing anger and aggression.
   c. **Planning/intervention:** Describe nursing interventions for clients demonstrating maladaptive expressions of anger.
   d. **Evaluation:** Evaluate achievement of the projected outcomes in the intervention with clients demonstrating maladaptive expression of anger.

arren (1990) reports the following statistics:

"In the United States in 1980, there was one violent crime very 24 seconds. There was one murder every 23 minutes, a total of 82,088 forcible rapes, one robbery every 58 seconds, and one aggravated assault every 48 seconds. In the case of murder, the victim was well known to the assailant well over 50 percent of the time, and in these cases angry arguments usually preceded the murderous event." (p. 1)

Anger need not be a negative expression. It is a normal human emotion that, when handled appropriately and expressed assertively, can provide an individual with a positive force to solve problems and make decisions concerning life situations. Anger becomes a problem when it is not expressed and when it is expressed aggressively. Violence occurs when individuals lose control of their anger. Violent acts are becoming commonplace in the United States. They are reported daily on the evening news, and health care workers see the results on a regular basis in the emergency departments of general hospitals.

This chapter addresses the concepts of anger and aggression. Predisposing factors to the maladaptive expression of anger are discussed, and the nursing process as a vehicle for delivery of care to assist clients in the management of anger and aggression is described.

ANGER AND AGGRESSION, DEFINED

Anger

Anger is the emotional response to one's perception of a situation (Milliken, 1993). Warren (1990) outlines some fundamental points about anger:

1. Anger is not a primary emotion, but it is typically experienced as an almost automatic inner response to hurt, frustration, or fear.

2. Anger is physiological arousal. It instills feelings of power and generates preparedness.
3. Anger and aggression are significantly different.
4. The expression of anger is learned.
5. The expression of anger can come under personal control.

Anger is a very powerful emotion. When it is denied or buried, it can precipitate a number of physical problems such as migraine headaches, ulcers, colitis, and even coronary heart disease. When turned inward on oneself, anger can result in depression and low self-esteem. When it is expressed inappropriately, it commonly interferes with relationships. When suppressed, anger may turn into resentment, which often manifests itself in negative, passive-aggressive behavior.

Anger creates a state of preparedness by arousing the sympathetic nervous system. The activation of this system results in increased heart rate and blood pressure, increased secretion of epinephrine (resulting in additional physiological arousal), and increased levels of serum glucose, among others. Anger prepares the body, physiologically, to fight. When anger goes unresolved, this physiological arousal can be the predisposing factor to a number of health problems. Even if the situation that created the anger is removed by miles or years, it can be replayed through the memory, reactivating the sympathetic arousal when this occurs.

Table 15.1 lists anger's positive and negative functions.

Aggression

The term *anger* often takes on a negative connotation because of its link with **aggression.** Warren (1990) defines aggression in the following manner:

"Aggression is a behavior intended to threaten or injure the victim's security or self-esteem. It means 'to go against,' 'to assault,' or 'to attack.' It is a response which aims at inflicting

▬ TABLE 15.1   THE FUNCTIONS OF ANGER

POSITIVE FUNCTIONS OR CONSTRUCTIVE USES	NEGATIVE FUNCTIONS OR DESTRUCTIVE USES
Anger energizes and mobilizes the body for self-defense.	Without cognitive input, anger may result in impulsive behavior, disregarding possible negative consequences.
Communicated assertively, anger can promote conflict resolution.	Communicated passive-aggressively or aggressively, conflict escalates, and the problem that created the conflict goes unresolved.
Anger arousal is a personal signal of threat or injustice against the self. The signal elicits coping responses to deal with the distress.	Anger can lead to aggression when the coping response is displacement. Anger can be destructive if it is discharged against an object or person unrelated to the true target of the anger.
Anger is constructive when it provides a feeling of control over a situation and the individual is able to assertively take charge of a situation.	Anger can be destructive when the feeling of control is exaggerated and the individual uses the power to intimidate others.
Anger is constructive when it is expressed assertively, serves to increase self-esteem, and leads to mutual understanding and forgiveness.	Anger can be destructive when it masks honest feelings, weakens self-esteem, and leads to hostility and rage.

SOURCES: Adapted from Kalman & Waughfield (1993) and Weisinger (1985).

pain or injury on objects or persons. Whether the damage is caused by words, fists, or weapons, the behavior is virtually always designed to punish. It is frequently accompanied by bitterness, meanness, and ridicule. An aggressive person is often vengeful." (p. 81)

Aggression is one way individuals express anger. It is sometimes used to try to force someone into compliance with the aggressor's wishes, but at other times the only objective seems to be the infliction of punishment and pain. In virtually all instances, aggression is a negative function or destructive use of anger.

PREDISPOSING FACTORS TO ANGER AND AGGRESSION

A number of factors have been implicated in the way individuals express anger. Some theorists view aggression as purely biological and some suggest that it results from individuals' interactions with their environments. Very likely, it is a combination of both.

Modeling

Role **modeling** is one of the strongest forms of learning. Children model their behavior at a very early age after their primary caregivers, usually parents. How parents or significant others express anger becomes the child's method of anger expression.

Whether role modeling is positive or negative depends on the behavior of the models. Much has been written about the abused child becoming physically abusive as an adult (Kempe & Helfer, 1980; Owens & Straus, 1975; Widom, 1989).

Role models are not always in the home, however. Evidence supports the role of television violence as a predisposing factor to later aggressive behavior (NIMH, 1982). Centerwall (1992) suggests that monitoring what children view and regulation of violence in the media are necessary to prevent this type of violent modeling.

Operant Conditioning

Operant conditioning occurs when a specific behavior is reinforced. A positive reinforcement is a response to the specific behavior that is pleasurable or produces the desired results. A negative reinforcement is a response to the specific behavior that prevents an undesirable result from occurring.

Anger responses can be learned through operant conditioning. For example, when a child wants something and has been told "no" by a parent, he or she may have a temper tantrum. If, when the temper tantrum begins, the parent lets the child have what is wanted, the anger has been positively reinforced (or rewarded).

An example of learning by negative reinforcement follows: A mother asks the child to pick up her toys and the child becomes angry and has a temper tantrum. If, when the temper tantrum begins, the mother thinks, "Oh, it's not worth all this!" and picks up the toys herself, the anger has been negatively reinforced (the child was rewarded by not having to pick up her toys).

Neurophysiological Disorders

Some research has implicated temporal lobe epilepsy in episodic aggression and violent behavior (Monroe, 1985; Weiger & Bear, 1988). Clients with episodic dyscontrol often respond to anticonvulsant medication.

Tumors in the brain, particularly in the areas of the limbic system and the temporal lobes; trauma to the brain, resulting in cerebral changes; and diseases, such as encephalitis (or medications that may effect this syndrome), have all been implicated in the predisposition to aggression and violent behavior. Tonkonogy (1991) suggests that subtle damage to the amygdaloid nucleus may be associated with violence.

Biochemical Factors

Violent behavior may be associated with hormonal dysfunction caused by Cushing's disease or hyperthyroidism (Tardiff, 1994). Studies have not supported a correlation between violence and increased levels of androgens or alterations in hormone levels associated with hypoglycemia or premenstrual syndrome.

Some research indicates that various neurotransmitters (e.g., epinephrine, norepinephrine, dopamine, acetylcholine, and serotonin) may play a role in the facilitation and inhibition of aggressive impulses (Goldstein, 1974).

Socioeconomic Factors

High rates of violence exist within the subculture of poverty in the United States. This has been attributed to lack of resources, break-up of families, alienation, discrimination, and frustration (Tardiff, 1994). An ongoing controversy exists as to whether economic inequality or absolute poverty is most responsible for violent behavior within this subculture. That is, does violence occur because individuals perceive themselves as disadvantaged relative to other persons, or does violence occur because of the deprivation itself? Messner and Tardiff (1986) found that absolute poverty was a greater determinant of violent behavior, citing deprivation, disruption of families, and unemployment as influencing factors.

Environmental Factors

Physical crowding may be related to violence through increased contact and decreased defensible space (Tardiff, 1994). Bell and Baron (1981) concluded that there is a relationship between heat and aggression. They found that moderately uncomfortable temperature produced an increase in aggression, while extremely hot temperatures decreased aggression.

A number of epidemiological studies have found a strong link between use of alcohol and violent behavior. Many street drugs, particularly cocaine, amphetamines, hallucinogens, and minor tranquilizers/sedatives, have also been associated with violent behavior (Tardiff, 1994).

Availability of firearms has been linked to commission of violent crimes. Evidence exists to support the effectiveness of gun control legislation in decreasing the rate of homicides involving firearms (Cook, 1982).

THE NURSING PROCESS

Assessment

Nurses must be aware of the symptoms associated with anger and aggression in order to make an accurate assessment. The best intervention is prevention, so risk factors for assessing violence potential are also presented.

Anger

Alexander (1991a) identifies a cluster of characteristics that describe anger:

> Intense distress
> Frowning
> Gritting of the teeth
> Pacing
> Eyebrow displacement (raised, lowered, knitted)
> Clenched fists
> Increased energy
> Fatigue
> Withdrawal
> Flushed face
> Emotional overcontrol
> Change in tone of voice (either lowered, with words spoken between clenched teeth, or yelling and shouting)

Anger has been identified as a stage in the grieving process. Individuals who become fixed in this stage may become depressed. In this instance, the anger is turned inward as a way for the individual to maintain control over the pent-up anger. Because of the negative connotation to the word *anger*, some clients will not acknowledge that what they are feeling is anger. These individuals will need assistance to recognize their true feelings and to understand that anger is a perfectly acceptable emotion, when it is expressed appropriately.

Aggression

Alexander (1991b) states that aggression can arise from such feeling states as anger, anxiety, tension, guilt, frustration, or hostility. Aggressive behaviors can be classified as mild (e.g., sarcasm), moderate (e.g., slamming doors), severe (e.g., threats of physical violence against others), or extreme (e.g., physical acts of violence against others). Alexander (1991b) identifies aggression by the following defining characteristics:

> Sarcasm
> Verbal or physical threats
> Change in voice tone (raised or quavering voice tone and pitch; rapid or hesitant speech)
> Degrading comments
> Pacing
> Throwing or striking objects or people
> Suspiciousness
> Suicidal ideation
> Homicidal ideation
> Self-mutilation
> Invasion of personal space
> Increase in agitation or irritability
> Disturbed thought process and perception
> Misinterpretation of stimuli
> Anger disproportionate to an event

Warren (1990) states, "Aggression has long-term negative consequences almost all of the time. Even the short-term gains it occasionally produces are usually canceled out over the long term."

Assessing Risk Factors

Prevention is the key issue in the management of aggressive or violent behavior. The individual who becomes violent usually feels an underlying helplessness. Haven and Piscitello (1989) identify three factors that are important considerations: (1) past history of violence, (2) client diagnosis, and (3) current behaviors.

Blair and New (1991) report the results of several studies that clearly implicate a history of assault as the most widely recognized risk factor for violence in a treatment setting. The second most frequently correlated factor with assaultive behavior is diagnosis. The diagnoses that have the highest association with violent behavior are substance abuse/intoxication (either as a primary or secondary diagnosis), schizophrenia, posttraumatic stress disorder, organic brain disorders, epilepsy, and temporal lobe abnormalities.

Some behaviors that may seen obvious, yet at times go unheeded, can be considered risk factors to violence. These predictive behaviors have been termed by Lanza (1988) the **"preassaultive tension state,"** and described by Haven and Piscitello (1989) as excessive motor activity—agitation and pacing, pounding, and slamming; tense posture; grim, defiant affect; clenched teeth; arguing; demanding;

clenched fists; talking in a rapid, raised voice; and challenging and threatening staff. Keen observation skills and background knowledge for accurate assessment are critical factors in predicting potential for violent behavior.

Diagnosis/Outcome Identification

The North American Nursing Diagnosis Association (NANDA) does not include a separate nursing diagnosis for anger. The nursing diagnosis of dysfunctional grieving may be used when anger is expressed inappropriately and the etiology is related to a loss.

The following nursing diagnoses may be considered for clients demonstrating inappropriate expression of anger or aggression:

Ineffective individual coping related to negative role modeling and dysfunctional family system evidenced by yelling, name calling, hitting others, and temper tantrums as expressions of anger.

Risk for violence: self-directed or directed at others related to having been nurtured in an atmosphere of violence.

Outcome Criteria

The following criteria may be used for measurement of outcomes in the care of the client needing assistance with management of anger and aggression.

THE CLIENT:

1. Is able to recognize when he or she is angry, and seeks out staff to talk about his or her feelings.
2. Is able to take responsibility for own feelings of anger.
3. Demonstrates the ability to exert internal control over feelings of anger.
4. Is able to diffuse anger before losing control.
5. Uses the tension generated by the anger in a constructive manner.
6. Does not cause harm to self or others.
7. Is able to use steps of the problem-solving process rather than becoming violent as a means of seeking solutions.

Planning/Implementation

In Table 15.2, a plan of care is presented for the client who expresses anger inappropriately. Outcome criteria, appropriate nursing interventions, and rationales are included for each diagnosis.

Evaluation

Evaluation consists of reassessment to determine if the nursing interventions have been successful in achieving the objectives of care. The following type of information may be gathered to determine the success of working with a client exhibiting inappropriate expression of anger.

Is the client able to recognize when he or she is angry now?

Can the client take responsibility for these feelings and keep them in check without losing control?

Does the client seek out staff to talk about feelings when they occur?

Is the client able to transfer tension generated by the anger into constructive activities?

Has harm to client and others been avoided?

Is the client able to solve problems adaptively without undue frustration and without becoming violent?

SUMMARY

Statistics show that violence is rampant in the United States. The precursor to violence is anger, which is a normal human emotion and need not necessarily be a negative response. When used appropriately, anger can provide positive assistance with problem solving and decision making in everyday life situations. Violence occurs when individuals lose control of their anger.

This chapter explores the concepts of anger and aggression. Anger is viewed as the emotional response to one's perception of a situation. It is a very powerful emotion and, when denied or buried, can precipitate a number of psychophysiological disorders. When it is turned inward on the self, it can result in depression. When expressed inappropriately, anger commonly interferes with interpersonal relationships. When it is suppressed, it often turns to resentment. Anger generates a physiological arousal comparable to the stress response discussed in Chapter 1.

Aggression is one way in which individuals express anger. It is behavior intended to threaten or injure the victim's security or self-esteem. It can be physical or verbal, but it is virtually always designed to punish. Aggression is a negative function or destructive use of anger.

Various predisposing factors to the way individuals express anger have been implicated. Some theorists suggest that the etiology is purely biological, whereas others believe it depends on psychological and environmental factors. Some possible predisposing factors include role modeling, operant conditioning, neurophysiological disorders (e.g., brain tumors, trauma, or diseases), biochemical factors (e.g., increased levels of androgens or other alterations in hormone levels and neurotransmitter involvement), socioeconomic factors (e.g., living in poverty), and environmental factors (e.g., physical crowding, uncomfortable temperature, use of alcohol or drugs, and availability of firearms).

Table 15.2 Care Plan for the Individual Who Expresses Anger Inappropriately

NURSING DIAGNOSES: INEFFECTIVE INDIVIDUAL COPING
RELATED TO: Negative role modeling and dysfunctional family system
EVIDENCED BY: Yelling, name calling, hitting others, and temper tantrums as expressions of anger

Outcome Criteria	Nursing Interventions	Rationale
Client will be able to recognize anger in self and take responsibility before losing control.	1. Remain calm when dealing with an angry client.	1. Anger expressed by the nurse will most likely incite increased anger in the client.
	2. Set verbal limits on behavior. Clearly delineate the consequences of inappropriate expression of anger and always follow through.	2. Consistency in enforcing the consequences is essential if positive outcomes are to be achieved. Inconsistency creates confusion and encourages testing of limits.
	3. Have the client keep a diary of angry feelings, what triggered them, and how they were handled.	3. This provides a more objective measure of the problem.
	4. Avoid touching the client when he or she becomes angry.	4. The client may view touch as threatening and could become violent.
	5. Help the client determine the true source of the anger.	5. Many times anger is being displaced onto a safer object or person. If resolution is to occur, the first step is to identify the source of the problem.
	6. It may be constructive to ignore initial derogatory remarks by the client.	6. Lack of feedback often extinguishes an undesirable behavior.
	7. Help the client find alternate ways of releasing tension, such as physical outlets, and more appropriate ways of expressing anger, such as seeking out staff when feelings emerge.	7. Client will likely need assistance to problem solve more appropriate ways of behaving.
	8. Role model appropriate ways of expressing anger assertively, such as, "I dislike being called names. I get angry when I hear you saying those things about me."	8. Role modeling is one of the strongest methods of learning.

NURSING DIAGNOSIS: RISK FOR VIOLENCE: SELF-DIRECTED OR DIRECTED AT OTHERS
RELATED TO: Having been nurtured in an atmosphere of violence

Outcome Criteria	Nursing Interventions	Rationale
The client will not harm self or others.	1. Observe client for escalation of anger (called the preassaultive tension state): increased motor activity, pounding, slamming, tense posture, defiant affect, clenched teeth and fists, arguing, demanding, and challenging or threatening staff.	1. Violence may be prevented if risks are identified in time.
	2. When these behaviors are observed, attempt to defuse the anger beginning with the least restrictive means.	2. Client rights must be honored while preventing harm to client and others on the unit.
	3. Techniques for dealing with aggression include:	3. Aggression control techniques promote safety and reduce risk of harm to client and others.

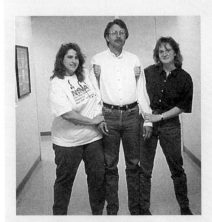

Figure 15.1 Walking a client to the seclusion room.

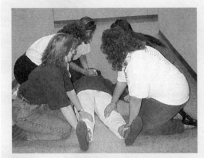

Figure 15.2 Staff restraint of a client in supine position. The client's head is controlled to prevent biting.

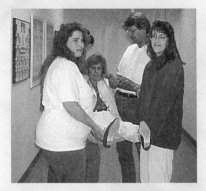

Figure 15.3 Transporting a client to the seclusion room.

a. Talking down. Say, "John, you seem very angry. Let's go to your room and talk about it." (Ensure that client does not position self between door and nurse.)

b. Physical outlets. "Maybe it would help if you punched your pillow or the punching bag for a while. I'll stay here with you if you want."

c. Medication. If agitation continues to escalate, offer client choice of taking medication voluntarily. If he or she refuses, reassess the situation to determine if harm to self or others is imminent.

d. Call for assistance. Remove self and other clients from the immediate area. Push "panic" button, call for assault team, or institute measures established by institution. Sufficient staff to indicate a show of strength may be enough to deescalate the situation, and client may agree to take the medication.

e. Restraints. If client is not calmed by "talking down" or by medication, use of mechanical restraints and/or seclusion may be necessary. Be sure to have sufficient staff available to assist. Figures 15.1, 15.2, and 15.3 illustrate ways in which staff can safely and appropriately deal with an out-of-control client. Follow protocol for restraints/seclusion established by the institution. Most states require that the physician reevaluate and issue a new order for restraints every 3 hours, except between midnight and 8 AM. If the client has previously refused medication, administer after restraints have been applied. Most states consider this intervention appropriate in emergency situations or if a client would likely harm self or others.

f. Observation and documentation. Observe the client in restraints every 15 minutes (or according to institutional policy). Ensure that circulation to extremities is not compromised (check temperature, color, pulses). Assist client with needs related to nutrition, hydration, and elimination. Position client so that comfort is facilitated and aspiration can be prevented. Document all observations.

a. Promotes a trusting relationship and may prevent the client's anxiety from escalating.

b. Provides effective way for client to release tension associated with high levels of anger.

c. Provides the least restrictive method of controlling client behavior.

d. Client and staff safety are of primary concern.

e. Clients who do not have internal control over their own behavior may require external controls, such as mechanical restraints, in order to prevent harm to self or others.

f. Client well-being is a nursing priority.

Continued on following page

TABLE 15.2 *Continued*

g. Ongoing assessment. As agitation decreases, assess client's readiness for restraint removal or reduction. With assistance from other staff members, remove one restraint at a time, while assessing client's response. This minimizes the risk of injury to client and staff.	g. Gradual removal of the restraints allows for testing of the client's self-control. Client and staff safety are of primary concern.
h. Staff debriefing. It is important when a client loses control for staff to follow-up with a discussion about the situation. Tardiff (1994) states, "The violent episode should be discussed in terms of what happened, what would have prevented it, why seclusion or restraint was used (if it was), and how the client or the staff felt in terms of the use of seclusion and restraint." It is also important to discuss the situation with other clients who witnessed the episode. It is important that they understand what happened. Some clients may fear that they could be secluded or restrained at some time for no apparent reason.	h. Debriefing diminishes the emotional impact of the intervention and provides an opportunity to clarify the need for the intervention, offer mutual feedback, and promote client's self-esteem (Norris & Kennedy, 1992).

Nurses must be aware of the symptoms associated with anger and aggression in order to make an accurate assessment. Prevention is the key issue in the management of aggressive or violent behavior. Three elements have been identified as key risk factors in the potential for violence: (1) past history of violence, (2) client diagnosis, and (3) current behaviors. Nursing diagnoses and outcome criteria for working with clients expressing anger or aggression were discussed, and a care plan outlining appropriate interventions was presented.

REVIEW QUESTIONS

SELF-EXAMINATION/LEARNING EXERCISE

Situation: John, age 27, was brought to the emergency department by two police officers. He smelled strongly of alcohol, was loud and verbally abusive to staff, slurred his words, and had difficulty standing and walking without assistance. Blood alcohol level was measured at 293 mg/dL. John's girlfriend reported that they were at a party and he became violent, hitting her and threatening to kill others who tried to protect her. She reported that he gets drunk almost every day and has beat her up a number of times. When told that he would be admitted to detox, he started cursing and hitting the staff who were trying to help him. He was admitted to the Detox Center of the Alcohol Treatment Unit with a diagnosis of Alcohol Intoxication. He was restrained for the protection of self and others. His diagnosis was later changed to Alcohol Dependence, following conclusion of the withdrawal syndrome.

Please answer the following questions related to this situation.

1. The nurses on the unit wrote a priority nursing diagnosis of Risk for Violence Toward Others for John. Using the assessment data provided, list the risk factors on which they based their diagnosis.

2. Which is the most appropriate *long-term* goal for the nursing diagnosis of Risk for Violence Toward Others?

    a. The client will not verbalize anger or hit anyone.
    b. The client will verbalize anger rather than hit others.
    c. The client will not harm self or others.
    d. The client will be restrained if he becomes verbally or physically abusive.

3. Which is the most appropriate *short-term* goal for the nursing diagnosis of Risk for Violence Toward Others?

    a. The client will not verbalize anger or hit anyone.
    b. The client will verbalize anger rather than hit others.
    c. The client will not harm self or others.
    d. The client will be restrained if he becomes verbally or physically abusive.

4. John is sitting in the dayroom watching TV with the other clients when the nurse approaches with his 5:00 PM dose of haloperidol. John says, "I feel in control now. I don't need any drugs." The nurse's best response is based on which of the following statements?

    a. John must have the medication, or he will become violent.
    b. John knows that if he will not take the medication orally, he will be restrained and given an intramuscular injection.
    c. John has the right to refuse the medication.
    d. John must take the medication at this time in order to maintain adequate blood levels.

5. Later that evening, the nurse hears John yelling in the dayroom. The nurse observes his increased agitation, clenched fists, and loud demanding voice. He is challenging and threatening staff and the other clients. The nurse's priority intervention would be:

    a. Call for assistance.
    b. Draw up a syringe of p.r.n haloperidol.
    c. Ask John if he would like to talk about his anger.
    d. Tell John if he does not calm down he will have to be restrained.

6. John is placed in restraints in the seclusion room. Describe care of the client in restraints.

7. When John has been in restraints several hours, he tells the nurse he can maintain control and is ready to have the restraints removed. How does the nurse proceed?

   a. She removes the restraints.
   b. She calls for assistance to remove the restraints.
   c. She removes one restraint.
   d. She tells John he will have to wait until the doctor comes in.

8. Which of these procedures is important in following up an episode of violence on the unit? (More than one answer may apply.)

   a. Document all observations and occurrences.
   b. Conduct a debriefing with staff.
   c. Discuss what occurred with other clients who witnessed the incident.
   d. Warn the client that it could happen again if he becomes violent.

9. Later in the day when John is calm, he apologizes to the nurse. "I hope I didn't hurt anyone." The nurse's best response is:

   a. "This is our job. We know how to handle violent clients."
   b. "We understand you were out of control and didn't really mean to hurt anyone."
   c. "It is fortunate that no one was hurt. You will not be placed in restraints as long as you can control your behavior."
   d. "It is an unpleasant situation to have to restrain someone, but we have to think of the other clients. We can't have you causing injury to others. I just hope it won't happen again."

10. John and his girlfriend had an argument during her visit. Which behavior by John would indicate he is learning to adaptively problem solve his frustrations?

    a. John says to the nurse, "Give me some of that medication before I end up in restraints!"
    b. When his girlfriend leaves, John goes to the exercise room and punches on the punching bag.
    c. John says to the nurse, "I guess I'm going to have to dump that broad!"
    d. John says to his girlfriend, "You'd better leave before I do something I'm sorry for."

REFERENCES

Alexander, D.I. (1991a). Anger. In G.K. McFarland & M.D. Thomas (Eds.), *Psychiatric mental health nursing: Application of the nursing process.* Philadelphia: J.B. Lippincott.

Alexander, D.I. (1991b). Aggression. In G.K. McFarland & M.D. Thomas (Eds.), *Psychiatric mental health nursing: Application of the nursing process.* Philadelphia: J.B. Lippincott.

Bell, P.A., & Baron, R.A. (1981). Ambient temperature and human violence. In P.F. Brain & D. Benton (Eds.), *Multidisciplinary approaches to aggression research.* Amsterdam: Elsevier.

Blair, D.T., & New. S.A. (1991). Assaultive behavior: Know the risks. *Journal of Psychosocial Nursing, 29*(11):25–30.

Centerwall, B.S. (1992). Television and violence: The scale of the problem and where to go from here. *Journal of the American Medical Association, 267,* 3059–3063.

Cook, P.J. (1982). The role of firearms in violent crime: An interpretive review of the literature. In M.E. Wolfgang & N.A. Weiner (Eds.), *Criminal violence.* Beverly Hills: Sage.

Goldstein, M. (1974). Brain research and violent behavior. *Archives of Neurology, 30*(1), 1–35.

Haven, E., & Piscitello, V. (1989). The patient with violent behavior. In S. Lewis, R. Grainger, W. McDowell, R.J. Gregory, & R. Messner (Eds.), *Manual of psychosocial nursing interventions: Promoting mental health in medical-surgical settings.* Philadelphia: W.B. Saunders.

Kalman, N., & Waughfield, C.G. (1993). *Mental health concepts* (3rd ed.). Albany, NY: Delmar Publishers.

Kempe, C.H., & Helfer, R.E. (1980). *The battered child* (3rd ed.). Chicago: University of Chicago Press.

Lanza, M.L. (1988). Factors relevant to patient assault. *Issues in Mental Health Nursing, 9,* 239–257.

Messner, S., & Tardiff, K. (1986). Economic inequality and levels of homicide: An analysis of urban neighborhoods. *Criminology, 24,* 297–317.

Milliken, M.E. (1993). *Understanding human behavior: A guide for health care providers* (5th ed.). Albany, NY: Delmar Publishers.

Monroe, R.R. (1985). Episodic behavioral disorders and limbic ictus. *Comprehensive Psychiatry, 26,* 466–479.

National Institute of Mental Health (NIMH). (1982). *Television and behavior: Ten years of scientific progress and implications for the eighties, Vol. 1, Summary report* (DHHS Publ No. 82-1195.) Rockville, MD: NIMH.

Norris, M.K., & Kennedy, C.W. (1992). How patients perceive the seclusion process. *Journal of Psychosocial Nursing and Mental Health Services, 30*(3): 7–13.

Owens, D.J., & Straus, M.A. (1975). The social structure of violence in childhood and approval of violence as an adult. *Aggressive Behavior, 1,* 193–211.

Tardiff, K. (1994). Violence. In R.E. Hales, S.C. Yudofsky, & J.A. Talbott (Eds.), *The American psychiatric press textbook of psychiatry* (2nd ed.). Washington, DC: American Psychiatric Press.

Tonkonogy, J.M. (1991). Violence and temporal lobe lesion: Head CT and MRI data. *Journal of Neuropsychiatry and Clinical Neurosciences, 3,* 189–196.

Warren, N.C. (1990). *Make anger your ally.* Colorado Springs, CO: Focus on the Family Publishing.

Weiger, B., & Bear, D. (1988). An approach to the neurology of aggression. *Journal of Psychiatric Research, 22,* 85–89.

Weisinger, H. (1985). *The anger work-out book.* New York: William Morrow.

Widom, C.S. (1989). The cycle of violence. *Science, 244,* 160–171.

Bibliography

Blair, D.T. (1991). Assaultive behavior: Does provocation begin in the front office? *Journal of Psychosocial Nursing, 29*(5), 21–26.

Green, R.G., & Donnerstein, E.I. (1983). *Aggression: Theoretical and empirical reviews.* Vols. 1 & 2. New York: Academic Press.

Jones, M.K. (1985). Patient violence. *Journal of Psychosocial Nursing, 23*(6), 12–17.

Lanza, M.L. (1983). Origins of aggression. *Journal of Psychosocial Nursing, 21*(6), 11–16.

Lerner, H.G. (1985). *The dance of anger.* New York: Harper & Row.

Murray, M.G., & Snyder, J.C. (1991). When staff are assaulted: A nursing consultation support service. *Journal of Psychosocial Nursing, 29*(7), 24–29.

Potter-Efron, R., & Potter-Efron, P. (1995). *Letting go of anger.* Oakland, CA: New Harbinger Publications.

Stearns, F.R. (1972). *Anger: Psychology, physiology, pathology.* Springfield, IL: Charles C. Thomas.

Stilling, L. (1992). The pros and cons of physical restraints and behavior controls. *Journal of Psychosocial Nursing, 30*(3), 18–20.

Talley, S., & King, M.C. (1984). *Psychiatric emergencies: Nursing assessment and intervention.* New York: Macmillan.

Valzelli, L. (1981). *Psychobiology of aggression and violence.* New York: Raven Press.

Vincent, M., & White, K. (1994). Patient violence toward a nurse: Predictable and preventable? *Journal of Psychosocial Nursing, 32*(2), 30–32.

THE SUICIDAL CLIENT

KEY TERMS

egoistic suicide   altruistic suicide   anomic suicide

OBJECTIVES

After reading this chapter, the student will be able to:

1. Discuss epidemiological statistics and risk factors related to suicide.
2. Describe predisposing factors implicated in the etiology of suicide.
3. Differentiate between facts and fables regarding suicide.
4. Apply the nursing process to individuals exhibiting suicidal behavior.

uicide is not a diagnosis or a disorder; it is a behavior. The Judeo-Christian belief has been that life is a gift from God and that taking it is strictly forbidden (Ghosh & Victor, 1994). A recent, and more secular, view has influenced how some individuals view suicide in our society. Growing support for an individual's right to choose death over pain has been evidenced. Some individuals are striving to advance the cause of physician-assisted suicides for the terminally ill. Can suicide be a rational act? Most people in our society do not yet believe that it can.

More than 90 percent of suicides are by individuals who are psychiatrically ill at the time of suicide (Black & Winokur, 1990). This chapter explores suicide from an epidemiological and etiological perspective. Care of the suicidal client is presented in the context of the nursing process.

EPIDEMIOLOGICAL FACTORS

Approximately 30,000 persons in the United States end their lives each year by suicide. These statistics have established suicide as the ninth leading cause of death among adults (Ghosh & Victor, 1994) and the third leading cause of death among adolescents (Kestenbaum & Trautman, 1992). Many more people attempt suicide than succeed, and countless others seriously contemplate the act without carrying it out. Suicide has become a major health care problem in the United States today.

Over the years confusion has existed over the reality of various notions regarding suicide. Some facts and fables relating to suicide are presented in Table 16.1.

RISK FACTORS

Marital Status

The suicide rate for single persons is twice that of married persons. The single, the divorced, and the widowed have rates four to five times greater than those of the married (Slaby, Lieb, & Tancredi, 1986).

Gender

Women attempt suicide more, but more men succeed. Successful suicides number about 70 percent for men and 30 percent for women. This has to do with the lethality of the means. Although women tend to overdose, men use more lethal means such as firearms. Interestingly, female medical students have suicide rates three to four times that of their nonmedical agemates (Slaby, Lieb, & Tancredi, 1986).

TABLE 16.1   FACTS AND FABLES ABOUT SUICIDE

FABLES	FACTS
People who talk about suicide do not commit suicide. Suicide happens without warning.	Eight out of ten people who kill themselves have given definite clues and warnings about their suicidal intentions. Very subtle clues may be ignored or disregarded by others.
You cannot stop a suicidal person. He or she is fully intent on dying.	Most suicidal people are very ambivalent about their feelings regarding living or dying. Most are "gambling with death" and see it as a cry for someone to save them.
Once a person is suicidal, he or she is suicidal forever.	People who want to kill themselves are only suicidal for a limited time. If they are saved from feelings of self-destruction, they can go on to lead normal lives.
Improvement after severe depression means that the suicidal risk is over.	Most suicides occur within about 3 months after the beginning of "improvement," when the individual has the energy to carry out suicidal intentions.
Suicide is inherited, or "runs in families."	Suicide is not inherited. It is an individual matter and can be prevented. However, suicide by a close family member increases an individual's risk factor for suicide.
All suicidal individuals are mentally ill, and suicide is the act of a psychotic person.	Although suicidal persons are extremely unhappy, they are not necessarily psychotic or otherwise mentally ill. They are merely unable at that point in time to see an alternative solution to what they consider an unbearable problem.
Suicidal threats and gestures should be considered manipulative or attention-seeking behavior, and should not be taken seriously.	All suicidal behavior must be approached with the gravity of the potential act in mind. Attention should be given to the possibility that the individual is issuing a cry for help.
People usually commit suicide by taking an overdose of drugs.	Gunshot wounds are the leading cause of death among suicide victims.
If an individual has attempted suicide, he or she will not do it again.	Fifty to 80% of all people who ultimately kill themselves have a history of a previous attempt.

SOURCES: From Shneidman & Farberow (1965); Freedman et al. (1976); and Slaby, Lieb, & Tancredi (1986).

Age

Suicide risk and age are positively correlated. This is particularly true with men. Although rates among women remain fairly constant throughout life, rates among men show a higher age correlation. The rates rise sharply during adolescence, peak between 30 and 40, and level off until age 65, when they rise again for the remaining years (Murphy, 1994).

Suicide has been identified as the third leading cause of death (following motor vehicle accidents and homicides) among the 15- to 24-year-old age group (Murray & Zentner, 1997). The suicide rate among adolescents has tripled over the past 30 years (Murphy, 1994). A major factor contributing to this increase is the rise in depressive disorders among youths (Ghosh & Victor, 1994). Other risk factors associated with adolescent suicide include religion (less likely if Catholic or Jewish), having parents with psychiatric illness (particularly drug or alcohol abuse), a history of suicide in the family, paternal unemployment, and paternal or maternal absence (Slaby, Lieb, & Tancredi, 1986).

Religion

Protestants have significantly higher rates of suicide than Catholics and Jews (Slaby, Lieb, & Tancredi, 1986). A strong feeling of cohesiveness within a religious organization seems to be an important factor.

Socioeconomic Status

Individuals in the very highest and lowest social classes have higher suicide rates than those in the middle classes (Kaplan & Sadock, 1998). With regard to occupation, suicide rates are higher among physicians, musicians, dentists, law enforcement officers, lawyers, and insurance agents than they are in the general population.

Ethnicity

With regard to ethnicity, most studies demonstrate that whites are at highest risk for suicide, followed by Native Americans, African Americans, Hispanic Americans, and Asian Americans (Ghosh & Victor, 1994).

Other Risk Factors

Individuals with mood disorders (major depression and bipolar disorder) are far more likely to commit suicide than those in any other psychiatric or medical risk group. Kaplan and Sadock (1998) report, "Almost 95 percent of all people who commit or attempt suicide have a diagnosed mental disorder. Depressive disorders account for 80 per-

cent of this figure." Suicide risk may increase early during treatment with antidepressants, as the return of energy brings about an increased ability to act out self-destructive wishes. Other psychiatric disorders that may account for suicidal behavior include psychoactive substance abuse disorders, schizophrenia, organic brain disorders, personality disorders, and panic disorders (Murphy, 1994).

Severe insomnia is associated with increased suicide risk, even in the absence of depression. Use of alcohol, and particularly a combination of alcohol and barbiturates, increases the risk of suicide. Psychosis, especially with command hallucinations, poses a higher than normal risk. Individuals with a predominantly homosexual orientation have an increased risk of suicide, especially if depressed, aging, or alcoholic (Slaby, Lieb, & Tancredi, 1986). Affliction with a chronic painful or disabling illness increases the risk of suicide.

Higher risk is also associated with a family history of suicide, especially in a same-sex parent, and with previous attempts. Fifty to 80 percent of those who ultimately commit suicide have a history of a previous attempt (Slaby, Lieb, & Tancredi, 1986). Loss of a loved one through death or separation and lack of employment or increased financial burden increase risk.

PREDISPOSING FACTORS: THEORIES OF SUICIDE

Psychological Theories

Anger Turned Inward. Freud (1957) believed that suicide was a response to the intense self-hatred that an individual possessed. The anger had originated toward a love object but was ultimately turned inward against the self. Freud believed that suicide occurred as a result of an earlier repressed desire to kill someone else. He interpreted suicide to be an aggressive act toward the self that often was really directed toward others.

Hopelessness. Ghosh and Victor (1994) identify hopelessness as a central underlying factor in the predisposition to suicide. Beck and associates (1990) also found a high correlation between hopelessness and suicide.

Desperation and Guilt. Hendin (1991) identified desperation as another important factor in suicide. With desperation, an individual feels helpless to change, but he or she feels also that life is impossible without such change. Guilt and self-recrimination are other aspects of desperation. These affective components were found to be prominent in Vietnam veterans with posttraumatic stress disorder exhibiting suicidal behaviors (Ghosh & Victor, 1994).

History of Aggression and Violence. Recent studies have indicated that violent behavior often goes hand-in-hand with suicidal behavior (Ghosh & Victor, 1994). Some studies have correlated the suicidal behavior in violent individuals to conscious rage, therefore citing rage as an important psychological factor underlying the suicidal behavior (Hendin, 1991).

Shame and Humiliation. Some individuals have viewed suicide as a "face-saving" mechanism—a way to prevent public humiliation following a social defeat such as a sudden loss of status or income. Often these individuals are too embarrassed to seek treatment or other support systems.

Developmental Stressors. Rich, Warsradt, and Nemiroff (1991) have associated developmental level with certain life stressors and their correlation to suicide. The stressors of conflict, separation, and rejection are associated with suicidal behavior in adolescence and early adulthood. The principal stressor associated with suicidal behavior in the 40- to 60-year-old group is economic problems. Medical illness plays an increasingly significant role after age 60 and becomes the leading predisposing factor to suicidal behavior in individuals over age 80.

Sociological Theory

Durkheim (1951) studied the individual's interaction with the society in which he or she lived. He believed that the more cohesive the society, and the more that the individual felt an integrated part of the society, the less likely he or she was to commit suicide. Durkheim described three social categories of suicide:

Egoistic suicide is the response of the individual who feels separate and apart from the mainstream of society. Integration is lacking, and the individual does not feel a part of any cohesive group (such as a family or a church).

Altruistic suicide is the opposite of egoistic suicide. The individual who is prone to altruistic suicide is excessively integrated into the group. The group is often governed by cultural, religious, or political ties, and allegiance is so strong that the individual will sacrifice his or her life for the group.

Anomic suicide occurs in response to changes that occur in an individual's life (e.g., divorce, loss of job) that disrupt feelings of relatedness to the group. An interruption in the customary norms of behavior instills feelings of "separateness" and fears of being without support from the formerly cohesive group.

Biological Theories

Genetics. Twin studies have shown a much higher concordance rate for monozygotic twins than for dizygotic twins. These results suggest a possible existence of genetic predisposition toward suicidal behavior (Ghosh & Victor, 1994).

Neurochemical Factors. A number of studies have been conducted to determine whether there is a correlation between neurochemical functioning in the central nervous system (CNS) and suicidal behavior. Some studies have revealed a deficiency of serotonin (measured as a decrease in the levels of 5-HIAA of the cerebrospinal fluid) in depressed clients who attempted suicide (Kaplan & Sadock, 1998). Postmortem studies focusing on other neurotransmitters have revealed increases in beta-adrenergic receptor binding and reductions in corticotropin-releasing factor binding sites in clients who committed suicide (Mann, Stanley, & McBride, 1986; Nemeroff, Owens, & Bissette, 1988).

APPLICATION OF THE NURSING PROCESS WITH THE SUICIDAL CLIENT

Assessment

Bassuk, Schoonover, and Gill (1982) suggest consideration of the following items when conducting a suicidal assessment: demographics, presenting symptoms/medical-psychiatric diagnosis, suicidal ideas or acts, interpersonal support system, analysis of the suicidal crisis, psychiatric/medical/ family history, and coping strategies. Table 16.2 presents some guidelines for determining the degree of suicide potential.

Demographics

The following demographics are assessed:

Age. Suicide is highest in persons over 50. Adolescents are also at high risk.

Gender. Males are at higher risk than females.

Ethnicity. Caucasians are at higher risk than are Native Americans, who are at higher risk than African Americans.

Martial Status. Single, divorced, and widowed are at higher risk than married.

Socioeconomical Status. Individuals in the highest and lowest socioeconomical classes are at higher risk than those in the middle classes.

Occupation. Professional health care personnel and business executives are at highest risk.

Method. Use of firearms presents a significantly higher risk than overdose of substances.

Religion. Protestants are at greater risk than Catholics or Jews.

Family History. Higher risk if has family history of suicide.

Presenting Symptoms/Medical-Psychiatric Diagnosis

Assessment data must be gathered regarding any psychiatric or physical condition for which the client is being treated. Mood disorders (major depression and bipolar disorders) are the most common disorders that precede suicide. Other chronic and terminal physical illnesses have also precipitated suicidal acts.

TABLE 16.2   ASSESSING THE DEGREE OF SUICIDAL RISK

BEHAVIOR OR SYMPTOM	INTENSITY OF RISK		
	LOW	MODERATE	HIGH
Anxiety	Mild	Moderate	High or panic
Depression	Mild	Moderate	Severe
Isolation; withdrawal	Some feelings of isolation; no withdrawal	Some feelings of helplessness, hopelessness, and withdrawal	Hopeless, helpless, withdrawn, and self-deprecating
Daily functioning	Fairly good in most activities	Moderately good in some activities	Not good in any activities
Resources	Several	Some	Few or none
Coping strategies being used	Generally constructive	Some that are constructive	Predominantly destructive
Significant others	Several who are available	Few or only one available	Only one or none available
Psychiatric help in past	None, or positive attitude toward	Yes, and moderately satisfied with results	Negative view of help received
Lifestyle	Stable	Moderately stable	Unstable
Alcohol or drug use	Infrequently to excess	Frequently to excess	Continual abuse
Previous suicide attempts	None, or of low lethality	One or more of moderate lethality	Multiple attempts of high lethality
Disorientation; disorganization	None	Some	Marked
Hostility	Little or none	Some	Marked
Suicidal plan	Vague, fleeting thoughts but no plan	Frequent thoughts, occasional ideas about a plan	Frequent or constant thought with a specific plan

SOURCE: From Hatten & Valente (1984), with permission.

Suicidal Ideas or Acts

How serious is the intent? Does the person have a plan? If so, does he or she have the means? How lethal is the means? These are all questions that must be answered by the person conducting the suicidal assessment.

Individuals may leave both behavioral and verbal clues as to the intent of their act. Examples of behavioral clues include giving away prized possessions, getting financial affairs in order, writing suicide notes, or sudden lifts in mood (may indicate a decision to carry out the intent).

Verbal clues may be both direct and indirect. Examples of direct statements include:

"I want to die."
"I'm going to kill myself."

Examples of indirect statements include:

"This is the last time you'll see me."
"I won't be around much longer for the doctor to have to worry about."
"I don't have anything worth living for anymore."

Other assessments include determining whether the individual has a plan and, if so, whether he or she has the means to carry out that plan. If the person states the suicide will be carried out with a gun, does he or she have access to a gun? Bullets? If pills are planned, what kind of pills? Are they accessible?

Interpersonal Support System

Does the individual have support persons on whom he or she can rely during a crisis situation? Lack of a meaningful network of satisfactory relationships may implicate an individual at high risk for suicide during an emotional crisis.

Analysis of the Suicidal Crisis

The Precipitating Stressor. Life stresses accompanied by an increase in emotional disturbance include the loss of a loved person either by death or by divorce, problems in major relationships, changes in roles, or serious physical illness. When compared with the general population, suicide attempters have experienced a greater number of situational crises in the previous 6 months, with the peak in the month prior to the suicidal act (Bassuk, Schoonover, & Gill, 1982).

Relevant History. Has the individual experienced numerous failures or rejections that would increase his or her vulnerability for a dysfunctional response to the current situation?

Life-Stage Issues. The ability to tolerate losses and disappointments is often compromised if those losses and disappointments occur during various stages of life in which the individual struggles with developmental issues (e.g., adolescence, midlife).

Psychiatric/Medical/Family History

The individual should be assessed with regard to previous psychiatric treatment for depression, alcoholism, or for previous suicide attempts. Medical history should be obtained to determine presence of chronic, debilitating, or terminal illness. Is there a history of depressive disorder in the family, and has a close relative committed suicide in the past?

Coping Strategies

How has the individual handled previous crisis situations? How does this situation differ from previous ones?

Diagnosis/Outcome Identification

Nursing diagnoses for the suicidal client may include the following:

1. Risk for self-directed violence related to feelings of hopelessness and desperation.
2. Hopelessness related to absence of support systems and perception of worthlessness.

The following criteria may be used for measurement of outcomes in the care of the suicidal client.

THE CLIENT:

1. Has experienced no physical harm to self.
2. Sets realistic goals for self.
3. Expresses some optimism and hope for the future.

Planning/Implementation

Colvin (1980) suggests that the most important aspect of care for the suicidal person is the provision of a caring, therapeutic environment. She states that the nurse may provide this type of environment by instituting the following eight-point plan:

1. **Establish a Therapeutic Relationship.** A therapeutic relationship conveys acceptance of the individual aside from the unacceptable act of suicide. If even one person is able to establish rapport with the client, this may well be the best protection against suicide.
2. **Communicate the Potential for Suicide to Team Members.** This is an around-the-clock team effort. Any clues of potential suicide, no matter how insignificant they may seem, should be reported to all team members, including the physician. Subtle clues may well reveal intent, and after-the-fact is too late to make the determination that the client was indeed serious about suicide.
3. **Stay With the Person.** Provide watchful care and give the person a sense of assurance that control will be provided until he or she can regain self-control. The nurse's presence will convey support for the suicidal person throughout the current crisis.
4. **Accept the Person.** Show unconditional positive regard. That is, convey to the individual: "I care about you and accept you for no other reason than the fact that you are a fellow human being." Unless the suicide potential is extremely acute, do not completely isolate this person from others and strip him or her of all personal possessions. This only serves to intensify feelings of worthlessness. Do, however, make the environment safe. Remove sharp items, belts, ties, smoking materials, and substances with which the individual could harm himself or herself.
5. **Listen to the Person.** After the client comes to realize that the nurse is interested in and accepts him or her, the nurse should encourage the client to identify, examine, and share the source of the current emotional pain. The suicide risk may decrease if the individual feels that someone hears and understands what he or she is feeling. Explore with the client others who might be available to provide comfort. Perhaps communication patterns with significant others may need improvement.
6. **Secure a No-Suicide Contract.** Have the client promise (verbally or in writing) that he or she will not attempt suicide for a specified length of time. When that time has elapsed, secure another promise. This gives the nurse and other professionals some time to help the client. This may also offer the client a sense of relief for getting the idea of suicide out in the open and discussing it in a nonjudgmental environment with a trusted individual.
7. **Give the Person a Message of Hope.** The suicidal person views life as hopeless, without any possibility for improvement. He or she undoubtedly has many ambivalent feelings regarding living or dying, but without hope for betterment, sees life as not worth living. After listening to the client's expression of emotional pain, encourage him or her to accept a message of optimism that life can be better. Discuss possible alternatives available to solve painful issues, and convey to the client that although the process may be very difficult, a measure of hope does exist.
8. **Give the Person Something to Do.** Meaningful activities that release tension and anger can benefit the individual by allowing a medium for expression of hostility and aggression in a constructive manner. Large motor activities such as volleyball, pounding clay, or repairing, sanding, and refinishing furniture are best for this. It is also important that the individual resume independent participation in activities of daily living. Activities such as those that promote achievement and a sense of belonging increase feelings of self-worth, as the individual once again becomes involved in the interactions of living.

Evaluation

Evaluation of the suicidal client is an ongoing process accomplished through continuous reassessment of the client, as well as determination of goal achievement. Once the immediate crisis has been resolved, extended psychotherapy may be indicated. The long-term goals of individual or group psychotherapy for the suicidal client would be for him or her to:

1. Develop and maintain a more positive self-concept.
2. Learn more effective ways to express feelings to others.
3. Achieve successful interpersonal relationships.
4. Feel accepted by others and achieve a sense of belonging.

A suicidal person feels worthless and hopeless. These goals serve to instill a sense of self-worth, while offering a measure of hope and a meaning for living.

SUMMARY

Suicide is the ninth leading cause of death among adults and the third leading cause of death among adolescents in the United States today. In assessing risk factors, it is important to consider marital status, gender, age, religion, socioeconomic status, ethnicity, occupation, family history, physical condition, support systems, precipitating stressors, coping strategies, seriousness of intent, and lethality and availability of method.

Predisposing factors include internalized anger, hopelessness, desperation and guilt, history of aggression and violence, shame and humiliation, developmental stressors, sociological influences, genetics, and neurochemical factors.

An eight-point plan is described for providing a caring therapeutic environment for the suicidal client:

1. Establish a therapeutic relationship.
2. Communicate the potential for suicide to team members.
3. Stay with the person.
4. Accept the person.
5. Listen to the person.
6. Secure a no-suicide contract.
7. Give the person a message of hope.
8. Give the person something to do.

Once the crisis intervention is complete, the individual may require long-term psychotherapy, in which he or she would work to develop and maintain a more positive self-concept, learn more effective ways to express feelings, improve interpersonal relationships, and achieve a sense of belonging and a measure of hope for living.

REVIEW QUESTIONS

SELF-EXAMINATION/LEARNING EXERCISE

Select the answer that is most appropriate for each of the following questions:

1. Which of the following individuals is at highest risk for suicide?
   a. Nancy, age 33, Asian American, Catholic, middle socioeconomic group, alcoholic.
   b. John, age 72, white, Methodist, low socioeconomic group, diagnosis of metastatic cancer of the pancreas.
   c. Carol, age 15, African American, Baptist, high socioeconomic group, no physical or mental health problems.
   d. Mike, age 55, Jewish, middle socioeconomic group, suffered myocardial infarction a year ago.

2. Some biological factors may be associated with the predisposition to suicide. Which of the following biological factors have been implicated?
   a. Genetics and decreased levels of serotonin.
   b. Heredity and increases levels of norepinephrine.
   c. Temporal lobe atrophy and decreased levels of acetylcholine.
   d. Structural alterations of the brain and increased levels of dopamine.

3. Theresa, age 27, was admitted to the psychiatric unit from the medical intensive care unit, where she was treated for taking a deliberate overdose of her antidepressant medication, trazodone (Desyrel). She says to the nurse, "My boyfriend broke up with me. We had been together for 6 years. I love him so much. I know I'll never get over him." Which is the best response by the nurse?
   a. "You'll get over him in time, Theresa."
   b. "Forget him. There are other fish in the sea."
   c. "You must be feeling very sad about your loss."
   d. "Why do you think he broke up with you, Theresa?"

4. The nurse identifies the primary nursing diagnosis for Theresa as Risk for Self-Directed Violence, related to feelings of hopelessness from loss of relationship. Which is the outcome criterion that would most accurately measure achievement of this diagnosis?
   a. The client has experienced no physical harm to herself.
   b. The client sets realistic goals for herself.
   c. The client expresses some optimism and hope for the future.
   d. The client has reached a stage of acceptance in the loss of the relationship with her boyfriend.

5. Freudian psychoanalytic theory would explain Theresa's suicide attempt in which of the following ways?
   a. She feels hopeless about her future without her boyfriend.
   b. Without her boyfriend, she feels separate and apart from the mainstream of society.
   c. She is feeling intense guilt because her boyfriend broke up with her.
   d. She is angry at her boyfriend for breaking up with her and has turned the anger inward on herself.

6. Theresa says to the nurse, "When I get out of here, I'm going to try this again, and next time I'll choose a no-fail method." Which is the best response by the nurse?
   a. "You are safe here. We will make sure nothing happens to you."
   b. "You're just lucky your roommate came home when she did."
   c. "What exactly do you plan to do?"
   d. "I don't understand. You have so much to live for."

7. In determining degree of suicidal risk with Theresa, the nurse assesses the following behavioral manifestations: severely depressed, withdrawn, statements of worthlessness, difficulty accomplishing activities of daily living, no close support systems. The nurse identifies Theresa's risk for suicide as:

    a. Low
    b. Moderate
    c. High
    d. Unable to determine

8. Theresa is placed on suicide precautions on the psychiatric unit. Which of the following interventions is most appropriate in this instance?

    a. Obtain an order from the physician to place Theresa in restraints to prevent any attempts to harm herself.
    b. Check on Theresa every 15 minutes or assign a staff person to stay with her on a one-to-one basis.
    c. Obtain an order from the physician to give Theresa a sedative to calm her and reduce suicide ideas.
    d. Do not allow Theresa to participate in any unit activities while she is on suicide precautions.

9. All of the following interventions are appropriate for Theresa while she is on suicide precautions *except:*

    a. Remove all sharp objects, belts, and other potentially dangerous articles from Theresa's environment.
    b. Explain to Theresa the procedures and rationale for suicide precautions.
    c. Obtain a promise from Theresa that she will not do anything to harm herself for the next 12 hours.
    d. Put all of Theresa's possessions in storage and explain to her that she may have them back when she is off suicide precautions.

10. Success of long-term psychotherapy with Theresa could be measured by which of the following behaviors?

    a. Theresa has a new boyfriend.
    b. Theresa has an increased sense of self-worth.
    c. Theresa does not take antidepressants anymore.
    d. Theresa told her old boyfriend how angry she was with him for breaking up with her.

REFERENCES

Bassuk, E.L., Schoonover, S.C., & Gill, A.D. (Eds.). (1982). *Lifelines: Clinical perspectives on suicide.* New York: Plenum Press.

Beck, A.T., Brown, G., & Berchick, R.J. (1990). Relationship between hopelessness and ultimate suicide: A replication with psychiatric outpatients. *American Journal of Psychiatry, 147,* 190–195.

Black, D.W., & Winokur, G. (1990). Suicide and psychiatric diagnosis. In S.J. Blumenthal & D.J. Kupfer (Eds.), *Suicide over the life cycle: Risk factors, assessment, and treatment of suicidal patients.* Washington, DC: American Psychiatric Press.

Colvin, L. (1980). Depression and suicidal behavior. In J. Lancaster (Ed.), *Adult psychiatric nursing.* Garden City, NY: Medical Examination Publishing Co.

Durkheim, E. (1951). *Suicide: A study of sociology.* Glencoe, IL: Free Press.

Freedman, A.M., et al. (1976). *Modern synopsis of psychiatry II.* Baltimore: Williams & Wilkins.

Freud, S. (1957). *Mourning and melancholia,* Vol. 14 (standard ed.). London: Hogarth Press. (Original work published 1917.)

Ghosh, T.B., & Victor, B.S. (1994). Suicide. In R.E. Hales, S.C. Yudofsky, & J.A. Talbott (Eds.), *The American Psychiatric Press textbook of psychiatry* (2nd ed.). Washington, DC: American Psychiatric Press.

Hatten, C.L., & Valente, S.M. (1984). *Suicide: Assessment and intervention* (2nd ed.). Norwalk, CT: Appleton-Century-Crofts.

Hendin, H. (1991). Psychodynamics of suicide, with particular reference to the young. *American Journal of Psychiatry, 148,* 1150–1158.

Kaplan, H.I., & Sadock B.J. (1998). *Synopsis of psychiatry: Behavioral sciences/chemical psychiatry* (8th ed.). Baltimore: Williams & Wilkins.

Kestenbaum, C.J., & Trautman, P.D. (1992). Normal development and major problems of adolescents. In F.I. Kass, J.M. Oldham, & H. Pardes (Eds.), *The Columbia University College of Physicians and Surgeons complete home guide to mental health.* New York: Henry Holt and Company.

Mann, J.J., Stanley, M., & McBride, P.A. (1986). Increased serotonin and beta-adrenergic receptor binding in the frontal cortices of suicide victims. *Archives of General Psychiatry, 43,* 954–959.

Murphy, G.E. (1994). Suicide and attempted suicide. In G. Winokur, & P.J. Clayton (Eds.). *The medical basis of psychiatry* (2nd ed.). Philadelphia: W.B. Saunders.

Murray, R.B., & Zentner, J.P. (1997). *Health assessment and promotion strategies through the life span* (6th ed.). Stamford, CT: Appleton & Lange.

Nemeroff, C.B., Owens, M.J., & Bissette, G. (1988). Reduced corticotropin releasing factor binding sites in the frontal cortex of suicide victims. *Archives of General Psychiatry, 45,* 577–579.

Rich, C.L., Warsradt, G.M., & Nemiroff, R.A. (1991). Suicide, stressors, and the life cycle. *American Journal of Psychiatry, 148,* 524–527.

Shneidman, E.S., & Farberow, N.L. (1965). *Some facts about suicide.* Washington, DC: Superintendent of Documents.

Slaby, A.E., Lieb, J., & Tancredi, L. (1986). *The handbook of psychiatric emergencies* (3rd ed.). New York: Medical Examination Publishing.

Bibliography

Anderson, D.B. (1991). Never too late: Resolving the grief of suicide. *Journal of Psychosocial Nursing and Mental Health Services, 29*(3), 29–31.

Busteed, E.L., & Johnstone, C. (1983). The development of suicide precautions for an inpatient psychiatric unit. *Journal of Psychosocial Nursing and Mental Health Services, 21*(5), 15–19.

Capodanno, A.E., & Targum, S.D. (1983, May). Assessment of suicide risk: Some limitations in the prediction of infrequent events. *Journal of Psychosocial Nursing and Mental Health Services, 21*(5), 11–14.

Fitzpatrick, J.J. (1983). Suicidology and suicide prevention: Historical perspectives from the nursing literature. *Journal of Psychosocial Nursing and Mental Health Services, 21*(5), 20–28.

Neville, D., & Barnes, S. (1985). The suicidal phone call. *Journal of Psychosocial Nursing and Mental Health Services, 23*(8), 14–18.

Suicide—Part I. (November 1996). *The Harvard Mental Health Letter, 13*(5): 1–5.

Suicide—Part II. (December 1996). *The Harvard Mental Health Letter, 13*(6): 1–5.

Tuskan, J.J., & Thase, M.E. (1983). Suicides in jails and prisons. *Journal of Psychosocial Nursing, 21*(5), 29–33.

BEHAVIOR THERAPY

CHAPTER OUTLINE

OBJECTIVES

INTRODUCTION

CLASSICAL CONDITIONING

OPERANT CONDITIONING

TECHNIQUES FOR MODIFYING CLIENT BEHAVIOR

ROLE OF THE NURSE IN BEHAVIOR THERAPY

SUMMARY

REVIEW QUESTIONS

KEY TERMS

classical conditioning
operant conditioning
unconditioned response
conditioned response
unconditioned stimulus
conditioned stimulus
stimulus generalization
stimuli

positive reinforcement
negative reinforcement
aversive stimulus
discriminative stimulus
shaping
modeling
Premack principle
extinction

contingency contracting
token economy
time out
reciprocal inhibition
overt sensitization
covert sensitization
systematic desensitization
flooding

OBJECTIVES

After reading this chapter, the student will be able to:

1. Discuss the principles of classical and operant conditioning as foundations for behavior therapy.
2. Identify various techniques used in the modification of client behavior.

3. Implement the principles of behavior therapy using the steps of the nursing process.

behavior is considered to be maladaptive when it is age-inappropriate, when it interferes with adaptive functioning, or when it is misunderstood by others in terms of cultural inappropriateness. The behavioral approach to therapy is that people have become what they are through learning processes or, more correctly, through the interaction of the environment with their genetic endowment (Chambless & Goldstein, 1979). The basic assumption is that problematic behaviors occur when there has been inadequate learning and therefore can be corrected through the provision of appropriate learning experiences. The principles of behavior therapy as we know it today are based on the early studies of **classical conditioning** by Pavlov (1927) and **operant conditioning** by Skinner (1938).

CLASSICAL CONDITIONING

Classical conditioning is a process of learning that was introduced by the Russian physiologist Pavlov. In his experiments with dogs, during which he hoped to learn more about the digestive process, he inadvertently discovered that organisms can learn to respond in specific ways if they are conditioned to do so.

In his trials he found that, as expected, the dogs salivated when they began to eat the food that was offered to them. This was a reflexive response that Pavlov called an **unconditioned response.** However, he also noticed that with time, the dogs began to salivate when the food came into their range of view, before it was even presented to them for consumption. Pavlov, concluding that this response was not reflexive but had been learned, called it a **conditioned response.** He carried the experiments even further by introducing an unrelated stimulus, one that had had no previous connection to the animal's food. He simultaneously presented the food with the sound of a bell. The animal responded with the expected reflexive salivation to the food. After a number of trials with the combined stimuli (food and bell), Pavlov found that the reflexive salivation began to occur when the dog was presented with the sound of the bell in the absence of food.

This was an important discovery in terms of how learning can occur. Pavlov found that unconditioned responses (salivation) occur in response to unconditioned stimuli (eating food). He also found that, over time, an unrelated stimulus (sound of the bell) introduced with the **unconditioned stimulus** can elicit the same response alone—that is, the conditioned response. The unrelated stimulus is called the **conditioned stimulus.** A graphic of Pavlov's classical conditioning model is presented in Figure 17.1. An example of the application of Pavlov's classical conditioning model to humans is shown in Figure 17.2. The process by which the fear response is elicited from similar stimuli (all individuals in white uniforms) is called **stimulus generalization.**

Sequence of Conditioning Operations:

1. UCS --→ UCR
   Unconditioned Stimulus   Unconditioned Response
   (eating food)   (salivation)

2. UCS --→ CR
   Unconditioned Stimulus   Conditioned Response
   (sight of food)   (salivation)

3. CS --→ NR
   Conditioned Stimulus   No Response or
   (bell)   Response Unrelated to Salivation

4. UCS + CS ----------------------------------→ CR
   Unconditioned + Conditioned Stimuli   Conditioned Response
   (food)   (bell)   (salivation)

5. CS --→ CR
   Conditioned Stimulus   Conditioned Response
   (bell)   (salivation)

Figure 17.1   Pavlov's model of classical conditioning.

OPERANT CONDITIONING

The focus of operant conditioning differs from that of classical conditioning. With classical conditioning, the focus is on behavioral responses that are elicited by specific objects or events. With operant conditioning, additional attention is given to the consequences of the behavioral response.

Operant conditioning was introduced by Skinner (1953), an American psychologist whose work was largely influenced by Thorndike's (1911) law of effect—that is, that the connection between a stimulus and a response is strengthened or weakened by the consequences of the re-

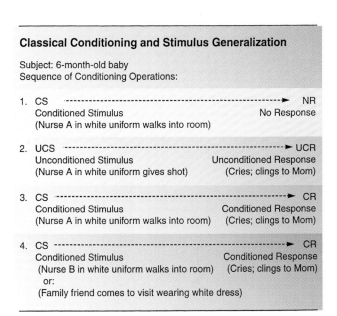

Classical Conditioning and Stimulus Generalization

Subject: 6-month-old baby
Sequence of Conditioning Operations:

1. CS --→ NR
   Conditioned Stimulus   No Response
   (Nurse A in white uniform walks into room)

2. UCS ---------------------------------------→ UCR
   Unconditioned Stimulus   Unconditioned Response
   (Nurse A in white uniform gives shot) (Cries; clings to Mom)

3. CS --→ CR
   Conditioned Stimulus   Conditioned Response
   (Nurse A in white uniform walks into room) (Cries; clings to Mom)

4. CS --→ CR
   Conditioned Stimulus   Conditioned Response
   (Nurse B in white uniform walks into room) (Cries; clings to Mom)
   or:
   (Family friend comes to visit wearing white dress)

Figure 17.2   Example: classical conditioning and stimulus generalization.

sponse. A number of terms must be defined in order to understand the concept of operant conditioning.

Stimuli are environmental events that interact with and influence an individual's behavior. Stimuli may precede or follow a behavior. A stimulus that follows a behavior (or response) is called a reinforcing stimulus or *reinforcer*: The function is called *reinforcement*. When the reinforcing stimulus increases the probability that the behavior will recur, it is called a *positive reinforcer*, and the function is called **positive reinforcement. Negative reinforcement** is increasing the probability that a behavior will recur by removal of an undesirable reinforcing stimulus. A stimulus that follows a behavioral response and decreases the probability that the behavior will recur is called an **aversive stimulus** or *punisher*. Examples of these reinforcing stimuli are presented in Table 17.1.

Stimuli that precede a behavioral response and predict that a particular reinforcement will occur are called **discriminative stimuli.** Discriminative stimuli are under the control of the individual. The individual is said to be able to *discriminate* between stimuli and to *choose* according to the type of reinforcement he or she has come to associate with a specific stimulus. The following is an example of the concept of discrimination:

EXAMPLE

Mrs. M was admitted to the hospital from a nursing home 2 weeks ago. She has no family, and no one visits her. She is very lonely. Nurse A and Nurse B have taken care of Mrs. M on a regular basis during her hospital stay. When she is feeling particularly lonely, Mrs. M calls Nurse A to her room, for she has learned that Nurse A will stay and talk to her for a while, but Nurse B only takes care of her physical needs and leaves. She no longer seeks out Nurse B for emotional support and comfort.

After several attempts, Mrs. M is able to discriminate between stimuli. She can predict with assurance that calling Nurse A (and not Nurse B) will result in the reinforcement she desires.

TECHNIQUES FOR MODIFYING CLIENT BEHAVIOR

Shaping

In **shaping** the behavior of another, reinforcements are given for increasingly closer approximations to the desired response. For example, in training a mute child to talk, the teacher may first reward the child for (a) watching the teacher's lips, then (b) for making any sound in imitation of the teacher, then (c) for forming sounds similar to the word uttered by the teacher, and so on, until only correct imitations are rewarded (Chambless & Goldstein, 1979).

Modeling

Modeling refers to the learning of new behaviors by imitating the behavior in others. Models are more likely to be imitated when they are perceived as prestigious, influential, or physically attractive and when the behavior is followed by positive reinforcement (Bandura, 1969). Modeling occurs in various ways. Children imitate the behavior patterns of their parents, teachers, friends, and others. Adults and children alike model many of their behaviors after individuals observed on television and in movies. Unfortunately, modeling can result in maladaptive behaviors as well as adaptive ones.

In the practice setting clients may imitate the behaviors of practitioners who are charged with their care. This can occur naturally in the therapeutic community environment. It can also occur in a therapy session in which the client watches a model demonstrate appropriate behaviors in a role play of the client's problem. The client is then instructed to imitate the model's behaviors in a similar role play and is positively reinforced for appropriate imitation (Sundel & Sundel, 1982).

Premack Principle

This technique, named for its originator, states that a frequently occurring response (R_1) can serve as a positive reinforcement for a response (R_2) that occurs less frequently (Premack, 1959). This is accomplished by allowing R_1 to occur only after R_2 has been performed. For example, 13-year-old Jennie has been neglecting her homework for the past few weeks. She spends a lot of time on the telephone talking to her friends. Applying the **Premack principle,** being allowed to talk on the telephone to her friends could serve as a positive reinforcement for completing her homework. A schematic of the Premack principle for this situation is presented in Figure 17.3.

▬ TABLE 17.1 EXAMPLES OF REINFORCING STIMULI

TYPE	STIMULUS	BEHAVIORAL RESPONSE	REINFORCING STIMULUS
Positive	Messy room	Child cleans her messy room.	Child gets allowance for cleaning room.
Negative	Messy room	Child cleans her messy room.	Child does not receive scolding from the mother.
Aversive	Messy room	Child does not clean her messy room.	Child receives scolding from the mother.

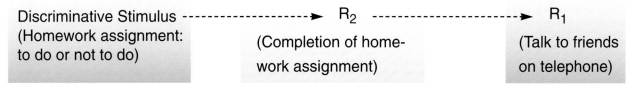

Figure 17.3 Example: Premack principle.

Extinction

Extinction is the gradual decrease in frequency or disappearance of a response when the positive reinforcement is withheld. A classic example of this technique is its use with children who have temper tantrums. The tantrum behaviors continue as long as the parent gives attention to them but decrease and often disappear when the parent simply leaves the child alone in the room.

Contingency Contracting

In **contingency contracting,** a contract is drawn up among all parties involved. The behavior change that is desired is stated, explicitly, in writing. The contract specifies the behavior change desired and the reinforcers to be given for performing the desired behaviors. The negative consequences or punishers that will be rendered for not fulfilling the terms of the contract are also delineated (Sundel & Sundel, 1982). The contract is specific about how reinforcers and punishment will be presented; however, flexibility is important so that renegotiations can occur if necessary.

Token Economy

Token economy is a type of contingency contracting (although there may or may not be a written and signed contract involved) in which the reinforcers for desired behaviors are presented in the form of *tokens.* Essential to this type of technique is the prior determination of items and situations of significance to the client that can be employed as reinforcements. With this therapy, tokens are awarded when desired behaviors are performed and may be exchanged for designated privileges. For example, a client may be able to "buy" a snack or cigarettes for 2 tokens, a trip to the coffee shop or library for 5 tokens, or even a trip outside the hospital (if that is a realistic possibility) for another designated number of tokens. The tokens themselves provide immediate positive feedback, and clients should be allowed to make the decision of whether to spend the token as soon as it is presented or to accumulate tokens that may be exchanged later for a more desirable reward.

Time Out

Time out is an aversive stimulus or punishment during which the client is removed from the environment where the unacceptable behavior is being exhibited. The client is usually isolated so that reinforcement from the attention of others is absent.

Reciprocal Inhibition

Also called counterconditioning, **reciprocal inhibition** decreases or eliminates a behavior by introducing a more adaptive behavior, but one that is incompatible with the unacceptable behavior (Wolpe, 1958). An example is the introduction of relaxation exercises to an individual who is phobic. Relaxation is practiced in the presence of anxiety so that, in time, the individual is able to manage the anxiety in the presence of the phobic stimulus by engaging in relaxation exercises. Relaxation and anxiety are incompatible behaviors.

Overt Sensitization

Overt sensitization is a type of aversion therapy that produces unpleasant consequences for undesirable behavior. For example, disulfiram (Antabuse) is a drug that is given to individuals who wish to stop drinking alcohol. If an individual consumes alcohol while on Antabuse therapy, symptoms of severe nausea and vomiting, dyspnea, palpitations, and headache will occur. Instead of the euphoric feeling normally experienced from the alcohol (the positive reinforcement for drinking), the individual receives a severe punishment that is intended to extinguish the unacceptable behavior (drinking alcohol).

Covert Sensitization

Covert sensitization relies on the individual's imagination to produce unpleasant symptoms, rather than on medication. The technique is under the client's control and can be used whenever and wherever it is required. The individual learns, through mental imagery, to visualize nauseating scenes and even to induce a mild feeling of nausea. This mental image is visualized when the individual is about to succumb to an attractive but undesirable behavior. It is most effective when paired with relaxation exercises that are performed instead of the undesirable behavior. The primary advantage of covert sensitization is that the individual does not have to perform the undesired behaviors but simply imagines them (Sundel & Sundel, 1982).

Systematic Desensitization

Systematic desensitization is a technique for assisting individuals to overcome their fear of a phobic stimulus. It is "systematic" in that there is a hierarchy of anxiety-producing events through which the individual progresses during therapy. An example of a hierarchy of events associated with a fear of elevators may be as follows:

1. Discuss riding an elevator with the therapist.
2. Look at a picture of an elevator.
3. Walk into the lobby of a building and see the elevators.
4. Push the button for the elevator.
5. Walk into an elevator with a trusted person; disembark before the doors close.
6. Walk into an elevator with a trusted person; allow doors to close; then open the doors and walk out.
7. Ride one floor with a trusted person, then walk back down the stairs.
8. Ride one floor with a trusted person and ride the elevator back down.
9. Ride the elevator alone.

As each of these steps is attempted, it is paired with relaxation exercises as an antagonistic behavior to anxiety. Generally, the desensitization procedures occur in the therapy setting by instructing the client to engage in relaxation exercises. When relaxation has been achieved, the client uses mental imagery to visualize the step in the hierarchy being described by the therapist. If the client becomes anxious, the therapist suggests relaxation exercises again, and presents a scene that is lower in the hierarchy. Therapy continues until the individual is able to progress through the entire hierarchy with manageable anxiety. The effects of relaxation in the presence of imagined anxiety-producing stimuli transfer to the real situation, once the client has achieved relaxation capable of suppressing or inhibiting anxiety responses (Sundel & Sundel, 1982).

However, some clients are not successful in extinguishing phobic reactions through imagery. For these clients, *real-life desensitization* may be required. In these instances, the therapist arranges for the client to be exposed to the hierarchy of steps in the desensitation process, but in real-life situations. Relaxation exercises may or may not be a part of real-life desensitization (Sherman, 1973).

Flooding

This technique, sometimes called *implosive therapy*, is also used to desensitize individuals to phobic stimuli. It differs from systematic desensitization in that, instead of working up a hierarchy of anxiety-producing stimuli, the individual is "flooded" with a continuous presentation (through mental imagery) of the phobic stimulus until it no longer elicits anxiety (Sundel & Sundel, 1982). **Flooding** is believed to produce results faster than systematic desensitization; however, some therapists report that clients are more likely to revert to previous phobic behaviors with flooding than with systematic desensitization (Mikulas, 1972). Some questions have also been raised in terms of the psychological discomfort that this therapy produces for the client as well as the possibility of increased anxiety when faced with the phobic stimulus in real-life situations (Sundel & Sundel, 1982).

ROLE OF THE NURSE IN BEHAVIOR THERAPY

The nursing process is the vehicle for delivery of nursing care with the client requiring assistance with behavior modification. The steps of the nursing process are illustrated in the following example case study.*

---

*Adapted from Spitzer et al. (1989).

CASE STUDY

ASSESSMENT

Jordan, age 6, has been admitted to the child psychiatric unit following evaluation by a child psychiatrist. The parents' already shaky marriage was being severely tested by conflict over their son's behavior at home and at school. The mother complained bitterly that the father, frequently away from home on business, "overindulged" their son. In point of fact, the son would argue and throw temper tantrums and insist on continuing games, books, and so forth, whenever his father put him to bed, so that a 7:30 PM bedtime was delayed until 10:30, 11:00, or even 11:30 at night. Similarly, the father had been known to cook four or five different meals for his son's dinner if Jordan stubbornly insisted that he would not eat what had been prepared. At school several teachers had complained that the child was stubborn and spiteful, often spoke out of turn, and refused to comply with classroom rules.

On questioning by the psychiatric nurse, the parents denied that their son had ever been destructive of property, lied excessively, or stolen. When interviewed, the child was observed to be cheerful and able to sit quietly in his chair, listening attentively to the questions that were asked of him. His answers, however, were brief, and he tended to minimize the extent of the problems he was having with his parents and teachers.

During his first 3 days on the unit, the following assessments were made:

1. Jordan loses his temper when he cannot have his way. He screams, stomps his feet, and sometimes kicks the furniture.
2. Jordan refuses to follow directions given by staff. He merely responds, "No, I won't."
3. Jordan likes to engage in behaviors that annoy the staff and other children: belching loudly, scraping his fingernails across the blackboard, making loud noises when the other children are trying to

Continued on following page

CASE STUDY *(Continued)*

watch television, opening his mouth when it is full of food.

4. Jordan blames others when he makes a mistake. He spilled his milk at lunchtime while racing to get to a specific seat he knew Tony wanted. He blamed the accident on Tony, saying, "He made me do it! He tripped me!"

Upon completion of the initial assessments, the psychiatrist diagnosed Jordan with oppositional defiant disorder.

DIAGNOSIS/OUTCOME IDENTIFICATION

Nursing diagnoses and outcome criteria for Jordan include:

NURSING DIAGNOSES	OUTCOME CRITERIA
Noncompliance with Therapy	Jordan participates in and cooperates during therapeutic activities.
Defensive Coping	Jordan accepts responsibility for own behaviors and interacts with others without becoming defensive.
Impaired Social Interaction	Jordan interacts with staff and peers using age-appropriate, acceptable behaviors.

PLANNING/INTERVENTION

A contract for Jordan's care was drawn up by the admitting nurse and others on the treatment team. Jordan's contract was based on a system of token economies. He discussed with the nurse the kinds of privileges he would like to earn. They included:

Getting to wear his own clothes (5 tokens)
Having a can of pop for a snack (2 tokens)
Getting to watch 30 minutes of TV (5 tokens)
Getting to stay up later on Friday nights with the other clients (7 tokens)
Getting to play the video games (3 tokens)
Getting to walk with the nurse to the gift shop to spend some of his money (8 tokens)
Getting to talk to his parents/grandparents on the phone (5 tokens)
Getting to go outside the therapeutic environment for recreational activities such as movies, the zoo, and picnics (10 tokens)

Tokens were awarded for appropriate behaviors:

Gets out of bed when the nurse calls him (1 token)
Gets dressed for breakfast (1 token)
Presents himself for *all* meals in an appropriate manner, that is, no screaming, no belching, no opening his mouth when it is full of food, no throwing of food, staying in his chair during the meal, putting his tray away in the appropriate place when he is finished (2 tokens × 3 meals = 6 tokens)
Completes hygiene activities (1 token)
Accepts blame for own mistakes (1 token)

Does not fight; uses no obscene language; does not "sass" staff (1 token)
Remains quiet while others are watching TV (1 token)
Participates and is not disruptive in unit meetings and group therapy sessions (2 tokens)
Displays no temper tantrums (1 token)
Follows unit rules (1 token)
Goes to bed at designated hour without opposition (1 token)

Tokens are awarded at bedtime for absence of inappropriate behaviors during the day. For example, if Jordan has no temper tantrums during the day, he is awarded 1 token. Likewise, if Jordan has a temper tantrum (or exhibits other inappropriate behavior), he must pay back the token amount designated for that behavior. No other attention is given to inappropriate behaviors other than withholding and payback of tokens.

EXCEPTION: If Jordan is receiving reinforcement from peers for inappropriate behaviors, staff has the option of imposing time out or isolation until the behavior is extinguished.

The contract may be renegotiated at any time between Jordan and staff. Additional privileges or responsibilities may be added as they develop and are deemed appropriate.

All staff members are consistent with the terms of the contract and do not allow Jordan to manipulate. There are no exceptions without renegotiation of the contract.

NOTE: Parents meet regularly with the social worker from the treatment team. Effective parenting techniques are discussed, as are other problems identified within the marriage relationship. Parenting instruction coordinates with the pattern of behavior modification Jordan is receiving on the psychiatric unit. The importance of follow-through is emphasized, along with strong encouragement that the parents maintain a united front in disciplining Jordan. Oppositional behaviors are nurtured by divided management.

EVALUATION

Reassessment is conducted to determine if the nursing actions have been successful in achieving the objectives of Jordan's care. Evaluation can be facilitated by gathering information using the following questions:

Does Jordan participate in and cooperate during therapeutic activities?
Does he follow the rules of the unit (including mealtimes, hygiene, and bedtime) without opposition?
Does Jordan accept responsibility for his own mistakes?
Is he able to complete a task without becoming defensive?
Does he refrain from interrupting when others are talking or making noise in situations where quiet is in order?
Does he attempt to manipulate the staff?
Is he able to express anger appropriately without tantrum behaviors?
Does he demonstrate acceptable behavior in interactions with peers?

SUMMARY

The basic assumption of behavior therapy is that problematic behaviors occur when there has been inadequate learning and, therefore, can be corrected through the provision of appropriate learning experiences. The antecedents of today's principles of behavior therapy are largely the products of laboratory efforts by Pavlov and Skinner.

Pavlov introduced a process that came to be known as classical conditioning. He demonstrated in his trials with laboratory animals that a neutral stimulus could acquire the ability to elicit a conditioned response through pairing with an unconditioned stimulus. Previous responses had been reflexive in nature. Pavlov considered the conditioned response to be a new, learned response.

Skinner, in his model of operant conditioning, gave additional attention to the consequences of the response as an approach to learning new behaviors. His work was largely influenced by Thorndike's law of effect, that is, that the connection between a stimulus and a response is strengthened or weakened by the consequences of the response.

Various techniques for modifying client behavior have been applied. Those most widely used include shaping, modeling, the Premack principle, extinction, contingency contracting, token economy, time out, reciprocal inhibition, overt and covert sensitization, systematic desensitization, and flooding.

Nurses are important members of the treatment team in the implementation of behavior therapy. Because nurses are the only members of the team who manage client behavior on a 24-hour basis, it is essential that they have input into the treatment plan. The nursing process provides a systematic method of directing care for clients who need assistance with modification of maladaptive behaviors. It is a dynamic process that allows each plan of care to be individualized for the personal requirements of each client.

REVIEW QUESTIONS

SELF-EXAMINATION/LEARNING EXERCISE

Select the correct answer for each of the following questions:

1. A positive reinforcer:

   a. Increases the probability that a behavior will recur.
   b. Decreases the probability that a behavior will recur.
   c. Has nothing to do with modifying behavior.
   d. Always results in positive behavior.

2. A negative reinforcer:

   a. Increases the probability that a behavior will recur.
   b. Decreases the probability that a behavior will recur.
   c. Has nothing to do with modifying behavior.
   d. Always results in unacceptable behavior.

3. An aversive stimulus or punisher:

   a. Increases the probability that a behavior will recur.
   b. Decreases the probability that a behavior will recur.
   c. Has nothing to do with modifying behavior.
   d. Always results in unacceptable behavior.

Situation: B.J. has been out with his friends. He is late getting home. He knows his wife will be angry and will yell at him for being late. He stops at the florist's and buys a dozen red roses for her. Questions 4, 5, and 6 are related to this situation.

4. Which of the following behaviors represents positive reinforcement on the part of the wife?

   a. She meets him at the door, accepts the roses, and says nothing further about his being late.
   b. She meets him at the door, yelling that he is late, and makes him spend the night on the couch.
   c. She meets him at the door, expresses delight with the roses, and kisses him on the cheek.
   d. She meets him at the door and says, "How could you? You know I'm allergic to roses!"

5. Which of the following behaviors represents negative reinforcement on the part of the wife?

   a. She meets him at the door, accepts the roses, and says nothing further about his being late.
   b. She meets him at the door, yelling that he is late, and makes him spend the night on the couch.
   c. She meets him at the door, expresses delight with the roses, and kisses him on the cheek.
   d. She meets him at the door and says, "How could you? You know I'm allergic to roses!"

6. Which of the following behaviors represents an aversive stimulus on the part of the wife?

   a. She meets him at the door, accepts the roses, and says nothing further about his being late.
   b. She meets him at the door, yelling that he is late, and makes him spend the night on the couch.
   c. She meets him at the door, expresses delight with the roses, and kisses him on the cheek.
   d. She meets him at the door and says, "How could you? You know I'm allergic to roses!"

7. Fourteen-year-old Sally has been spending many hours after school watching TV. She has virtually stopped practicing her piano lessons. Her parents have told her that she may watch TV only after she has practiced the piano for 1 hour. This is an example of which behavior modification technique?

   a. Shaping.
   b. Extinction.
   c. Contingency contracting.
   d. The Premack principle.

8. Nancy has a fear of dogs. In helping her overcome this fear, the therapist is using systematic desensitization. List the following steps in the order in which the therapist would proceed.

   Having Nancy:
   a. Look at a real dog.
   b. Look at a stuffed toy dog.
   c. Pet a real dog.
   d. Pet the stuffed toy dog.
   e. Walk past a real dog.
   f. Look at a picture of a dog.

REFERENCES

Bandura, A. (1969). *Principles of behavior modification.* New York: Holt, Rinehart & Winston.

Chambless, D.L., & Goldstein, A.J. (1979). Behavioral psychotherapy. In R.J. Corsini (Ed.), *Current psychotherapies* (2nd ed.). Itasca, IL: F.E. Peacock.

Mikulas, W.L. (1972). *Behavior modification: An overview.* New York: Harper & Row.

Pavlov, I.P. (1927). *Conditioned reflexes.* London: Oxford University Press.

Premack, D. (1959). Toward empirical behavior laws: I. Positive reinforcement. *Psychological Review, 66,* 219–233.

Sherman, R.A. (1973). *Behavior modification: Theory and practice.* Monterey, CA: Brooks/Cole.

Skinner, B.F. (1938) *The behavior of organisms.* New York: Appleton-Century-Crofts.

Skinner, B.F. (1953). *Science and human behavior.* New York: Macmillan.

Spitzer, R.L., Gibbon, M., Skodol, A.E. Williams, J.B.W., and First, M.B. (1989). *DSM-III-R case book.* Washington, DC: American Psychiatric Press, Inc.

Sundel, M., & Sundel, S.S. (1982). *Behavior modification in the human services: A systematic introduction to concepts and applications* (2nd ed.). Englewood Cliffs, NJ: Prentice-Hall.

Thorndike, E.L. (1911). *Animal intelligence.* New York: Macmillan.

Wolpe, J. (1958). *Psychotherapy by reciprocal inhibition.* Stanford, CA: Stanford University Press.

Bibliography

Gelder, M. (1997). The future of behavior therapy. *Journal of Psychotherapy Practice and Research, 6:*285–293.

Hersen, M., & Last, C.G. (1985). *Behavior therapy casebook.* New York: Springer.

O'Donohue, W. *Learning and behavior therapy.* (1997) Boston: Allyn and Bacon.

Raue, P.J., Goldfried, M.R., & Barkham, M. (1997). The therapeutic alliance in psychodynamic-interpersonal and cognitive-behavioral therapy. *Journal of Consulting and Clinical Psychology, 65:*582–587.

Spiegler, M.D. & Guevremont, D.C. (1998). *Contemporary behavior therapy* (3rd ed.). Monterey, CA: Brooks/Cole Publishing Company.

Wolpe, J. & Plaud, J.J. (1997). Pavlov's contributions to behavior therapy: The obvious and not so obvious. *American Journal of Psychology, 52:*966–972.

COGNITIVE THERAPY

CHAPTER OUTLINE

KEY TERMS

automatic thoughts
schemas
arbitrary inference
overgeneralizations
dichotomous thinking

selective abstraction
magnification
minimization
catastrophic
    thinking

personalization
Socratic questioning
decatastrophizing
distraction

OBJECTIVES

After reading this chapter, the student will be able to:

1. Discuss historical perspectives associated with cognitive therapy.
2. Identify various indications for cognitive therapy.
3. Describe goals, principles, and basic concepts of cognitive therapy.
4. Discuss a variety of cognitive therapy techniques.
5. Apply techniques of cognitive therapy within the context of the nursing process.

right and Beck (1994) state, "The writing of Epictetus (around 100 AD): '*Men are disturbed not by things, but by the views which they take of them*,' captures the essence of the perspective that our ideas or thoughts are a controlling factor in our emotional lives." This concept provides the foundation upon which the cognitive model is established. In cognitive therapy, the therapist's objective is to use a variety of methods to create change in the client's thinking and belief system in an effort to bring about lasting emotional and behavioral change (Beck, 1995).

This chapter examines the historical development of the cognitive model, defines the goals of therapy, and describes various techniques of the cognitive approach. A discussion of the role of the nurse in the implementation of cognitive behavioral techniques with clients is presented.

HISTORICAL BACKGROUND

Cognitive therapy has its roots in the early 1960s research on depression conducted by Aaron Beck (1963, 1964). Beck had been trained in the Freudian psychoanalytic view of depression as "anger turned inward." In his clinical research, he began to observe a common theme of negative cognitive processing in the thoughts and dreams of his depressed clients (Beck & Weishaar, 1995).

A number of theorists have both taken from and expanded upon Beck's original concept. The common theme is the rejection of the passive listening of the psychoanalytic method in favor of active, direct dialogues with clients (Beck & Weishaar, 1995). The work of contemporary behaviorists (Bandura, 1977; Meichenbaum, 1977) has also influenced the evolution of cognitive therapy. Behavioral techniques such as expectancy of reinforcement and modeling are used within the cognitive domain.

Richard Lazarus (1966), upon whose premise of *personal appraisal* and *coping* the conceptual format of this book is founded, has also contributed a great deal to the cognitive approach to therapy. The model for cognitive therapy is based on cognition, and more specifically, the personal cognitive appraisal by an individual of an event, and the emotions or behaviors that result from that appraisal. Personality—which undoubtedly influences our cognitive appraisal of an event—is viewed as having been shaped by the interaction between innate predisposition and environment (Beck & Freeman, 1990). Whereas some therapies may be directed toward improvement in coping strategies or the adaptiveness of behavioral response, cognitive therapy is aimed at modifying distorted cognitions about a situation.

INDICATIONS FOR COGNITIVE THERAPY

Cognitive therapy was originally developed for use with depression. Today it is used for a broad range of emo-

tional disorders. The proponents of cognitive therapy suggest that the emphasis of therapy must be varied and individualized for clients according to their specific diagnosis, symptoms, and level of functioning. In addition to depression, cognitive therapy may be used with the following clinical conditions: panic disorder, generalized anxiety disorder, social phobias, obsessive-compulsive disorder, posttraumatic stress disorder, eating disorders, substance abuse, personality disorders, schizophrenia, couples' problems, bipolar disorder, hypochondriasis, and somatoform disorder (Kaplan & Sadock, 1998; Wright & Beck, 1994; Beck, 1995).

GOALS AND PRINCIPLES OF COGNITIVE THERAPY

Beck, Rush, and Shaw (1979) define the goals of cognitive therapy in the following way:

THE CLIENT WILL:
1. Monitor his or her negative, automatic thoughts.
2. Recognize the connections between cognition, affect, and behavior.
3. Examine the evidence for and against distorted automatic thoughts.
4. Substitute more realistic interpretations for these biased cognitions.
5. Learn to identify and alter the dysfunctional beliefs that predispose him or her to distort experiences.

Cognitive therapy is highly structured and short term, lasting from 12 to 16 weeks (Beck & Weishaar, 1995). Kaplan and Sadock (1998) suggest that if a client does not improve within 25 weeks of therapy, a reevaluation of the diagnosis should be made. Although therapy must be tailored to the individual, the following principles underlie cognitive therapy for all clients (Beck, 1995).

Principle 1. **Cognitive therapy is based on an ever-evolving formulation of the client and his or her problems in cognitive terms.** The therapist identifies the event that precipitated the distorted cognition. Current thinking patterns that serve to maintain the problematic behaviors are reviewed. The therapist then hypothesizes about certain developmental events and enduring patterns of cognitive appraisal that may have predisposed the client to specific emotional and behavioral responses.

Principle 2. **Cognitive therapy requires a sound therapeutic alliance.** A trusting relationship between therapist and client must exist for cognitive therapy to succeed. The therapist must convey warmth, empathy, caring, and genuine positive regard. Development of a working relationship between therapist and client is an individual process, and clients with various disorders will require varying degrees of effort to achieve this therapeutic alliance.

Principle 3. **Cognitive therapy emphasizes collaboration and active participation.** Teamwork is emphasized between therapist and client. They decide together what to work on during each session, how often they should meet, and what homework assignments should be completed between sessions.

Principle 4. **Cognitive therapy is goal-oriented and problem-focused.** At the beginning of therapy, the client is encouraged to identify what he or she perceives to be the problem or problems. With guidance from the therapist, goals are established as outcomes of therapy. Assistance in problem solving is provided as required as the client comes to recognize and correct distortions in thinking.

Principle 5. **Cognitive therapy initially emphasizes the present.** Resolution of distressing situations that are based in the present usually lead to symptom reduction. It is therefore of more benefit to begin with current problems and delay shifting attention to the past until (1) the client expresses the desire to do so, (2) work on current problems produces little or no change, or (3) the therapist decides it is important to determine how dysfunctional ideas affecting the client's current thinking originated.

Principle 6. **Cognitive therapy is educative, aims to teach the client to be his or her own therapist, and emphasizes relapse prevention.** From the beginning of therapy, the client is taught about the nature and course of his or her disorder, about the cognitive model (i.e., how thoughts influence emotions and behavior), and about the process of cognitive therapy. The client is taught how to set goals, plan behavioral change, and intervene on his or her own behalf.

Principle 7. **Cognitive therapy aims to be time-limited.** Clients often are seen weekly for a couple of months, followed by a number of biweekly sessions, then possibly a few monthly sessions. Some clients will want periodic "booster" sessions every few months.

Principle 8. **Cognitive therapy sessions are structured.** Each session has a set structure that includes (1) reviewing the client's week, (2) collaboratively setting the agenda for this session, (3) reviewing the previous week's session, (4) reviewing the previous week's homework, (5) discussing this week's agenda items, (6) establishing homework for next week, (7) summarizing this week's session. This format focuses attention on what is important and maximizes the use of therapy time.

Principle 9. **Cognitive therapy teaches clients to identify, evaluate, and respond to their dysfunctional thoughts and beliefs.** Through gentle questioning and review of data, the therapist helps the client identify his or her dysfunctional thinking, evaluate the validity of the thoughts, and devise a plan of action. This is done by helping the client to examine evidence that supports or contradicts the accuracy of the thought, rather than directly challenging or confronting the belief.

Principle 10. **Cognitive therapy uses a variety of techniques to change thinking, mood, and behavior.** Techniques from various therapies may be used within the cognitive framework. Emphasis in treatment is guided by the client's particular disorder and directed toward modification of the client's dysfunctional cognitions that are contributing to the maladaptive behavior associated with the disorder. Examples of disorders and the dysfunctional thinking for which cognitive therapy may be of benefit are discussed later in this chapter.

BASIC CONCEPTS

Wright and Beck (1994) state, "The general thrust of cognitive therapy is that emotional responses are largely dependent on cognitive appraisals of the significance of environmental cues." Basic concepts include **automatic thoughts** and **schemas** or core beliefs.

Automatic Thoughts. Automatic thoughts are those that occur rapidly in response to a situation and without rational analysis. These thoughts are often negative and based on erroneous logic. Beck, Rush, and Shaw (1979) call these thoughts *cognitive errors*. Following are some examples of common cognitive errors:

1. **Arbitrary Inference.** In a type of thinking error known as **arbitrary inference,** the individual automatically comes to a conclusion about an incident without the facts to support it, even sometimes despite contradictory evidence to support it.

   EXAMPLE:

   Two months ago, Mrs. B. sent a wedding gift to the daughter of an old friend. She has not yet received acknowledgment of the gift. Mrs. B. thinks, "They obviously think I have poor taste."

2. **Overgeneralization (Absolutistic Thinking).** Sweeping conclusions are **overgeneralizations** made based on one incident—a type of "all-or-nothing" kind of thinking.

   EXAMPLE:

   Frank submitted an article to a nursing journal and it was rejected. Frank thinks, "No journal will ever be interested in anything I write."

3. **Dichotomous Thinking.** An individual who is using **dichotomous thinking** views situations in all-or-nothing, black-or-white, good-or-bad terms.

   EXAMPLE:

   Frank submits an article to a nursing journal and the editor returns it and asks Frank to rewrite parts of it. Frank thinks, "I'm a bad writer," instead of recognizing that revision is a common part of the publication process.

4. **Selective Abstraction.** A **selective abstraction** (sometimes referred to as *mental filter*) is a conclusion that is based on only a selected portion of the evidence. The selected portion is usually the negative evidence or what the individual views as a failure, rather than any successes that have occurred.

EXAMPLE:

Jackie just graduated from high school with a 3.98/4.00 grade point average. She won a scholarship to the large state university near her home. She was active in sports and activities in high school and well-liked by all her peers. However, she is very depressed and dwells on the fact that she did not earn a scholarship to a prestigious Ivy League college to which she had applied.

5. **Magnification.** Exaggerating the negative significance of an event is known as **magnification.**

EXAMPLE:

Nancy hears that her colleague at work is having a cocktail party over the weekend and she is not invited. Nancy thinks, "She doesn't like me."

6. **Minimization.** Undervaluing the positive significance of an event is called **minimization.**

EXAMPLE:

Mrs. M is feeling lonely. She calls her granddaughter Amy, who lives in a nearby town, and invites her to visit. Amy apologizes that she must go out of town on business and would not be able to visit at that time. While Amy is out of town, she calls Mrs. M twice, but Mrs. M still feels unloved by her granddaughter.

7. **Catastrophic Thinking.** Always thinking that the worst will occur without considering the possibility of more likely, positive outcomes is considered **catastrophic thinking.**

EXAMPLE:

On Janet's first day in her secretarial job, her boss asked her to write a letter to another firm and put it on his desk for his signature. She did so and left for lunch. When she returned, the letter was on her desk with a typographical error circled in red and a note from her boss to redo the letter. Janet thinks, "This is it! I will surely be fired now!"

8. **Personalization.** In **personalization,** the person takes complete responsibility for situations without considering that other circumstances may have contributed to the outcome.

EXAMPLE:

Jack, who sells vacuum cleaners door-to-door, has just given a two-hour demonstration to Mrs. W. At the end of the demonstration, Mrs. W tells Jack that she appreciates his demonstration, but she won't be purchasing a vacuum cleaner from him. Jack thinks, "I'm a lousy salesman" (when in fact, Mrs. W's husband lost his job last week and they have no extra money to buy a new vacuum cleaner at this time).

Schemas (Core Beliefs). Beck and Weishaar (1995) define schemas as:

> "cognitive structures that consist of the individual's fundamental beliefs and assumptions, which develop early in life from personal experiences and identification with significant others. These concepts are reinforced by further learning experiences and, in turn, influence the formation of other beliefs, values, and attitudes." (p. 237)

These schemas, or core beliefs, may be adaptive or maladaptive. They may be general or specific, and they may be latent, becoming evident only when triggered by a specific stressful stimulus. Schemas differ from automatic thoughts in that they are deeper cognitive structures that serve to screen information from the environment. For this reason they are often more difficult to modify than automatic thoughts. However, the same techniques are employed at the schema level as at the level of automatic thoughts. Schemas can be positive or negative, and they generally fall into two broad categories: those associated with *helplessness* and those associated with *unlovability* (Beck, 1995). Some examples of types of schemas are presented in Table 18.1.

TECHNIQUES OF COGNITIVE THERAPY

The three major components of cognitive therapy are didactic, or educational, aspects, cognitive techniques, and behavioral interventions (Wright & Beck, 1994; Kaplan & Sadock, 1998).

Didactic (Educational) Aspects

One of the basic principles of cognitive therapy is to prepare the client to eventually become his or her own cognitive therapist. The therapist provides information to the client about what cognitive therapy is, how it works, and the structure of the cognitive process. Explanation about expectations of both client and therapist is provided. Reading assignments are given in order to reinforce learning. Some therapists audiotape or videotape sessions to teach clients about cognitive therapy. A full explanation about the relationship between depression (or anxiety, or whatever maladaptive response the client is experiencing)

TABLE 18.1   EXAMPLES OF SCHEMAS (OR CORE BELIEFS)

SCHEMA CATEGORY	MALADAPTIVE/NEGATIVE	ADAPTIVE/POSITIVE
Helplessness	No matter what I do, I will fail. I must be perfect. If I make one mistake, I will lose everything.	If I try and work very hard, I will succeed. I am not afraid of a challenge. If I make a mistake, I will try again.
Unlovability	I'm stupid. No one would love me. I'm nobody without a man.	I'm a lovable person. People respect me for myself.

and distorted thinking patterns is an essential part of cognitive therapy.

Cognitive Techniques

Strategies used in cognitive therapy include recognizing and modifying automatic thoughts (cognitive errors) and recognizing and modifying schemas (core beliefs). Wright and Beck (1994) identify the following techniques commonly used in cognitive therapy.

Recognizing Automatic Thoughts and Schemas

1. **Socratic Questioning.** In **Sococratic questioning** (also called *guided discovery*), the therapist questions the client about his or her situation. With Socratic questioning, the client is asked to describe feelings associated with specific situations. Questions are stated in a way that may stimulate in the client recognition of possible dysfunctional thinking and produce dissonance about the validity of the thoughts.

2. **Imagery and Role Play.** When Socratic questioning does not produce the desired results, the therapist may choose to guide the client through imagery exercises or role play in an effort to elicit automatic thoughts. Through guided imagery, the client is asked to "relive" the stressful situation by imagining the setting in which it occurred. Where did it occur? Who was there? What happened just prior to the stressful situation? What feelings did the client experience in association with the situation?

   Role play is not used as commonly as imagery. It is a technique that should be used only when the relationship between client and therapist is exceptionally strong and there is little likelihood of maladaptive transference occurring. With role play, the therapist assumes the role of an individual within a situation that produces a maladaptive response in the client. The situation is played out in an effort to elicit recognition of automatic thinking on the part of the client.

3. **Thought Recording.** This technique, one of the most frequently used methods of recognizing automatic thoughts, is taught to and discussed with the client in the therapy session. Thought recording is assigned as homework for the client outside of therapy. In thought recording, the client is asked to keep a written record of situations that occur and the automatic thoughts that are elicited by the situation. This is called a "two-column thought recording." Some therapists ask their clients to keep a "three-column recording," which includes a description of the emotional response also associated with the situation, as illustrated in Table 18.2.

Modifying Automatic Thoughts and Schemas

1. **Generating Alternatives.** To help the client see a broader range of possibilities than had originally been considered, the therapist guides the client in generating alternatives.

2. **Examining the Evidence.** With this technique, the client and therapist set forth the automatic thought as the hypothesis, and they study the evidence both for and against the hypothesis.

3. **Decatastrophizing.** With the technique of **decatastrophizing,** the therapist assists the client to examine the validity of a negative automatic thought.

TABLE 18.2   THREE-COLUMN THOUGHT RECORDING

SITUATION	AUTOMATIC THOUGHTS	EMOTIONAL RESPONSE
My girlfriend broke up with me.	I'm a stupid person. No one would ever want to marry me.	Sadness, depression
I was turned down for a promotion.	Stupid boss!! He doesn't know how to manage people. It's not fair!	Anger

Even if some validity exists, the client is then encouraged to review ways to cope adaptively, moving beyond the current crisis situation.

4. **Reattribution.** It is believed that depressed clients attribute life events in a negatively distorted manner; that is, they have a tendency "to blame themselves for adverse life events, and to believe that these negative situations will last indefinitely" (Wright & Beck, 1994). Through Socratic questioning and testing of automatic thoughts, this technique is aimed at reversing the negative attribution of depressed clients from internal and enduring to the more external and transient manner of nondepressed individuals.

5. **Daily Record of Dysfunctional Thoughts (DRDT).** In this common tool used in cognitive therapy to modify automatic thoughts, two more columns are added to the three-column thought record presented earlier. Clients are then asked to rate the intensity of the thoughts and emotions on a 0-to-100 percent scale. The fourth column of the DRDT asks the client to describe a more rational cognition than the automatic thought identified in the second column and rate the intensity of the belief in the rational thought. In the fifth column, the client records any changes that have occurred as a result of modifying the automatic thought and the new rate of intensity associated with it. Table 18.3 presents an example of a DRDT as an extension to the three-column thought recording presented in Table 18.2.

6. **Cognitive Rehearsal.** This technique uses mental imagery to uncover potential automatic thoughts in advance of their occurrence in a stressful situation. A discussion is held to identify ways to modify these dysfunctional cognitions. The client is then given "homework" assignments to try these newly learned methods in real situations.

Behavioral Interventions

In cognitive therapy, it is believed that an interactive relationship exists between cognitions and behavior; that is, that cognitions affect behavior and behavior influences cognitions. With this concept in mind, a number of interventions are structured for clients to assist in identifying and modifying maladaptive cognitions and behaviors. The following procedures, which are behavior-oriented, are directed toward helping clients learn more adaptive behavioral strategies that will in turn have a more positive effect on cognitions (Wright & Beck, 1994; Kaplan & Sadock, 1998):

1. **Activity Scheduling.** With this intervention, clients are asked to keep a daily log of their activities on an hourly basis and rate each activity, for mastery and pleasure, on a zero-to-ten scale. The schedule is then shared with the therapist and used to identify important areas needing concentration during therapy.

2. **Graded Task Assignments.** This intervention is used with clients who are facing a situation that they perceive as overwhelming. The task is broken down into subtasks that clients can complete one step at a time. Each subtask will have a goal and a time interval attached to it. Successful completion of each subtask helps to increase self-esteem and decrease feelings of helplessness.

3. **Behavioral rehearsal.** Somewhat akin to, and often used in conjunction with, cognitive rehearsal, this technique uses role play to "rehearse" a modification of maladaptive behaviors that may be contributing to dysfunctional cognitions.

4. **Distraction.** When dysfunctional cognitions have been recognized, activities are identified that can be used to **distract** clients and divert them from the intrusive thoughts or depressive ruminations that are contributing to the maladaptive responses.

TABLE 18.3 DAILY RECORD OF DYSFUNCTIONAL THOUGHTS

SITUATION	AUTOMATIC THOUGHT	EMOTIONAL RESPONSE	RATIONAL RESPONSE	OUTCOME: EMOTIONAL RESPONSE
My girlfriend broke up with me.	I'm a stupid person. No one would ever want to marry me. (95%)	Sadness; depression (90%)	I'm not stupid. Lots of people like me. Just because one person doesn't want to date me doesn't mean that no one would want to. (75%)	Sadness, depression (50%)
I was turned down for a promotion.	Stupid boss!! He doesn't know how to manage people. It's not fair! (90%)	Anger (95%)	I guess I have to admit the other guy's education and experience fit the position better than mine. The boss was being fair because he filled the position based on qualifications. I'll try for the next promotion that fits my qualifications better. (70%)	Anger (20%) Disappointment (80%) Hope (80%)

5. **Miscellaneous Techniques.** Relaxation exercises, assertiveness training, role modeling, and social-skills training are additional types of behavioral interventions that are used in cognitive therapy to assist clients to modify dysfunctional cognitions. Thought-stopping techniques (described in Chapter 13) may also be used to restructure dysfunctional thinking patterns.

ROLE OF THE NURSE IN COGNITIVE THERAPY

Many of the techniques used in cognitive therapy are well within the scope of nursing practice, from generalist through specialist levels. Unfortunately, most nurses are not introduced to the major concepts of cognitive therapy during their nursing education. Cognitive therapy requires an understanding of educational principles and the ability to use problem-solving skills to guide clients' thinking through a reframing process. The scope of contemporary psychiatric nursing practice is expanding, and although psychiatric nurses have been using some of these techniques in various degrees within their practices for years, it is important that knowledge and skills related to this type of therapy be further promoted. The value of cognitive therapy as a useful and cost-effective tool has been observed in a number of inpatient and community mental health settings.

The following case study is used to present the role of the nurse in cognitive therapy in the context of the nursing process.

CASE STUDY

ASSESSMENT

Sam is a 45-year-old white male admitted to the psychiatric unit of a general medical center by his family physician, Dr. Jones, who reported that Sam had become increasingly despondent over the last month. His wife reported that he had made statements such as, "Life is not worth living" and "I think I could just take all those pills Dr. Jones prescribed at one time, then it would all be over." He was admitted at 6:40 PM, via wheelchair from admissions, accompanied by his wife. He reports no known allergies. Vital signs upon admission were temperature, 97.9°F; P, 80; respirations, 16; and BP, 132/77. He is 5 feet 11 inches tall and weighs 160 pounds. He was referred to the psychiatrist on call, Dr. Smith. Orders include suicide precautions, level I; regular diet; chemistry profile and routine urinalysis in AM; Desyrel, 200 mg tid; Dalmane, 30 mg hs p.r.n. for sleep.

Family dynamics: Sam says he loves his wife and children and does not want to hurt them, but feels they no longer need him. He states, "They would probably be better off without me." His wife appears to be very concerned about his condition, though in his despondency, he seems oblivious to her feelings. His mother lives in a neighboring state, and he sees her infrequently. He admits that he is somewhat bitter toward her for allowing him and his siblings to "suffer from the physical and emotional brutality of our father." His siblings and their families live in distant states, and he sees them rarely, during holiday gatherings. He feels closest to the older of his two brothers.

Medical/psychiatric history: Sam's father died 5 years ago at age 65 of a myocardial infarction. Sam and both his brothers have a history of high cholesterol and triglycerides from approximately age 30. During his regular physical examination 1 month ago, Sam's family doctor recognized symptoms of depression and prescribed Elavil. Sam's mother has a history of depressive episodes. She was hospitalized once about 7 years ago for depression, and she has taken various antidepressant medications over the years. Her family physician has also prescribed Valium for her on numerous occasions for her "nerves." No other family members have a history of psychiatric problems.

Past experiences: Sam was the first child in a family of four. He is 2 years older than his sister and 4 years older than the third child, a brother. He was 6 years old when his youngest sibling, also a boy, was born. Sam's father was a career Army man, who moved his family many times during their childhood years. Sam attended 15 schools from the time he entered kindergarten until he graduated from high school.

Sam reports that his father was very autocratic and had many rules that he expected his children to obey without question. Infraction resulted in harsh discipline. Because Sam was the oldest child, his father believed he should assume responsibility for the behavior of his siblings. Sam describes the severe physical punishment he received from his father when he or his siblings allegedly violated one of the rules. It was particularly intense when Sam's father had been drinking, which he did most evenings and weekends.

Sam's mother was very passive. Sam believes she was afraid of his father, particularly when he was drinking, so she quietly conformed to his lifestyle and offered no resistance, even though she did not agree with his disciplining of the children. Sam reports that he observed his father physically abusing his mother on a number of occasions, most often when he had been drinking.

Sam states that he had very few friends when he was growing up. With all the family moves, he gave up trying to make new friends because it became too painful to give them up when it was time to leave. He took a paper route when he was 13 years old and then worked in fast-food restaurants from age 15 on. He was a hard worker and never seemed to have difficulty finding work in any of the places where the family relocated. He states that he appreciated the independence and the opportunity of being away from home as much as his job would allow. "I guess I can honestly say I hated my father, and working was my way of getting away from all the stress that was going on in that house. I guess my dad hated me, too, because he never was satisfied with

Continued on following page

C A S E   S T U D Y *(Continued)*

anything I did. I never did well enough for him in school, on the job, or even at home. When I think of my dad now, the memories I have are of being criticized and beaten with a belt."

On graduation from high school, Sam joined the Navy, where he learned a skill that he used after discharge to obtain a job in a large aircraft plant. He also attended the local university at night, where he earned his accounting degree. When he completed his degree, he was reassigned to the administration department of the aircraft company, and he has been in the same position for 12 years without a promotion.

Precipitating event: Over the last 12 years, Sam has watched while a number of his peers were promoted to management positions. Sam has been considered for several of these positions but has never been selected. Last month a management position became available for which Sam felt he was qualified. He applied for this position, believing he had a good chance of being promoted. However, when the announcement was made, the position had been given to a younger man who had been with the company only 5 years. Sam seemed to accept the decision, but over the last few weeks he has become more and more withdrawn. He speaks to very few people at the office and is becoming more and more behind in his work. At home, he eats very little, talks to family members only when they ask a direct question, withdraws to his bedroom very early in the evening, and does not come out until time to leave for work the next morning. Today, he refused to get out of bed or to go to work. His wife convinced him to talk to their family doctor, who admitted him to the hospital.

Client's perception of the stressor: Sam states that all his life he has "not been good enough at anything. I could never please my father. Now I can't seem to please my boss. What's the use of trying? I came to the hospital because my wife and my doctor are afraid I might try to kill myself. I must admit the thought has crossed my mind more than once. I seem to have very little motivation for living. I just don't care any more."

DIAGNOSES/OUTCOME IDENTIFICATION

The following nursing diagnoses were formulated for Sam:

1. Risk for self-directed violence related to depressed mood and expressions of having nothing to live for.
2. Chronic low self-esteem related to lack of positive feedback and learned helplessness evidenced by a sense of worthlessness, lack of eye contact, social isolation, and negative/pessimistic outlook.

The following may be used as criteria for measurement of outcomes in the planning of care for Sam. The client will:

1. Not harm self
2. Acquire a feeling of hope for the future
3. Demonstrate increased self-esteem and perception of self as worthwhile person.

PLANNING/IMPLEMENTATION

Table 18.4 presents a nursing care plan for Sam employing some techniques associated with cognitive therapy that are within the scope of nursing practice. Rationale are presented for each intervention:

EVALUATION

Reassessment is conducted to determine if the nursing interventions have been successful in achieving the objectives of Sam's care. Evaluation can be facilitated by gathering information using the following questions:

1. Has self-harm to Sam been avoided?
2. Have Sam's suicidal ideations subsided?
3. Does Sam know where to seek help in a crisis situation?
4. Has Sam discussed the recent loss with staff and family?
5. Is Sam able to verbalize personal hope for the future?
6. Can Sam identify positive attributes about himself?
7. Does Sam demonstrate motivation to move on with his life without a fear of failure?

SUMMARY

The premise upon which cognitive therapy is founded maintains that "how one thinks largely determines how one feels and behaves" (Beck & Weishaar, 1995). The concept was initiated in the 1960s by Aaron Beck in his work with depressed clients. Since that time, it has been expanded for use with a number of emotional illnesses.

Cognitive therapy is short-term, highly structured, and goal-oriented therapy, which consists of three major components: didactic, or educational, aspects; cognitive techniques; and behavioral interventions. The therapist teaches the client about the relationship between his or her illness and the distorted thinking patterns. Explanation about cognitive therapy and how it works is provided.

The therapist helps the client to recognize his or her negative automatic thoughts (sometimes called *cognitive errors*). Once these automatic thoughts have been identified, various cognitive and behavioral techniques are employed to assist the client to modify the dysfunctional thinking patterns. Independent homework assignments are an important part of the cognitive therapist's strategy.

Many of the cognitive therapy techniques are within the scope of nursing practice. The role of the nurse was presented in this chapter in the context of the nursing process with a sample case study. As the role of the psychiatric nurse continues to expand, the knowledge and skills associated with a variety of therapies will need to be broadened. Cognitive therapy is likely to be one in which nurses will become more involved.

TABLE 18.4   CARE PLAN FOR "SAM" (AN EXAMPLE OF INTERVENTION WITH COGNITIVE THERAPY)

NURSING DIAGNOSIS: RISK FOR SELF-DIRECTED VIOLENCE
RELATED TO: Depressed mood
EVIDENCED BY: Expressions of having nothing to live for

OUTCOME CRITERIA	NURSING INTERVENTIONS*	RATIONALE*
Sam will not harm himself.	1. Acknowledge Sam's feelings of despair. 2. Convey warmth, accurate empathy, and genuineness. 3. Through Socratic questioning, challenge irrational pessimism. Ask Sam to discuss what problems suicide would solve. Then try to get him to think of reasons for *not* attempting suicide. 4. Begin a serious discussion of alternatives.	1. Cognitive therapists actively pursue the client's point of view. 2. Cognitive therapists use these skills to understand the client's personal view of the world and to establish rapport. 3. Cognitive therapists use problem-solving techniques to help the suicidal client think beyond the immediate future. 4. Cognitive therapists use this strategy to decrease feelings of hopelessness in suicidal clients.

*Interventions and rationale for this diagnosis adapted from Harvard Medical School (1996) and Beck & Weishaar (1995).

NURSING DIAGNOSIS: CHRONIC LOW SELF-ESTEEM
RELATED TO: Lack of positive feedback and learned helplessness
EVIDENCED BY: A sense of worthlessness, lack of eye contact, social isolation, and negative/pessimistic outlook

OUTCOME CRITERIA	NURSING INTERVENTIONS	RATIONALE
Sam will demonstrate increased self-esteem and perception of himself as a worthwhile person.	1. Ask Sam to keep a three-column automatic thought recording. 2. Help Sam to recognize that his worth as a person is not tied to his promotion at work. The world will go on and he can survive this loss. 3. Help Sam to identify ways in which he could feel better about himself. For example, Sam states that he would like to update his computer skills, but he is afraid he is too old. Challenge his negative thinking about his age by using the cognitive therapy technique of "examining the evidence." 4. Ask Sam to expand on his three-column automatic thought recording and make a DRDT. 5. Discourage Sam's ruminating about his failures. May need to withdraw attention if he persists. Focus on past accomplishments and offer support in undertaking new tasks. Offer recognition of successful endeavors and positive reinforcement of attempts made.	1. Cognitive therapists use this tool to help clients identify automatic thoughts (cognitive errors). 2. Cognitive therapists use the technique of "decatastrophizing" to help clients get past a crisis situation. 3. Cognitive therapists use the technique of "generating alternatives" to help clients recognize that a broader range of possibilities may exist than may be evident at the moment. 4. Cognitive therapists use this tool to help clients examine their automatic thoughts and come up with more rational responses. 5. Cognitive therapy employs some techniques of behavior therapy. Lack of attention to undesirable behavior may discourage its repetition. Recognition and positive reinforcement enhance self-esteem and encourage repetition of desirable behaviors.

REVIEW QUESTIONS

SELF-EXAMINATION/LEARNING EXERCISE

Match the automatic thoughts on the left to the examples in the right-hand column:

_____ 1. Overgeneralization

_____ 2. Magnification

_____ 3. Catastrophic thinking

_____ 4. Personalization

a. Janet failed her first test in nursing school. She thinks, "Well, that's it! I'll never be a nurse."

b. When Jack is not accepted at the law school of his choice, he thinks, "I'm so stupid. No law school will ever accept me."

c. Nancy's new in-laws came to dinner for the first time. When Nancy's mother-in-law left some food on her plate, Nancy thought, "I must be a lousy cook."

d. Barbara burned the toast. She thinks, "I'm a totally incompetent person."

Situation: Opal is a 43-year-old woman who is suffering from depression and suicidal ideation. Select the most appropriate answer to following questions about Opal related to cognitive therapy techniques:

5. Opal says, "I'm such a worthless person. I don't deserve to live." The therapist responds, "I would like for you to think about what problems committing suicide would solve." This therapist is using:

   a. Imagery
   b. Role play
   c. Problem solving
   d. Thought recording

6. The purpose of the thought-recording technique is to help Opal:

   a. Identify automatic thoughts
   b. Modify automatic thoughts
   c. Identify rational alternatives
   d. All of the above

7. The purpose of the daily record of dysfunctional thoughts is to help Opal:

   a. Identify automatic thoughts
   b. Modify automatic thoughts
   c. Identify rational alternatives
   d. All of the above

8. Opal tells the therapist, "I thought I would just die when my husband told me he was leaving me. If I had been a better wife, he wouldn't have fallen in love with another woman. It's all my fault." The therapist asks Opal to think back to the day her husband told her he was leaving and to describe the situation and her feelings. This technique is called:

   a. Imagery
   b. Role play
   c. Problem solving
   d. Thought recording

9. The therapist wants to use the technique of "examining the evidence." Which of the following statements reflects this technique:

   a. "How do you think you could have been a better wife?"
   b. "Okay, you say it's all your fault. Let's discuss why it might be your fault, and then we will look at why it may not be."
   c. "Let's talk about what would make you a happier person."
   d. "Would you have wanted him to stay if he didn't really want to?"

10. The therapist teaches Opal that when the idea of herself as a worthless person starts to form in her mind, she should immediately start to whistle the tune of "Dixie." This is an example of the cognitive therapy technique of:

    a. Behavioral rehearsal
    b. Social skills training
    c. Distraction
    d. Generating alternatives

REFERENCES

Bandura, A. (1977). *Social learning theory.* Englewood Cliffs, NJ: Prentice Hall.

Beck, A.T. (1963). Thinking and depression, I. Idiosyncratic content and cognitive distortions. *Archives of General Psychiatry, 9,* 324–333.

Beck, A.T., (1964). Thinking and depression, II. Theory and therapy. *Archives of General Psychiatry, 10,* 561–571.

Beck, J.S. (1995). *Cognitive therapy: Basics and beyond.* New York: The Guilford Press.

Beck, A.T., & Freeman, A. (1990). *Cognitive therapy of personality disorders.* New York: Plenum.

Beck, A.T., Rush, A.H., & Shaw, B.F. (1979). *Cognitive therapy of depression.* New York: Guilford Press.

Beck, A.T., & Weishaar, M.E. (1995). Cognitive therapy. In R.J. Corsini and D. Wedding (Eds.), *Current psychotherapies* (5th ed.). Itasca, IL: F.E. Peacock Publishers.

Harvard Medical School. (1996). *The Harvard Mental Health Letter,13* (6). Boston, MA: The Harvard Medical School Health Publications Group.

Kaplan, H.I., & Sadock, B.J. (1998). *Synopsis of psychiatry: Behavioral sciences/clinical psychiatry* (8th ed.). Baltimore: Williams & Wilkins.

Lazarus, R.S. (1966). *Psychological stress and the coping process.* New York: McGraw-Hill.

Meichenbaum, D. (1977). *Cognitive-behavior modification: An integrative approach.* New York: Plenum.

Wright, J.H., & Beck, A.T. (1994). Cognitive therapy. In R.E. Hales, S.C. Yudofsky, & J.A. Talbott (Eds.), *Textbook of psychiatry* (2nd ed.). Washington, D.C.: American Psychiatric Press.

Bibliography

Blair, D.T. (1996). Cognitive behavioral therapies within the biological paradigm. *Journal of Psychosocial Nursing, 34*(12), 26–33.

Blair, D. T., & Ramones, V.A. (1997). Education as psychiatric intervention: The cognitive-behavioral context. *Journal of Psychosocial Nursing, 35*(12), 29–36.

Castonguay, L.G., Goldfried, M.R., & Wiser, S. (1996). Predicting the effect of cognitive therapy for depression: A study of unique and common factors. *Journal of Consulting and Clinical Psychology, 64*(3), 497–504.

Fowler, D., Garety, P., & Kuipers, E. (1995). *Cognitive behavior therapy for psychosis.* New York: Wiley.

Goisman, R.M. (1997). Cognitive-behavioral therapy today. *The Harvard Mental Health Letter, 13*(11), 4–7.

Jacobson, N.S., Dobson, K.S., & Truax, P.A. (1996). A component analysis of cognitive-behavioral treatment for depression. *Journal of Consulting and Clinical Psychology, 64*(2), 295–304.

Karasu, T.B. (1990). *Psychotherapy for depression.* Northvale, NJ: Jason Aronson.

Lineham, M.M. (1993). *Cognitive-behavioral treatment of borderline personality disorder.* New York: Guilford Press.

Schweitzer, P.B., Nesse, R.M., Fantone, R.F., & Curtis, G.C. (1995). Outcomes of group cognitive behavioral training in the treatment of panic disorder and agoraphobia. *Journal of the American Psychiatric Nurses Association, 1*(3), 83–91.

Shear, M.K., Pilkonis, P.A., Cloitre, M., & Leon, A.C. (1994). Cognitive behavioral treatment compared with nonprescriptive treatment of panic disorder. *Archives of General Psychiatry, 51*(5), 395–401.

PSYCHOPHARMACOLOGY

KEY TERMS

hypertensive crisis
priapism
agranulocytosis
extrapyramidal symptoms
tardive dyskinesia

neuroleptic malignant
 syndrome
retrograde ejaculation
gynecomastia
amenorrhea

akinesia
akathisia
dystonia
oculogyric crisis

OBJECTIVES

After reading this chapter, the student will be able to:

1. Discuss historical perspectives related to psychopharmacology.
2. Describe indications, actions, contraindications, precautions, side effects, and nursing implications for the following classifications of drugs:
   a. Antianxiety agents
   b. Antidepressants
   c. Antimanics
   d. Antipsychotics
   e. Antiparkinsonian agents
   f. Sedative-hypnotics
   g. Central nervous system stimulants
3. Apply the steps of the nursing process to the administration of psychotropic medications.

*T*he middle of the 20th century identifies a pivotal period in the treatment of the mentally ill. It was during this time that the phenothiazines were introduced into the United States. Before that time they had been used in France as preoperative medications. As Dr. Henri Laborit of the Hospital Boucicaut in Paris states,

> "It was our aim to decrease the anxiety of the patients to prepare them in advance for their postoperative recovery. With these new drugs, the phenothiazines, we were seeing a profound psychic and physical relaxation . . . a real indifference to the environment and to the upcoming operation. It seemed to me these drugs must have an application in psychiatry." (Public Broadcasting System, 1984)

Indeed they have had a significant application in psychiatry. Not only have they given many individuals a chance, without which they would have been unable to function, but also they have provided researchers and clinicians with information to study the origins and etiologies of mental illness. Knowledge gained from learning how these drugs work has promoted advancement in understanding how behavioral disorders develop. Dr. Arnold Scheibel, Director of the UCLA Brain Research Institute, states, "[When these drugs came out] there was a sense of disbelief that we could actually do something substantive for the patients . . . see them for the first time as sick individuals and not as something bizarre that we could literally not talk to." (Public Broadcasting System, 1984.)

This chapter explores historical perspectives in the use of psychotropic medications in the treatment of the mentally ill. Seven classifications of medications are discussed, and their implications for psychiatric nursing are presented in the context of the steps of the nursing process.

HISTORICAL PERSPECTIVES*

Historically, reaction to and treatment of the mentally ill ranged from benign involvement to intervention some would consider inhumane. Mentally ill individuals were feared because of common beliefs associating them with demons or the supernatural. They were looked upon as loathsome and often were mistreated.

Beginning in the late 18th century, a type of "moral reform" in the treatment of the mentally ill began to occur. This resulted in the establishment of community and state hospitals concerned with the needs of the mentally ill. Considered a breakthrough in the humanization of care, these institutions, however well intentioned, fostered the concept of custodial care. Clients were ensured the provision of food and shelter but received little or no hope of change for the future. As they became increasingly dependent

upon the institution to fill their needs, the likelihood of their return to the family or community diminished.

The early part of the 20th century saw the advent of the somatic therapies in psychiatry. Mentally ill individuals were treated with insulin shock therapy, wet sheet packs, ice baths, electronconvulsive therapy, and psychosurgery. Before 1950, no important chemical agents existed in psychiatric practice except sedatives and amphetamines, which had limited use owing to their toxicity and addicting effects (Burgess, 1985). Since the 1950s, the development of psychopharmacology has expanded to include widespread use of antipsychotic, antidepressant, and antianxiety medications. Research into how these drugs work has provided an understanding of the etiology of many psychiatric disorders.

Psychotropic medications are not intended to "cure" the mental illness. Most physicians who prescribe these medications for their clients use them as an adjunct to individual or group psychotherapy. Although their contribution to psychiatric care cannot be minimized, it must be emphasized that psychotropic medications relieve physical and behavioral symptoms. They do not resolve emotional problems.

Nurses must understand the legal implications associated with administration of psychotropic medications. Laws differ from state to state, but most adhere to the client's right to refuse treatment. Exceptions exist in emergency situations when it has been determined that clients are likely to harm themselves or others.

This chapter presents information necessary for nurses to safely administer psychotropic medications in seven classifications: antianxiety agents, antidepressants, antimanics, antipsychotics, antiparkinsonian agents, sedative-hypnotics, and central nervous system (CNS) stimulants. Nursing care in the administration of psychotropic medications is presented in the context of the nursing process.

APPLYING THE NURSING PROCESS IN PSYCHOPHARMACOLOGICAL THERAPY

An assessment tool for obtaining a drug history is provided in Table 19.1. This tool may be adapted for use by staff nurses admitting clients to the hospital, or by nurse practitioners who may wish to use it with prescriptive privileges. It may also be used when a client's signature of informed consent is required prior to pharmacological therapy.

Antianxiety Agents

Background Assessment Data

Indications. Antianxiety drugs are also called *anxiolytics* and *minor tranquilizers.* They are used in the treatment of anxiety disorders, anxiety symptoms, acute alcohol withdrawal, skeletal muscle spasms, convulsive disorders, status epilepticus, and preoperative sedation. Their use

---

*From Townend (1995), pp. 1–2.

▰ TABLE 19.1 MEDICATION ASSESSMENT TOOL

Date _____ Client's Name _____ Age _____

Marital Status _____ Children _____ Occupation _____

Presenting Symptoms (subjective and objective) _____

_____

_____

Diagnosis (*DSM-IV*) _____

Current Vital Signs: Blood Pressure   Sitting _____ / _____ Standing _____ / _____ Pulse _____ Respirations _____

Current/Past Use of Prescription Drugs (Indicate with c or p beside name of drug whether current or past use):

Name	Dosage	How Long Used	Why Prescribed	By Whom	Side Effects/Results

Current/Past Use of Over-the-Counter Drugs (Indicate with c or p beside name of drug):

Name	Dosage	How Long Used	Why Prescribed	By Whom	Side Effects/Results

Current/Past Use of Street Drugs, Alcohol, Nicotine, and/or Caffeine: (Indicate with c or p beside name of drug):

Name	Amount Used	How Often Used	When Last Used	Effects Produced

Any allergies to food or drugs? _____

Any special diet considerations? _____

Do you have (or have you ever had) any of the following? If yes, provide explanation on the back of this sheet.

	Yes	No			Yes	No			Yes	No
1. Difficulty swallowing	___	___	12. Chest pain	___	___	23. Sexual dysfunction	___	___
2. Delayed wound healing	___	___	13. Blood clots/pain in legs	___	___	24. Lumps in your breasts	___	___
3. Constipation problems	___	___	14. Fainting spells	___	___	25. Blurred or double vision	___	___
4. Urination problems	___	___	15. Swollen ankles/legs/hands	___	___	26. Ringing in the ears	___	___
5. Recent change in elimination patterns	___	___	16. Asthma	___	___	27. Insomnia	___	___
			17. Varicose veins	___	___	28. Skin rashes	___	___
6. Weakness or tremors	___	___	18. Numbness/tingling	___	___	29. Diabetes	___	___
7. Seizures	___	___	(state location)			30. Hepatitis (or other	___	___
8. Headaches	___	___	19. Ulcers	___	___	liver disease)		
9. Dizziness	___	___	20. Nausea/vomiting	___	___	31. Kidney disease	___	___
10. High blood pressure	___	___	21. Problems with diarrhea	___	___	32. Glaucoma	___	___
11. Palpitations	___	___	22. Shortness of breath	___	___			

Are you pregnant or breast-feeding? _____ Date of last menses _____ Types of contraception used _____

Describe any restrictions/limitations that might interfere with your use of medication for your current problem.

Prescription orders: Patient teaching related to medications prescribed:

Lab work ordered:

Nurse's signature   Client's Signature

and efficacy for periods greater than 4 months have not been evaluated.

Examples of commonly used antianxiety agents are presented in Table 19.2.

Action. Antianxiety drugs depress subcortical levels of the CNS, particularly the limbic system and reticular formation. They may potentiate the effects of the powerful inhibitory neurotransmitter gamma-aminobutyric acid (GABA) in the brain, thereby producing a calming effect. All levels of CNS depression can be affected, from mild sedation to hypnosis to coma.

EXCEPTION: Buspirone (BuSpar) does not depress the CNS. Although its action is unknown, the drug is believed to produce the desired effects through interactions with serotonin, dopamine, and other neurotransmitter receptors.

Contraindications/Precautions. Antianxiety drugs are contraindicated in individuals with known hypersensitivity to any of the drugs within the classification (i.e., anxiolytics) or group (e.g., benzodiazepines). They should not be taken in combination with other CNS depressants and are contraindicated in pregnancy and lactation, narrow-angle glaucoma, shock, and coma.

Caution should be taken in administering these drugs to elderly or debilitated clients and clients with hepatic or renal dysfunction. (The dosage usually has to be decreased.) Caution is also required with individuals who have a history of drug abuse or addiction and with those who are depressed or suicidal. In depressed clients, CNS depressants can exacerbate symptoms.

Interactions. Increased effects of antianxiety agents can occur when taken concomitantly with alcohol, barbiturates, narcotics, antipsychotics, antidepressants, antihistamines, neuromuscular blocking agents, cimetidine, or disulfiram. Decreased effects can be noted with cigarette smoking and caffeine consumption.

Diagnosis

The following nursing diagnoses may be considered for clients receiving therapy with antianxiety agents:

TABLE 19.2   ANTIANXIETY AGENTS

Chemical Class	Generic (Trade) Name	Controlled Categories	Half-Life	Daily Adult Dosage Range	Available Forms (mg)
Antihistamines	Hydroxyzine (Atarax)		3 hr	100–400 mg	tabs: 10, 25, 50, 100 syrup: 10 mg/5 ml
	(Vistaril)		3 hr	100–400 mg	caps: 25, 50, 100 oral susp: 25 mg/5 ml inj: 25, 50, 100
Benzodiazepines	Alprazolam (Xanax)	CIV	6–26 hr	0.75–4 mg	tabs: 0.25, 0.5, 1.0, 2.0 oral solu: 0.5 mg/5 ml
	Chlordiazepoxide (Librium)	CIV	5–30 hr	15–100 mg	tabs & caps: 5, 10, 25 inj: 100
	Clonazepam (Klonopin)	CIV	18–50 hr	4.5–20 mg	tabs: 0.5, 1, 2
	Clorazepate (Tranxene)	CIV	30–100 hr	15–60 mg	tabs: 3.75, 7.5, 15
	Diazepam (Valium)	CIV	20–80 hr	4–40 mg	tabs: 2, 5, 10 oral solu: 5 mg/ml, 5 mg/5 ml inj: 5 mg/ml
	Lorazepam (Ativan)	CIV	10–20 hr	2–6 mg	tabs: 0.5, 1.0, 2.0 oral solu: 2 mg/ml inj: 2 mg/ml, 4 mg/ml
	Oxazepam (Serax)	CIV	5–20 hr	30–120 mg	tabs & caps: 10, 15, 30
Metathiazanones	Chlormezanone (Trancopal)		24 hr	100–800 mg	tabs: 100, 200
Propanediols	Meprobamate (Equanil)	CIV	6–16 hr	400–2400 mg	tabs: 200, 400
	(Miltown)	CIV	6–16 hr	400–2400 mg	tabs: 200, 400, 600
Miscellaneous	Buspirone (BuSpar)		2–11 hr	15–60 mg	tabs: 5, 10

1. Risk for injury related to seizures; panic anxiety; abrupt withdrawal after long-term use; effects of intoxication or overdose.
2. Risk for activity intolerance related to side effects of sedation and lethargy.
3. Risk for acute confusion related to action of the medication on the CNS.

Planning/Implementation

The plan of care should include monitoring for the following side effects from antianxiety agents. Nursing implications related to each side effect are designated by an asterisk (*).

1. Drowsiness, confusion, lethargy (most common side effects)
   * Instruct the client not to drive or operate dangerous machinery while taking the medication.
2. Tolerance; physical and psychological dependence (does not apply to buspirone)
   * Instruct the client on long-term therapy not to quit taking the drug abruptly. Abrupt withdrawal can be life-threatening. Symptoms include depression, insomnia, increased anxiety, abdominal and muscle cramps, tremors, vomiting, sweating, convulsions, and delirium.
3. Ability to potentiate the effects of other CNS depressants
   * Instruct the client not to drink alcohol or take other medications that depress the CNS while taking this medication.
4. Possibility of aggravating symptoms in depressed persons
   * Assess the client's mood daily.
   * Take necessary precautions for potential suicide.
5. Orthostatic hypotension
   * Monitor lying and standing blood pressure and pulse every shift.
   * Instruct the client to arise slowly from a lying or sitting position.
6. Paradoxical excitement (client develops symptoms opposite of the medication's desired effect)
   * Withhold drug and notify the physician.
7. Dry mouth
   * Have the client take frequent sips of water, suck on ice chips or hard candy, or chew sugarless gum.
8. Nausea and vomiting
   * Have the client take the drug with food or milk.
9. Blood dyscrasias
   * Symptoms of sore throat, fever, malaise, easy bruising, or unusual bleeding should be reported to the physician immediately.
10. Delayed onset (buspirone only)
    * Ensure that the client understands there is a lag time of 10 days to 2 weeks between onset of ther-

apy with buspirone and subsiding of anxiety symptoms. Client should continue to take the medication during this time.

NOTE: This medication is not recommended for p.r.n. administration because of this delayed therapeutic onset. There is no evidence that buspirone creates tolerance or physical dependence as do the CNS depressant anxiolytics.

Client/Family Education. The client should:

* Not drive or operate dangerous machinery. Drowsiness and dizziness can occur.
* Not stop taking the drug abruptly, as this can produce serious withdrawal symptoms, such as depression, insomnia, anxiety, abdominal and muscle cramps, tremors, vomiting, sweating, convulsions, delirium.
* (With buspirone only): Be aware of lag time between start of therapy and subsiding of symptoms. Relief is usually evident within 10 to 14 days. The client must take the medication regularly, as ordered, so that it has sufficient time to take effect.
* Not consume other CNS depressants (including alcohol).
* Not take nonprescription medication without approval from physician.
* Rise slowly from sitting or lying position to prevent sudden drop in blood pressure.
* Report symptoms of sore throat, fever, malaise, easy bruising, unusual bleeding, or motor restlessness to physician immediately.
* Be aware of risks of taking this drug during pregnancy. (Congenital malformations have been associated with use during the first trimester.) The client should notify the physician of the desirability to discontinue the drug if pregnancy is suspected or planned.
* Be aware of possible side effects. The client should refer to written materials furnished by health care providers regarding the correct method of self-administration.
* Carry card or piece of paper at all times stating the names of medications being taken.

Outcome Criteria/Evaluation

The following criteria may be used for evaluating the effectiveness of therapy with antianxiety agents.

THE CLIENT:

1. Demonstrates a reduction in anxiety, tension, and restless activity.
2. Experiences no seizure activity.
3. Experiences no physical injury.
4. Is able to tolerate usual activities without excessive sedation.
5. Exhibits no evidence of confusion.

6. Tolerates the medication without gastrointestinal distress.
7. Verbalizes understanding of the need for, side effects of, and regimen for self-administration.
8. Verbalizes possible consequences of abrupt withdrawal from the medication.

Antidepressants

Background Assessment Data

Indications. Antidepressant medications are used in the treatment of dysthymic disorder; major depression with melancholia or psychotic symptoms; depression associated with organic disease, alcoholism, schizophrenia, or mental retardation; depressive phase of bipolar disorder; and depression accompanied by anxiety. These drugs elevate mood and alleviate other symptoms associated with moderate-to-severe depression.

Examples of commonly used antidepressant medications are presented in Table 19.3.

Action. These drugs ultimately work to increase the concentration of norepinephrine, serotonin, and/or dopamine in the body. This is accomplished in the brain by blocking the reuptake of these neurotransmitters by the neurons (tricyclics, tetracyclics, selective serotonin reuptake inhibitors, and others). It also occurs when an enzyme, monoamine oxidase (MAO), that is known to inactivate norepinephrine, serotonin, and dopamine is inhibited at various sites in the nervous system (MAO inhibitors [MAOIs]).

Contraindications/Precautions. Antidepressant drugs are contraindicated in individuals with hypersensitivity. They are also contraindicated in the acute recovery phase following myocardial infarction and in individuals with angle-closure glaucoma.

Caution should be used in administering these drugs to elderly or debilitated clients and those with hepatic, renal, or cardiac insufficiency. (The dosage usually must be decreased.) Caution is also required with psychotic clients, with clients who have benign prostatic hypertrophy, and with individuals who have a history of seizures (may decrease seizure threshold).

NOTE: As these drugs take effect, and mood begins to lift, the individual may have increased energy with which to implement a suicide plan. Suicide potential often increases as level of depression decreases. The nurse should be particularly alert to sudden lifts in mood.

Interactions

Tricyclic Antidepressants. Hyperpyretic crisis, **hypertensive crisis,** severe seizures, and tachycardia may occur when used with MAOIs. Use of these drugs may prevent therapeutic response to some antihypertensives (clonidine, guanethidine). Additive CNS depression occurs with concurrent use of CNS depressants. Additive sympathomimetic and anticholinergic effects occur with use of other drugs possessing these same properties.

MAO Inhibitors. Hypertensive crisis may occur with concurrent use of amphetamines, methyldopa, levodopa, dopamine, epinephrine, norepinephrine, reserpine, vasoconstrictors, or ingestion of tyramine-containing foods (Table 19.4). Hypertension or hypotension, coma, convulsions, and death may occur with meperidine or other narcotic analgesics when used with MAOIs. Additive hypotension may result with concurrent use of antihypertensives or spinal anesthesia and MAOIs. Additive hypoglycemia may result with concurrent use of insulin or oral hypoglycemic agents and MAOIs.

Selective Serotonin Reuptake Inhibitors (SSRIs). Concurrent use with cimetidine may result in increased concentrations of SSRIs. Hypertensive crisis can occur if used within 14 days of MAOIs. Impairment of mental and motor skills may be potentiated with use of alcohol. Concurrent use with diazepam may result in prolonged half-life or increased concentrations of diazepam. Use with warfarin may result in tendency for increased bleeding.

Diagnosis

The following nursing diagnoses may be considered for clients receiving therapy with antidepressant medications:

1. Risk for self-directed violence related to depressed mood.
2. Risk for injury related to side effects of sedation, lowered seizure threshold, orthostatic hypotension, **priapism,** photosensitivity, arrhythmias, and hypertensive crisis.
3. Social isolation related to depressed mood.
4. Constipation related to side effects of the medication.

Planning/Implementation

The plan of care should include monitoring for the following side effects from antidepressant medications. Nursing implications are designated by an asterisk (*). A general profile of the side effects of antidepressant medications is presented in Table 19.5.

1. May occur with all chemical classes
   a. Dry mouth
      * Offer the client sugarless candy, ice, frequent sips of water.
      * Strict oral hygiene is very important.
   b. Sedation
      * Request an order from the physician for the drug to be given at bedtime.
      * Request that the physician decrease the dosage or perhaps order a less sedating drug.

TABLE 19.3 ANTIDEPRESSANT MEDICATIONS

CHEMICAL CLASS	GENERIC (TRADE) NAME	DAILY ADULT DOSAGE RANGE*	THERAPEUTIC PLASMA RANGES	AVAILABLE FORMS (MG)
Tricyclics	Amitriptyline (Elavil; Endep)	75–300 mg	110–250 ng/ml (including metabolite)	tabs: 10, 25, 50, 75, 100, 150 inj: 10 mg/ml
	Amoxapine (Asendin)	100–600 mg	200–600 ng/ml (including metabolite)	tabs: 25, 50, 100, 150
	Clomipramine (Anafranil)	75–300 mg	80–100 ng/ml	caps: 25, 50, 75
	Desipramine (Norpramin)	75–300 mg	125–300 ng/ml	tabs: 10, 25, 50, 75, 100, 150
	Doxepin (Sinequan; Adapin)	75–300 mg	100–200 ng/ml (including metabolite)	caps: 10, 25, 50, 75, 100, 150 oral conc: 10 mg/ml
	Imipramine (Tofranil)	75–300 mg	200–350 ng/ml (including metabolite)	tabs: 10, 25, 50 caps: 75, 100, 125, 150 inj: 25 mg/2 ml
	Nortriptyline (Aventyl; Pamelor)	75–150 mg	50–150 ng/ml	caps: 10, 25, 50, 75 oral solution: 10 mg/5 ml
	Protriptyline (Vivactil)	15–60 mg	100–200 ng/ml	tabs: 5, 10
	Trimipramine (Surmontil)	75–300 mg	180 ng/ml (including metabolite)	caps: 25, 50, 100
Heterocyclics	Bupropion (Wellbutrin)	200–450 mg	Not well established	tabs: 75, 100
	Maprotiline (Ludiomil)	75–225 mg	200–300 ng/ml	tabs: 25, 50, 75
	Mirtazapine (Remeron)	15–45 mg	Not well established	tabs: 15, 30
	Trazodone (Desyrel)	150–600 mg	800–1600 ng/ml	tabs: 50, 100, 150, 300
Selective Serotonin Reuptake Inhibitors	Citalopram (Celexa)	20–40 mg	Not well established	tabs: 20, 40
	Fluoxetine (Prozac)	20–80 mg	Not well established	caps: 10, 20
	Fluvoxamine (Luvox)	50–300 mg	Not well established	tabs: 50, 100
	Paroxetine (Paxil)	20–50 mg	Not well established	tabs; caps: 10, 20, 30, 40
	Sertraline (Zoloft)	50–200 mg	Not well established	tabs: 50, 100
Nonselective Reuptake Inhibitors	Venlafaxine (Effexor)	75–375 mg	Not well established	tabs: 25, 37.5, 50, 75, 100
	Nefazodone (Serzone)	200–600 mg	Not well established	tabs: 100, 150, 200, 250
Monoamine Oxidase Inhibitors	Isocarboxazid (Marplan)	10–30mg	Not well established	tabs: 10
	Phenelzine (Nardil)	45–90 mg	Not well established	tabs: 15
	Tranylcypromine (Parnate)	30–60 mg	Not well established	tabs: 10

[handwritten: so sedative to help people sleep]

[handwritten: not used too often]

[handwritten: Can't eat food c tyramine, will ↑ BP – hypertension ER situation used as last resort.]

*Dosage requires slow titration; onset of therapeutic response may be 1 to 4 weeks.

* Instruct the client not to drive or use dangerous equipment while experiencing sedation.
c. Nausea
* Medication may be taken with food to minimize GI distress.
2. Most commonly occur with tricyclics

a. Blurred vision
* Offer reassurance that this symptom should subside after a few weeks
* Instruct the client not to drive until vision is clear.
* Clear small items from routine pathway to prevent falls.

■ TABLE 19.4 DIET AND DRUG RESTRICTIONS FOR CLIENTS ON MAOI THERAPY

FOODS CONTAINING TYRAMINE

High Tyramine Content (avoid while on MAOI therapy)	Moderate Tyramine Content (may eat occasionally while on MAOI therapy)	Low Tyramine Content (limited quantities permissible while on MAOI therapy)
Aged cheeses (cheddar, Swiss, camembert, blue cheese, Parmesan, provolone, Romano, brie)	Gouda cheese, processed American cheese, mozzarella	Pasteurized cheeses (cream cheese, cottage cheese, ricotta)
Raisins, fava beans, flat Italian beans, Chinese pea pods	Yogurt, sour cream	Figs
Red wines (Chianti, burgundy, cabernet sauvignon)	Avocados, bananas	Distilled spirits (in moderation)
Smoked and processed meats (salami, bologna, pepperoni, summer sausage)	Beer, white wine, coffee, colas, tea, hot chocolate	
Caviar, pickled herring, corned beef, chicken or beef liver	Meat extracts, such as bullion	
Soy sauce, brewer's yeast, meat tenderizer (MSG)	Chocolate	

DRUG RESTRICTIONS

Ingestion of the following substances while on MAOI therapy could result in life-threatening hypertensive crisis. A 14-day interval is recommended between use of these drugs and an MAOI.

Other antidepressants (tricyclic; SSRIs)

Sympathomimetics (epinephrine, dopamine, norepinephrine, ephedrine, pseudoephedrine, phenylephrine, phenylpropanolamine, over-the-counter cough and cold preparations)

Stimulants (amphetamines, cocaine, methyldopa, diet drugs)

Antihypertensives (methyldopa, guanethidine, reserpine)

Meperidine and (possibly) other opioid narcotics (morphine, codeine)

Antiparkinsonian agents (levodopa)

SOURCE: Adapted from Kurtz & Robinson (1988); and Gerald & O'Bannon (1988).

b. Constipation
  * Order foods high in fiber; increase fluid intake if not contraindicated; and encourage the client to increase physical exercise, if possible.
c. Urinary retention
  * Instruct the client to report hesitancy or inability to urinate.
  * Monitor intake and output.
  * Try various methods to stimulate urination, such as running water in the bathroom or pouring water over the perineal area.
d. Orthostatic hypotension
  * Instruct the client to rise slowly from a lying or sitting position.
  * Monitor blood pressure (lying and standing) frequently, and document and report significant changes.
  * Avoid long hot showers or tub baths.
e. Reduction of seizure threshold
  * Observe clients with history of seizures closely.
  * Institute seizure precautions as specified in hospital procedure manual.

* Bupropion (Wellbutrin) should be administered in doses of no more than 150 mg and should be given at least 4 hours apart. Bupropion has been associated with a relatively high incidence of seizure activity in anorectic and cachectic clients.
f. Tachycardia; arrhythmias
  * Carefully monitor blood pressure and pulse rate and rhythm, and report any significant change to the physician.
g. Photosensitivity
  * Ensure that client wears protective sunscreens, clothing, and sunglasses while outdoors.
h. Weight gain
  * Provide instructions for reduced-calorie diet.
  * Encourage increased level of activity, if appropriate.
3. Most commonly occur with SSRIs
  a. Insomnia; agitation
    * Administer or instruct client to take dose early in the day.
    * Instruct client to avoid caffeinated food and drinks.

TABLE 19.5 SIDE EFFECT PROFILES OF ANTIDEPRESSANT MEDICATIONS

| | CNS SIDE EFFECTS* | | CARDIOVASCULAR SIDE EFFECTS | | OTHER SIDE EFFECTS | | |
DRUG	SEDATION	INSOMNIA/ AGITATION	ORTHOSTATIC HYPOTENSION	CARDIAC ARRHYTHMIA	GASTROINTEST- INAL DISTRESS	WEIGHT GAIN (>6 KG)	ANTICHO- LINERGIC†
Amitriptyline	4+	0	4+	3+	0	4+	4+
Desipramine	1+	1+	2+	2+	0	1+	1+
Doxepin	4+	0	2+	2+	0	3+	3+
Imipramine	3+	1+	4+	3+	1+	3+	3+
Nortriptyline	1+	0	2+	2+	0	1+	1+
Protriptyline	1+	1+	2+	2+	0	0	2+
Trimipramine	4+	0	2+	2+	0	3+	1+
Amoxapine	2+	2+	2+	3+	0	1+	2+
Maprotiline	4+	0	0	1+	0	2+	2+
Mirtazapine	4+	0	0	1+	0	2+	2+
Trazodone	4+	0	1+	1+	1+	1+	0
Bupropion	0	2+	0	1+	1+	0	0
Fluoxetine	0	2+	0	0	3+	0	0
Fluvoxamine	0	2+	0	0	3+	0	0
Paroxetine	0	2+	0	0	3+	0	0
Sertraline	0	2+	0	0	3+	0	0
Monoamine oxidase inhibitors (MAOIs)	1+	2+	2+	0	1+	2+	1+

*Key: 0 = Absent or rare.
1+ = Infrequent.
2+, 3+ = Relatively common.
4+ = Frequent.
†Dry mouth, blurred vision, urinary hesitancy, constipation.
SOURCE: Adapted from Depression Guideline Panel (1993); *Facts & Comparisons* (1998); and Bernstein (1995).

* Teach relaxation techniques to use before bedtime.
  b. Headache
    * Administer analgesics, as prescribed.
    * Request that the physician order another SSRI or another class of antidepressants
  c. Weight loss
    * Ensure that client is provided with caloric intake sufficient to maintain desired weight.
    * Caution must be used in prescribing these drugs for anorectic clients.
    * Weigh client daily or every other day, at the same time and on the same scale, if possible.
  d. Sexual dysfunction
    * Men may report abnormal ejaculation or impotence.
    * Women may experience delay or loss of orgasm.
    * If side effect become intolerable, a switch to another antidepressant may be necessary.
4. Most commonly occur with MAOIs
  a. Hypertensive crisis
    * Hypertensive crisis occurs if the individual consumes foods containing tyramine while receiving MAOI therapy (see Table 19.4).

    * Watch for symptoms of hypertensive crisis—severe occipital headache, palpitations, nausea and vomiting, nuchal rigidity, fever, sweating, marked increase in blood pressure, chest pain, and coma.
    * Discontinue drug immediately; monitor vital signs; administer short-acting antihypertensive medication, as ordered by physician; use external cooling measures to control hyperpyrexia.
5. Miscellaneous side effects
  a. Priapism with trazodone (Desyrel)
    * Priapism is a rare side effect, but it has occurred in some men taking trazodone.
    * If the client complains of prolonged or inappropriate penile erection, withhold medication dosage and notify the physician immediately.
    * Priapism can become very problematic, requiring surgical intervention, and, if not treated successfully, can result in impotence.

Client/Family Education. The client should:

* Continue to take the medication even though the symptoms have not subsided. The therapeutic effect may not be seen for as long as 4 weeks. If after this

length of time no improvement is noted, the physician may prescribe a different medication.

* Use caution when driving or operating dangerous machinery. Drowsiness and dizziness can occur. If these side effects become persistent or interfere with activities of daily living, the client should report them to the physician. Dosage adjustment may be necessary.

* Not stop taking the drug abruptly. To do so might produce withdrawal symptoms, such as nausea, vertigo, insomnia, headache, malaise, and nightmares.

* If taking a tricyclic, use sunscreens and wear protective clothing when spending time outdoors. The skin may be sensitive to sunburn.

* Report occurrence of any of the following symptoms to the physician immediately: sore throat, fever, malaise, unusual bleeding, easy bruising, persistent nausea/vomiting, severe headache, rapid heart rate, difficulty urinating, anorexia/ weight loss, seizure activity, stiff or sore neck, and chest pain.

* Rise slowly from a sitting or lying position to prevent a sudden drop in blood pressure.

* Take frequent sips of water, chew sugarless gum, or suck on hard candy if dry mouth is a problem. Good oral care (frequent brushing, flossing) is very important.

* Not consume the following foods or medications while taking MAOIs: aged cheese, wine (especially chianti), beer, chocolate, colas, coffee, tea, sour cream, beef/chicken livers, canned figs, soy sauce, overripe and fermented foods, pickled herring, preserved sausages, yogurt, yeast products, broad beans, cold remedies, diet pills. To do so could cause a life-threatening hypertensive crisis.

* Avoid smoking while receiving tricyclic therapy. Smoking increases the metabolism of tricyclics, requiring an adjustment in dosage to achieve the therapeutic effect.

* Not drink alcohol while taking antidepressant therapy. These drugs potentiate the effects of each other.

* Not consume other medications (including over-the-counter medications) without the physician's approval while receiving antidepressant therapy. Many medications contain substances that, in combination with antidepressant medication, could precipitate a life-threatening hypertensive crisis.

* Notify physician immediately if inappropriate or prolonged penile erections occur while taking trazodone (Desyrel). If the erection persists longer than 1 hour, seek emergency room treatment. This condition is rare but has occurred in some men who have taken trazodone. If measures are not instituted immediately, impotence can result.

* Not "double up" on medication if a dose of bupropion (Wellbutrin) is missed, unless advised to do so by the physician. Taking bupropion in divided doses will decrease the risk of seizures and other adverse effects.

* Be aware of possible risks of taking antidepressants during pregnancy. Safe use during pregnancy and lactation has not been fully established. These drugs are believed to readily cross the placental barrier; if so, the fetus could experience adverse effects of the drug. Inform the physician immediately if pregnancy occurs, is suspected, or is planned.

* Be aware of the side effects of antidepressants. Refer to written materials furnished by health care providers for safe self-administration.

* Carry a card or other identification at all times describing the medications being taken.

Outcome Criteria/Evaluation

The following criteria may be used for evaluating the effectiveness of therapy with antidepressant medications:

THE CLIENT:

1. Has not harmed self.
2. Has not experienced injury caused by side effects such as priapsim, hypertensive crisis, or photosensitivity.
3. Exhibits vital signs within normal limits.
4. Manifests symptoms of improvement in mood (brighter affect, interaction with others, improvement in hygiene, clear thought and communication patterns).
5. Stays out of room and willingly participates in activities on the unit.

Antimanic Agents

Background Assessment Data

The drug of choice for treatment and management of bipolar disorder, mania, is lithium carbonate. However, in recent years, a number of investigators and clinicians in practice have achieved satisfactory results with several other medications, either alone or in combination with lithium. Table 19.6 provides information about the indication, action, and contraindications and precautions of various medications being used as mood stabilizers.

Interactions

Lithium carbonate. Lithium may prolong neuromuscular blockage. Encephalopathic syndrome may occur with haloperidol. Diuretics, methyldopa, probenecid, indomethacin, and other nonsteroidal anti-inflammatory agents may increase the risk of lithium toxicity. Aminophylline, phenothiazines, sodium bicarbonate, and sodium chloride may hasten excretion, leading to decreased effect. Lithium may decrease the effectiveness of phenothiazines. Hypothyroid effects may be additive with potassium iodide.

Clonazepam. Additive CNS depression may occur with other CNS depressants. Absence status may occur with concurrent use of valproic acid. A decrease in the ef-

■ TABLE 19.6   ANTIMANIC AGENTS

CLASSIFICATION: GENERIC (TRADE)	INDICATIONS	MECHANISM OF ACTION	CONTRAINDICATIONS/ PRECAUTIONS	DAILY ADULT DOSAGE RANGE	THERAPEUTIC PLASMA RANGE
Antimanic					
Lithium carbonate (Eskalith, Lithane)	Prevention and treatment of manic episodes of bipolar disorder. Also used for bipolar depression.	Not fully understood but may enhance reuptake of norepinephrine and serotonin, decreasing the levels in the body, resulting in decreased hyperactivity (may take 1–3 wk for symptoms to subside).	Hypersensitivity. Cardiac or renal disease, dehydration; sodium depletion; brain damage; pregnancy and lactation. Caution with thyroid disorders, diabetes, urinary retention, history of seizures, and with the elderly.	Acute mania: 1800–2400 mg Maintenance: 300–1200 mg	Acute mania: 1.0–1.5 mEq/l Maintenance: 0.6–1.2 mEq/l
Anticonvulsants					
Clonazepam (Klonopin)	Absence, akinetic, and myoclonic seizures. Unlabeled use: bipolar mania.	Action in the treatment of bipolar disorder is unclear.	Hypersensitivity. Glaucoma, liver disease, lactation. Caution in elderly, liver/renal disease, pregnancy.	2–20 mg	20–80 ng/ml
Carbamazepine (Tegretol)	Grand mal and psychomotor seizures. Unlabeled uses: Bipolar mania, rage reactions, resistant schizophrenia.	Action in the treatment of bipolar disorder is unclear.	Hypersensitivity. With MAOIs, lactation. Caution with elderly, liver/renal/cardiac disease, pregnancy.	400–1200 mg	6–12 μg/ml
Valproic acid (Depakene; Depakote)	Absence seizures. Unlabeled use: bipolar mania.	Action in the treatment of bipolar disorder is unclear.	Hypersensitivity; liver disease. Caution in elderly, renal/cardiac diseases, pregnancy and lactation.	500–1500 mg	50–100 μg/ml
Calcium Channel Blocker					
Verapamil (Calan; Isoptin)	Angina, hypertension, arrhythmias. Unlabeled use: bipolar mania, migraine headache prophylaxis.	Action in the treatment of bipolar disorder is unclear.	Hypersensitivity; heart block, hypotension, cardiogenic shock, congestive heart failure, pregnancy, lactation. Caution in liver or renal disease, cardiomyopathy, intracranial pressure, the elderly.	240–320 mg	80–300 ng/ml

fectiveness of clonazepam can occur with phenobarbital, phenytoin, and carbamazepine. Concurrent use of disulfiram may result in increased clonazepam effects, and possible toxicity.

Carbamazepine. An increase in the effects of carbamazepine can occur with concurrent use of erythromycin, verapamil, isoniazid, propoxyphene, troleandomycin, and cimetidine. Decreased effects of carbamazepine can occur with concurrent use of phenytoin, primidone, and phenobarbital. A decrease in the effects of phensuximide, doxycycline, theophylline, oral anticoagulants, oral contraceptives, phenytoin, ethosuximide, valproic acid, and haloperidol can occur when used concomitantly with carbamazepine. Concurrent use of lithium and carbamazepine increases risk of neurotoxicity.

Valproic Acid. A potentiation of the CNS depressant effects can occur with concurrent use of CNS depressants. Use of valproic acid with phenytoin or clonazepam may result in seizures. Increased effects of phenobarbital, primidone, or MAOIs may result when used with valproic acid. Concomitant use of valproic acid with aspirin or warfarin may lead to prolonged bleeding time.

Verapamil. Additive depression of myocardial contractility and atrioventricular conduction can occur when verapamil is used with beta-adrenergic blockers. The effects of verapamil may be decreased when used with rifampin, calcium salts, and vitamin D, and may be increased when used with cimetidine. Effects may be increased or decreased when used with other highly protein-bound drugs. The interaction of verapamil with cardiac glycosides may increase serum digitoxin/digoxin levels and result in toxicity.

Diagnosis

The following nursing diagnoses may be considered for clients receiving therapy with antimanic agents:

1. Risk for injury related to manic hyperactivity.
2. Risk for violence: self-directed or directed at others related to unresolved anger turned inward on the self or outward on the environment.
3. Risk for injury related to lithium toxicity.
4. Risk for activity intolerance related to side effects of drowsiness and dizziness.

Planning/Implementation

The plan of care should include monitoring for side effects of therapy with antimanic agents and intervening when required to prevent the occurrence of adverse events related to medication administration. Side effects and nursing implications for antimanic agents are presented in Table 19.7.

Lithium Toxicity. The margin between the therapeutic and toxic levels of lithium carbonate is very narrow. The usual ranges of therapeutic serum concentrations are:

* For acute mania: 1.0 to 1.5 mEq/l

* For maintenance: 0.6 to 1.2 mEq/l

Serum lithium levels should be monitored once or twice a week after initial treatment until dosage and serum levels are stable, then monthly during maintenance therapy.

Blood samples should be drawn 12 hours after the last dose.

Symptoms of lithium toxicity begin to appear at blood levels greater than 1.5 mEq/l and are dosage determinate. Symptoms include:

* **At serum levels of 1.5 to 2.0 mEq/l:** blurred vision, ataxia, tinnitus, persistent nausea and vomiting, severe diarrhea.
* **At serum levels of 2.0 to 3.5 mEq/l:** excessive output of dilute urine, increasing tremors, muscular irritability, psychomotor retardation, mental confusion, giddiness.
* **At serum levels above 3.5 mEq/l:** impaired consciousness, nystagmus, seizures, coma, oliguria/anuria, arrhythmias, myocardial infarction, cardiovascular collapse.

Lithium levels should be monitored prior to medication administration. The dosage should be withheld and the physician notified if the level reaches 1.5 mEq/l or at the earliest observation or report by the client of even the mildest symptom. If left untreated, lithium toxicity can be life threatening.

Lithium is similar in chemical structure to sodium, behaving in the body in much the same manner and competing at various sites in the body with sodium. If sodium intake is reduced or the body is depleted of its normal sodium (e.g., due to excessive sweating, fever, diuresis), lithium is reabsorbed by the kidneys, increasing the possibility of toxicity. Therefore, the client must consume a diet adequate in sodium as well as 2500 to 3000 ml of fluid per day. Accurate records of intake, output, and client's weight should be kept on a daily basis.

Client/Family Education (for Lithium). The client should:

* Take medication on a regular basis, even when feeling well. Discontinuation can result in return of symptoms.
* Not drive or operate dangerous machinery until lithium levels are stabilized. Drowsiness and dizziness can occur.
* Not skimp on dietary sodium intake. He or she should choose foods from the food pyramid and avoid "junk" foods. The client should drink 6 to 8 large glasses of water each day and avoid excessive use of beverages containing caffeine (coffee, tea, colas), which promote increased urine output.
* Notify the physician if vomiting or diarrhea occur. These symptoms can result in sodium loss and an increased risk of toxicity.
* Carry card or other identification noting that he or she is taking lithium.
* Be aware of appropriate diet should weight gain become a problem. Include adequate sodium and other nutrients while decreasing number of calories.

TABLE 19.7   SIDE EFFECTS AND NURSING IMPLICATIONS OF ANTIMANIC AGENTS

MEDICATION	SIDE EFFECTS	NURSING IMPLICATIONS
Antimanic		
Lithium carbonate (Eskalith, Lithane)	Drowsiness, dizziness, headache	● Ensure that client does not participate in activities that require alertness.
	✳ Dry mouth; thirst	● Provide sugarless candy, ice, frequent sips of water. ● Strict oral hygiene is very important.
	GI upset; nausea/vomiting	● Administer medications with meals to minimize GI upset.
	✳ Fine hand tremors	● Report to physician, who may decrease dosage. ● Some physicians prescribe a small dose of beta-blocker propranolol to counteract this effect.
	Hypotension; arrhythmias; pulse irregularities	● Monitor vital signs two or three times a day. ● Physician may decrease dose of medication.
	Polyuria; dehydration	● May subside after initial week or two. ● Monitor daily intake and output and weight. ● Monitor skin turgor daily.
	Weight gain	● Provide instructions for reduced calorie diet. ● Emphasize importance of maintaining adequate intake of sodium.
	Drowsiness; dizziness	● Ensure that client does not operate dangerous machinery or participate in activities that require alertness.
Anticonvulsants		
Clonazepam (Klonopin)	Nausea/vomiting	● May give with food or milk to minimize GI upset.
Carbamazepine (Tegretol)	Blood dyscrasias	● Ensure that client understands the importance of regular blood tests while receiving anticonvulsant therapy.
Valproic acid (Depakene; Depakote)	Prolonged bleeding time (with valproic acid)	● Ensure that platelet counts and bleeding time are determined before initiation of therapy with valproic acid. Monitor for spontaneous bleeding or bruising.
Calcium Channel Blocker		
Verapamil (Calan; Isoptin)	Drowsiness; dizziness	● Ensure that client does not operate dangerous machinery or participate in activities that require alertness.
	Hypotension; bradycardia	● Take vital signs just before initiation of therapy and before daily administration of the medication. Physician will provide acceptable parameters for administration. Report marked changes immediately.
	Nausea	● May be given with food to minimize GI upset.
	Constipation	● Encourage increased fluid (if not contraindicated) and fiber in diet.

* Be aware of risks of becoming pregnant while receiving lithium therapy. Use information furnished by health care providers regarding methods of contraception. Notify the physician as soon as possible if pregnancy is suspected or planned.
* Be aware of side effects and symptoms associated with toxicity. Notify the physician if any of the following symptoms occur: persistent nausea and vomiting, severe diarrhea, ataxia, blurred vision, tinnitus, excessive output of urine, increasing tremors, or mental confusion.
* Refer to written materials furnished by health care providers while receiving self-administered mainte-

nance therapy. Keep appointments for outpatient follow-up; have serum lithium level checked every 1 to 2 months, or as advised by physician.

Client/Family Education (for Anticonvulsants). The client should:

* Not stop taking the drug abruptly. The Physician will administer orders for tapering the drug when therapy is to be discontinued.
* Report the following symptoms to the physician immediately: unusual bleeding, spontaneous bruising, sore throat, fever, malaise, dark urine, and yellow skin or eyes.

* Not drive or operate dangerous machinery until reaction to the medication has been established.
* Avoid consuming alcoholic beverages and nonprescription medications without approval from physician.
* Carry card at all times identifying the name of medications being taken.

Client/Family Education (for Calcium Channel Blocker). The client should:

* Take medication with meals if gastrointestinal (GI) upset occurs.
* Use caution when driving or when operating dangerous machinery. Dizziness, drowsiness, and blurred vision can occur.
* Not abruptly discontinue taking drug. To do so may precipitate cardiovascular problems.
* Report occurrence of any of the following symptoms to physician immediately: irregular heartbeat, shortness of breath, swelling of the hands and feet, pronounced dizziness, chest pain, profound mood swings, severe and persistent headache.
* Rise slowly from a sitting or lying position to prevent a sudden drop in blood pressure.
* Not consume other medications (including over-the-counter medications) without physician's approval.
* Carry card at all times describing medications being taken.

Outcome Criteria/Evaluation

The following criteria may be used for evaluating the effectiveness of therapy with antimanic agents:

THE CLIENT:

1. Is maintaining stability of mood.
2. Has not harmed self or others.
3. Has experienced no injury from hyperactivity.
4. Is able to participate in activities without excessive sedation or dizziness.
5. Is maintaining appropriate weight.
6. Exhibits no signs of lithium toxicity.
7. Verbalizes importance of taking medication regularly and reporting for regular laboratory blood tests.

Antipsychotics

Background Assessment Data

Indications. Antipsychotic drugs are also called *major tranquilizers* and *neuroleptics*. They are used in the treatment of acute and chronic psychoses, particularly when accompanied by increased psychomotor activity. Selected agents are used as antiemetics (chlorpromazine, per- phenazine, prochlorperazine) in the treatment of intractable hiccoughs (chlorpromazine, perphenazine) and for the control of tics and vocal utterances in Tourette's disorder (haloperidol, pimozide).

Examples of commonly used antipsychotic agents are presented in Table 19.8.

Action. The exact mechanism of action is not known. These drugs are thought to work by blocking postsynaptic dopamine receptors in the basal ganglia, hypothalamus, limbic system, brainstem, and medulla. Newer medications may exert antipsychotic properties by blocking action on receptors specific to dopamine, serotonin, and other neurotransmitters. Antipsychotic effects may also be related to inhibition of dopamine-mediated transmission of neural impulses at the synapses (see Chapter 4).

Contraindications/Precautions. These drugs are contraindicated in clients with known hypersensitivity (cross-sensitivity may exist among phenothiazines). They should not be used when CNS depression is evident, when blood dyscrasias exist, in clients with Parkinson's disease, or those with liver, renal, or cardiac insufficiency.

Caution should be taken in administering these drugs to clients who are elderly, severely ill, or debilitated and to diabetic clients or clients with respiratory insufficiency, prostatic hypertrophy, or intestinal obstruction. Antipsychotics may lower seizure threshold. Individuals should avoid exposure to extremes in temperature while taking antipsychotic medication. Safety in pregnancy and lactation has not been established.

Interactions. Additive anticholinergic effects are observed when antipsychotics are taken concurrently with other drugs that produce these properties (e.g., antihistamines, antidepressants, antiparkinsonian agents). Additive hypotensive effects may occur with beta-adrenergic blocking agents (e.g., propranolol, metoprolol). Antacids and antidiarrheals may decrease absorption of antipsychotics. Barbiturates may increase metabolism and decrease effectiveness of antipsychotics. Additive CNS depression can occur with alcohol, antihistamines, antidepressants, sedative-hypnotics, and anxiolytics.

Diagnosis

The following nursing diagnoses may be considered for clients receiving antipsychotic therapy:

1. Risk for violence directed at others related to panic anxiety and mistrust of others.
2. Risk for injury related to medication side effects of sedation, photosensitivity, reduction of seizure threshold, **agranulocytosis, extrapyramidal symptoms, tardive dyskinesia,** and **neuroleptic malignant syndrome.**
3. Risk for activity intolerance related to medication side effects of sedation, blurred vision, weakness.

TABLE 19.8 ANTIPSYCHOTIC AGENTS

CHEMICAL CLASS	GENERIC NAME	TRADE NAME	DOSAGE RANGE (MG/DAY)	AVAILABLE FORMS (MG)
Phenothiazines	Acetophenazine	Tindal	60–120 mg	tabs: 20
	Chlorpromazine	Thorazine	40–800 mg	tabs: 10, 25, 50, 100, 200 caps (SR): 30, 75, 150 syrup: 10/5 ml supp: 25, 100 conc: 30/ml, 100/ml inj: 25/ml
	Fluphenazine	Prolixin	1–40 mg	tabs: 1, 2.5, 5, 10 elixir: 0.5/ml conc: 5/ml inj: 2.5/ml inj (long-acting): 25/ml
	Mesoridazine	Serentil	30–400 mg	tabs: 10, 25, 50, 100 conc: 25/ml inj: 25/ml
	Perphenazine	Trilafon	12–64 mg	tabs: 2, 4, 8, 16 conc: 16/5 ml inj: 5/ml
	Prochlorperazine	Compazine	15–150 mg	tabs: 5, 10, 25 caps: 10, 15, 30 supp: 2.5, 5, 25 syrup: 5/5 ml inj: 5/ml
	Promazine	Sparine	40–1200 mg	tabs: 25, 50, 100 syrup: 10/5 ml inj: 25/ml, 50/ml
	~~Thioridazine~~ Duckboxed	~~Mellaril~~	150–800 mg	tabs: 10, 15, 25, 50, 100, 150, 200 conc: 30/ml, 100/ml susp: 25/5 ml, 100/5 ml
	Triflupromazine	Vesprin	60–150 mg	inj: 10/ml, 20/ml
Thioxanthene	Thiothixene	Navane	8–30 mg	caps: 1, 2, 5, 10, 20 conc: 5/ml inj: 2/ml, 5/ml
Benzisoxazole	Risperidone	Risperdal	4–6 mg	tabs: 1, 2, 3, 4
Butyrophenone	Haloperidol	Haldol	1–100 mg	tabs: 0.5, 1, 2, 5, 10, 20 conc: 2/ml inj: 5/ml inj (long-acting): 50/ml, 100/ml
Dibenzoxazepine	Loxapine	Loxitane	20–250 mg	caps: 5, 10, 25, 50 conc: 25/ml inj: 50/ml
Dihydroindolone	Molindone	Moban	15–225 mg	tabs: 5, 10, 25, 50, 100 conc: 20/ml
Dibenzodiazepine	Clozapine	Clozaril	300–900 mg	tabs: 25, 100
Thienobenzodiazepine	Olanzapine	Zyprexa	10–15 mg	tabs: 5, 7.5, 10
Dibenzothiazepine	Quetiapine	Seroquel	50–400 mg	tabs: 25, 100, 200

4. Noncompliance with medication regimen related to suspiciousness and mistrust of others.

Planning/Implementation

The plan of care should include monitoring for the following side effects from antipsychotic medications. Nursing implications related to each side effect are designated by an asterisk (*). A profile of side effects comparing various antipsychotic medications is presented in Table 19.9.

1. Anticholinergic effects
   a. Dry mouth
      * Provide the client with sugarless candy, ice, and frequent sips of water.
      * Ensure that the client practices strict oral hygiene.

TABLE 19.9   COMPARISON OF SIDE EFFECTS AMONG ANTIPSYCHOTIC AGENTS

Chemical Class	Generic Name	Trade Name	Side Effect Profiles*				
			Extrapyramidal Symptoms	Sedation	Anticholinergic	Orthostatic Hypotension	Seizures
Phenothiazines	Acetophenazine	Tindal	4	3	3	2	2
	Chlorpromazine	Thorazine	3	4	3	4	4
	Fluphenazine	Prolixin	5	2	2	2	2
	Mesoridazine	Serentil	2	4	4	4	2
	Perphenazine	Trilafon	4	2	2	2	3
	Prochlorperazine	Compazine	4	3	2	2	4
	Promazine	Sparine	3	3	4	3	4
	Thioridazine	Mellaril	2	4	4	4	1
	Triflupromazine	Vesprin	3	4	4	3	4
Thioxanthenes	Thiothixene	Navane	4	2	2	2	2
Benzisoxazole	Risperidone	Risperdal	1	1	1	3	1
Butyrophenone	Haloperidol	Haldol	5	1	1	1	1
Dibenzoxazepine	Loxapine	Loxitane	4	3	2	3	4
Dihydroindolone	Molindone	Moban	4	1	2	2	2
Dibenzodiazepine	Clozapine	Clozaril	1	5	5	4	4
Thienobenzodiazepine	Olanzapine	Zyprexa	1	3	2	1	1
Dibenzothiazepine	Quetiapine	Seroquel	1	3	2	1	1

*Key: 1 = Very low
2 = Low
3 = Moderate
4 = High
5 = Very high

SOURCE: Adapted from Puzantian & Stimmel (1994); *Facts and Comparisons* (1998); Marder (1997); and Jibson & Tandon (1996).

b. Blurred vision
  * Explain that symptom will most likely subside after a few weeks.
  * Advise client not to drive a car until vision clears.
  * Clear small items from pathway to prevent falls.
c. Constipation
  * Order foods high in fiber; encourage increase in physical activity and fluid intake if not contraindicated.
d. Urinary retention
  * Instruct client to report any difficulty urinating; monitor intake and output.

2. Nausea; GI upset
  * Tablets or capsules may be administered with food to minimize GI upset.
  * Concentrate forms may be diluted and administered with fruit juice or other liquid. They should be mixed immediately before administration.

3. Skin rash
  * Report appearance of any rash on skin to the physician.
  * Avoid spilling any of the liquid concentrate on skin; contact dermatitis can occur.

4. Sedation
  * Discuss with the physician the possibility of administering the drug at bedtime.
  * Discuss with the physician a possible decrease in dosage or an order for a less sedating drug. Instruct client not to drive or use dangerous equipment while experiencing sedation.

5. Orthostatic hypotension
  * Instruct the client to rise slowly from a lying or sitting position; monitor blood pressure (lying and standing) each shift; document and report significant changes.

6. Photosensitivity
  * Make sure that the client wears protective sunscreens, clothing, and sunglasses while spending time outdoors.

7. Hormonal effects
  a. Decreased libido; **retrograde ejaculation; gynecomastia** (men)
    * Provide an explanation of the effects and reassurance of their reversibility. If necessary, discuss with the physician the possibility of ordering an alternate medication.
  b. Amenorrhea (women)
    * Offer reassurance of reversibility, and instruct the client to continue the use of contraception, as **amenorrhea** does not indicate cessation of ovulation.
  c. Weight gain
    * Weigh client every other day; order calorie-controlled diet; provide opportunity for phys-

ical exercise; provide diet and exercise instruction.

8. Reduction of seizure threshold
  * Closely observe clients with history of seizures.
  * **NOTE:** This is particularly important with clients taking clozapine (Clozaril). Reportedly, seizures affect 1 to 5 percent of individuals who take this drug, depending on the dosage (Pokalo, 1991).

9. Agranulocytosis
  * Relatively rare with most of the antipsychotic drugs. It usually occurs within the first 3 months of treatment. Observe for symptoms of sore throat, fever, and malaise. A complete blood count should be monitored if these symptoms appear.
  * **EXCEPTION:** With clozapine (Clozaril), agranulocytosis occurs in 1 to 2 percent of all clients taking the drug (Pokalo, 1991). It is a potentially fatal blood disorder in which the client's white blood cell (WBC) count can drop to extremely low levels. Individuals receiving clozapine therapy are required to have blood levels drawn weekly to continue therapy. They are given a 1-week supply of medication at a time. If the WBC count falls below 3000 mm^3 or the granulocyte count falls below 1500 mm^3, clozapine therapy is discontinued. The disorder is reversible if discovered in the early stages. However, this additional required technology of weekly blood tests has made this drug cost prohibitive for some people.

10. Salivation (with clozapine)
  * A significant number of clients receiving clozapine (Clozaril) therapy experience extreme salivation. Offer support to the client, as this may be an embarrassing situation. It may even be a safety issue (e.g., risk of aspiration), if the problem is very severe.

11. Extrapyramidal symptoms
  * Observe for symptoms and report; administer antiparkinsonian drugs, as ordered (Table 19.10).
  a. Pseudoparkinsonism (tremor, shuffling gait, drooling, rigidity)
    * Symptoms may appear 1 to 5 days following initiation of antipsychotic medication. They occur most often in women, the elderly, and dehydrated clients.
  b. **Akinesia** (muscular weakness)
    * Same as above.
  c. **Akathisia** (continuous restlessness and fidgeting)
    * This occurs most frequently in women; symptoms may occur 50 to 60 days following initiation of therapy.

TABLE 19.10 ANTIPARKINSONIAN AGENTS USED TO TREAT EXTRAPYRAMIDAL SIDE EFFECTS OF ANTIPSYCHOTIC DRUGS

Indication	Used to treat parkinsonism of various causes and drug-induced extrapyramidal reactions.
Action	Restores the natural balance of acetylcholine and dopamine in the CNS. The imbalance is a deficiency in dopamine that results in excessive cholinergic activity.
Contraindications/ Precautions	Antiparkinsonian agents are contraindicated in individuals with hypersensitivity. Anticholinergics should be avoided by individuals with angle-closure glaucoma; pyloric, duodenal, or bladder neck obstructions; prostatic hypertrophy; or myasthenia gravis. Caution should be used in administering these drugs to clients with hepatic, renal, or cardiac insufficiency; elderly and debilitated clients; those with a tendency toward urinary retention; or those exposed to high environmental temperatures.
Common side effects	Anticholinergic effects (dry mouth, blurred vision, constipation, paralytic ileus, urinary retention, tachycardia, elevated temperature, decreased sweating), nausea/GI upset, sedation, dizziness, orthostatic hypotension, exacerbation of psychoses.

Chemical Class	Generic (Trade) Name	Daily Dosage Range	Available Forms (mg)
Anticholinergics	Benztropine (Cogentin)	0.5–6 mg	tabs: 0.5, 1, 2; inj: 1/ml
	Biperiden (Akineton)	2–8 mg	tabs: 2; inj: 5/ml
	Ethopropazine (Parsidol)	50–600 mg	tabs: 10, 50
	Procyclidine (Kemadrin)	5–20 mg	tabs: 5
	Trihexyphenidyl (Artane)	1–15 mg	tabs: 2, 5; elixir: 2/5 ml
Antihistamines	Diphenhydramine (Benadryl)	75–200 mg	tabs/caps: 25, 50; elixir: 12.5/5 ml inj: 10/ml, 50/ml
Dopaminergic agonists	Amantadine (Symmetrel)	100–300 mg	caps: 100; syrup: 50/5 ml
	Bromocriptine (Parlodel)	2.5–100 mg	tabs: 2.5; caps: 5

d. **Dystonia** (involuntary muscular movements [spasms] of face, arms, legs, and neck)
   * This occurs most often in men and in clients younger than 25 years of age.
e. **Oculogyric crisis** (uncontrolled rolling back of the eyes)
   * This may appear as part of the syndrome described as dystonia. It may be mistaken for seizure activity. Dystonia and oculogyric crisis should be treated as an emergency situation. The physician should be contacted, and intravenous benztropine mesylate (Cogentin) is commonly administered. Stay with the client and offer reassurance and support during this frightening time.
12. Tardive dyskinesia (bizarre facial and tongue movements, stiff neck, and difficulty swallowing)
   * All clients receiving long-term (months or years) antipsychotic therapy are at risk.
   * Symptoms are potentially irreversible.
   * Drug should be withdrawn at the first sign, which is usually vermiform movements of the tongue; prompt action may prevent irreversibility.
13. Neuroleptic malignant syndrome
   * This is a rare, but potentially fatal, complication of treatment with neuroleptic drugs. Routine assessments should include temperature and observation for parkinsonian symptoms.
   * Onset can occur within hours or even years after

drug initiation, and progression is rapid over the following 24 to 72 hours.
   * Symptoms include severe parkinsonian muscle rigidity, hyperpyrexia up to 107°F, tachycardia, tachypnea, fluctuations in blood pressure, diaphoresis, and rapid deterioration of mental status to stupor and coma.
   * Discontinue neuroleptic medication immediately.
   * Monitor vital signs, degree of muscle rigidity, intake and output, and level of consciousness.
   * The physician may order bromocriptine (Parlodel) or dantrolene (Dantrium) to counteract the effects of neuroleptic malignant syndrome.

Client/Family Education. The client should:

* Use caution when driving or operating dangerous machinery. Drowsiness and dizziness can occur.
* Not stop taking the drug abruptly after long-term use. To do so might produce withdrawal symptoms such as nausea, vomiting, gastritis, headache, tachycardia, insomnia, and tremulousness.
* Use sunscreens and wear protective clothing when spending time outdoors. Skin is more susceptible to sunburn, which can occur in as few as 30 minutes.
* Report weekly (if receiving clozapine therapy) to have blood levels drawn and to obtain a weekly supply of the drug.
* Report the occurrence of any of the following symptoms to physician immediately: sore throat, fever,

malaise, unusual bleeding, easy bruising, persistent nausea/vomiting, severe headache, rapid heart rate, difficulty urinating, muscle twitching, tremors, darkly colored urine, pale stools, yellow skin or eyes, muscular incoordination, skin rash, or seizures.

* Rise slowly from a sitting or lying position to prevent a sudden drop in blood pressure.

* Take frequent sips of water, chew sugarless gum, or suck on hard candy if dry mouth is a problem. Good oral care (frequent brushing, flossing) is very important.

* Consult the physician regarding smoking while receiving neuroleptic therapy. Smoking increases the metabolism of neuroleptics, requiring an adjustment in dosage to achieve a therapeutic effect.

* Dress warmly in cold weather and avoid extended exposure to very high or low temperatures. Body temperature is harder to maintain with this medication.

* Not drink alcohol while receiving neuroleptic therapy. These drugs potentiate each other's effects.

* Not consume other medications (including over-the-counter medications) without the physician's approval. Many medications contain substances that interact with neuroleptics in a way that may be harmful.

* Be aware of possible risks of taking neuroleptics during pregnancy. Safe use during pregnancy and lactation has not been established. Neuroleptics are thought to readily cross the placental barrier; if so, a fetus could experience adverse effects of the drug. The client should inform the physician immediately if pregnancy occurs, is suspected, or is planned.

* Be aware of side effects of neuroleptic drugs. Refer to written materials furnished by health care providers for safe self-administration.

* Continue to take the medication, even if feeling well and as though it is not needed. Symptoms may return if medication is discontinued.

* Carry card or other identification at all times describing medications being taken.

Outcome Criteria/Evaluation

The following criteria may be used for evaluating the effectiveness of therapy with antipsychotic medications.

THE CLIENT:

1. Has not harmed others.
2. Has not experienced injury caused by side effects of lowered seizure threshold or photosensitivity.
3. Maintains a WBC within normal limits.
4. Exhibits no symptoms of extrapyramidal side effects, tardive dyskinesia, or neuroleptic malignant syndrome.
5. Maintains weight within normal limits.
6. Tolerates activity unaltered by the effects of sedation or weakness.
7. Takes medication willingly.
8. Verbalizes understanding of medication regimen and the importance of regular administration.

Sedative-Hypnotics

Background Assessment Data

Indications. Sedative-hypnotics are used in the short-term management of various anxiety states and to treat insomnia. Selected agents are used as anticonvulsants and preoperative sedatives (phenobarbital, pentobarbital, secobarbital) and to reduce anxiety associated with drug withdrawal (chloral hydrate).

Examples of commonly used sedative-hypnotics are presented in Table 19.11.

Action. Sedative-hypnotics cause generalized CNS depression. They may produce tolerance with chronic use and have the potential for psychological or physical dependence.

Contraindications/Precautions. Sedative-hypnotics are contraindicated in individuals with hypersensitivity to the drug or to any drug within the chemical class.

Caution should be used in administering these drugs to clients with hepatic dysfunction or severe renal impairment. They should be used with caution in clients who may be suicidal or who may have been addicted to drugs previously. Hypnotic use should be short term. Elderly clients may be more sensitive to CNS depressant effects, and dosage reduction may be required.

Interactions. Additive CNS depression can occur when sedative-hypnotics are taken concomitantly with alcohol, antihistamines, antidepressants, phenothiazines, or any other CNS depressants. Barbiturates induce hepatic drug-metabolizing enzymes and can decrease the effectiveness of drugs metabolized by the liver. Sedative-hypnotics should not be used with MAOIs.

Diagnosis

The following nursing diagnoses may be considered for clients receiving therapy with sedative hypnotics:

1. Risk for injury related to abrupt withdrawal from long-term use or decreased mental alertness caused by residual sedation.
2. Sleep pattern disturbance related to situational crises, physical condition, or severe level of anxiety.
3. Risk for activity intolerance related to side effects of lethargy, drowsiness, dizziness.
4. Risk for acute confusion related to action of the medication on the central nervous system.

▰ TABLE 19.11 SEDATIVE-HYPNOTIC AGENTS

CHEMICAL GROUP	GENERIC (TRADE) NAME	DAILY DOSAGE RANGE	CONTROLLED CATEGORIES	HALF-LIFE (HR)	AVAILABLE FORMS (MG)
Barbiturates	Amobarbital (Amytal)	60–200 mg	CII	14–42	inj: powder, 250/vial, 500/vial
	Aprobarbital (Alurate)	60–200 mg	CIII	14–34	elixir: 40/5 ml
	Butabarbital (Butisol)	45–100 mg	CIII	66–140	tabs: 15, 30, 50, 100 elixir: 30/5 ml
	Pentobarbital (Nembutal)	60–100 mg	CII	15–50	caps: 50, 100 supp: 30, 60, 120, 200 inj: 50/ml
	Phenobarbital (Luminal)	30–320 mg	CIV	53–118	tabs: 15, 16, 30, 60, 100 caps: 16 elixir: 15/5 ml; 20/5 ml inj mg/ml: 30, 60, 65, 130
	Secobarbital (Seconal)	100–300 mg	CII	15–40	caps: 100 inj: 50/ml
Benzodiazepines	Estazolam (ProSom)	1–2 mg	CIV	10–24	tabs: 1, 2
	Flurazepam (Dalmane)	15–30 mg	CIV	40–150	caps: 15, 30
	Quazepam (Doral)	7.5–15 mg	CIV	25–41	tabs: 7.5, 15
	Temazepam (Restoril)	15–30 mg	CIV	10–15	caps: 7.5, 15, 30
	Triazolam (Halcion)	0.25–0.5 mg	CIV	1.5–5	tabs: 0.125, 0.25
Miscellaneous	Chloral hydrate (Noctec)	500–1000 mg	CIV	8	caps: 500 syrup: 250/5 ml; 500/5 ml supp: 324, 500, 648
	Ethchlorvynol (Placidyl)	250–500 mg	CIV	10–20	caps: 200, 500, 750
	Glutethimide (Doriden)	250–500 mg	CII	10–12	tabs: 250
	Methyprylon (Noludar)	200–400 mg	CIII	13–61	tabs: 50 caps: 300
	Zolpidem (Ambien)	5–10 mg	CIV	2–3	tabs: 5, 10

Planning/Implementation

Refer to this section in the discussion of antianxiety medications.

Outcome Criteria/Evaluation

The following criteria may be used for evaluating the effectiveness of therapy with sedative-hypnotic medications:

THE CLIENT:

1. Demonstrates a reduction in anxiety, tension, and restless activity.
2. Falls asleep within 30 minutes of taking the medication and remains asleep for 6 to 8 hours without interruption.
3. Is able to participate in usual activities without residual sedation.
4. Experiences no physical injury.
5. Exhibits no evidence of confusion.
6. Verbalizes understanding of taking the medication on a short-term basis.
7. Verbalizes understanding of potential for development of tolerance and dependence with long-term use.

Central Nervous System Stimulants

Background Assessment Data

Indications. CNS stimulants are used in the management of narcolepsy, attention-deficit disorder with hyperactivity in children, and as adjunctive therapy to caloric restriction in the treatment of exogenous obesity.

Examples of commonly used CNS stimulants are presented in Table 19.12.

Action. CNS stimulants increase levels of neurotransmitters (probably norepinephrine, dopamine, and serotonin) in the CNS. They produce CNS and respiratory stimulation, dilated pupils, increased motor activity and mental alertness, diminished sense of fatigue, and brighter spirits.

Contraindications/Precautions. CNS stimulants are contraindicated in individuals with hypersensitivity to sympathomimetic amines. They should not be used in advanced arteriosclerosis, symptomatic cardiovascular disease, hypertension, hyperthyroidism, glaucoma, agitated or hyperexcitability states, in clients with a history of drug abuse, during or within 14 days of receiving therapy with MAOIs, in children under 3 years of age, and in pregnancy.

Caution is advised in using CNS stimulants during lactation; with psychotic children; in Tourette's disorder; in

▰ TABLE 19.12   CNS STIMULANTS

CHEMICAL GROUP	GENERIC (TRADE) NAME	DAILY DOSAGE RANGE	CONTROLLED CATEGORIES	AVAILABLE FORMS (MG)
Amphetamines	Amphetamine sulfate	5–60 mg	CII	tabs: 5, 10
	Dextroamphetamine sulfate (Dexedrine)	5–60 mg	CII	tabs: 5, 10 caps (SR): 5, 10, 15
	Methamphetamine (Desoxyn)	5–25 mg	CII	tabs: 5 tabs (LA): 5, 10, 15
Anorexigenics	Benzphetamine (Didrex)	25–150 mg	CIII	tabs: 25, 50
	Diethylpropion (Tenuate)	75–100 mg	CIV	tabs: 25 tabs (SR): 75
	Mazindol (Mazanor)	1–3 mg	CIV	tabs: 1, 2
	Phendimetrazine (Prelu-2)	35–105 mg	CIII	tabs/caps: 35 caps (SR): 105
	Phentermine (Fastin)	15–37.5 mg	CIV	tabs: 8, 30, 37.5 caps: 15, 18.75, 30, 37.5
Miscellaneous	Methylphenidate (Ritalin)	10–60 mg	CII	tabs: 5, 10, 20 tabs (SR): 20
	Pemoline (Cylert)	37.5–112.5 mg	CIV	tabs: 18.75, 37.5, 75

SR = sustained-release or slow-release; LA = long-acting.

clients with anorexia or insomnia; in elderly, debilitated, or asthenic clients; and in clients with a history of suicidal or homicidal tendencies. Prolonged use may result in tolerance and physical or psychological dependence.

Interactions. Use of CNS stimulants within 14 days following administration of MAOIs may result in hypertensive crisis, headache, hyperpyrexia, intracranial hemorrhage, and bradycardia. Insulin requirements may be altered with CNS stimulants. Urine alkalinizers decrease excretion, enhancing the effects of amphetamines; urine acidifiers increase excretion, decreasing the effects. Decreased effects of both drugs can occur when administered concurrently with phenothiazines.

Diagnosis

The following nursing diagnoses may be considered for clients receiving therapy with CNS stimulants:

1. Risk for injury related to overstimulation and hyperactivity.
2. Risk for self-directed violence related to abrupt withdrawal after extended use.
3. Altered in nutrition less than body requirements related to side effects of anorexia and weight loss.
4. Altered in nutrition more than body requirements related to excess intake in relation to metabolic needs.
5. Sleep pattern disturbance related to overstimulation resulting from use of the medication.

Planning/Implementation

The plan of care should include monitoring for the following side effects from CNS stimulants. Nursing impli-

cations related to each side effect are designated by an asterisk (*).

1. Overstimulation, restlessness, insomnia
   * Assess mental status for changes in mood, level of activity, degree of stimulation, and aggressiveness.
   * Ensure that the client is protected from injury.
   * Keep stimuli low and environment as quiet as possible to discourage overstimulation.
   * To prevent insomnia, administer the last dose at least 6 hours before bedtime. Administer sustained-release forms in the morning.
2. Palpitations, tachycardia
   * Monitor and record vital signs at regular intervals (two or three times a day) throughout therapy. Report significant changes to the physician immediately.
3. Anorexia, weight loss
   * If this drug is being taken by children with behavior disorders (and not as an anorexigenic): To reduce anorexia, the medication may be administered immediately after meals. The client should be weighed regularly (at least weekly) during hospitalization and at home while receiving therapy with CNS stimulants because of the potential for anorexia/weight loss and temporary interruption of growth and development.
4. Tolerance, physical and psychological dependence
   * Tolerance develops rapidly. If anorexigenic effects begin to diminish, the client should notify the physician immediately. The client should be on reduced-calorie diet and program of regular exercise in addition to the medication.
   * In children with behavior disorders, a drug "holi-

day" should be attempted periodically under direction of the physician to determine the effectiveness of the medication and the need for continuation.

* The drug should not be withdrawn abruptly. To do so could initiate the following syndrome of symptoms: nausea, vomiting, abdominal cramping, headache, fatigue, weakness, mental depression, suicidal ideation, increased dreaming, and psychotic behavior.

Client/Family Education. The client should:

* Use caution in driving or operating dangerous machinery. Drowsiness, dizziness, and blurred vision can occur.
* Not stop taking the drug abruptly. To do so could produce serious withdrawal symptoms.
* Avoid taking medication late in the day to prevent insomnia. Take no later than 6 hours before bedtime.
* Not take other medications (including over-the-counter drugs) without physician's approval. Many medications contain substances that, in combination with CNS stimulants, can be harmful.
* Diabetic clients should monitor blood sugar two or three times a day or as instructed by the physician. Be aware of need for possible alteration in insulin requirements owing to changes in food intake, weight, and activity.
* Avoid consumption of large amounts of caffeinated products (coffee, tea, colas, chocolate), as they may enhance the stimulant effect of these medications.
* Follow a reduced-calorie diet provided by the dietitian, as well as a program of regular exercise. Do not exceed the recommended dose if the appetite suppressant effect diminishes. Contact the physician.
* Notify physician if restlessness, insomnia, anorexia, or dry mouth become severe or if rapid, pounding heartbeat becomes evident.
* Be aware of possible risks of taking CNS stimulants during pregnancy. Safe use during pregnancy and lactation has not been established. Inform the physician immediately if pregnancy is suspected or planned.
* Be aware of potential side effects of CNS stimulants. Refer to written materials furnished by health care providers for safe self-administration.
* Carry a card or other identification at all times describing medications being taken.

Outcome Criteria/Evaluation

The following criteria may be used for evaluating the effectiveness of therapy with CNS stimulants.

The client:

1. Does not exhibit excessive hyperactivity.
2. (The overweight client) is losing a safe 2 lb per week.
3. Has not experienced injury.
4. (The behavior disorder client) is maintaining expected parameters of growth and development.
5. Verbalizes understanding of safe self-administration and the importance of not withdrawing medication abruptly.

SUMMARY

Psychotropic medications are intended to be used as adjunctive therapy to individual or group psychotherapy. *Antianxiety agents* are used in the treatment of anxiety disorders and to alleviate acute anxiety symptoms. The benzodiazepines are the most commonly used group. They are CNS depressants and have a potential for physical and psychological dependence. They should not be discontinued abruptly following long-term use, as they can produce a life-threatening withdrawal syndrome. The most common side effects are drowsiness, confusion, and lethargy.

Antidepressants elevate mood and alleviate other symptoms associated with moderate-to-severe depression. These drugs work to increase the concentration of norepinephrine and serotonin in the body. The tricyclics and related drugs accomplish this by blocking the reuptake of these chemicals by the neurons. Another group of antidepressants inhibit MAO, an enzyme that is known to inactivate norepinephrine and serotonin. They are called MAO inhibitors. A third category of drugs block neuronal reuptake of serotonin and have minimal or no effect on reuptake of norepinephrine or dopamine. They are called selective serotonin reuptake inhibitors (SSRIs). Antidepressant medications may take up to 4 weeks to produce the desired effect. The most common side effects are anticholinergic effects, sedation, and orthostatic hypotension. They also reduce the seizure threshold. MAO inhibitors can cause hypertensive crisis if products containing tyramine are consumed while taking these medications.

The *antimanic agent* of choice is lithium carbonate. Its mechanism of action is not fully understood, but it is thought to enhance the reuptake of norepinephrine and serotonin in the brain, thereby lowering the levels in the body, resulting in decreased hyperactivity. The most common side effects are dry mouth, GI upset, polyuria, and weight gain. There is a very narrow margin between the therapeutic and toxic levels of lithium. Serum levels must be drawn regularly to monitor for toxicity. Symptoms of lithium toxicity begin to appear at serum levels of approximately 1.5 mEq/l. If left untreated, lithium toxicity can be life-threatening.

Several other medications are being used for stabilizing mood. Two groups, anticonvulsants (carbamazepine, clonazepam, and valproic acid) and the calcium channel blocker, verapamil, have been used with some effectiveness. Their action in the treatment of bipolar mania is not known.

Antipsychotic drugs are used in the treatment of acute and chronic psychoses. Their action is unknown but is thought to decrease the activity of dopamine in the brain. The phenothiazines are the most commonly used group. Their most common side effects include anticholinergic effects, sedation, weight gain, reduction in seizure threshold, photosensitivity, and extrapyramidal symptoms. A newer generation of antipsychotic medications, which includes clozapine, risperidone, olanzapine, and quetiapine, may have an effect on dopamine, serotonin, and other neurotransmitters. They show promise of greater efficacy with fewer side effects.

Antiparkinsonian agents are used to counteract the extrapyramidal symptoms associated with antipsychotic medications. Antiparkinsonian drugs work to restore the natural balance of acetylcholine and dopamine in the brain. The most common side effects of these drugs are the anticholinergic effects. They may also cause sedation and orthostatic hypotension.

Sedative-hypnotics are used in the management of anxiety states and to treat insomnia. These CNS depressants have the potential for physical and psychological dependence. They are indicated for short-term use only. Side effects and nursing implications are similar to those described for antianxiety medications.

CNS stimulants are prescribed for attention-deficit disorder with hyperactivity, narcolepsy, and endogenous obesity. These drugs have the potential for physical and psychological dependence. Tolerance develops quickly, and they should not be withdrawn abruptly, as they can produce serious withdrawal symptoms. The most common side effects are restlessness, anorexia, and insomnia.

REVIEW QUESTIONS

SELF-EXAMINATION/LEARNING EXERCISE

Select the answer that is most appropriate for each of the following questions.

1. Antianxiety medications produce a calming effect by:
   a. Depressing the CNS.
   b. Decreasing levels of norepinephrine and serotonin in the brain.
   c. Decreasing levels of dopamine in the brain.
   d. Inhibiting production of the enzyme MAO.

2. Nancy has a new diagnosis of panic disorder. Dr. S has written a p.r.n. order for alprazolam (Xanax) for when Nancy is feeling anxious. She says to the nurse, "Dr. S prescribed buspirone for my friend's anxiety. Why did he order something different for me?" The nurse's answer is based on which of the following?
   a. Buspirone is not an antianxiety medication.
   b. Alprazolam and buspirone are essentially the same medication, so either one is appropriate.
   c. Buspirone has delayed onset of action and cannot be used on a p.r.n. basis.
   d. Alprazolam is the only medication that really works for panic disorder.

3. Education for the client who is taking MAOIs should include which of the following?
   a. Fluid and sodium replacement when appropriate, frequent drug blood levels, signs and symptoms of toxicity.
   b. Lifetime of continuous use, possible tardive dyskinesia, advantages of an injection every 2 to 4 weeks.
   c. Short-term use, possible tolerance to beneficial effects, careful tapering of the drug at end of treatment.
   d. Tyramine-restricted diet, prohibitive concurrent use of over-the-counter medications without physician notification.

4. There is a very narrow margin between the therapeutic and toxic levels of lithium carbonate. Symptoms of toxicity are most likely to appear if the serum levels exceed
   a. 0.15 mEq/l.
   b. 1.5 mEq/l.
   c. 15.0 mEq/l.
   d. 150 mEq/l.

5. Initial symptoms of lithium toxicity include:
   a. Constipation, dry mouth, drowsiness, oliguria.
   b. Dizziness, thirst, dysuria, arrhythmias.
   c. Ataxia, tinnitus, blurred vision, diarrhea.
   d. Fatigue, vertigo, anuria, weakness.

6. Antipsychotic medications are thought to decrease psychotic symptoms by:
   a. Blocking reuptake of norepinephrine and serotonin.
   b. Blocking the action of dopamine in the brain.
   c. Inhibiting production of the enzyme MAO.
   d. Depressing the CNS.

7. Part of the nurse's continual assessment of the client taking antipsychotic medications is to observe for extrapyramidal symptoms. Examples include:
   a. Muscular weakness, rigidity, tremors, facial spasms.
   b. Dry mouth, blurred vision, urinary retention, orthostatic hypotension.
   c. Amenorrhea, gynecomastia, retrograde ejaculation.
   d. Elevated blood pressure, severe occipital headache, stiff neck.

8. If the foregoing extrapyramidal symptoms should occur, which of the following would be a priority nursing intervention?

    a. Notify the physician immediately.
    b. Administer p.r.n. trihexyphenidyl (Artane).
    c. Withhold the next dose of antipsychotic medication.
    d. Explain to the client that these symptoms are only temporary and will disappear shortly.

9. Carol has been taking fenfluramine (Pondimin) for 12 weeks. She has lost 25 lb and wants to lose 75 more. She says to the nurse, "This medication isn't helping anymore. It doesn't curb my appetite like it did at first. I'm afraid I'm going to start gaining weight again." The most appropriate response by the nurse is:

    a. "Go ahead and stop the medication if you feel it isn't helping."
    b. "You must be eating more than your diet allows if you aren't losing weight."
    c. "Continue to take the medication as prescribed and come in to see the physician as soon as you can."
    d. "Try doubling the dose and see if that helps."

10. The rationale for the correct answer in question 9 is:

    a. The client should not take medication purposelessly.
    b. Anorexigenics do not work without diet and exercise.
    c. The drug must be tapered to prevent serious withdrawal symptoms.
    d. Some individuals require higher dosages than others to achieve the desired effect.

REFERENCES

Bernstein, J.G. (1995). *Handbook of drug therapy in psychiatry* (3rd ed.). St. Louis: Mosby.

Burgess, A.W. (1985). *Psychiatric nursing in the hospital and the community* (4th ed.). Englewood Cliffs, NJ: Prentice-Hall.

Depression Guideline Panel. (1993). *Depression in primary care: Vol. 2. Treatment of major depression. Clinical practice guideline, No. 5.* Rockville, MD: U.S. Department of Health and Human Services, Public Health Service, Agency for Health Care Policy and Research. AHCPR Pub. No. 93-0551.

Facts and comparisons. (1998). St. Louis: Wolters Kluwer.

Gerald, M.C., & O'Bannon, F.V. (1988). *Nursing pharmacology and therapeutics* (2nd ed.). Norwalk, CT: Appleton & Lange.

Kurtz, N.M., & Robinson, D.S. (1988). Monoamine oxidase inhibitors. In A. Georgotas & R. Cancro (Eds.), *Depression and mania.* New York: Elsevier Science Publishing.

Jibson, M.D., & Tandon, R. (1996). A summary of research findings on the new antipsychotic drugs. *The Psychiatric Nursing Forum, 2*: i–viii.

Marder, S.R. (1997, May). Comparative data on newer antipsychotic drugs. *Current Approaches to Psychoses, 6*: 2–4.

Pokalo, C.L. (1991). Clozapine: Benefits and controversies. *Journal of Psychosocial Nursing, 29*(2), 33–36.

Puzantian, T., & Stimmel, G.L. (1994). *Review of psychotropic drugs.* New York: The McMahon Group.

Sage, D.L. (Producer) (1984). *The Brain: Madness.* Washington, DC: Public Broadcasting System.

Townsend, M.C. (1995). *Drug guide for psychiatric nursing* (2nd ed.). Philadelphia: F.A. Davis.

Bibliography

Bowden, C. (1996, Spring). The efficacy of divalproex sodium and lithium in the treatment of acute mania. *The Psychiatric Nursing Forum, 2*: i–viii.

Davis, K.M., & Matthew, E. (1998). Pharmacologic management of depression in the elderly. *The Nurse Practitioner, 23*(6): 16–45.

Drug Watch. (1998). How ethnicity and culture affect antipsychotic response. *American Journal of Nursing, 98*(5): 56.

Glod, C.A. (1997). Factors in antidepressant selection: Sorting out the issues. *APNA News, 9*(3): 3.

Hanrahan, N. (1997) Case study of movement disorders associated with antipsychotic medications. *APNA News, 9*(3): 2.

Preston, J., & Johnson, J. (1997). *Clinical psychopharmacology made ridiculously simple* (3rd ed.). Miami, FL: MedMaster, Inc.

Townsend, M.C. (1997). *Nursing diagnoses in psychiatric nursing: A pocket guide for care plan construction* (4th ed.). Philadelphia: F.A. Davis.

ELECTROCONVULSIVE THERAPY

CHAPTER OUTLINE

OBJECTIVES

INTRODUCTION

ELECTROCONVULSIVE THERAPY, DEFINED

HISTORICAL PERSPECTIVES

INDICATIONS

CONTRAINDICATIONS

MECHANISM OF ACTION

SIDE EFFECTS

RISKS ASSOCIATED WITH ELECTROCONVULSIVE THERAPY

THE ROLE OF THE NURSE IN ELECTROCONVULSIVE THERAPY

SUMMARY

REVIEW QUESTIONS

KEY TERMS

electroconvulsive therapy

insulin coma therapy

pharmacoconvulsive therapy

OBJECTIVES

After reading this chapter, the student will be able to:

1. Define *electroconvulsive therapy*.
2. Discuss historical perspectives related to electroconvulsive therapy.
3. Discuss indications, contraindications, mechanism of action, and side effects of electroconvulsive therapy.
4. Identify risks associated with electroconvulsive therapy.
5. Describe the role of the nurse in the administration of electroconvulsive therapy.

lectroconvulsive therapy (ECT) has had very bad press. In the movie *One Flew Over the Cuckoo's Nest*, it is depicted as a physically and emotionally brutal procedure imposed on unwilling clients in order to calm them. Today, ECT remains one of the most controversial treatments for psychological disorders and continues to be the subject of impassioned debate among various factions of society, within both the professional and lay communities.

Despite its controversial image, ECT has been used continuously for more than 50 years, longer than any other physical treatment available for mental illness. It has achieved this longevity because when administered properly, for the right illness, it can help as much as or more than any other treatment (Sackeim, 1985).

This chapter explores the historical perspectives, indications and contraindications, mechanism of action, side effects, and risks associated with ECT. The role of the nurse in the care of the client receiving ECT is presented in the context of the nursing process.

ELECTROCONVULSIVE THERAPY, DEFINED

Electroconvulsive therapy is the induction of a grand mal (generalized) seizure through the application of electrical current to the brain. The stimulus is applied through electrodes that are placed either bilaterally in the frontotemporal region or unilaterally on the same side as the dominant hand (American Psychiatric Association [APA], 1990). Controversy exists over optimal placement of the electrodes in terms of possible greater efficacy, with bilateral placement versus the potential in some clients for less confusion and acute amnesia with unilateral placement.

The amount of electrical stimulus applied is a point of controversy among clinicians. Dose of stimulation is based upon the client's seizure threshold, which is highly variable among individuals. The duration of the seizure should be at least 25 seconds (Kaplan & Sadock, 1998). Movements are very minimal owing to the administration of a muscle relaxant before the treatment. The tonic phase of the seizure usually lasts 10 to 15 seconds and may be identified by a rigid plantar extension of the feet. The clonic phase follows and is usually characterized by rhythmic movements of the muscles that decrease in frequency and finally disappear. Because of the muscle relaxant, movements may be observed merely as a rhythmic twitching of the toes.

Most clients require an average of 6 to 12 treatments, but some may require up to 20 treatments (Kaplan & Sadock, 1998). Treatments are usually administered every other day, three times per week. Treatments are performed on an inpatient basis for those who require close observation and care (e.g., clients who are suicidal, agitated, delusional, catatonic, or acutely manic). Those at less risk may have the option of receiving therapy at an outpatient treatment facility.

HISTORICAL PERSPECTIVES

The first electroconvulsive therapy treatment was performed in April 1938 by Italian psychiatrists Ugo Cerletti and Lucio Bini in Rome. Other somatic therapies had been tried before that time, in particular **insulin coma therapy** and **pharmacoconvulsive therapy.**

Insulin coma therapy was introduced by the German psychiatrist Manfred Sakel in 1933. His therapy was used for clients with schizophrenia. The insulin injection treatments would induce a hypoglycemic coma, which Sakel claimed was effective in alleviating schizophrenic symptoms. This therapy required vigorous medical and nursing intervention through the stages of induced coma. Some fatalities occurred when clients failed to respond to efforts directed at termination of the coma. The efficacy of insulin coma therapy has been questioned, and its use has been discontinued in the treatment of mental illness.

Pharmacoconvulsive therapy was introduced in Budapest in 1934 by Ladislas Meduna (Endler & Persad, 1988). He induced convulsions with intramuscular injections of camphor in oil in clients with schizophrenia. He based his treatment on clinical observation and on his theory that there was a biological antagonism between schizophrenia and epilepsy. Thus, by inducing seizures he hoped to reduce schizophrenic symptoms. Because he discovered that camphor was unreliable for inducing seizures, he began using pentylenetetrazol (Cardiazol/Metrazol). Some successes were reported in terms of reduction of psychotic symptoms, and, until the advent of ECT in 1938, pentylenetetrazol was the most frequently used procedure for producing seizures in psychotic clients. There was a brief resurgence of pharmacoconvulsive therapy in the late 1950s, when flurothyl (Indoklon), a potent inhalant convulsant, was introduced as an alternative for individuals who were unwilling to consent to ECT for the treatment of depression and schizophrenia (Cherkin, 1974). Pharmacoconvulsive therapy is no longer used in psychiatry.

Periodic recognition of the important contribution of ECT in the treatment of mental illness has been evident in the United States. An initial acceptance was observed from 1940 to 1955, followed by a 20-year period in which ECT was considered objectionable by both the psychiatric profession and the lay public. A second wave of acceptance began around 1975 and has been increasing to the present. The period of nonacceptability coincided with the introduction of tricyclic and monoamine oxidase inhibitor antidepressant drugs and ended with the realization among many psychiatrists that the widely heralded replacement of ECT with these chemical agents had failed to materialize (Abrams, 1988). Some individuals showed improvement with ECT after failing to respond to other forms of therapy.

An estimated 50,000 to 100,000 people per year receive ECT treatments in the United States. The typical client is white, female, middle-aged and from a middle- to upper-income background, receiving treatment in a private or university hospital for major depression, usually after drug therapy has proved ineffective. Largely because of the expense involved, as well as the need for a team of highly skilled medical specialists, many public hospitals are not able to offer this service to their clients.

INDICATIONS

Major Depression

Electroconvulsive therapy has been shown to be effective in the treatment of severe depression. It appears to be particularly effective in depressed clients who are also experiencing psychotic symptoms and those with psychomotor retardation and neurovegetative changes, such as disturbances in sleep, appetite, and energy. These symptoms would be associated with the diagnoses of major depressive disorder, major depressive disorder with psychotic or melancholic symptoms, and bipolar disorder depression (Kaplan & Sadock, 1998). Electroconvulsive therapy is not often used as the treatment of choice for depressive disorders but is considered only after a trial of therapy with antidepressant medication has proved ineffective.

Mania

Electroconvulsive therapy is also indicated in the treatment of acute manic episodes of bipolar affective disorder (Endler & Persad, 1988). At present it is rarely used for this purpose, having been superseded by the widespread use of antipsychotic drugs and/or lithium. However, it has been shown to be effective in the treatment of manic clients who do not tolerate or fail to respond to lithium or other drug treatment, or when life is threatened by dangerous behavior or exhaustion.

Schizophrenia

Electroconvulsive therapy can induce a remission in some clients who present with acute schizophrenia, particularly if it is accompanied by catatonic or affective (depression or mania) symptomatology (Kaplan & Sadock, 1998). It does not appear to be of value to individuals with chronic schizophrenic illness.

Other Conditions

Electroconvulsive therapy has also been tried with clients experiencing a variety of neuroses, obsessive-compulsive

disorders, and personality disorders (Kendell, 1981). Little evidence exists to support the efficacy of ECT in the treatment of these conditions.

CONTRAINDICATIONS

The only absolute contraindication for ECT is increased intracranial pressure (from brain tumor, recent cardiovascular accident, or other cerebrovascular lesion). Electroconvulsive therapy is associated with a physiological rise in cerebrospinal fluid pressure during the treatment, resulting in increased intracranial pressure that could lead to brainstem herniation (Crowe, 1984).

Various other conditions, not considered absolute contraindications but rendering clients at high risk for the treatment, have been identified (Endler & Persad, 1988; Kaplan & Sadock, 1998; Silver, Yudofsky, & Hurowitz, 1994). They are largely cardiovascular in nature and include myocardial infarction or cerebrovascular accident within the preceding 3 months, aortic or cerebral aneurysm, severe underlying hypertension, and congestive heart failure. Clients with cardiovascular problems are placed at risk because of the response of the body to the seizure itself. The initial vagal response results in a sinus bradycardia and drop in blood pressure. This is followed immediately by tachycardia and a hypertensive response. These changes can be life threatening to an individual with an already compromised cardiovascular system. Other factors that place clients at risk for ECT include severe osteoporosis, acute and chronic pulmonary disorders, and high-risk or complicated pregnancy.

MECHANISM OF ACTION

The exact mechanism by which ECT effects a therapeutic response is unknown. Several theories exist, but the one to which the most credibility has been given is the biochemical theory. A number of researchers have demonstrated that electric stimulation results in significant increases in the circulating levels of several neurotransmitters (Endler & Persad, 1988). These neurotransmitters include serotonin, norepinephrine, and dopamine, the same biogenic amines that are affected by antidepressant drugs.

SIDE EFFECTS

The most common side effects of ECT are temporary memory loss and confusion. Critics of the therapy argue that these changes represent irreversible brain damage. Proponents insist they are temporary and reversible. In a review of a number of studies dealing with this question, Kendell (1981) could find no evidence of memory deficits persisting beyond 3 months. Other researchers have suggested that varying degrees of memory loss may be evident in some clients up to 6 to 9 months following ECT (Squire, 1977; Weiner et al., 1986).

The controversy continues regarding the choice of unilateral versus bilateral ECT. Studies have shown that unilateral placement of the electrodes decreases the amount of memory disturbance. However, unilateral ECT often requires a greater number of treatments to match the efficacy of bilateral ECT in the relief of depression (Endler & Persad, 1988).

RISKS ASSOCIATED WITH ELECTROCONVULSIVE THERAPY

Mortality

Studies indicate that the mortality rate from ECT falls somewhere between 0.01 and 0.04 percent (Abrams, 1988). Although the occurrence is rare, the major cause of death with ECT is cardiovascular complications, such as acute myocardial infarction, acute coronary insufficiency, ventricular fibrillation, myocardial rupture, cardiac arrest, cardiovascular collapse, stroke, and ruptured cerebral or aortic aneurysm. Assessment and management of cardiovascular disease *prior to* treatment is vital in the reduction of morbidity and mortality rates associated with ECT.

Permanent Memory Loss

Freeman and associates (1980) conducted a study of cognitive dysfunction in a group of individuals who had received a course of ECT treatments an average of 10 years previously. These clients were given a battery of cognitive memory tasks, on several of which they were found to be significantly impaired; a few even scored in the organic impairment range. The authors concluded that a small subgroup of clients receiving ECT might suffer permanent memory impairment.

Brain Damage

Brain damage from ECT remains a concern for those who continue to believe in its usefulness and efficacy as a treatment for depression. Critics of the procedure remain adamant in their belief that ECT always results in some degree of immediate brain damage (Endler & Persad, 1988). However, evidence is based largely on animal studies in which the subjects received excessive electrical dosages and the seizures were unmodified by muscle paralysis and oxygenation (Abrams, 1988). Although this is an area for continuing study, there is no evidence to substantiate that ECT produces any permanent changes

in brain structure or functioning (Kaplan & Sadock, 1998).

THE ROLE OF THE NURSE IN ELECTROCONVULSIVE THERAPY

Nurses routinely assist with ECT, providing support before, during, and after the treatment to the client, family, and medical professionals who are conducting the therapy. The nursing process provides a systematic approach to the provision of care for the client receiving ECT.

Assessment

A complete physical examination must be completed by the appropriate medical professional prior to the initiation of ECT. This evaluation should include a thorough assessment of cardiovascular and pulmonary status as well as laboratory blood and urine studies. A skeletal history and X-ray assessment should also be considered.

The nurse may be responsible for ensuring that informed consent has been obtained from the client. If the depression is severe and the client is clearly unable to consent to the procedure, permission may be obtained from family or other legally responsible individual. Consent is secured only after the client or responsible individual acknowledges understanding of the procedure, including possible side effects and potential risks involved.

Nurses may also be required to assess:

- The client's mood and level of interaction with others
- Evidence of suicidal ideation, plan, and means
- Level of anxiety and fears associated with receiving ECT
- Thought and communication patterns
- Baseline memory for short- and long-term events
- Client and family knowledge of indications for, side effects of, and potential risks involved with ECT
- Current and past use of medications
- Baseline vital signs and history of allergies
- The client's ability to carry out activities of daily living

Diagnosis/Outcome Identification

Selection of appropriate nursing diagnoses for the client undergoing ECT is based on continual assessment before, during, and after treatment. Following are selected potential nursing diagnoses with outcome criteria for evaluation.

NURSING DIAGNOSES	OUTCOME CRITERIA
Anxiety (moderate to severe) related to impending therapy	Client verbalizes a decrease in anxiety following explanation of procedure and expression of fears.
Knowledge deficit related to necessity for and side effects or risks of ECT	Client verbalizes understanding of need for and side effects/risks of ECT following explanation.
Risk for injury related to risks associated with ECT	Client undergoes treatment without sustaining injury
Risk for aspiration related to altered level of consciousness immediately following treatment	Client experiences no aspiration during ECT.
Decreased cardiac output related to vagal stimulation occurring during the ECT	Client demonstrates adequate tissue perfusion during and after treatment (absence of cyanosis or severe change in mental status).
Altered thought processes related to side effects of temporary memory loss and confusion	Client maintains reality orientation following ECT treatment.
Self-care deficit related to incapacitation during postictal stage	Client's self-care needs are fulfilled at all times.
Risk for activity intolerance related to post-ECT confusion and memory loss	Client gradually increases participation in therapeutic activities to the highest level of personal capability.

Planning/Implementation

Electroconvulsive therapy treatments are usually performed in the morning. The client is given nothing by mouth (NPO) for 4 to 8 hours before the treatment. Some institutional policies require that the client be placed on NPO status at midnight prior to the treatment day. The treatment team routinely consists of the psychiatrist, anesthesiologist, and two or more nurses.

Nursing interventions before the treatment include:

● Ensure that the physician has obtained informed consent and that a signed permission form is on the chart.
● Ensure that the most recent laboratory reports (complete blood count, urinalysis) and results of electrocardiogram (ECG) and X-ray examination are available.
● Approximately 1 hour before treatment is scheduled, take vital signs and record them. Have the client void and remove dentures, eyeglasses or contact lenses, jewelry, and hairpins. Following institutional requirements, the client should change into hospital gown or, if permitted, into own loose clothing or pajamas. Client should remain in bed with siderails up.
● Approximately 30 minutes before treatment, administer the pretreatment medication as prescribed by the physician. The usual order is for atropine sulfate or glycopyrrolate (Robinul) given intramuscularly. Either of these medications may be ordered to decrease secretions and counteract the effects of vagal stimulation induced by the ECT.
● Stay with the client to help allay fears and anxiety. Maintain a positive attitude about the procedure, and encourage the client to verbalize feelings.

In the treatment room the client is placed on the treatment table in a supine position. The anesthesiologist administers intravenously a short-acting anesthetic, such as thiopental sodium (Pentothal) or methohexital sodium (Brevital). A muscle relaxant, usually succinylcholine chloride (Anectine), is given intravenously to prevent severe muscle contractions during the seizure, thereby reducing the possibility of fractured or dislocated bones. Because succinylcholine paralyzes respiratory muscles as well, the client is oxygenated with pure oxygen during and after the treatment, except for the brief interval of electrical stimulation, until spontaneous respirations return (Kaplan & Sadock, 1998). A blood pressure cuff may be placed on the lower leg and inflated above systolic pressure prior to the injection of the succinylcholine. This is to ensure that the seizure activity can be observed in this one limb that is unaffected by the muscle relaxant.

An airway/bite block is placed in the client's mouth and he or she is positioned to facilitate airway patency. Electrodes are placed (either bilaterally or unilaterally) on the temples to deliver the electrical stimulation.

Nursing interventions during the treatment include:

● Ensure patency of airway. Provide suctioning if needed.
● Assist anesthesiologist with oxygenation as required.
● Observe readouts on machines monitoring vital signs and cardiac functioning.
● Provide support to the client's arms and legs during the seizure.
● Observe and record the type and amount of movement induced by the seizure.

After the treatment the anesthesiologist continues to oxygenate the client with pure oxygen until spontaneous respirations return. Most clients awaken within 10 or 15 minutes of the treatment and are confused and disoriented; however, some clients will sleep for 1 to 2 hours following the treatment. All clients require close observation in this immediate posttreatment period.

Nursing interventions in the posttreatment period include:

- Monitor pulse, respirations, and blood pressure every 15 minutes for the first hour, during which time the client should remain in bed.
- Position the client on side to prevent aspiration.
- Orient the client to time and place.
- Describe what has occurred.
- Provide reassurance that any memory loss the client may be experiencing is only temporary.
- Allow the client to verbalize fears and anxieties related to receiving ECT.
- Stay with the client until he or she is fully awake, oriented, and able to perform self-care activities without assistance.
- Provide the client with a highly structured schedule of routine activities in order to minimize confusion.

Evaluation

Evaluation of the effectiveness of nursing interventions is based on the achievement of the projected outcomes. Reassessment may be based on answers to the following questions:

- Was the client's anxiety maintained at a manageable level?
- Was the client/family teaching completed satisfactorily?
- Did the client/family verbalize understanding of the procedure, its side effects, and risks involved?
- Did the client undergo treatment without experiencing injury or aspiration?
- Has the client maintained adequate tissue perfusion during and following treatment? Have vital signs remained stable?
- With consideration to the individual client's condition and response to treatment, is the client reoriented to time, place, and situation?
- Have all of the client's self-care needs been fulfilled?
- Is the client participating in therapeutic activities to his or her maximum potential? What is the client's level of social interaction?

Careful documentation is an important part of the evaluation process. Some routine observations may be evaluated on flow sheets specifically identified for ECT. However, progress notes with detailed descriptions of client behavioral changes are essential to evaluate improvement and help determine the number of treatments that will be administered. Continual reassessment, planning, and evaluation ensure that the client will receive adequate and appropriate nursing care throughout the course of therapy.

SUMMARY

Electroconvulsive therapy is the induction of a grand mal seizure through the application of electrical current to the brain. It is a safe and effective treatment alternative for individuals with depression, mania, or schizoaffective disorder who do not respond to other forms of therapy.

Electroconvulsive therapy is contraindicated for individuals with increased intracranial pressure. Individuals with cardiovascular problems are at high risk for complications from ECT. Other factors that place clients at risk include severe osteoporosis, acute and chronic pulmonary disorders, and high-risk or complicated pregnancy.

The exact mechanism of action of ECT is unknown, but it is thought that the electrical stimulation results in significant increases in the circulating levels of the neurotransmitters serotonin, norepinephrine, and dopamine.

The most common side effects with ECT are temporary memory loss and confusion. Although it is rare, death must be considered a risk associated with ECT. When it does occur, the most common cause is cardiovascular complications. Other possible risks include permanent memory loss and brain damage, for which there is little substantiating evidence.

The nurse assists with ECT using the steps of the nursing process before, during, and after treatment. Important nursing interventions include ensuring client safety, managing client anxiety, and providing adequate client education. Nursing input into the ongoing evaluation of client behavior is an important factor in determining the therapeutic effectiveness of ECT.

REVIEW QUESTIONS

SELF-EXAMINATION/LEARNING EXERCISE

Select the answer that is most appropriate for each of the following questions.

1. Electroconvulsive therapy is most commonly prescribed for:

    a. Bipolar disorder, manic.
    b. Paranoid schizophrenia.
    c. Major depression.
    d. Obsessive-compulsive disorder.

2. Which of the following best describes the *average* number of ECT treatments given and the timing of administration?

    a. 1 treatment per month for 6 months.
    b. 1 treatment every other day for a total of 6 to 10.
    c. 1 treatment three times per week for a total of 20 to 30.
    d. 1 treatment every day for a total of 10 to 15.

3. Which of the following conditions is considered to be the only *absolute* contraindication for ECT?

    a. Increased intracranial pressure.
    b. Recent myocardial infarction.
    c. Severe underlying hypertension.
    d. Congestive heart failure.

4. Electroconvulsive therapy is thought to effect a therapeutic response by

    a. Stimulation of the CNS.
    b. Decreasing the levels of acetylcholine and monoamine oxidase.
    c. Increasing the levels of serotonin, norepinephrine, and dopamine.
    d. Altering sodium metabolism within nerve and muscle cells.

5. The most common side effects of ECT are:

    a. Permanent memory loss and brain damage.
    b. Fractured and dislocated bones.
    c. Myocardial infarction and cardiac arrest.
    d. Temporary memory loss and confusion.

Situation: Sam has just been admitted to the inpatient psychiatric unit with a diagnosis of major depression. Sam has been treated with antidepressant medication for 6 months without improvement. His psychiatrist has suggested a series of ECT treatments. Sam says to the nurse on admission, "I don't want to end up like McMurphy in *One Flew Over the Cuckoo's Nest!* I'm scared!" The following questions pertain to Sam.

6. Sam's priority nursing diagnosis at this time would be:

    a. Anxiety related to knowledge deficit about ECT.
    b. Potential for injury related to risks associated with ECT.
    c. Knowledge deficit related to negative media presentation of ECT.
    d. Altered thought processes related to side effects of ECT.

7. Which of the following statements would be most appropriate by the nurse in response to Sam's expression of concern?

    a. "I guarantee you won't end up like McMurphy, Sam."
    b. "The doctor knows what he is doing. There's nothing to worry about."
    c. "I know you are scared, Sam, and we're going to talk about what you can expect from the therapy."
    d. "I'm going to stay with you as long as you are scared."

8. The priority nursing intervention before starting Sam's therapy is to:

    a. Take vital signs and record.
    b. Have the patient void.
    c. Administer succinylcholine.
    d. Ensure that the consent form has been signed.

9. Atropine sulfate is administered to Sam for what purpose?

    a. To alleviate anxiety.
    b. To decrease secretions.
    c. To relax muscles.
    d. As a short-acting anesthetic.

10. Succinylcholine is administered to Sam for what purpose?

    a. To alleviate anxiety.
    b. To decrease secretions.
    c. To relax muscles.
    d. As a short-acting anesthetic.

REFERENCES

Abrams, R. (1988). *Electroconvulsive therapy.* New York: Oxford University Press.

American Psychiatric Association. (1990). *The practice of electroconvulsive therapy: Recommendations for treatment, training, and privileging.* A Task Force Report of the American Psychiatric Association. Washington, DC: American Psychiatric Association.

Cherkin, A. (1974). Effects of flurothyl (Indoklon) upon memory in the chick. In M. Fink, S. Kety, & J. McGaugh (Eds.), *Psychobiology of convulsive therapy.* New York: John Wiley & Sons.

Crowe, R.R. (1984, July 19). Electroconvulsive therapy—A current perspective. *New England Journal of Medicine, 163–166.*

Endler, N.S., & Persad, E. (1988). *Electroconvulsive therapy—The myths and the realities.* Toronto: Hans Huber Publishers.

Freeman, C.P., et al. (1980). ECT: Patients who complain. *British Journal of Psychiatry, 137,* 17–25.

Kaplan, H.I., & Sadock, B.J. (1998). *Synopsis of psychiatry: Behavioral sciences/clinical psychiatry* (8th ed.). Baltimore: Williams & Wilkins.

Kendell, R.E. (1981). The present status of electroconvulsive therapy. *British Journal of Psychiatry, 139,* 265–283.

Sackeim, H.A. (1985, June). The case for ECT. *Psychology Today,* 36–40.

Silver, J.M., Yudofsky, S.C., & Hurowitz, G.I. (1994). Psychopharmacology and electroconvulsive therapy. In R.E. Hales, S.C. Yudofsky, & J.A. Talbott (Eds.), *Textbook of Psychiatry* (2nd ed.). Washington, DC: American Psychiatric Press.

Squire, L.R. (1977, September). ECT and memory loss. *American Journal of Psychiatry, 134*(9), 997–1001.

Weiner, R.D., Rogers, H.J., Davidson, J.R., & Squire, L.R. (1986). Effects of stimulus parameters on cognitive side effects. *Annals of New York Academy of Science, 462,* 315–325.

Bibliography

Abrams, R., Swartz, C.M., & Vedak, C. (1991, August). Antidepressant effects of high-dose right unilateral electroconvulsive therapy. *Archives of General Psychiatry, 48,* 746–748.

Culver, C.M., et al. (1980, May). ECT and special problems of informed consent. *American Journal of Psychiatry, 137*(5), 586–591.

Fink, M. (1977, September). Myths of shock therapy. *American Journal of Psychiatry, 134*(9), 991–996.

Fink, M. (1979). *Convulsive therapy: Theory and practice.* New York: Raven Press.

Fink, M., & Jenike, M.A. (1985, September). Electroshock—Exploding the myths. *RN,* 58–66.

Fink, M., Kety, S., & McGaugh, J. (1974). *Psychobiology of convulsive therapy.* New York: John Wiley & Sons.

Frankel, F.H. (1977, September). Current perspectives on ECT: A discussion. *American Journal of Psychiatry, 134*(9), 1014–1019.

Friedberg, J. (1977, September). Shock treatment, brain damage, and memory loss: A neurological perspective. *American Journal of Psychiatry, 134*(9), 1010–1014.

Greenblatt, M. (1977, September). Efficacy of ECT in affective and schizophrenic illness. *American Journal of Psychiatry, 134*(9), 1001–1005.

Mulaik, J.S. (1979, February). Nurses' questions about electroconvulsive therapy. *Journal of Psychosocial Nursing,* 15–19.

Rosenfeld, A.H. (1985, June). Depression: Dispelling despair. *Psychology Today,* 29–34.

Salzman, C. (1977, September). ECT and ethical psychiatry. *American Journal of Psychiatry, 134*(9), 1006–1009.

Weiner, R.D., & Coffey, C.E. (1988). Indications for use of electroconvulsive therapy. In A.J. Allen & R.E. Hales (Eds.), *Review of psychiatry,* Vol. 7. Washington, DC: American Psychiatric Press.

Yudofsky, S.C. (1982, July). Electroconvulsive therapy in the eighties: Technique and technologies. *American Journal of Psychotherapy, 36*(3), 391–397.

COMPLEMENTARY THERAPIES

KEY TERMS

allopathic medicine
alternative medicine
complementary medicine
acupressure

acupuncture
chi
meridians
acupoints

chiropractic medicine
subluxation
yoga

OBJECTIVES

After reading this chapter, the student will be able to:

1. Describe the philosophies behind various complementary therapies, including herbal medicine, acupressure and acupuncture, diet and nutrition, chiropractic medicine, therapeutic touch and massage, yoga, and pet therapy.

2. Discuss the historical background of various complementary therapies.
3. Describe the techniques used in various complementary therapies.

he connection between mind and body, and the influence of each on the other, is well recognized by all clinicians, and particularly by psychiatrists. Traditional medicine as it is currently practiced in the United States is based solely on scientific methodology. Traditional medicine, also known as **allopathic medicine,** is the type of medicine historically taught in U.S. medical schools.

The term **alternative medicine** has come to be recognized as practices that differ from the usual traditional practices in the treatment of disease. A recent national survey by the American Medical Association's Council on Scientific Affairs revealed that 33 percent of those polled reported at least one alternative treatment during the previous 12 months ("Hocus Pocus," 1997). More than $15 billion a year is spent on alternative medical therapies in the United States (Kaplan & Sadock, 1998).

In 1991, an Office of Alternative Medicine (OAM) was established by the National Institutes of Health (NIH) to study nontraditional therapies and to evaluate their usefulness and their effectiveness. The mission statement of the OAM states:

"The NIH Office of Alternative Medicine facilitates research and evaluation of unconventional medical practices and disseminates this information to the public." ("Complementary and Alternative Medicine," 1998.)

Although the OAM has not endorsed the methodologies, they have established a list of alternative therapies to be used in practice and for investigative purposes. This list is presented in Table 21.1.

Some health insurance companies and health maintenance organizations (HMOs) appear to be bowing to public pressure by including alternative providers in their networks of providers for treatments such as acupuncture and massage therapy. Chiropractic care has been covered by some third-party payers for many years. Individuals who seek alternative therapy, however, are often reimbursed at lower rates than those who choose traditional practitioners.

Credit, Hartunian, and Nowak (1998) view these treatments not as *alternative,* but as **complementary medicine,** in partnership with traditional medical practice. They acknowledge the superiority of traditional medical intervention in certain medical situations. However, they do not discount "the body's ability to heal itself with the help of natural, noninvasive therapies that are effective and without harmful side effects" (p. 3).

Client education is an important part of complementary care. Positive lifestyle changes are encouraged, and practitioners serve as educators as well as treatment specialists (Credit et al., 1998). Complementary medicine is viewed as *holistic* health care, which deals with not only the physical perspective but also the emotional and spiritual components of the individual. Dr. Tom Coniglione, former professor of medicine at the Oklahoma University Health Sciences Center, states:

"We must look at treating the 'total person' in order to be more efficient and balanced within the medical community. Even finding doctors who are well-rounded and balanced has become a criteria in the admitting process for medical students. Medicine has changed from just looking at the 'scientist perspective of organ and disease' to the total perspective of lifestyle and real impact/results to the patient. This evolution is a progressive and very positive shift in the right direction." (Coniglione, 1998.)

Terms such as *harmony* and *balance* are often associated with complementary care. In fact, restoring harmony and balance between body and mind is often the goal of complementary health care approaches (Credit et al., 1998).

This chapter examines various complementary therapies by describing the therapeutic approach and identifying the conditions for which the therapy is intended. Although most are not founded in scientific principles, they have been shown to be effective in the treatment of certain disorders and merit further examination as a viable component of holistic health care.

TYPES OF COMPLEMENTARY THERAPIES

Herbal Medicine

The use of plants to heal is probably as old as humankind. Virtually every culture in the world has relied on herbs and plants to treat illness. Clay tablets from about 4000 BC reveal that the Sumerians had apothecaries for dispensing medicinal herbs; and the *Pen Tsao,* a Chinese text written around 3000 BC, contained some 1000 herbal formulas that had probably been used as remedies for thousands of years (Guinness, 1993). When the Pilgrims came to America in the 1600s, they brought with them a variety of herbs to be established and used for medicinal purposes. The new settlers soon discovered that the Native Americans also had their own varieties of plants for healing.

Many people are seeking a return to herbal remedies, because they view these remedies as being less potent than prescription drugs and as being free of adverse side effects. However, because the Food and Drug Administration (FDA) classifies herbal remedies as dietary supplements or food additives, their labels cannot indicate medicinal uses. They are not subjected to FDA approval and lack uniform standards of quality control. Several organizations have been established to attempt regulation and control of the herbal industry. They include the Council for Responsible Nutrition, the American Herbal Association, and the American Botanical Council. The Commission E of the German Federal Health Agency is the group responsible for researching and regulating the safety and efficacy of herbs and plant medicines in Germany. Recently, all 380 German Commission E monographs of herbal medicines have been translated into English and compiled into one text. This should prove to be an invaluable reference for practitioners of holistic medicine.

TABLE 21.1 CLASSIFICATION OF ALTERNATIVE MEDICINE PRACTICES FROM THE NIH OFFICE OF ALTERNATIVE MEDICINE

Alternative Systems of Medical Practice
Acupuncture
Anthroposophically extended medicine
Ayurveda
Community-based health care practices
Environmental medicine
Homeopathic medicine
Latin American rural practices
Native American practices
Natural products
Naturopathic medicine
Past life therapy
Shamanism
Tibetan medicine
Traditional Oriental medicine

Bioelectromagnetic Applications
Blue light treatment and artificial lighting
Electroacupuncture
Electromagnetic fields
Electrostimulation and neuromagnetic stimulation devices
Magnetoresonance spectroscopy

Diet, Nutrition, Lifestyle Changes
Changes in lifestyle
Diet
Gerson therapy
Macrobiotics
Megavitamins
Nutritional supplements

Herbal Medicine
Echinacea (purple coneflower)
Ginger rhizome
Ginkgo biloba extract
Ginseng root
Wild chrysanthemum flower
Witch hazel
Yellowdock

Manual Healing
Acupressure
Alexander technique
Biofield therapeutics
Chiropractic medicine
Feldenkrais method
Massage therapy
Osteopathy
Reflexology
Rolfing
Therapeutic touch
Trager method
Zone therapy

Mind/Body Control
Art therapy
Biofeedback
Counseling
Dance therapy
Guided imagery
Humor therapy
Hypnotherapy
Meditation
Music therapy
Prayer therapy
Psychotherapy
Relaxation techniques
Support groups
Yoga

Pharmacological and Biological Treatments
Antioxidizing agents
Cell treatment
Chelation therapy
Metabolic therapy
Oxidizing agents (ozone, hydrogen peroxide)

This list of complementary and alternative medical health care practices was developed by the ad hoc Advisory Panel to the Office of Alternative Medicine (OAM), National Institutes of Health (NIH). It was further refined at a workshop for alternative medicine researchers and practitioners. It was designed for the purposes of discussion and study and is considered neither complete nor authoritative.

Until the time that more extensive testing has been completed on humans and animals, the use of herbal medicines must be approached with caution and responsibility. *The notion that because something is "natural" it is therefore completely safe is a myth.* In fact, some of the plants from which even prescription drugs are derived are highly toxic in their natural state (Guinness, 1993). Also, because of lack of regulation and standardization, ingredients in these herbal remedies may be adulterated. Their method of manufacture may also alter potency. For example, dried herbs lose potency rapidly because of exposure to air. Guinness (1993) offers the following points for practitioners and individuals contemplating the use of herbal medicines:

1. **Be Careful of Your Sources.** Owing to the lack of government scrutiny, the purity and potency of the herbal medicines cannot be guaranteed. The buyer must be careful to select reputable brands.
2. **Choose the Most Reliable Forms.** Tinctures and freeze-dried products have been prepared to retard spoilage and prevent loss of potency.
3. **More Is Not Better.** Always take the recommended dosages at the suggested intervals. Adverse effects can occur from overdosing with herbal medicines, just as they do with prescription pharmaceuticals.
4. **Monitor Your Reactions.** Discontinue the herbal medication at the first sign of allergic or other adverse reaction. Discontinue it after a reasonable

length of time if there seems to be no significant indication that it is producing the desired effect.

5. **Take No Risks.** Do not self-medicate with herbal remedies for serious illnesses or injuries. Do not take herbal medications without a physician's approval if you are pregnant or lactating, very young or very old, or taking other medications.

Table 21.2 lists a variety of information about common herbal remedies, with possible implications for psychiatric and mental health nursing. It gives the botanical name, medicinal uses, and safety profile of the herbs.

Acupressure and Acupuncture

Acupressure and **acupuncture** are healing techniques based on the ancient philosophies of traditional Chinese medicine dating back to 3000 BC. The main concept behind Chinese medicine is that healing energy (**chi**) flows through the body along specific pathways called **meridians.** It is believed that these meridians of chi connect various parts of the body in a manner similar to the way in which lines on a road map link various locations. The pathways link a conglomerate of points, called **acupoints.** Therefore, it is possible to treat a part of the body distant to another, because they are linked by a meridian. Credit and associates (1998) state, "The goal of traditional Chinese medicine is to keep the body in balance and harmony through the free flow of chi. Disease is a result of blockages in this energy current."

In acupressure, the fingers, thumbs, palms, or elbows are used to apply pressure to the acupoints. This pressure is thought to dissolve any obstructions in the flow of healing energy and to restore the body to a healthier functioning. In acupuncture, hair-thin, sterile, disposable, stainless-steel needles are inserted into acupoints to dissolve the obstructions along the meridians. The needles may be left in place for a specified length of time or they may be rotated or a mild electric current may be applied. An occasional tingling or numbness is experienced, but little to no pain is associated with the treatment (Credit et al., 1998).

The Western medical philosophy regarding acupressure and acupuncture is that they stimulate the body's own pain-killing chemicals, the morphinelike substances known as *endorphins.* The treatment has been found to be effective in the treatment of asthma, headaches, dysmenorrhea, cervical pain, insomnia, anxiety, depression, substance abuse, stroke rehabilitation, nausea of pregnancy, postoperative and chemotherapy-induced nausea and vomiting, tennis elbow, fibromyalgia, low back pain, and carpal tunnel syndrome (Kaplan & Sadock, 1998; National Institutes of Health, 1997).

Acupuncture is gaining wide acceptance in the United States by both patients and physicians. This treatment can be administered at the same time other techniques are being used, such as conventional Western techniques, although it is essential that all health care providers have knowledge of all treatments being received. Acupuncture should be administered by a physician or an acupuncturist who is board certified by the National Commission for the Certification of Acupuncturists (NCCA), which requires more than 1000 hours of acupuncture training. Currently 34 states have set licensure standards for acupuncturists (Institute for Natural Resources, 1998).

Diet and Nutrition

The value of nutrition in the healing process has long been underrated. Lutz & Przytulski (1994) state:

> "Today many diseases are linked to lifestyle behaviors such as smoking, lack of adequate physical activity, and poor nutritional habits. Health care providers, in their role as educators, emphasize the relationship between lifestyle and risk of contracting disease. People are increasingly managing their health problems and making personal commitments to lead healthier lives. Nutrition is, in part, a preventive science. How and what one eats is a lifestyle choice." (p. 5)

Individuals select the foods they eat based on a number of factors, not the least of which is enjoyment. Eating must serve social and cultural, as well as nutritional, needs. The U.S. Departments of Agriculture and Health and Human Services (USDA/USDHHS, 1995) have collaborated on a set of guidelines to help individuals understand what types of foods to eat in order to promote health and prevent disease. Following is a list of these guidelines.

1. Eat a Variety of Foods

No single food can supply all nutrients in the amounts needed for good health. A variety of foods should be selected from the food guide pyramid (Figure 21.1). Most of the daily servings of food should be selected from the food groups that are closest to the base of the pyramid. A range of servings is suggested for each group of foods. Smaller, sedentary persons should select the lower number of servings. The higher numbers of servings are meant for larger, more active individuals. Table 21.3 provides a summary of information about essential vitamins and minerals.

2. Balance the Food You Eat With Physical Activity—Maintain or Improve Your Weight

Many individuals gain weight with age, increasing their chances of developing a number of health problems associated with excess weight. These include high blood pressure, heart disease, stroke, diabetes, certain types of

TABLE 21.2   HERBAL REMEDIES

COMMON NAMES (BOTANICAL NAME)	MEDICINAL USES/POSSIBLE ACTION	SAFETY PROFILE
Black cohosh (*Cimicifuga racemosa*)	May provide relief of menstrual cramps; improved mood; calming effect. Extracts from the roots are thought to have action similar to estrogen.	Generally considered safe in low doses. Toxic in large doses, causing dizziness, nausea, headaches, stiffness, and trembling. Should not be taken with heart problems, concurrently with antihypertensives, or during pregnancy.
Cascara sagrada (*Rhamnus purshiana*)	Relief of constipation.	Generally recognized as safe; sold as over-the-counter drug in the United States. Should not be used during pregnancy.
Chamomile (*Matricaria chamomilla*)	As a tea, it is effective as a mild sedative in the relief of insomnia. May also aid digestion, relieve menstrual cramps, and settle upset stomach.	Generally recognized as safe when consumed in reasonable amounts.
Echinacea (*Echinacea angustifolia* and *Echinacea purpurea*)	Stimulates immune system; may have value in fighting infections and easing the symptoms of colds and flu.	Considered safe in reasonable doses. Observe for side effects of allergic reaction.
Fennel (*Foeniculum vulgare* or *Foeniculum officinale*)	Used to ease stomachaches and to aid digestion. Taken in a tea or in extracts to stimulate the appetites of people with anorexia (1–2 tsp. seeds steeped in boiling water for making tea).	Generally recognized as safe when consumed in reasonable amounts.
Feverfew (*Tanacetum parthenium*)	Prophylaxis and treatment of migraine headaches. Effective in either the fresh leaf or freeze-dried forms (2–3 fresh leaves [or equivalent] per day).	A small percentage of individuals may experience the adverse effect of temporary mouth ulcers. Considered safe in reasonable doses.
Ginger (*Zingiber officinale*)	Ginger tea to ease stomachaches and to aid digestion. Two powdered ginger-root capsules have been shown to be effective in preventing motion sickness.	Generally recognized as safe
Ginkgo (*Ginkgo biloba*)	Used to treat senility, short-term memory loss, and peripheral insufficiency. Has been shown to dilate blood vessels. Usual dosage is 120 mg/day.	Safety has been established with recommended dosages. Possible side effects include headache, gastrointestinal (GI) problems, and dizziness. Contraindicated in pregnancy and lactation and in patients with bleeding disorders.
Ginseng (*Panax ginseng*)	The ancient Chinese saw this herb as one that increased wisdom and longevity. Current studies support a possible positive effect on the cardiovascular system. Action not known.	Generally considered safe. Side effects may include headache, insomnia, anxiety, skin rashes, diarrhea.
Hops (*Humulus lupulus*)	Used in cases of nervousness, mild anxiety, and insomnia. Also may relieve the cramping associated with diarrhea. May be taken as a tea, in extracts, or capsules.	Generally recognized as safe when consumed in recommended dosages.
Kava-Kava (*Piper methylsticum*)	Used to reduce anxiety while promoting mental acuity. Dosage range: 70–400 mg day.	Generally considered safe. May cause scaly skin rash when taken at the higher dosage range for long periods. Concurrent use with alcohol may produce additive tranquilizing effects.
Passion flower (*Passiflora incarnata*)	Used in tea, capsules, or extracts to treat nervousness and insomnia. Depresses the central nervous system to produce a mild sedative effect.	Generally recognized as safe in recommended doses.
Peppermint (*Mentha piperita*)	Used as a tea to relieve upset stomachs and headaches and as a mild sedative. Pour boiling water over 1 tbsp. dried leaves and steep to make a tea.	Considered to be safe when consumed in normal quantities.

Continued on following page

TABLE 21.2 **HERBAL REMEDIES** *(Continued)*

COMMON NAMES (BOTANICAL NAME)	MEDICINAL USES/POSSIBLE ACTION	SAFETY PROFILE
Psyllium (*Plantago ovata* and *Plantago major*)	Psyllium seeds are a popular bulk laxative commonly used for chronic constipation.	Approved as an over-the-counter drug in the United States.
Scullcap (*Scutellaria lateriflora*)	Used as a sedative for mild anxiety and nervousness.	Considered safe in reasonable amounts.
St. John's Wort (*Hypericum perforatum*)	● Used in the treatment of mild to moderate depression. May block reuptake of serotonin/norepinephrine and have a mild MAO inhibiting effect. Effective dose: 900 mg/day. ● May also have antiviral, antibacterial, and antiinflammatory properties. Currently being tested in high doses as an anti-HIV drug.	Generally recognized as safe when taken at recommended dosages. Side effects include mild GI irritation that is lessened with food; photosensitivity when taken in high dosages over long periods. Should not be taken with other psychoactive medications.
Valerian (*Valeriana officinals*)	Used to treat insomnia. Produces restful sleep without morning "hangover." The root may be used to make a tea, or capsules are available at a common dosage of 400 mg. Mechanism of action is similar to benzodiazepines, but without addicting properties.	Generally recognized as safe when taken at recommended dosages. Side effects may include mild headache or upset stomach. Taking doses higher than recommended may result in severe headache, nausea, morning grogginess, blurry vision. Should not be taken concurrently with other sedatives.

SOURCES: Adapted from Guinness (1993); Kaplan & Sadock (1998); Institute for Natural Resources (1998); and Yeager (1998).

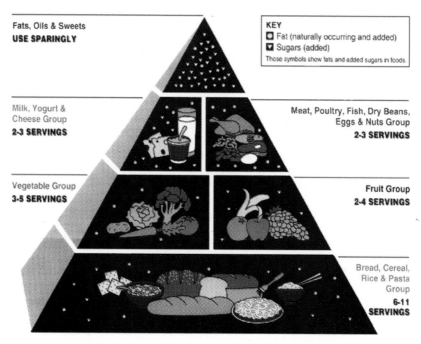

Figure 21.1 The Food Guide Pyramid.

TABLE 21.3   ESSENTIAL VITAMINS AND MINERALS

VITAMIN/ MINERAL	FUNCTION	RDA*	FOOD SOURCES	COMMENTS
Vitamin A	Prevention of night blindness; calcification of growing bones; resistance to infection	Men: 1000 μg; Women: 800 μg	Liver, butter, cheese, whole milk, egg yolk, fish liver oil, green leafy vegetables, carrots	May be of benefit in prevention of cancer, because of its antioxidant properties, which are associated with control of free radicals that damage DNA and cell membranes.
Vitamin D	Promotes absorption of calcium and phosphorus in the small intestine; prevention of rickets	Men: 5 μg; Women: 5 μg	Fortified milk and dairy products, egg yolk, fish liver oils, liver, oysters; formed in the skin by exposure to sunlight	Without vitamin D, very little dietary calcium can be absorbed.
Vitamin E	An antioxidant that prevents cell membrane destruction	Men: 10 mg; Women: 8 mg	Vegetable oils, wheat germ, whole grain or fortified cereals, green leafy vegetables	As an antioxidant, may have implications in the prevention of Alzheimer's disease, heart disease, breast cancer.
Vitamin K	Synthesis of prothrombin and other clotting factors; normal blood coagulation	Men: 80 μg; Women: 65 μg	Formed in intestines by bacteria; also found in green leafy vegetables, meats, dairy products	
Vitamin C	Formation of collagen in connective tissues; a powerful antioxidant; facilitates iron absorption; aids in the release of epinephrine from the adrenal glands during stress	Men and women: 60 mg	Citrus fruits, tomatoes, potatoes, green leafy vegetables, strawberries	As an antioxidant, may have implications in the prevention of cancer, cataracts, heart disease. It may stimulate the immune system to fight various types of infection.
Vitamin B_1 (thiamine)	Essential for normal functioning of nervous tissue; coenzyme in carbohydrate metabolism	Men: 1.5 mg; Women: 1.1 mg	Whole grains, legumes, nuts, egg yolk, meat, green leafy vegetables	Large doses may improve mental performance in people with Alzheimer's disease.
Vitamin B_2 (riboflavin)	Coenzyme in the metabolism of protein and carbohydrate	Men: 1.7 mg; Women: 1.3 mg	Meat, dairy products, whole or enriched grains, legumes	May help in the prevention of cataracts; high dose therapy may be effective in migraine prophylaxis (Schoenen Jacquy, & Lenaerts, 1998).
Vitamin B_3 (niacin)	Coenzyme in the metabolism of protein and carbohydrate	Men: 19 mg; Women: 15 mg	Milk, eggs, meats, legumes, whole grain and enriched cereals	High doses of niacin have been successful in decreasing levels of cholesterol in some individuals.
Vitamin B_6 (pyridoxine)	Coenzyme in the synthesis and catabolism of amino acids; essential for metabolism of tryptophan to niacin	Men: 2 mg; Women: 1.6 mg	Meat, fish, grains, legumes, bananas, figs	May decrease depression in some individuals by increasing levels of serotonin; deficiencies may contribute to memory problems; also used in the treatment of migraines and premenstrual discomfort.

Continued on following page

TABLE 21.3   ESSENTIAL VITAMINS AND MINERALS *(Continued)*

VITAMIN/ MINERAL	FUNCTION	RDA*	FOOD SOURCES	COMMENTS
Vitamin B_{12}	Necessary in the formation of DNA and the production of red blood cells; associated with folic acid metabolism	Men and Women: 2 μg	Found in animal products (e.g., meats, eggs, dairy products)	Deficiency may contribute to memory problems. Vegetarians can get this vitamin from fortified foods. Intrinsic factor must be present in the stomach for absorption of vitamin B_{12}.
Folic acid (folate)	Necessary in the formation of DNA and the production of red blood cells	Men: 200 μg; Women: 180 μg	Meat, green leafy vegetables, beans, peas, oranges, cantaloupe	Important in women of childbearing age to prevent fetal neural tube defects; may contribute to prevention of heart disease and colon cancer.
Calcium	Necessary in the formation of bones and teeth; neuron and muscle functioning; blood clotting	Men and Women: 800 mg	Dairy products, green leafy vegetables, sardines, oysters, salmon	Calcium has been associated with preventing headaches, muscle cramps, osteoporosis, and premenstrual problems. Requires vitamin D for absorption.
Phosphorus	Necessary in the formation of bones and teeth; a component of DNA, RNA, ADP, and ATP; helps control acid-base balance in the blood	Men and Women: 800 mg	Milk, cheese, fish, meat	
Magnesium	Protein synthesis and carbohydrate metabolism; muscular relaxation following contraction; bone formation	Men: 350 mg; Women: 280 mg	Green vegetables, legumes, seafood, milk	May aid in prevention of asthmatic attacks and migraine headaches. Deficiencies may contribute to insomnia, premenstrual problems.
Iron	Synthesis of hemoglobin and myoglobin; cellular oxidation	Men and Women: 10 mg (Lactating women and those of childbearing age: 15 mg)	Meats, egg yolks, shellfish, dark green leafy vegetables, dried fruit	Iron deficiencies can result in headaches and feeling chronically fatigued.
Iodine	Aids in the synthesis of T_3 and T_4	Men and Women: 150 μg	Iodized salt, seafood	Exerts strong controlling influence on overall body metabolism.
Selenium	Works with vitamin E to protect cellular compounds from oxidation	Men: 70 μg; Women: 55 μg	Seafood, low-fat meats, whole grains, dairy products, legumes	As an antioxidant combined with vitamin E, may have some anticancer effect. Deficiency has also been associated with depressed mood.

Continued on following page

TABLE 21.3   ESSENTIAL VITAMINS AND MINERALS *(Continued)*

VITAMIN/ MINERAL	FUNCTION	RDA*	FOOD SOURCES	COMMENTS
Zinc	Involved in synthesis of DNA and RNA; energy metabolism and protein synthesis; wound healing; increased immune functioning; necessary for normal smell and taste sensation.	Men: 15 mg; Women: 12 mg	Meat, seafood, grains, legumes	An important source for the prevention of infection and improvement in wound healing.

*Recommended dietary allowances.
DNA = Deoxyribonucleic acid. Present in cell nucleus, carrier of genetic information.
RNA = Ribonucleic acid. Controls protein synthesis in all living cells.
ADP = Adenosine diphosphate. } Compounds of adenosine and phosphates involved in energy production.
ATP = Adenosine triphosphate.
SOURCES: Adapted from Yeager (1998); Lutz & Przytulski (1994); Scanlon & Sanders (1995); Institute for Natural Resources (1998).

cancer, arthritis, breathing problems, and other illnesses. Thirty minutes or more of moderate physical activity, such as walking, regularly 3 to 5 days a week can help to increase calorie expenditure and assist in maintaining a healthy weight.

3. Choose a Diet With Plenty of Grain Products, Vegetables, and Fruits

Consumption of these foods is associated with a substantially lower risk for many chronic diseases, including certain types of cancer. These foods are emphasized in this guideline because they are an excellent source of vitamins, minerals, complex carbohydrates (starch and dietary fiber) and, depending upon how they are prepared, are also low in fat.

4. Choose a Diet Low in Fat, Saturated Fat, and Cholesterol

Heart disease and some types of cancer (e.g., breast and colon) have been linked to high-fat diets. Some dietary fat is required for good health. Fats supply energy and essential fatty acids, and they promote absorption of the fat-soluble vitamins A, D, E, and K. However, fats should comprise no more than 30 percent of the total daily calorie intake. Choose foods with mono- and polyunsaturated fat sources, and keep daily cholesterol intake below 300 mg.

5. Choose a Diet Moderate in Sugars

Many foods that contain sugars supply unnecessary calories and few nutrients. A significant health problem from eating too much sugar is tooth decay. Scientific evidence indicates that diets high in sugars do not cause hyperac-

tivity or diabetes. A recent study by Dr. W.B. Grant of the Atmospheric Sciences Division of NASA's Langley Research Center reports that sugar may be the highest dietary risk factor for heart disease in women 35 and older ("Accent on Today's Woman," 1998). He states that, "fructose metabolizes into triglycerides, then is incorporated into very low density lipoprotein cholesterol." Sugar should be used in moderation by most healthy people and sparingly by people with low calorie needs.

6. Choose a Diet Moderate in Salt and Sodium

Sodium and sodium chloride (salt) occur naturally in foods, usually in small amounts. Most foods are prepared with some salt, and some has already been added during processing. In studies with many diverse populations, it has been established that a high intake of salt is associated with high blood pressure. It is therefore important for individuals at risk for high blood pressure to consume less salt in their diets (as well as to increase their physical activity and control their weight).

7. If You Drink Alcoholic Beverages, Do So in Moderation

High levels of alcohol intake raise the risk for high blood pressure, stroke, heart disease, certain cancers, accidents, violence, suicides, birth defects, and overall mortality. Too much alcohol may cause cirrhosis of the liver, inflammation of the pancreas, and damage to the brain and heart. Heavy drinkers also are at risk of malnutrition because alcohol contains calories that may substitute for those in more nutritious foods. The USDA/USDHHS (1995) report defines "moderation" as:

" . . . no more than one drink per day for women and no more than two drinks per day for men. Count as a drink:

● 12 ounces of regular beer (150 calories)
● 5 ounces of wine (100 calories)
● 1.5 ounces of 80-proof distilled spirits (100 calories)"

Good nutrition can help with adaptation to the inevitable stresses of life by promoting a healthy body and a feeling of well-being. Knowledge of good nutrition is learned and not necessarily something that comes naturally. Nurses are in an ideal situation for providing individuals with this type of information.

Chiropractic Medicine

Chiropractic medicine is probably the most widely used form of alternative healing in the United States. It was developed in the late 1800s by a self-taught healer named David Palmer. It was later reorganized and expanded by his son Joshua, a trained practitioner. Palmer's objective was to find a cure for disease and illness that did not rely on drugs, which he considered harmful (Guinness, 1993). Palmer's theory behind chiropractic medicine was that energy flows from the brain to all parts of the body through the spinal cord and spinal nerves. When vertebrae of the spinal column become displaced, they may press on a nerve and interfere with the normal nerve transmission. Palmer named the displacement of these vertebrae **subluxation,** and he alleged that the way to restore normal function was to manipulate the vertebrae back into their normal positions. These manipulations are called *adjustments* (Guinness, 1993).

Adjustments are usually performed by hand, although some chiropractors have special treatment tables equipped to facilitate these manipulations (Figure 21.2). Other processes used to facilitate the outcome of the spinal adjustment by providing muscle relaxation include massage tables, application of heat or cold, and ultrasound treatments.

The chiropractor takes a medical history and performs a clinical examination, which usually includes X-rays of the spine. Today's chiropractors may practice "straight" therapy, that is, the only process provided is that of subluxation adjustments. "Mixer" is a term applied to chiropractors who combine adjustments with adjunct therapies, such as exercise, heat treatments, or massage.

Individuals seek treatment from chiropractors for many types of ailments and illnesses, the most common being back pain. In addition, chiropractors treat clients with headaches, sciatica, shoulder pain, tennis and golfer's elbow, leg and foot pain, hand and wrist pain, allergies, asthma, stomach disorders, and menstrual problems (Guinness, 1993). Some chiropractors are employed by professional sports teams as their team physicians.

Chiropractors are licensed to practice in all 50 states and treatment is covered by government and most private insurance plans. They treat approximately 20 million people in the United States annually (Kaplan & Sadock, 1998).

Therapeutic Touch and Massage

Therapeutic Touch

The technique of therapeutic touch was developed in the 1970s by Dolores Krieger, a nurse associated with the New York University School of Nursing. This therapy is based on the philosophy that the human body projects a field of energy around it. When this field of energy becomes blocked, pain or illness occurs. Practitioners of therapeutic touch use this technique to correct the blockages, thereby relieving the discomfort and improving health.

Based on the premise that the energy field extends beyond the surface of the body, the practitioner need not actually touch the client's skin. The therapist's hands are passed over the client's body, remaining two to four inches from the skin. The goal is to repattern the energy field (Credit et al., 1998). This is done by performing slow, rhythmic, sweeping hand motions over the entire body. Heat should be felt where the energy is blocked. The therapist "massages" the energy field in that area, smoothing it out, and thus correcting the obstruction. Therapeutic touch is thought to reduce pain and anxiety and promote relaxation and health maintenance. It has been useful in the treatment of chronic health conditions.

Massage

Massage is the technique of manipulating the muscles and soft tissues of the body. Chinese physicians prescribed massage for the treatment of disease more than 5000 years ago. The Eastern style of massage focuses on balancing the body's vital energy (chi) as it flows through pathways (meridians), as described earlier in the discussion of acupressure and accupuncture. The western style of massage affects muscles, connective tissues, such as tendons and ligaments, and the cardiovascular system. The Swedish massage, which is probably the best-known Western style, uses a variety of gliding and kneading strokes, along with deep circular movements and vibrations, to relax the muscles, improve circulation, and increase mobility (Guinness, 1993).

Massage has been shown to be beneficial in the following conditions: anxiety, chronic back and neck pain, arthritis, sciatica, migraine headaches, muscle spasms, insomnia, pain of labor and delivery, stress-related disorders, and whiplash. Massage is contraindicated in certain conditions, such as high blood pressure, acute infection, osteoporosis, phlebitis, skin conditions, varicose veins, or over the site of a recent injury, bruise, or burn.

Massage therapists require specialized training in a program accredited by the American Massage Therapy

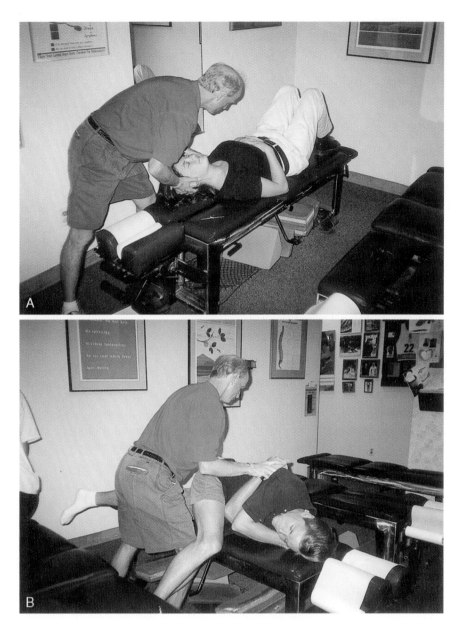

Figure 21.2 Chiropractic adjustments.

Association and must pass the National Certification Examination for Therapeutic Massage and Bodywork.

Yoga

It is thought that **yoga** was developed in India some 5000 years ago. It is attributed to an Indian physician and Sanskrit scholar, Patanjali. The ultimate goal of yoga is to unite the human soul with the universal spirit (Guinness, 1993). Yoga has been found to be especially helpful in relieving stress and in improving overall physical and psychological wellness. Proper breathing is a major component of yoga. It is believed that yoga breathing, a deep, diaphramatic breathing, increases oxygen to brain and body tissues, thereby easing stress and fatigue, and boosting energy.

Another component of yoga is meditation (see Chap-

ter 12). Individuals who practice the meditation and deep breathing associated with yoga find that they are able to achieve a profound feeling of relaxation.

The most familiar type of yoga practiced in the Western countries is hatha yoga. Hatha yoga uses body postures, along with the meditation and breathing exercises, to achieve a balanced, disciplined workout that releases muscle tension, tones the internal organs, and energizes the mind, body, and spirit, so that natural healing can occur (Credit et al., 1998). The complete routine of poses is designed to work all parts of the body, stretching and toning muscles, while also keeping joints flexible. Studies have shown that yoga has provided beneficial effects to some individuals with back pain, stress, migraine, insomnia, high blood pressure, rapid heart rates, and limited mobility (Guiness, 1993).

Pet Therapy

The therapeutic value of pets is no longer just theory. Evidence has shown that animals can directly influence a person's mental and physical well-being. A wave of pet-therapy programs have been established across the country and the numbers are increasing regularly.

A number of studies have provided information about the positive results of human interaction with pets. Some of these include:

1. One year following heart attack, clients who have pets have one-fifth the death rate as those who do not (Friedmann & Thomas, 1995).
2. Petting a dog or cat has been shown to lower blood pressure (Sobel & Ornstein, 1996).
3. Bringing a pet into a nursing home or hospital has been shown to enhance a client's mood and social interaction (Sobel & Ornstein, 1996).

Some researchers believe that animals actually may retard the aging process among those who live alone. Loneliness often results in premature death, and having a pet mitigates the effects of loneliness and isolation.

It may never be known precisely why animals affect humans the way they do, but for those who have pets to love, it comes as no surprise. They provide unconditional, non-judgmental love and affection, which can be the perfect antidote for a depressed mood or a stressful situation. The role of animals in the human healing process still requires more research, but its validity is now widely accepted in both the medical and lay communities.

SUMMARY

Alternative medicine includes those practices that differ from the usual traditional ones in the treatment of disease. Complementary therapies are those that work in partnership with traditional medical practice. This chapter has presented an overview of several complementary therapies and provided information concerning the appropriateness of their use.

Complementary therapies assist the practitioner to view the client in a holistic manner. Most complementary therapies consider the mind and body connection and strive to enhance the body's own natural healing powers. The Office of Alternative Medicine of the National Institutes of Health has established a list of alternative therapies to be used in practice and for investigative purposes. More than $15 billion a year is spent on alternative medical therapies in the United States.

This chapter examined herbal medicine, acupressure, acupuncture, diet and nutrition, chiropractic medicine, therapeutic touch, massage, yoga, and pet therapy. Nurses must be familiar with these therapies, as more and more clients seek out the healing properties of these complementary care strategies.

REVIEW QUESTIONS

SELF-EXAMINATION/LEARNING EXERCISE

Match the following herbs with the uses for which they have been associated:

_____ 1. Chamomile
_____ 2. Echinacea
_____ 3. Feverfew
_____ 4. Ginkgo
_____ 5. Psyllium
_____ 6. St. John's Wort
_____ 7. Valerian

a. For mild to moderate depression
b. To improve memory
c. To relieve upset stomach
d. For insomnia
e. To stimulate the immune system
f. For migraine headache
g. For constipation

8. Which of the following applies to vitamin C?

   a. Coenzyme in protein metabolism; found in meat and dairy products.
   b. Necessary in formation of DNA; found in beans and other legumes.
   c. A powerful antioxidant; found in tomatoes and strawberries.
   d. Necessary for blood clotting; found in whole grains and bananas.

9. Which of the following applies to calcium?

   a. Coenzyme in carbohydrate metabolism; found in whole grains and citrus fruits.
   b. Facilitates iron absorption; found in vegetable oils and liver.
   c. Prevents night blindness; found in egg yolk and cantaloupe.
   d. Important for nerve and muscle functioning; found in dairy products and oysters.

10. Subluxation is a term used by chiropractic medicine to describe

    a. Displacement of vertebrae in the spine.
    b. Adjustment of displaced vertebrae in the spine.
    c. Interference with the flow of energy from the brain.
    d. Pathways along which energy flows throughout the body.

REFERENCES

Accent on today's woman: Sugar blues. (1998, August 2). *The Sunday Oklahoman.*

Complementary and alternative medicine. (1998, Spring). *Complementary & Alternative Medicine Newsletter, V*(2). Silver Spring, MD: Office of Alternative Medicine Clearinghouse.

Coniglione, T. (1998, June). Our doctors must begin looking at the total person. *InBalance.* Oklahoma City, OK: The Balanced Healing Medical Center.

Credit, L.P., Hartunian, S.G., & Nowak, M.J. (1998). *Your guide to complementary medicine.* Garden City Park, NY: Avery Publishing Group.

Friedmann, E., & Thomas, S.A. (1995). Pet ownership, social support, and one-year survival after acute myocardial infarction in the cardiac arrhythmia suppression trial. *American Journal of Cardiology, 76*(17): 1213.

Guinness, A.E. (Ed.). (1993). *Family guide to natural medicine.* Pleasantville, NY: The Reader's Digest Association.

Hocus pocus comes of age. (1997, November). *MoneyWorld,* p. 17.

Institute for Natural Resources. (1998). *Alternative medicine: An objective view* (2nd ed.). Berkeley, CA: INR.

Kaplan, H.I., & Sadock, B.J. (1998). *Synopsis of psychiatry: Behavioral sciences/clinical psychiatry* (8th ed.). Baltimore: Williams & Wilkins.

Lutz, C.A., & Przytulski, K.R. (1994). *Nutrition and diet therapy.* Philadelphia: F.A. Davis.

National Institutes of Health. (1997, November). *NIH consensus report on acupuncture, 15*(5).

Scanlon, V.C., & Sanders, T. (1995). *Essentials of anatomy and physiology* (2nd ed.). Philadelphia: F.A. Davis.

Schoenen, J., Jacquy, J., & Lenaerts, M. (1998, February). Effectiveness of high-dose riboflavin in migraine prophylaxis: A randomized controlled trial. *Neurology, 50:* 466–469.

Sobel, D.S., & Ornstein, R. (1996). *The healthy mind, healthy body handbook.* Los Altos, CA: DR$_X$.

U.S. Department of Agriculture & U.S. Department of Health and Human Services. (1995). *Nutrition and your health: Dietary guidelines for Americans* (4th ed.). Washington, DC: USDA & USDHHS.

Yeager, S. (1998). *New foods for healing.* Emmaus, PA: Rodale Press.

UNIT THREE

Nursing Care of Clients with Alterations in Biopsychosocial Adaptation

DISORDERS USUALLY FIRST DIAGNOSED IN INFANCY, CHILDHOOD, OR ADOLESCENCE

KEY TERMS

autistic disorder
impulsivity
aggression

temperament
negativism
palilalia

echolalia
clinging

OBJECTIVES

After reading this chapter, the student will be able to:

1. Identify psychiatric disorders usually first diagnosed in infancy, childhood, or adolescence.
2. Discuss predisposing factors implicated in the etiology of mental retardation, autistic disorder, attention-deficit/hyperactivity disorder, conduct disorder, oppositional defiant disorder, Tourette's disorder, and separation anxiety disorder.
3. Identify symptomatology and use the infor-

mation in the assessment of clients with the aforementioned disorders.
4. Identify nursing diagnoses common to clients with these disorders and select appropriate nursing interventions for each.
5. Discuss relevant criteria for evaluating nursing care of clients with selected infant, childhood, and adolescent psychiatric disorders.
6. Describe treatment modalities relevant to selected disorders of infancy, childhood, and adolescence.

his chapter examines various disorders in which the symptoms usually first become evident during infancy, childhood, or adolescence. That is not to say that some of the disorders discussed in this chapter do not appear later in life or that symptoms associated with other disorders, such as major depression or schizophrenia, do not appear in childhood or adolescence. The basic concepts of care are applied to treatment in those instances, with consideration of the variances in age and developmental level.

Developmental theories were discussed at length in Chapter 3. Any nurse working with children or adolescents should be knowledgeable about "normal" stages of growth and development. In any case, the developmental process is one that is fraught with frustrations and difficulties at best. Behavioral responses are individual and idiosyncratic. They are, indeed, *human* responses.

Whether or not a child's behavior indicates emotional problems is often difficult to determine. The *DSM-IV* (American Psychiatric Association [APA], 1994) includes the following criteria among many of its diagnostic categories. An emotional problem exists if the behavioral manifestations:

● Are not age-appropriate.
● Deviate from cultural norms.
● Create deficits or impairments in adaptive functioning.

This chapter focuses on the nursing process in care of clients with mental retardation, autistic disorder, attention-deficit/hyperactivity disorder, conduct disorder, oppositional defiant disorder, Tourette's disorder, and separation anxiety disorder.

MENTAL RETARDATION

Mental retardation is defined by deficits in general intellectual functioning and adaptive functioning (APA, 1994). General intellectual functioning is measured by an individual's performance on intelligence quotient (IQ) tests. Adaptive functioning refers to the person's ability to adapt to the requirements of daily living and the expectations of his or her age and cultural group. The *DSM-IV* diagnostic criteria for mental retardation are presented in Table 22.1.

Predisposing Factors

The *DSM-IV* (APA, 1994) states that the etiology of mental retardation may be primarily biological or primarily psychosocial, or some combination of both. In approximately 30 to 40 percent of individuals seen in clinical settings, the etiology cannot be determined. Five major predisposing factors have been identified:

TABLE 22.1   DIAGNOSTIC CRITERIA FOR MENTAL RETARDATION

A. Significantly subaverage general intellectual functioning: an IQ of approximately 70 or below on an individually administered IQ test (for infants, a clinical judgment of significantly subaverage intellectual functioning).
B. Concurrent deficits or impairments in adaptive functioning (i.e., the person's effectiveness in meeting the standards expected for his or her age by his or her cultural group) in at least two of the following areas: communication, self-care, home living, social/interpersonal skills, use of community resources, self-direction, functional academic skills, work, leisure, health, and safety.
C. The onset is before age 18 years.

SOURCE: From APA (1994), with permission.

Heredity Factors. Heredity factors are implicated as the cause in approximately 5 percent of the cases. These factors include inborn errors of metabolism, such as Tay-Sachs disease, phenylketonuria, and hyperglycinemia. Also included are chromosomal disorders, such as Down's syndrome and Klinefelter's syndrome, and single-gene abnormalities, such as tuberous sclerosis and neurofibromatosis.

Early Alterations in Embryonic Development. Prenatal factors that result in early alterations in embryonic development account for approximately 30 percent of mental retardation cases. Damages may occur in response to toxicity associated with maternal ingestion of alcohol or other drugs. Maternal illnesses and infections during pregnancy (e.g., rubella and cytomegalovirus) can also result in congenital mental retardation, as can complications of pregnancy, such as toxemia and uncontrolled diabetes (Kaplan, Sadock, & Grebb, 1994).

Pregnancy and Perinatal Factors. Approximately 10 percent of cases of mental retardation are the result of factors that occur during pregnancy (e.g., fetal malnutrition, viral and other infections, and prematurity) or during the birth process. Examples of the latter include trauma to the head incurred during the process of birth, placenta previa or premature separation of the placenta, and prolapse of the cord.

General Medical Conditions Acquired in Infancy or Childhood. These conditions account for approximately 5 percent of cases of mental retardation. They include infections, such as meningitis and encephalitis; poisonings, such as from insecticides, medications, and lead; and physical trauma, such as head injuries, asphyxiation, and hyperpyrexia (Kaplan & Sadock, 1998).

Environmental Influences and Other Mental Disorders. Fifteen to 20 percent of cases of mental retardation are attributed to deprivation of nurturance and social, linguistic, and other stimulation, and to severe mental disorders, such as autistic disorder (APA, 1994).

Recognition of the cause and period of inception provides information regarding what to expect in terms of behavior and potential. However, each child is different, and consideration must be given on an individual basis in every case.

Application of the Nursing Process

Background Assessment Data (Symptomatology)

The degree of severity of mental retardation is identified by the client's IQ level. Four levels have been delineated: mild, moderate, severe, and profound. The various behavioral manifestations and abilities associated with each of these levels of retardation are outlined in Table 22.2.

Nurses should assess and focus on each client's strengths and individual abilities. Knowledge regarding level of independence in the performance of self-care activities is essential to the development of an adequate plan for the provision of nursing care.

Diagnosis/Outcome Identification

Selection of appropriate nursing diagnoses for the mentally retarded client depends largely on the degree of severity of the condition and the client's capabilities. Possible nursing diagnoses include:

Risk for injury related to altered physical mobility or aggressive behavior.

Self-care deficit related to altered physical mobility or lack of maturity.

Impaired verbal communication related to developmental alteration.

Impaired social interaction related to speech deficiencies or difficulty adhering to conventional social behavior.

Altered growth and development related to isolation from significant others; inadequate environmental stimulation; hereditary factors.

Anxiety (moderate to severe) related to hospitalization and absence of familiar surroundings.

Defensive coping related to feelings of powerlessness and threat to self-esteem.

■ TABLE 22.2   DEVELOPMENTAL CHARACTERISTICS OF MENTAL RETARDATION BY DEGREE OF SEVERITY

LEVEL (IQ)	ABILITY TO PERFORM SELF-CARE ACTIVITIES	COGNITIVE/EDUCATIONAL CAPABILITIES	SOCIAL/COMMUNICATION CAPABILITIES	PSYCHOMOTOR CAPABILITIES
Mild (50–70)	Capable of independent living, with assistance during times of stress.	Capable of academic skills to sixth-grade level. As adult can achieve vocational skills for minimal self-support.	Capable of developing social skills. Functions well in a structured, sheltered setting.	Psychomotor skills usually not affected, although may have some slight problems with coordination.
Moderate (35–49)	Can perform some activities independently. Requires supervision.	Capable of academic skill to second-grade level. As adult may be able to contribute to own support in sheltered workshop.	May experience some limitation in speech communication. Difficulty adhering to social convention may interfere with peer relationships.	Motor development is fair. Vocational capabilities may be limited to unskilled gross motor activities.
Severe (20–34)	May be trained in elementary hygiene skills. Requires complete supervision.	Unable to benefit from academic or vocational training. Profits from systematic habit training.	Minimal verbal skills. Wants and needs often communicated by acting-out behaviors.	Poor psychomotor development. Only able to perform simple tasks under close supervision.
Profound (below 20)	No capacity for independent functioning. Requires constant aid and supervision.	Unable to profit from academic or vocational training. May respond to minimal training in self-help if presented in the close context of a one-to-one relationship.	Little, if any, speech development. No capacity for socialization skills.	Lack of ability for both fine and gross motor movements. Requires constant supervision and care. May be associated with other physical disorders.

SOURCES: Adapted from APA (1994) and Kaplan, Sadock, & Grebb (1994).

Ineffective individual coping related to inadequate coping skills secondary to developmental delay.

The following criteria may be used for measurement of outcomes in the care of the mentally retarded client.

THE CLIENT:

1. Has experienced no physical harm.
2. Has had self-care needs fulfilled.
3. Interacts with others in a socially appropriate manner.
4. Has maintained anxiety at a manageable level.
5. Is able to accept direction without becoming defensive.
6. Demonstrates adaptive coping skills in response to stressful situations.

Planning/Implementation

Table 22.3 provides a plan of care for the child with mental retardation using selected nursing diagnoses, outcome criteria, and appropriate nursing interventions and rationales.

Although this plan of care is directed toward the individual client, it is essential that family members or primary caregivers participate in the ongoing care of the mentally retarded client. They need to receive information regarding the scope of the condition, realistic expectations and client potentials, methods for modifying behavior as required, and community resources from whom they may seek assistance and support.

Evaluation

Evaluation of care given to the mentally retarded client should reflect positive behavioral changes. Evaluation is accomplished by determining if the goals of care have been met through implementation of the nursing actions selected. The nurse reassesses the plan and makes changes where required. Reassessment data may include information gathered by asking the following questions:

1. Have nursing actions providing for the client's safety been sufficient to prevent injury?
2. Have all of the client's self-care needs been fulfilled? Can he or she fulfill some of these needs independently?
3. Has the client been able to communicate needs and desires so that he or she can be understood?
4. Has the client learned to interact appropriately with others?
5. When regressive behaviors surface, can the client accept constructive feedback and discontinue the inappropriate behavior?
6. Has anxiety been maintained at a manageable level?
7. Has the client learned new coping skills through behavior modification? Does the client demonstrate evidence of increased self-esteem because of the accomplishment of these new skills and adaptive behaviors?
8. Have primary caregivers been taught realistic expectations of the client's behavior and methods for attempting to modify unacceptable behaviors?
9. Have primary caregivers been given information regarding various resources from which they can seek assistance and support within the community?

AUTISTIC DISORDER

Autistic disorder is characterized by a withdrawal of the child into the self and into a fantasy world of his or her own creation. The child has markedly abnormal or impaired development in social interaction and communication and a markedly restricted repertoire of activity and interests (APA, 1994). Activities and interests are restricted and may be considered somewhat bizarre.

The disorder is relatively rare and occurs four to five times more often in boys than in girls. Onset of the disorder occurs prior to age 3 and in most cases it runs a chronic course, with symptoms persisting into adulthood.

Predisposing Factors

Although the exact underlying pathology associated with autistic disorder is unknown, several theories have evolved that speculate about etiology. Attention has been focused on the relationship between autistic children and their social environment and on basic biological factors (Schreibman & Charlop, 1989). Both topics are discussed here, although little evidence exists to support the notion that psychosocial factors or parenting abnormalities cause autistic disorder (Popper & Steingard, 1994).

Social Environment

The proponents of these theories have suggested that autistic disorder is caused by the parents and the social environment they provide. Some of the specific causative factors proposed in these theories are parental rejection, child responses to deviant parental personality characteristics, family break-up, family stress, insufficient stimulation, and faulty communication patterns (Schreibman & Charlop, 1989).

Mahler, Pine, and Bergman (1975) suggested that the autistic child is fixed in the presymbiotic phase of development. In this phase, the child creates a barrier between self and others. The normal symbiotic relationship between mother and child, followed by the progression to separation/individuation, does not occur. Ego development is inhibited and the child fails to achieve a sense of self.

TABLE 22.3   CARE PLAN FOR THE CHILD WITH MENTAL RETARDATION

NURSING DIAGNOSIS: RISK FOR INJURY

RELATED TO: Altered physical mobility or aggressive behavior

OUTCOME CRITERIA	NURSING INTERVENTIONS	RATIONALE
Client will not experience injury.	1. Create a safe environment for the client. 2. Ensure that small items are removed from area where client will be ambulating and that sharp items are out of reach. 3. Store items that client uses frequently within easy reach. 4. Pad siderails and headboard of client with history of seizures. 5. Prevent physical aggression and acting-out behaviors by learning to recognize signs that client is becoming agitated.	1–5. Client safety is a nursing priority.

NURSING DIAGNOSIS: SELF-CARE DEFICIT

RELATED TO: Altered physical mobility or lack of maturity

OUTCOME CRITERIA	NURSING INTERVENTIONS	RATIONALE
Client will be able to participate in aspects of self-care.	1. Identify aspects of self-care that may be within the client's capabilities. Work on one aspect of self-care at a time. Provide simple, concrete explanations. Offer positive feedback for efforts. 2. When one aspect of self-care has been mastered to the best of the client's ability, move on to another. Encourage independence but intervene when client is unable to perform.	1. Positive reinforcement enhances self-esteem and encourages repetition of desirable behaviors. 2. Client comfort and safety are nursing priorities.

NURSING DIAGNOSIS: IMPAIRED VERBAL COMMUNICATION

RELATED TO: Developmental alteration

OUTCOME CRITERIA	NURSING INTERVENTIONS	RATIONALE
Client will be able to communicate needs and desires to staff.	1. Maintain consistency of staff assignments over time. 2. Anticipate and fulfill client's needs until satisfactory communication patterns are established. Learn (from family, if possible) special words client uses that are different from the norm. Identify nonverbal gestures or signals that client may use to convey needs if verbal communication is absent. Practice these communications skills repeatedly.	1. Consistency of staff assignments facilitates trust and the ability to understand client's actions and communications. 2. Some children with mental retardation, particularly at the severe level, can learn only by systematic habit training.

Continued on following page

TABLE 22.3 *(Continued)*

NURSING DIAGNOSIS: IMPAIRED SOCIAL INTERACTION
RELATED TO: Speech deficiencies or difficulty adhering to conventional social behavior

OUTCOME CRITERIA	NURSING INTERVENTIONS	RATIONALE
Client will be able to interact with others using behaviors that are socially acceptable and appropriate to developmental level.	1. Remain with client during initial interactions with others on the unit. 2. Explain to other clients the meaning behind some of the client's nonverbal gestures and signals. Use simple language to explain to client which behaviors are acceptable and which are not. Establish a procedure for behavior modification with rewards for appropriate behaviors and aversive reinforcement for inappropriate behaviors.	1. Presence of a trusted individual provides a feeling of security. 2. Positive, negative, and aversive reinforcements can contribute to desired changes in behavior. These privileges and penalties are individually determined as staff learns the likes and dislikes of the client.

These older theories have lost a great deal of credibility through years of research. Many of their claims about the cause of autism have been proved false. Most clinicians now believe that autism is not caused by bad parenting, and no known psychological factors in the development of the child have been shown to be the primary cause of autism (Johnson & Dorman, 1998).

Biological Factors

Genetics. Recent research has revealed strong evidence that genetic factors may play a significant role in the etiology of autism (Popper & Steingard, 1994). Some studies have shown that siblings of autistic children have a 50 times greater chance of being autistic than the general population. Studies with both monozygotic and dizygotic twins have provided strong evidence of a genetic involvement. The understanding of how genetic factors influence the development of autistic disorder has only just begun. Future research is indicated to delineate these factors more clearly.

Neurological Factors. Popper and Steingard (1994) identify early developmental problems such as postnatal neurological infections, congenital rubella, phenylketonuria, and fragile X syndrome as possible implications in the predisposition to autistic disorder. Several studies have also implicated various structural and functional abnormalities in the brain. These include ventricular enlargement, left temporal abnormalities, increased glucose metabolism, and an elevated blood serotonin level. Magnetic resonance imaging (MRI) and positron emission tomography (PET) have shown abnormalities in the structure of the autistic brain, with significant differences within the cerebellum, including the size and numbers of Purkinje cells (Johnson & Dorman, 1998). Popper and Steingard (1994) state: "No evidence exists that any single neurological dysfunction represents a primary deficit in the majority of autistic individuals."

Application of the Nursing Process
Background Assessment Data (Symptomatology)

Impairment in Social Interaction. Autistic children do not form interpersonal relationships with others. They do not respond to, or show interest in, people. As infants they may have an aversion to affection and physical contact. As toddlers, the attachment to a significant adult may be either absent or manifested as exaggerated adherence behaviors. In childhood, there is failure to develop cooperative play, imaginative play, and friendships. Those children with minimal handicaps may eventually progress to the point of recognizing other children as part of their environment, if only in a passive manner.

Impairment in Communication and Imaginative Activity. Both verbal and nonverbal skills are affected. Language may be totally absent, or characterized by immature structure or idiosyncratic utterances whose meaning is clear only to those who are familiar with the child's past experiences. Nonverbal communication, such as facial expression or gestures, is often absent or socially inappropriate. The pattern of imaginative play is often restricted and stereotypical.

Restricted Activities and Interests. Even minor changes in the environment are often met with resistance, or sometimes with hysterical responses. Attachment to, or extreme fascination with, objects that move or spin (e.g., fans) is common. Routine may become an obsession, with minor alterations in routine leading to marked distress. Stereotyped body movements (hand-clapping, rocking, whole-body swaying) and verbalizations (repetition of words or phrases) are typical. Diet abnormalities may include eating only a few specific foods or consuming an excessive amount of fluids.

Behaviors that are self-injurious, such as head-banging or biting the hands or arms, may be evident.

The *DSM-IV* (APA, 1994) diagnostic criteria for autistic disorder are presented in Table 22.4.

Diagnosis/Outcome Identification

Based on data collected during the nursing assessment, possible nursing diagnoses for the client with autistic disorder include:

Risk for self-mutilation related to neurological alterations.

Impaired social interaction related to inability to trust; neurological alterations.

Impaired verbal communication related to withdrawal

<table>
<tr><td>▰ TABLE 22.4 DIAGNOSTIC CRITERIA FOR AUTISTIC DISORDER</td></tr>
</table>

A. A total of six (or more) items from (1), (2), and (3), with at at least two from (1), and one each from (2) and (3):
  1. Qualitative impairment in social interaction, as manifested by at least two of the following:
    (a) Marked impairment in the use of multiple nonverbal behaviors such as eye-to-eye gaze, facial expression, body postures, and gestures to regulate social interaction.
    (b) Failure to develop peer relationships appropriate to developmental level.
    (c) Lack of social or emotional reciprocity.
  2. Qualitative impairments in communication as manifested by at least one of the following:
    (a) Delay in, or total lack of, the development of spoken language (not accompanied by an attempt to compensate through alternative modes of communication such as gesture or mime).
    (b) In individuals with adequate speech, marked impairment in the ability to initiate or sustain a conversation with others.
    (c) Stereotyped and repetitive use of language or idiosyncratic language.
    (d) Lack of varied, spontaneous make-believe play or social imitative play appropriate to developmental level.
  3. Restricted repetitive and stereotyped patterns of behavior, interests, and activities, as manifested by at least one of the following:
    (a) Encompassing preoccupation with one or more stereotyped and restricted patterns of interest that is abnormal either in intensity or focus.
    (b) Apparently inflexible adherence to specific, nonfunctional routines or rituals.
    (c) Stereotyped and repetitive motor mannerisms (e.g., hand or finger flapping or twisting, or complex whole-body movements).
    (d) Persistent preoccupation with parts of objects.
B. Delays or abnormal functioning in at least one of the following areas, with onset prior to age 3 years: (1) social interaction, (2) language as used in social communication, or (3) symbolic or imaginative play.

SOURCE: From APA (1994), with permission.

into the self; inadequate sensory stimulation; neurological alterations.

Personal identity disturbance related to fixation in presymbiotic phase of development; inadequate sensory stimulation; neurological alterations.

The following criteria may be used for measurement of outcomes in the care of the client with autistic disorder.

THE CLIENT:
1. Exhibits no evidence of self-harm.
2. Interacts appropriately with at least one staff member.
3. Demonstrates trust in at least one staff member.
4. Is able to communicate so that he or she can be understood by at least one staff member.
5. Demonstrates behaviors that indicate he or she has begun the separation/individuation process.

Planning/Implementation

Table 22.5 provides a plan of care for the child with autistic disorder, including selected nursing diagnoses, outcome criteria, and appropriate nursing interventions and rationales.

Evaluation

Evaluation of care for the autistic child reflects whether or not the nursing actions have been effective in achieving the established goals. The nursing process calls for reassessment of the plan. Questions for gathering reassessment data may include:

1. Has the child been able to establish trust with at least *one* caregiver?
2. Have the nursing actions directed toward preventing mutilative behaviors been effective in protecting the client from self-harm?
3. Has the child attempted to interact with others? Has he or she received positive reinforcement for these efforts?
4. Has eye contact improved?
5. Has the child established a means of communicating his or her needs and desires to others? Have all self-care needs been met?
6. Does the child demonstrate an awareness of self as separate from others? Can he or she name own body parts and body parts of caregiver?
7. Can he or she accept touch from others? Does he or she willingly and appropriately touch others?

ATTENTION-DEFICIT/HYPERACTIVITY DISORDER

The essential feature of attention-deficit/hyperactivity disorder (ADHD) is a persistent pattern of inattention and/or hyperactivity-**impulsivity** that is more frequent and severe

TABLE 22.5 CARE PLAN FOR THE CHILD WITH AUTISTIC DISORDER

NURSING DIAGNOSIS: RISK FOR SELF-MUTILATION
RELATED TO: Neurological alterations

OUTCOME CRITERIA	NURSING INTERVENTIONS	RATIONALE
Client will not harm self.	1. Work with the child on a one-to-one basis. 2. Try to determine if the self-mutilative behavior occurs in response to increasing anxiety, and if so, to what the anxiety may be attributed. 3. Try to intervene with diversion or replacement activities and offer self to the child as anxiety level starts to rise. 4. Protect the child when self-mutilative behaviors occur. Devices such as a helmet, padded hand mitts, or arm covers may provide protection when the risk for self-harm exists.	1. One-to-one interaction facilitates trust. 2. Mutilative behaviors may be averted if the cause can be determined and alleviated. 3. Diversion and replacement activities may provide needed feelings of security and substitute for self-mutilative behaviors. 4. Client safety is a priority nursing intervention.

NURSING DIAGNOSIS: IMPAIRED SOCIAL INTERACTION
RELATED TO: Inability to trust; neurological alterations

OUTCOME CRITERIA	NURSING INTERVENTIONS	RATIONALE
Client will initiate social interactions with caregiver.	1. Assign a limited number of caregivers to the child. Ensure that warmth, acceptance, and availability are conveyed. 2. Provide child with familiar objects, such as familiar toys or a blanket. Support child's attempts to interact with others. 3. Give positive reinforcement for eye contact with something acceptable to the child (e.g., food, familiar object). Gradually replace with social reinforcement (e.g., touch, smiling, hugging).	1. Warmth, acceptance, and availability, along with consistency of assignment, enhance the establishment and maintenance of a trusting relationship. 2. Familiar objects and presence of a trusted individual provide security during times of distress. 3. Being able to establish eye contact is essential to the child's ability to form satisfactory interpersonal relationships.

NURSING DIAGNOSIS: IMPAIRED VERBAL COMMUNICATION
RELATED TO: Withdrawal into the self; inadequate sensory stimulation; neurological alterations

OUTCOME CRITERIA	NURSING INTERVENTIONS	RATIONALE
Client will establish a means of communicating needs and desires to others.	1. Maintain consistency in assignment of caregivers. 2. Anticipate and fulfill the child's needs until communication can be established. 3. Seek clarification and validation. 4. Give positive reinforcement when eye contact is used to convey nonverbal expressions.	1. Consistency facilitates trust and enhances the caregiver's ability to understand the child's attempts to communicate. 2. Anticipating needs helps to minimize frustration while the child is learning communication skills. 3. Validation ensures that the intended message has been conveyed. 4. Positive reinforcement increases self-esteem and encourages repetition.

NURSING DIAGNOSIS: PERSONAL IDENTITY DISTURBANCE
RELATED TO: Fixation in presymbiotic phase of development; inadequate sensory stimulation; neurological alterations

OUTCOME CRITERIA	NURSING INTERVENTIONS	RATIONALE
Client will name own body parts as separate and individual from those of others.	1. Assist child to recognize separateness during self-care activities, such as dressing and feeding. 2. Assist the child in learning to name own body parts. This can be facilitated by the use of mirrors, drawings, and pictures of the child. Encourage appropriate touching of, and being touched by, others.	1. Recognition of body parts during dressing and feeding increases the child's awareness of self as separate from others. 2. All of these activities may help increase the child's awareness of self as separate from others.

than is typically observed in individuals at a comparable level of development (APA, 1994). These children are highly distractible and unable to contain stimuli. Motor activity is excessive, and movements are random and impulsive. Onset of the disorder is difficult to diagnose in children younger than age 4 because their characteristic behavior is much more variable than that of older children. Frequently the disorder is not recognized until the child enters school. It is four to nine times more common in boys than in girls, and may occur in as many as 3 to 5 percent of school-age children. The disorder is further categorized into the following subtypes (APA, 1994):

1. **Attention-Deficit/Hyperactivity Disorder, Combined Type.** This subtype is used if at least six symptoms of inattention and at least six symptoms of hyperactivity-impulsivity have persisted for at least 6 months. Most children and adolescents with the disorder have the combined type. It is not known whether the same is true of adults with the disorder.

2. **Attention Deficit/Hyperactivity Disorder, Predominantly Inattentive Type.** This subtype is used if at least six symptoms of inattention (but fewer than six symptoms of hyperactivity-impulsivity) have persisted for at least 6 months.

3. **Attention Deficit/Hyperactivity Disorder, Predominantly Hyperactive-Impulsive Type.** This subtype is used if at least six symptoms of hyperactivity-impulsivity (but fewer than six symptoms of inattention) have persisted for at least 6 months. Inattention may often still be a significant clinical feature in such cases.

Predisposing Factors

Biological Influences

Genetics. A number of studies have revealed supportive evidence of genetic influences in the etiology of ADHD. Results have indicated that a large number of parents of hyperactive children showed signs of hyperactivity during their own childhood; that hyperactive children are more likely than normal children to have siblings who are also hyperactive; and that full siblings of hyperactive children are more likely than half-siblings to show hyperactive behavior patterns (Whalen, 1989).

Biochemical Theory. Shaywitz and associates (1983) have implicated a deficit of the catecholamines dopamine and norepinephrine in the overactivity attributed to ADHD. This deficit of neurotransmitters is thought to lower the threshold for stimuli input. The controversy surrounding this theory relates to cause and effect. Does the deficit of neurotransmitters result in hyperactive behavior, or does the stress associated with these problem behaviors result in altered neurotransmitter metabolism? Obviously, more investigation is required for validation of this theory.

Prenatal, Perinatal, and Postnatal Factors. A recent study is consistent with an earlier finding that links maternal smoking during pregnancy and hyperkinetic-impulsive behavior in offspring (Nichols & Chen, 1981). Intrauterine exposure to toxic substances, including alcohol, can produce effects on behavior. Fetal alcohol syndrome includes hyperactivity, impulsivity, and inattention, as well as physical anomalies (Popper & Steingard, 1994).

Perinatal influences that may contribute to ADHD are prematurity, signs of fetal distress, precipitated or prolonged labor, and perinatal asphyxia and low Apgar scores (Clunn, 1991). Postnatal factors that have been implicated include cerebral palsy, epilepsy, and other central nervous system (CNS) abnormalities resulting from trauma, infections, or other neurological disorders (Clunn, 1991; Popper & Steingard, 1994).

Environmental Influences

Environmental Lead. Studies continue to provide evidence of the adverse effects on cognitive and behavioral development in children with elevated body levels of lead. Lead is pervasive in our environment, even though the government has placed tighter restrictions on the substance in recent years. A possible causal link between elevated lead levels and behavior associated with ADHD is still being investigated.

Diet Factors. The possible link between food dyes and additives, such as artificial flavorings and preservatives, was introduced in the mid-1970s by a San Francisco pediatrician (Feingold, 1976). Striking improvement in behavior is often reported by parents and teachers when hyperactive children are placed on a diet free of dyes and additives; however, results have been inconsistent.

Another diet factor that has been receiving much attention in its possible link to ADHD is sugar. A number of studies have been conducted in an effort to determine the effect of sugar on hyperactive behavior. The results have been less than revealing.

What has been clear is that the etiological roles of both food additives and sugar have been greatly exaggerated. There are no reliable indications to date that either of these diet components plays a significant role in the development or exacerbation of hyperactivity (Whalen, 1989).

Psychosocial Influences

Disorganized or chaotic environments, a disruption in family equilibrium, or a disruption in bonding during the first 3 years of life may predispose some individuals to ADHD (Garfinkel & Wender, 1989; Kaplan & Sadock, 1998). Other psychosocial influences that have been implicated include family history of alcoholism, hysterical and sociopathic behaviors, and parental history of hyperactivity. Developmental learning disorders may also predispose to ADHD (Clunn, 1991).

Application of the Nursing Process

Background Assessment Data (Symptomatology)

A major portion of the hyperactive child's problems relate to difficulties in performing age-appropriate tasks. They are highly distractible and have extremely limited attention spans. They often shift from one uncompleted activity to another. Impulsivity, or deficit in inhibitory control, is also common.

Hyperactive children have difficulty forming satisfactory interpersonal relationships. They demonstrate behaviors that inhibit acceptable social interaction. They are disruptive and intrusive in group endeavors. They have difficulty complying with social norms. Some ADHD children are very **aggressive** or oppositional, while others exhibit more regressive and immature behaviors. Low frustration tolerance and outbursts of temper are not uncommon.

Children with ADHD have boundless energy, exhibiting excessive levels of activity, restlessness, and fidgeting. They have been described as "perpetual motion machines," continuously running, jumping, wiggling, or squirming. They experience a greater than average number of accidents, from minor mishaps to more serious incidents that may lead to physical injury or the destruction of property.

The *DSM-IV* diagnostic criteria for ADHD are presented in Table 22.6.

Diagnosis/Outcome Identification

Based on the data collected during the nursing assessment, possible nursing diagnoses for the child with ADHD include:

Risk for injury related to impulsive and accident-prone behavior and the inability to perceive self-harm.
Impaired social interaction related to intrusive and immature behavior.
Self-esteem disturbance related to dysfunctional family system and absence of parent-infant bonding.
Noncompliance with task expectations related to low frustration tolerance and short attention span.

The following criteria may be used for measurement of outcomes in the care of the child with ADHD.

THE CLIENT:

1. Has experienced no physical harm.
2. Interacts with others appropriately.
3. Verbalizes positive aspects about self.
4. Demonstrates fewer demanding behaviors.
5. Cooperatives with staff in an effort to complete assigned tasks.

Planning/Implementation

Table 22.7 provides a plan of care for the child with ADHD using nursing diagnoses common to the disorder, outcome criteria, and appropriate nursing interventions and rationales.

Evaluation

Evaluation of the care of a client with ADHD involves examining client behaviors following implementation of the nursing actions to determine if the goals of therapy have been achieved. Collecting data by using the following types of questions may provide appropriate information for evaluation.

1. Have the nursing actions directed at client safety been effective in protecting the child from injury?

TABLE 22.6   DIAGNOSTIC CRITERIA FOR ATTENTION-DEFICIT/HYPERACTIVITY DISORDER

A. Either (1) or (2):

   1. Six (or more) of the following symptoms of inattention have persisted for at least 6 months to a degree that is maladaptive and inconsistent with developmental level:

   Inattention
   (a) Often fails to give close attention to details or makes careless mistakes in school work, work, or other activities.
   (b) Often has difficulty sustaining attention in tasks or play activities.
   (c) Often does not seem to listen when spoken to directly.
   (d) Often does not follow through on instructions and fails to finish schoolwork, chores, or duties in the workplace (not because of oppositional behavior or failure to understand instructions).
   (e) Often has difficulty organizing tasks and activities.
   (f) Often avoids, dislikes, or is reluctant to engage in tasks that require sustained mental effort (such as schoolwork or homework).
   (g) Often loses things necessary for tasks or activities (e.g., toys, school assignments, pencils, books, or tools).
   (h) Is often easily distracted by extraneous stimuli.
   (i) Is often forgetful in daily activities.

   2. Six (or more) of the following symptoms of hyperactivity-impulsivity have persisted for at least 6 months to a degree that is maladaptive and inconsistent with developmental level:

   Hyperactivity
   (a) Often fidgets with hands or feet or squirms in seat.
   (b) Often leaves seat in classroom or in other situations in which remaining seated is expected.
   (c) Often runs about or climbs excessively in situations in which it is inappropriate (in adolescents or adults, may be limited to subjective feelings of restlessness).
   (d) Often has difficulty playing or engaging in leisure activities quietly.
   (e) Is often "on the go" or often acts as if "driven by a motor."
   (f) Often talks excessively.

   Impulsivity
   (g) Often blurts out answers before questions have been completed.
   (h) Often has difficulty awaiting turn.
   (i) Often interrupts or intrudes on others (e.g., butts into conversations or games).

B. Some hyperactive-impulsive or inattentive symptoms that caused impairment were present before age 7 years.

C. Some impairment from the symptoms is present in two or more settings (e.g., at school or work and at home).

D. There is clear evidence of clinically significant impairment in social, academic, or occupational functioning.

E. The symptoms do not occur exclusively during the course of a pervasive developmental disorder, schizophrenia, or other psychotic disorder and are not better accounted for by another mental disorder (e.g., mood disorder, anxiety disorder, dissociative disorder, or a personality disorder).

   Subtypes:
   1. **Attention-Deficit/Hyperactivity Disorder, Combined Type:** If both criteria A1 and A2 are met for the past 6 months.
   2. **Attention-Deficit/Hyperactivity Disorder, Predominantly Inattentive Type:** If criterion A1 is met but criterion A2 is not met for the past 6 months.
   3. **Attention-Deficit/Hyperactivity Disorder, Predominantly Hyperactive-Impulsive Type:** If criterion A2 is met but criterion A1 is not met for the past 6 months.

SOURCE: From APA (1994), with permission.

2. Has the child been able to establish a trusting relationship with the primary caregiver?

3. Is the client responding to limits set on unacceptable behaviors?

4. Is the client able to interact appropriately with others?

5. Is the client able to verbalize positive statements about self?

6. Is the client able to complete tasks independently or with a minimum of assistance? Can he or she follow through after listening to simple instructions?

7. Is the client able to apply self-control to decrease motor activity?

Psychopharmacological Intervention

Central nervous system stimulants are sometimes given to children with ADHD. Those commonly used include dextroamphetamine (Dexadrine), methylphenidate (Ritalin), and pemoline (Cylert). The actual mechanism by which these medications improve behavior associated with ADHD is not known. In most individuals, they produce stimulation, excitability, and restlessness. In children with ADHD, the effects include an increased attention span, control of hyperactive behavior, and improvement in learning ability.

Side effects include insomnia, anorexia, weight loss,

TABLE 22.7   CARE PLAN FOR THE CHILD WITH ATTENTION-DEFICIT/HYPERACTIVITY DISORDER

NURSING DIAGNOSIS: RISK FOR INJURY
RELATED TO: Impulsive and accident-prone behavior and the inability to perceive self-harm

OUTCOME CRITERIA	NURSING INTERVENTIONS	RATIONALE
Client will be free of injury.	1. Ensure that client has a safe environment. Remove objects from immediate area on which client could injure self as the result of random, hyperactive movements. 2. Identify deliberate behaviors that put the child at risk for injury. Institute consequences for repetition of this behavior. 3. If there is risk of injury associated with specific therapeutic activities, provide adequate supervision and assistance or limit client's participation if adequate supervision is not possible.	1. Objects that are appropriate to the normal living situation can be hazardous to the child whose motor activities are out of control. 2. Behavior can be modified with negative reinforcement. 3. Client safety is a nursing priority.

NURSING DIAGNOSIS: IMPAIRED SOCIAL INTERACTION
RELATED TO: Intrusive and immature behavior

OUTCOME CRITERIA	NURSING INTERVENTIONS	RATIONALE
Client will observe limits set on intrusive behavior and will demonstrate ability to interact appropriately with others.	1. Develop a trusting relationship with the child. Convey acceptance of the child separate from the unacceptable behavior. 2. Discuss with client which behaviors are and are not acceptable. Describe in a matter-of-fact manner the consequences of unacceptable behavior. Follow through. 3. Provide group situations for client.	1. Unconditional acceptance increases feelings of self-worth. 2. Negative reinforcement can alter undesirable behaviors. 3. Appropriate social behavior is often learned from the positive and negative feedback of peers.

NURSING DIAGNOSIS: SELF-ESTEEM DISTURBANCE
RELATED TO: Dysfunctional family system

OUTCOME CRITERIA	NURSING INTERVENTIONS	RATIONALE
Client will demonstrate increased feelings of self-worth by verbalizing positive statements about self and exhibiting fewer demanding behaviors.	1. Ensure that goals are realistic. 2. Plan activities that provide opportunities for success. 3. Convey unconditional acceptance and positive regard. 4. Offer recognition of successful endeavors and positive reinforcement for attempts made. Give immediate positive feedback for acceptable behavior.	1. Unrealistic goals set client up for failure, which diminishes self-esteem. 2. Success enhances self-esteem. 3. Affirmation of client as worthwhile human being may increase self-esteem. 4. Positive reinforcement enhances self-esteem and may increase the desired behaviors.

NURSING DIAGNOSIS: NONCOMPLIANCE (WITH TASK EXPECTATIONS)
RELATED TO: Low frustration tolerance and short attention span

OUTCOME CRITERIA	NURSING INTERVENTIONS	RATIONALE
Client will be able to complete assigned tasks independently or with a minimum of assistance.	1. Provide an environment for task efforts that is as free of distractions as possible. 2. Provide assistance on a one-to-one basis, beginning with simple, concrete instructions. 3. Ask client to repeat instructions to you. 4. Establish goals that allow client to complete a part of the task, rewarding each step-completion with a break for physical activity. 5. Gradually decrease the amount of assistance given to task performance, while assuring the client that assistance is still available if seemed necessary.	1. Client is highly distractible and is unable to perform in the presence of even minimal stimulation. 2. Client lacks the ability to assimilate information that is complicated or has abstract meaning. 3. Repetition of the instructions helps to determine client's level of comprehension. 4. Short-term goals are less overwhelming to clients with a short attention span. The positive reinforcement (physical activity) increases self-esteem and provides incentive for client to pursue the task to completion. 5. This encourages the client to perform independently while providing a feeling of security with the presence of a trusted individual.

tachycardia, and temporary decrease in rate of growth and development. Physical tolerance can occur (less with pemoline than with dextroamphetamine or methylphenidate).

Route and Dosage Information

DEXTROAMPHETAMINE (DEXADRINE)

● Orally (PO) (children 3 to 5 years old): Initial dosage: 2.5 mg/day. This may be increased in increments of 2.5 mg/day at weekly intervals until the desired response is achieved.
● PO (children age 6 years or older): Initial dosage: 5 mg daily or twice a day. This may be increased in increments of 5 mg/day at weekly intervals until the desired response is achieved. Dosage will rarely exceed 40 mg/day. First dose of tablets or elixir forms may be given on awakening; additional doses at intervals of 4 to 6 hours. Sustained-release forms may be used for once-a-day dosage, given in the morning.

METHYLPHENIDATE (RITALIN)

● PO (children age 6 and older): Initial dosage 5 mg before breakfast and lunch. Dosage may be increased gradually in increments of 5 to 10 mg/day at weekly intervals. Maximum daily dosage: 60 mg. Sustained-release form may be used for once-a-day dosage, given in the morning.

PEMOLINE (CYLERT)

● PO (Children age 6 and older): Initial dosage: 37.5 mg/day, administered as a single dose each morning. Dosage may be gradually increased at 1-week intervals in increments of 18.75 mg/day until the desired effect is achieved. Effective dosage usually ranges from 56.25 to 75 mg/day. Maximum recommended dose: 112.5 mg/day.

Nursing Implications

● Assess the client's mental status for changes in mood, level of activity, degree of stimulation, and aggressiveness.
● Ensure that the client is protected from injury. Keep stimuli low and environment as quiet as possible to discourage overstimulation.
● To reduce anorexia, the medication may be administered immediately after meals. The client should be weighed regularly (at least weekly) during hospitalization and at home while on therapy with CNS stimulants because of the potential for anorexia and weight loss and the temporary interruption of growth and development.
● To prevent insomnia, administer last dose at least 6 hours before bedtime. Administer sustained-release forms in the morning.

- In children with behavior disorders, a drug "holiday" should be attempted periodically under direction of the physician to determine effectiveness of the medication and need for continuation.
- Ensure that the parents are aware of the delayed effects of pemoline. Therapeutic response may not be seen for 2 to 4 weeks. The drug should not be discontinued for lack of immediate results.
- Inform parents that over-the-counter (OTC) medications should be avoided while the child is receiving stimulant medication. Some OTC medications, particularly cold and hay fever preparations, contain sympathomimetic agents that could compound the effects of the stimulant and create a drug interaction that may be toxic to the child.
- Ensure that parents are aware that the drug should not be withdrawn abruptly. Withdrawal should be gradual and under the direction of the physician.

CONDUCT DISORDER

With this disorder there is a repetitive and persistent pattern of behavior in which the basic rights of others or major age-appropriate societal norms or rules are violated (APA, 1994). Physical aggression is common. The *DSM-IV* divides this disorder into two subtypes based on the age at onset:

1. **Childhood-Onset Type.** This subtype is defined by the onset of at least one criterion characteristic of conduct disorder prior to age 10. Individuals with this subtype are usually boys, frequently display physical aggression, and have disturbed peer relationships. They may have had oppositional defiant disorder during early childhood, usually meet the full criteria for conduct disorder by puberty, and are likely to develop antisocial personality disorder in adulthood.
2. **Adolescent-Onset Type.** This subtype is defined by the absence of any criteria characteristic of conduct disorder prior to age 10. They are less likely to display aggressive behaviors and tend to have more normal peer relationships than those with childhood-onset type. They are also less likely to have persistent conduct disorder or develop antisocial personality disorder than those with childhood-onset type. The ratio of boys to girls is lower in adolescent-onset type than in childhood-onset type.

Predisposing Factors

Biological Influences

Genetics. Studies with monozygotic and dizygotic twins as well as with nontwin siblings have revealed a sig-

nificantly higher number of conduct disorders among those who have family members with the disorder (Baum, 1989). Although genetic factors appear to be involved in the etiology of conduct disorders, little is yet known about the actual mechanisms involved in genetic transmission. A reasonable assumption is that environmental factors play an important role in the manifestation of the disorder in those who are genetically susceptible.

Temperament. The term **temperament** refers to personality traits that become evident very early in life and may be present at birth. Evidence suggests a genetic component in temperament and an association between temperament and behavioral problems later in life (Plomin, 1983). In a study of children who had been identified as temperamentally difficult in early childhood, Rutter (1987) found a significantly higher degree of aggressive behavior at age 6 than in children who had not been described as difficult.

Biochemical Factors. Various studies have reported a possible correlation between elevated plasma levels of testosterone and aggressive behavior (Baum, 1989). There are, however, insufficient data available at this time to identify a positive relationship. Olweus and colleagues (1980) suggest that testosterone may increase in response to aversive, stressful, or physically strenuous events. Thus, although these hormonal differences are not sufficient to account for aggressive and antisocial behavior, they may serve a mediating role in individual responses to particular environmental circumstances (Baum, 1989).

Psychosocial Influences

Impaired Social Cognition. Studies indicate that children rejected by their peers (i.e., actively disliked as opposed to neglected) have been observed to behave more aggressively, and to engage in lower rates of task-appropriate behaviors and higher rates of task-inappropriate behaviors (Dodge et al., 1982). These children may suffer from cognitive deficits that result in aggressive and inappropriate behavior. These inappropriate responses are in turn causally related to peer rejection, which contributes to a cycle of maladaptive behavior.

Family Influences

The following factors related to family dynamics have been implicated as contributors in the predisposition to this disorder (Clunn, 1991; Popper & Steingard, 1994):

- Parental rejection
- Inconsistent management with harsh discipline
- Early institutional living
- Frequent shifting of parental figures
- Large family size
- Absent father

- Parents with antisocial personality disorder and/or alcohol dependence
- Association with a delinquent subgroup

In addition to those aspects of family dynamics described above, Baum (1989) reports on various studies that implicate additional family influences in the predisposition to conduct disorder. They include:

- Marital conflict and divorce
- Inadequate communication patterns
- Parental permissiveness

Application of the Nursing Process

Background Assessment Data (Symptomatology)

The classic characteristic of conduct disorder is the use of physical aggression in the violation of the rights of others. The behavior pattern manifests itself in virtually all areas of the child's life (home, school, with peers, and in the community). Stealing, lying, and truancy are common problems. The child lacks feelings of guilt or remorse.

The use of tobacco, liquor, or nonprescribed drugs, as well as the participation in sexual activities, occurs earlier than for the peer group's expected age. Projection is a common defense mechanism.

Low self-esteem is manifested by a "tough guy" image. Characteristics include poor frustration tolerance, irritability, and frequent temper outbursts. Symptoms of anxiety and depression are not uncommon.

Level of academic achievement may be low in relation to age and IQ. Manifestations associated with ADHD (e.g., attention difficulties, impulsiveness, and hyperactivity) are very common in children with conduct disorder.

The *DSM-IV* diagnostic criteria for conduct disorder are presented in Table 22.8.

Diagnosis/Outcome Identification

Based on the data collected during the nursing assessment, possible nursing diagnoses for the client with conduct disorder include:

Risk for violence directed toward others related to characteristics of temperament, peer rejection, negative parental role models, dysfunctional family dynamics.
Impaired social interaction related to negative parental role models, impaired social cognition leading to inappropriate social behaviors.

TABLE 22.8 DIAGNOSTIC CRITERIA FOR CONDUCT DISORDER

A. A repetitive and persistent pattern of behavior in which the basic rights of others or major age-appropriate societal norms or rules are violated, as manifested by the presence of three (or more) of the following criteria in the past 12 months, with at least one criterion present in the past 6 months:

Aggression to people and animals
1. Often bullies, threatens, or intimidates others.
2. Often initiates physical fights.
3. Has used a weapon that can cause serious physical harm to others (e.g., a bat, brick, broken bottle, knife, gun).
4. Has been physically cruel to people.
5. Has been physically cruel to animals.
6. Has stolen while confronting a victim (e.g., mugging, purse snatching, extortion, armed robbery).
7. Has forced someone into sexual activity.

Destruction of property
8. Has deliberately engaged in fire setting with the intention of causing serious damage.
9. Has deliberately destroyed others' property (other than by fire setting).

Deceitfulness or theft
10. Has broken into someone else's house, building, or car.
11. Often lies to obtain goods or favors or to avoid obligations (i.e., "cons" others).
12. Has stolen items of nontrivial value without confronting a victim (e.g., shoplifting, but without breaking and entering; forgery).

Serious violations of rules
13. Often stays out at night despite parental prohibitions, beginning before age 13 years.
14. Has run away from home overnight at least twice while living in parental or parental surrogate home (or once without returning for a lengthy period).
15. Is often truant from school, beginning before age 13 years.

B. The disturbance in behavior causes clinically significant impairment in social, academic, or occupational functioning.

C. If the individual is age 18 years or older, criteria are not met for antisocial personality disorder.

Subtypes:
1. **Childhood-Onset Type:** Onset of at least one criterion characteristic of conduct disorder prior to age 10 years.
2. **Adolescent-Onset Type:** Absence of any criteria characteristic of conduct disorder prior to age 10 years.

SOURCE: From APA (1994), with permission.

Defensive coping related to low self-esteem and dysfunctional family system.

Self-esteem disturbance related to lack of positive feedback and unsatisfactory parent-child relationship.

The following criteria may be used for measurement of outcomes in the care of the client with conduct disorder:

THE CLIENT:

1. Has not harmed self or others.
2. Interacts with others in a socially inappropriate manner.
3. Accepts direction without becoming defensive.
4. Demonstrates evidence of increased self-esteem by discontinuing exploitative and demanding behaviors toward others.

Planning/Implementation

Table 22.9 provides a plan of care for the child with conduct disorder using nursing diagnoses common to the disorder, outcome criteria, and appropriate nursing interventions and rationales.

Evaluation

Following the planning and implementation of care, evaluation is made of the behavioral changes in the child with conduct disorder. This is accomplished by determining if the goals of therapy have been achieved. Reassessment, the next step in the nursing process, may be initiated by gathering information using the following questions.

1. Have the nursing actions directed toward managing the client's aggressive behavior been effective?
2. Have interventions prevented harm to others or others' property?
3. Is the client able to express anger in an appropriate manner?
4. Has the client developed more adaptive coping strategies to deal with anger and feelings of aggression?
5. Does the client demonstrate the ability to trust others? Is he or she able to interact with staff and peers in an appropriate manner?
6. Is the client able to accept responsibility for his or her own behavior? Is there less blaming of others?
7. Is the client able to accept feedback from others without becoming defensive?
8. Is the client able to verbalize positive statements about self?
9. Is the client able to interact with others without engaging in manipulation?

OPPOSITIONAL DEFIANT DISORDER

This disorder is characterized by a pattern of negativistic, defiant, disobedient, and hostile behavior toward authority figures that occurs more frequently than is typically observed in individuals of comparable age and developmental level, and interferes with social, academic, or occupational functioning (APA, 1994). The disorder typically begins by 8 years of age, and usually not later than early adolescence. It is more prevalent in boys than in girls before puberty, but the rates are more closely equal after puberty. In a significant proportion of cases, oppositional defiant disorder is a developmental antecedent to conduct disorder (APA, 1994).

Predisposing Factors

Biological Influences

Because the behaviors associated with oppositional defiant disorder are very similar to those of conduct disorder, with the exception of violation of the rights of others, it is reasonable to speculate that they may share at least *some* of the same biological influences. What role, if any, genetics, temperament, or biochemical alterations play in the etiology of oppositional defiant disorder has not been determined.

Family Influences

Opposition during various developmental stages is both normal and healthy. Children first exhibit oppositional behaviors at around 10 or 11 months of age, again as a toddler between 18 and 36 months of age, and finally during adolescence. Pathology is only considered when the developmental phase is prolonged, or when there is overreaction in the child's environment to his or her behavior.

About 10 percent of children exhibit these behaviors in a more intense form than others (Kaplan & Sadock, 1985). Some parents interpret average or increased level of developmental oppositionalism as hostility and a deliberate effort on the part of the child to be in control. If power and control are issues for parents, or if they exercise authority for their own needs, a power struggle can be established between the parents and the child that sets the stage for the development of oppositional defiant disorder.

Popper and Steingard (1994) suggest that the following familial influences may play an etiological role in the development of oppositional defiant disorder:

1. Parental problems in disciplining, structuring, and limit setting.
2. Identification by the child with an impulse-disordered parent who sets a role model for oppositional and defiant interactions with other people.

TABLE 22.9 CARE PLAN FOR CHILD/ADOLESCENT WITH CONDUCT DISORDER

NURSING DIAGNOSIS: RISK FOR VIOLENCE DIRECTED TOWARD OTHERS

RELATED TO: Characteristics of temperament, peer rejection, negative parental role models, dysfunctional family dynamics

OUTCOME CRITERIA	NURSING INTERVENTIONS	RATIONALE
Client will not harm others or others' property.	1. Observe client's behavior frequently through routine activities and interactions. Become aware of behaviors that indicate a rise in agitation. 2. Redirect violent behavior with physical outlets for suppressed anger and frustration. 3. Encourage client to express anger and act as a role model for appropriate expression of anger. 4. Ensure that a sufficient number of staff are available to indicate a show of strength if necessary. 5. Administer tranquilizing medication, if ordered, or use mechanical restraints or isolation room only if situation cannot be controlled with less restrictive means.	1. Recognition of behaviors that precede the onset of aggression may provide the opportunity to intervene before violence occurs. 2. Excess energy is released through physical activities, inducing a feeling of relaxation. 3. Discussion of situations that create anger may lead to more effective ways of dealing with them. 4. This conveys an evidence of control over the situation and provides physical security for staff. 5. It is the client's right to expect the use of techniques that ensure safety of the client and others by the least restrictive means.

NURSING DIAGNOSIS: IMPAIRED SOCIAL INTERACTION

RELATED TO: Negative parental role models; impaired social cognition leading to inappropriate social behavior

OUTCOME CRITERIA	NURSING INTERVENTIONS	RATIONALE
Client will be able to interact with staff and peers using age-appropriate, acceptable behaviors.	1. Develop a trusting relationship with the client. Convey acceptance of the person separate from the unacceptable behavior. 2. Discuss with client which behaviors are and are not acceptable. Describe in matter-of-fact manner the consequence of unacceptable behavior. Follow through. 3. Provide group situations for client.	1. Unconditional acceptance increases feeling of self-worth. 2. Aversive reinforcement can alter undesirable behaviors. 3. Appropriate social behavior is often learned from the positive and negative feedback of peers.

NURSING DIAGNOSIS: DEFENSIVE COPING

RELATED TO: Low self-esteem and dysfunctional family system

OUTCOME CRITERIA	NURSING INTERVENTIONS	RATIONALE
Client will accept responsibility for own behaviors and interact with others without becoming defensive.	1. Explain to client the correlation between feelings of inadequacy and the need for acceptance from others, and how these feelings provoke defensive behaviors, such as blaming others for own behaviors. 2. Provide immediate, matter-of-fact, nonthreatening feedback for unacceptable behaviors.	1. Recognition of the problem is the first step in the change process toward resolution. 2. Client may not realize how these behaviors are being perceived by others.

Continued on following page

TABLE 22.9 *(Continued)*

	3. Help identify situations that provoke defensiveness and practice through role-play more appropriate responses.	3. Role-playing provides confidence to deal with difficult situations when they actually occur.
	4. Provide immediate positive feedback for acceptable behaviors.	4. Positive feedback encourages repetition, and immediacy is significant for these children who respond to immediate gratification.

NURSING DIAGNOSIS: SELF-ESTEEM DISTURBANCE
RELATED TO: Lack of positive feedback and unsatisfactory parent/child relationship

OUTCOME CRITERIA	NURSING INTERVENTIONS	RATIONALE
Client will demonstrate increased feelings of self-worth by verbalizing positive statements about self and exhibiting fewer manipulative behaviors.	1. Ensure that goals are realistic.	1. Unrealistic goals set client up for failure, which diminishes self-esteem.
	2. Plan activities that provide opportunities for success.	2. Success enhances self-esteem.
	3. Convey unconditional acceptance and positive regard.	3. Affirmation of client as a worthwhile human being may increase self-esteem.
	4. Set limits on manipulative behavior. Take caution not to reinforce manipulative behaviors by providing desired attention. Identify the consequences of manipulation. Administer consequences matter-of-factly when manipulation occurs.	4. Negative consequences may work to decrease unacceptable behaviors.
	5. Help client understand that he or she uses manipulation to try to increase own self-esteem. Interventions should reflect other actions to accomplish this goal.	5. When the client feels better about self, the need to manipulate others will diminish.

3. Parental unavailability (e.g., separation, evening work hours).

Application of the Nursing Process

Background Assessment Data (Symptomatology)

The focal issue of oppositional defiant disorder is passive-aggression and is exhibited by obstinacy, procrastination, disobedience, carelessness, **negativism,** dawdling, provocation, resistance to change, violation of minor rules, blocking out communications from others, and resistance to authority (Kaplan & Sadock, 1985). Other symptoms that may be evident are enuresis, encopresis, elective mutism, running away, school avoidance, school underachievement, eating and sleeping problems, temper tantrums, fighting, and argumentativeness.

The oppositional attitude is directed toward adults, most particularly the parents. Symptoms of the disorder may or may not be evident in school or elsewhere in the community (APA, 1994).

Usually these children do not see themselves as being oppositional but view the problem as arising from others whom they believe are making unreasonable demands on them. Interpersonal relationships are fraught with difficulty, including those with peers. These children are often friendless, perceiving human relationships as negative and unsatisfactory. School performance is usually poor because of their refusal to participate and resistance to external demands.

The *DSM-IV* (1994) diagnostic criteria for oppositional defiant disorder is presented in Table 22.10.

Diagnosis/Outcome Identification

Based on the data collected during the nursing assessment, possible nursing diagnoses for the client with oppositional defiant disorder include:

Noncompliance with therapy related to negative temperament, denial of problems, underlying hostility.
Defensive coping related to retarded ego development, low self-esteem, unsatisfactory parent-child relationship.

▰ TABLE 22.10 DIAGNOSTIC CRITERIA FOR OPPOSITIONAL DEFIANT DISORDER

A. A pattern of negativistic, hostile, and defiant behavior lasting at least 6 months, during which four (or more) of the following are present:
  1. Often loses temper
  2. Often argues with adults
  3. Often actively defies or refuses to comply with adult requests or rules
  4. Often deliberately annoys people
  5. Often blames others for his or her mistakes or misbehavior
  6. Is often touchy or easily annoyed by others
  7. Is often angry and resentful
  8. Is often spiteful or vindictive
B. The disturbance in behavior causes clinically significant impairment in social, academic, or occupational functioning.
C. The behaviors do not occur exclusively during the course of a psychotic or mood disorder.
D. Criteria are not met for conduct disorder, and if the individual is age 18 years or older, criteria are not met for antisocial personality disorder.

SOURCE: From APA (1994), with permission.

Self-esteem disturbance related to lack of positive feedback, retarded ego development.
Impaired social interaction related to negative temperament, underlying hostility, manipulation of others.

The following criteria may be used for measurement of outcomes in the care of the client with oppositional defiant disorder.

THE CLIENT:

1. Complies with treatment by participating in therapies without negativism.
2. Accepts responsibility for his or her part in the problem.
3. Takes direction from staff without becoming defensive.
4. Does not manipulate other people.
5. Verbalizes positive aspects about self.
6. Interacts with others in an appropriate manner.

Planning/Implementation

Table 22.11 provides a plan of care for the child with oppositional defiant disorder using nursing diagnoses common to the disorder, outcome criteria, and appropriate nursing interventions and rationales.

Evaluation

The evaluation step of the nursing process calls for reassessment of the plan of care to determine if the nursing actions have been effective in achieving the goals of therapy. The following questions can be used with the child or adolescent with oppositional defiant disorder to gather information for the evaluation.

1. Is the client cooperating with schedule of therapeutic activities? Is level of participation adequate?
2. Is attitude toward therapy less negative?
3. Is the client accepting responsibility for problem behavior?
4. Is the client verbalizing the unacceptableness of his or her passive-aggressive behavior?
5. Is he or she able to identify which behaviors are unacceptable and substitute more adaptive behaviors?
6. Is the client able to interact with staff and peers without defending behavior in an angry manner?
7. Is the client able to verbalize positive statements about self?
8. Is increased self-worth evident with fewer manifestations of manipulation?
9. Is the client able to make compromises with others when issues of control emerge?
10. Is anger and hostility expressed in an appropriate manner? Can the client verbalize ways of releasing anger adaptively?
11. Is he or she able to verbalize true feelings instead of allowing them to emerge through use of passive-aggressive behaviors?

TOURETTE'S DISORDER

The essential feature of this disorder is the presence of multiple motor tics and one or more vocal tics (APA, 1994). They may appear simultaneously or at different periods during the illness. The disturbance causes marked distress or interferes with social, occupational, or other important areas of functioning. The onset of the disorder is before age 18 and is more common in boys than in girls. The duration of the disorder is usually lifelong, but the symptoms usually diminish during adolescence and adulthood.

Predisposing Factors

Biological Factors

Genetics. Tics are noted in two thirds of relatives of Tourette's disorder clients (Popper & Steingard, 1994). Twin studies with both monozygotic and dizygotic twins suggest an inheritable component. Evidence suggests that Tourette's disorder may be transmitted in an autosomal dominant fashion (Kaplan & Sadock, 1998).

Biochemical Factors. Abnormalities in levels of dopamine, serotonin, dynorphin, gamma-aminobutyric acid (GABA), acetylcholine, and norepinephrine have been associated with Tourette's disorder (Popper & Steingard, 1994).

TABLE 22.11 CARE PLAN FOR THE CHILD/ADOLESCENT WITH OPPOSITIONAL DEFIANT DISORDER

NURSING DIAGNOSIS: NONCOMPLIANCE WITH THERAPY
RELATED TO: Negative temperament; denial of problems; underlying hostility

OUTCOME CRITERIA	NURSING INTERVENTIONS	RATIONALE
Client will participate in and cooperate during therapeutic activities.	1. Set forth a structured plan of therapeutic activities. Start with minimum expectations and increase as client begins to manifest evidence of compliance. 2. Establish a system of rewards for compliance with therapy and consequences for noncompliance. Ensure that the rewards and consequences are concepts of value to the client. 3. Convey acceptance of the client separate from the undesirable behaviors being exhibited. ("It is not *you*, but your *behavior*, that is unacceptable.")	1. Structure provides security and one or two activities may not seem as overwhelming as the whole schedule of activities presented at one time. 2. Positive, negative, and aversive reinforcements can contribute to desired changes in behavior. 3. Unconditional acceptance enhances self-worth and may contribute to a decrease in the need for passive-aggression toward others.

NURSING DIAGNOSIS: DEFENSIVE COPING
RELATED TO: Retarded ego development; low self-esteem; unsatisfactory parent-child relationship

OUTCOME CRITERIA	NURSING INTERVENTIONS	RATIONALE
Client will accept responsibility for own behaviors and interact with others without becoming defensive.	1. Help client recognize that feelings of inadequacy provoke defensive behaviors, such as blaming others for problems and the need to "get even." 2. Provide immediate, nonthreatening feedback for passive-aggressive behavior. 3. Help identify situations that provoke defensiveness and practice through role-play more appropriate responses. 4. Provide immediate positive feedback for acceptable behaviors.	1. Recognition of the problem is the first step toward initiating change. 2. Because client denies responsibility for problems, he or she is denying the inappropriateness of behavior. 3. Role-playing provides confidence to deal with difficult situations when they actually occur. 4. Positive feedback encourages repetition, and immediacy is significant for these children who respond to immediate gratification.

NURSING DIAGNOSIS: SELF-ESTEEM DISTURBANCE
RELATED TO: Lack of positive feedback; retarded ego development

OUTCOME CRITERIA	NURSING INTERVENTIONS	RATIONALE
Client will demonstrate increased feelings of self-worth by verbalizing positive statements about self and exhibiting fewer manipulative behaviors.	1. Ensure that goals are realistic. 2. Plan activities that provide opportunities for success. 3. Convey unconditional acceptance and positive regard. 4. Set limits on manipulative behavior. Take caution not to reinforce manipulative behaviors by providing desired attention. Identify the consequences of manipulation. Administer consequences matter-of-factly when manipulation occurs.	1. Unrealistic goals set client up for failure, which diminishes self-esteem. 2. Success enhances self-esteem. 3. Affirmation of client as worthwhile human being may increase self-esteem. 4. Aversive reinforcement may work to decrease unacceptable behaviors.

| | 5. Help client understand that he or she uses manipulation to try to increase own self-esteem. Interventions should reflect other actions to accomplish this goal. | 5. When client feels better about self, the need to manipulate others will diminish. |

NURSING DIAGNOSIS: IMPAIRED SOCIAL INTERACTION
RELATED TO: Negative temperament; underlying hostility; manipulation of others

OUTCOME CRITERIA	NURSING INTERVENTIONS	RATIONALE
Client will be able to interact with staff and peers using age-appropriate, acceptable behaviors.	1. Develop a trusting relationship with the client. Convey acceptance of the person separate from the unacceptable behavior. 2. Explain to the client about passive-aggressive behavior. Explain how these behaviors are perceived by others. Describe which behaviors are not acceptable and role play more adaptive responses. Give positive feedback for acceptable behaviors. 3. Provide peer group situations for the client.	1. Unconditional acceptance increases feelings of self-worth and may serve to diminish feelings of rejection that have accumulated over a long period. 2. Role-playing is a way to practice behaviors that do not come readily to the client, making it easier when the situation actually occurs. Positive feedback enhances repetition of desirable behaviors. 3. Appropriate social behavior is often learned from the positive and negative feedback of peers. Groups also provide an atmosphere for using the behaviors rehearsed in role-play.

Neurotransmitter pathways through the basal ganglia, globus pallidus, and subthalamic regions appear to be involved.

Structural Factors. Neuroimaging brain studies have been consistent in finding dysfunction in the area of the basal ganglia. Enlargement has been found in the caudate nucleus and decreased cerebral blood flow in the left lenticular nucleus (Riddle, Rasmussen, & Woods, 1992; Singer, Reiss, & Brown, 1993).

Environmental Factors

Additional retrospective findings may be implicated in the etiology of Tourette's disorder, such as increased prenatal complications and low birth weight. Greater emotional stress during pregnancy and more nausea and vomiting during the first trimester of pregnancy have been noted in the mothers of these children (Leckman, Dolnansky, & Hardin 1990). It is speculated that these environmental factors may temper the genetic predisposition to Tourette's disorder.

Application of the Nursing Process

Background Assessment Data (Symptomatology)

The motor tics of Tourette's disorder may involve the head, torso, and upper and lower limbs. Initial symptoms may begin with a single motor tic, most commonly eye blinking, or with multiple symptoms. The *DSM-IV* identifies simple

motor tics as eye blinking, neck jerking, shoulder shrugging, facial grimacing, and coughing. Common complex motor tics include touching, squatting, hopping, skipping, deep knee bends, retracing steps, and twirling when walking.

Vocal tics include various words or sounds such as clicks, grunts, yelps, barks, sniffs, snorts, coughs, and in about 10 percent of cases, a complex vocal tic involving the uttering of obscenities (APA, 1994). Vocal tics may include repeating certain words or phrases out of context, repeating one's own sounds or words **(palilalia)**, or repeating what others say **(echolalia).**

The movements and vocalizations are experienced as compulsive and irresistible but can be suppressed for varying lengths of time. They are exacerbated by stress and attenuated during periods in which the individual becomes totally absorbed by an activity. Tics are usually markedly diminished during sleep (APA, 1994).

The age at onset of Tourette's disorder can be as early as age 2 years but occurs most commonly during childhood or early adolescence, with the median age being 7 years. It affects four to five individuals per 10,000. The *DSM-IV* diagnostic criteria for Tourette's disorder are presented in Table 22.12.

Diagnosis/Outcome Identification

Based on data collected during the nursing assessment, possible nursing diagnoses for the client with Tourette's disorder include:

TABLE 22.12 DIAGNOSTIC CRITERIA FOR TOURETTE'S DISORDER

A. Both multiple motor and one or more vocal tics have been present at some time during the illness, although not necessarily concurrently. (A *tic* is a sudden, rapid, recurrent, nonrhythmic, stereotyped motor movement or vocalization.)
B. The tics occur many times a day (usually in bouts) nearly every day or intermittently throughout a period of more than 1 year, and during this period there was never a tic-free period of more than 3 consecutive months.
C. The disturbance causes marked distress or significant impairment in social, occupational, or other important areas of functioning.
D. The onset is before age 18 years.
E. The disturbance is not due to the direct physiological effects of a substance (e.g., stimulants) or a general medical condition (e.g., Huntington's disease or postviral encephalitis).

SOURCE: From APA (1994), with permission.

Risk for violence directed at self or others related to low tolerance for frustration.

Impaired social interaction related to impulsiveness, oppositional and aggressive behavior.

Self-esteem disturbance related to shame associated with tic behaviors.

The following criteria may be used for measurement of outcomes in the care of the client with Tourette's disorder.

THE CLIENT:

1. Has not harmed self or others.
2. Interacts with staff and peers in an appropriate manner.
3. Demonstrates self-control by managing tic behavior.
4. Follows rules of unit without becoming defensive.
5. Verbalizes positive aspects about self.

Planning/Implementation

Table 22.13 provides a plan of care for the child or adolescent with Tourette's disorder using selected nursing diagnoses, outcome criteria, and appropriate nursing interventions and rationales.

Evaluation

Evaluation of care for the child with Tourette's disorder reflects whether or not the nursing actions have been effective in achieving the established goals. The nursing process calls for reassessment of the plan. Questions for gathering reassessment data may include:

1. Has the client refrained from causing harm to self or others during times of increased tension?

2. Has the client developed adaptive coping strategies for dealing with frustration to prevent resorting to self-destruction or aggression to others?
3. Is the client able to interact appropriately with staff and peers?
4. Is the client able to suppress tic behaviors when he or she chooses to do so?
5. Does the client set a time for "release" of the suppressed tic behaviors?
6. Does the client verbalize positive aspects about self, particularly as they relate to his or her ability to manage the illness?
7. Does the client comply with treatment in a nondefensive manner?

Psychopharmacological Intervention

Medications are used to reduce the severity of the tics in clients with Tourette's disorder. Pharmacotherapy is most effective when it is combined with other forms of therapy, such as education and supportive intervention, individual counseling or psychotherapy, and family therapy (McSwiggan-Hardin, 1995). Some cases of the disorder are mild, and clients choose not to use medication until the symptoms become severe and more intense intervention is warranted. A number of medications have been used to treat Tourette's disorder. The most common ones are discussed here.

Haloperidol (Haldol). Haloperidol has been the drug of choice for Tourette's disorder. The dosage is 0.05 to 0.075 mg/kg/day in two to three divided doses. Children taking haloperidol can develop the same side effects associated with the neuroleptic as prescribed for psychotic disorders (see Chapter 19). Children should be monitored closely for efficacy of the drug as well as adverse effects. Because of the potential for adverse effects, haloperidol should be reserved for children with severe symptoms or with symptoms that impede their ability to function in school, socially, or within their family setting (McSwiggan-Hardin, 1995).

Pimozide (Orap). Pimozide is a neuroleptic with a response rate and side effect profile similar to those of haloperidol. It is used in the management of severe motor or vocal tics that have failed to respond to more conventional treatment. Pimozide is not recommended for children under age 12. Dosage is initiated at 1 to 2 mg/day and increased weekly up to 3 to 5 mg/day.

Clonidine (Catapres). Clonidine is an alpha-adrenergic agonist that is approved for use as an antihypertensive agent. Results of studies on the efficacy of clonidine in the treatment of Tourette's disorder have been mixed. Some physicians use clonidine as a first choice because of the few side effects and relative safety associated with it. Common side effects include dry mouth, sedation, and dizziness or hypotension.

TABLE 22.13   CARE PLAN FOR THE CHILD OR ADOLESCENT WITH TOURETTE'S DISORDER

NURSING DIAGNOSIS: RISK FOR VIOLENCE DIRECTED AT SELF OR OTHERS
RELATED TO: Low tolerance for frustration

OUTCOME CRITERIA	NURSING INTERVENTIONS	RATIONALE
Client will not harm self or others.	1. Observe client's behavior frequently through routine activities and interactions. Become aware of behaviors that indicate a rise in agitation. 2. Monitor for self-destructive behavior and impulses. A staff member may need to stay with the client to prevent self-mutilation. 3. Provide hand coverings and other restraints that prevent the client from self-mutilative behaviors. 4. Redirect violent behavior with physical outlets for frustration.	1. Stress commonly increases tic behaviors. Recognition of behaviors that precede the onset of aggression may provide the opportunity to intervene before violence occurs. 2. Client safety is a nursing priority. 3. Provide immediate external controls against self-aggressive behaviors. 4. Excess energy is released through physical activities and a feeling of relaxation is induced.

NURSING DIAGNOSIS: IMPAIRED SOCIAL INTERACTION
RELATED TO: Impulsiveness; oppositional and aggressive behavior

OUTCOME CRITERIA	NURSING INTERVENTIONS	RATIONALE
Client will be able to interact with staff and peers using age-appropriate, acceptable behaviors.	1. Develop a trusting relationship with the client. Convey acceptance of the person separate from the unacceptable behavior. 2. Discuss with client which behaviors are and are not acceptable. Describe in matter-of-fact manner the consequences of unacceptable behavior. Follow through. 3. Provide group situations for client.	1. Unconditional acceptance increases feelings of self-worth. 2. Negative reinforcement can alter undesirable behaviors. 3. Appropriate social behavior is often learned from the positive and negative feedback of peers.

NURSING DIAGNOSIS: SELF-ESTEEM DISTURBANCE
RELATED TO: Shame associated with tic behaviors

OUTCOME CRITERIA	NURSING INTERVENTIONS	RATIONALE
Client will verbalize positive aspects about self not associated with tic behaviors.	1. Convey unconditional acceptance and positive regard. 2. Set limits on manipulative behavior. Take caution not to reinforce manipulative behaviors by providing desired attention. Identify the consequences of manipulation. Administer consequences matter-of-factly when manipulation occurs. 3. Help client understand that he or she uses manipulation to try to increase own self-esteem. Interventions should reflect other actions to accomplish this goal.	1. Communication of client as a worthwhile human being may increase self-esteem. 2. Aversive consequences may work to decrease unacceptable behaviors. 3. When client feels better about self, the need to manipulate others will diminish.

Continued on following page

TABLE 22.13 *(Continued)*

4. If client chooses to suppress tics in the presence of others, provide a specified "tic time," during which he or she "vents" tics, feelings, and behaviors (alone or with staff).	4. Allows for release of tics and assists in sense of control and management of symptoms (Rosner & Pollice, 1991).
5. Ensure that client has regular one-to-one time with RN staff.	5. Provides opportunity for educating about illness and teaching management tactics. Assists in exploring feelings around illness and incorporating illness into a healthy sense of self (Rosner & Pollice, 1991).

SEPARATION ANXIETY DISORDER

The essential feature of this disorder is excessive anxiety concerning separation from the home or from those to whom the person is attached (APA, 1994). The anxiety is beyond that which would be expected for the individual's developmental level and interferes with social, academic, occupational, or other areas of functioning. Onset may occur anytime before age 18 years and is more common in girls than in boys.

Predisposing Factors

Biological Influences

Genetics. Studies have been conducted in which the children of adult clients diagnosed as having separation anxiety disorder were studied. A second method, studying parents and other relatives of children diagnosed as having separation anxiety disorder, has also been used (Klein & Last, 1989). The results of these studies have shown that a greater number of children with relatives who manifest anxiety problems develop anxiety disorders themselves than do children with no such family patterns. The results are significant enough to speculate that there is a hereditary influence in the development of separation anxiety disorder, but the mode of genetic transmission has not been determined.

Temperament. It is well established that children differ from birth or shortly thereafter on a number of temperamental characteristics (Berger, 1985; Thomas & Chess, 1977). These studies indicate that from a hereditary perspective, individual differences in temperaments may be related to the acquisition of fear and anxiety disorders in childhood. This may be referred to as *anxiety proneness* or *vulnerability* and may denote an inherited "disposition" toward developing anxiety disorders.

Environmental Influences

Stressful Life Events. Studies have shown a relationship between life events and the development of anxiety disorders (Klein & Last, 1989). It is thought that perhaps children who already are vulnerable or predisposed to developing anxiety disorders may be affected significantly by stressful life events. More research is needed before firm conclusions can be drawn.

Family Influences

Various theories expound on the idea that anxiety disorders in children are related to an overattachment to the mother (Last, 1989). Kaplan and Sadock (1985) attribute the major determinants of anxiety disorders to transactions relating to separation conflicts between parent and child. The *DSM-IV* (APA, 1994) suggests that children with separation anxiety disorders come from families that are close-knit.

Some parents may instill anxiety in their children by overprotecting them from expectable dangers or by exaggerating the dangers of the present and the future (Kaplan & Sadock, 1998). Some parents may also transfer their fears and anxieties to their children through role modeling. For example, a parent who becomes fearful in the presence of a small, harmless dog and retreats with dread and apprehension teaches the young child by example that this is an appropriate response.

Application of the Nursing Process

Background Assessment Data (Symptomatology)

Age at onset of this disorder may be as early as preschool age, rarely as late as adolescence. In most cases, the child has difficulty separating from the mother. Occasionally the separation reluctance is directed toward the father, siblings, or another significant individual to whom the child is attached. Anticipation of separation may result in tantrums, crying, screaming, complaints of physical problems, and **"clinging"** behaviors.

Reluctance or refusal to attend school is especially common in adolescence. Younger children may "shadow," or follow around, the person from whom they are afraid to be separated. During middle childhood or adolescence they may refuse to sleep away from home (e.g., at a friend's house or at camp). Interpersonal peer relationships are usually not a problem with these children. They are generally well liked by their peers and are reasonably socially skilled (Last, 1989).

Worrying is common and relates to the possibility of harm coming to self or to the attachment figure. Younger children may even have nightmares to this effect.

Specific phobias are not uncommon (e.g., fear of the dark, ghosts, animals). Depressed mood is frequently present and often precedes the onset of the anxiety symptoms, which commonly occur following a major stressor. The *DSM-IV* diagnostic criteria for separation anxiety disorder are presented in Table 22.14.

Diagnosis/Outcome Identification

Based on the data collected during the nursing assessment, possible nursing diagnoses for the client with separation anxiety disorder include:

Anxiety (severe) related to family history, temperament, overattachment to parent, negative role modeling.
Ineffective individual coping related to unresolved separation conflicts and inadequate coping skills evidenced by numerous somatic complaints.
Impaired social interaction related to reluctance to be away from attachment figure.

The following criteria may be used for measurement of outcomes in the care of the client with separation anxiety disorder.

THE CLIENT:

1. Is able to maintain anxiety at manageable level.
2. Demonstrates adaptive coping strategies for dealing with anxiety when separation from attachment figure is anticipated.
3. Interacts appropriately with others and spends time away from attachment figure to do so.

Planning/Implementation

Table 22.15 provides a plan of care for the child or adolescent with separation anxiety disorder, using nursing diagnoses common to this disorder, outcome criteria, and appropriate nursing interventions and rationales.

Evaluation

Evaluation of the child or adolescent with separation anxiety disorder requires reassessment of the behaviors for which the family sought treatment. Both the client and the family members will have to change their behavior. The following types of questions may provide assistance in gathering data required for evaluating whether the nursing interventions have been effective in achieving the goals of therapy.

1. Is the client able to maintain anxiety at a manageable level—that is, without temper tantrums, screaming, "clinging"?
2. Have complaints of physical symptoms diminished?
3. Has the client demonstrated the ability to cope in more adaptive ways in the face of escalating anxiety?

TABLE 22.14 DIAGNOSTIC CRITERIA FOR SEPARATION ANXIETY DISORDER

A. Developmentally inappropriate and excessive anxiety concerning separation from home or from those to whom the individual is attached, as evidenced by three (or more) of the following:
   1. Recurrent excessive distress when separation from home or major attachment figures occurs or is anticipated
   2. Persistent and excessive worry about losing, or about possible harm befalling, major attachment figures
   3. Persistent and excessive worry that an untoward event will lead to separation from a major attachment figure (e.g., getting lost or being kidnapped)
   4. Persistent reluctance or refusal to go to school or elsewhere because of fear of separation.
   5. Persistently and excessively fearful or reluctant to be alone or without major attachment figures at home or without significant adults in other settings
   6. Persistent reluctance or refusal to go to sleep without being near a major attachment figure or to sleep away from home
   7. Repeated nightmares involving the theme of separation
   8. Repeated complaints of physical symptoms (such as headaches, stomachaches, nausea, or vomiting) when separation from major attachment figures occurs or is anticipated
B. The duration of the disturbance is at least 4 weeks.
C. The onset is before age 18 years.
D. The disturbance causes clinically significant distress or impairment in social, academic (occupational), or other important areas of functioning.
E. The disturbance does not occur exclusively during the course of a pervasive developmental disorder, schizophrenia, or other psychotic disorder and, in adolescents and adults, is not better accounted for by panic disorder with agoraphobia.

SOURCE: From APA (1994), with permission.

TABLE 22.15   CARE PLAN FOR THE CLIENT WITH SEPARATION ANXIETY DISORDER

NURSING DIAGNOSIS: ANXIETY (SEVERE)

RELATED TO: Family history; temperament; overattachment to parent; negative role-modeling

OUTCOME CRITERIA	NURSING INTERVENTIONS	RATIONALE
Client will maintain anxiety at no higher than moderate level in the face of events that formerly have precipitated panic.	1. Establish an atmosphere of calmness, trust, and genuine positive regard.	1. Trust and unconditional acceptance are necessary for satisfactory nurse-client relationship. Calmness is important because anxiety is easily transmitted from one person to another.
	2. Assure client of his or her safety and security.	2. Symptoms of panic anxiety are very frightening.
	3. Explore the child's or adolescent's fears of separating from the parents. Explore with the parents possible fears they may have of separation from the child.	3. Some parents may have an underlying fear of separation from the child, of which they are unaware and which they are unconsciously transferring to the child.
	4. Help parents and child initiate realistic goals (e.g., child to stay with sitter for 2 hours with minimal anxiety; or, child to stay at friend's house without parents until 9 PM without experiencing panic anxiety).	4. Parents may be so frustrated with child's clinging and demanding behaviors that assistance with problem solving may be required.
	5. Give, and encourage parents to give, positive reinforcement for desired behaviors.	5. Positive reinforcement encourages repetition of desirable behaviors.

NURSING DIAGNOSIS: INEFFECTIVE INDIVIDUAL COPING

RELATED TO: Unresolved separation conflicts and inadequate coping skills

EVIDENCED BY: Numerous somatic complaints

OUTCOME CRITERIA	NURSING INTERVENTIONS	RATIONALE
Client will demonstrate use of more adaptive coping strategies (than physical symptoms) in response to stressful situations.	1. Encourage child or adolescent to discuss specific situations in life that produce the most distress and describe his or her response to these situations. Include parents in the discussion.	1. Client and family may be unaware of the correlation between stressful situations and the exacerbation of physical symptoms.
	2. Help the child or adolescent who is perfectionistic to recognize that self-expectations may be unrealistic. Connect times of unmet self-expectations to the exacerbation of physical symptoms.	2. Recognition of maladaptive patterns is the first step in the change process.
	3. Encourage parents and child to identify more adaptive coping strategies that the child could use in the face of anxiety that feels overwhelming. Practice through role-play.	3. Practice facilitates the use of the desired behavior when the individual is actually faced with the stressful situation.

NURSING DIAGNOSIS: IMPAIRED SOCIAL INTERACTION

RELATED TO: Reluctance to be away from attachment figure

OUTCOME CRITERIA	NURSING INTERVENTIONS	RATIONALE
Client will be able to spend time with staff and peers without excessive anxiety.	1. Develop a trusting relationship with client.	1. This is the first step in helping the client learn to interact with others.

2. Attend groups with the child and support efforts to interact with others. Give positive feedback.

3. Convey to the child the acceptability of his or her not participating in group in the beginning. Gradually encourage small contributions until client is able to participate more fully.

4. Help client set small personal goals (e.g., "Today I will speak to one person I don't know.").

2. Presence of a trusted individual provides security during times of distress. Positive feedback encourages repetition.

3. Small successes will gradually increase self-confidence and decrease self-consciousness, so that client will feel less anxious in the group situation.

4. Simple, realistic goals provide opportunities for success that increase self-confidence and may encourage the client to attempt more difficult objectives in the future.

TEST YOUR CRITICAL THINKING SKILLS

Jimmy, age 9, has been admitted to the child psychiatric unit with a diagnosis of attention-deficit/hyperactivity disorder. He has been unmanageable at school and at home, and was recently suspended from school for continuous disruption of his class. He refuses to sit in his chair or do his work. He yells out in class, interrupts the teacher and the other students, and lately has become physically aggressive when he cannot have his way. He was suspended after hitting his teacher when she asked him to return to his seat.

Jimmy's mother describes him as a restless and demanding baby, who grew into a restless and demanding toddler. He has never gotten along well with his peers. Even as a small child, he would take his friends' toys away from them or bite them if they tried to hold their own with him. His 5-year-old sister is afraid of him and refuses to be alone with him.

During the nurse's intake assessment, Jimmy paced the room or rocked in his chair. He talked incessantly on a superficial level and jumped from topic to topic. He told the nurse that he did not know why he was there. He acknowledged that he had some problems at school but said that was only because the other kids picked on him and the teacher did not like him. He said he got into trouble at home sometimes but that was because his parents liked his little sister better than they liked him.

The physician has ordered methylphenidate 5 mg twice a day for Jimmy. His response to this order is, "I'm not going to take drugs. I'm not sick!"

Answer the following questions related to Jimmy:

1. What are the pertinent assessment data to be noted by the nurse?
2. What is the primary nursing diagnosis for Jimmy?
3. Aside from client safety, to what problems would the nurse want to direct intervention with Jimmy?

R E S E A R C H   N O T E

Adult psychiatric status of hyperactive boys grown up. *American Journal of Psychiatry* (1998, April), 155, 493–498.
Mannuzza, S., Klein, R.G., Bessler, A., Malloy, P., & LaPadula, M.

Description of the Study: In this study, 85 Caucasian boys with ADHD were compared, at mean ages of 7 to 24, with 73 control subjects. At a mean age of 24, the groups were interviewed by trained clinicians who were using structured tools and who were blind as to group status.

Results of the Study: It was found that as adults, 12 percent of the boys with ADHD, as compared to 3 percent of the control subjects, had antisocial disorders and 19 percent of ADHD boys, as compared to 10 percent of the control subjects, had a substance-use disorder. Only 4 percent of boys with ADHD still had ADHD as adults. The prevalence of mood and anxiety disorders was similar for the two groups.

Comments: The authors concluded that the results of this study were consistent with earlier studies which indicated that children with ADHD are at higher risk for antisocial personality disorder and substance-use disorder as adults than children who do not have ADHD.

5. Does the client verbalize an intention to return to school?
6. Have nightmares and fears of the dark subsided?
7. Is the client able to interact with others away from the attachment figure?
8. Has the precipitating stressor been identified? Have strategies for coping more adaptively to similar stressors in the future been established?

SUMMARY

Child and adolescent psychiatric nursing is a specialty that has been given little attention. Most basic nursing

4. Have the parents identified their role in the separation conflict? Are they able to discuss more adaptive coping strategies?

INTERNET REFERENCES

- Additional information about attention-deficit/hyperactivity disorder may be located at the following websites:
  a. http://www.chadd.org
  b. http://www.laurus.com

- Additional information about autism may be located at the following websites:
  a. http://www.autism-society.org/autism.html/
  b. http://www.laurus.com

- Additional information about medications to treat attention-deficit/hyperactivity disorder may be located at the following websites:
  a. http://www.fadavis.com
  b. http://www.laurus.com

curricula include minimal instruction in child psychiatric nursing, and the topic is often ignored on state board examinations (Clunn, 1991). Even though nurses work in many areas that place them in ideal positions to identify emotionally disturbed children, many of them do not have sufficient knowledge of child psychopathology to recognize maladaptive behaviors.

This chapter has presented some of the most prevalent disorders identified by the *DSM-IV* (APA, 1994) as first becoming evident in infancy, childhood, or adolescence. An explanation of various etiological factors was presented for each disorder to assist in the comprehension of underlying dynamics. These included biological, environmental, and family influences.

The nursing process was presented as the vehicle for delivery of care. Symptomatology for each of the disorders provided background assessment data. Nursing diagnoses identified specific behaviors that were targets for change. Both client and family were considered in the planning and implementation. Behavior modification is the focus of nursing intervention with children and adolescents. With families, attention is given to education and referrals to community resources from which they can derive support. Reassessment data provide information for evaluation of nursing interventions in achieving the desired outcomes.

Child psychiatry is an area in which nursing can make a valuable contribution. Nurses who choose this field have an excellent opportunity to serve in the promotion of emotional wellness for children and adolescents.

A discussion of psychopharmacological intervention was included for the disorders for which this form of treatment is relevant.

REVIEW QUESTIONS

SELF-EXAMINATION/LEARNING EXERCISE

Select the answer that is most appropriate for each of the following questions.

1. In an effort to help the mild-to-moderately mentally retarded child develop satisfying relationships with others, which of the following nursing interventions is most appropriate?
   a. Interpret the child's behavior for others.
   b. Set limits on behavior that is socially inappropriate.
   c. Allow the child to behave spontaneously, for he or she has no concept of right or wrong.
   d. This child is not capable of forming social relationships.

2. The autistic child has difficulty with trust. With this in mind, which of the following nursing actions would be *most* appropriate?
   a. Encourage all staff to hold the child as often as possible, conveying trust through touch.
   b. Assign a different staff member each day so the child will learn that everyone can be trusted.
   c. Assign the same staff person as often as possible to promote feelings of security and trust.
   d. Avoid eye contact, as it is extremely uncomfortable for the child and may even discourage trust.

3. Which of the following nursing diagnoses would be considered the *priority* in planning care for the autistic child?
   a. Risk for self-mutilation evidenced by banging head against wall.
   b. Impaired social interaction evidenced by unresponsiveness to people.
   c. Impaired verbal communication evidenced by absence of verbal expression.
   d. Personal identity disturbance evidenced by inability to differentiate self from others.

4. Which of the following activities would be most appropriate for the child with ADHD?
   a. Monopoly
   b. Volleyball
   c. Pool
   d. Checkers

5. With regard to the literature (even though the results are inconclusive), which of the following foods might it be wise to omit when helping the hyperactive child select a snack?
   a. Peanut butter and crackers
   b. Popcorn and apple juice
   c. Peanuts and raisins
   d. Cookies and Koolaid

6. Which of the following groups are most commonly used for drug management of the hyperactive child?
   a. CNS depressants (e.g., diazepam [Valium])
   b. CNS stimulants (e.g., methylphenidate [Ritalin])
   c. Anticonvulsants (e.g., phenytoin [Dilantin])
   d. Major tranquilizers (e.g., haloperidol [Haldol])

7. The nursing history and assessment of an adolescent with a conduct disorder might reveal all of the following behaviors *except:*
   a. Manipulation of others for fulfillment of own desires
   b. Chronic violation of rules
   c. Feelings of guilt associated with the exploitation of others
   d. Inability to form close peer relationships

8. Certain family dynamics often predispose adolescents to the development of conduct disorder. Which of the following patterns is thought to be a contributing factor?
   a. Parents who are overprotective
   b. Parents who have high expectations for their children
   c. Parents who consistently set limits on their children's behavior
   d. Parents who are alcohol dependent

9. Which of the following is *least* likely to predispose a child to Tourette's disorder?
   a. Absence of parental bonding
   b. Family history of the disorder
   c. Abnormalities of brain neurotransmitters
   d. Structural abnormalities of the brain

10. Which of the following is the drug of choice for Tourette's disorder?
    a. Methylphenidate (Ritalin)
    b. Haloperidol (Haldol)
    c. Imipramine (Tofranil)
    d. Pemoline (Cylert)

REFERENCES

American Psychiatric Association. (1994). *Diagnostic and statistical manual of mental disorders* (4th ed.). Washington, DC: American Psychiatric Association.

Baum, C.G. (1989). Conduct disorders. In T.H. Ollendick & M. Hersen (Eds.), *Handbook of child psychopathology* (2nd ed.). New York: Plenum Press.

Berger, M. (1985). Temperament and individual differences. In M. Rutter & L. Hersov (Eds.), *Child and adolescent psychiatry: Modern approaches.* Oxford: Blackwell Scientific.

Clunn, P. (1991). *Child psychiatric nursing.* St. Louis: Mosby-Year Book.

Dodge, K.A., et al. (1982). Behavior patterns of socially rejected and neglected preadolescents: The roles of social approach and aggression. *Journal of Abnormal Child Psychology, 10,* 389–410.

Feingold, B.F. (1976). Hyperkinesis and learning disabilities linked to the ingestion of artificial food colors and flavors. *Journal of Learning Disabilities, 9,* 551–559.

Garfinkel, B.D., & Wender, P.H. (1989). Attention-deficit hyperactivity disorder. In H.I. Kaplan & B.J. Sadock (Eds.), *Comprehensive Textbook of Psychiatry,* Vol. 2 (5th ed.). Baltimore: Williams & Wilkins.

Johnson, C. & Dorman, B. (1998). *What is autism?* Autism Society of America (on-line). Available: http://www.autism-society.org/autism.html

Kanner, L. (1973). To what extent is early infantile autism determined by constitutional inadequacies? *Childhood psychosis: Initial studies and new insights.* Washington, DC: V.H. Winston.

Kaplan, H.I., & Sadock, B.J. (1985). *Modern synopsis of comprehensive textbook of psychiatry* (4th ed.). Baltimore: Williams & Wilkins.

Kaplan H.I., & Sadock, B.J. (1998). *Synopsis of psychiatry: Behavioral sciences/clinical psychiatry* (8th ed.). Baltimore: Williams & Wilkins.

Kaplan, H.I., Sadock, B.J., & Grebb, J.A. (1994). *Synopsis of psychiatry* (7th ed.). Baltimore: Williams & Wilkins.

Klein, R.G., & Last, C.G. (1989). *Anxiety disorders in children.* Newbury Park: Sage Publications.

Last, C. (1989). Anxiety disorders. In T.H. Ollendick & M. Hersen (Eds.), *Handbook of child psychopathology* (2nd ed.). New York: Plenum Press.

Leckman, J.F., Dolnansky, E.S., & Hardin, M.T. (1990). Perinatal factors in the expression of Tourette's syndrome: An exploratory study. *Journal of the American Academy of Child and Adolescent Psychiatry, 29,* 220–226.

Mahler, M., Pine, F., & Bergman, A. (1975). *Psychological birth of the human infant.* New York: Basic Books.

McSwiggan-Hardin, M.T. (1995). Tic disorders. In B.S. Johnson (Ed.), *Child, adolescent and family psychiatric nursing.* Philadelphia: J.B. Lippincott.

Nichols, P.L., & Chen, T.C. (1981). *Minimal brain dysfunction: A prospective study.* Hillsdale, N.J.: Lawrence Erlbaum.

Olweus, D., Mattsson, A., Shalling, D., & Low, H. (1980). Testosterone, aggression, physical, and personality dimensions in normal adolescent males. *Psychosomatic Medicine, 42,* 253–269.

Plomin, R. (1983). Childhood temperament. In B.B. Lahey & A.E. Kazdin (Eds.), *Advances in clinical child psychology* (Vol. 6). New York: Plenum Press.

Popper, C.W., & Steingard, R.J. (1994). Disorders usually first diagnosed in infancy, childhood, or adolescence. In R.E. Hales, S.C. Yudofsky, & J.A. Talbott (Eds.), *The American Psychiatric Press textbook of psychiatry* (2nd ed.). Washington, DC: The American Psychiatric Press.

Riddle, M.A., Rasmussen, A.M., & Woods, S.W. (1992). SPECT imaging of cerebral blood flow in Tourette's syndrome. In T.N. Chase, A.J. Friedhoff, & D.J. Cohen (Eds.), *Tourette's syndrome: Genetics, neurobiology, and treatment.* New York: Raven.

Rosner, T.A., & Pollice, S.A. (1991). Tourette's syndrome. *Journal of Psychosocial Nursing, 29*(1), 4–9.

Rutter, M. (1987). Temperament, personality, and personality disorder. *British Journal of Psychiatry, 100,* 443–58.

Schreibman, L., & Charlop, M.H. (1989). Infantile autism. In T.H. Ollendick & M. Hersen (Eds.), *Handbook of child psychopathology* (2nd ed.). New York: Plenum Press.

Shaywitz, S.E., Shaywitz, B.A., Cohen, D.J., & Young, J.G. (1983). Monoaminergic mechanisms in hyperactivity. In M. Rutter (Ed.), *Developmental neuropsychiatry.* New York: Guilford Press.

Singer, H.S., Reiss, A.L., & Brown, J.E. (1993). Volumetric MRI changes in the basal ganglia of children with Tourette's syndrome. *Neurology, 43,* 950–956.

Thomas, A., & Chess, S. (1977). *Temperament and development.* New York: Brunner/Mazel.

Whalen, C.K. (1989). Attention deficit and hyperactivity disorders. In T.H. Ollendick & M. Hersen (Eds.), *Handbook of child psychopathology* (2nd ed.). New York: Plenum Press.

Bibliography

Barkley, R.A. (1998, February). How should attention deficit disorder be described? *The Harvard Mental Health Letter, 14*(8), 8.

Canuso, R. (1997, April). Rethinking behavior disorders: Whose attention has a deficit? *Journal of Psychosocial Nursing, 35*(4), 24–29.

Devine, P. (1983, March). Mental retardation: An early subspecialty in psychiatric nursing. *Journal of Psychosocial Nursing and Mental Health Services, 21*(3), 21–30.

Dizon, M.A.B. (1984, March). Secure attachment—Anxious attachment. *Journal of Psychosocial Nursing and Mental Health Services, 22*(3): 27–31.

Doenges, M., Townsend, M., & Moorhouse, M. (1998). *Psychiatric care plans: Guidelines for client care* (3rd ed.). Philadelphia: F.A. Davis.

Gilliam, J.E. (1981). *Autism: Diagnosis, instruction, management, and research.* Springfield, IL: Charles C. Thomas.

Glod, C.A. (1997, June). Attention deficit hyperactivity disorder throughout the lifespan: Diagnosis, etiology, and treatment. *Journal of American Psychiatric Nurses' Association, 3*(3), 89–92.

Harvard Medical School. (1997, March). Autism—Part I. *The Harvard Mental Health Letter, 13*(9), 1–4.

Harvard Medical School. (1997, April). Autism—Part II. *The Harvard Mental Health Letter, 13*(10), 1–4.

Rutter, M., et al. (1964). Temperamental characteristics in infancy and the later development of behavioural disorders. *British Journal of Psychiatry, 110*,651–661.

Schopler, E., & Mesibon, G.B. (1988). *Diagnosis and assessment in autism.* New York: Plenum Press.

Townsend, M.C. (1997). *Nursing diagnoses in psychiatric nursing: A pocket guide for care plan construction* (4th ed.). Philadelphia: F.A. Davis.

Weisz, J.R., Weersing, V.R., & Valeri, S.M. (1997, February). How effective is psychotherapy for children and adolescents? *The Harvard Mental Health Letter, 13*(8), 4–6.

DELIRIUM, DEMENTIA, AND AMNESTIC DISORDERS

KEY TERMS

delirium
dementia
primary dementia
secondary dementia

aphasia
apraxia
sundowning
ataxia

amnesia
confabulation
pseudodementia

OBJECTIVES

After reading this chapter, the student will be able to:

1. Define and differentiate among *delirium*, *dementia*, and *amnestic disorder*.
2. Discuss predisposing factors implicated in the etiology of delirium, dementia, and amnestic disorders.
3. Identify symptomatology and use the information to assess clients with delirium, dementia, and amnestic disorders.
4. Identify nursing diagnoses common to clients with delirium, dementia, and amnestic disorders, and select appropriate nursing interventions for each.
5. Identify topics for client and family teaching, relevant to cognitive disorders.
6. Discuss relevant criteria for evaluating nursing care of clients with delirium, dementia, and amnestic disorders.
7. Describe various treatment modalities relevant to care of clients with delirium, dementia, and amnestic disorders.

*T*his chapter discusses disorders in which a clinically significant deficit in cognition or memory exists, representing a significant change from a previous level of functioning. The *DSM-IV* (APA, 1994) describes the etiology of these disorders as a general medical condition or a substance, or a combination of these factors.

These disorders were previously identified as *organic mental syndromes and disorders.* With the publication of the *DSM-IV,* the name has been changed to prevent the implication that *nonorganic* mental disorders do not have a biological basis.

These disorders constitute a large and growing public health problem that is expected to persist well into the next century. Government estimates suggest that up to 4 million Americans suffer from severe dementia, and an additional 1 to 5 million have mild or moderate dementia (Wise & Gray, 1994). Ten times as many people are affected now as were at the turn of the century, and the number of people with severe dementia is expected to increase 60 percent by the year 2000. Unless cures or means of prevention are found for the common causes of dementia, 7.4 million Americans will be affected by the year 2040 (Cook-Deegan et al., 1988). This proliferation is not the result of an "epidemic" but rather because more people now survive into the high-risk period for dementia, which is middle age and beyond.

This chapter presents predisposing factors, symptomatology, and nursing interventions for care of the client with delirium, dementia, and amnestic disorders. The objective is to provide these individuals with the dignity and quality of life they deserve, while offering guidance and support to their families or primary caregivers.

DELIRIUM

A **delirium** is characterized by a disturbance of consciousness and a change in cognition that develop rapidly over a short period (APA, 1994). Symptoms of delirium include difficulty sustaining and shifting attention. The person is extremely distractible and must be repeatedly reminded to focus attention. Disorganized thinking prevails and is reflected by speech that is rambling, irrelevant, pressured, and incoherent, and that unpredictably switches from subject to subject. Reasoning ability and goal-directed behavior are impaired. Disorientation to time and place is common, and impairment of recent memory is invariably evident. Misperceptions of the environment, including illusions and hallucinations, prevail.

Level of consciousness is often affected, with a disturbance in the sleep-wake cycle. The state of awareness may range from that of hypervigilance to stupor or semicoma. Sleep may fluctuate between hypersomnolence and insomnia. Vivid dreams and nightmares are common.

Psychomotor activity may fluctuate between agitated, purposeless movements, such as restlessness, hyperactivity, and striking out at nonexistent objects, and a vegetative state resembling catatonic stupor. Various forms of tremor are frequently present.

Emotional instability may be manifested by fear, anxiety, depression, irritability, anger, euphoria, or apathy. These various emotions may be evidenced by crying, calls for help, cursing, muttering, moaning, acts of self-destruction, and fearful attempts to flee or attacks upon others who are falsely viewed as threatening. Autonomic manifestations, such as tachycardia, sweating, flushed face, dilated pupils, and elevated blood pressure, are common.

The symptoms of delirium usually begin quite abruptly, such as following a head injury or seizure. At other times, they may be preceded by several hours or days of prodromal symptoms, such as restlessness, difficulty thinking clearly, insomnia or hypersomnolence, and nightmares. The slower onset is more common if the underlying etiology is systemic illness or metabolic imbalance.

The duration of delirium is usually brief (e.g., 1 week; rarely more than 1 month) and subsides completely upon recovery from the underlying determinant. If the underlying condition persists, the syndrome of delirium may gradually shift to a more stable syndrome, such as dementia, or progress to coma. The individual then recovers (with or without chronic brain damage), becomes chronically vegetative, or dies (Wise & Gray, 1994).

Predisposing Factors

The *DSM-IV* (APA, 1994) differentiates between the disorders of delirium by their etiology, although they share a common symptom presentation. Categories of delirium include:

1. Delirium due to a general medical condition.
2. Substance-induced delirium.
3. Substance-intoxication delirium.
4. Substance-withdrawal delirium.
5. Delirium due to multiple etiologies.

Delirium Due to a General Medical Condition

In this type of delirium, evidence must exist (from history, physical examination, or laboratory findings) to show that the symptoms of delirium are a direct result of the physiological consequences of a general medical condition (APA, 1994). Such conditions include systemic infections, metabolic disorders (e.g., hypoxia, hypercarbia, and hypoglycemia), fluid or electrolyte imbalances, hepatic or renal disease, thiamine deficiency, postoperative states, hypertensive encephalopathy, postictal states, and sequelae of head trauma (APA, 1994).

rofibrillary tangles occur in the greatest numbers (Cohen & Eisdorfer, 1987). This decrease in production of acetylcholine reduces the amount of the neurotransmitter that is released to cells in the cortex and hippocampus, resulting in a disruption of the cognitive processes (Cook-Deegan et al., 1988).

2. **Accumulation of Aluminum.** Several studies have reported higher concentrations of aluminum in the brains of Alzheimer's clients than in those of healthy older persons without dementia (Cohen & Eisdorfer, 1987). However, high concentrations of aluminum have also been reported in the brains of clients with other types of dementias. Therefore, aluminum as a contributing factor is probably not specific to Alzheimer's disease. The current consensus is that aluminum compounds accumulate only in a brain that is already damaged (Harvard Medical School, 1995a&b). More research is necessary to determine the role of aluminum in the etiology of all dementias.

3. **Alterations in the Immune System.** Several studies have shown that antibodies are produced in the Alzheimer's brain. What the antibodies are produced in response to is unknown. The reactions are actually *auto*antibody production—a reaction against the self—suggesting a possible alteration in the body's immune system as an etiological factor in Alzheimer's disease.

4. **Head Trauma.** The etiology of Alzheimer's disease has been associated with serious head trauma (Williams, 1995). Studies have shown that some individuals who had experienced head trauma had subsequently (after years) developed Alzheimer's disease. This hypothesis is currently being investigated as a possible cause.

5. **Genetic Factors.** There is clearly a familial pattern with some forms of Alzheimer's disease. Some families exhibit a pattern of inheritance that suggests possible autosomal-dominant gene transmission (Cook-Deegan et al., 1988). Some studies indicate that early-onset cases are more likely to be familial than late-onset cases, and that from one third to one half of all cases may be of the genetic form. Some researchers believe that there is a link between Alzheimer's disease and the alteration of a gene found on chromosome 21. People with Down's syndrome, who carry an extra copy of chromosome 21, have been found to be unusually susceptible to Alzheimer's disease (Harvard Medical School, 1995a&b).

Vascular Dementia

In this disorder, the clinical syndrome of dementia is due to significant cerebrovascular disease. The blood vessels of the brain are affected, and progressive intellectual de-

terioration occurs. Vascular dementia is second most common cause of dementia about 20 percent of cases (Harvard 1995a&b).

Vascular dementia differs from Alzh that it has a more abrupt onset and runs course. Progression of the symptoms rather than as a gradual deterioration; t dementia seems to clear up and the i fairly lucid thinking. Memory may see client may become optimistic that impr ring, only to experience further decline fluctuating pattern of progression. Thi of decline appears to be an intense sourc client with this disorder (Cohen & Eisd

In vascular dementia, clients suffer small strokes that destroy many areas pattern of deficits is variable, depending of the brain have been affected (APA, cal neurological signs are commonly s dementia, including weaknesses of t stepped gait, and difficulty with speech

Life expectancy is somewhat shorter f cular dementia than for those with A (Cook-Deegan et al., 1988), and the dis mon in men than in women (APA, 19 can be subtyped when the dementia is symptoms of delirium, delusions, or dep

Etiology. The cause of vascular de related to an interruption of blood f Symptoms result from death of nerv nourished by diseased vessels. Various ditions that interfere with blood circula plicated.

1. **Arterial Hypertension.** High thought to be one of the most si the etiology of multiple small stro farcts. Hypertension causes thic eration of cerebral arterioles, m teries vulnerable to rupture (Phi

2. **Cerebral Emboli.** Dementia c farcts related to occlusion of blo within the bloodstream. These from diseased heart valves, dama heart, dislodging of clots in large of fat from large bones, or large air or other gases (APA, 1994; C 1988).

3. **Cerebral Thrombosis.** Multi may occur in persons whose blo mal or even below normal if ath have occurred in the lining o (Phipps et al., 1995). This condit small and barely perceptible infa personality changes and cogniti

Substance-Induced Delirium

This disorder is characterized by the symptoms of delirium that are attributed to medication side effects or exposure to a toxin. The *DSM-IV* (APA, 1994) lists the following examples of medications that, when given in therapeutic doses, have resulted in substance-induced delirium: analgesics, anticonvulsants, antiparkinsonian agents, neuroleptics, sedative/hypnotics, anxiolytics, antidepressants, cardiovascular medications, anticoagulants, antineoplastics, respiratory drugs, hormones, and diuretics.

Substance-Intoxication Delirium

With this disorder, the symptoms of delirium may arise within minutes to hours after taking relatively high doses of certain drugs such as cannabis, cocaine, and hallucinogens (APA, 1994). It may take longer periods of sustained intoxication to produce delirium symptoms with alcohol, anxiolytics, or narcotics.

Substance-Withdrawal Delirium

Withdrawal delirium symptoms develop after reduction or termination of sustained, usually high-dose use of certain substances, such as alcohol, sedatives, hypnotics, or anxiolytics (APA, 1994). The duration of the delirium is directly related to the half-life of the substance involved, and may last from a few hours to 2 to 4 weeks.

Delirium Due to Multiple Etiologies

This diagnosis is used when the symptoms of delirium are brought on by more than one etiology. For example, the delirium may be related to more than one general medical condition or it may be due to the combined effects of a general medical condition and substance use (APA, 1994.)

DEMENTIA

Dementia is defined as a syndrome of acquired, persistent intellectual impairment with compromised function in multiple spheres of mental activity, such as memory, language, visuospatial skills, emotion or personality, and cognition (Wise & Gray, 1994).

Dementia can be classified as either primary or secondary. Devanand and Mayeux (1992) define **primary dementias** as those, such as Alzheimer's disease, in which the dementia itself is the major sign of some organic brain disease not directly related to any other organic illness. **Secondary dementias** are those caused by or related to another disease or condition, such as HIV disease or a cerebral trauma. In dementia, impairment is evident in abstract thinking, judgment, and impulse control. The conventional rules of social conduct are often disregarded. Behavior may be uninhibited and inappropriate. Personal appearance and hygiene are often neglected.

Language may or may not be affected. Some individuals may have difficulty naming objects, or the language may seem vague and imprecise. In severe forms of dementia, the individual may not speak at all (**aphasia**).

Personality change is common in dementia and may be manifested by either an alteration or accentuation of premorbid characteristics. For example, an individual who was previously very socially active may become apathetic and socially isolated. A previously neat person may become markedly untidy in his or her appearance. Conversely, an individual who may have had difficulty trusting others prior to the illness may exhibit extreme fear and paranoia as manifestations of the dementia.

The reversibility of a dementia is a function of the underlying pathology and of the availability and timely application of effective treatment (APA, 1994). Truly reversible dementia occurs in only 2 to 3 percent of cases (Cook-Deegan et al., 1988). In most clients, dementia runs a progressive, irreversible course.

As the disease progresses, **apraxia,** the inability to carry out motor activities despite intact motor function, may develop. The individual may be irritable, moody, or exhibit sudden outbursts over trivial issues. The ability to work or care for personal needs independently will no longer be possible. These individuals can no longer be left alone, as they do not comprehend their limitations and are therefore at serious risk for accidents. Wandering away from the home or care setting often becomes a problem.

Several etiologies have been described for the syndrome of dementia (see section on Predisposing Factors), but dementia of the Alzheimer's type (DAT) accounts for about 70 percent of all cases of dementia (Harper, 1988). The progressive nature of symptoms associated with DAT has been described according to stages (Devanand & Mayeux, 1992; Hall, 1991, Hall, 1994; Harper, 1988; Harvard Medical School, 1995a&b).

Stage 1. No Apparent Symptoms. In the first stage of the illness, there is no apparent decline in memory.

Stage 2. Forgetfulness. In this stage, the individual may lose things or forget names of people. Losses in short-term memory are common. The individual is aware of the intellectual decline and may feel ashamed and become anxious and depressed, which in turn may worsen the symptom. Maintaining organization with lists and a structured routine provide some compensation.

Stage 3. Early Confusion. As the symptom of confusion begins, there is interference with work performance. The individual may get lost while driving his or her car. Concentration may be interrupted.

Stage 4. Late Confusion. At this stage, the individual may forget major events in personal history, such as his or her own child's birthday; experience declining ability to perform tasks, such as shopping and managing personal finances; or be unable to understand current news events. He or she may deny that a problem exists by covering up memory loss with **confabulation** (creating imaginary events to fill in memory gaps). Depression and social withdrawal are common.

Stage 5. Early Dementia. In the early stages of dementia, individuals lose the ability to perform activities of daily living (ADLs) independently, such as hygiene, dressing, grooming, and toileting. Many forget addresses, phone numbers, and names of close relatives. Others require some assistance to manage on an ongoing basis. Frustration, withdrawal, and self-absorption are common.

Stage 6. Middle Dementia. At this stage, the individual may be unable to recall recent major life events or even the name of his or her spouse. Disorientation to surroundings is common, and the person may be unable to recall the day, season, or year. Urinary and fecal incontinence are common. Sleeping becomes a problem. Psychomotor symptoms include wandering, obsessiveness, agitation, and aggression. Symptoms seem to worsen in the late afternoon and evening, a phenomenon termed **sundowning**. Communication becomes more difficult, with increasing loss of language skills. Institutional care is usually required at this stage.

Stage 7. Late Dementia. In the end stages of DAT, the individual is unable to recognize family members. He or she is most commonly bedfast and aphasic. Problems of immobility, such as decubiti and contractures, may occur.

Cook-Deegan and associates (1988) describe the late stages of dementia in the following manner:

"The late stages of the disease often begin with the onset of incontinence. Gradually the apraxia progresses until these persons are unable to walk without help. Many are bedfast. They will need to be bathed, fed, dressed, and toileted. They will be essentially mute; language will consist only of one or two words or cries. Behavior problems disappear due to the severity of the overall impairment. Seizures are common. These people become feeble and emaciated. They may refuse to eat or be unable to swallow without choking, so that artificial feeding may be required. They are at risk of developing bedsores, infections, and pneumonia. Pneumonia is a common cause of death. There is significant variability in the symptoms from person to person and some symptoms never appear in some individuals."

Predisposing Factors

The *DSM-IV* (APA, 1994) differentiates between the disorders of dementia by their etiology, although they share

a common symptom presenta[tion...] tia include:

1. Dementia of the Alzhe[imer's type]
2. Vascular dementia.
3. Dementia due to HIV[...]
4. Dementia due to head [...]
5. Dementia due to Parki[nson's]
6. Dementia due to Hunt[ington's]
7. Dementia due to Pick's [...]
8. Dementia due to Creu[tzfeldt...]
9. Dementia due to other [...]
10. Substance-induced per[sisting...]
11. Dementia due to multi[...]

Dementia of the Alzhe[imer's Type]

This disorder is characterized [...] toms identified as dementia i[...] seven stages described previou[sly...] is slow and insidious, and th[...] generally progressive and de[...] further categorizes this disord[er...] toms occurring at age 65 or [...] symptoms occurring after age [...] sentation of other symptoms [...] mentia: with delirium, delusio[ns...]

A definitive diagnosis of thi[s...] autopsy examination of brain [...] 1988), although refinement of [...] ables clinicians to use specific cl[...] disease at an accuracy rate appr[...] Gray, 1994). Gross examinat[ion...] pathology of the brain that inc[...] tical sulci, and enlarged cere[...] these changes can be viewed in [...] mography (CT) scan or pneum[...]

Microscopic examinations [...] rillary tangles and senile plaq[ues...] with Alzheimer's disease. The[se...] as a part of the normal aging [...] with Alzheimer's disease, they[...] increased numbers and their [...] the hippocampus and certain [...] In aging clients who do not [...] and tangles are much less fre[quent...] dispersed (Cook-Deegan et al[...]

Etiology. The exact cause [...] known. Several hypotheses ha[ve...] ing amounts and quality of s[...] potheses include:

1. **Acetylcholine Alterati[on...]** that in the brains of Alzh[eimer's...] required to produce ac[...] reduced. The reduction [...] areas of the brain where

---

Dementia Due to Human Immunodeficiency Virus

Infection with the human immunodeficiency virus–type 1 (HIV-1) produces a dementing illness called HIV-1–associated dementia complex (Wise & Gray, 1994). A less severe form, known as HIV-1–associated minor cognitive/motor disorder, also occurs. The severity of symptoms is correlated to the degree of brain pathology. The immune dysfunction associated with HIV disease can lead to brain infections by other organisms, and the HIV-1 also appears to cause dementia directly. In the early stages, neuropsychiatric symptoms may be manifested by barely perceptible changes in a person's normal psychological presentation. Severe cognitive changes, particularly confusion, changes in behavior, and sometimes psychoses, are not uncommon in the later stages.

Dementia Due to Head Trauma

Symptoms of posttraumatic or postconcussion syndrome include headache, irritability, dizziness, diminished concentration, and hypersensitivity to certain stimuli. Intellectual function and memory may also be impaired (Patrick et al., 1991). Traumatic brain injury also increases the risk for developing psychiatric disorders such as depression, mania, and psychosis (McAllister, 1992).

Dementia Due to Parkinson's Disease

Dementia occurs in about one fifth of clients with Parkinson's disease (Fraser, 1987). In this disease, there is a loss of nerve cells located in the substantia nigra, and dopamine activity is diminished, resulting in involuntary muscle movements, slowness, and rigidity. Tremor in the upper extremities is characteristic. In some instances, the cerebral changes that occur in dementia of Parkinson's disease closely resemble those of Alzheimer's disease.

Dementia Due to Huntington's Disease

Huntington's disease is transmitted as a mendelian dominant gene. Damage is seen in the areas of the basal ganglia and the cerebral cortex. The onset of symptoms (i.e., involuntary twitching of the limbs or facial muscles) is usually between age 30 and 40. The client usually declines into a profound state of dementia and **ataxia** within 5 to 10 years of onset (Fraser, 1987).

Dementia Due to Pick's Disease

The cause of Pick's disease is unknown, but a genetic factor appears to be involved. The clinical picture is strikingly similar to that of Alzheimer's disease. In fact, diagnosis of Pick's disease is most often made on autopsy of a client with clinically diagnosed Alzheimer's disease (Cook-Deegan et al., 1988). Onset of symptoms is usually in middle age, and women are affected more frequently than men (Fraser, 1987). Studies reveal that pathology results from atrophy in the frontal and temporal lobes of the brain.

Dementia Due to Creutzfeldt-Jacob Disease

Creutzfeldt-Jacob disease is an uncommon neurodegenerative disease caused by a transmissible agent known as a "slow virus" or prion (APA, 1994). Five to 15 percent of cases have a genetic component. The clinical presentation is typical of the syndrome of dementia, along with involuntary movements, muscle rigidity, and ataxia. Symptoms may develop at any age in adults, but typically occur between ages 40 and 60 years. The clinical course is extremely rapid, with progressive deterioration and death within 1 year (Wise & Gray, 1994).

Dementia Due to Other General Medical Conditions

A number of other general medical conditions can cause dementia. Some of these include endocrine conditions (hypoglycemia, hypothyroidism), pulmonary disease, hepatic or renal failure, cardiopulmonary insufficiency, fluid and electrolyte imbalances, nutritional deficiencies, frontal or temporal lobe lesions, central nervous system (CNS) or systemic infections, uncontrolled epilepsy, and other neurological conditions such as multiple sclerosis (APA, 1994).

Substance-Induced Persisting Dementia

The features associated with this type of dementia are those associated with dementias in general; however, evidence must exist from history, physical examination, or laboratory findings to show that the deficits are etiologically related to the persisting effects of substance use (APA, 1994). The term "persisting" is used to indicate that the dementia persists long after the effects of substance intoxication or substance withdrawal have subsided. The *DSM-IV* identifies the following types of substances with which persisting dementia is associated:

1. Alcohol
2. Inhalants
3. Sedatives, hypnotics, and anxiolytics
4. Medications
   a. Anticonvulsants
   b. Intrathecal methotrexate
5. Toxins
   a. Lead
   b. Mercury

c. Carbon monoxide
d. Organophosphate insecticides
e. Industrial solvents

The diagnosis is made according to the specific etiological substance involved. For example, if the substance known to cause the dementia is alcohol, the diagnosis is Alcohol-Induced Persisting Dementia. If the exact substance presumed to be causing the dementia is unknown, the diagnosis would be Unknown Substance–Induced Persisting Dementia.

Dementia Due to Multiple Etiologies

This diagnosis is used when the symptoms of dementia are attributed to more than one etiology. For example, the dementia may be related to more than one medical condition or to the combined effects of a general medical condition and the long-term use of a substance (APA, 1994).

The etiological factors associated with delirium and dementia are summarized in Table 23.1.

AMNESTIC DISORDERS

Amnestic disorders are characterized by an inability to learn new information (short-term memory deficit), despite normal attention, and an inability to recall previously learned information (long-term memory deficit). Events from the very remote past are often more easily recalled than recently occurring ones. The syndrome differs from dementia in that there is no impairment in abstract thinking or judgment, no other disturbances of higher cortical function, and no personality change.

Profound **amnesia** may result in disorientation to place and time, but rarely to self (APA, 1994). The individual may engage in confabulation.

Some individuals will continue to deny that they have a problem despite evidence to the contrary. Others may acknowledge that a problem exists but appear unconcerned. Apathy, lack of initiative, and emotional blandness are common. The person may appear friendly and agreeable, but the emotionality is superficial.

The onset of symptoms may be acute or insidious, depending on the pathological process causing the amnestic disorder. Duration and course of the illness may be quite variable and are also correlated with extent and severity of the cause.

Predisposing Factors

Amnestic disorders share a common symptom presentation of memory impairment but are differentiated in the *DSM-IV* (APA, 1994) according to etiology:

1. Amnestic disorder due to a general medical condition
2. Substance-induced persisting amnestic disorder

TABLE 23.1 ETIOLOGICAL FACTORS IMPLICATED IN THE DEVELOPMENT OF DELIRIUM AND/OR DEMENTIA

BIOLOGICAL FACTORS	EXOGENOUS FACTORS
Hypoxia: any condition leading to a deficiency of oxygen to the brain	Birth trauma: prolonged labor, damage from use of forceps, other obstetric complications
Nutritional deficiencies: vitamins (particularly the B and C); protein; fluid and electrolyte imbalances	Cranial trauma: concussion, contusions, hemorrhage, hematomas
Metabolic disturbances: porphyria; encephalopathies related to hepatic, renal, pancreatic, or pulmonary insufficiencies; hypoglycemia	Volatile inhalant compounds: gasoline, glue, paint, paint thinners, spray paints, cleaning fluids, typewriter correction fluid, varnishes, and lacquers
Endocrine dysfunction: thyroid, parathyroid, adrenal, pancreas, pituitary	Heavy metals: lead, mercury, manganese
Cardiovascular disease: stroke, cardiac insufficiency, atherosclerosis	Other metallic elements: aluminum
Primary brain disorders: epilepsy, Alzheimer's disease, Pick's disease, Huntington's chorea, multiple sclerosis, Parkinson's disease	Organic phosphates: various insecticides
Infections: encephalitis, meningitis, pneumonia, septicemia, neurosyphilis (dementia paralytica), HIV disease, acute rheumatic fever, Creutzfeldt-Jacob disease	Substance abuse/dependence: alcohol, amphetamines, caffeine, cannabis, cocaine, hallucinogens, inhalants, nicotine, opioids, phencyclidine, sedatives, hypnotics, anxiolytics
Intracranial neoplasms	Other medications: anticholinergics, antihistamines, antidepressants, antipsychotics, antiparkinsonians, antihypertensives, steroids, digitalis
Congenital defects: prenatal infections, such as first-trimester maternal rubella	

Amnestic Disorder Due to a General Medical Condition

In this type of amnestic disorder, evidence must exist from the history, physical examination, or laboratory findings to show that the memory impairment is the direct physiological consequence of a general medical condition (APA, 1994). The diagnosis is specified further by indicating whether the symptoms are *transient* (present for no more than 1 month) or *chronic* (present for more than 1 month).

General medical conditions that may be associated with amnestic disorder include head trauma, cerebrovascular disease, cerebral neoplastic disease, cerebral anoxia, herpes simplex encephalitis, poorly controlled insulin-dependent diabetes, and surgical intervention to the brain (APA, 1994; Wise & Gray, 1994).

Transient amnestic syndromes can occur from epileptic seizures, electroconvulsive therapy, severe migraine, and drug overdose (Wise & Gray, 1994).

Substance-Induced Persisting Amnestic Disorder

In this disorder, evidence must exist from the history, physical examination, or laboratory findings that the memory impairment is related to the persisting effects of substance use (e.g., a drug of abuse, a medication, or toxin exposure) (APA, 1994). The term "persisting" is used to indicate that the symptoms exist long after the effects of substance intoxication or withdrawal have subsided. The *DSM-IV* identifies the following substances with which amnestic disorder can be associated:

1. Alcohol
2. Sedatives, hypnotics, and anxiolytics
3. Medications
   a. Anticonvulsants
   b. Intrathecal methotrexate
4. Toxins
   a. Lead
   b. Mercury
   c. Carbon monoxide
   d. Organophosphate insecticides
   e. Industrial solvents

The diagnosis is made according to the specific etiological substance involved. For example, if the substance known to be the cause of the amnestic disorder is alcohol, the diagnosis would be Alcohol-Induced Persisting Amnestic Disorder.

APPLICATION OF THE NURSING PROCESS

Assessment

Nursing assessment of the client with delirium, dementia, or persisting amnesia is based on knowledge of the symptomatology associated with the various disorders described in the beginning of this chapter. Subjective and objective data are gathered by various members of the health care team. Clinicians report use of a variety of methods for obtaining assessment information (Cook-Deegan et al., 1988; Cohen & Eisdorfer, 1987).

The Client History

Nurses play a significant role in acquiring the client history, including the specific mental and physical changes that have occurred and the age at which the changes began. If the client is unable to relate information adequately, the data should be obtained from family members or others who would be aware of the client's physical and psychosocial history. From the client history, nurses should assess the following areas of concern: type, frequency, and severity of mood swings, personality and behavioral changes, and catastrophic emotional reactions; cognitive changes, such as problems with attention span, thinking process, problem solving, and memory (recent and remote); language difficulties; orientation to person, place, time, and situation; and appropriateness of social behavior.

The nurse also should obtain information regarding current and past medication usage, history of other drug and alcohol use, and possible exposure to toxins. Knowledge regarding the history of related symptoms or specific illnesses, such as Huntington's disease, Alzheimer's disease, Pick's disease, or Parkinson's disease, in other family members may be useful.

Physical Assessment

Assessment of physical systems by both the nurse and the physician has two main emphases: signs of damage to the nervous system and evidence of diseases of other organs that could affect mental function (Cook-Deegan et al., 1988). Diseases of various organ systems can induce confusion, loss of memory, and behavioral changes. These causes must be considered in diagnosing cognitive disorders. In the neurological examination, the client is asked to perform maneuvers or answer questions that are designed to elicit information about the condition of specific parts of the brain or peripheral nerves. Testing will assess mental status and alertness, muscle strength, reflexes, sensory-perception, language skills, and coordination (Cohen & Eisdorfer, 1987). A battery of psychological tests may be ordered as part of the diagnostic examination. The results of these tests may be used to make a differential diagnosis between dementia and **pseudodementia** (depression).

Depression is the most common mental illness in the elderly, but it is often misdiagnosed and treated inadequately. Cognitive symptoms of depression may mimic dementia, and because of the prevalence of dementia in the elderly, diagnosticians are often too eager to make this diagnosis. A comparison of symptoms of dementia and pseudodementia (depression) is presented in Table 23.2. Nurses can assist in this assessment by carefully observing and documenting these sometimes subtle differences.

Diagnostic Laboratory Evaluations

The nurse also may be required to help the client fulfill the physician's orders for special diagnostic laboratory evaluations. Many of these tests are routinely included with the physical examination and may include evaluation of blood and urine samples to test for various infections, hepatic and renal dysfunction, diabetes or hypoglycemia, electrolyte imbalances, metabolic and endocrine disorders, nutritional deficiencies, and presence of toxic substances, including alcohol and other drugs.

Other diagnostic evaluations may be made by electroencephalogram (EEG), which measures and records the brain's electrical activity. With CT scan, an image of the size and shape of the brain can be obtained. A relatively new technology called *positron emission tomography* (PET) reveals the metabolic activity of the brain, an evaluation some researchers believe will be important in the diagnosis of Alzheimer's disease. Magnetic resonance imaging (MRI) is used to obtain a computerized image of soft tissue in the body. It provides a sharp, detailed picture of the tissues of the brain (Cohen & Eisdorfer, 1987). A lumbar puncture may be performed to examine the cerebrospinal fluid for evidence of CNS infection or hemorrhage.

Diagnosis/Outcome Identification

Using information collected during the assessment, the nurse completes the client database, from which the selection of appropriate nursing diagnoses is determined. Possible nursing diagnoses for clients with cognitive disorders include:

Risk for trauma related to impairments in cognitive and psychomotor functioning.

Risk for self-directed violence related to depressed mood secondary to awareness in decline of mental and/or physical capability.

Risk for violence directed toward others related to impairment of impulse control; hallucinations.

Altered thought processes related to cerebral degeneration evidenced by disorientation, confusion, memory deficits, and inaccurate interpretation of the environment.

Self-esteem disturbance related to loss of independent functioning evidenced by expressions of shame and self-degradation and progressive social isolation.

Self-care deficit related to disorientation, confusion, memory deficits evidenced by inability to fulfill activities of daily living (ADLs).

The following criteria may be used for measurement of outcomes in the care of the client with cognitive disorders.

THE CLIENT:

1. Has not experienced physical injury.
2. Has not harmed self or others.
3. Has maintained reality orientation to the best of his or her capability.
4. Discusses positive aspects about self and life.
5. Fulfills activities of daily living with assistance.

Planning/Implementation

Table 23.3 provides a plan of care for the client with a cognitive disorder (irrespective of etiology). Selected nursing diagnoses are presented, along with outcome criteria, appropriate nursing interventions, and rationales for each.

Client/Family Education

The role of client teacher is important in the psychiatric area, as it is in all areas of nursing. A list of topics for

TABLE 23.2   A COMPARISON OF DEMENTIA AND PSEUDODEMENTIA (DEPRESSION)

SYMPTOM ELEMENT	DEMENTIA	PSEUDODEMENTIA (DEPRESSION)
Progression of symptoms	Slow	Rapid
Memory	Progressive deficits; recent memory loss greater than remote; may confabulate for memory "gaps"; no complaints of loss	More like forgetfulness; no evidence of progressive deficit; recent and remote loss equal; complaints of deficits; no confabulation (will more likely answer "I don't know")
Orientation	Disoriented to time and place; may wander in search of the familiar	Oriented to time and place; no wandering
Task performance	Consistently poor performance, but struggles to perform	Performance is variable; little effort is put forth
Symptom severity	Worse as the day progresses	Better as the day progresses
Affective distress	Appears unconcerned	Communicates severe distress
Appetite	Unchanged	Diminished
Attention and concentration	Impaired	Intact

Table 23.3   Care Plan for the Client With a Cognitive Disorder

NURSING DIAGNOSIS: RISK FOR TRAUMA
RELATED TO: Impairments in cognitive and psychomotor functioning

OUTCOME CRITERIA	NURSING INTERVENTIONS	RATIONALE
Client will not experience injury.	The following measures may be instituted: a. Arrange furniture and other items in the room to accommodate client's disabilities. b. Store frequently used items within easy access. c. Keep bed in unelevated position. Pad siderails and headboard if client has history of seizures. Keep bedrails up when client is in bed. d. Assign room near nurses' station; observe frequently. e. Assist client with ambulation. f. Keep a dim light on at night. g. If client is a smoker, cigarettes and lighter or matches should be kept at the nurses' station and dispensed only when someone is available to stay with client while he or she is smoking. h. Frequently orient client to place, time, and situation. i. If client is prone to wander, provide an area within which wandering can be carried out safely. j. Soft restraints may be required if client is very disoriented and hyperactive.	To ensure client safety.

NURSING DIAGNOSIS: ALTERED THOUGHT PROCESSES
RELATED TO: Cerebral degeneration
EVIDENCED BY: Disorientation, confusion, memory deficits, and inaccurate interpretation of the environment

OUTCOME CRITERIA	NURSING INTERVENTIONS	RATIONALE
Client will interpret the environment accurately and maintain reality orientation to the best of his or her cognitive ability.	1. Frequently orient client to reality. Use clocks and calendars with large numbers that are easy to read. Notes and large, bold signs may be useful as reminders. Allow client to have personal belongings. 2. Keep explanations simple. Use face-to-face interaction. Speak slowly and do not shout. 3. Discourage rumination of delusional thinking. Talk about real events and real people. 4. Monitor for medication side effects.	1. All of these items serve to help maintain orientation and aid in memory and recognition. 2. These interventions facilitate comprehension. Shouting may create discomfort and in some instances may provoke anger. 3. Rumination promotes disorientation. Reality orientation increases sense of self-worth and personal dignity. 4. Physiological changes in the elderly can alter the body's response to certain medications. Toxic effects may intensify altered thought processes.

NURSING DIAGNOSIS: SELF-CARE DEFICIT
RELATED TO: Disorientation, confusion, and memory deficits
EVIDENCED BY: Inability to fulfill ADLs

OUTCOME CRITERIA	INTERVENTIONS	RATIONALE

Client will accomplish ADLs to the best of his or her ability. Unfullfilled needs will be met by caregivers.	1. Provide a simple, structured environment:
	  a. Identify self-care deficits and provide assistance as required. Promote independent actions as able.
	  b. Allow plenty of time for client to perform tasks.
	  c. Provide guidance and support for independent actions by talking the client through the task one step at a time.
	  d. Provide a structured schedule of activities that does not change from day to day.
	  e. ADLs should follow home routine as closely as possible.
	  f. Provide for consistency in assignment of daily caregivers.
	2. Perform ongoing assessment of client's ability to fulfill nutritional needs, ensure personal safety, follow medication regimen, and communicate need for assistance with those activities that he or she cannot accomplish independently.
	3. Assess prospective caregivers' ability to anticipate and fulfill client's unmet needs. Provide information to assist caregivers with this responsibility. Ensure that caregivers are aware of available community support systems from whom they can seek assistance when required. Examples include adult day-care centers, housekeeping and homemaker services, respite care services, or perhaps the local chapter of a national support organization:
	  a. For Parkinson's disease information:
	  National Parkinson Foundation Inc.
	  1501 NW 9th Avenue
	  Miami, FL 33136
	  1-800-327-4545
	  b. For Alzheimer's disease information:
	  Alzheimer's Association
	  919 N. Michigan Avenue, Suite 1000
	  Chicago, IL 60611
	  1-800-272-3900
		1. To minimize confusion.
		
		2. Client safety and security are nursing priorities.
		
		3. To facilitate transition to discharge from treatment center.

client/family education relevant to cognitive disorders is presented in Table 23.4.

Evaluation

In the final step of the nursing process, reassessment occurs to determine if the nursing interventions have been effective in achieving the intended goals of care. Evaluation of the client with cognitive disorders is based on a series of short-term goals rather than on long-term goals. Resolution of identified problems is unrealistic for this client. Instead, outcomes must be measured in terms of slowing down the process rather than stopping or curing the problem (Devanand & Mayeux, 1992). Evaluation questions may include:

1. Has the client experienced injury?
2. Does the client maintain orientation to time, person, place, and situation most of the time?
3. Is the client able to fulfill basic needs? Have those needs unmet by the client been fulfilled by caregivers?
4. Is confusion minimized by familiar objects and a structured, routine schedule of activities?
5. Do the prospective caregivers have information regarding the progression of the client's illness?
6. Do caregivers have information regarding where to go for assistance and support in the care of their loved one?
7. Have the prospective caregivers received instruction in how to promote the client's safety, minimize confusion and disorientation, and cope with difficult client behaviors (hostility, anger, depression, agitation)?

TABLE 23.4 TOPICS FOR CLIENT/FAMILY EDUCATION RELATED TO COGNITIVE DISORDERS

Nature of the Illness
1. Possible causes
2. What to expect
3. Symptoms

Management of the Illness
1. Ways to ensure client safety
2. How to maintain reality orientation
3. Providing assistance with ADLs
4. Nutritional information
5. Difficult behaviors
6. Medication administration
7. Matters related to hygiene and toileting

Support Services
1. Financial assistance
2. Legal assistance
3. Caregiver support groups
4. Respite care
5. Home health care

MEDICAL TREATMENT MODALITIES

Delirium

The first step in the treatment of delirium should be the determination and correction of the underlying causes (Popkin, 1994). Additional attention must be given to fluid and electrolyte status, hypoxia, anoxia, and diabetic problems. Staff members should remain with the client at all times to monitor behavior and provide reorientation and assurance. The room should maintain a low level of stimuli.

Some physicians prefer not to prescribe medications for the delirious client, reasoning that additional agents may only compound the syndrome of brain dysfunction (Popkin, 1994). However, the agitation and aggression demonstrated by the delirious client may require chemical and/or mechanical restraint. Low-dose neuroleptics—usually haloperidol (Haldol)—are commonly used in daily amounts between 2 and 15 mg orally (or half as much intramuscularly). Dosages should be adjusted lower for the elderly client. It is helpful to administer the medication at night to facilitate sleep and help restore the disrupted sleep-wake cycle (Popkin, 1994).

Dementia

Once a definitive diagnosis of dementia has been made, a primary consideration in the treatment of the disorder is the etiology. Focus must be directed to the identification and resolution of potentially reversible processes. Popkin (1994) states:

"Data indicate that as few as 7% of dementias are actually reversed. Yet the obligation to be circumspect remains; to miss a potentially reversible etiology borders on negligence." (p. 29)

The need for general supportive care, with provisions for security, stimulation, patience, and nutrition, has been recognized and accepted. A number of pharmaceutical agents have been tried, with varying degrees of success, in the treatment of clients with dementia. Some of these drugs are described in the following section according to the symptomatology for which they are indicated. (See Chapter 19 for side effects and nursing implications of the psychotropics.)

Cognitive Impairment

The angiotensin-converting enzyme inhibitor physostigmine (Antilirium) has been shown to enhance the ability to assimilate new information into long-term memory (Fraser, 1987). Use of vasodilators, such as cyclandelate (Cyclan), has resulted in improvements in orientation, communication, and socialization in clients with vascular dementia (Frazer, 1987). Probably the most extensively studied and widely prescribed drug for dementia is ergoloid mesylate (Hydergine). Its precise mode of action is unclear, but it is thought to enhance brain cell metabolism. However, this medication has not demonstrated consistent beneficial effects (Wise & Gray, 1994).

Two relatively new medications for improvement of cognition and functional autonomy in mild to moderate dementia of the Alzheimer's type have been introduced. Tacrine (Cognex) and donepezil (Aricept) act by elevating acetylcholine concentrations in the cerebral cortex by slowing the degradation of acetylcholine released by still-intact cholinergic neurons. Because the action relies on functionally intact cholinergic neurons, the effects of these drugs may lessen as the disease process advances, and there is no evidence that these medications alter the course of the underlying dementing process.

Agitation, Aggression, Hallucinations, Thought Disturbances, and Wandering

Antipsychotic medications are used to control these behaviors in clients with dementia. Commonly used drugs include thiothixene (Navane), chlorpromazine (Thorazine), thioridazine (Mellaril), and haloperidol (Haldol). The usual adult dosage must be decreased in the elderly client. Paradoxical effects are not uncommon. Haloperidol is extremely effective in calming a disturbed client; however, it is generally not suitable for continual use as it tends to accumulate and produce heavy sedation. Extrapyramidal side effects are most common with haloperidol. Thioridazine is considered an excellent choice for tranquilization of the demented elderly person both during the day and at night (Fraser, 1987).

Depression

Depression has been observed in 15 to 20 percent of early dementia clients (Cohen & Eisdorfer, 1987). Recognizing the symptoms of depression in these individuals is often a challenge. Depression, which affects thinking, memory, sleep, appetite, and interferes with daily life, is sometimes difficult to distinguish from dementia. Clearly, the existence of depression in the client with dementia complicates and worsens the individual's functioning. Antidepressant medication is sometimes used in treatment of depression in dementia. The tricyclics have been the most commonly used group. Examples of tricyclics are amitriptyline (Elavil), desipramine (Norpramine), doxepin (Adapin), and imipramine (Tofranil). The dosage for elderly individuals is usually one fourth to one half of the usual daily adult dose. The newer generation of antidepressants, including trazodone (Desyrel); bupropion (Wellbutrin); and the selective serotonin reuptake inhibitors (SSRIs), fluoxetine (Prozac), paroxitine (Paxil), and sertraline (Zoloft), are also available. Their long-term advantages and disadvantages have not yet been fully evaluated for use in older persons with dementia.

Anxiety

The progressive loss of mental functioning is a significant source of anxiety in the early stages of dementia. It is important that clients be encouraged to verbalize their feelings and fears associated with this loss. These interventions may be useful in reducing the anxiety of clients with dementia. Antianxiety medications may be helpful but should not be used routinely or for prolonged periods. The least toxic and most effective of the antianxiety medications are the benzodiazepines. Examples include diazepam (Valium), chlordiazepoxide (Librium), alprazolam (Xanax), lorazepam (Ativan), and oxazepam (Serax). Barbiturates are not appropriate as antianxiety agents, as they frequently induce confusion and paradoxical excitement in elderly individuals.

Sleep Disturbances

Sleep problems are common in clients with dementia and often intensify as the disease progresses. Wakefulness and nighttime wandering create much distress and anguish in family members who are charged with protection of their loved one. Indeed, sleep disturbances are among the problems that most frequently cause families to place the

---

TEST YOUR CRITICAL THINKING SKILLS

Joe,[1] a 62-year-old accountant, began having difficulty remembering details necessary to perform his job. He was also having trouble at home, failing to keep his finances straight and forgetting to pay bills. It became increasingly difficult for him to function properly at work, and eventually he was forced to retire. Cognitive deterioration continued, and behavioral problems soon began. He became stubborn, verbally and physically abusive, and suspicious of most everyone in his environment. His wife and son convinced him to see a physician, who recommended hospitalization for testing.

At Joe's initial evaluation, he was fully alert and cooperative but obviously anxious and fidgety. He thought he was at his accounting office and the year was "1960 or something." He could not say the names of his parents or siblings, nor did he know who was currently president of the United States. He could not perform simple arithmetic calculations, write a proper sentence, or draw a house. He interpreted proverbs concretely and had difficulty finding similarities between related objects.

Laboratory serum studies revealed no abnormalities, but a CT scan showed marked cortical atrophy. The physician's diagnosis was dementia of the alzheimer's type, early onset.

Answer the following questions related to Joe:

1. Identify the pertinent assessment data from which nursing care will be devised.
2. What is the primary nursing diagnosis for Joe?
3. How would outcomes be identified?

[1]Adapted from Spitzer et al. (1989).

RESEARCH NOTE

In sickness and in health: An exploration of the perceived quality of the marital relationship, coping, and depression in caregivers of spouses with Alzheimer's Disease. *Journal of Psychosocial Nursing and Mental Health Services* (1998, January), 36(1), 16–21.
Knop, D.S., Bergman-Evans, B., & McCabe, B.W.

Description of the Study: The purpose of this study was to determine if there is a correlation between a caregiver's perception of past and present marital relationship and coping skills used and level of depression in individuals caring for spouses with Alzheimer's disease. The sample included 63 caregivers between the ages of 55 and 88, the majority of whom were female. Instrument used included questions from the Jalowiec Coping Scale, the Center for Epidemiologic Studies Depression Scale, and a demographic data sheet that obtained information about the caregiver's perception of quality of the marital relationship (past and present).

Results of the Study: Forty-six percent of the caregivers rated the quality of their past relationships as favorable. Only 20 percent rated the quality of their present relationships as favorable. A positive correlation was found between favorable past and present marital relationship and confrontive coping skills (that is, the ability to make decisions and confront problems of daily living). An inverse correlation was found between negative past marital relationship and emotive coping skills (the use of emotionality, e.g., anxiety, to deal with problems). An inverse correlation was also found between unfavorable past marital relationship and level of depression in caregivers (although somewhat less so in the caregivers who used confrontive coping than in those who used emotive coping skills).

Comments: The authors concluded that a caregiver's perception of the quality of past and present marital relationship may influence that individual's response to the caregiving experience. It is important to identify and confront unresolved marital issues that may influence not only the quality of care the caregiver provides but also the mental health of the caregiver. Questions to identify this type of information should be incorporated into the interview process.

client in a long-term care facility (Cohen & Eisdorfer, 1987). Some physicians treat sleep problems with sedative-hypnotic medications. The benzodiazepines may be useful for some clients but are indicated for relatively brief periods only. Examples include flurazepam (Dalmane), temazepam (Restoril), and triazolam (Halcion). As previously stated, barbiturates should not be used in elderly clients. Sleep problems are usually ongoing, and most clinicians prefer to use medications only to help an individual through a short-term stressful situation. Behavioral approaches to sleep problems, such as rising at the same time each morning, eliminating or minimizing afternoon naps, regular physical exercise, proper nutrition, stimulating activities, and retiring at the same time each night, may eliminate the need for sleep aids, particularly in the early stages of dementia (Cohen & Eisdorfer, 1987).

SUMMARY

This chapter examined a group of disorders that constitute a large and growing public health concern. Cognitive disorders include delirium, dementia, and amnestic disorders.

A delirium is a disturbance of consciousness and a change in cognition that develop rapidly over a short period. Level of consciousness is often affected and psychomotor activity may fluctuate between agitated purposeless movements and a vegetative state resembling catatonic stupor. The symptoms of delirium usually begin quite abruptly and are often reversible and of brief duration. Delirium may be caused by a general medical condition, by substance intoxication or withdrawal, or by ingestion of a medication or toxin.

Dementia is a syndrome of acquired, persistent intellectual impairment with compromised function in multiple spheres of mental activity, such as memory, language, visuospatial skills, emotion or personality, and cognition. Symptoms are insidious and develop slowly over time. In most clients, dementia runs a progressive, irreversible course. It may be caused by genetics, cardiovascular disease, infections, neurophysiological disorders, and other general medical conditions.

Amnestic disorders are characterized by an inability to learn new information despite normal attention and an inability to recall previously learned information. Very remote past events are often more easily recalled than recent ones. The onset of symptoms may be acute or insidious, depending on the pathological process causing the amnestic disorder. Duration and course of the illness may be quite variable and are also correlated with extent and severity of the cause.

Nursing care of the client with a cognitive disorder is presented around the six steps of the nursing process. Objectives of care for the client experiencing an acute syndrome are aimed at eliminating the etiology, promoting client safety, and a return to highest possible functioning. Objectives of care for the client experiencing a chronic,

INTERNET REFERENCES

- Additional information about Alzheimer's disease may be located at the following websites:
  a. http://www.alz.org
  b. http://www.alzheimers.org/adear
  c. http://www.brain.nwu.edu/
- Information on caregiving can be located at the following website:
  a. http://www.aarp.org
- Additional information about medications to treat Alzheimer's disease may be located at the following websites:
  a. http://www.fadavis.com
  b. http://www.laurus.com

progressive disorder are aimed at preserving the dignity of the individual, promoting deceleration of the symptoms, and maximizing functional capabilities.

Nursing interventions are also directed toward helping the client's family or primary caregivers learn about a chronic, progressive cognitive disorder. Education is pro-vided about the disease process, expectations of client be-havioral changes, methods for facilitating care, and sources of assistance and support, as they struggle, both physically and emotionally, with the demands brought on by a disease process that is slowly taking their loved one away from them.

REVIEW QUESTIONS

SELF-EXAMINATION/LEARNING EXERCISE

Situation: Mrs. G is 67 years old. She is brought to the hospital by her husband. He explains that she has become increasingly confused and forgetful. Yesterday, she started a fire in the kitchen when she put some bacon on to fry and went off and forgot it on the stove. Her husband reports that sometimes she seems okay, and sometimes she is completely disoriented. The physician has made an admitting diagnosis of dementia, etiology unknown.

Select the answer that is most appropriate for each of the following questions related to the above situation:

1. Because the etiology of Mrs. G's symptoms is unknown, the physician will attempt to rule out the possibility that a reversible condition exists. An example of a treatable (reversible) form of dementia is one that is caused by:

    a. Multiple sclerosis
    b. Multiple small brain infarcts
    c. Electrolyte imbalances
    d. HIV disease

2. The physician rules out all reversible etiological factors and diagnoses Mrs. G with dementia of the Alzheimer's type. The cause of this disorder is:

    a. Multiple small brain infarcts.
    b. Chronic alcohol abuse.
    c. Cerebral abscess.
    d. Unknown.

3. The *primary* nursing intervention in working with Mrs. G would be:

    a. Ensuring that she receives food she likes, to prevent hunger.
    b. Ensuring that the environment is safe, to prevent injury.
    c. Ensuring that she meets the other patients, to prevent social isolation.
    d. Ensuring that she takes care of her own ADLs, to prevent dependence.

4. Some medications have been indicated to decrease the agitation, violence, and bizarre thoughts associated with dementia. A drug suggested for this use is:

    a. Haloperidol (Haldol).
    b. Tacrine (Cognex).
    c. Ergoloid (Hydergine).
    d. Diazepam (Valium).

5. Mrs. G says to the nurse, "I have a date tonight. I always have a date on Christmas." The most appropriate response is:

    a. "Don't be silly. It's not Christmas, Mrs. G."
    b. "Today is Tuesday, Oct. 21, Mrs. G. We will have supper soon, and then your daughter will come to visit."
    c. "Who is your date with, Mrs. G?"
    d. "I think you need some more medication, Mrs. G. I'll bring it to you now."

6. In addition to disturbances in her cognition and orientation, Mrs. G may also show changes in her:

    a. Hearing, speech, and vision.
    b. Energy, creativity, and coordination.
    c. Personality, speech, and mobility.
    d. Appetite, affect, and attitude.

7. Mrs. G has trouble sleeping and wanders around at night. Which of the following nursing actions would be *best* to promote sleep in Mrs. G?

   a. Ask the doctor to prescribe flurazepam (Dalmane).
   b. Ensure that Mrs. G gets an afternoon nap so she will not be overtired at bedtime.
   c. Make Mrs. G a cup of tea with honey before bedtime.
   d. Ensure that Mrs. G gets regular physical exercise during the day.

8. Mrs. G's daughter says to the nurse, "I read an article about Alzheimer's and it said the disease is hereditary. Does that mean I'll get it when I'm old?" The nurse bases her response on the knowledge that which of the following factors is *not* associated with increased incidence of dementia of the Alzheimer's type?

   a. Multiple small strokes.
   b. Family history of Alzheimer's disease.
   c. Head trauma.
   d. Advanced age.

9. The physician determines that Mrs. G's dementia is related to cardiovascular disease and changes her diagnosis to vascular dementia. In explaining this disorder to Mrs. G's family, which of the following statements by the nurse is correct?

   a. "She will probably live longer than if her dementia was of the Alzheimer's type."
   b. "Vascular dementia shows step-wise progression. This is why she sometimes seems okay."
   c. "Vascular dementia is caused by plaques and tangles that form in the brain."
   d. "The cause of vascular dementia is unknown."

10. Which of the following interventions is most appropriate in helping Mrs. G with her ADLs?

    a. Perform ADLs for her while she is in the hospital.
    b. Provide her with a written list of activities she is expected to perform.
    c. Tell her that if her morning care is not completed by 9 AM it will be performed for her by the nurse's aide so that Mrs. G can attend group therapy.
    d. Encourage her and give her plenty of time to perform as many of her ADLs as possible independently.

REFERENCES

American Psychiatric Association. (1994). *Diagnostic and statistical manual of mental disorders* (4th ed.). Washington, DC: American Psychiatric Association.

Cohen, D., & Eisdorfer, C. (1987). *The loss of self.* New York: NAL/Dutton.

Cook-Deegan, R.M., et al. (1988). *Confronting Alzheimer's disease and other dementias.* Philadelphia: J.B. Lippincott.

Devanand, D.P., & Mayeux, R. (1992). Alzheimer's disease and other organic causes of mental disorders. In F.I. Kass, J.M. Oldham, & H. Pardes (Eds.), *The Columbia University College of Physicians and Surgeons Complete Home Guide to Mental Health.* New York: Henry Holt.

Fraser, M. (1987). *Dementia: Its nature and management.* Chichester, Great Britain: John Wiley & Sons.

Hall, G.R. (1991, October) This hospital patient has Alzheimer's. *American Journal of Nursing, 91*(10), 44–50.

Hall, G.R. (1994, March). Caring for people with Alzheimer's disease using the conceptual model of progressively lowered stress threshold in the clinical setting. *Nursing Clinics of North America, 29*(1), 129–141.

Harper, M.S. (1988). Behavioral, social and mental health aspects of home care for older Americans. *Home Health Care Services Quarterly, 9*(4), 61–124.

Harvard Medical School. (1995a, February). Update on Alzheimer's Disease—Part I. *The Harvard Mental Health Letter.* Boston, MA: Harvard Medical School Publications Group.

Harvard Medical School. (1995b, March). Update on Alzheimer's Disease—Part II. *The Harvard Mental Health Letter.* Boston, MA: Harvard Medical School Publications Group.

McAllister, T.W. (1992). Neuropsychiatric sequelae of head injuries. *Psychiatric Clinics of North America, 15,* 395–413.

Patrick, M.L., Woods, S.L., Craven, R.F., Rokosky, J.S., & Bruno, P.M. (1991). *Medical-surgical nursing: Pathophysiological concepts* (2nd ed.). Philadelphia: J.B. Lippincott.

Phipps, W.J., Cassmeyer, V.L., Sands, J.K., & Lehman, M.K. (1995). *Medical-surgical nursing: Concepts and clinical practice* (5th ed.). St. Louis: C.V. Mosby.

Popkin, M.K. (1994). Syndromes of brain dysfunction presenting with cognitive impairment or behavioral disturbance: Delirium, dementia, and mental disorders due to a general medical condition. In G. Winokur & P.J. Clayton (Eds.), *The medical basis of psychiatry* (2nd ed.). Philadelphia: W.B. Saunders.

Spitzer, R.L., Gibbon, M., Skodol, A.E., Williams, J.B., & First, M.B. (1989). *DSM-III-R Casebook.* Washington, DC: American Psychiatric Press.

Thompson, J.M., McFarland, G.K., Hirsch, J.E., Tucker, S.M., & Bowers, A.C. (1986). *Clinical nursing.* St. Louis: C.V. Mosby.

Wertheimer, J., & Marois, M. (1984). *Senile dementia: Outlook for the future.* New York: Alan R. Liss.

Williams, M.E. (1995). *Complete guide to aging and health.* New York: Harmony Books.

Wise, M.G., & Gray, K.F. (1994). Delirium, dementia, and amnestic disorders. In R.E. Hales, S.C. Yudofsky, & J.A. Talbott (Eds.), *The*

American Psychiatric Press textbook of psychiatry (2nd ed.). Washington, D.C.: American Psychiatric Press.

Bibliography

Alzheimer's disease. (March, 1994). *Nursing Clinics of North America, 29*(1).

Briley, M., et al. (1986). *New concepts in Alzheimer's disease.* London: The Macmillan Press LTD.

Clark, M., et al. (1984, December 3). A slow death of the mind. *Newsweek,* 56–62.

Gillick, M.R. (1998). *Tangled minds: Understanding Alzheimer's disease and other dementias.* New York: NAL/Dutton.

Gruetzner, H. (1992). *Alzheimer's: A caregiver's guide and source book.* New York: John Wiley & Sons.

Hodgson, H. (1997). *The Alzheimer's caregiver: Dealing with the realites of dementia.* Minnetonka, MN: Chronimed Publishing.

Mace, N., & Rabins, P.V. (1991). *The 36-hour day* (rev. ed.). Baltimore: Johns Hopkins University Press.

Mahendra, B. (1987). *Dementia: A survey of the syndrome of dementia* (2nd ed.). Boston: MTP Press.

SUBSTANCE-RELATED DISORDERS

CHAPTER OUTLINE

OBJECTIVES

INTRODUCTION

SUBSTANCE-USE DISORDERS

SUBSTANCE-INDUCED DISORDERS

CLASSES OF PSYCHOACTIVE SUBSTANCES

PREDISPOSING FACTORS

THE DYNAMICS OF SUBSTANCE-RELATED DISORDERS

APPLICATION OF THE NURSING PROCESS

THE IMPAIRED NURSE

CODEPENDENCY

TREATMENT MODALITIES FOR SUBSTANCE-RELATED DISORDERS

SUMMARY

REVIEW QUESTIONS

KEY TERMS

dependence
abuse
amphetamines
phencyclidine
opioids
cannabis

Wernicke's encephalopathy
Korsakoff's psychosis
ascites
esophageal varices
hepatic encephalopathy
detoxification

substitution therapy
peer assistance programs
codependence
Alcoholics Anonymous
disulfiram (Antabuse)

OBJECTIVES

After reading this chapter, the student will be able to:

1. Define *abuse, dependence, intoxication,* and *withdrawal.*
2. Discuss predisposing factors implicated in the etiology of substance-related disorders.
3. Identify symptomatology and use the information in assessment of clients with various substance-use disorders and substance-induced disorders.
4. Identify nursing diagnoses common to clients with substance-use disorders and substance-induced disorders, and select appropriate nursing interventions for each.
5. Identify topics for client and family teaching relevant to substance-use disorders and substance-induced disorders.

6. Describe relevant outcome criteria for evaluating nursing care of clients with substance-use disorders and substance-induced disorders.
7. Discuss the issue of substance-related disorders within the profession of nursing.
8. Define codependency and identify behavioral characteristics associated with the disorder.
9. Discuss treatment of codependency.
10. Describe various modalities relevant to treatment of individuals with substance-use disorders and substance-induced disorders.

he substance-related disorders are composed of two groups: the substance-use disorders (**dependence** and **abuse**) and the substance-induced disorders (intoxication, withdrawal, delirium, dementia, amnesia, psychosis, mood disorder, anxiety disorder, sexual dysfunction, and sleep disorders). This chapter discusses dependence, abuse, intoxication, and withdrawal. The remainder of the substance-induced disorders are included in the chapters with which they share symptomatology (e.g., substance-induced mood disorders are included in Chapter 26).

Drugs are a pervasive part of our society. Certain mood-altering substances are quite socially acceptable and are used moderately by many adult Americans. They include alcohol, caffeine, and nicotine. Society has even developed a relative indifference to an occasional abuse of these substances, despite documentation of their negative impact on health.

A wide variety of substances are produced for medicinal purposes. These include central nervous system (CNS) stimulants (e.g., **amphetamines**), CNS depressants (e.g., sedatives, tranquilizers), as well as numerous over-the-counter preparations designed to relieve nearly every kind of human ailment, real or imagined.

Some illegal substances have achieved a degree of social acceptance by various subcultural groups within our society. These drugs, such as marijuana and hashish, are by no means harmless, and the long-term effects are still being studied. On the other hand, the dangerous effects of other illegal substances (e.g., lysergic acid diethylamide [LSD], **phencyclidine,** cocaine, and heroin) have been well documented.

This chapter discusses the physical and behavioral manifestations and personal and social consequences related to the abuse of or dependency on alcohol, other CNS depressants, CNS stimulants, **opioids,** hallucinogens, and cannabinols. Wide cultural variations in attitudes exist regarding substance consumption and patterns of use. A high prevalence of substance use occurs between the ages of 18 and 24. Substance-related disorders are diagnosed more commonly in men than in women, but the gender ratios vary with the class of the substance (APA, 1994).

The concept of codependency is described in this chapter, as are aspects of treatment for the disorder. The issue of substance impairment within the profession of nursing is also explored. Nursing care for substance abuse, dependence, intoxication, and withdrawal is presented in the context of the six steps of the nursing process. Various medical and other treatment modalities are also discussed.

SUBSTANCE-USE DISORDERS

Substance Abuse

Bennett and Woolf (1991) defined substance abuse as psychoactive drug use of any class or type, used alone or in combination, that poses significant hazards to health. The *DSM-IV* (APA, 1994) identifies substance abuse as a maladaptive pattern of substance use manifested by recurrent and significant adverse consequences related to repeated use of the substance.

DSM-IV Criteria for Substance Abuse

Substance abuse is described as a maladaptive pattern of substance use, leading to clinically significant impairment or distress, that has never met the criteria for substance dependence for this class of substance and is manifested by at least one of the following:

1. Recurrent substance use resulting in a failure to fulfill major role obligations at work, school, or home (e.g., repeated absences or poor work performance related to substance use; substance-related absences, suspensions, or expulsions from school; neglect of children or household).
2. Recurrent substance use in situations in which it is physically hazardous (e.g., driving an automobile or operating a machine when impaired by substance use).
3. Recurrent substance-related legal problems (e.g., arrests for substance-related disorderly conduct).
4. Continued substance use despite having persistent or recurrent social or interpersonal problems caused or exacerbated by the effects of the substance (e.g., arguments with spouse about consequences of intoxication, physical fights).

Substance Dependence

Physical Dependence

This disorder is evidenced by a cluster of cognitive, behavioral, and physiological symptoms indicating a loss of control over use of the substance and a continual use of the substance despite significant substance-related problems (APA, 1994). As this condition develops, the repeated administration of the substance necessitates its continued use to prevent the appearance of unpleasant effects characteristic of the withdrawal syndrome associated with that particular drug (Bratter & Forrest, 1985). The development of physical dependence is promoted by the phenomenon of *tolerance*. Tolerance is defined as the need for increasingly larger or more frequent doses of a substance in order to obtain the desired effects originally produced by a lower dose.

Psychological Dependence

An individual is considered to be psychologically dependent on a substance when its use is *perceived by the user to be necessary* to maintain an optimal state of personal well-being, interpersonal relations, or skill performance (Bratter & Forrest, 1985).

DSM-IV Criteria for Substance Dependence

At least three of the following characteristics must be present for a diagnosis of substance dependence:

1. Evidence of tolerance, as defined by either of the following:
   a. A need for markedly increased amounts of the substance to achieve intoxication or desired effects.
   b. Markedly diminished effect with continued use of the same amount of the substance.
2. Evidence of withdrawal symptoms, as manifested by either of the following:
   a. The characteristic withdrawal syndrome for the substance.
   b. The same (or a closely related) substance is taken to relieve or avoid withdrawal symptoms.
3. The substance is often taken in larger amounts or over a longer period than was intended.
4. There is a persistent desire or unsuccessful efforts to cut down or control substance use.
5. A great deal of time is spent in activities necessary to obtain the substance (e.g., visiting multiple doctors or driving long distances), use the substance (e.g., chain smoking), or recover from its effects.
6. Important social, occupational, or recreational activities are given up or reduced because of substance use.
7. The substance use is continued despite knowledge of having a persistent or recurrent physical or psychological problem that is likely to have been caused or exacerbated by the substance (e.g., current cocaine use despite recognition of cocaine-induced depression, or continued drinking despite recognition that an ulcer was made worse by alcohol consumption).

SUBSTANCE-INDUCED DISORDERS

Substance Intoxication

Substance intoxication is defined as the development of a reversible substance-specific syndrome caused by the recent ingestion of (or exposure to) a substance (APA, 1994). The behavior changes can be attributed to the physiological effects of the substance on the CNS and develop during or shortly after use of the substance. This category does not apply to nicotine.

DSM-IV Criteria for Substance Intoxication

1. The development of a reversible substance-specific syndrome caused by recent ingestion of (or exposure to) a substance.

NOTE: Different substances may produce similar or identical syndromes.

2. Clinically significant maladaptive behavior or psychological changes that are due to the effect of the substance on the CNS (e.g., belligerence, mood lability, cognitive impairment, impaired judgment, impaired social or occupational functioning) and develop during or shortly after use of the substance.
3. The symptoms are not due to a general medical condition and are not better accounted for by another mental disorder.

Substance Withdrawal

Substance withdrawal is the development of a substance-specific maladaptive behavioral change, with physiological and cognitive concomitants, that is due to the cessation of, or reduction in, heavy and prolonged substance use (APA, 1994). Withdrawal is usually, but not always, associated with substance dependence.

DSM-IV Criteria for Substance Withdrawal

1. The development of a substance-specific syndrome caused by the cessation of (or reduction in) heavy and prolonged substance use.
2. The substance-specific syndrome causes clinically significant distress or impairment in social, occupational, or other important areas of functioning.
3. The symptoms are not due to a general medical condition and are not better accounted for by another mental disorder.

CLASSES OF PSYCHOACTIVE SUBSTANCES

The following 11 classes of psychoactive substances are associated with substance-use and substance-induced disorders. They include:

1. Alcohol
2. Amphetamines and related substances
3. Caffeine
4. **Cannabis**
5. Cocaine
6. Hallucinogens
7. Inhalants
8. Nicotine
9. Opioids
10. Phencyclidine (PCP) and related substances
11. Sedatives, hypnotics, or anxiolytics

PREDISPOSING FACTORS

A number of factors have been implicated in the predisposition to abuse of substances. At present, there is no single theory that can adequately explain the etiology of this problem. No doubt the interaction between various elements forms a complex collection of determinants that influence a person's susceptibility to abuse substances.

Biological Factors

Genetics

An apparent hereditary factor is involved in the development of substance-use disorders. This is especially evident with alcoholism, less so with other substances. Some studies have indicated that the development of alcoholism in first-degree relatives of alcoholics may be as high as 50 percent (Estes & Heinemann, 1986). Studies with monozygotic and dizygotic twins have also supported the genetic hypothesis. Monozygotic (one egg, genetically identical) twins have a two-times higher rate for the concordance of alcoholism compared with dizygotic (two eggs, genetically nonidentical) twins (Frances & Franklin, 1994). Other studies have shown that male biological offspring of alcoholic fathers have a four-times greater incidence of alcoholism than offspring of nonalcoholic fathers. This is true whether the child was reared by the biological parents or by nonalcoholic surrogate parents (Frances & Franklin, 1994).

Biochemical

A second biological hypothesis relates to the possibility that alcohol may produce morphine-like substances in the brain that are responsible for alcohol addiction. These substances are formed by the reaction of biologically active amines (e.g., dopamine, serotonin) with products of alcohol metabolism, such as acetaldehyde (Bennett & Woolf, 1991). Examples of these morphine-like substances include tetrahydropapaveroline and salsolinol. Some tests with animals have shown that injection of these compounds into the brain in small amounts results in patterns of alcohol addiction in animals who had previously avoided even the most dilute alcohol solutions (Estes & Heinemann, 1986).

Psychological Factors

Developmental Influences

The psychodynamic approach to the etiology of substance abuse proposes that the predisposition relates to severe ego impairment and disturbances in the sense of self (Leigh, 1985). The person retains a highly dependent nature, with characteristics of poor impulse control, low frustration tolerance, and low self-esteem. Freud (Jones, 1959) described this person as fixed in the oral stage of development and as one who seeks satisfaction through oral gratification (e.g., ingestion of substances). Having once experienced the gratification of a supportive, drug-induced pattern of ego functioning, users attempt to repeat this satisfying experience as a solution to their own conflicts (Milkman & Frosch, 1980).

Personality Factors

Research suggests that certain personality traits may play an important part in both the development and maintenance of alcohol dependence (Barnes, 1980). Characteristics that have been identified include impulsivity, negative self-concept, weak ego, low social conformity, neuroticism, and introversion. Substance abuse has also been associated with antisocial personality and depressive response styles (Leigh, 1985). This may be explained by the inability of the individual with antisocial personality to anticipate the aversive consequences of his or her behavior. It is likely an effort on the part of the depressed person to treat the symptoms of discomfort associated with dysphoria. Achievement of relief then provides the positive reinforcement to continue abusing the substance.

Sociocultural Factors

Social Learning

The effects of modeling, imitation, and identification on behavior can be observed from early childhood onward. In relation to drug consumption, the family appears to be an important influence. Various studies have shown that children and adolescents are more likely to use substances if they have parents who provide a model for substance use (Leigh, 1985). Peers often exert a great deal of influence in the life of the child or adolescent who is being encouraged to use substances for the first time. Modeling may continue to be a factor in the use of substances once the individual enters the work force. This is particularly true in the work setting that provides plenty of leisure time with coworkers and where drinking is valued and is used to express group cohesiveness (Cosper, 1979).

Conditioning

Another important learning factor is the effect of the substance itself. Many substances create a pleasurable experience that encourages the user to repeat it. Thus, it is the intrinsically reinforcing properties of addictive drugs that "condition" the individual to seek out their use again and again. The environment in which the substance is taken also contributes to the reinforcement. If the environment is pleasurable, substance use is usually increased. Aversive stimuli within an environment are thought to be associated with a decrease in substance use within that environment (Leigh, 1985).

Cultural and Ethnic Influences

Factors within an individual's culture help to establish patterns of substance use by molding attitudes, influencing patterns of consumption based on cultural acceptance, and determining the availability of the substance. For centuries, the French and Italians have considered wine an essential part of the family meal, even for the children. The incidence of alcohol dependency is low, and acute intoxication from alcohol is not common. However, the possibility of chronic physiological effects associated with lifelong alcohol consumption cannot be ignored.

Historically, a high incidence of alcohol dependency has existed within the Native American culture (Westermeyer & Baker, 1986). Drinking was a primary group activity, and failure to drink would be considered a social offense. Native American students in U.S. universities report personal conflict with the attempt to conform to the dominant white society while retaining their own cultural identity. Baker (1982) has suggested that this cognitive dissonance may be a predisposing factor to alcohol abuse among Native Americans who have left their own culture.

The incidence of alcohol dependence is higher among northern Europeans than southern Europeans. The Finns and the Irish use excessive alcohol consumption for the release of aggression, and the English "pub" is known for its attraction as a social meeting place (Ahlstrom-Laakso, 1976).

Incidence of alcohol dependence among people of Asian cultures is relatively low. This may be a result of a possible genetic intolerance of the substance. Some Asians develop unpleasant symptoms, such as flushing, headaches, and palpitations, upon drinking of alcohol. Research indicates that this is due to an isoenzyme variant that quickly converts alcohol to acetaldehyde, as well as the absence of an isoenzyme that is needed to oxidize acetaldehyde. This results in a rapid accumulation of acetaldehyde, which produces the unpleasant symptoms (Madden, 1984).

THE DYNAMICS OF SUBSTANCE-RELATED DISORDERS

Alcohol Abuse and Dependence

A Profile of the Substance

Alcohol is a natural substance formed by the reaction of fermenting sugar with yeast spores. Although there are many alcohols, the kind in alcoholic beverages is known scientifically as ethyl alcohol, and chemically as C_2H_5OH.

Its abbreviation, ETOH, is sometimes seen in medical records and in various other documents and publications.

By strict definition, alcohol is classified as a food because it contains calories; however, it has no nutritional value. Different alcoholic beverages are produced by using different sources of sugar for the fermentation process. For example, beer is made from malted barley, wine from grapes or berries, whiskey from malted grains, and rum from molasses. Distilled beverages (e.g., whiskey, scotch, gin, vodka, and other "hard" liquors) derive their name from further concentration of the alcohol through a process called distillation.

The alcohol content varies by type of beverage. For example, most American beers contain 3 to 6 percent alcohol, wines average 10 percent to 20 percent, and distilled beverages range from 40 percent to 50 percent alcohol. The average-sized drink, regardless of beverage, will contain a similar amount of alcohol. That is, 12 oz of beer, 3 to 5 oz of wine, and a cocktail with 1 oz of whiskey would all contain approximately 0.5 oz of alcohol, and if consumed at the same rate, would have an equal effect on the body.

Alcohol exerts a depressant effect on the CNS, resulting in behavioral and mood changes. The effects of alcohol on the CNS are proportional to the alcoholic concentration in the blood. Most states consider that an individual is legally intoxicated with a blood alcohol level of 0.10 g/dl (100 mg %). The body burns alcohol at the rate of about one-half ounce per hour, so behavioral changes would not be expected to occur in an individual who slowly consumed only one averaged-sized drink per hour. Other factors do influence these effects, however, such as individual size and whether or not the stomach contains food at the time the alcohol is consumed. Alcohol is thought to have a more profound effect when an individual is emotionally stressed or fatigued (National Institute on Alcohol Abuse and Alcoholism [NIAAA], 1997).

Historical Aspects

The use of alcohol can be traced back to the Neolithic age (Blum, 1984). Beer and wine are known to have been used around 6400 BC. Although alcohol has little therapeutic value, with the introduction of distillation by the Arabs in the Middle Ages, alchemists believed that alcohol was the answer to all of their ailments. The word "whiskey," meaning "water of life," became widely known.

In America, Native Americans had been drinking beer and wine prior to the arrival of the first white settlers. Refinement of the distillation process made beverages with high alcohol content readily available. By the early 1800s, one renowned physician of the time, Benjamin Rush, had begun to identify the widespread excessive, chronic alcohol consumption as a disease and an addiction (Keller, 1979). The strong religious mores on which this country was founded soon led to a driving force aimed at prohibiting the sale of alcoholic beverages. By the middle of the 19th century, 13 states had passed prohibition laws. The most notable prohibition of major proportions was that in effect in the United States from 1920 to 1933. The mandatory restrictions on national social habits resulted in the creation of profitable underground markets that led to flourishing criminal enterprises. Furthermore, millions of dollars in federal, state, and local revenues from taxes and import duties on alcohol were lost. It is difficult to measure the value of this dollar loss against the human devastation and social costs that occur as a result of alcohol abuse in the United States today.

Patterns of Use/Abuse

Approximately 70 percent of adults in the United States drink alcohol. Of these individuals, 10 percent are described as heavy drinkers and 5 to 10 percent as problem drinkers (Frances & Franklin, 1994).

Why do people drink? Drinking patterns in the United States show that people use alcoholic beverages to enhance the flavor of food with meals; at social gatherings to encourage relaxation and conviviality among the guests; and to promote a feeling of celebration at special occasions such as weddings, birthdays, and anniversaries. Alcoholic beverages (wine) are also used as part of the sacred ritual in some religious ceremonies. Therapeutically, alcohol is the major ingredient in many over-the-counter and prescription medicines that are prepared in concentrated form. Therefore, alcohol can be harmless and enjoyable, sometimes even beneficial, if it is used responsibly and in moderation. Like any other mind-altering drug, however, alcohol has the potential for abuse. Indeed, it is the most widely abused drug in the United States today (Frances & Franklin, 1994). Schenk (1995) states:

> "Alcoholism is said to be the third major health problem in the United States. Conservative estimates are that about 90 million people use alcohol and at least 9 to 10 million persons are alcoholics or 'problem drinkers.' In addition, alcoholism adversely affects the mental health or functioning of another 30 million friends and relatives of alcohol abusers." (p. 484)

Jellinek (1952) outlined four phases through which the alcoholic's pattern of drinking progresses. Some variability among individuals is to be expected within this model of progression.

Phase I. The Prealcoholic Phase. This phase is characterized by the use of alcohol to relieve the everyday stress and tensions of life. As a child, the individual may have observed parents or other adults drinking alcohol and enjoying the effects. The child learns that use of alcohol is an acceptable method of coping with stress. Tolerance develops, and the amount required to achieve the desired effect increases steadily.

Phase II. The Early Alcoholic Phase. This phase begins with blackouts—brief periods of amnesia that occur during or immediately following a period of drinking. Now the alcohol is no longer a source of pleasure or relief for the individual but rather a drug that is *required* by the individual. Common behaviors include sneaking drinks or secret drinking, preoccupation with drinking and maintaining the supply of alcohol, rapid gulping of drinks, and further blackouts. The individual feels enormous guilt and becomes very defensive about his or her drinking. Excessive use of denial and rationalization is evident.

Phase III. The Crucial Phase. In this phase, the individual has lost control, and physiological dependence is clearly evident. This loss of control has been described as the inability to choose whether or not to drink. Binge drinking, lasting from a few hours to several weeks, is common. These episodes are characterized by sickness, loss of consciousness, squalor, and degradation. In this phase, the individual is extremely ill. Anger and aggression are common manifestations. Drinking is the total focus, and he or she is willing to risk losing everything that was once important in an effort to maintain the addiction. By this phase of the illness, it is not uncommon for the individual to have experienced the loss of job, marriage, family, friends, and most especially, self-respect.

Phase IV. The Chronic Phase. This phase is characterized by emotional and physical disintegration. The individual is usually intoxicated more than he or she is sober. Emotional disintegration is evidenced by profound helplessness and self-pity. An impairment in reality testing may result in psychosis. Life-threatening physical manifestations may be evident in virtually every system of the body. Abstention from alcohol results in a terrifying syndrome of symptoms that include hallucinations, tremors, convulsions, severe agitation, and panic. Depression and ideas of suicide are not uncommon.

Effects on the Body

Alcohol can induce a general, nonselective, reversible depression of the CNS. About 20 percent of a single dose of alcohol is absorbed directly and immediately into the bloodstream through the stomach wall. Unlike other "foods," it does not have to be digested. The blood carries it directly to the brain, where the alcohol acts on the brain's central control areas, slowing down or depressing brain activity (NIAAA, 1997). The other 80 percent of the alcohol in one drink is processed only slightly slower through the upper intestinal tract and into the bloodstream. Only moments after alcohol is consumed, it can be found in all tissues, organs, and secretions of the body. Rapidity of absorption is influenced by various factors. For example, absorption is delayed when the drink is sipped, rather than gulped; when the stomach contains food, rather than being empty; and when the drink is wine or beer, rather than distilled beverages.

At low doses, alcohol produces relaxation, loss of inhibitions, lack of concentration, drowsiness, slurred speech, and sleep. Chronic abuse results in multisystem physiological impairments. These complications include (but are not limited to) those outlined below.

Peripheral Neuropathy. This disorder, characterized by peripheral nerve damage, results in pain, burning, tingling, or prickly sensations of the extremities. Researchers believe it is the direct result of deficiencies in the B vitamins, particularly thiamine. Nutritional deficiencies are common in chronic alcoholics because of insufficient intake of nutrients as well as the toxic effect of alcohol that results in malabsorption of nutrients. The process is reversible with abstinence from alcohol and restoration of nutritional deficiencies. Otherwise, permanent muscle wasting and paralysis can occur.

Alcoholic Myopathy. This syndrome may occur as an acute or chronic condition. In the acute condition, the individual experiences pain, tenderness, and edema in the skeletal muscles of the extremities, pelvic and shoulder girdle, and the muscles of the thoracic cage following acute excesses of alcoholic ingestion (Estes & Heinemann, 1986). Laboratory studies show elevations of the enzymes creatine phosphokinase (CPK), lactate dehydrogenase (LDH), aldolase, and aspartate aminotransferase (AST). The symptoms of chronic alcoholic myopathy include a gradual wasting and weakness in skeletal muscles. Neither the pain and tenderness nor the elevated muscle enzymes seen in acute myopathy are evident in the chronic condition.

Alcoholic myopathy is thought to be a result of the same B vitamin deficiency that contributes to peripheral neuropathy. Improvement is observed with abstinence from alcohol and the return to a nutritious diet with vitamin supplements.

Wernicke's Encephalopathy. Wernicke's encephalopathy represents the most serious form of thiamine deficiency in alcoholics. Symptoms include paralysis of the ocular muscles, diplopia, ataxia, somnolence, and stupor. If thiamine replacement therapy is not undertaken quickly, death will ensue.

Korsakoff's Psychosis. Korsakoff's psychosis is identified by a syndrome of confusion, loss of recent memory, and confabulation in alcoholics. It is frequently encountered in clients recovering from Wernicke's encephalopathy. In the United States, the two disorders are usually considered together and are called *Wernicke-Korsakoff syndrome*. Treatment is with parenteral or oral thiamine replacement.

Alcoholic Cardiomyopathy. The effects of alcohol on the heart is an accumulation of lipids in the myocardial cells, resulting in enlargement and a weakened condition. The clinical findings of alcoholic cardiomyopathy generally relate to congestive heart failure or arrhythmia (Estes & Heinemann, 1986). Symptoms include decreased exercise tolerance, tachycardia, dyspnea, edema, palpitations, and nonproductive cough. Laboratory studies may show elevation of the enzymes CPK, AST, alanine aminotransferase (ALT), and LDH. Changes may be observed by electrocardiogram (ECG), and congestive heart failure may be evident on chest X-ray films.

The treatment is total permanent abstinence from alcohol. Treatment of the congestive heart failure may include rest, oxygen, digitalization, sodium restriction, and diuretics. Prognosis is encouraging if treated in the early stages. The death rate is high for individuals with advanced symptomatology.

Esophagitis. This inflammation and pain in the esophagus occurs because of the toxic effects of alcohol on the esophageal mucosa and also because of frequent vomiting associated with alcohol abuse.

Gastritis. The effects of alcohol on the stomach include inflammation of the stomach lining characterized by epigastric distress, nausea, vomiting, and distention. Alcohol breaks down the stomach's protective mucosal barrier, allowing hydrochloric acid to erode the stomach wall. Damage to blood vessels may result in hemorrhage.

Pancreatitis. This condition may be categorized as *acute* or *chronic*. Acute pancreatitis usually occurs 1 or 2 days after a binge of excessive alcohol consumption. Symptoms include constant, severe epigastric pain, nausea and vomiting, and abdominal distention. The chronic condition leads to pancreatic insufficiency resulting in steatorrhea, malnutrition, weight loss, and diabetes mellitus.

Alcoholic Hepatitis. This disease often follows a severe prolonged bout of drinking and is usually superimposed on an already damaged liver (Bratter & Forrest, 1985). It is characterized by a syndrome of inflammation and necrosis. Clinical manifestations include an enlarged liver and spleen, abdominal pain, vomiting, weakness, low-grade fever, fatigability, loss of appetite, elevated white blood cell count, and jaundice. Ascites and weight loss may be evident in more severe cases. With treatment, which includes strict abstinence from alcohol, proper nutrition, and rest, the individual can experience complete recovery. Fatality or progression to cirrhosis occurs in the majority of the most severe cases.

Cirrhosis of the Liver. Cirrhosis is the end-stage of alcoholic liver disease and is believed to be caused by the direct toxic effect of alcohol on the liver (Bratter & Forrest, 1985). There is widespread destruction of liver cells, which are replaced by fibrous (scar) tissue. Clinical manifestations are similar to those described for alcoholic hepatitis. In more advanced stages, the liver may have shrunk to the point where it cannot be palpated (Bratter & Forrest, 1985). Treatment includes abstention from alcohol, correction of malnutrition, and supportive care to prevent complications of the disease. Complications of cirrhosis include:

1. **Portal Hypertension.** Elevation of blood pressure through the portal circulation results from defective blood flow through the cirrhotic liver.
2. **Ascites. Ascites,** a condition in which an excessive amount of serous fluid accumulates in the abdominal cavity, occurs in response to portal hypertension. The increased pressure results in the seepage of fluid from the surface of the liver into the abdominal cavity.
3. **Esophageal Varices. Esophageal varices** are veins in the esophagus that become distended because of excessive pressure from defective blood flow through the cirrhotic liver. As this pressure increases, these varicosities can rupture, resulting in hemorrhage and sometimes death.
4. **Hepatic Encephalopathy.** This serious complication of **hepatic encephalopathy** occurs in response to the inability of the diseased liver to convert ammonia to urea for excretion. The continued rise in serum ammonia results in progressively impaired mental functioning, apathy, euphoria or depression, sleep disturbance, increasing confusion, and progression to coma and eventual death. Treatment requires complete abstention from alcohol, temporary elimination of protein from the diet, and reduction of intestinal ammonia using neomycin or lactulose (Bratter & Forrest, 1985).

Leukopenia. The production, function, and movement of the white blood cells is impaired in chronic alcoholics. This places the individual at high risk for contracting infectious diseases as well as for complicated recovery.

Thrombocytopenia. Platelet production and survival is impaired owing to toxic effects of alcohol. This places the alcoholic at risk for hemorrhage. Abstinence from alcohol rapidly reverses this deficiency.

Sexual Dysfunction. Alcohol has both short- and long-term effects on sexual functioning. In the short-term, enhanced libido and failure of erection are common. Long-term effects include gynecomastia, sterility, impotence, and decreased libido (Blum, 1984).

Alcohol Intoxication

Symptoms of alcohol intoxication include disinhibition of sexual or aggressive impulses, mood lability, impaired judgment, impaired social or occupational functioning, slurred speech, incoordination, unsteady gait, nystagmus, and flushed face. Intoxication usually occurs at blood alcohol levels between 100 and 200 mg/dl. Death has been reported at levels ranging from 400 to 700 mg/dl.

Alcohol Withdrawal

Within 4 to 12 hours of cessation of or reduction in heavy and prolonged (several days or longer) alcohol use, the following symptoms may appear: coarse tremor of hands, tongue, or eyelids; nausea or vomiting; malaise or weakness; tachycardia; sweating, elevated blood pressure; anxiety; depressed mood or irritability; transient hallucinations or illusions; headache; and insomnia. A complicated withdrawal syndrome may progress to *alcohol withdrawal delirium*. Onset of delirium is usually on the second or third day following cessation of or reduction in prolonged, heavy alcohol use. Symptoms include those described under the syndrome of delirium (Chapter 23).

Sedative, Hypnotic, or Anxiolytic Abuse and Dependence

A Profile of the Substance

The sedative-hypnotic compounds are drugs of diverse chemical structures that are all capable of inducing varying degrees of CNS depression, from tranquilizing relief of anxiety to anesthesia, coma, and even death. They are generally categorized as (1) barbiturates, (2) nonbarbiturate hypnotics, and (3) antianxiety agents. Effects produced by these substances depend on size of dose and potency of drug administered.

Table 24.1 presents a selected list of drugs included in these categories. Generic names are followed in parentheses by the trade names. Common street names for each category are also included.

Several principles have been identified that apply fairly uniformly to all CNS depressants (Julien, 1981):

1. **The effects of CNS depressants are additive with one another and with the behavioral state of the user.** For example, when these drugs are used in combination with each other or in combination with alcohol, the depressive effects are compounded. These intense depressive effects are often unpredictable and can even be fatal. Similarly, a person who is mentally depressed or physically fatigued may have an exaggerated response to a dose of the drug that would only slightly affect a person in a normal or excited state.
2. **No specific antagonist will block the action of the CNS depressants.** CNS stimulants may temporarily arouse the individual, but what is needed is a drug that actually displaces the depressant from its receptors in the brain, thus immediately terminating the action of the depressant. This would save thousands of lives each year of people who attempt suicide with CNS depressants.
3. **Low doses of CNS depressants produce an initial excitatory response.** CNS depressants relieve inhibitions and induce a feeling of euphoria. This is thought to occur because, at low doses, inhibitory synapses in the brain are depressed slightly earlier than are excitatory synapses. At higher doses, how-

⬛ TABLE 24.1 SEDATIVE, HYPNOTIC, AND ANXIOLYTIC DRUGS

CATEGORIES	GENERIC (TRADE) NAMES	COMMON STREET NAMES
Barbiturates	Pentobarbital (Nembutal)	Yellow jackets, yellow birds
	Secobarbital (Seconal)	GBs, red birds, red devils
	Amobarbital (Amytal)	Blue birds, blue angels
	Secobarbital/amobarbital (Tuinal)	Tooies, jelly beans
Nonbarbiturate hypnotics	Methaqualone (Quaalude)	Ludes, sopers, love drug
	Ethchlorvynol (Placidyl)	Dyls
	Glutethimide (Doriden)	Gorilla pills, CBs, Cibas, D
	Chloral hydrate (Noctec)	Peter, Mickey
	Triazolam (Halcion)	Sleepers
	Flurazepam (Dalmane)	Sleepers
	Temazepam (Restoril)	Sleepers
Antianxiety agents	Diazepam (Valium)	Vs (color designates strength)
	Chlordiazepoxide (Librium)	Green and whites; roaches
	Meprobamate (Equanil; Miltown)	Dolls, dollies
	Oxazepam (Serax)	
	Alprazolam (Xanax)	
	Lorazepam (Ativan)	

ever, excitatory synapses are also depressed, and sleep follows.

4. **CNS depressants are capable of producing physiological dependency.** If large doses of CNS depressants are repeatedly administered over a prolonged duration, a period of hyperexcitability occurs on withdrawal of the drug. The response can be quite severe, even leading to convulsions and death.

5. **CNS depressants are capable of producing psychological dependence.** CNS depressants have the potential to generate within the individual a psychic drive for periodic or continuous administration of the drug to achieve a maximum level of functioning or feeling of well-being.

6. **Cross-tolerance and cross-dependence may exist between various CNS depressants.** Cross-tolerance is exhibited when one drug results in a lessened response to another drug. Cross-dependence is a condition in which one drug can prevent withdrawal symptoms associated with physical dependence on a different drug.

Historical Aspects

Anxiety and insomnia, two of the most common human afflictions, were treated during the 19th century with opiates, bromide salts, chloral hydrate, paraldehyde, and alcohol (Blum, 1984). Because the opiates were known to produce physical dependence, the bromides carried the risk of chronic bromide poisoning, and chloral hydrate and paraldehyde had an objectionable taste and smell, alcohol became the prescribed depressant drug of choice. However, some people refused to use alcohol either because they did not like the taste or for moral reasons, and

others tended to take more than was prescribed. So a search for a better sedative drug continued.

Although barbituric acid was first synthesized in 1864, it was not until 1903 that the first barbiturate derivative (barbital) was introduced into medicine as a sedative drug (Julien, 1981). The second barbiturate to be introduced was phenobarbital (Luminol) in 1912. Since that time, more than 2500 barbiturate derivatives have been synthesized, but currently only 12 remain in medical use (Kee & Hayes, 1993). Illicit use of the drugs for recreational purposes grew throughout the 1930s and 1940s.

Efforts to create depressant medications that were not barbiturate derivatives accelerated. By the mid-1950s the market for depressants had been expanded by the appearance of the nonbarbiturates glutethimide, ethchlorvynol, methyprylon, and meprobamate. Introduction of the benzodiazepines occurred around 1960 with the marketing of chlordiazepoxide (Librium), followed shortly by its derivative diazepam (Valium). The use of these drugs, and others within their group, has grown so rapidly that they have become some of the most widely prescribed medications in clinical use today. Their margin of safety is greater than that of barbiturates and the other nonbarbiturates. However, prolonged use of even moderate doses is likely to result in physical and psychological dependence, with a characteristic syndrome of withdrawal that can be very severe.

Patterns of Use/Abuse

In the early 1980s, 15 percent of the United States population used a benzodiazepine during a 1-year period (Frances & Franklin, 1994). Sixty-one million prescriptions for benzodiazepines were written in 1985 (Kuhn, 1991). The ratios of female-to-male use and white-to-black use are approximately 3 to 1. Of all the drugs used in clinical practice, the sedative, hypnotic, and anxiolytic drugs are among the most widely prescribed (Bennett & Woolf, 1991).

The *DSM-IV* (APA, 1994) describes two patterns of development of dependence and abuse. The first pattern is one of an individual whose physician originally prescribed the CNS depressant as treatment for anxiety or insomnia. Independently, the individual has increased the dosage or frequency from that which was prescribed. Use of the medication is justified on the basis of treating symptoms, but as tolerance grows, more and more of the medication is required to produce the desired effect. Substance-seeking behavior is evident as the individual seeks prescriptions from several physicians in order to maintain sufficient supplies.

The second pattern, which the *DSM-IV* reports is more frequent than the first, involves young people in their teens or early 20s who, in the company of their peers, use substances that were obtained illegally. The initial objective is to achieve a feeling of euphoria. The drug is usually used intermittently during recreational gatherings. This pattern of intermittent use leads to regular use and extreme levels of tolerance. Combining use with other substances is not uncommon. Physical and psychological dependence leads to intense substance-seeking behaviors, most often through illegal channels.

Effects on the Body

The sedative-hypnotic compounds induce a general depressant effect. That is, they depress the activity of the brain, the nerves, the muscles, and the heart tissue. They reduce the rate of metabolism in a variety of tissues throughout the body, and in general, they depress any system that uses energy (Julien, 1981). Large doses are required to produce these effects. In lower doses these drugs appear to be more selective in their depressant actions. Specifically, in lower doses these drugs appear to exert their action on the centers within the brain that are concerned with arousal (e.g., the ascending reticular activating system, in the reticular formation, and the diffuse thalamic projection system).

As stated previously, the sedative-hypnotics are capable of producing all levels of CNS depression from mild sedation to death. The level is determined by dosage and potency of the drug used. In Figure 24.1, a continuum of the CNS depressant effects is presented to demonstrate how increasing doses of sedative-hypnotic drugs affect behavioral depression.

The primary action of sedative-hypnotics is on nervous tissue. However, large doses may have an effect on other organ systems. Following is a discussion of the physiological effects of sedative, hypnotic, and anxiolytic agents.

The Effects of Sleep and Dreaming. With barbiturates, the amount of sleep time spent in dreaming is decreased. Some investigators believe that this decrease (or absence) of rapid-eye-movement sleep with loss of dreaming may be harmful and may even be capable of precipitating psychotic episodes in some individuals (Julien, 1981). Rebound insomnia is not uncommon with abrupt withdrawal from long-term use of these drugs as sleeping aids.

Respiratory Depression. Barbiturates are capable of inhibiting the reticular activating system, resulting in respiratory depression (Kaplan, Sadock, & Grebb, 1994). Additive effects can occur with the concurrent use of other CNS depressants, effecting a life-threatening situation.

Cardiovascular Effects. Hypotension may be a problem with large doses. High dosages of barbiturates may impair cardiac contractility or induce cardiac arrhythmias (Kaplan, Sadock, & Grebb, 1994).

Renal Function. In doses high enough to produce anesthesia, barbiturates may suppress urine function. At the usual sedative-hypnotic dosage, however, there is no evidence that they have any direct action on the kidneys.

Hepatic Effects. The barbiturates may produce jaundice with doses large enough to produce acute intoxication. Barbiturates stimulate the production of liver enzymes, resulting in a decrease in the plasma levels of both the barbiturates and other drugs metabolized in the liver (Kaplan, Sadock, & Grebb, 1994). Preexisting liver disease may predispose an individual to additional liver damage with excessive barbiturate use.

Body Temperature. High doses of barbiturates can greatly decrease body temperature. It is not significantly altered with normal dosage levels.

Sexual Functioning. As with alcohol, these other CNS depressants have a tendency to produce a biphasic response. There is an initial increase in libido, presumably

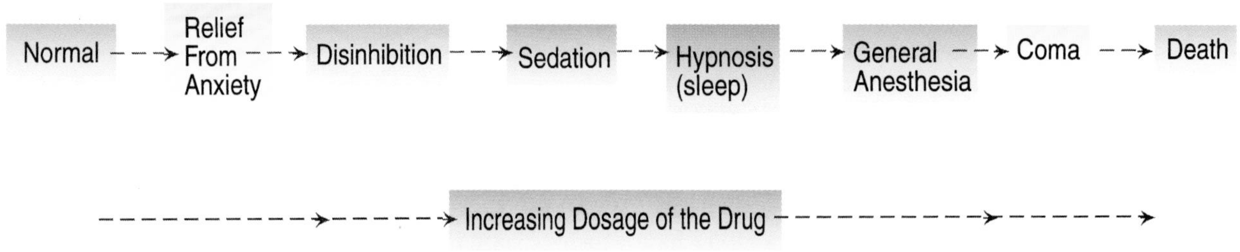

Normal - - -> Relief From Anxiety - - -> Disinhibition - - -> Sedation - - -> Hypnosis (sleep) - - -> General Anesthesia - - -> Coma - - -> Death

- - - - - - - - - -> - - - - -> Increasing Dosage of the Drug - - - - - - - - - -> - - - - ->

Figure 24.1 Continuum of behavioral depression.

from the primary disinhibitory effects of the drug. This initial response is then followed by a decrease in the ability to maintain an erection.

Sedative, Hypnotic, or Anxiolytic Intoxication

The *DSM-IV* (APA, 1994) describes sedative, hypnotic, or anxiolytic intoxication as the presence of clinically significant maladaptive behavioral or psychological changes that develop during, or shortly after, use of one of these substances. These maladaptive changes may include inappropriate sexual or aggressive behavior, mood lability, impaired judgment, or impaired social or occupational functioning. Other symptoms that may develop with excessive use of sedatives, hypnotics, or anxiolytics include slurred speech, incoordination, unsteady gait, nystagmus, impairment in attention or memory, and stupor or coma.

Sedative, Hypnotic, or Anxiolytic Withdrawal

Withdrawal from sedatives, hypnotics, or anxiolytics produces a characteristic syndrome of symptoms that develops after a marked decrease in or cessation of intake after several weeks or more of regular use (APA, 1994). Onset of the symptoms depends on the drug from which the individual is withdrawing. A short-acting anxiolytic (e.g., lorazepam or oxazepam) may produce symptoms within 6 to 8 hours of decreasing blood levels, while withdrawal symptoms from substances with longer half-lives (e.g., diazepam) may not develop for more than a week.

Severe withdrawal is most likely to occur when a substance has been used at high dosages for prolonged periods. However, withdrawal symptoms also have been reported with moderate dosages taken over relatively short duration. Withdrawal symptoms associated with sedatives, hypnotics, or anxiolytics include autonomic hyperactivity (e.g., sweating or pulse rate greater than 100), increased hand tremor, insomnia, nausea or vomiting,

hallucinations, illusions, psychomotor agitation, anxiety, or grand mal seizures.

CNS Stimulant Abuse and Dependence

A Profile of the Substance

The CNS stimulants are identified by the behavioral stimulation and psychomotor agitation that they induce. They differ widely in their molecular structures and in their mechanisms of action. The degree of CNS stimulation caused by a certain drug depends on both the area in the brain or spinal cord that is affected by the drug and the cellular mechanism fundamental to the increased excitability (Byers, 1991).

Groups within this category are classified according to similarities in mechanism of action. The *psychomotor stimulants* induce stimulation by augmentation or potentiation of the neurotransmitters norepinephrine, epinephrine, or dopamine. The *general cellular stimulants* (caffeine and nicotine) exert their action directly on cellular activity. Caffeine inhibits the enzyme phosphodiesterase, allowing increased levels of adenosine $3',5'$-cyclic phosphate (cAMP), a chemical substance that promotes increased rates of cellular metabolism. Nicotine stimulates ganglionic synapses. This results in increased acetylcholine, which stimulates nerve impulse transmission to the entire autonomic nervous system. A selected list of drugs included in these categories is presented in Table 24.2.

The two most prevalent and widely used stimulants are caffeine and nicotine. Caffeine is readily available in every supermarket and grocery store as a common ingredient in coffee, tea, colas, and chocolate. Nicotine is the primary psychoactive substance found in tobacco products. When used in moderation, these stimulants tend to relieve fatigue and increase alertness. They have become a generally accepted part of our culture.

The more potent stimulants, because of their potential for physiological dependency, are under regulation by the Controlled Substances Act. These controlled stimulants are available for therapeutic purposes by prescription

---

◢ TABLE 24.2 CNS STIMULANTS

CATEGORIES	GENERIC (TRADE) NAMES	COMMON STREET NAMES
Amphetamines	Amphetamine sulfate (Benzedrine)	Bennies, splash, peaches
	Dextroamphetamine (Dexedrine)	Dexies, uppers, diet pills
	Methamphetamine (Desoxyn)	Meth, speed, water, crystal
	1-Amphetamine + d-amphetamine (Biphetamine)	Black beauties, speed
Nonamphetamine stimulants	Phenmetrazine (Preludin)	Diet pills
	Methylphenidate (Ritalin)	Speed, uppers
	Pemoline (Cylert)	
Cocaine	Cocaine hydrochloride	Coke, blow, toot, snow, lady, flake
Caffeine	Coffee, tea, colas, chocolate	Java, mud, brew, cocoa
Nicotine	Cigarettes, cigars, pipe tobacco, snuff	Weeds, fags, butts, chaw, cancer sticks

only. They are also clandestinely manufactured in vast quantities for distribution on the illicit market.

Historical Aspects

Cocaine is the most potent stimulant derived from natural origin. It is extracted from the leaves of the coca plant, which has been cultivated in the Andean highlands of South America since prehistoric times. Natives of the region chew the leaves of the plant for refreshment and relief from fatigue.

The coca leaves must be mixed with lime to release the cocaine alkaloid. The chemical formula for the pure form of the drug was obtained in 1960. Physicians began using the drug as an anesthetic in eye, nose, and throat surgeries. These therapeutic uses are now obsolete. In recent years, however, it has been used in the United States in a morphine-cocaine elixir designed to relieve the suffering associated with terminal illness (Drug Enforcement Administration [DEA], 1979).

Cocaine has achieved a degree of acceptability within some social circles. It is illicitly distributed as a white crystalline powder, often mixed with other ingredients to increase its volume and therefore create more profits. The drug is most commonly "snorted," and chronic users may manifest symptoms that resemble the congested nose of a common cold. The intensely pleasurable effects of the drug create the potential for extraordinary psychological dependency.

Another form of cocaine commonly used in the United States, called "crack," is a cocaine alkaloid that is extracted from its powdered hydrochloride salt by mixing it with sodium bicarbonate and allowing it to dry into small "rocks" (APA, 1994). Because this type of cocaine can be easily vaporized and inhaled, its effects have an extremely rapid onset.

Amphetamine was first prepared in 1887. Various derivatives of the drug soon followed, and clinical use of the drug began in 1927. Amphetamines were used quite extensively for medical purposes through the 1960s, but recognition of their abuse potential has sharply decreased clinical use. Today, they are prescribed only to treat narcolepsy (a rare disorder resulting in an uncontrollable desire for sleep), hyperactivity disorders in children, and certain cases of obesity. Clandestine production of amphetamines for distribution on the illicit market has become a thriving business.

The earliest history of caffeine is unknown and is shrouded by legend and myth. Caffeine was first discovered in coffee in 1820 and 7 years later in tea. Both beverages have been widely accepted and enjoyed as a "pick-me-up" by many cultures.

Tobacco was used by the aborigines from remote times. Introduced in Europe in the mid-16th century, its use grew rapidly and soon became prevalent in the Orient. Tobacco came to America with the settlement of the earliest colonies. Today, it is grown in many countries of the world, and although smoking is decreasing in most industrialized nations, it is increasing in the developing areas (APA, 1994).

Patterns of Use/Abuse

Because of their pleasurable effects, CNS stimulants have a high abuse potential. Approximately 30 million Americans admit to having tried some form of cocaine, and about 1 million are so addicted to the drug that they will do *anything* to get it (House, 1990). Many individuals who abuse or are dependent on CNS stimulants began using the substance for the appetite-suppressant effect in an attempt at weight control (APA, 1994). Higher and higher doses are consumed in an effort to maintain the pleasurable effects. With continued use, the pleasurable effects diminish, and there is a corresponding increase in dysphoric effects. There is a persistent craving for the substance, however, even in the face of unpleasant adverse effects from the continued drug taking.

CNS stimulant abuse and dependence are usually characterized by either episodic or chronic daily, or almost daily, use. Individuals who use the substances on an episodic basis often "binge" on the drug, with very high dosages followed by a day or two of recuperation. This recuperation period is characterized by extremely intense and unpleasant symptoms (called a "crash").

The daily user may take large or small doses, and may use the drug several times a day or only at a specific time during the day. The amount consumed usually increases over time as tolerance occurs. Chronic users tend to rely on CNS stimulants to feel more powerful, more confident, and more decisive. They often fall into a pattern of taking "uppers" in the morning and "downers," such as alcohol or sleeping pills, at night.

The average American consumes two cups of coffee (about 200 mg of caffeine) per day. Caffeine is consumed in various amounts by 90 percent of the population. At a level of 500 to 600 mg of daily caffeine consumption, symptoms of anxiety, insomnia, and depression are not uncommon. It is also at this level that caffeine dependence and withdrawal can occur. Caffeine consumption is prevalent among children as well as adults. Table 24.3 lists some common sources of caffeine.

Next to caffeine, nicotine, an active ingredient in tobacco, is the most widely used psychoactive substance in our society. Thirty-two percent of the U.S. population smoke or use smokeless forms of the drug (Kaplan & Sadock, 1998). Since 1964, when the results of the first public health report on smoking were issued, the percentage of total smokers has been on the decline. However, the percentage of women and teenage smokers has declined more slowly than that of adult men. Approximately 400,000 people die annually because of tobacco use, and an estimated 60 percent of the direct health care

TABLE 24.3 COMMON SOURCES OF CAFFEINE

SOURCE	CAFFEINE CONTENT
Food and Beverages	
5–6 oz. brewed coffee	90–125 mg
5–6 oz. instant coffee	60–90 mg
5–6 oz. decaffeinated coffee	3 mg
5–6 oz. brewed tea	70 mg
5–6 oz. instant tea	45 mg
8–12 oz. cola drinks	60 mg
5–6 oz. cocoa	20 mg
8 oz. chocolate milk	2–7 mg
1 oz. chocolate bar	22 mg
Prescription Medications	
APCs (aspirin, phenacetin, caffeine)	32 mg
Cafergot	100 mg
Darvon compound	32 mg
Fiorinal	40 mg
Migral	50 mg
Over-the-Counter Analgesics	
Anacin, Empirin, Midol, Vanquish	32 mg
Excedrin	60 mg
Over-the-Counter Stimulants	
No Doz Tablets	100 mg
Vivarin	200 mg
Caffedrine	250 mg

SOURCE: Adapted from Kaplan, Sadock, & Grebb (1994); Pilette (1983); Blum (1984); and Bennett & Woolf (1991).

costs in the United States go to treat tobacco-related illnesses (Kaplan & Sadock, 1998).

Effects on the Body

The CNS stimulants are a group of pharmacological agents that are capable of exciting the entire nervous system. This is accomplished by increasing the activity or augmenting the capability of the neurotransmitter agents known to be directly involved in bodily activation and behavioral stimulation. Physiological responses vary markedly according to the potency and dosage of the drug.

Central Nervous System Effects. Stimulation of the CNS results in tremor, restlessness, anorexia, insomnia, agitation, and increased motor activity. Amphetamines, nonamphetamine stimulants, and cocaine produce increased alertness, decrease in fatigue, elation and euphoria, and subjective feelings of greater mental agility and muscular power. Chronic use of these drugs may result in compulsive behavior, paranoia, hallucinations, and aggressive behavior (Blum, 1984).

Cardiovascular/Pulmonary Effects. Amphetamines can induce increased systolic and diastolic blood pressure, increased heart rate, and cardiac arrhythmias (Blum, 1984). These drugs also relax bronchial smooth muscle.

Cocaine intoxication typically produces a rise in myocardial demand for oxygen and an increase in heart rate.

Severe vasoconstriction may occur and can result in myocardial infarction, ventricular fibrillation, and sudden death (House, 1990). Inhaled cocaine can cause pulmonary hemorrhage, chronic bronchiolitis, and pneumonia. Nasal rhinitis is a result of chronic cocaine snorting.

Caffeine ingestion can result in increased heart rate, palpitations, extrasystoles, arrhythmias, and in very large doses, cardiac standstill (Pilette, 1983). Caffeine induces dilation of pulmonary and general systemic blood vessels and constriction of cerebral blood vessels.

Nicotine stimulates the release of epinephrine from the adrenal gland, resulting in constriction of peripheral blood vessels, decreased body temperature, and increased blood pressure (Bennett & Woolf, 1991). Contractions of gastric smooth muscle associated with hunger are inhibited, thereby producing a mild anorectic effect.

Gastrointestinal and Renal Effects. Gastrointestinal (GI) effects of amphetamines are somewhat unpredictable (Blum, 1984); however, a decrease in GI tract motility commonly results in constipation (Bennett & Woolf, 1991). Contraction of the bladder sphincter makes urination difficult. Caffeine exerts a diuretic effect on the kidneys. Nicotine stimulates the hypothalamus to release antidiuretic hormone, reducing the excretion of urine. Because nicotine increases the tone and activity of the bowel, it may occasionally cause diarrhea.

Most CNS stimulants induce a small rise in metabolic rate and various degrees of anorexia. Amphetamines and cocaine can cause a rise in body temperature.

Sexual Functioning. CNS stimulants apparently promote the coital urge in both men and women. Women, more than men, report that stimulants make them feel sexier and have more orgasms. In fact, some men may experience sexual dysfunction with the use of stimulants. For the majority of individuals, however, these drugs exert a powerful aphrodisiac effect and may be one reason for relapse or continued abuse of the substance (Goldstein, 1994).

CNS Stimulant Intoxication

CNS stimulant intoxication produces maladaptive behavioral and psychological changes that develop during, or shortly after, use of these drugs. Amphetamine and cocaine intoxication typically produces euphoria or affective blunting; changes in sociability; hypervigilance; interpersonal sensitivity; anxiety, tension, or anger; stereotyped behaviors; or impaired judgment. Physical effects include tachycardia or bradycardia, pupillary dilation, elevated or lowered blood pressure, perspiration or chills, nausea or vomiting, weight loss, psychomotor agitation or retardation, muscular weakness, respiratory depression, chest pain, cardiac arrhythmias, confusion, seizures, dyskinesias, dystonias, or coma (APA, 1994).

Intoxication from caffeine usually occurs following

consumption in excess of 250 mg. Symptoms include restlessness, nervousness, excitement, insomnia, flushed face, diuresis, GI disturbance, muscle twitching, rambling flow of thought and speech, tachycardia or cardiac arrhythmia, periods of inexhaustibility, and psychomotor agitation (APA, 1994).

CNS Stimulant Withdrawal

CNS stimulant withdrawal is the presence of a characteristic withdrawal syndrome that develops within a few hours to several days after cessation of, or reduction in, heavy and prolonged use (APA, 1994). Withdrawal from amphetamines and cocaine cause dysphoria, fatigue, vivid unpleasant dreams, insomnia or hypersomnia, increased appetite, and psychomotor retardation or agitation (APA, 1994).

The *DSM-IV* does not include a diagnosis of caffeine withdrawal. However, Kaplan, Sadock, and Grebb (1994), state that a number of well-controlled research studies indicate that caffeine withdrawal exists. They cite the following symptoms as typical: headache, marked fatigue or drowsiness, anxiety or depression, and nausea or vomiting.

Withdrawal from nicotine results in dysphoric or depressed mood; insomnia; irritability, frustration, or anger; anxiety; difficulty concentrating; restlessness; decreased heart rate; and increased appetite or weight gain (APA, 1994). A mild syndrome of nicotine withdrawal can appear when a smoker switches from regular cigarettes to low-nicotine cigarettes (Kaplan, Sadock, & Grebb, 1994).

Opioid Abuse and Dependence

A Profile of the Substance

The term *opioid* refers to a group of compounds that includes opium, opium derivatives, and synthetic substitutes. Opioids exert both a sedative and an analgesic effect, and their major medical uses are for the relief of pain, the treatment of diarrhea, and the relief of coughing.

These drugs have addictive qualities; that is, they are capable of inducing tolerance and physiological and psychological dependence.

Opioids are popular drugs of abuse in that they desensitize an individual to both psychological and physiological pain and induce a sense of euphoria. Lethargy and indifference to the environment are common manifestations.

Opioid abusers usually spend much of their time nourishing their habit. Individuals who are opioid dependent are seldom able to hold a steady job that will support their need. They must therefore secure funds from friends, relatives, or whomever they have not yet alienated with their dependency-related behavior. Obtaining funds illegally is not uncommon. Common criminal methods are burglary, robbery, prostitution, and selling drugs (Goldstein, 1994).

Methods of administration of opioid drugs include oral, sorting, and smoking and by subcutaneous, intramuscular, and intravenous injection. A selected list of opioid substances is presented in Table 24.4.

Under close supervision, opioids are indispensable in the practice of medicine. They are the most effective agents known for the relief of intense pain. However, they also induce a pleasurable effect on the CNS that promotes their abuse. The physiological and psychological dependence that occurs with opioids, as well as the development of profound tolerance, contribute to the addict's ongoing quest for more of the substance, regardless of the means.

Historical Aspects

Opium is the Greek word for "juice." It is produced from the milk exudate of the unripe seed capsules of the poppy plant (Kaplan & Sadock, 1985). References to the use of opiates have been found in the Egyptian, Greek, and Arabian cultures as early as 3000 BC (Julien, 1981). The drug became widely used both medicinally and recreationally throughout Europe during the 16th and 17th centuries. Most of the opium supply came from China, where the drug was introduced by Arabic traders in the late 17th

---

TABLE 24.4 OPIOIDS AND RELATED SUBSTANCES

CATEGORIES	GENERIC (TRADE) NAMES	COMMON STREET NAMES
Opioids of natural origin	Opium (ingredient in various antidiarrheal agents)	Black stuff, poppy, tar, big O
	Morphine (Astramorph)	M, white stuff, Miss Emma
	Codeine (ingredient in various analgesics and cough suppressants)	Terp, robo, romo, syrup
Opioid derivatives	Heroin	H, horse, junk, brown, smack, scag, TNT, Harry
	Hydromorphone (Dilaudid)	DLs, 4s, lords, little D
	Oxycodone (in Percodan)	Perks, perkies
	Hydrocodone (Hycodan)	
Synthetic opiate-like drugs	Meperidine (Demerol)	Doctors
	Methadone (Dolophine)	Dollies, done
	Propoxyphene (Darvon)	Pinks and grays
	Pentazocine (Talwin)	Ts

century. Morphine, the primary active ingredient of opium, was isolated in 1803 by the European chemist Frederich Serturner. Since that time, morphine, rather than crude opium, has been used throughout the world for the medical treatment of pain and diarrhea (Julien, 1981). This process was facilitated in 1853 by the development of the hypodermic syringe, which made it possible to deliver the undiluted morphine quickly into the body for rapid relief from pain (Blum, 1984).

This development also created a new variety of opiate user in the United States: one who was able to self-administer the drug by injection. During this time, there was also a large influx of Chinese immigrants into the United States, who introduced opium smoking to this country. By the early part of the 20th century, opium addiction was widespread.

In response to the concerns over widespread addiction, the U.S. government passed the Harrison Narcotic Act in 1914, which created strict controls on the accessibility of opiates. Until that time, these substances had been freely available to the public without a prescription. The Harrison Act banned the use of opiates for other than medicinal purposes and drove the use of heroin underground. To this day, the beneficial uses of these substances are widely acclaimed within the medical profession, but the illicit trafficking of the drugs for recreational purposes continues to resist most efforts aimed at control.

Patterns of Use/Abuse

The development of opioid abuse and dependence may follow one of two typical behavior patterns. The first occurs in the individual who has obtained the drug by prescription from a physician for the relief of a medical problem. Abuse and dependency occur when the individual increases the amount and frequency of use, justifying the behavior as symptom treatment. He or she becomes obsessed with obtaining more and more of the substance, seeking out several physicians in order to replenish and maintain supplies.

The second pattern of behavior associated with abuse and dependency of opioids occurs among individuals who use the drugs for recreational purposes and obtain them from illegal sources. Opioids may be used alone to induce the euphoric effects or in combination with stimulants or other drugs to enhance the euphoria or to counteract the depressant effects of the opioid. Tolerance develops and dependency occurs, leading the individual to procure the substance by whatever means is required in an effort to support the habit. Blum (1984) has stated:

"The classic user (of opioids) was once a young, ghetto male, wearing long sleeves to cover the needle marks. He was unemployed, malnourished, had a short attention span, and of course, noticeable miosis. The major exceptions were members of the medical profession who became dependent on Demerol (or morphine) rather than heroin, and generally attempted to keep working to maintain their proximity to hospital supplies.

Now increasing numbers of young people on all social levels are becoming involved with opioids. Some are students; others work, deal drugs, or steal. However, despite this increase in the number of users, there are still relatively few users of illicit opioids, compared with the tremendous number of people using other drugs."

Effects on the Body

Opiates are sometimes classified as *narcotic analgesics.* They exert their major effects primarily on the CNS, the eyes, and the gastrointestinal tract (Bennett & Woolf, 1991). Chronic morphine use or acute morphine toxicity is manifested by a syndrome of sedation, chronic constipation, decreased respiratory rate, and pinpoint pupils. Intensity of symptoms is largely dose dependent. The following physiological effects are common with opioid use.

Central Nervous System. All opioids, opioid derivatives, and synthetic opioid-like drugs affect the CNS. Common manifestations include euphoria, mood changes, and mental clouding (Bennett & Woolf, 1991). Other common CNS effects include drowsiness and pain reduction. Pupillary constriction occurs in response to stimulation of the oculomotor nerve. CNS depression of the respiratory centers within the medulla results in respiratory depression. The antitussive response is due to suppression of the cough center within the medulla. The nausea and vomiting commonly associated with opiate ingestion are related to the stimulation of the centers within the medulla that trigger this response.

Gastrointestinal Effects. These drugs exert a profound effect on the GI tract. Both stomach and intestinal tone are increased, whereas peristaltic activity of the intestines is diminished. These effects lead to a marked decrease in the movement of food through the GI tract. This is a notable therapeutic effect in the treatment of severe diarrhea. In fact, no drugs have yet been developed that are more effective than the opioids for this purpose. However, constipation, and even fecal impaction, may be a serious problem for the chronic opioid user.

Cardiovascular Effects. In therapeutic doses, opioids have minimal effect on the action of the heart. Morphine is used extensively to relieve pulmonary edema and the pain of myocardial infarction in cardiac clients (Blum, 1984; Bennett & Woolf, 1991). At high doses, opioids induce hypotension, which may be caused by direct action on the heart or by opioid-induced histamine release.

Sexual Functioning. A number of studies with opioids, particularly heroin and methadone, have indicated that these drugs cause decreased libido (in both men and women), retarded ejaculation, impotence, and orgasm failure (Blum, 1984). Sexual side effects from opioids appear to be largely influenced by dosage.

Opioid Intoxication

Opioid intoxication constitutes clinically significant maladaptive behavioral or psychological changes that develop during, or shortly after, opioid use (APA, 1994). Symptoms include initial euphoria followed by apathy, dysphoria, psychomotor agitation or retardation, and impaired judgment. Physical symptoms include pupillary constriction (or dilation due to anoxia from severe overdose), drowsiness, slurred speech, and impairment in attention or memory (APA, 1994). Symptoms are consistent with the half-life of most opioid drugs and usually last for several hours. Severe opioid intoxication can lead to respiratory depression, coma, and even death.

Opioid Withdrawal

Opioid withdrawal produces a syndrome of symptoms that develops after cessation of, or reduction in, heavy and prolonged use of an opiate or related substance. Symptoms include dysphoric mood, nausea or vomiting, muscle aches, lacrimation or rhinorrhea, pupillary dilation, piloerection, sweating, abdominal cramping, diarrhea, yawning, fever, and insomnia. With short-acting drugs such as heroin, withdrawal symptoms occur within 6 to 24 hours after the last dose, peak within 1 to 3 days, and gradually subside over a period of 5 to 7 days (APA, 1994). With longer-acting drugs such as methadone, withdrawal symptoms begin within 1 to 3 days after the last dose and are complete in 10 to 14 days (Kaplan, Sadock, & Grebb, 1994). Withdrawal from the ultra–short-acting meperidine begins quickly, reaches a peak in 8 to 12 hours, and is complete in 4 to 5 days (Kaplan, Sadock, & Grebb, 1994).

Hallucinogen Abuse and Dependence

A Profile of the Substance

Hallucinogenic substances are capable of distorting an individual's perception of reality. They have the ability to alter sensory perception and induce hallucinations, and for this reason have been referred to as "mind expanding" (Julien, 1981). Some of the manifestations have been likened to a psychotic break. The hallucinations experienced by an individual with schizophrenia are most often auditory, however, whereas substance-induced hallucinations are usually visual (Holbrook, 1991). Perceptual distortions have been reported by some users as a sense of depersonalization (observing oneself having the experience), as one of being at peace with self and the universe, and as spiritual in nature. Others, who describe their experiences as "bad trips," report feelings of panic and a fear of dying or going insane. These feelings of terror can recur at any time, even without the drug, and the experience can have lasting effects (Blum, 1984). These adverse reactions are referred to as "flashbacks."

Recurrent use can produce tolerance, encouraging users to resort to higher and higher dosages. No evidence of physical dependence is detectable when the drug is withdrawn; however, recurrent use appears to induce a psychological dependence on the insight-inducing experiences that a user may associate with episodes of hallucinogen use (Kaplan, Sadock, & Grebb, 1994). This psychological dependence varies according to the drug, the dose, and the individual user. Hallucinogens are highly unpredictable in the effects they may induce each time they are used.

Many of the hallucinogenic substances have structural similarities. Some are produced synthetically, whereas others are natural products of plants and fungi. A selected list of hallucinogens is presented in Table 24.5.

Historical Aspects

Archeological data obtained with carbon-14 dating suggest that hallucinogens have been used as part of religious ceremonies and at social gatherings by Native Americans for as long as 7000 years (Goldstein, 1994). Use of the peyote cactus as part of religious ceremonies in the southwestern part of the United States still occurs today, although this ritual use has greatly diminished.

LSD was first synthesized in 1938 by Dr. Albert Hoffman (Holbrook, 1991). It was used as a clinical research tool to investigate the biochemical etiology of schizophrenia. It soon, however, reached the illicit market, and its abuse began to overshadow the research effort.

The abuse of hallucinogens reached a peak in the late 1960s, waned during the 1970s, and returned to favor in the 1980s with the so-called designer drugs (e.g., 3,4-methylene-dioxyamphetamine [MDMA] and methoxyamphetamine [MDA]). One of the most commonly abused hallucinogens today is PCP, even though many of its effects are perceived as undesirable. A number of deaths have been directly attributed to the use of PCP, and numerous accidental deaths have occurred as a result of overdose and of the behavioral changes the drug precipitates (Holbrook, 1991).

Several therapeutic uses of LSD have been proposed, including the treatment of chronic alcoholism and the reduction of intractable pain such as occurs in malignant disease and in phantom limb sensations (McKenry & Salerno, 1989). A great deal more research is required, however, regarding the therapeutic uses of LSD. At this time, there is no real evidence of the safety and efficacy of the drug in humans.

Patterns of Use/Abuse

Use of hallucinogens is usually episodic. Because cognitive and perceptual abilities are so markedly affected by these substances, the user must set aside time from nor-

▄ TABLE 24.5 HALLUCINOGENS

CATEGORIES	GENERIC (TRADE) NAMES	COMMON STREET NAMES
Naturally occurring hallucinogens	Mescaline (the primary active ingredient of the peyote cactus)	Cactus, mesc, mescal, half moon, big chief, bad seed, peyote
	Psilocybin and psilocyn (active ingredients of psilocybe mushrooms)	Magic mushroom, God's flesh, rooms
	Ololiugui (morning glory seeds)	Heavenly blue, pearly gates, flying saucers
Synthetic compounds	Lysergic acid diethylamide [LSD] (synthetically produced from a fungal substance found on rye or a chemical substance found in morning glory seeds)	Acid, cube, big D, California sunshine, microdots, blue dots, sugar, orange wedges, peace tablets, purple haze, cupcakes
	Dimethyltryptamine [DMT] and diethyltryptamine [DET] (chemical analogues of tryptamine)	Businessman's trip
	2,5-dimethoxy-4-methylamphetamine [STP, DOM]	STP (serenity, tranquility, peace)
	Phencyclidine [PCP]	Angel dust, hog, peace pill, rocket fuel
	3,4-Methylene-dioxyamphetamine [MDMA]	XTC, ecstasy, Adam
	Methoxy-amphetamine [MDA]	Love drug

mal daily activities for indulging in the consequences. The *DSM-IV* reports that a community survey conducted in the United States in 1991 revealed that 8 percent of the population had used hallucinogens or PCP at least one or more times in their lifetime (APA, 1994). The use of LSD does not lead to the development of either physical or psychological dependence (Holbrook, 1991). However, tolerance does develop quickly and to a high degree. In fact, an individual who uses LSD repeatedly for a period of 3 to 4 days may develop complete tolerance to the drug. Recovery from the tolerance also occurs very rapidly (in 2 to 3 days), so that the individual is able to achieve the desired effect from the drug repeatedly and often.

PCP is usually taken episodically, in binges that can last for several days. However, some chronic users take the substance on a daily basis (APA, 1994). Physical dependence does not occur with PCP; however, psychological dependence characterized by craving for the drug has been reported in chronic users, as has the slow development of tolerance (Holbrook, 1991). Tolerance apparently develops only with frequent use, such as on a daily basis.

Psilocybin is an ingredient of the psilocybe mushroom indigenous to the United States and Mexico. Ingestion of these mushrooms produces an effect similar to that of LSD but of a shorter duration. This hallucinogenic chemical can now be produced synthetically.

Mescaline is the only hallucinogenic compound used legally for religious purposes today by members of the Native American Church of the United States. It is the primary active ingredient of the peyote cactus. Neither physical nor psychological dependence occurs with the use of mescaline, although tolerance does develop slowly with repeated use (Holbrook, 1991).

Among the very potent hallucinogens of the current drug culture are those that are categorized as derivatives of amphetamines. These include 2,5-dimethoxy-4-

methylamphetamine (DOM, STP), MDMA, and MDA. At lower doses, these drugs produce the "high" associated with CNS stimulants. At higher doses, hallucinogenic effects occur. These drugs have existed for many years but were only *rediscovered* in the mid-1980s. Because of the rapid increase in recreational use, the DEA imposed an emergency classification of MDMA as a schedule I drug in 1985.

Effects on the Body

The effects produced by the various hallucinogenics are highly unpredictable. The variety of effects may be related to dosage, the mental state of the individual, and the environment in which the substance is used. Some common effects have been reported (Kauffman et al., 1985):

PHYSIOLOGICAL EFFECTS

- Nausea and vomiting
- Chills
- Pupil dilation
- Increased pulse, blood pressure, and temperature
- Mild dizziness
- Trembling
- Loss of appetite
- Insomnia
- Sweating
- A slowing of respirations
- Elevation in blood sugar

PSYCHOLOGICAL EFFECTS

- Heightened response to color, texture, and sounds
- Heightened body awareness
- Distortion of vision
- Sense of slowing of time
- All feelings magnified: love, lust, hate, joy, anger, pain, terror, despair

- Fear of losing control
- Paranoia, panic
- Euphoria, bliss
- Projection of self into dreamlike images
- Serenity, peace
- Depersonalization
- Derealization
- Increased libido

The effects of hallucinogens are not always pleasurable for the user. Two types of toxic reactions are known to occur. The first is the *panic reaction*, or "bad trip." Symptoms include an intense level of anxiety, fear, and stimulation. The individual hallucinates and fears going insane. Paranoia and acute psychosis may be evident.

The second type of toxic reaction to hallucinogens is the *flashback*. This phenomenon refers to the transient, spontaneous repetition of a previous LSD-induced experience that occurs in the absence of the substance. Various studies have reported that a range from 15 to 80 percent of hallucinogen users report having experienced flashbacks (Kaplan, Sadock, & Grebb, 1994).

Hallucinogen Intoxication

Symptoms of hallucinogen intoxication develop during, or shortly after (within minutes to a few hours), hallucinogen use (APA, 1994). Maladaptive behavioral or psychological changes include marked anxiety or depression, ideas of reference, fear of losing one's mind, paranoid ideation, and impaired judgment. Perceptual changes occur in a state of full wakefulness and alertness and include intensification of perceptions, depersonalization, derealization, illusions, hallucinations, and synesthesias (APA, 1994). Physical symptoms include pupillary dilation, tachycardia, sweating, palpitations, blurring of vision, tremors, and incoordination (APA, 1994).

Symptoms of PCP intoxication develop within an hour of using the substance (or less when it is smoked, snorted, or used intravenously) (APA, 1994). Specific symptoms are dose related and include belligerence, assaultiveness, impulsiveness, unpredictability, psychomotor agitation, and impaired judgment. Physical symptoms include vertical or horizontal nystagmus, hypertension or tachycardia, numbness or diminished responsiveness to pain, ataxia, dysarthria, muscle rigidity, seizures or coma, and hyperacusis.

Cannabis Abuse and Dependence

A Profile of the Substance

Cannabis is second only to alcohol as the most widely abused drug in the United States. The major psychoactive ingredient of this class of substances is delta-9-tetrahydrocannabinol (THC). It occurs naturally in the plant *Cannabis sativa*, which grows readily in warm climates. Marijuana, the most prevalent type of cannabis preparation, is composed of the dried leaves, stems, and flowers of the plant. Hashish is a more potent concentrate of the resin derived from the flowering tops of the plant. Hash oil is a very concentrated form of THC made by boiling hashish in a solvent and filtering out the solid matter (Holbrook, 1991). Cannabis products are usually smoked in the form of loosely rolled cigarettes. Cannabis can also be taken orally when it is prepared in food, but about two to three times as much cannabis must be taken orally to be as potent as cannabis taken by the inhalation of its smoke (Kaplan, Sadock, & Grebb, 1994).

All the cannabis drugs act as CNS depressants (McKenry & Salerno, 1989). By depressing higher brain centers, they release lower centers from inhibitory influences. There has been some controversy in the past over the classification of these substances. They are not narcotics, although they are legally classified as controlled substances. They are not hallucinogens, although in very high dosages they can induce hallucinations. They are not sedative-hypnotics, although they most closely resemble these substances. Like sedative-hypnotics, their action occurs in the ascending reticular activating system. With increasing dosage, they can produce increasing levels of sedation, hypnosis, and anesthesia.

Both tolerance and physical dependence have been reported to develop with the chronic use of marijuana (Holbrook, 1991). Tolerance tends to be lost rapidly, however, so it may never be evident in the casual or infrequent user. The capacity to lead to psychological dependence is not nearly as strong as that of either tobacco or alcohol (Kaplan & Sadock, 1985). Common cannabis preparations are presented in Table 24.6.

Historical Aspects

Products of *Cannabis sativa* have been used therapeutically for nearly 5000 years (Blum, 1984). Cannabis was first employed in China and India as an antiseptic and an analgesic. Its use later spread to the Middle East, Africa, and Eastern Europe.

In the United States, medical interest in the use of cannabis arose during the early part of the 19th century.

TABLE 24.6 CANNABINOIDS

CATEGORY	COMMON PREPARATIONS	STREET NAMES
Cannabis	Marijuana	Joint, weed, pot, grass, Mary Jane, Texas tea, locoweed, MJ, hay, stick
	Hashish	Hash, bhang, ganja, charas

Many articles were published espousing its use for many and varied reasons. The drug was almost as commonly used for medicinal purposes as aspirin is today and could be purchased without a prescription in any drug store. It was purported to have antibacterial and anticonvulsant capabilities, to decrease intraocular pressure, decrease pain, help in the treatment of asthma, increase appetite, and generally raise one's morale (Schuckit, 1979).

The drug went out of favor primarily because of the huge variation in potency within batches of medication caused by the variations in the THC content of different plants. Other medications were favored for their greater degree of solubility and faster onset of action than cannabis products. In the late 1920s, an association between marijuana and criminal activity was reported (Holbrook, 1991). A federal law put an end to its legal use in 1937. In the 1960s, marijuana became the symbol of the "antiestablishment" generation, at which time it reached its peak as a drug of abuse.

Research continues in regard to the possible therapeutic uses of cannabis. It has been shown to be an effective agent for relieving intraocular pressure in clients with glaucoma. However, lifelong use is often necessary, and the long-term safety and efficacy of these drugs has not been established (Frances & Franklin, 1994).

The use for which cannabis products appear to have the most promising future is in the treatment of nausea and vomiting that accompany cancer chemotherapy. It has been shown in a number of studies to be effective for this purpose when other antinausea medications fail.

Advocates who praise the therapeutic usefulness and support the legalization of the cannabinoids persist within the United States today. Blum (1984) predicted that if marijuana were legalized, more than 1 million Americans would probably be smoking pot daily by the year 2001, including more children, at earlier ages. He also suggested that the potency of the cannabis used would increase. Goldstein (1994) states:

> "Alaska, Oregon, California, and eight other states began a move in the 1970s to adopt more lenient laws concerning possession of small amounts [of marijuana] for personal use; but that trend was reversed by voters and legislatures before long-term results could be evaluated. However, in the few instances in which adequate data were obtained, there was clearly an increase in consumption during the few years of relaxed prohibition." (p. 248)

A great deal more research is required to determine the long-term effects of the drug. Until results indicate otherwise, it is safe to assume that the harmful effects of the drug largely outweigh the benefits.

Patterns of Use/Abuse

In a report from the Substance Abuse and Mental Health Services Administration (1995), it was estimated that 9.8 million people in the United States had used marijuana or hashish in the past month. Marijuana is the most commonly abused illicit drug, and the rate continues to grow. Since 1992, the rate of use among adolescents has more than doubled. However, frequency of use (defined as use on at least 51 days during the past year) dropped from 8.4 million in 1985 to 5.3 million in 1995.

Many people incorrectly regard cannabis as a substance of low abuse potential. This lack of knowledge has promoted use of the substance by some individuals who believe it is harmless. Tolerance, although it tends to decline rapidly, does occur with chronic use. As tolerance develops, physical dependence also occurs, resulting in a mild withdrawal syndrome upon cessation of drug use. The syndrome is characterized by irritability, restlessness, anorexia, insomnia, tremor, sweating, nausea, vomiting, and diarrhea (Goldstein, 1994).

One controversy that exists regarding marijuana is whether or not its use leads to the use of other illicit drugs. In describing the results of longitudinal studies of drug-use progression, Frances and Franklin (1994) stated:

> "Marijuana use was found to be a key stepping-stone to other illicit drugs, and progression to harder drugs was directly related to the intensity of marijuana use. Marijuana introduces youth to drug subcultures and lowers inhibition to use of other drugs." (p. 399)

Effects on the Body

Following is a summary of some of the effects that have been attributed to marijuana in recent years. Undoubtedly, as research continues, evidence of additional physiological and psychological effects will be made available.

Cardiovascular Effects. Cannabis ingestion induces tachycardia and orthostatic hypotension (Holbrook, 1991). With the decrease in blood pressure, myocardial oxygen supply is decreased. Tachycardia in turn increases oxygen demand.

Respiratory Effects. Marijuana produces a greater amount of "tar" than its equivalent weight in tobacco. Because of the method by which marijuana is smoked—that is, the smoke is held in the lungs for as long as possible to achieve the desired effect—larger amounts of tar are deposited in the lungs, promoting deleterious effects to the lungs.

Although the initial reaction to the marijuana is bronchodilatation, thereby facilitating respiratory function, chronic use results in obstructive airway disorders (Holbrook, 1991). Frequent marijuana users often have laryngitis, bronchitis, cough, and hoarseness. Cannabis smoke contains more carcinogens than tobacco smoke; therefore, lung damage and cancer are real risks for heavy users (Goldstein, 1994).

Reproductive Effects. Some studies have shown a decrease in levels of serum testosterone and abnormalities in

TABLE 24.7 PSYCHOACTIVE SUBSTANCES: A PROFILE SUMMARY

CLASS OF DRUGS	SYMPTOMS OF USE	THERAPEUTIC USES	SYMPTOMS OF OVERDOSE	TRADE NAMES	COMMON NAMES
CNS Depressants Alcohol	Relaxation, loss of inhibitions, lack of concentration, drowsiness, slurred speech, sleep	Antidote for methanol consumption; ingredient in many pharmacological concentrates	Nausea, vomiting; shallow respirations; cold, clammy skin; weak, rapid pulse; coma; possible death	Ethyl alcohol, beer, gin, rum, vodka, bourbon, whiskey, liqueurs, wine, brandy, sherry, champagne	Booze, alcohol, liquor, drinks, cocktails, highballs, nightcaps, moonshine, white lightening, firewater
Other (barbiturates and nonbarbiturates)	Same as alcohol	Relief from anxiety and insomnia; as anticonvulsants and anesthetics	Anxiety, fever, agitation, hallucinations, disorientation, tremors, delirium, convulsions, possible death	Seconal, Nembutal, Amytal Valium, Librium Noctec Equanil, Miltown	Red birds, yellow birds, blue birds Blues/yellows; green & whites Mickies Downers
CNS Stimulants Amphetamines and related drugs	Hyperactivity, agitation, euphoria insomnia, loss of appetite	Management of narcolepsy, hyperkinesia, and weight control	Cardiac arrhythmias, headache, convulsions, hypertension, rapid heart rate, coma, possible death	Dexedrine, Didrex, Tenuate Preludin, Ritalin, Plegine, Cylert, Ionamin, Sanorex	Uppers, pep pills, wakeups, bennies, eye-openers, speed, black beauties, sweet As
Cocaine	Euphoria, hyperactivity, restlessness, talkativeness, increased pulse, dilated pupils, rhinitis	Topical anesthetic	Hallucinations, convulsions, pulmonary edema, respiratory failure, coma, cardiac arrest, possible death	Cocaine hydrochloride	Coke, flake, snow, dust, happy dust, gold dust, girl, cecil, C, toot, blow, crack
Opioids	Euphoria, lethargy, drowsiness, lack of motivation, constricted pupils	As analgesics; methadone in substitution therapy; heroin has no therapeutic use	Shallow breathing, slowed pulse, clammy skin, pulmonary edema, respiratory arrest, convulsions, coma, possible death	Heroin Morphine Codeine Dilaudid Demerol Dolophine Percodan Talwin Opium	Snow, stuff, H, harry, horse M, morph, Miss Emma Schoolboy Lords, Doctors Dollies Perkies Ts Big O, black stuff
Hallucinogens	Visual hallucinations, disorientation, confusion, paranoid delusions, euphoria, anxiety, panic, increased pulse	LSD has been proposed in the treatment of chronic alcoholism, and in the reduction of intractable pain	Agitation, extreme hyperactivity, violence, hallucinations, psychosis, convulsions, possible death	LSD PCP Mescaline DMT STP	Acid, cube, big D Angel dust, hog, peace pill Mesc Businessman's trip Serenity and peace

TABLE 24.7   PSYCHOACTIVE SUBSTANCES: A PROFILE SUMMARY

CLASS OF DRUGS	SYMPTOMS OF USE	THERAPEUTIC USES	SYMPTOMS OF OVERDOSE	TRADE NAMES	COMMON NAMES
Cannabinols	Relaxation, talkativeness, lowered inhibitions, euphoria, mood swings	Marijuana has been used for relief of nausea and vomiting associated with antineoplastic chemotherapy and to reduce eye pressure in glaucoma	Fatigue, paranoia, delusions, hallucinations, possible psychosis	Cannabis Hashish	Marijuana, pot, grass, joint, Mary Jane, MJ Hash, rope, Sweet Lucy

sperm count, motility, and structure correlated with heavy marijuana use (Blum, 1984). In women, heavy marijuana use has been correlated with failure to ovulate, difficulty with lactation, and an increased risk of spontaneous abortion.

Central Nervous System Effects. Acute CNS effects of marijuana are dose related. Many people report a feeling of being "high," the equivalent of being "drunk" on alcohol. Symptoms include feelings of euphoria, relaxed inhibitions, disorientation, depersonalization, and relaxation. At higher doses, sensory alterations may occur, including impairment in judgment of time and distance, recent memory, and learning ability. Physiological symptoms may include tremors, muscle rigidity, and conjunctival redness. Toxic effects are generally characterized by panic reactions. Very heavy usage has been shown to precipitate an acute psychosis that is self-limited and short-lived once the drug is removed from the body (Blum, 1984).

Heavy long-term cannabis use is also associated with a syndrome called *amotivational syndrome*. When this syndrome occurs, the individual is totally preoccupied with using the substance. Symptoms include lethargy, apathy, social and personal deterioration, and lack of motivation. This syndrome appears to be more common in countries in which the most potent preparations are used and where the substance is more freely available than it is in the United States.

Sexual Functioning. Marijuana is reported to enhance the sexual experience in both men and women. The intensified sensory awareness and the subjective slowness of time perception are thought to increase sexual satisfaction. Marijuana also enhances the sexual functioning by releasing inhibitions for certain activities that would normally be restrained.

Cannabis Intoxication

Cannabis intoxication is evidenced by the presence of clinically significant maladaptive behavioral or psychological changes that develop during, or shortly after,

cannabis use (APA, 1994). Symptoms include impaired motor coordination, euphoria, anxiety, a sensation of slowed time, and impaired judgment. Physical symptoms include conjunctival injection, increased appetite, dry mouth, and tachycardia. The impairment of motor skills lasts for 8 to 12 hours and interferes with the operation of motor vehicles. Moreover, these effects are additive to those of alcohol, which is commonly used in combination with cannabis (Kaplan, Sadock, & Grebb, 1994).

Tables 24.7 and 24.8 include summaries of the psychoactive substances, including symptoms of intoxication, withdrawal, use, overdose, possible therapeutic uses, and trade and common names by which they may be referred. The dynamics of substance use disorders using the transactional model of stress/adaptation are presented in Figure 24.2.

APPLICATION OF THE NURSING PROCESS

Assessment

In the preintroductory phase of relationship development, the nurse must examine his or her feelings about working with a client who abuses substances. If these behaviors are viewed as morally wrong and the nurse has internalized these attitudes from very early in life, it may be very difficult to suppress judgmental feelings. The role that alcohol or other substances has played (or plays) in the life of the nurse will most certainly affect the way in which he or she approaches interaction with the substance-abusing client.

How are attitudes examined? Some individuals may have sufficient ability for introspection to be able to recognize on their own whether they have unresolved issues related to substance abuse. For others, it may be more helpful to discuss these issues in a group situation, where insight may be gained from feedback regarding the perceptions of others.

Whether alone or in a group, the nurse may gain a greater understanding about attitudes and feelings related

TABLE 24.8   SUMMARY OF SYMPTOMS ASSOCIATED WITH THE SYNDROMES OF INTOXICATION AND WITHDRAWAL

CLASS OF DRUGS	INTOXICATION	WITHDRAWAL	COMMENTS
Alcohol	Aggressiveness, impaired judgment, impaired attention, irritability, euphoria, depression, emotional lability, slurred speech, incoordination, unsteady gait, nystagmus, flushed face	Tremors, nausea/vomiting, malaise, weakness, tachycardia, sweating, elevated blood pressure, anxiety, depressed mood, irritability, hallucinations, headache, insomnia, seizures	Alcohol withdrawal begins within 4–6 hr after last drink. May progress to delirium tremens on 2nd or 3rd day. Use of Librium or Serax is common for substitution therapy.
Amphetamines and related substances	Fighting, grandiosity, hypervigilance, psychomotor agitation, impaired judgment, tachycardia, pupillary dilation, elevated blood pressure, perspiration or chills, nausea and vomiting	Anxiety, depressed mood, irritability, craving for the substance, fatigue, insomnia or hypersomnia, psychomotor agitation, paranoid and suicidal ideation	Withdrawal symptoms usually peak within 2–4 days, although depression and irritability may persist for months. Antidepressants may be used.
Caffeine	Restlessness, nervousness, excitement, insomnia, flushed face, diuresis, gastrointestinal complaints, muscle twitching, rambling flow of thought and speech, cardiac arrhythmia, periods of inexhaustibility, psychomotor agitation	Headache	Caffeine is contained in coffee, tea, colas, cocoa, chocolate, some over-the-counter analgesics, "cold" preparations, and stimulants.
Cannabis	Euphoria, anxiety, suspiciousness, sensation of slowed time, impaired judgment, social withdrawal, tachycardia, conjunctival redness, increased appetite, hallucinations	Restlessness, irritability, insomnia, loss of appetite	Intoxication occurs immediately and lasts about 3 hours. Oral ingestion is more slowly absorbed and has longer-lasting effects.
Cocaine	Euphoria, fighting, grandiosity, hypervigilance, psychomotor agitation, impaired judgment, tachycardia, elevated blood pressure, pupillary dilation, perspiration or chills, nausea/vomiting, hallucinations, delirium	Depression, anxiety, irritability, fatigue, insomnia or hypersomnia, psychomotor agitation, paranoid or suicidal ideation, apathy, social withdrawal	Large doses of the drug can result in convulsions or death from cardiac arrhythmias or respiratory paralysis.
Inhalants	Belligerence, assaultiveness, apathy, impaired judgment, dizziness, nystagmus, slurred speech, unsteady gait, lethargy, depressed reflexes, tremor, blurred vision, stupor or coma, euphoria, irritation around eyes, throat, and nose		Intoxication occurs within 5 minutes of inhalation. Symptoms last 60–90 min. Large doses can result in death from CNS depression or cardiac arrhythmia.
Nicotine		Craving for the drug, irritability, anger, frustration, anxiety, difficulty concentrating, restlessness, decreased heart rate, increased appetite, weight gain, tremor, headaches, insomnia	Symptoms begin within 24 hours of last drug use and decrease in intensity over days, weeks, or sometimes longer.
Opioids	Euphoria, lethargy, somnolence, apathy, dysphoria, impaired judgment, pupillary constriction, drowsiness, slurred speech, constipation, nausea, decreased respiratory rate and blood pressure	Craving for the drug, nausea/vomiting, muscle aches, lacrimation or rhinorrhea, pupillary dilation, piloerection or sweating, diarrhea, yawning, fever, insomnia	Withdrawal symptoms appear within 6–8 hours after last dose, reach a peak in the 2nd or 3rd day, and disappear in 7–10 days.

Table 24.8 Summary of Symptoms Associated with the Syndromes of Intoxication and Withdrawal

Class of Drugs	Intoxication	Withdrawal	Comments
Phencyclidine and related substances	Belligerence, assaultiveness, impulsiveness, psychomotor agitation, impaired judgment, nystagmus, increased heart rate and blood pressure, diminished pain response, ataxia, dysarthria, muscle rigidity, seizures, hyperacusis, delirium		Delirium can occur within 24 hours after use of phencyclidine, or may occur up to a week following recovery from an overdose of the drug.
Sedatives, hypnotics, anxiolytics	Disinhibition of sexual or aggressive impulses, mood lability, impaired judgment, slurred speech, incoordination, unsteady gait, impairment in attention or memory disorientation, confusion	Nausea/vomiting, malaise, weakness, tachycardia, sweating, anxiety, irritability, orthostatic hypotension, tremor, insomnia, seizures	Withdrawal may progress to delirium, usually within 1 week of last use. Long-acting barbiturates or benzodiazepines may be used in withdrawal substitution therapy.

to substance abuse by responding to the following types of questions. The questions are specific to alcohol, but could be adapted for any substance.

What are my drinking patterns?

If I drink, why do I drink? When, where, and how much?

If I don't drink, why is it that I abstain?

Am I comfortable with my drinking patterns?

If I decided not to drink any more, would that be a problem for me?

What did I learn from my parents about drinking?

Have my attitudes changed as an adult?

What are my feelings about people who become intoxicated?

Does it seem more acceptable for some individuals than for others?

Do I ever use terms like "sot," "drunk," or "boozer," to describe some individuals who overindulge, yet overlook it in others?

Do I ever overindulge myself?

Has the use of alcohol (by myself or others) affected my life in any way?

Do I see alcohol/drug abuse as a sign of weakness? A moral problem? An illness?

Unless nurses fully understand and accept their own attitudes and feelings, they cannot be empathetic toward clients' problems. Clients in recovery need to know they are accepted for themselves, regardless of past behaviors. Nurses must be able to separate the client from the behavior and to accept that individual with unconditional positive regard.

Assessment Tools

Nurses are often the individuals who perform the admission interview. A variety of assessment tools are appropri-

ate for use in chemical dependency units. A nursing history and assessment tool was presented in Chapter 7 of this text. With some adaptation, it is an appropriate instrument for creating a database on clients who abuse substances. Table 24.9 presents a drug history and assessment that could be used in conjunction with the general biopsychosocial assessment.

Other screening tools exist for determining whether an individual has a problem with substances. Two such tools developed by the APA for the diagnosis of alcoholism include the Michigan Alcoholism Screening Test and the CAGE Questionnaire (Tables 24.10 and 24.11). Some psychiatric units administer these surveys to all clients who are admitted, in an effort to determine if there is a secondary alcoholism problem in addition to the psychiatric problem for which the client is being admitted (sometimes called dual diagnosis). It would be possible to adapt these tools to use in diagnosing problems with other drugs as well.

Diagnosis/Outcome Identification

The next step in the nursing process is to identify appropriate nursing diagnoses by analyzing the data collected during the assessment phase. The individual who abuses or is dependent on substances will undoubtedly have many unmet physical and emotional needs. Possible nursing diagnoses for clients with substance-related disorders include:

Ineffective denial related to weak, underdeveloped ego evidenced by "I don't have a problem with (substance). I can quit any time I want to."

Ineffective individual coping related to inadequate coping skills and weak ego evidenced by use of substances as coping mechanism.

Altered nutrition: Less than body requirements/fluid volume deficit related to drinking or taking drugs

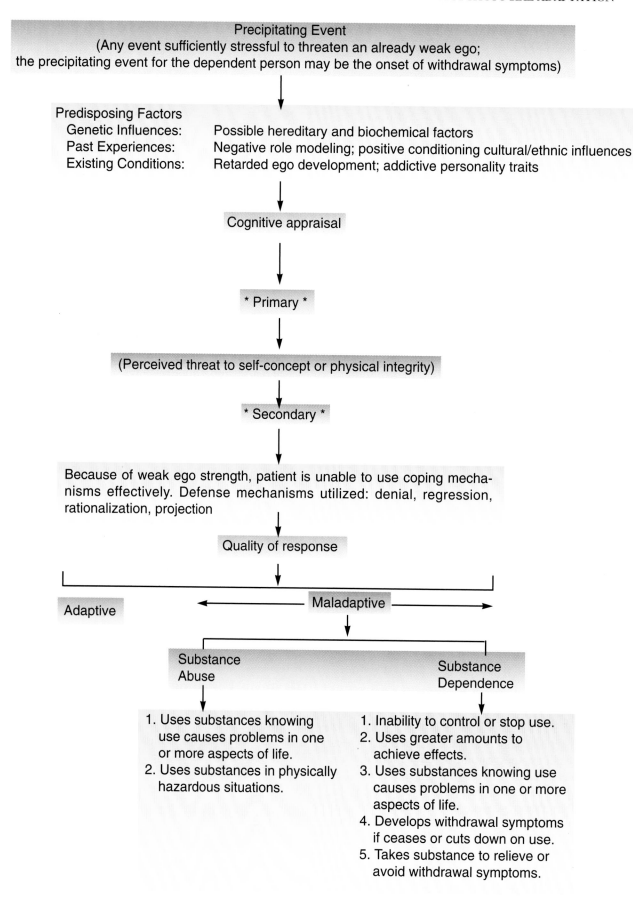

Figure 24.2   The dynamics of substance-use disorders using the transactional model of stress/adaptation.

TABLE 24.9   DRUG HISTORY AND ASSESSMENT

1. When you were growing up, did anyone in your family drink alcohol or take other kinds of drugs?
2. If so, how did the substance use affect the family situation?
3. When did you have your first drink/drugs?
4. How long have you been drinking/taking drugs on a regular basis?
5. What is your pattern of substance use?
   a. When do you use substances?
   b. What do you use?
   c. How much do you use?
   d. Where are you and with whom when you use substances?
6. When did you have your last drink/drug? What was it and how much did you consume?
7. Does using the substance(s) cause problems for you? Describe. Include family, friends, job, school, other.
8. Have you ever experienced injury due to substance use?
9. Have you ever been arrested or incarcerated for drinking/drugs?
10. Have you ever tried to stop drinking/drugs? If so, what was the result? Did you experience any physical symptoms, such as tremors, headache, insomnia, sweating, seizures?
11. Have you ever experienced loss of memory for times when you have been drinking/taking drugs?
12. Describe a typical day in your life for me.
13. Are there any changes you would like to make in your life? If so, what?
14. What plans or ideas do you have for seeing that these changes occur?

*To be used in conjunction with general biopsychosocial nursing history and assessment tool (Chapter 7).

instead of eating, evidenced by loss of weight, pale conjunctiva and mucous membranes, poor skin turgor, electrolyte imbalance, anemias, and other signs and symptoms of malnutrition/dehydration.

Risk for infection related to malnutrition and altered immune condition.

Self-esteem disturbance related to weak ego, lack of positive feedback evidenced by criticism of self and others and use of substances as coping mechanism (self-destructive behavior).

Knowledge deficit (effects of substance abuse on the body) related to denial of problems with substances evidenced by abuse of substances.

For the client in substance withdrawal, possible nursing diagnoses include:

Risk for injury related to CNS agitation (withdrawal from CNS depressants).

Risk for self-directed violence related to depressed mood (withdrawal from CNS stimulants).

The following criteria may be used for measurement of outcomes in the care of the client with substance-related disorders.

THE CLIENT:

1. Has not experienced physical injury.
2. Has not caused harm to self or others.
3. Accepts responsibility for own behavior.
4. Acknowledges association between personal problems and use of substance(s).
5. Demonstrates more adaptive coping mechanisms that can be used in stressful situations (instead of taking substances).
6. Shows no signs or symptoms of infection or malnutrition.
7. Exhibits evidence of increased self-worth by attempting new projects without fear of failure and by demonstrating less defensive behavior toward others.
8. Verbalizes importance of abstaining from use of substances in order to maintain optimal wellness.

Planning/Implementation

Table 24.12 provides a plan of care for the client with a substance-related disorder. Selected nursing diagnoses are presented, along with outcome criteria, appropriate nursing interventions, and rationales for each.

Some institutions are using a case management model to coordinate care (see Chapter 7 for a more detailed explanation). In case management models, the plan of care may take the form of a critical pathway. Table 24.13 presents an example of a critical pathway of care for a client experiencing the alcohol withdrawal syndrome.

Implementation with clients who abuse substances is a long-term process, often beginning with **detoxification** and progressing to total abstinence. Smith and coworkers (1984) identified the following common major treatment objectives for hospitalized clients with substance-use disorders.

SHORT-TERM OBJECTIVES

1. Support withdrawal from substances and prevent physical complications.
2. Monitor toxic state, provide physical nursing care, and administer **substitution therapy** as ordered.
3. Provide psychological support and promote a restful environment.

INTERMEDIATE OBJECTIVES

1. Interpret symptoms, course of treatment, and expected outcomes for client and family.
2. Promote understanding of substance abuse and dependency and participation in treatment program.

LONG-TERM OBJECTIVES

1. Encourage participation in the treatment program and promote understanding of underlying problems associated with substance use.

TABLE 24.10 MICHIGAN ALCOHOLISM SCREENING TEST

Answer the following questions by placing an X under yes or no.*

	Yes	No
1. Do you enjoy a drink now and then?	0	0
2. Do you feel you are a normal drinker? (By normal we mean you drink less than or as much as most people.)		2
3. Have you ever awakened the morning after some drinking the night before and found that you could not remember a part of the evening?	2	
4. Does your wife, husband, parent, or other near relative ever worry or complain about your drinking?	1	
5. Can you stop drinking without a struggle after one or two drinks?		2
6. Do you ever feel guilty about your drinking?	1	
7. Do friends or relatives think you are a normal drinker?		2
8. Are you able to stop drinking when you want to?		2
9. Have you ever attended a meeting of Alcoholics Anonymous (AA)?	5	
10. Have you gotten into physical fights when drinking?	1	
11. Has your drinking ever created problems between you and your wife, husband, a parent, or other relative?	2	
12. Has your wife, husband, or another family member ever gone to anyone for help about your drinking?	2	
13. Have you ever lost friends because of your drinking?	2	
14. Have you ever gotten into trouble at work or school because of drinking?	2	
15. Have you ever lost a job because of drinking?	2	
16. Have you ever neglected your obligations, your family, or your work for 2 or more days in a row because you were drinking?	2	
17. Do you drink before noon fairly often?	1	
18. Have you ever been told you have liver trouble? Cirrhosis?	2	
19. After heavy drinking have you ever had delirium tremens (DTs) or severe shaking or heard voices or seen things that really were not there?	5	
20. Have you ever gone to anyone for help about your drinking?	5	
21. Have you ever been in a hospital because of drinking?	5	
22. Have you ever been a patient in a psychiatric hospital or on a psychiatric ward of a general hospital where drinking was part of the problem that resulted in hospitalization?	2	
23. Have you ever been seen at a psychiatric or mental health clinic or gone to any doctor, social worker, or clergyman for help with any emotional problem, where drinking was part of the problem?	2	
24. Have you ever been arrested for drunk driving, driving while intoxicated, or driving under the influence of alcoholic beverages? (If yes, how many times?)	2 ea	
25. Have you ever been arrested, or taken into custody, even for a few hours, because of other drunk behavior? (If yes, how many times?)	2 ea	

*Items are scored under the response that would indicate a problem with alcohol.
Method of scoring: 0–3 points = no problem with alcohol
4 points = possible problem with alcohol
5 or more = indicates problem with alcohol
Source: From Selzer (1971), with permission.

2. Monitor for signs of acute stress or possible resumption of substance use.
3. Assist client to explore alternative coping strategies to achieve satisfaction (Table 22.14).
4. Assist with plans for follow-up therapy.

Client/Family Education

The role of client teacher is important in the psychiatric area, as it is in all areas of nursing. A list of topics for client/family education relevant to substance-related disorders is presented in Table 24.15.

TABLE 24.11 THE CAGE QUESTIONNAIRE

1. Have you ever felt you should Cut down on your drinking?
2. Have people Annoyed you by criticizing your drinking?
3. Have you ever felt bad or Guilty about your drinking?
4. Have you ever had a drink first thing in the morning to steady your nerves or get rid of a hangover (Eye-opener)?

Scoring: 2 or 3 "yes" answers strongly suggest a problem with alcohol.
Source: From Mayfield, McLeod, & Hall (1974), with permission.

TABLE 24.12 CARE PLAN FOR THE CLIENT WITH A SUBSTANCE-RELATED DISORDER

NURSING DIAGNOSIS: INEFFECTIVE DENIAL

RELATED TO: Weak, underdeveloped ego

EVIDENCED BY: Statements indicating no problem with substance use

OUTCOME CRITERIA	NURSING INTERVENTIONS	RATIONALE
Client will demonstrate acceptance of responsibility for own behavior and acknowledge association between substance use and personal problems.	1. Develop trust. Convey an attitude of acceptance. Ensure that client understands it is not the *person* but the *behavior* that is unacceptable 2. Correct any misconceptions, such as, "I don't have a drinking problem. I can quit any time I want to." Do this in a matter-of-fact, non-judgmental manner. 3. Identify recent maladaptive behaviors or situations that have occurred in the client's life, and discuss how use of substances may be a contributing factor. Say, "The lab report shows your blood alcohol level was 250 when you were involved in that automobile accident." 4. Do not allow client to rationalize or blame others for behaviors associated with substance use.	1. Unconditional acceptance promotes dignity and self-worth, qualities that this individual has been trying to achieve with substances. 2. These interventions help the client see the condition as an illness that requires help. 3. The first step in decreasing use of denial is for the client to see the relationship between substance use and personal problems. To confront issues with a caring attitude preserves self-esteem. 4. This only serves to prolong the denial.

NURSING DIAGNOSIS: INEFFECTIVE INDIVIDUAL COPING

RELATED TO: Inadequate coping skills and weak ego

EVIDENCED BY: Use of substances as a coping mechanism

OUTCOME CRITERIA	NURSING INTERVENTIONS	RATIONALE
Client will be able to verbalize adaptive coping mechanisms to use, instead of substance abuse, in response to stress (and demonstrate, as applicable).	1. Set limits on manipulative behavior. Administer consequences when limits are violated. Obtain routine urine samples for laboratory analysis of substances. 2. Explore options available to assist with stress rather than resorting to substance use (see Table 24.14). Practice these techniques. 3. Give positive reinforcement for ability to delay gratification and respond to stress with adaptive coping strategies.	1. Because of weak ego and delayed development, client is unable to establish own limits or delay gratification. Client may obtain substances from various sources while in the hospital. 2. Because gratification has been closely tied to oral needs, it is unlikely that client is aware of more adaptive coping strategies. 3. Because of weak ego, client needs lots of positive feedback to enhance self-esteem and enhance ego development.

NURSING DIAGNOSIS: ALTERED NUTRITION: LESS THAN BODY REQUIREMENTS/FLUID VOLUME DEFICIT

RELATED TO: Use of substances instead of eating

EVIDENCED BY: Loss of weight, pale conjunctiva and mucous membranes, poor skin turgor, electrolyte imbalance, anemias (and/or other signs and symptoms of malnutrition and dehydration)

OUTCOME CRITERIA	NURSING INTERVENTIONS	RATIONALE
Client will be free of signs or symptoms of malnutrition and dehydration.	1. Parenteral support may be required initially.	1. To correct fluid and electrolyte imbalance, hypoglycemia, and some vitamin deficiencies.

Continued on following page

TABLE 24.12 *(Continued)*

2. Encourage cessation of smoking	2. To facilitate repair of damage to GI tract.
3. Consult dietitian. Determine the number of calories required based on body size and level of activity. Document intake and output and calorie count, and weigh client daily.	3. These interventions are necessary to maintain an ongoing nutritional assessment.
4. Ensure that the amount of protein in the diet is correct for the individual client's condition. Protein intake should be adequate to maintain nitrogen equilibrium, but should be drastically decreased or eliminated if there is potential for hepatic coma.	4. Diseased liver may be incapable of properly metabolizing proteins, resulting in an accumulation of ammonia in the blood that circulates to the brain and can result in altered consciousness.
5. Sodium may need to be restricted.	5. To minimize fluid retention (e.g., ascites and edema).
6. Provide foods that are nonirritating to the clients with esophageal varices.	6. To avoid irritation and bleeding of these swollen blood vessels.
7. Provide small frequent feeding of client's favorite foods. Supplement nutritious meals with multiple vitamin and mineral tablet.	7. To encourage intake and facilitate client's achievement of adequate nutrition.

Evaluation

The final step of the nursing process involves reassessment to determine if the nursing interventions have been effective in achieving the intended goals of care. Evaluation of the client with a substance-related disorder may be accomplished by using information gathered from the following reassessment questions:

1. Has detoxification occurred without complications?
2. Is the client still in denial?
3. Does the client accept responsibility for his or her own behavior? Has he or she acknowledged a personal problem with substances?
4. Has a correlation been made between personal problems and the use of substances?
5. Does the client still make excuses or blame others for use of substances?
6. Has the client remained substance-free during hospitalization?
7. Does the client cooperate with treatment?
8. Does the client refrain from manipulative behavior and violation of limits?
9. Is the client able to verbalize alternative adaptive coping strategies to substitute for substance use? Has the use of these strategies been demonstrated? Does positive reinforcement encourage repetition of these adaptive behaviors?
10. Has nutritional status been restored? Does the client consume a diet adequate for his or her size and level of activity? Is the client able to discuss the importance of adequate nutrition?
11. Has the client remained free of infection during hospitalization?
12. Is the client able to verbalize the effects of substance abuse on the body?
13. Does the client verbalize that he or she wants to recover and lead a life free of substances?

THE IMPAIRED NURSE

Substance abuse and dependency is a problem that has the potential for impairment in an individual's social, occupational, psychological, and physical functioning. This becomes an especially serious problem when the impaired person is responsible for the lives of others on a daily basis. Hughes and Smith (1994) report, "The American Nurses' Association has estimated that 6 percent to 8 percent of nurses use alcohol or other drugs to an extent sufficient to impair their professional performance." Narcotic addiction among nurses has been reported to be at least 30 times greater than it is among the general population (Caroselli-Karinja & Zboray, 1987). A survey of 44 state boards of nursing revealed that 67 percent of cases handled by the boards were related to substance abuse (Sullivan, Bissell, & Williams, 1988).

For years, the impaired nurse was protected, promoted, transferred, ignored, or fired. These types of responses promoted the growth of the problem. A humane system of intervention and treatment is necessary to redeem the future for the chemically dependent nurse, while significantly reducing cost and risk for health care employers (Sullivan, Bissell, & Williams, 1988).

How does one identify the impaired nurse? It is still easiest to overlook what *might* be a problem. Denial, on the part of the impaired nurse as well as nurse colleagues,

TABLE 24.13 CRITICAL PATHWAY OF CARE FOR CLIENT IN ALCOHOL WITHDRAWAL

Estimated Length of Stay: 7 days—variations from designated pathway should be documented in progress notes

Nursing Diagnosis and Categories of Care	Time Dimension	Goals and/or Actions	Time Dimension	Goals and/or Actions	Time Dimension	Discharged Outcome
Risk for injury related to CNS agitation					Day 7	Client shows no evidence of injury obtained during ETOH withdrawal.
Referrals	Day 1	Psychiatrist Assess need for: Neurologist Cardiologist Internist			Day 7	Discharge with follow-up appointments as required.
Diagnostic studies	Day 1	Blood alcohol level Drug screen SMAC 27 Urinalysis Chest X-ray ECG	Day 4	Repeat of selected diagnostic studies as necessary		
Additional assessments	Day 1 Day 1–5 ongoing ongoing	VS q4h I&O Restraints p.r.n. Assess withdrawal symptoms: tremors, nausea/ vomiting, tachycardia, sweating, high blood pressure, seizures, insomnia, hallucinations	Day 2–3 Day 6 Day 4	VS q8h if stable DC I&O Marked decrease in objective symptoms	Day 4–7 Day 7	VS b.i.d.; remain stable Discharge; absence of objective withdrawal symptoms
Medications	Day 1 Day 2 Day 1–6 Day 1–7	Librium 200 mg Librium 160 mg Librium p.r.n. Maalox a.c. and h.s.	Day 3 Day 4	Librium 120 mg Librium 80 mg	Day 5 Day 6 Day 7	Librium 40 mg DC Librium Discharge; no withdrawal symptoms
Client education			Day 5	Discuss goals of AA and need for outpatient therapy	Day 7	Discharge with information regarding AA attendance or outpatient treatment
Altered nutrition: Less than body requirements					Day 7	Nutritional condition has stabilized.
Referrals	Day 1	Consult dietitian	Day 1–7	Fulfill nutritional needs		
Diet	Day 1	Bland as tolerated; fluids as tolerated	Day 2–3	Frequent, small, meals; easily digested foods; advance as tolerated	Day 4–7	High-protein, high-carbohydrate diet

Continued on following page

Table 24.13 *(Continued)*

Estimated Length of Stay: 7 days—variations from designated pathway should be documented in progress notes

Nursing Diagnosis and Categories of Care	Time Dimension	Goals and/or Actions	Time Dimension	Goals and/or Actions	Time Dimension	Discharge Outcome
Additional assessments	Day 1–7	Weight I&O Skin turgor Color of mucous membranes				
Medications	Day 1–4	Thiamine 100-mg injections	Day 2–7	Multiple vitamin tablet		
Client education			Day 5	Principles of nutrition; foods for maintenance of wellness	Day 6–7	Client demonstrates ability to select appropriate foods for healthy diet

is still the strongest defense for dealing with substance-abuse problems. Some states have mandatory reporting laws that require observers to report substance-abusing nurses to the board of nursing (Sullivan, Bissell, & Williams, 1988). They are difficult laws to enforce, and hospitals are not always compliant with mandatory reporting. Some hospitals may choose not to report to the state board of nursing if the impaired nurse is actively seeking treatment and is not placing clients in danger.

Murphy and Violette (1985) identified some clues for recognizing substance impairment in nurses. They are not easy to detect and will vary according to the substance being used. The impaired nurse may appear happy or sad, may have an increased appetite or no appetite at all. He or she may be verbal and energetic, or slow-thinking with impaired concentration. This nurse may volunteer to work additional shifts and have an excellent work attendance record (since work is the source of the substance supply). However, the impaired nurse may leave the floor a lot or spend a great deal of time in the restroom. When an impaired nurse is on duty, there may be more accidents, more incidents reported, and more clients who complain of unrelieved pain and insomnia, even though many narcotic analgesics and sedatives have been documented as administered. As the impairment progresses, clues may be reflected by inaccurate drug counts, increased vial breakage and drug wastage, and discrepancies in documentation. Lapses in memory may occur, and personal appearance and job performance will likely be affected.

If suspicious behavior occurs, it is important to keep careful, objective records. Confrontation with the impaired nurse will undoubtedly result in hostility and de-

nial. Confrontation should occur in the presence of a supervisor or other nurse and should include the offer of assistance in seeking treatment. If a report is made to the state board of nursing, it should be a factual documentation of specific events and actions, not a diagnostic statement of impairment.

What will the state board do? Sullivan, Bissell, & Williams (1988) identify three ways in which a state board may respond to a nurse's impaired practice.

1. They may refuse to restore or grant a license.
2. They may rely on a host of experts to testify about whether the nurse's addiction poses a hazard, thus providing some degree of assurance of client safety as well as someone with whom to share the responsibility if the nurse fails.
3. They may institute or cooperate with a strict and thorough monitoring system designed to discover relapse. Strict monitoring is expensive and intrusive, but it can reduce the public's risk to an acceptable level.

Several state boards of nursing have passed diversionary laws that allow impaired nurses to avoid disciplinary action by agreeing to seek treatment. Some of these state boards administer the treatment programs themselves, and others refer the nurse to community resources or state nurses' association assistance programs.

In 1982, the ANA House of Delegates adopted a national resolution to provide assistance to impaired nurses. Since that time, the majority of state nurses' associations have developed (or are developing) programs for nurses who are impaired by substances or psychiatric illness. The individuals who administer these efforts are nurse mem-

⬛ TABLE 24.14   MOTIVES FOR, AND ALTERNATIVES TO, THE USE OF DRUGS

LEVEL OF EXPERIENCE	EXAMPLES OF MOTIVES FOR TAKING DRUGS	EXAMPLES OF POSSIBLE ALTERNATIVES TO TAKING DRUGS
Physical	Desire for physical satisfaction; physical relaxation; relief from sickness; desire for more energy; maintenance of physical dependency	Athletics; dance; exercise; hiking; diet; health training; carpentry or outdoor work
Sensory	Desire to stimulate sight, sound, touch, taste; need for sensual-sexual stimulation; desire to magnify sensorium	Sensory awareness training; sky diving; experiencing sensory beauty of nature; lovemaking; swimming; running; mountaineering
Emotional	Relief from psychological pain; attempt to solve personal perplexities; relief from bad mood; escape from anxiety; desire for emotional insight; liberation of feeling; emotional relaxation	Individual counseling; group therapy; instruction in psychology of personal development; sensitivity training
Interpersonal	To gain peer acceptance; to break through interpersonal barriers; to "communicate," especially nonverbally; defiance of authority figures; cement two-person relationships; relaxation of interpersonal hangups	Sensitivity and encounter groups; group therapy; instruction in social customs; confidence training; social-interpersonal counseling; emphasis on assisting others in distress via education
Social/Cultural/ Environmental	To promote social change; find identifiable subculture; tune out intolerable environmental conditions (e.g., poverty); change awareness of the masses	Social service; community action in positive social change; helping the poor, aged, infirm, young; tutoring handicapped; ecology action
Political	To promote political change; identify with antiestablishment subgroup; to change drug legislation; out of desperation with the social-political order; to gain wealth, affluence, or power	Political service; political action; nonpartisan projects such as ecological lobbying; field work with politicians and public officials
Intellectual	To escape mental boredom; out of intellectual curiosity; to solve cognitive problems; to gain new understanding in the world of ideas; to study better; to research one's own awareness; for science	Intellectual excitement through reading; or through discussion; creative games and puzzles; self-hypnosis; training in concentration; synectics—training in intellectual breakthroughs; memory training
Creative/ Aesthetic	To improve creativity in the arts; to enhance enjoyment of art already produced (e.g., music); to enjoy imaginative mental productions	Nongraded instruction in producing and/or appreciating art, music, drama, crafts, handiwork, cooking, sewing, gardening, writing, singing, and so forth
Philosophical	To discover meaningful values; to grasp the nature of the universe; to find meaning in life; to help establish personal identity; to organize a belief structure	Discussions, seminars, courses in the meaning of life; study of ethics, morality, the nature of reality; relevant philosophical literature; guided exploration of value systems
Spiritual/Mystical	To transcend orthodox religion; to develop spiritual insights; to reach higher levels of consciousness; to have divine visions; to communicate with God; to augment yogic practices; to get a spiritual shortcut; to attain enlightenment; to attain spiritual powers	Exposure to nonchemical methods of spiritual development; study of world religions; introduction to applied mysticism, meditation; yogic techniques
Miscellaneous	Adventure, risk, drama, "kicks," unexpressed motives; prodrug general attitudes	"Outward Bound" survival training; combinations of alternatives above; pronaturalness attitudes; brain wave training; meaningful employment

SOURCES: From Cohen (1972) and Julien (1981), with permission.

bers of the state associations, as well as nurses who are in recovery themselves. For this reason, they are called **peer assistance programs.**

The peer assistance programs strive to intervene early, to reduce hazards to clients, and to increase prospects for the nurse's recovery. Most states provide either a hot-line number that the impaired nurse or intervening colleague may call or phone numbers of peer assistance committee members, which are made available for the same purpose. Typically, a contract is drawn up detailing the method of treatment, which may be obtained from various sources, such as employee assistance programs, Alcoholics Anonymous, Narcotics Anonymous, private counseling, or outpatient clinics. Guidelines for monitoring the course of treatment are established. Peer support is provided through regular contact with the impaired nurse, usually

▰▰ **TABLE 24.15 TOPICS FOR CLIENT/FAMILY EDUCATION RELATED TO SUBSTANCE-USE DISORDERS**

Nature of the illness
1. Effects of (substance) in the body
   a. Alcohol
   b. Other CNS depressants.
   c. CNS stimulants
   d. Hallucinogens
   e. Narcotics
   f. Cannabinols
2. Ways in which use of (substance) affects life

Management of the Illness
1. Activities to substitute for (substance) in time of stress
2. Relaxation techniques
   a. Progressive relaxation
   b. Tense and relax
   c. Deep breathing
   d. Autogenics
3. Problem-solving skills
4. The essentials of good nutrition

Support Services
1. Financial assistance
2. Legal assistance
3. Alcoholics Anonymous (or other support group specific to another substance)
4. One-to-one support person

for a period of 2 years. Peer assistance programs serve to assist impaired nurses to recognize their impairment, to obtain necessary treatment, and to regain accountability within their profession.

CODEPENDENCY

Codependence is a term that has been given much attention in the last few years. The concept arose out of a need to define the dysfunctional behaviors that are evident among members of the family of a chemically dependent person. The term has been expanded to include all individuals from families that harbor secrets of physical or emotional abuse, other cruelties or pathological conditions—families that admonish their members, "Don't talk, don't trust, don't feel" (Black, 1982). This inability to relate results in unmet needs for autonomy and self-esteem, and a profound sense of powerlessness. The codependent person is able to achieve a sense of control only through fulfilling the needs of others. Cermak (1986) has stated, "Power through sacrifice of self lies at the core of codependence."

A number of authors have proposed various definitions for codependence. Examples include the following:

"An exaggerated dependent pattern of learned behaviors, beliefs, and feelings that make life painful. It is a dependence on people and things outside the self, along with neglect of

the self to the point of having little self-identity." (Smalley, 1984)

"A dysfunctional pattern of living learned from our family of origin as well as our culture, producing arrested identity development and resulting in an overreaction to things outside of us and an underreaction to things inside of us. Left untreated, it can deteriorate into an addiction." (Friel & Friel, 1988)

"A recognizable pattern of personality traits, predictably found within most members of chemically dependent families, which are capable of creating sufficient dysfunction to warrant the diagnosis of Mixed Personality Disorder as outlined in DSM-III." (Cermak, 1986)

The traits associated with a codependent personality are varied. The *DSM-IV* (APA, 1994) states that personality traits only become disorders when they are "inflexible and maladaptive and cause significant functional impairment or subjective distress." To date, no diagnostic criteria exist for the diagnosis of codependent personality disorder. Cermak (1986) has proposed the following criteria in the style of the *DSM-IV*.

A. Continued investment of self-esteem in the ability to control both oneself and others in the face of serious adverse consequences.

B. Assumption of responsibility for meeting others' needs to the exclusion of acknowledging one's own.

C. Anxiety and boundary distortions around intimacy and separation.

D. Enmeshment in relationships with personality-disordered, chemically dependent, other codependent, or impulse-disordered individuals.

E. Three or more of the following:
   1. Excessive reliance on denial.
   2. Constriction of emotions (with or without dramatic outbursts).
   3. Depression.
   4. Hypervigilance.
   5. Compulsions.
   6. Anxiety.
   7. Substance abuse.
   8. Has been (or is) the victim of recurrent physical [emotional] or sexual abuse.
   9. Stress-related medical illnesses.
   10. Has remained in a primary relationship with an active substance abuser [or individual with other pathological condition] for at least 2 years without seeking outside help.

   NOTE: Bracketed items added by author.

A codependent individual is confused about his or her own identity. In a relationship, the codependent person derives self-worth from that of the partner, whose feelings and behaviors determine how the codependent should feel and behave. In order for the codependent to feel good, his or her partner must be happy and behave in appropriate ways. If the partner is not happy, the codependent feels responsible for *making* him or her happy (Cermak, 1986). The codependent's home life is fraught with stress. Ego boundaries are weak and behaviors are often enmeshed with those of the pathological partner. Denial that problems exist is common. Feelings are kept in control, and anxiety may be released in the form of stress-related illnesses or compulsive behaviors such as eating, spending, working, or use of substances.

The Codependent Nurse

Hall and Wray (1989) have identified certain characteristics associated with codependence that they apply to nursing. A shortage of nurses combined with the increasing ranks of seriously ill clients may result in nurses providing care and fulfilling everyone's needs but their own. Also, a disproportionate percentage of mental health workers come from chemically dependent homes or backgrounds, which puts them at risk for having any unresolved codependent tendencies activated (Cermak, 1986). Hall and Wray identify the following classic characteristics of the codependent nurse:

1. **Caretaking.** This occurs when nurses attempt to meet others' needs to the point of neglecting their own. They are attracted to people who need them, yet resent receiving so little in return. Their emotional needs go unmet, yet they continue to deny that these needs exist.
2. **Perfectionism.** Low self-esteem and fear of failure drive codependent nurses to strive for an unrealistic level of achievement. They are highly critical of themselves and others. They reject praise from others and achieve personal satisfaction only out of feeling needed.
3. **Denial.** Codependent nurses refuse to acknowledge that any personal problems or painful issues exist. This is often facilitated through use of compulsive behaviors, such as work or spending excessively, or addictions, such as to food or substances.
4. **Poor Communication.** Codependent nurses rarely express their true feelings. Their interactive style often reflects a tendency to say and do what they believe others want, to preserve harmony and maintain control.

Treating Codependence

Cermak (1986) has identified four stages in the recovery process for individuals with codependent personality:

Stage I: The Survival Stage. In this first stage, codependent persons must begin to let go of the denial that problems exist or that their personal capabilities are unlimited. This initiation of abstinence from blanket denial may be a very emotional and painful period.

Stage II: The Reidentification Stage. Reidentification occurs when the individuals are able to glimpse their true selves through a break in the denial system. They accept the label of codependent and take responsibility for their own dysfunctional behavior. Codependents tend to enter reidentification only after being convinced that it is more painful not to. They accept their limitations and are ready to face the issues of codependence.

Stage III: The Core Issues Stage. In this stage, the recovering codependent must face the fact that relationships cannot be managed by force of will. Each partner must be independent and autonomous. The goal of this stage is to detach from the struggles of life that exist because of prideful and willful efforts to control those things that are beyond the individual's power to control.

Stage IV: The Reintegration Stage. This is a stage of self-acceptance and willingness to change when codependents relinquish the power *over others* that was not rightfully theirs but reclaim the *personal* power that they do possess. Integrity is achieved out of awareness, honesty, and being in touch with one's spiritual consciousness. Control is achieved through self-discipline and self-confidence.

Self-help groups have been found to be useful in the treatment of codependency. Groups developed for families of chemically dependent people, such as Al-Anon, may be of assistance. Groups specific to the problem of codependency also exist. Two of these groups are:

Co-Dependents Anonymous (CoDA)
P.O. Box 33577
Phoenix, AZ 85067-3577

Co-Dependents Anonymous for Helping Professionals (CODAHP)
P.O. Box 42253
Mesa, AZ 85274-2253

Both of these groups apply the Twelve Steps and Twelve Traditions developed by Alcoholics Anonymous to codependency (Tables 24.16 and 24.17).

TREATMENT MODALITIES FOR SUBSTANCE-RELATED DISORDERS

Alcoholics Anonymous

Alcoholics Anonymous (AA) is a major self-help organization for the treatment of alcoholism. It was founded in 1935 by a stockbroker named Bill Wilson and a physician, Dr. Bob Smith, both alcoholics who discovered that they could remain sober through mutual support. This they accomplished not as professionals, but as peers who were able to share their common experiences. Soon they were working with other alcoholics, who in turn worked with others. The movement grew and, remarkably, individuals who had been treated unsuccessfully by professionals

▰ TABLE 24.16 THE TWELVE STEPS OF ALCOHOLICS ANONYMOUS

1. We admitted we were powerless over alcohol—that our lives have become unmanageable.
2. Came to believe that a Power greater than ourselves could restore us to sanity.
3. Made a decision to turn our will and our lives over to the care of God as we understood Him.
4. Made a searching and fearless moral inventory of ourselves.
5. Admitted to God, to ourselves, and to another human being the exact nature of our wrongs.
6. Were entirely ready to have God remove all these defects of character.
7. Humbly asked Him to remove our shortcomings.
8. Made a list of all persons we had harmed and became willing to make amends to them all.
9. Made direct amends to such people whenever possible except when to do so would injure them or others.
10. Continued to take personal inventory and when we were wrong promptly admitted it.
11. Sought through prayer and meditation to improve our conscious contact with God as we understood Him, praying only for knowledge of His will for us and the power to carry that out.
12. Having a spiritual awakening as the result of these steps, we tried to carry this message to alcoholics and to practice these principles in all our affairs.

SOURCE: From Alcoholics Anonymous (1953), with permission. (*Note:* Permission to reprint does not mean that AA has reviewed or approved contents of this publication.)

were able to maintain sobriety through helping one another (Curlee-Salisbury, 1986).

Today AA chapters exist in virtually every community in the United States. The self-help groups are based on the concept of peer support—acceptance and understanding from others who have experienced the same problems in their lives. The only requirement for membership is a desire on the part of the alcoholic person to stop drinking (Estes, Smith-DiJulio, & Heinemann, 1980). Each new member is assigned a support person from whom he or she may seek assistance when the temptation to drink occurs.

According to a survey by the General Service Office of Alcoholics Anonymous in 1989 (AA, 1990), changing trends in the membership are becoming apparent. The numbers of female and younger (30 and below) members are increasing, as are the numbers of members addicted to more than one substance. Female membership grew from 22 percent in 1968 to 35 percent in 1989. Members 30 years old and younger, who comprised 7 percent of the membership in 1968, increased to 22 percent. The 1989 survey reported that 46 percent of the membership claimed addiction to at least one other drug besides alcohol.

The sole purpose of AA is to help members stay sober. When sobriety has been achieved, they in turn are expected to help other alcoholic persons. The Twelve Steps that embody the philosophy of AA provide specific guidelines on how to attain and maintain sobriety.

Alcoholics Anonymous accepts alcoholism as an illness and promotes total abstinence as the only cure, emphasizing that the alcoholic person can never safely return to social drinking. They encourage the members to seek sobriety, taking one day at a time. The Twelve Traditions are the statements of principles that govern the organization.

Alcoholics Anonymous has been the model for various other self-help groups associated with abuse or dependency problems. Some of these groups and the memberships for which they are organized are listed in Table 24.18. Nurses need to be fully and accurately informed about available self-help groups as an important and necessary treatment resource on the health care continuum so that they can use them as a referral source for clients with substance-related disorders.

▰ TABLE 24.17 THE TWELVE TRADITIONS OF ALCOHOLICS ANONYMOUS

1. Our common welfare should come first; personal recovery depends upon AA unity.
2. For our group purpose there is but one ultimate authority—a loving God as He may express Himself in our group conscience. Our leaders are but trusted servants; they do not govern.
3. The one requirement for AA membership is a desire to stop drinking.
4. Each group should be autonomous except in matters affecting other groups or AA as a whole.
5. Each group has but one primary purpose—to carry its message to the alcoholic who still suffers.
6. An AA group ought never endorse, finance, or lend the AA name to any related facility or outside enterprise, lest problems of money, property, and prestige divert us from our primary purpose.
7. Every AA group ought to be fully self-supporting, declining outside contributions.
8. Alcoholics Anonymous should remain forever nonprofessional, but our service centers may employ special workers.
9. Alcoholics Anonymous, as such, ought never be organized; but we may create service boards of committees directly responsible to those they serve.
10. Alcoholics Anonymous has no opinion on outside issues; hence, the Alcoholics Anonymous name ought never be drawn into public controversy.
11. Our public relations policy is based on attraction rather than promotion; we need always maintain personal anonymity at the level of press, radio, and films.
12. Anonymity is the spiritual foundation of all our traditions, ever reminding us to place principles before personalities.

SOURCE: From Alcoholics Anonymous (1953), with permission. (*Note:* Permission to reprint does not mean that AA has reviewed or approved contents of this publication.)

TABLE 24.18 ADDICTION SELF-HELP GROUPS

GROUP	MEMBERSHIP
Adult Children of Alcoholics	Adults who grew up with an alcoholic in the home
Al-Anon	Families of alcoholics
Alateen	Adolescent children of alcoholics
Children Are People	School-age children with an alcoholic family member
Cocaine Anonymous	Cocaine addicts
Families Anonymous	Parents of children who abuse substances
Fresh Start	Nicotine addicts
Narcotics Anonymous	Narcotics addicts
Nar-Anon	Families of narcotics addicts
Overeaters Anonymous	Food addicts
Pills Anonymous	Polysubstance addicts
Potsmokers Anonymous	Marijuana smokers
Smokers Anonymous	Nicotine addicts
Women for Sobriety	Female alcoholics

Pharmacotherapy

Disulfiram (Antabuse)

Disulfiram (Antabuse) is a drug that can be administered to individuals who abuse alcohol as a deterrent to drinking. Ingestion of alcohol while disulfiram is in the body results in a syndrome of symptoms that can produce a good deal of discomfort for the individual. It can even result in death if the blood alcohol level is high. The reaction varies according to the sensitivity of the individual and how much alcohol was ingested.

Disulfiram works by inhibiting the enzyme aldehyde dehydrogenase, thereby blocking the oxidation of alcohol at the stage when acetaldehyde is converted to acetate. This results in an accumulation of acetaldehyde in the blood, which is thought to produce the symptoms associated with the disulfiram-alcohol reaction. These symptoms persist as long as alcohol is being metabolized. The rate of alcohol elimination does not appear to be affected (Townsend, 1995).

Symptoms of disulfiram-alcohol reaction can occur within 5 to 10 minutes of ingestion of alcohol. Mild reactions can occur at blood alcohol levels as low as 5 to 10 mg/dl. Symptoms are fully developed at approximately 50 mg/dl, and may include flushed skin, throbbing in the head and neck, respiratory difficulty, dizziness, nausea and vomiting, sweating, hyperventilation, tachycardia, hypotension, weakness, blurred vision, and confusion. With a blood alcohol level of approximately 125 to 150 mg/dl, severe reactions can occur, including respiratory depression, cardiovascular collapse, arrhythmias, myocardial infarction, acute congestive heart failure, unconsciousness, convulsions, and death.

Disulfiram should not be administered until it has been ascertained that the client has abstained from alcohol for at least 12 hours. If disulfiram is discontinued, it is important for the client to understand that the sensitivity to alcohol may last for as long as 2 weeks. Consuming alcohol or alcohol-containing substances during this 2-week period could result in the disulfiram-alcohol reaction.

The client receiving disulfiram therapy should be aware of the large number of alcohol-containing substances. These products, such as liquid cough and cold preparations, vanilla extract, aftershave lotions, colognes, mouthwash, nail polish removers, and isopropyl alcohol, if ingested or even rubbed on the skin, are capable of producing the symptoms described. The individual must read labels carefully and must inform any doctor, dentist, or other health care professional from whom assistance is sought that he or she is taking disulfiram. In addition, it is important that the client carry a card explaining participation in disulfiram therapy, possible consequences of the therapy, and symptoms that may indicate an emergency situation.

Obviously, the client must be assessed carefully before beginning disulfiram therapy. A thorough medical screening is performed before starting therapy, and written informed consent is usually required. The drug is contraindicated for clients who are at high risk for alcohol ingestion. It is also contraindicated for psychotic clients and clients with severe cardiac, renal, or hepatic disease.

Disulfiram therapy is not a cure for alcoholism. It provides a measure of control for the individual who desires to avoid impulse drinking. Clients receiving disulfiram therapy are encouraged to seek other assistance with their problem, such as AA or other support group, to aid in the recovery process.

Other Medication for Treatment of Alcoholism

The narcotic antagonist naltrexone (ReVia) was approved by the Food and Drug Administration (FDA) in 1994 for the treatment of alcohol dependence. Naltrexone, which was approved in 1984 for the treatment of heroin abuse, works on the same receptors in the brain that produce the feelings of pleasure when heroin or other opiates bind to them, but it does not produce the "narcotic high" and is not habit-forming. Although alcohol does not bind to these same brain receptors, studies have shown that naltrexone works equally well against it (O'Mallye et al., 1992; Volpicelli et al., 1992). In comparison to the placebo-treated clients, subjects on naltrexone therapy showed significantly lower overall relapse rates and fewer drinks per drinking day among those clients who did resume drinking. A recent study with an oral form of nalmefene (Revex) has produced similar results (Mason et al., 1994).

The efficacy of selective serotonin reuptake inhibitors (SSRIs) in the decrease of alcohol craving among alcohol-dependent individuals has yielded mixed results (NIAAA, 1997). A greater degree of success was observed with moderate drinkers than with heavy drinkers.

Counseling

Counseling on a one-to-one basis is often used to help the substance-abusing client. The relationship is goal-directed, and the length of the counseling may vary from weeks to years. The focus is on current reality, active development of a working treatment relationship, environmental manipulation, and strengthening ego assets (Estes, Smith-DiJulio, & Heinemann, 1980). The counselor must be warm, kind, and nonjudgmental, yet able to set limits firmly.

Weinberg (1986) identifies the following stages in the counseling relationship:

Stage I: Assessment. In this stage, factual data are collected to determine whether the client does indeed have a problem with substances; that is, that substances are regularly impairing effective functioning in a significant life area.

Stage II: Problem Recognition and Acceptance. In this stage the person accepts that the use of substances causes problems in significant life areas and that he or she is not able to prevent it from occurring. The client states a desire to make changes. During this stage the denial defense must be eliminated. The strength of the denial system is determined by the duration and extent of substance-related adverse effects in the person's life. Thus, those individuals with rather minor substance-related problems of recent origin have less difficulty with this stage than those with long-term extensive impairment. Also in stage II, the individual works to gain self-control and abstain from substances.

Stage III: Sobriety and Beyond. The question that is discussed in this stage of counseling is: During the times that you usually used substances, what will you do now instead? The client must have a concrete and workable plan for getting through the early weeks of abstinence. Anticipatory guidance through role play helps the individual practice how he or she will respond when substances are readily obtainable and the impulse to partake is strong.

Counseling often includes the family or specific family members. In family counseling the therapist tries to help each member see how he or she has affected, and been affected by, the substance-abuse behavior. Family strengths are mobilized, and family members are encouraged to move in a positive direction. Referrals are often made to self-help groups such as Al-Anon, Nar-Anon, Alateen, Families Anonymous, and Adult Children of Alcoholics.

Group Therapy

Group therapy with substance abusers has long been regarded as a powerful agent of change. Vannicelli (1986) identifies three unique opportunities that group work can provide for substance abusers:

1. To share and to identify with others who are going through similar problems.
2. To understand their own attitudes about substance use and their defenses about giving up the substance, by confronting similar attitudes and defenses in others.
3. To learn to communicate needs and feelings more directly.

Some groups may be task-oriented education groups in which the leader is charged with presenting material associated with substance abuse and its various effects on the person's life. Other educational groups that may be helpful with individuals who abuse substances include assertiveness techniques and relaxation training. Teaching groups differ from psychotherapy groups, whose focus is more on helping individuals understand and manage difficult feelings and situations and gain understanding about where they fit in with the difficulties they experience (Vannicelli, 1986).

Therapy groups and self-help groups such as AA are complementary to each other. Whereas the self-help group focus is on achieving and maintaining sobriety, in the therapy group the individual may learn more adaptive ways of coping, how to deal with problems that may have arisen or were exacerbated by the former substance use, and ways to improve quality of life and to function more effectively without substances.

Psychopharmacology for Substance Intoxication and Substance Withdrawal

Various medications have been used to decrease the intensity of symptoms in an individual who is withdrawing from, or who is experiencing the effects of excessive use of, alcohol and other drugs. Substitution therapy may be required to reduce the life-threatening effects of intoxication or withdrawal from some substances. The severity of the withdrawal syndrome depends on the particular drug used, how long it has been used, the dose used, and the rate at which the drug is eliminated from the body (Bennett & Woolf, 1991).

Alcohol

Benzodiazepines are the most widely used group of drugs for substitution therapy in alcohol withdrawal. Chlordiazepoxide (Librium), oxazepam (Serax), and diazepam (Valium) are the most commonly used agents. Because of its ability to decrease the cardiovascular hyperactivity associated with alcohol withdrawal, the benzodiazepine alprazolam (Xanax) is also frequently being used (NIAAA, 1997). The approach to treatment with benzodiazepines for alcohol withdrawal is to start with relatively high doses and reduce the dosage by 20 to 25 percent each day until withdrawal is complete. In clients with liver disease, accumulation of the longer-acting agents (chlordiazepoxide and diazepam) may be problematic, and the use of the shorter-acting benzodiazepine (oxazepam) is more appropriate. Recent studies have also indicated that control of withdrawal symptoms with benzodiazepines on an "as-needed basis," rather than a fixed schedule, resulted in the need for lower doses of the medication and less time in treatment (NIAAA, 1997).

Some physicians may order anticonvulsant medication (e.g., phenytoin, phenobarbital, or magnesium sulfate) for management of withdrawal seizures. This is not a universal intervention, and it is likely that most clients are adequately protected against seizures by the benzodiazepine used to stop the progression of withdrawal symptoms. If seizures do occur, diazepam or lorazepam (Ativan) administered intravenously is probably indicated (Bennett & Woolf, 1991).

Multivitamin therapy, in combination with daily injections or oral administration of thiamine, is common protocol. Thiamine is commonly deficient in chronic alcoholics. Replacement therapy is required to prevent neuropathy, confusion, and encephalopathy.

Opioids

Examples of opioids are heroin, morphine, opium, meperidine, codeine, and methadone. Withdrawal symptoms generally begin within 8 to 12 hours after the last opioid dose and become most intense by 36 to 48 hours (Bennett & Woolf, 1991). The acute phase of withdrawal is over in approximately 10 days; however, symptoms of irritability and restlessness may persist for 2 to 3 months.

Opioid intoxication is treated with narcotic antagonists such as naloxone (Narcan), nalorphine (Nalline), or levallorphan (Lorfan). Withdrawal therapy includes rest, adequate nutritional support, and methadone substitution. Methadone is given on the first day in a dose sufficient to suppress withdrawal symptoms. The dose is then gradually tapered so that methadone substitution is complete in 21 days. Propoxyphene (Darvon) has also been tried in opioid substitution therapy, but usually with less than satisfactory results (Bennett & Woolf, 1991).

Clonidine (Catapres) has been used to suppress opiate withdrawal symptoms. Although it is not as effective as substitution with an opioid, it is nonaddicting and can serve as a bridge to enable the client to stay opiate-free long enough to initiate naltrexone (Trexan) therapy, which is used to facilitate termination of methadone maintenance (Bennett & Woolf, 1991).

Depressants

Substitution therapy for CNS depressant withdrawal (particularly barbiturates) is most commonly with the long-acting barbiturate phenobarbital (Luminal). The dosage required to suppress withdrawal symptoms is given. When stabilization has been achieved, the dose is gradually decreased by 30 mg/day until withdrawal is complete. Long-acting benzodiazepines are commonly used for substitution therapy when the abused substance is a nonbarbiturate CNS depressant (Bennett & Woolf, 1991).

TEST YOUR CRITICAL THINKING SKILLS

Kelly, age 23, is a first-year law student. She is engaged to a surgical resident at the local university hospital. She has been struggling to do well in law school because she wants to make her parents, two prominent local attorneys, proud of her. She had never aspired to do anything but go into law, and that is also what her parents expected her to do.

Kelly's mid-term grades were not as high as she had hoped, so she increased the number of hours of study time, staying awake all night several nights a week to study. She started drinking large amounts of coffee to stay awake, but still found herself falling asleep as she tried to study at the library and in her apartment. As final exams approached, she began to panic that she would not be able to continue the pace of studying she felt she needed in order to make the grades she hoped for.

One of Kelly's classmates told her that she needed some "speed" to give her that extra energy to study. Her classmate said, "All the kids do it. Hardly anyone I know gets through law school without it." She gave Kelly the name of a source.

Kelly contacted the source, who supplied her with enough amphetamines to see her through final exams. Kelly was excited, because she had so much energy, did not require sleep, and was able to study the additional hours she thought she needed for the exams. However, when the results were posted, Kelly had failed two courses and would have to repeat them in summer school if she was to continue with her class in the fall. She continued to replenish her supply of amphetamines from her "contact" until he told her he could not get her anymore. She became frantic and stole a prescription blank from her fiance and forged his name for more pills.

She started taking more and more of the medication in order to achieve the "high" she wanted to feel. Her behavior became erratic. Yesterday, her fiance received a call from a pharmacy to clarify an order for amphetamines that Kelly had written. He insisted that she admit herself to the chemical dependency unit for detoxification.

On the unit, she appears tired, depressed, moves very slowly, and wants to sleep all the time. She keeps saying to the nurse, "I'm a real failure. I'll never be an attorney like my parents. I'm too dumb. I just wish I could die."

Answer the following questions related to Kelly:

1. What is the primary nursing diagnosis for Kelly?
2. Describe important nursing interventions to be implemented with Kelly.
3. In addition to physical safety, what would be the primary short-term goal the nurses would strive to achieve with Kelly?

Stimulants

Treatment of stimulant intoxication usually begins with minor tranquilizers such as chlordiazepoxide and progresses to major tranquilizers such as haloperidol (Haldol). Phenothiazines are avoided owing to a reduction in seizure threshold and anticholinergic side effects (Schuckit, 1979). Intravenous phentolamine (Regitine) may be administered for severe hypertension. Repeated seizures are treated with intravenous diazepam.

Withdrawal from CNS stimulants is not the medical emergency observed with CNS depressants. Treatment is usually aimed at reducing drug craving and managing severe depression. The client is placed in a quiet atmosphere and allowed to sleep and eat as much as is needed or desired. Suicide precautions may need to be instituted. Therapy with tricyclic antidepressants (e.g., desipramine [Norpramine]) has been successful in treating the symptoms of cocaine withdrawal (Bennett & Woolf, 1991).

R E S E A R C H   N O T E

Severity of depression, cognitions, and functioning among depressed inpatients with and without coexisting substance abuse. *Journal of the American Psychiatric Nurses Association* **(1995, April), 1(2),55–60.**
Zauszniewski, J.A.

Description of the Study: This study was conducted with 63 depressed adult inpatients representing African-American and European-American cultures. Of the 63 depressed patients, 31 also met *DSM-III-R* criteria for substance abuse and 32 did not. Those who met the substance-abuse criteria used substances that included alcohol, amphetamines, cannabis, cocaine, opioids, and phencyclidine. The individuals participated in face-to-face structured interviews with trained interviewers who gathered demographic data, which included age, gender, marital status, educational level, and annual income. They also responded to self-rating evaluations that measured severity of depression (Beck Depression Inventory), adaptive functioning (Community Living Skills Scale), and depressive cognitions (Cognitive Triad Index [negative view of the self, the world, and the future]).

Results of the Study: It was found that there was a statistical difference between the two groups in all three areas measured. The depressed individuals who also met criteria for substance abuse scored higher in severity of depression, adaptive functioning, and cognitive distortions related to clinical depression.

Comments: The author reminds us of the high rate of depression among alcohol abusers, as well as the fact that depression may be alcohol induced, and that depressed persons may turn to the use of substances for relief of their symptoms. Results of this study reinforce the importance of helping clients to change their negative cognitions (negative view of self, world, and future) to more healthy and adaptive thought processes, as an integral part of holistic nursing, when working with clients who have dual diagnoses of depression and substance abuse.

I N T E R N E T   R E F E R E N C E S

- Additional information on addictions may be located at the following websites:
  a. http://www.recovery-works.com
  b. http://www.ncbi.nlm.nih.gov
  c. http://www.liebertpub.com
  d. http://www.drugs.indiana.edu
- Additional information on self-help organizations may be located at the following websites:
  a. http://www.ca.org (Cocaine Anonymous)
  b. http://www.alcoholics-anonymous.org (AA)
  c. http://www/delphi.com (Narcotics Anonymous)
- Additional information about medications for treatment of alcohol and drug dependence may be located at the following websites:
  a. http://www.fadavis.com
  b. http://www.laurus.com

Hallucinogens and Cannabinols

Substitution therapy is not required with these drugs. When adverse reactions, such as anxiety or panic, occur, benzodiazepines (e.g., diazepam or chlordiazepoxide) may be prescribed to prevent harm to the client or others. Should psychotic reactions occur, they may be treated with antipsychotics, such as the phenothiazines or haloperidol.

SUMMARY

An individual is considered to be dependent on a substance when he or she is unable to control its use, even knowing that it interferes with normal functioning; when more and more of the substance is required to produce the desired effects; and when characteristic withdrawal symptoms develop upon cessation or drastic decrease in use of the substance. Abuse is considered when there is continued use of the substance despite having a persistent or recurrent problem that is caused or exacerbated by its use or when the substance is used in physically hazardous situations.

Substance intoxication is defined as the development of a reversible syndrome of maladaptive behavioral or psychological changes that are due to the direct physiological effects of a substance on the CNS and develop during or shortly after ingestion of (or exposure to) a substance. Substance withdrawal is the development of a substance-specific maladaptive behavioral change, with physiological and cognitive concomitants, that is due to the cessation of, or reduction in, heavy and prolonged substance use.

The etiology of substance-use disorders is unknown. Various contributing factors have been implicated, such as genetics, biochemical changes, developmental influences, personality factors, social learning, conditioning, and cultural and ethnic influences.

Six classes of substances are presented in terms of a profile of the substance, historical aspects, patterns of use and abuse, and effects on the body. These six classes include alcohol, other CNS depressants, CNS stimulants, opioids, hallucinogens, and cannabinols.

The nursing process is presented as the vehicle for delivery of care of the client with a substance-related disorder. The nurse must first examine his or her own feelings regarding personal and others' substance use. Only the nurse who can be accepting and nonjudgmental of substance-abuse behaviors will be effective in working with these clients.

Substance abuse by members of the nursing profession is discussed. Many state boards of nursing and state nurses' associations have established avenues for peer assistance to provide help to impaired members of the profession.

Individuals who are reared in families with chemically dependent persons learn patterns of dysfunctional behavior that carry over into adult life. These dysfunctional behavior patterns have been termed *codependence*. Codependent persons sacrifice their own needs for the fulfillment of others' in order to achieve a sense of control. Many nurses also have codependent traits.

Treatment modalities for substance-related disorders include self-help groups, deterrent therapy, individual counseling, and group therapy. Substitution pharmacotherapy is frequently implemented with clients experiencing substance intoxication or substance withdrawal. Treatment modalities are implemented on an inpatient basis or in outpatient settings, depending on the severity of the impairment.

REVIEW QUESTIONS

SELF-EXAMINATION/LEARNING EXERCISE

For each of the following situations, select the answer that is most appropriate.

Situation: Mr. White is admitted to the hospital after an extended period of binge alcohol drinking. His wife reports that he has been a heavy drinker for a number of years. Lab reports reveal he has a blood alcohol level of 250 mg/dl. He is placed on the chemical dependency unit for detoxification.

1. When would the first signs of alcohol withdrawal symptoms be expected to occur?

    a. Several hours after the last drink.
    b. Two to 3 days after the last drink.
    c. Four to 5 days after the last drink.
    d. Six to 7 days after the last drink.

2. Symptoms of alcohol withdrawal include:

    a. Euphoria, hyperactivity, and insomnia.
    b. Depression, suicidal ideation, and hypersomnia.
    c. Diaphoresis, nausea and vomiting, and tremors.
    d. Unsteady gait, nystagmus, and profound disorientation.

3. Which of the following medications is the physician most likely to order for Mr. White during his withdrawal syndrome?

    a. Haloperidol (Haldol).
    b. Chlordiazepoxide (Librium).
    c. Propoxyphene (Darvon).
    d. Phenytoin (Dilantin).

Situation: Dan, age 32, has been admitted for inpatient treatment of his alcoholism. He began drinking when he was 15 years old. Through the years, the amount of alcohol he consumes has increased. He and his wife report that for the last 5 years he has consumed at least a pint of bourbon a day. He also drinks beer and wine. He has been sneaking drinks at work, and his effectiveness has started to decline. His boss has told him he must seek treatment or be fired. This is his second week in treatment. The first week he experienced an uncomplicated detoxification.

4. Dan states, "I don't have a problem with alcohol. I can handle my booze better than anyone I know. My boss is a jerk! I haven't missed any more days than my coworkers." The nurse's best response is:

    a. "Maybe your boss is mistaken, Dan."
    b. "You are here because your drinking was interfering with your work, Dan."
    c. "Get real, Dan! You're a boozer and you know it!"
    d. "Why do you think your boss sent you here, Dan?"

5. The defense mechanism that Dan is using is:

    a. Denial.
    b. Projection.
    c. Displacement.
    d. Rationalization.

6. Dan's drinking buddies come for a visit, and when they leave, the nurse smells alcohol on Dan's breath. Which of the following would be the best intervention with Dan at this time?

    a. Search his room for evidence.
    b. Ask, "Have you been drinking alcohol, Dan?"
    c. Send a urine specimen from Dan to the lab for drug screening.
    d. Tell Dan, "These guys cannot come to the unit to visit you again."

7. Dan begins attendance at AA meetings. Which of the statements by Dan reflects the purpose of this organization?

    a. "They claim they will help me stay sober."

    b. "I'll dry out in AA, then I can have a social drink now and then."

    c. "AA is only for people who have reached the bottom."

    d. "If I lose my job, AA will help me find another."

The following general questions relate to substance abuse.

8. From which of the following symptoms might the nurse identify a chronic cocaine user?

    a. Clear, constricted pupils.

    b. Red, irritated nostrils.

    c. Muscle aches.

    d. Conjunctival redness.

9. An individual who is addicted to heroin is likely to experience which of the following symptoms of withdrawal?

    a. Increased heart rate and blood pressure.

    b. Tremors, insomnia, and seizures.

    c. Incoordination and unsteady gait.

    d. Nausea and vomiting, diarrhea, and diaphoresis.

10. A polysubstance abuser makes the statement, "The green and whites do me good after speed." How might the nurse interpret the statement?

    a. The client abuses amphetamines and sedative/hypnotics.

    b. The client abuses alcohol and cocaine.

    c. The client is psychotic.

    d. The client abuses narcotics and marijuana.

REFERENCES

Ahlstrom-Laakso, S. (1976). European drinking habits. In Everett et al. (Eds.), *Cross-cultural approaches to the study of alcohol.* The Hague: Mouton.

Alcoholics Anonymous. (1953). *Twelve steps and twelve traditions.* New York: Alcoholics Anonymous World Services.

Alcoholics Anonymous. (1990). *Analysis of the 1989 survey of the membership of AA.* New York: Alcoholics Anonymous World Services.

American Nurses' Association. (1984). *Addictions and psychological dysfunctions in nursing.* Kansas City, MO: American Nurses' Association.

American Psychiatric Association. (1994). *Diagnostic and statistical manual of mental disorders* (4th ed.). Washington, DC: American Psychiatric Association.

Baker, J.M. (1982). Alcoholism and the American Indian. In N.J. Estes & M.E. Heineman (Eds.), *Alcoholism: Development, consequences, and interventions* (2nd ed.). St. Louis: C.V. Mosby.

Barnes, G.E. (1980). Characteristics of the clinical alcoholic personality. *Journal of Studies on Alcohol, 41*, 894–910.

Bennett, E.G., & Woolf, D. (1991). *Substance abuse: Pharmacologic, developmental, and clinical perspectives* (2nd ed.). Albany, NY: Delmar Publishers.

Black, C. (1982). *It will never happen to me.* Denver: M.A.C., Printing and Publications Division.

Blum, K. (1984). *Handbook of abusable drugs.* New York: Gardner Press.

Bratter, T.E., & Forrest, G.G. (1985). *Alcoholism and substance abuse.* New York: The Free Press.

Byers, V.L. (1991). Central nervous system stimulants. In M.M. Kuhn (Ed.), *Pharmacotherapeutics: A nursing process approach* (2nd ed.). Philadelphia: F.A. Davis.

Caroselli-Karinja, M.F., & Zboray, S.D. (1987, June). The impaired nurse. *Journal of Psychosocial Nursing, 24*(6), 14–19.

Cermak, T.L. (1986). *Diagnosing and treating co-dependence.* Minneapolis: Johnson Institute Books.

Cohen, A.Y. (1972). The journey beyond trips: Alternative to drugs. In D.E. Smith & G.R. Gay (Eds.), *It's so good, don't even try it once: Heroin in perspective.* Englewood Cliffs, NJ: Prentice-Hall.

Cosper, R. (1979). Drinking as conformity: A critique of the sociological literature on occupational differences in drinking. *Journal of Studies on Alcohol, 40*, 868–891.

Curlee-Salisbury, J. (1986). Perspectives on Alcoholics Anonymous. In N.J. Estes & M.E. Heinemann (Eds.), *Alcoholism: Development, consequences, and interventions* (3rd ed.). St. Louis: C.V. Mosby.

Drug Enforcement Administration. (1979). *Drugs of abuse.* Washington, DC: U.S. Department of Justice.

Estes, N.J., & Heinemann, M.E. (1986). *Alcoholism: Development, consequences, and interventions* (3rd ed.). St. Louis: C.V. Mosby.

Estes, N.J., Smith-DiJulio, K., & Heinemann, M.E. (1980). *Nursing diagnosis of the alcoholic person.* St. Louis: C.V. Mosby.

Frances, R.J., & Franklin, J.E. (1994). Alcohol and other psychoactive substance use disorders. In R.E. Hales, S.C. Yudofsky, & J.A. Talbott (Eds.), *Textbook of Psychiatry* (2nd ed). Washington, DC: American Psychiatric Press.

Friel, J., & Friel, L. (1988). *Adult children: Secrets of dysfunctional families.* Deerfield Beach, FL: Health Communications.

Goldstein, A. (1994). *Addiction: From biology to drug policy.* New York: W.H. Freeman.

Hall, S.F., & Wray, L.M. (1989, November). Codependency: Nurses who give too much. *American Journal of Nursing, 89*(11), 1456–1460.

Holbrook, J.M. (1991). Hallucinogens. In E.G. Bennett & D. Woolf (Eds.), *Substance abuse* (2nd ed.). Albany, NY: Delmar Publishers.

House, M.A. (1990, April). Cocaine. *American Journal of Nursing, 90*(4), 41–45.

Hughes, T.L., & Smith, L.L. (1994). Is your colleague chemically dependent? *American Journal of Nursing, 94*(9), 31–35.

Jellinek, E.M. (1952). Phases of alcohol addiction. *QJ Stud Alcohol, 13*, 673–684.

Jones, E. (1959). *Collected papers of Sigmund Freud.* New York: Basic Books.

Julien, R.M. (1981). *A primer of drug action* (3rd ed.). San Francisco: W.H. Freeman.

Kaplan, H.I., & Sadock, B.J. (1985). *Modern synopsis of comprehensive textbook of psychiatry* (4th ed.). Baltimore: Williams & Wilkins.

Kaplan, H.I. & Sadock, B.J. (1998). *Synopsis of psychiatry: Behavorial science/clinical psychiatry* (8th ed.). Baltimore: Williams and Wilkins.

Kaplan, H.I., Sadock, B.J., & Grebb, J.A. (1994). *Kaplan and Sadock's synopsis of psychiatry* (7th ed.). Baltimore: Williams & Wilkins.

Kauffman, J.E., et al. (1985). The biological basics: Drugs and their effects. In T.E. Bratter & G.G. Forrest (Eds.), *Alcoholism and substance abuse.* New York: The Free Press.

Kee, J.L., & Hayes, E.R. (1993). *Pharmacology: A nursing process approach.* Philadelphia: W.B. Saunders.

Keller, M. (1979). A historical overview of alcohol and alcoholism. *Cancer Research, 39*, 2822–2829.

Kuhn, M.M. (1991). *Pharmacotherapeutics: A nursing process approach* (2nd ed.) Philadelphia: F.A. Davis.

Leigh, G. (1985). Psychosocial factors in the etiology of substance abuse. In T.E. Bratter & G.G. Forrest (Eds.), *Alcoholism and substance abuse: Strategies for clinical intervention.* New York: The Free Press.

Madden, J.S. (1984). *A guide to alcohol and drug dependence* (2nd ed.). Bristol, England: John Wright & Sons.

Mason, G.J., et al. (1994). Double-blind, placebo-controlled pilot study to evaluate the efficacy and safety of oral nalmefene HCl for alcohol dependence. *Alcoholism, Clinical and Experimental Research 18*(5), 1162–1167.

Mayfield, D., McLeod, G., & Hall, P. (1974). The CAGE questionnaire: Validation of a new alcoholism screening instrument. *American Journal of Psychiatry, 131*, 1121–1123.

McKenry, L.M., & Salerno, E. (1989). *Pharmacology in nursing.* St. Louis: C.V. Mosby.

Milkman, H., & Frosch, W. (1980). Theory of drug use. In Lettieri et al. (Eds.), *Theories on drug abuse: Selected contemporary perspectives.* Rockville, MD: National Institute on Alcohol Abuse & Alcoholism.

Murphy, S.S., & Violette, R.W. (1985, August). More clues to drug abuse. *RN, 48*(8), 19–21.

National Institute on Alcohol Abuse and Alcoholism (NIAAA). (1997). *Ninth special report to the U.S. Congress on alcohol and health.* Rockville, MD: The Institute.

O'Malley, S.S., et al. (1992). Naltrexene and coping skills therapy for alcohol dependence: A controlled study. *Archives of General Psychiatry 49*(11), 881–887.

Pilette, W.L. (1983, August). Caffeine: Psychiatric grounds for concern. *Journal of Psychosocial Nursing and Mental Health Services, 21*(8), 19–24.

Schenk, E.A. (1995). Substance abuse. In W.J. Phipps, V.L. Cassmeyer, J.K. Sands, & M.K. Lehman (Eds.), *Medical-surgical nursing: Concepts and clinical practice* (5th ed.). St Louis: C.V. Mosby.

Schuckit, M.A. (1979). *Drug and alcohol abuse: A clinical guide to diagnosis and treatment.* New York: Plenum medical Book Company.

Seltzer, M.L. (1971). The Michigan Alcoholism Screening Test: The quest for a new diagnostic instrument. *American Journal of Psychiatry, 127*, 1653–1658.

Smalley, S. (1984). Paper presented at the Conference of International Doctors in AA. Minneapolis, MN.

Smith, S.F., Karasik, D.A., & Meyer, B.J. (1984). *Psychiatric and psychosocial nursing.* Los Altos, CA: National Nursing Review, Inc.

Substance Abuse and Mental Health Services Administration Office of Applied Studies. (1995). *Preliminary estimates from the 1995 national household survey on drug abuse.* Washington, DC: U.S. Government Printing Office.

Sullivan, E., Bissell, L., & Williams, E. (1988). *Chemical dependency in nursing: The deadly diversion.* Menlo Park, CA: Addison-Wesley.

Townsend, M.C. (1995). *Drug guide for psychiatric nursing* (2nd ed.). Philadelphia: F.A. Davis.

Vannicelli, M. (1986). Group psychotherapy with alcoholics: Special techniques. In N.J. Estes & M.E. Heinemann (Eds.), *Alcoholism: Development, consequences, and interventions* (3rd ed.). St. Louis: C.V. Mosby.

Volpicelli, J.R., Alterman, A.I., Hayashida, M., & O'Brien, C.P. (1992). Naltrexone in the treatment of alcohol dependence. *Archives of General Psychiatry 49*(11), 876–880.

Weinberg, J.R. (1986). Counseling the person with alcohol problems. In N.J. Estes & M.E. Heinemann (Eds.), *Alcoholism: Development, consequences, and interventions* (3rd ed.). St. Louis: C.V. Mosby.

Westermeyer, J., & Baker, J.M. (1986). Alcoholism and the American Indian. In N.J. Estes & M.E. Heinemann (Eds.), *Alcoholism: Development, consequences, and interventions* (3rd ed.). St. Louis: C.V. Mosby.

Bibliography

Finke, L., Williams, J., & Stanley, R. (1996). Nurses referred to a peer assistance program for alcohol and drug problems. *Archives of Psychiatric Nursing, 10*, 319.

Goldfarb, J., Houlihan, L., & Meyer, K. (1997, November/December). The home detox alternative. *Behavioral Health Management*, 24–27.

Harvard Medical School. (1992, October). Addiction—Part I. *Harvard Mental Health Letter 9*(4), 1.

Harvard Medical School. (1992, November). Addiction—Part II. *Harvard Mental Health Letter 9*(5), 1.

Mynatt, S. (1996). A Model of contributing risk factors to chemical dependency in nurses. *Journal of Psychosocial Nursing, 34*, 13.

Smith, L.L., & Hughes, T.L. (1996, February). Re-entry: When a chemically dependent colleague returns to work. *American Journal of Nursing, 96*(2), 32–37.

Townsend, M.C. (1997). *Nursing diagnoses in psychiatric nursing: A pocket guide for care plan construction* (4th ed.). Philadelphia: F.A. Davis.

Wegscheider-Cruse, S. (1989). *Another chance: Hope and health for the alcoholic family* (2nd ed.). Palo Alto, CA: Science and Behavior Books, Inc.

Woititz, J.G., (1990). *Adult children of alcoholics.* Deerfield Beach, FL: Health Communications, Inc.

Yates, J.G., & McDaniel, J.L. (1994, April). Are you losing yourself in codependency? *American Journal of Nursing, 94*(4), 32–36.

SCHIZOPHRENIA AND OTHER PSYCHOTIC DISORDERS

CHAPTER OUTLINE

KEY TERMS

catatonic behavior
neuroleptic
delusions
hallucinations
double-bind
    communication
religiosity
paranoia

magical thinking
associative looseness
neologism
clang association
word salad
circumstantiality
tangentiality
perseveration

illusion
echolalia
echopraxia
autism
waxy flexibility
anhedonia
social skills training

OBJECTIVES

After reading this chapter, the student will be able to:

1. Discuss the concepts of schizophrenia and related psychotic disorders.
2. Identify predisposing factors in the development of these disorders.
3. Describe various types of schizophrenia and related psychotic disorders.
4. Identify symptomatology associated with these disorders and use this information in client assessment.
5. Formulate nursing diagnoses and goals of care for clients with schizophrenia and other psychotic disorders.

6. Identify topics for client and family teaching relevant to schizophrenia and other psychotic disorders.
7. Describe appropriate nursing interventions for behaviors associated with these disorders.
8. Describe relevant criteria for evaluating nursing care of clients with schizophrenia and related psychotic disorders.
9. Discuss various modalities relevant to treatment of schizophrenia and related psychotic disorders.

he term *schizophrenia* was coined in 1908 by the Swiss psychiatrist Eugen Bleuler. The word was derived from the Greek "skhizo" (split) and "phren" (mind) (Birchwood et al., 1989).

Over the years, much debate has surrounded the concept of schizophrenia. Various definitions of the disorder have evolved, and numerous treatment strategies have been proposed, but none have proved to be uniformly effective or sufficient.

Although the controversy lingers, two general factors appear to be gaining acceptance among clinicians. The first is that schizophrenia is probably not a homogeneous disease entity with a single cause but results from a variable combination of genetic predisposition, biochemical dysfunction, physiological factors, and psychosocial stress. The second factor is that there is not now and probably never will be a single treatment that cures the disorder. Instead, effective treatment requires a comprehensive, multidisciplinary effort, including pharmacotherapy and various forms of psychosocial care, such as living skills and social skills training, rehabilitation, and family therapy.

Of all the mental illnesses responsible for suffering in society, schizophrenia probably causes more lengthy hospitalizations, more chaos in family life, more exorbitant costs to individuals and governments, and more fears than any other. Because it is such an enormous threat to life and happiness and because its causes are an unsolved puzzle, it has been studied more than any other mental disorder.

The following remarks were made by Dr. Laura Hall at a symposium on schizophrenia research cosponsored by the National Foundation for Brain Research and the National Alliance for the Mentally Ill (NAMI) in March 1996 before the U.S. Congress:

"Approximately 1.7 million American adults have the brain disorder schizophrenia. No more than 15 percent of them have a job. They make up more than half of the long-term residents of state and county mental hospitals. They, and others with severe mental illnesses, make up at least one-third of our nation's homeless population. Between 10 and 15 percent of individuals with schizophrenia commit suicide, usually before age 30. About 8 percent of people in our jails have schizophrenia and are usually housed there for want of appropriate treatment and housing facilities. People with schizophrenia are disproportionately the victims of crime."

This chapter explores various theories of predisposing factors that have been implicated in the development of schizophrenia. Symptomatology associated with different diagnostic categories of the disorder is discussed. Nursing care is presented in the context of the six steps of the nursing process. Various dimensions of medical treatment are explored.

NATURE OF THE DISORDER

Perhaps no psychological disorder is more crippling than schizophrenia. Characteristically, disturbances in thought processes, perception, and affect invariably result in a severe deterioration of social and occupational functioning (Hollandsworth, 1990).

Approximately 1 percent of the population will develop schizophrenia over the course of a lifetime (Birchwood et al., 1989). Societal economic costs are estimated in billions of dollars per year. Symptoms generally appear in late adolescence or early adulthood, although they may occur in middle or late adult life (American Psychiatric Association [APA], 1994). Some studies have indicated that symptoms occur earlier in men than in women. The premorbid personality usually indicates social and sexual maladjustment or schizoid, paranoid, or borderline personality characteristics (Cutting, 1985; Pfohl & Winokur, 1983).

This premorbid behavior is often a predictor in the pattern of development of schizophrenia, which can be viewed in four phases.

Phase I: The Schizoid Personality. The *DSM-IV* (APA, 1994) describes this individual as indifferent to social relationships and having a very limited range of emotional experience and expression. They do not enjoy close relationships and prefer to be "loners." They appear cold and aloof. Not all individuals who demonstrate the characteristics of schizoid personality will progress to schizophrenia. However, most individuals with schizophrenia show evidence of having had these characteristics in the premorbid condition.

Phase II: The Prodromal Phase. Characteristics of this phase include social withdrawal; impairment in role functioning; behavior that is peculiar or eccentric; neglect of personal hygiene and grooming; blunted or inappropriate affect; disturbances in communication; bizarre ideas; unusual perceptual experiences; and lack of initiative, interests, or energy. The length of this phase is highly variable, and may last for many years before deteriorating to the schizophrenic state.

Phase III: Schizophrenia. In the active phase of the disorder, psychotic symptoms are prominent. Following are the *DSM-IV* (APA, 1994) diagnostic criteria for schizophrenia:

1. **Characteristic Symptoms:** Two (or more) of the following, each present for a significant portion of time during a 1-month period (or less if successfully treated):
   a. Delusions
   b. Hallucinations
   c. Disorganized speech (e.g., frequent derailment or incoherence)
   d. Grossly disorganized or **catatonic behavior**
   e. Negative symptoms (i.e., affective flattening, alogia, or avolition)

2. **Social/Occupational Dysfunction:** For a significant portion of the time since the onset of the disturbance, one or more major areas of functioning such as work, interpersonal relations, or self-care are markedly below the level achieved before the onset (or when the onset is in childhood or adolescence, failure to achieve expected level of interpersonal, academic, or occupational achievement).

3. **Duration:** Continuous signs of the disturbance persist for at least 6 months. This 6-month period must include at least 1 month of symptoms (or less if successfully treated) that meet criterion 1 (i.e., active-phase symptoms) and may include periods of prodromal or residual symptoms. During these prodromal or residual periods, the signs of the disturbance may be manifested by only negative symptoms or two or more symptoms listed in criterion 1 present in an attenuated form (e.g., odd beliefs, unusual perceptual experiences).

4. **Schizoaffective and Mood Disorder Exclusion:** Schizoaffective disorder and mood disorder with psychotic features have been ruled out because either (1) no major depressive, manic, or mixed episodes have occurred concurrently with the active-phase symptoms; or (2) if mood episodes have occurred during active-phase symptoms, their total duration has been brief relative to the duration of the active and residual periods.

5. **Substance/General Medical Condition Exclusion:** The disturbance is not due to the direct physiological effects of a substance (e.g., a drug of abuse, a medication) or a general medical condition.

6. **Relationship to a Pervasive Developmental Disorder:** If there is a history of autistic disorder or another pervasive developmental disorder, the additional diagnosis of schizophrenia is made only if prominent delusions or hallucinations are also present for at least a month (or less if successfully treated).

Phase IV: Residual Phase. Schizophrenia is characterized by periods of remission and exacerbation. A residual phase usually follows an active phase of the illness. Symptoms during the residual phase are similar to those of the prodromal phase, with flat affect and impairment in role functioning being prominent. Residual impairment often increases between episodes of active psychosis.

A return to full premorbid functioning is not common (APA, 1994). However, several factors have been associated with a more positive prognosis. They include good premorbid adjustment, later age at onset, being female, abrupt onset of symptoms precipitated by a stressful event (as opposed to gradual insidious onset of symptoms), associated mood disturbance, brief duration of active-phase symptoms, good interepisode functioning, minimal residual symptoms, absence of structural brain abnormalities, normal neurological functioning, a family history of mood disorder, and no family history of schizophrenia (APA, 1994).

PREDISPOSING FACTORS

The cause of schizophrenia is still uncertain. Most likely no single factor can be implicated in the etiology; rather the disease probably results from a combination of influences including biological, psychological, and environmental factors.

Biological Influences

Refer to Chapter 4 for a more thorough review of the biological implications of psychiatric illness.

Genetics

The body of evidence for genetic vulnerability to schizophrenia is growing. Studies show that relatives of individuals with schizophrenia have a much higher probability of developing the disease than the general population. Whereas the lifetime risk for developing schizophrenia is about 1 percent in most population studies, the siblings or offspring of an identified client have a 5 to 10 percent risk of developing schizophrenia (Black & Andreasen, 1994).

How schizophrenia is inherited is uncertain. No reliable biological marker has as yet been found (Tsuang & Faraone, 1994). It is unknown which genes are important in the vulnerability to schizophrenia, or whether one or many genes are implicated. Some individuals have a strong genetic link to the illness, whereas others may have only a weak genetic basis. This theory gives further credence to the notion of multiple causation.

Twin Studies. The rate of schizophrenia among monozygotic (identical) twins is four times that of dizygotic (fraternal) twins, and approximately 50 times that of the general population (Kaplan & Sadock, 1998). Identical twins reared apart have the same rate of development of the illness as do those reared together. Because in about half of the cases only one of a pair of monozygotic twins develops schizophrenia, some investigators believe environmental factors interact with genetic ones.

Adoption Studies. In studies conducted by both American and Danish investigators, adopted children born of schizophrenic mothers were compared with adoptees whose mothers had no psychiatric disorder. It was found that the children who were born of schizophrenic mothers were more likely to develop the illness than the comparison control groups (Black & Andreasen, 1994). Studies also indicate that children born of nonschizophrenic parents, but reared by schizophrenic parents, do not seem to suffer more often from schizophrenia than general controls. These findings provide additional evidence for the genetic basis of schizophrenia.

Biochemical Influences

The oldest and most thoroughly explored biological theory in the explanation of schizophrenia attributes a pathogenic role to abnormal brain biochemistry (Birchwood et al., 1989). Notions of a "chemical disturbance" as an explanation for insanity were suggested by some theorists as early as the mid-19th century.

The Dopamine Hypothesis. This theory suggests that schizophrenia (or schizophrenia-like symptoms) may be caused by an excess of dopamine-dependent neuronal activity in the brain (Hollandsworth, 1990). This excess activity may be related to increased production or release of the substance at nerve terminals, increased receptor sensitivity, or reduced activity of dopamine antagonists (Birchwood et al., 1989).

Pharmacological support for this hypothesis exists. Amphetamines, which increase levels of dopamine, induce psychotomimetic symptoms (Kaplan & Sadock, 1998). The **neuroleptics** (e.g., chlorpromazine or haloperidol) lower brain levels of dopamine by blocking dopamine receptors, thus reducing schizophrenic symptoms, including those induced by amphetamines.

Postmortem studies of schizophrenic brains have reported a significant increase in the average number of dopamine receptors in approximately two thirds of the brains studied. This suggests that an increased dopamine response may not be important in *all* schizophrenic clients. Clients with acute manifestations (e.g., **delusions** and **hallucinations**) respond with greater efficacy to neuroleptic drugs than do clients with chronic manifestations (e.g., apathy, poverty of ideas, and loss of drive). The current position, in terms of the dopamine hypothesis, is that manifestations of acute schizophrenia may be related to increased numbers of dopamine receptors in the brain and respond to neuroleptic drugs that block these receptors. Manifestations of chronic schizophrenia are probably unrelated to numbers of dopamine receptors, and neuroleptic drugs are unlikely to be as effective in treating these chronic symptoms.

Other Biochemical Hypotheses. Various other biochemicals have been implicated in the predisposition to schizophrenia. Abnormalities in the neurotransmitters norepinephrine, serotonin, acetylcholine, and gamma-aminobutyric acid, and the neuroregulators, such as prostaglandins and endorphins, have been suggested. Cutting (1985) suggests that the body may manufacture a hallucinogen or psychotomimetic that usurps the usual neurotransmitter or neuroregulator pathways in the brains of individuals with schizophrenia.

Physiological Influences

A number of physical factors of possible etiological significance have been identified in the medical literature, although their specific mechanisms in the implication of schizophrenia are unclear.

Viral Infection. In postmortem studies, Stevens (1982) reported observations of degenerative changes within the neurons and an increase in the supporting glial cells of schizophrenic brains. These structural changes are similar to those characteristically reported in infectious inflammatory diseases such as viral encephalitis. Stevens considered these changes in the brains of individuals with schizophrenia to be consistent with a "healed inflammatory" process.

Anatomical Abnormalities. Computed tomography (CT) scan abnormalities occur in up to 40 percent of schizophrenic patients (Black & Andreasen, 1994). Ventricular enlargement is the most consistent finding; however, sulci enlargement and cerebellar atrophy are also reported. Magnetic resonance imaging (MRI) provides a greater ability to image in multiple planes. Black & Andreasen (1994) report on the use of MRI to explore possible abnormalities in specific subregions such as the amygdala, hippocampus, temporal lobes, and basal ganglia in the brains of people with schizophrenia.

Functional cerebral asymmetries of the brain occur normally as they relate to language comprehension and speech production. Computerized studies with schizophrenic populations have suggested that some individuals with the disorder exhibit a reversal of the normal anatomical asymmetry (Birchwood et al., 1989). The significance of these results in the etiology of schizophrenia is unclear, however, because of the relatively few studies that have addressed this issue to date.

Histological Changes. Scheibel and his associates (1991) at UCLA have studied cerebral changes at the microscopic level. In studying brains of clients with schizophrenia they found a "disordering" or disarray of the pyramidal cells in the area of the hippocampus. This they compared to the normal alignment of the cells in the brains of clients without the disorder. They have hypothesized that this alteration in hippocampal cells occurs during the second trimester of pregnancy and may be related to an influenza virus encountered by the mother during this period. Further research is required to determine the possible link between this birth defect and the development of schizophrenia.

Physical Conditions. Cutting (1985) cites various studies that report a well-established, positive link between schizophrenia and the following conditions: epilepsy (particularly temporal lobe), Huntington's chorea, birth trauma, head injury in adulthood, alcohol abuse, cerebral tumor (particularly in the limbic system), cerebrovascular accidents, systemic lupus erythematosus, myxedema, parkinsonism, and Wilson's disease.

Psychological Influences

Early conceptualizations of schizophrenia focused on family relationship factors as major influences in the development of the illness. This probably occurred in light of the conspicuous absence of information related to a biological connection.

In the past decade researchers have doubted these theories and are now focusing their studies more in terms of schizophrenia as a brain disorder. Can family interaction patterns cause schizophrenia? Cutting (1985) states: "These purely psychological causes are *theoretically* possible, even if difficult to prove in practice."

Kaplan and Sadock (1998) state:

"Clinicians should consider the psychosocial factors affecting schizophrenia. Although, historically, theorists have attributed the development of schizophrenia to psychosocial factors, contemporary clinicians can benefit from using the relevant theories and guidelines of these past observations and hypotheses." (p. 465)

The following psychosocial theories are presented for enlightenment and discussion.

Psychoanalytic Theories

Early theorists characterized the mothers of individuals with schizophrenia as cold, overprotective, and domineering (Birchwood et al., 1989). They were thought to have arrested the ego development of the child, who, upon encountering the real world in adolescence or early adulthood, was unable to deal with the demands and was forced to retreat into a form of thinking characteristic of early childhood. Freud (1961) coined the term *primary process thinking* to describe the narcissism and fantasy associated with schizophrenic thought processes.

Sullivan (1953), who did much of his work with clients who had schizophrenia, believed that the illness stemmed from a parent-child relationship fraught with intense anxiety. He described three components of the self-system (the good me, the bad me, and the not me) which are determined by one's early interpersonal experiences (see Chapter 3 for a discussion of Sullivan's theory). The intense anxiety produces feelings of horror, awe, dread, and loathing, leading the child to deny these feelings in an effort to relieve anxiety. These feelings, having then been denied, become "not me," but someone else. This withdrawal from emotions, or the "not me" portion of the self-system, is the basis for the later development of schizophrenia.

Mahler, Pine, and Bergman (1975) describe the important phases in the separation-individuation process of the infant from the maternal figure. In phase 2 (age 1 to 5 months), which is called the symbiotic phase, there is a type of "psychic fusion" of mother and child. The child does not view the self as separate but as an extension of the mother, who serves to fulfill every need. Fixation in this stage of development has been implicated in the predisposition to adult schizophrenia.

Erikson (1963) described eight stages of human development during which individuals struggle with various crises, the resolution of which contribute to emotional growth. In the first stage, which Erikson called "trust versus mistrust," the task is to develop trust in the mothering figure that is then generalized to other interpersonal relationships. Nonachievement and fixation at this level result in suspiciousness of others, dissatisfaction with the self, isolation, and difficulty with interpersonal relationships. This occurs when the child is rejected and deprived of nurturing and love from the primary caregiver—experiences that have been associated with vulnerability to serious mental disturbances in later life.

Family Theories

Dysfunctional Family System

Bowen (1978) describes the development of schizophrenia as it evolves out of a dysfunctional family system. When a conflictual marital relationship exists, a great deal of anxiety may be experienced within the family. Out of a need to reduce the anxiety, one parent (usually the mother) may become emotionally overinvested in the child. Her anxiety decreases out of her attachment to the child, and the problems within the marriage relationship, although unresolved, become stabilized. A symbiotic relationship may develop between mother and child (the psychic fusion, as described by Mahler), a relationship so intense that they may report thinking the same thoughts or expressing the same emotions. The child remains totally dependent on the parent into adulthood and is unable to respond to the demands of adult functioning.

Double-Bind Communication

Bateson and coworkers (1956) identified a pattern of communication that has been implicated in the development of schizophrenia. Communication between parents and offspring was described as frequently contradictory and placed the child in a "double-bind." **Double-bind communication** may occur when a statement is made and succeeded by a contradictory statement. It also occurs when a statement is made accompanied by nonverbal expression that is inconsistent with the verbal communication. These incompatible communications may interfere with ego development, thereby causing the individual to generate false ideas and exhibit extreme mistrust of all communications (Birchwood et al., 1989).

Double-bind communication gives mixed messages and creates confusion in the receiver.

EXAMPLES

1. Mother says, "I'm really happy you are going to the school dance tonight, Sally. I'll just stay here at home all alone."
2. Johnny falls and hurts his hand. His mother says, "Come and let Mommy kiss it for you." When Johnny goes to his mother she says, "Don't be a baby! Big boys don't cry! Shut up. You're not hurt!"
3. Jack, who is 27 years old, has never lived away from home. His parents have told him he should get his own apartment. When his parents go on a trip, his mother leaves prepared food for each day they will be gone and ensures that Jack's clothes have been washed and ironed before they leave.

Environmental Influences

Sociocultural Factors

Many studies have been conducted that have attempted to link schizophrenia to social class. Indeed epidemiological statistics have shown that greater numbers of individuals from the lower socioeconomic classes experience symptoms associated with schizophrenia than those from the higher socioeconomic groups (Black & Andreasen, 1994). Explanations for this occurrence include the conditions associated with living in poverty, such as congested housing accommodations, inadequate nutrition, absence of prenatal care, few resources for dealing with stressful situations, and feelings of hopelessness for changing one's lifestyle of poverty.

Some studies have attempted to refute this hypothesis and view the link between low socioeconomic status and schizophrenia as merely a shift downward because of the client's difficulty maintaining stable employment and relationships (Birchwood et al., 1989). These statistics may relate to the schizophrenic's tendency for social isolation, and the segregation of self from others in areas accessible to one who has experienced a passive downward shift in social status because of characteristics of the disease process itself. Proponents of this notion view poor social conditions as a consequence rather than a cause of schizophrenia.

Stressful Life Events

Studies have been conducted in an effort to determine whether psychotic episodes may be precipitated by stressful life events. The strongest evidence for the role of stressful life events in schizophrenia comes from the research of Brown and Birley (1968). In the individuals they studied, it was found that stressful events were most likely to have occurred in the 3-week period just before the onset of symptoms. Other investigators have supported the hypothesis that stressful life events can precipitate schizophrenic symptoms in a genetically predisposed individual (Goldstein, 1987; Liberman et al., 1984).

Birchwood and colleagues (1989) suggest that an individual's response to stressful life events may vary as a function of (1) the number or severity of life events and (2) the degree of vulnerability to the impact of life stress. They suggest that one's degree of vulnerability may be increased by a high level of autonomic arousal, an impoverished capacity to cope with stressful experiences, or a lack of support and ties with other people, including family.

The Transactional Model

The etiology of schizophrenia remains unclear. No single theory or hypothesis has been postulated that substantiates a clear-cut explanation for the disease. Indeed, it seems the more research that is conducted, the more evidence is compiled to support the concept of multiple causation. The transactional model recognizes the combined effects of biological, psychological, and environmental influences on an individual's susceptibility to psychotic illness. Liberman and coworkers (1984) support the concept of multiple causation. They state:

"Schizophrenic symptoms and impaired functioning occur when noxious social events combine with preexisting vulnerability to produce states of sensory overload, hyperarousal, and impaired processing of social stimuli. The appearance or increase in characteristic schizophrenic symptoms may occur in a susceptible individual when:

1. The underlying biological vulnerability increases.
2. Stressful life events intervene that overwhelm the individual's coping in social and instrumental roles.
3. The individual's social support network weakens or diminishes.
4. Previously acquired social problem-solving skills diminish due to disuse, reinforcement of the sick role, loss of motivation, or social isolation."

The dynamics of schizophrenia using the transactional model of stress/adaptation are presented in Figure 25.1.

TYPES OF SCHIZOPHRENIA AND OTHER PSYCHOTIC DISORDERS

The *DSM-IV* (APA, 1994) identifies various types of schizophrenia and other psychotic disorders. Differential diagnosis is made according to the total symptomatic clinical picture presented.

Disorganized Schizophrenia

This type was previously called *hebephrenic schizophrenia*. Onset of symptoms is usually before age 25, and the

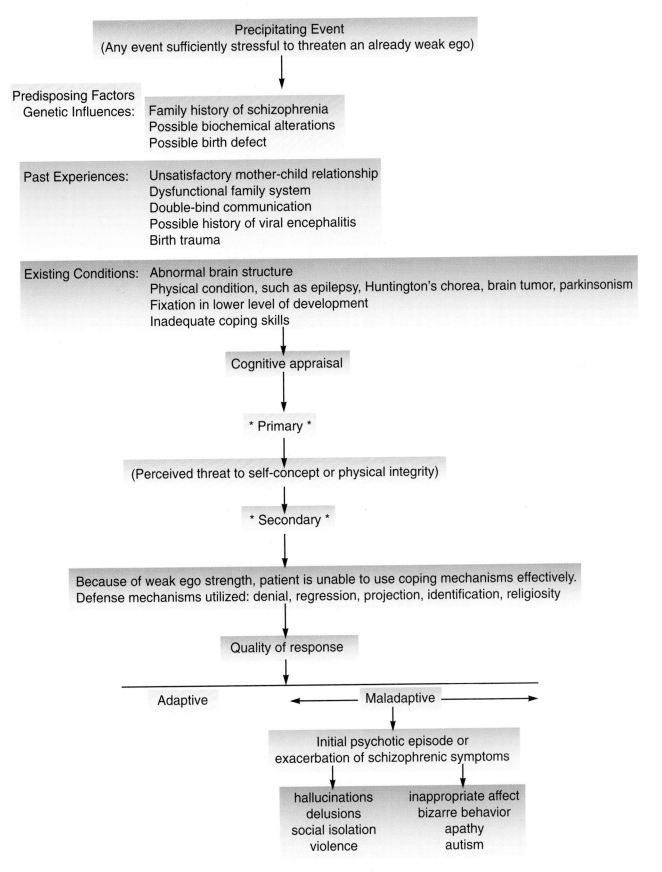

Figure 25.1 The dynamics of schizophrenia using the transactional model of stress/adaptation.

course is commonly chronic. Behavior is markedly regressive and primitive. Contact with reality is extremely poor. Affect is flat or grossly inappropriate, often with periods of silliness and incongruous giggling. Facial grimaces and bizarre mannerisms are common, and communication is consistently incoherent. Personal appearance is generally neglected, and social impairment is extreme.

Catatonic Schizophrenia

Catatonic schizophrenia is characterized by marked abnormalities in motor behavior and may be manifested in the form of *stupor* or *excitement* (Kaplan, Sadock, & Grebb, 1994).

Catatonic stupor is characterized by extreme psychomotor retardation. The individual exhibits a pronounced decrease in spontaneous movements and activity. Mutism (i.e., absence of speech) is common, and negativism (i.e., an apparently motiveless resistance to all instructions or attempts to be moved) may be evident. Waxy flexibility may be exhibited. This term describes a type of "posturing," or voluntary assumption of bizarre positions, in which the individual may remain for long periods of time. Efforts to move the individual may be met with rigid bodily resistance.

Catatonic excitement is manifested by a state of extreme psychomotor agitation. The movements are frenzied and purposeless, and are usually accompanied by continuous incoherent verbalizations and shouting. Clients in catatonic excitement require physical and medical control, as they are often destructive and violent to others and their excitement may cause them to injure themselves or to collapse from exhaustion.

Catatonic schizophrenia was very common only a few decades ago. However, since the advent of antipsychotic medications for use in psychiatry, the illness is now rare in Europe and North America (Kaplan, Sadock, & Grebb, 1994).

Paranoid Schizophrenia

Paranoid schizophrenia is characterized mainly by the presence of delusions of persecution or grandeur and auditory hallucinations related to a single theme. The individual is often tense, suspicious, and guarded, and may be argumentative, hostile, and aggressive. Onset of symptoms is usually later (perhaps in the late 20s or 30s), and less regression of mental faculties, emotional response, and behavior is seen than in the other subtypes of schizophrenia (Kaplan, Sadock, & Grebb, 1994). Social impairment may be minimal, and there is some evidence that prognosis, particularly with regard to occupational functioning and capacity for independent living, is promising (APA, 1994).

Undifferentiated Schizophrenia

Sometimes clients with schizophrenic symptoms do not meet the criteria for any of the subtypes, or they may meet the criteria for more than one subtype. These individuals may be given the diagnosis of undifferentiated schizophrenia. The behavior is clearly psychotic, that is, there is evidence of delusions, hallucinations, incoherence, and bizarre behavior. However, the symptoms cannot be easily classified into any of the previously listed diagnostic categories.

Residual Schizophrenia

This diagnostic category is used when the individual has a history of at least one previous episode of schizophrenia with prominent psychotic symptoms. Residual schizophrenia occurs in an individual who has a chronic form of the disease and is the stage that follows an acute episode (prominent delusions, hallucinations, incoherence, bizarre behavior, violence). In the residual stage, there is continuing evidence of the illness, although there are no prominent psychotic symptoms. Residual symptoms may include social isolation, eccentric behavior, impairment in personal hygiene and grooming, blunted or inappropriate affect, poverty of or overelaborate speech, illogical thinking, or apathy. Residual schizophrenia is sometimes referred to as *ambulatory schizophrenia* (Kaplan & Sadock, 1985).

Schizoaffective Disorder

This disorder is manifested by schizophrenic behaviors, with a strong element of symptomatology associated with the mood disorders, either mania or depression. The client may appear depressed, with psychomotor retardation and suicidal ideation; or symptoms may include euphoria, grandiosity, and hyperactivity. The decisive factor in the diagnosis of schizoaffective disorder, however, is the presence of characteristic schizophrenic symptoms (Kaplan & Sadock, 1985). For example, in addition to the dysfunctional mood, the individual exhibits bizarre delusions, prominent hallucinations, incoherent speech, catatonic behavior, or blunted or inappropriate affect. The prognosis for schizoaffective disorder is generally better than that for other schizophrenic disorders but worse than that for mood disorders alone (Kaplan, Sadock, & Grebb, 1994).

Brief Psychotic Disorder

The essential feature of this disorder is sudden onset of psychotic symptoms following a severe psychosocial stressor. These symptoms last at least 1 day but less than 1 month, and there is an eventual full return to the premorbid level of functioning (APA, 1994). The stressor is severe enough to bring about emotional turmoil or overwhelming perplexity or confusion in the individual. Evidence of impaired reality testing may include incoherent speech, delusions, hallucinations, bizarre behavior, and disorientation. Individuals with preexisting personality disorders (most commonly, histrionic, narcissistic, paranoid, schizotypal, and borderline personality disorders) appear to be susceptible to this disorder (Kaplan, Sadock, & Grebb, 1994).

Schizophreniform Disorder

The essential features of this disorder are identical to those of schizophrenia, with the exception that the duration, including prodromal, active, and residual phases, is at least 1 month but less than 6 months (APA, 1994). If the diagnosis is made while the individual is still symptomatic but has been so for less than 6 months, it is qualified as "provisional." The diagnosis is changed to schizophrenia if the clinical picture persists beyond 6 months.

Schizophreniform disorder is thought to have a good prognosis if at least two of the following features are present:

1. Onset of prominent psychotic symptoms within 4 weeks of first noticeable change in usual behavior or functioning.
2. Confusion, disorientation, or perplexity at the height of the psychotic episode.
3. Good premorbid social and occupational functioning.
4. Absence of blunted or flat affect (APA, 1994).

Delusional Disorder

The essential feature of this disorder is the presence of one or more nonbizarre delusions that persist for at least 1 month (APA, 1994). Hallucinations, if present at all, are not prominent, and behavior, apart from the delusions, is not bizarre. The subtype of delusional disorder is based on the predominant delusional theme.

Erotomanic Type

With this type of delusion, the individual believes that someone, usually of a higher status, is in love with him or her. Famous persons are often the subjects of erotomanic delusions. Sometimes the delusion is kept secret, but some individuals may follow, contact, or otherwise try to pursue the object of their delusion.

Grandiose Type

Individuals with grandiose delusions have irrational ideas regarding their own worth, talent, knowledge, or power.

They may believe that they have a special relationship with a famous person, or even assume the identity of a famous person (believing that the actual person is an imposter). Grandiose delusions of a religious nature may lead to assumption of the identity of a deity or religious leader.

Jealous Type

The content of jealous delusions centers on the idea that the person's sexual partner is unfaithful. The idea is irrational and without cause, but the deluded individual searches for evidence to justify the belief. The sexual partner is confronted (and sometimes physically attacked) regarding the imagined infidelity. The imagined "lover" of the sexual partner may also be the object of the attack. Attempts to restrict the autonomy of the sexual partner in an effort to stop the imagined infidelity are common.

Persecutory Type

In persecutory delusions, which are the most common type, individuals believe they are being malevolently treated in some way. Frequent themes include being conspired against, cheated, spied on, followed, poisoned or drugged, maliciously maligned, harassed, or obstructed in the pursuit of long-term goals (APA, 1994). The individual may obsess about and exaggerate a slight rebuff (either real or imagined) until it becomes the focus of a delusional system. Repeated complaints may be directed at legal authorities, lack of satisfaction from which may result in violence toward the object of the delusion.

Somatic Type

Individuals with somatic delusions believe they have some physical defect, disorder, or disease. The *DSM-IV* (APA, 1994) identifies the most common types of somatic delusions as those in which the individual believes that he or she:

1. Emits a foul odor from the skin, mouth, rectum, or vagina.
2. Has an infestation of insects in or on the skin.
3. Has an internal parasite.
4. Has misshapen and ugly body parts.
5. Has dysfunctional body parts.

Shared Psychotic Disorder

The essential feature of this disorder, also called *folie à deux*, is a delusional system that develops in a second person as a result of a close relationship with another person who already has a psychotic disorder with prominent delusions (APA, 1994). The person with the primary delusional disorder is usually the dominant person in the relationship, and the delusional thinking is gradually imposed on the more passive partner. This occurs within the context of a long-term close relationship, particularly when the couple has been socially isolated from other people. The course is usually chronic, and it is more common in women than in men.

Psychotic Disorder Due to a General Medical Condition

The essential features of this disorder are prominent hallucinations and delusions that can be directly attributed to a general medical condition (APA, 1994). The diagnosis is not made if the symptoms occur during the course of a delirium or chronic, progressing dementia. A number of medical conditions can cause psychotic symptoms. Common ones identified by the *DSM-IV* (APA, 1994) are presented in Table 25.1.

Substance-Induced Psychotic Disorder

The essential features of this disorder are the presence of prominent hallucinations and delusions that are judged to be directly attributable to the physiological effects of a substance (i.e., a drug of abuse, a medication, or toxin exposure) (APA, 1994). The diagnosis is made in the absence of reality testing and when history, physical examination, or laboratory findings indicate use of substances. When reality testing has been retained in the presence of substance-induced psychotic symptoms, the diagnosis

would be substance-related disorder (Kaplan, Sadock, & Grebb, 1994). Substances identified by the *DSM-IV* (APA, 1994) that are believed to induce psychotic disorders are presented in Table 25.2.

APPLICATION OF THE NURSING PROCESS

Background Assessment Data

In the first step of the nursing process, the nurse gathers a database from which nursing diagnoses are derived and a plan of care is formulated. This first step of the nursing process is extremely important, for without an accurate assessment, problem identification, objectives of care, and outcome criteria cannot be accurately determined.

Assessment of the client with schizophrenia may be a complex process, based on information gathered from a number of sources. Clients in an acute episode of their illness are seldom able to make a significant contribution to their history. Data may be obtained from family members, if possible; from old records, if available; or from other individuals who have been in a position to report on the progression of the client's behavior.

TABLE 25.1 GENERAL MEDICAL CONDITIONS THAT MAY CAUSE PSYCHOTIC SYMPTOMS

Neurological conditions	Neoplasms
	Cerebrovascular disease
	Huntington's disease
	Epilepsy
	Auditory nerve injury
	Deafness
	Migraine headache
	CNS infections
Endocrine conditions	Hyperthyroidism
	Hypothyroidism
	Hyperparathyroidism
	Hypoparathyroidism
	Hypoadrenocorticism
Metabolic conditions	Hypoxia
	Hypercarbia
	Hypoglycemia
Autoimmune disorders	Systemic lupus erythematosus
Others	Fluid or electrolyte imbalances
	Hepatic or renal diseases

TABLE 25.2 SUBSTANCES THAT MAY CAUSE PSYCHOTIC DISORDERS

Drugs of abuse	Alcohol
	Amphetamines and related substances
	Cannabis
	Cocaine
	Hallucinogens
	Inhalants
	Opioids
	Phencyclidine and related substances
	Sedatives, hypnotics, and anxiolytics
Medications	Anesthetics and analgesics
	Anticholinergic agents
	Anticonvulsants
	Antidepressant medications
	Antihistamines
	Antihypertensive agents
	Cardiovascular medications
	Antimicrobial medications
	Antiparkinsonian agents
	Chemotherapeutic agents
	Corticosteroids
	Disulfiram
	Gastrointestinal medications
	Muscle relaxants
	Nonsteroidal anti-inflammatory agents
Toxins	Anticholinesterase
	Organophosphate insecticides
	Nerve gases
	Carbon monoxide
	Carbon dioxide
	Volatile substances (e.g., fuel or paint)

The nurse must be familiar with behaviors common to the disorder in order to obtain an adequate assessment of the client with schizophrenia. The *DSM-III-R* (APA, 1987) previously presented behavioral disturbances in eight areas of functioning: content of thought, form of thought, perception, affect, sense of self, volition, impaired interpersonal functioning and relationship to the external world, and psychomotor behavior. These areas of functioning are employed to facilitate the presentation of background information on which to base the initial assessment of the client with schizophrenia. Additional impairments outside the limits of these eight areas are also presented.

Content of Thought

Delusions. Delusions are false personal beliefs that are inconsistent with the person's intelligence or cultural background. The individual continues to have the belief in spite of obvious proof that it is false or irrational. Delusions are subdivided according to their content. Some of the more common ones are listed here.

Delusion of Persecution. The individual feels threatened and believes that others intend harm or persecution toward him or her in some way (e.g., "The FBI has 'bugged' my room and intends to kill me." "I can't take a shower in this bathroom; the nurses have put a camera in there so that they can watch everything I do").

Delusion of Grandeur. The individual has an exaggerated feeling of importance, power, knowledge, or identity (e.g., "I am Jesus Christ").

Delusion of Reference. All events within the environment are referred by the psychotic person to himself or herself (e.g., "Someone is trying to get a message to me through the articles in this magazine [or newspaper or TV program]; I must break the code so that I can receive the message"). Ideas of reference are less rigid than delusions of reference. An example of an idea of reference would be irrationally thinking that one is being talked about or laughed at by other people.

Delusion of Control or Influence. The individual believes certain objects or persons have control over his or her behavior (e.g., "The dentist put a filling in my tooth; I now receive transmissions through the filling that control what I think and do").

Somatic Delusion. The individual has a false idea about the functioning of his or her body (e.g., "I'm 70 years old and I will be the oldest person ever to give birth; the doctor says I'm not pregnant, but I know I am").

Nihilistic Delusion. The individual has a false idea that the self, a part of the self, others, or the world is nonexistent (e.g., "The world no longer exists." "I have no heart.").

Religiosity. This is an excessive demonstration of or obsession with religious ideas and behavior. Because individuals vary greatly in their religious beliefs and level of spiritual commitment, **religiosity** is often difficult to assess. The individual with schizophrenia may use religious ideas in an attempt to provide rational meaning and structure to his or her behavior. Religious preoccupation in this vein may therefore be considered a manifestation of the illness. However, clients who derive comfort from their religious beliefs should not be discouraged from employing this means of support. An example of religiosity is the individual who believes the voice he or she hears is God and incessantly searches the Bible for interpretation.

Paranoia. Individuals with **paranoia** have extreme suspiciousness of others and of their actions or perceived intentions (e.g., "I won't eat this food; I know it has been poisoned").

Magical Thinking. The person believes that his or her thoughts or behaviors have control over specific situations or people (e.g., the mother who believes if she scolds her son in any way he will be taken away from her). **Magical thinking** is common in children (e.g., "Step on a crack and you break your mother's back." "An apple a day keeps the doctor away").

Form of Thought

Associative Looseness. Thinking is characterized by speech in which ideas shift from one unrelated subject to another. With **associative looseness**, the individual is unaware that the topics are unconnected. When the condition is severe, speech may be incoherent. (For example, "We wanted to take the bus, but the airport took all the traffic. Driving is the ticket when you want to get somewhere. No one needs a ticket to heaven. We have it all in our pockets.")

Neologisms. The psychotic person invents new words, or **neologisms,** that are meaningless to others but have symbolic meaning to the psychotic person (e.g., "She wanted to give me a ride in her new uniphorum").

Concrete Thinking. Concreteness, or literal interpretations of the environment, represents a regression to an earlier level of cognitive development. Abstract thinking is very difficult. For example, the client with schizophrenia would have great difficulty describing the abstract meaning of sayings such as "I'm climbing the walls" or "it's raining cats and dogs."

Clang Associations. Choice of words is governed by sounds. **Clang associations** often take the form of rhyming. For instance, "It is very cold. I am cold and bold. The gold has been sold."

Word Salad. A **word salad** is a group of words that are put together in a random fashion, without any logical connection (e.g., "Most forward action grows life double plays circle uniform").

Circumstantiality. With **circumstantiality** the individual is delayed in reaching the point of a communication because of unnecessary and tedious details. The point or goal is usually achieved but only with numerous interruptions by the interviewer to keep the person on track of the topic being discussed.

Tangentiality. **Tangentiality** differs from circumstantiality in that the person never really gets to the point of the communication. Unrelated topics are introduced, and the original discussion is lost.

Mutism. This is an individual's inability or refusal to speak.

Perseveration. The individual who exhibits **perseveration** persistently repeats the same word or idea in response to different questions.

Perception

Hallucinations. Hallucinations, or false sensory perceptions not associated with real external stimuli, may involve any of the five senses. Kaplan, Sadock, and Grebb (1994) identify the following types:

Auditory. This is a false perception of sound. Most commonly they are of voices, but the individual may report clicks, rushing noises, music, and other noises. Command hallucinations may place the individual or others in a potentially dangerous situation. "Voices" that issue commands for violence to self or others may or may not be heeded by the psychotic person. Auditory hallucinations are the most common type in psychiatric disorders.

Visual. A false visual perception. They may consist of formed images, such as of people, or of unformed images, such as flashes of light.

Tactile. A false perception of the sense of touch, often of something on or under the skin. One specific tactile hallucination is *formication*, the sensation that something is crawling on or under the skin.

Gustatory. A false perception of taste. Most commonly, gustatory hallucinations are described as unpleasant tastes.

Olfactory. A false perception of the sense of smell.

Illusions. **Illusions** are misperceptions or misinterpretations of real external stimuli (Kaplan, Sadock, & Grebb, 1994).

Affect

Affect describes the behavior associated with an individual's feeling state or emotional tone.

Inappropriate Affect. Affect is inappropriate when the individual's emotional tone is incongruent with the circumstances (e.g., a young woman who laughs when told of the death of her mother).

Bland or Flat Affect. Affect is described as bland when the emotional tone is very weak. The individual with flat affect appears to be void of emotional tone (or overt expression of feelings).

Apathy. The client with schizophrenia often demonstrates an indifference to or lack of interest in the environment. The bland or flat affect is a manifestation of the emotional apathy.

Sense of Self

Sense of self describes the uniqueness and individuality a person feels. Because of extremely weak ego boundaries, the schizophrenic person lacks this feeling of uniqueness and experiences a great deal of confusion regarding his or her identity.

Echolalia. The client with schizophrenia may repeat words that he or she hears, which is called **echolalia.** This is an attempt to identify with the person speaking. (For instance, the nurse says, "John, it's time for lunch." The client may respond, "It's time for lunch, it's time for lunch" or sometimes, "Lunch, lunch, lunch, lunch").

Echopraxia. The client who exhibits **echopraxia** may purposelessly imitate movements made by others.

Identification (on an Unconscious Level) and Imitation (on a Conscious Level). These ego defense mechanisms are used by individuals with schizophrenia in their confusion regarding their self-identity. Because they have difficulty knowing where their ego boundaries end and another person's begins, their behavior often takes on the form of that which they see in the other person.

Depersonalization. The unstable self-identity of an individual with schizophrenia may lead to feelings of unreality (e.g., feeling that one's extremities have changed in size; or a sense of seeming to perceive oneself from a distance [APA, 1987]).

Volition

Volition has to do with impairment in the ability to initiate goal-directed activity. In the individual with schizophrenia, this may take the form of inadequate interest, drive, or ability to follow a course of action to its logical conclusion (APA, 1987).

Emotional Ambivalence. Ambivalence in the client with schizophrenia refers to the coexistence of opposite emotions toward the same object, person, or situation. These opposing emotions may interfere with the person's ability to make even a very simple decision (e.g., whether to have coffee or tea with lunch). Underlying the ambivalence in the schizophrenic client is the difficulty he or she has in fulfilling a satisfying human relationship. This difficulty is based on the *need-fear dilemma*—the simultaneous need for and fear of intimacy.

Impaired Interpersonal Functioning and Relationship to the External World

Some clients with acute schizophrenia cling to others, intrude on strangers, and fail to recognize that excessive closeness makes other people uncomfortable and likely to pull away (APA, 1987). Impairment in social functioning may also be reflected in social isolation, emotional detachment, and lack of regard for social convention.

Autism. **Autism** describes the condition created by the person with schizophrenia who focuses inward on a fantasy world, while distorting or excluding the external environment.

Deteriorated Appearance. Personal grooming and self-care activities may become minimal. The client with schizophrenia may appear disheveled and untidy and may need to be reminded of the need for personal hygiene.

Psychomotor Behavior

Anergia. A deficiency of energy. The individual with schizophrenia may lack sufficient energy to carry out activities of daily living or to interact with others.

Waxy Flexibility. **Waxy flexibility** describes a condition in which the client with schizophrenia passively yields all moveable parts of the body to any efforts made at placing them in certain positions (Kaplan & Sadock, 1985). For example, once placed in position, the arm, leg, or head remains in that position for long periods, regardless of how uncomfortable it is for the client.

Posturing. This symptom is manifested by the voluntary assumption of inappropriate or bizarre postures.

Pacing and Rocking. Pacing back and forth and body rocking (a slow, rhythmic, backward-and-forward swaying of the trunk from the hips, usually while sitting) are common psychomotor behaviors of the client with schizophrenia (Kaplan & Sadock, 1985).

Associated Features

Anhedonia. **Anhedonia** is the inability to experience or even imagine any pleasant emotion (Kaplan & Sadock, 1985). This is a particularly distressing symptom that compels some clients to attempt suicide.

Regression. This is the retreat to an earlier level of development. Regression, a primary defense mechanism of schizophrenia, is a dysfunctional attempt to reduce anxiety. It provides the basis for changes in cognition, perception, affect, relationships, and behavior seen in clients with schizophrenia (Haber et al., 1987).

Positive and Negative Symptoms

Some clinicians find it useful to describe symptoms of schizophrenia as positive or negative. Positive symptoms tend to reflect an excess or distortion of normal functions, whereas negative symptoms reflect a diminution or loss of normal functions (APA, 1994). Most clients exhibit a mixture of both types of symptoms.

Positive symptoms are associated with normal brain structures on CT scan and relatively good responses to treatment. Individuals who exhibit mostly negative symptoms often show structural brain abnormalities on CT scans and respond poorly to treatment (Kaplan, Sadock, & Grebb, 1994).

Examples of positive and negative symptoms are presented in Table 25.3.

Diagnosis/Outcome Identification

From analysis of the assessment data, appropriate nursing diagnoses are formulated for the psychotic client and his or her family. From these identified problems, accurate planning of nursing care is executed. Possible nursing diagnoses for clients with psychotic disorders include:

Alteration in thought processes related to inability to trust, panic anxiety, possible hereditary or biochemical factors, evidenced by delusional thinking; inability to concentrate; impaired volition; inability to problem solve, abstract, or conceptualize; extreme suspiciousness of others.

TABLE 25.3 POSITIVE AND NEGATIVE SYMPTOMS OF SCHIZOPHRENIA

POSITIVE SYMPTOMS	NEGATIVE SYMPTOMS
Hallucinations	Affective flattening
Auditory	Unchanging facial expression
Visual	Poor eye contact
Olfactory	Reduced body language
Gustatory	Inappropriate affect
Tactile	Diminished emotional
Delusions	expression
Persecution	Alogia (poverty of speech)
Grandeur	Brief, empty responses
Reference	Decreased fluency of speech
Control or influence	Decreased content of speech
Somatic	Avolition/Apathy
Disorganized	Inability to initiate
thinking/speech	goal-directed activity
Loose associations	Little or no interest in work
Incoherent	or social activities
Clang associations	Impaired grooming/hygiene
Word salad	Anhedonia
Neologisms	Absence of pleasure in social
Concrete thinking	activities
Echolalia	Diminished intimacy/sexual
Tangentiality	interest
Circumstantiality	Social isolation
Disorganized behavior	
Disheveled appearance	
Inappropriate sexual	
behavior	
Restless, agitated	
behavior	
Waxy flexibility	

SOURCE: Adapted from *DSM-IV* (APA, 1994).

Sensory-perceptual alteration: Auditory/visual, related to panic anxiety, extreme loneliness and withdrawal into the self, evidenced by inappropriate responses, disordered thought sequencing, rapid mood swings, poor concentration, disorientation.

Social isolation related to inability to trust, panic anxiety, weak ego development, delusional thinking, regression, evidenced by withdrawal, sadness, dull affect, need-fear dilemma, preoccupation with own thoughts, expression of feelings of rejection or of aloneness imposed by others.

Risk for violence: Self-directed or directed at others related to extreme suspiciousness, panic anxiety, catatonic excitement, rage reactions, command hallucinations, evidenced by overt and aggressive acts, goal-directed destruction of objects in the environment, self-destructive behavior, or active aggressive suicidal acts.

Impaired verbal communication related to panic anxiety, regression, withdrawal, and disordered, unrealistic thinking, evidenced by loose association of ideas, neologisms, word salad, clang association, echolalia, verbalizations that reflect concrete thinking, and poor eye contact.

Self-care deficit related to withdrawal, regression, panic anxiety, perceptual or cognitive impairment, inability to trust, evidenced by difficulty carrying out tasks associated with hygiene, dressing, grooming, eating, and toileting.

Ineffective family coping: Disabling related to highly ambivalent family relationships, impaired family communication, evidenced by neglectful care of the client in regard to basic human needs or illness treatment, extreme denial or prolonged overconcern regarding client's illness.

Altered health maintenance related to disordered thinking, delusions, evidenced by reported or observed inability to take responsibility for meeting basic health practices in any or all functional pattern areas.

Impaired home-maintenance management related to regression, withdrawal, lack of knowledge/resources, impaired physical or cognitive functioning, evidenced by unsafe, unclean, disorderly home environment.

The following criteria may be used for measurement of outcomes in the care of the client with schizophrenia.

THE CLIENT:

1. Demonstrates an ability to relate satisfactorily with others.
2. Recognizes distortions of reality.
3. Has not harmed self or others.
4. Perceives self realistically.
5. Demonstrates the ability to perceive the environment correctly.
6. Maintains anxiety at a manageable level.
7. Relinquishes the need for delusions and hallucinations.

8. Demonstrates the ability to trust others.
9. Uses appropriate verbal communication in interactions with others.
10. Performs self-care activities independently.

Planning/Implementation

Table 25.4 provides a plan of care for the client with schizophrenia. Selected nursing diagnoses are presented, along with outcome criteria, appropriate nursing interventions, and rationales for each.

Some institutions are using a case management model to coordinate care (see Chapter 7 for more detailed explanation). In case management models, the plan of care may take the form of a critical pathway. Table 25.5 depicts an example of a critical pathway of care for a client experiencing an exacerbation of schizophrenic psychosis.

Client/Family Education

The role of client teacher is important in the psychiatric area, as it is in all areas of nursing. A list of topics for client/family education relevant to schizophrenia is presented in Table 25.6.

Evaluation

In the final step of the nursing process, a reassessment is conducted in order to determine if the nursing actions have been successful in achieving the objectives of care. Evaluation of the nursing actions for the client with exacerbation of schizophrenic psychosis may be facilitated by gathering information utilizing the following types of questions.

1. Has the client established trust with at least one staff member?
2. Is the anxiety level maintained at a manageable level?
3. Is delusional thinking still prevalent?
4. Is hallucinogenic activity evident? Does the client share content of hallucination, particularly if commands are heard?
5. Is the client able to interrupt escalating anxiety with adaptive coping mechanisms?
6. Is the client easily agitated?
7. Is the client able to interact with others appropriately?
8. Does the client voluntarily attend therapy activities?
9. Is verbal communication comprehensible?
10. Is the client compliant with medication? Does the client verbalize the importance of taking medication regularly and on a long-term basis? Does he or she verbalize understanding of possible side effects, and when to seek assistance from the physician?
11. Does the client spend time with others rather than isolating self?

TABLE 25.4   CARE PLAN FOR THE CLIENT WITH SCHIZOPHRENIA

NURSING DIAGNOSIS: ALTERATION IN THOUGHT PROCESSES

RELATED TO: Inability to trust, panic anxiety, possible hereditary or biochemical factors

EVIDENCED BY: Delusional thinking; inability to concentrate; impaired volition; inability to problem solve, abstract, or conceptualize; extreme suspiciousness of others

OUTCOME CRITERIA	NURSING INTERVENTIONS	RATIONALE

Client will eliminate pattern of delusional thinking. Client will demonstrate trust in others.	1. Convey that you accept client's need for the false belief but that you do not share the belief.
	2. Do not argue or deny the belief. Use "reasonable doubt" as a therapeutic technique: "I find that hard to believe."
	
	3. Reinforce and focus on reality. Discourage long ruminations about the irrational thinking. Talk about real events and real people.
	4. If client is highly suspicious, the following interventions may help:
	  a. Use same staff as much as possible; be honest and keep all promises.
	  b. Avoid physical contact; avoid laughing, whispering, or talking quietly where client can see but cannot hear what is being said; provide canned food with can opener or serve food family-style; avoid competitive activities; use assertive, matter-of-fact, yet friendly approach.
		1. Client must understand that you do not view the idea as real.
		
		2. Arguing or denying the belief serves no useful purpose, as delusional ideas are not eliminated by this approach, and the development of a trusting relationship may be impeded.
		3. Discussions that focus on the false ideas are purposeless and useless, and may even aggravate the psychosis.
		4. To decrease client's suspiciousness:
		
		  a. Promote trust.
		
		  b. Prevent the client from feeling threatened.

NURSING DIAGNOSIS: SENSORY-PERCEPTUAL ALTERATION: AUDITORY AND VISUAL

RELATED TO: Panic anxiety, extreme loneliness, and withdrawal into the self

EVIDENCED BY: Inappropriate responses, disordered thought sequencing, rapid mood swings, poor concentration, disorientation

OUTCOME CRITERIA	NURSING INTERVENTIONS	RATIONALE
Client will be able to define and test reality, eliminating the occurrence of hallucinations.	1. Observe client for signs of hallucinations (listening pose, laughing or talking to self, stopping in midsentence). 2. Avoid touching the client without warning. 3. An attitude of acceptance will encourage the client to share the content of the hallucination with you. 4. Do not reinforce the hallucination. Use "the voices" instead of words like "they" that imply validation. Let client know that you do not share the perception. Say, "Even though I realize the voices are real to you, I do not hear any voices."	1. Early intervention may prevent aggressive response to command hallucinations. 2. Client may perceive touch as threatening and may respond in an aggressive manner. 3. Encouraging the client to share is important to prevent possible injury to the client or others from command hallucinations. 4. Client must accept the perception as unreal before hallucinations can be eliminated.

Continued on following page

TABLE 25.4 *(Continued)*

	5. Help the client understand the connection between anxiety and hallucinations. 6. Try to distract the client from the hallucination.	5. If client can learn to interrupt escalating anxiety, hallucinations may be prevented. 6. Involvement in interpersonal activities and explanation of the actual situation will help bring the client back to reality.

NURSING DIAGNOSIS: SOCIAL ISOLATION

RELATED TO: Inability to trust, panic anxiety, weak ego development, delusional thinking, regression

EVIDENCED BY: Withdrawal; sad, dull affect; need-fear dilemma; preoccupation with own thoughts; expression of feelings of rejection or of aloneness imposed by others

OUTCOME CRITERIA	NURSING INTERVENTIONS	RATIONALE
Client will voluntarily spend time with other clients and staff members in group activities on the unit.	1. Convey an accepting attitude by making brief, frequent contacts. Show unconditional positive regard. 2. Offer to be with client during group activities that he or she finds frightening or difficult. 3. Give recognition and positive reinforcement for client's voluntary interactions with others.	1. Accepting attitude increases feelings of self-worth and facilitates trust. 2. The presence of a trusted individual provides emotional security for the client. 3. Positive reinforcement enhances self-esteem and encourages repetition of acceptable behaviors.

NURSING DIAGNOSIS: RISK FOR VIOLENCE: SELF-DIRECTED OR DIRECTED AT OTHERS

RELATED TO: Extreme suspiciousness, panic anxiety, catatonic excitement, rage reactions, command hallucinations

EVIDENCED BY: Overt and aggressive acts, goal-directed destruction of objects in the environment, self-destructive behavior or active aggressive suicidal acts

OUTCOME CRITERIA	NURSING INTERVENTIONS	RATIONALE
Client will not harm self or others.	1. Maintain low level of stimuli in client's environment (low lighting, few people, simple decor, low noise level). 2. Observe client behavior frequently. Do this while carrying out routine activities. 3. Remove all dangerous objects from client's environment. 4. Redirect violent behavior with physical outlets for the anxiety. 5. Staff should maintain a calm attitude toward client. 6. Have sufficient staff available to indicate a show of strength to client if it becomes necessary. 7. Administer tranquilizing medications as ordered by physician. If client is not calmed by "talking down" or by medication, use of mechanical restraints may be necessary.	1. Anxiety level rises in stimulating environment. Individuals may be perceived as threatening by a suspicious, agitated client. 2. Observation during routine activities avoids creating suspiciousness on the part of the client. Close observation is necessary so that intervention can occur if required to ensure client's (and others') safety. 3. Removal of dangerous objects prevents client, in an agitated, confused state, from harming self or others. 4. Physical exercise is a safe and effective way of relieving pent-up tension. 5. Anxiety is contagious and can be transmitted from staff to client. 6. This shows the client evidence of control over the situation and provides some physical security for staff. 7. The avenue of the "least restrictive alternative" must be selected when planning interventions for a violent client.

NURSING DIAGNOSIS: IMPAIRED VERBAL COMMUNICATION
RELATED TO: Panic anxiety; regression; withdrawal; disordered, unrealistic thinking
EVIDENCED BY: Loose association of ideas, neologisms, word salad, clang association, echolalia, verbalizations that reflect concrete thinking, poor eye contact

OUTCOME CRITERIA	NURSING INTERVENTIONS	RATIONALE
Client will be able to communicate appropriately and comprehensibly by discharge.	1. Attempt to decode incomprehensible communication patterns. Seek validation and clarification by stating, "Is it that you mean . . . ?" or "I don't understand what you mean by that. Would you please clarify it for me?"	1. These techniques reveal how the client is being perceived by others, while the responsibility for not understanding is accepted by the nurse.
	2. Facilitate trust and understanding by maintaining staff assignments as consistently as possible. The technique of *verbalizing the implied* is used with the client who is mute (unable or unwilling to speak). Example: "That must have been a very difficult time for you when your mother left. You must have felt very alone."	2. This approach conveys empathy and may encourage the client to disclose painful issues.
	3. Anticipate and fulfill client's needs until functional communication pattern returns.	3. Client safety and comfort are nursing priorities.
	4. Orient client to reality as required. Call the client by name. Validate those aspects of communication that help differentiate between what is real and not real.	4. These techniques may facilitate restoration of functional communication patterns in the client.

NURSING DIAGNOSIS: SELF-CARE DEFICIT
RELATED TO: Withdrawal, regression, panic anxiety, perceptual or cognitive impairment, inability to trust
EVIDENCED BY: Difficulty carrying out tasks associated with hygiene, dressing, grooming, eating, toileting

OUTCOME CRITERIA	NURSING INTERVENTIONS	RATIONALE
Client will demonstrate ability to meet self-care needs independently.	1. Provide assistance with self-care needs as required. Some clients who are severely withdrawn may require total care.	1. Client safety and comfort are nursing priorities.
	2. Encourage client to perform independently as many activities as possible. Provide positive reinforcement for independent accomplishments.	2. Independent accomplishment and positive reinforcement enhance self-esteem and promote repetition of desirable behaviors.
	3. Use concrete communication to show client what is expected. Example: "Pick up the spoon, scoop some mashed potatoes into it, and put it in your mouth."	3. Because concrete thinking prevails, explanations must be provided at the client's concrete level of comprehension.
	4. Creative approaches may need to be taken with the client who is not eating, such as allowing client to open own canned or packaged foods; family-style serving may also be an option.	4. These techniques may be helpful with the client who is paranoid and may be suspicious that he or she is being poisoned with food or medication.
	5. If toileting needs are not being met, establish a structured schedule for the client.	5. A structured schedule will help the client establish a pattern so that he or she can develop a habit of toileting self independently.

Continued on following page

TABLE 25.4 *(Continued)*

NURSING DIAGNOSIS: INEFFECTIVE FAMILY COPING, DISABLING
RELATED TO: Highly ambivalent family relationships, impaired family communication
EVIDENCED BY: Neglectful care of the client in regard to basic human needs or illness treatment, extreme denial, or prolonged overconcern regarding client's illness

OUTCOME CRITERIA	NURSING INTERVENTIONS	RATIONALE
Family will identify more adaptive coping strategies for dealing with client's illness and treatment regimen.	1. Identify level of family functioning. Assess communication patterns, interpersonal relationships between members, role expectations, problem-solving skills, and availability of outside support systems.	1. These factors will help to identify how successful the family is in dealing with stressful situations and areas where assistance is required.
	2. Provide information for the family about the client's illness, what will be required in the treatment regimen, and long-term prognosis.	2. Knowledge and understanding about what to expect may facilitate the family's ability to successfully integrate the client into the system.
	3. With family members, practice responses to bizarre behavior and communication patterns and response in the event that the client becomes violent.	3. A plan of action will assist the family to respond adaptively in the face of what they may consider to be a crisis situation.

12. Is the client able to carry out all activities of daily living independently?

13. Is the client able to verbalize resources from whom he or she may seek assistance outside the hospital?

14. Does the family have information regarding support groups in which they may participate, and from which they may seek assistance in dealing with their ill member?

15. If the client lives alone, does he or she have a source for assistance with home maintenance and health management?

TREATMENT MODALITIES FOR SCHIZOPHRENIA AND OTHER PSYCHOTIC DISORDERS

Psychological Treatments

Individual Psychotherapy

Black and Andreasen (1994) state:

> "Although insight-oriented psychotherapy may not be helpful for some patients, this in no way diminishes the value that a long-term, supportive relationship with an interested clinician has for the schizophrenic patient. Supportive therapy that is reality oriented and pragmatic can be enormously helpful. For example, the clinician can help a patient to develop new coping strategies, to test reality, to resolve concrete problems, and to identify common stressors and prodromal symptoms of relapse. A strong 'therapeutic alliance' may also help to boost medication compliance." (p. 448)

Strauss (1983) suggests that "reality-oriented individual therapy" is the most suitable approach to individual psychotherapy for schizophrenia. The primary focus in all cases must reflect efforts to decrease anxiety and increase trust.

Establishing a relationship is often particularly difficult, for the individual with schizophrenia is desperately lonely yet defends against closeness and trust and is likely to become suspicious, anxious, hostile, or regressed when someone attempts to draw close (Kaplan & Sadock, 1985). Successful intervention may be achieved with honesty, simple directness, and a manner that respects the client's privacy and human dignity. Exaggerated warmth and professions of friendship are likely to be met with confusion and suspicion.

Once a therapeutic interpersonal relationship has been established, reality orientation is maintained through exploration of the client's behavior within relationships. Education is provided to help the client identify sources of real or perceived danger and ways of reacting appropriately. Methods for improving interpersonal communication, emotional expression, and frustration tolerance are attempted.

Individual psychotherapy for clients with schizophrenia is seen as a long-term endeavor that requires from a therapist exquisite patience and freedom from the need to prove oneself by effecting change (Gomes-Schwartz, 1984). Some cases report treatment durations of many years before clients regain some degree of independent functioning.

Group Therapy

A number of studies on the efficacy of group therapy in the treatment of schizophrenia have reported meager but

TABLE 25.5   CRITICAL PATHWAY OF CARE FOR CLIENT WITH SCHIZOPHRENIC PSYCHOSIS

Estimated Length of Stay: 14 days—variations from designated pathway should be documented in progress notes

Nursing Diagnosis and Categories of Care	Time Dimension	Goals and/or Actions	Time Dimension	Goals and/or Actions	Time Dimension	Discharge Outcome
Alteration in thought processes/sensory-perceptual alteration			Day 7	Client is able to differentiate between what is real and what is not real.	Day 14	Client experiences no delusional thinking or hallucinations.
Referrals	Day 1	Psychiatrist Psychologist Social worker Clinical nurse specialist Music therapist Occupational therapist Recreational therapist			Day 14	Discharge with follow-up appointments as required.
Diagnostic studies	Day 1 Day 3–5	Drug screen. CT scan, MRI, PET, EEG. (These may be ordered to examine structure and function of the brain.)				
Additional assessments	Day 1 Day 1	VS every shift. Assess for: delusions, hallucinations, loose associations, inappropriate affect, excitement/ stupor, panic anxiety, suspiciousness.	Day 2–14 Day 2–5	Ongoing assessments. Establish trust with at least one person.	Day 2–14 Day 14	VS daily if stable. No evidence of delusions, hallucinations, loose associations, inappropriate affect, excitement/ stupor, panic anxiety, suspiciousness.
Medications	Day 1	Antipsychotic medication (scheduled and p.r.n.). May need order for concentrate and injectable form. Antiparkinsonian medication (p.r.n.).	Day 1–14	Assess for effectiveness and side effects of medications.	Day 14	Client is discharged with medications.
Client education			Day 7	Discuss correlation between increased anxiety and psychotic symptoms. Discuss ways to de-escalate anxiety.	Day 12–13	Reinforce teaching.

Continued on following page

TABLE 25.5 (*Continued*)

Estimated Length of Stay: 14 days—variations from designated pathway should be documented in progress notes

Nursing Diagnosis and Categories of Care	Time Dimension	Goals and/or Actions	Time Dimension	Goals and/or Actions	Time Dimension	Discharge Outcome
			Day 10	Discuss importance of taking medications regularly, even when feeling well. Discuss possible side effects of medications and when to see the doctor.	Day 14	Client verbalizes understanding of information presented prior to discharge.
Risk for violence: Self-directed or directed at others	Day 1	Environment is made safe for patient and others.	Ongoing	Client does not harm self or others.	Day 14	Client is discharged without harm to self or others.
Referrals	Day 1	Alert hostility management team of the admission of a potentially violent client. For relaxation therapy: Music therapist Clinical nurse specialist Stress management specialist Psychiatrist: May give order for mechanical restraints to be used if needed.			Day 14	Discharge with follow-up appointments as required.
Additional assessments	Day 1	Assess for signs of impending violent behavior: increase in psychomotor activity; angry affect; verbalized persecutory delusions or frightening hallucinations.	Day 2–14	Ongoing assessments.		
Medications	Day 1	P.r.n. antipsychotic medications when signs of agitation begin.	Day 1–14	Use of medications, isolation/seclusion, or mechanical restraints. If client refuses medications, administer following application of restraints.	Day 14	Client is discharged with medications.

Client education		Day 3–12	Teach relaxation techniques; discuss activities in which client could participate to relieve pent-up tension; discuss signs and symptoms of escalating anxiety.	Day 12–13 Day 14	Reinforce teaching. Client verbalizes understanding of information, presented prior to discharge.

CT = computed tomography; MRI = magnetic resonance imaging; PET = positron emission tomography; EEG = electroencephalogram.

positive results, particularly with outpatients and when combined with drug treatment (Cutting, 1985; Kaplan & Sadock, 1985). Kaplan and Sadock (1985) have stated:

"Results are more likely to be positive when treatment focuses on real-life plans, problems, and relationships; on social and work roles and interaction; on cooperation with drug therapy and discussion of the side effects; or on some practical recreational or work activity." (p. 224)

Group therapy in inpatient settings is less productive. Inpatient treatment usually occurs when symptomatology and social disorganization are at their most intense. At this time, the least amount of stimuli possible is most beneficial for the client. Because group therapy is, in fact, a multistimuli situation frequently high in intensity, it may be counterproductive early in treatment (Keith & Matthews, 1984).

Group therapy for schizophrenia has been most useful over the long-term course of the illness. The social interaction, sense of cohesiveness, identification, and reality testing achieved within the group setting have proven to be highly therapeutic processes for these clients. Groups led in a supportive manner, rather than in an interpretative way, appear to be most helpful for schizophrenic clients (Kaplan, Sadock, & Grebb, 1994).

Behavior Therapy

Behavior modification cannot cure schizophrenia in the sense of reversing the assumed biological or psychological defect (Kaplan & Sadock, 1985). It has, however, had a history of qualified success in reducing the frequency of bizarre, disturbing, and deviant behaviors and increasing appropriate behaviors.

Liberman (1970) has summarized the behavior modification features that have led to the most positive results as follows:

1. Clear definition and measurement of goals.
2. Attachment of clear positive and negative consequences to adaptive and maladaptive behavior.
3. Reinforcement for achieving small behavioral changes.

TABLE 25.6   TOPICS FOR CLIENT/FAMILY EDUCATION RELATED TO SCHIZOPHRENIA

Nature of the Illness
1. What to expect as the illness progresses
2. Symptoms associated with the illness
3. Ways for family to respond to behaviors associated with the illness

Management of the Illness
1. Connection of exacerbation of symptoms to times of stress
2. Appropriate medication management
3. Side effects of medications
4. Importance of not stopping medications
5. When to contact health care provider
6. Relaxation techniques
7. Social skills
8. Daily living skills

Support Services
1. Financial assistance
2. Legal assistance
3. Caregiver support groups
4. Respite care
5. Home health care

4. Use of instructions and prompts to elicit the desired behavior.

Regarding behavior therapy for schizophrenia, Kaplan, Sadock, & Grebb (1994) state:

"Adaptive behaviors are reinforced by praise or tokens that can be redeemed for desired items, such as hospital privileges and passes. Consequently, the frequency of maladaptive or deviant behavior—such as talking loudly, talking to oneself in public, and bizarre posturing—can be reduced. (p. 483)

The chief limitation of this type of therapy has been the inability of some individuals with schizophrenia to generalize what has been learned to the community setting once the client has been discharged from the hospital (Black & Andreasen, 1994).

Social Skills Training

Social skills training has become one of the most widely used psychosocial interventions in the treatment of schizophrenia. Bellack (1984) defines a social skill as the use of

> "...eye contact, interpersonal distance, voice intonation, posture, etc., with appropriate variation as to sex, age, status, degree of familiarity, and the cultural background of the interpersonal partner, as well as with the context of the interaction."

Social dysfunction is a hallmark of schizophrenia. Indeed, impairment in social functioning is included as one of the defining diagnostic criteria for schizophrenia in the *DSM-IV* (APA, 1994). Considerable attention is now being given to enhancement of social skills in these clients.

The educational procedure in social skills training focuses on role play. A series of brief scenarios are selected. These should be typical of situations clients experience in their daily lives and be graduated in terms of level of difficulty (Bellack, 1984). The therapist may serve as a role model for some behaviors. For example, "See how I sort of nod my head up and down and look at your face while you talk." The therapist's demonstration is followed by the client's role-playing. Immediate feedback is provided regarding the client's presentation. Only by countless repetitions does the response gradually becomes smooth and effortless.

Progress is geared toward the client's needs and limitations. The focus is on small units of behavior, and the training proceeds very gradually. Highly threatening issues are avoided, and emphasis is placed on functional skills that are relevant to daily living and are likely to secure positive reinforcement for the client (Bellack, 1984).

Social Treatment

Milieu Therapy

Some clinicians believe that milieu therapy can be an appropriate treatment for the client with schizophrenia. Research suggests that psychotropic medication is more effective at all levels of care when used along with milieu therapy and that milieu therapy is more successful if used in conjunction with these medications.

Kaplan and Sadock (1985) state:

> "Milieu therapy is enhanced by group meetings of clients and staff, separately and together, that focus on social functioning, rather than on psychopathology. In general, a therapeutic community encourages self-reliance and rewards the client progressively for efforts toward social readaptation. The client is expected to participate in planning his or her own treatment program and in helping other clients, and to assume responsibility in unit affairs and the outside world." (p. 222)

Individuals with schizophrenia who are treated with milieu therapy alone require longer hospital stays than do those treated with drugs and behavior therapy. Other economic considerations, such as the need for a high staff-to-client ratio, in addition to the longer admission, will likely limit the use of milieu therapy in the treatment of schizophrenia.

Family Therapy

Some therapists treat schizophrenia as an illness not of the client alone, but of the entire family. Even when families appear to cope well, there is a notable impact on the mental health status of relatives when a family member has the illness. Safier (1997) states:

> "When a family member has a serious mental illness, the family must deal with a major upheaval in their lives, a terrible event that causes great pain and grief for the loss of a once-promising child or relationship." (p. 5)

The importance of the expanded role of family in the aftercare of relatives with schizophrenia has been recognized, thereby stimulating interest in family intervention programs designed to support the family system, prevent or delay relapse, and help to maintain the client in the community.

These psychoeducational programs treat the family as a resource rather than a stressor, with the focus on concrete problem solving and specific helping behaviors for coping with stress. Many of these programs recognize a biological basis for the illness and the impact that stress has on the client's ability to function. By providing the family with information about the illness and suggestions for effective coping, psychoeducational programs reduce the likelihood of the client's relapse and the possible emergence of mental illness in previously nonaffected relatives.

Anderson and colleagues (1980) outlined several goals and strategies in family therapy for clients with schizophrenia. The goals include:

1. To increase family members' understanding of the illness.
2. To reduce family stress.
3. To enhance social networks for family interaction.
4. To diminish long-term issues contributing to family stress.

Strategies for intervention with families include:

1. Connection with, and introduction to, the family.
2. Teaching survival skills for living with a client with schizophrenia.
3. Monitoring the application of these skills.
4. Continued treatment or disengagement.

Family therapy typically consists of a brief program of family education about schizophrenia, and a more extended program of family contact designed to reduce overt manifestations of conflict and to alter patterns of family communication and problem solving. The response to this type of therapy has been very dramatic. Kaplan, Sadock, and Grebb (1994) report on the results of family therapy with schizophrenic clients and their families. In controlled studies, the reduction in relapse rate was significant: 25 to 50 percent annual relapse rate without family therapy and 5 to 10 percent with family therapy. Clearly, a more positive outcome in the treatment of the schizophrenic client can be achieved by including the family system in the program of care.

Organic Treatment

Psychopharmacology

Chlorpromazine (Thorazine) was first introduced in the United States in 1952. At that time, it was used in conjunction with barbiturates in surgical anesthesia. With increased use, the drug's psychic properties were recognized, and by 1954, it was marketed as an antipsychotic medication in the United States. The manufacture and sale of other antipsychotic drugs followed in rapid succession. (See Chapter 19 for a detailed discussion of antipsychotic medications.)

Antipsychotic medications are very effective in treating the symptoms of schizophrenia. Unfortunately, substantiated evidence of long-term recovery with antipsychotic medications is notably lacking.

Lickey and Gordon (1983) report that the most optimistic estimates suggest that approximately 10 percent of the clients fail to respond to drugs and remain chronically ill inside psychiatric hospitals for much of their lives. About 30 percent experience partial recovery; these people remain outside the hospital and are employed much of the time, but they still need some help in caring for themselves. Approximately 30 percent do not recover completely but are not obviously ill. Their occupational level may have decreased because of their illness or they may be socially isolated. The remaining 30 percent appear to recover completely. These people are almost continuously employed and stay out of institutions. Some are married. It is not obvious that they had previously suffered from schizophrenia.

Schatzberg and Cole (1986) state:

" . . . although psychotropic drugs exert profound and beneficial effects on cognition, mood, and behavior, they often do not change the underlying disease process, which is frequently highly sensitive to intrapsychic, intrapersonal, and psychosocial stressors." (p. 2)

As mentioned earlier, the efficacy of antipsychotic medications is enhanced by adjunct psychosocial therapy. Because the psychotic manifestations of the illness subside with use of the drugs, clients are generally more cooperative with the psychosocial therapies.

Antipsychotic drugs, also called neuroleptics or major tranquilizers, are effective in the treatment of acute and chronic manifestations of schizophrenia, as well as in maintenance therapy to prevent exacerbation of schizophrenic symptoms. However, because of a number of unpleasant and even dangerous side effects, the advisability of long-term use may be questionable. Common side effects include anticholinergic manifestations (dry mouth, blurred vision, constipation, urinary retention), nausea, gastrointestinal upset, skin rash, sedation, orthostatic hypotension, photosensitivity, decreased libido, retrograde ejaculation, gynecomastia, amenorrhea, weight gain, reduction in seizure threshold, agranulocytosis, extrapyramidal symptoms (pseudoparkinsonism, akinesia, akathisia, dystonia, oculogyric crisis), tardive dyskinesia, and neuroleptic malignant syndrome.

Antiparkinsonian agents may be prescribed to counteract the extrapyramidal symptoms associated with antipsychotic medications. These drugs are cholinergic blockers, producing the same anticholinergic side effects as the antipsychotic medications. Some physicians routinely prescribe the antiparkinsonian drug to be given on a scheduled basis with the antipsychotic medication. Others prefer to order the drug on an as-needed basis, to be administered only if the neurological symptoms appear, thus reducing the compounded anticholinergic effects of the two drugs together. When the drug is given as needed, it is extremely important for the nurse to be able to recognize the symptoms associated with extrapyramidal side effects so that he or she can administer the antiparkinsonian drug without delay (see Chapter 19).

For those clients with schizophrenia who do not respond to antipsychotic medications, a number of other pharmacological options have been tried, with various degrees of success. Use of the following medication alternatives have been reported (Kaplan, Sadock, & Grebb, 1994; Black & Andreasen, 1994):

1. Reserpine is most often used as an antihypertensive; has a very slow onset of action; and has produced tardive dyskinesia early in therapy in some individuals.
2. Lithium carbonate can ameliorate schizophrenic symptoms or suppress episodic violence in clients with schizophrenia but is seldom an adequate drug therapy alone.
3. Carbamazepine ameliorates symptoms in some treatment-resistant psychotic clients, but it alone is not an adequate therapy for schizophrenia.
4. Valium, in high dosages, was shown to control psychotic symptoms of paranoid schizophrenia for up to 4 weeks. Follow-up data are not available.
5. Propranolol may be useful in controlling temper outbursts in aggressive or violent psychotic clients.

The advent of antipsychotic medications in the 1950s was hailed as a medical breakthrough for psychiatry. At

TEST YOUR CRITICAL THINKING SKILLS

Sara, a 23-year-old single woman, has just been admitted to the psychiatric unit by her parents. They explain that over the past few months she has become more and more withdrawn. She stays in her room alone, but lately has been heard talking and laughing to herself.

Sara left home for the first time at age 18 to attend college. She performed well during her first semester, but when she returned after Christmas, she began to accuse her roommate of stealing her possessions. She started writing to her parents that her roommate wanted to kill her and that her roommate was turning everyone against her. She said she feared for her life. She started missing classes and stayed in her bed most of the time. Sometimes she locked herself in her closet. Her parents took her home, and she was hospitalized and diagnosed with paranoid schizophrenia. She has since been maintained on antipsychotic medication while taking a few classes at the local community college.

Sara tells the admitting nurse that she quit taking her medication 4 weeks ago because the pharmacist who fills the prescriptions is plotting to have her killed. She believes he is trying to poison her. She says she got this information from a television message. As Sara speaks, the nurse notices that she sometimes stops in midsentence and listens; sometimes she cocks her head to the side and moves her lips as though she is talking.

Answer the following questions related to Sara:

1. From the assessment data, what would be the most immediate nursing concern in working with Sara?
2. What would be the nursing diagnosis related to this concern?
3. What interventions must be accomplished before the nurse can be successful in working with Sara?

---

last the physician could do something substantive for the client with schizophrenia. No one knows exactly how the antipsychotic effect is achieved, or why it takes several weeks for these effects to be observed. Scientists cannot yet explain why clients do not become tolerant to antipsychotics, or why discontinuing the drug does not make the disease worse than it was before treatment (Lickey & Gordon, 1983). But by studying the action of antipsychotic drugs, progress has been made toward understanding what is wrong with the schizophrenic brain. Continual refinement of the research methods and investigation of other transmitter systems may reveal more precisely how the schizophrenic brain differs from the healthy one.

SUMMARY

Of all mental illness, schizophrenia undoubtedly results in the greatest amount of personal, emotional, and social costs. It presents an enormous threat to life and happiness, yet it remains a puzzle to the medical community. In fact, for many years there was little agreement as to a definition of the concept of schizophrenia. The *DSM-IV* (APA, 1994) identifies specific criteria for the diagnosis of the disorder, which were presented in this chapter.

The initial symptoms of schizophrenia most often occur in early adulthood, and development of the disorder can be viewed in four phases: the schizoid personality, the prodromal phase, the active phase of schizophrenia, and the residual phase.

The cause of schizophrenia remains unclear. Research continues, and many contemporary psychiatrists are giving more credence to the biological theories and placing less emphasis on psychosocial influences. The transactional view, however, supports the idea that no single factor can be implicated in the etiology, but that the disease

RESEARCH NOTE

Randomised controlled trial of intensive cognitive behaviour therapy for patients with chronic schizophrenia. *British Medical Journal* (1998, August), 317, 303–307. Tarrier, N., Yusupoff, L., Kinney, C., McCarthy, E., Gledhill, A., Haddock, G., & Morris, J.

Description of the Study: This study included a randomized sample of 87 patients with chronic schizophrenia who were taking antipsychotic medication, but who still had symptoms of schizophrenia. One third of the patients were to receive routine medication and patient monitoring, or routine care (RC); one third would receive routine care plus supportive counseling (SC); and one third would receive routine care and cognitive behavior therapy (CBT). Seventy-two patients completed the treatment study. The SC subjects developed an emotionally supportive relationship with a therapist. The CBT subjects received training in problem solving, coping with symptoms, and strategies to reduce risk of relapse. Sessions were provided twice weekly for 10 weeks. Prescribed medication protocols, that is, routine care, did not differ for the three groups. Outcomes were measured by number and severity of positive psychotic symptoms before treatment and 3 months after treatment and by rates of readmission to the hospital.

Results of the Study: After 3 months of treatment, the following results were achieved: 33 percent of the CBT subjects, 15 percent of the SC subjects, and 11 percent of the RC subjects showed 50 percent improvement in positive psychotic symptoms. Hospital admissions and readmissions of the CBT and SC subjects during the course of the study were substantially reduced in comparison to the RC subjects.

Comments: The authors suggest that the treatment effects of neuroleptic medication therapy for chronic schizophrenic patients may be significantly enhanced when combined with CBT. Supportive counseling was also effective, but to a lesser degree. Both CBT and SC, as adjunctive therapy to medication, were effective in reducing hospitalization of patients with chronic schizophrenia who are maintained on medications alone.

INTERNET REFERENCES

- Additional information about schizophrenia may be located at the following websites:
  a. http://www.schizophrenia.com
  b. http://www.nimh.nih.gov
  c. http://schizophrenia.nami.org
  d. http://mentalhealth.com
- Support and information for patients with schizophrenia and their families may be located at the following websites:
  a. http://www.mhhub.com/psychosis.html
  b. http://www.health-center.com/english/brain/schiz/fact.htm
- Additional information about medications to treat schizophrenia may be located at the following websites:
  a. http://www.mentalhealth.com/menu.htm/
  b. http://www.mediconsult.com
  c. http://www.fadavis.com
  d. http://www.laurus.com

most likely results from a combination of influences, including genetics, biochemical dysfunction, and physiological, psychological, or environmental factors.

Various types of schizophrenic and related psychotic disorders have been identified. They are differentiated by their total picture of clinical symptomatology. They include disorganized schizophrenia, catatonic schizophrenia, paranoid schizophrenia, undifferentiated schizophrenia, residual schizophrenia, schizoaffective disorder, brief psychotic disorder, schizophreniform disorder, delusional disorder, shared psychotic disorder, psychotic disorder due to a general medical condition, and substance-induced psychotic disorder.

Care of the client with schizophrenia was presented in the context of the six steps of the nursing process. Nursing assessment is based on knowledge of symptomatology related to thought content and form, perception, affect, sense of self, volition, impaired interpersonal functioning and relationship to the external world, and psychomotor behavior. Nursing diagnoses were formulated from the assessment data, and a plan of care was developed. A critical pathway of care for the client with schizophrenia was included as a guideline for nurses who follow a program of case management. Guidelines for evaluation of client outcomes were presented.

Various treatment modalities for schizophrenia were discussed, including individual psychotherapy, group therapy, behavior therapy, social skills training, milieu therapy, family therapy, and psychopharmacology. For the majority of clients, the most effective treatment appears to be a combination of psychotropic medication and psychosocial therapy.

REVIEW QUESTIONS

SELF-EXAMINATION/LEARNING EXERCISE

Situation: Tony, a 20-year-old college dropout who had become increasingly withdrawn, suspicious, and isolated during the past 2 months since his return from an out-of-state college, is brought to the emergency room. His family reports that he has been looking at them strangely as if he did not know them, refusing to talk to anyone, spending a lot of time in his room alone, refusing all help. The father brought the client to the hospital against his will following a verbal argument in the course of which the client had attempted to stab the father with a kitchen knife. The father had successfully subdued him and had removed the weapon. On arrival at the emergency room, the client was agitated and exhibiting acutely psychotic symptoms. He reports that "they" told him to kill his father before his father kills him. Verbalizations are often incoherent. Affect is flat, and he continuously scans the environment. He is admitted to the psychiatric unit with a diagnosis of schizophreniform disorder, provisional.

For the above situation, select the answer that is most appropriate for each of the following questions:

1. The *initial* nursing intervention for Tony is to:
   a. Give him an injection of Thorazine.
   b. Ensure a safe environment for him and others.
   c. Place him in restraints.
   d. Order him a nutritious diet.

2. The primary goal in working with Tony would be to:
   a. Promote interaction with others.
   b. Decrease his anxiety and increase trust.
   c. Improve his relationship with his parents.
   d. Encourage participation in therapy activities.

3. Orders from the physician include 100 mg chlorpromazine (Thorazine) STAT and then 50 mg b.i.d.; 2 mg benztropine (Cogentin) b.i.d. p.r.n. Why is chlorpromazine ordered?
   a. To reduce extrapyramidal symptoms.
   b. To prevent neuroleptic malignant syndrome.
   c. To decrease psychotic symptoms.
   d. To induce sleep.

4. Benztropine was ordered on a p.r.n. basis. Which of the following assessments by the nurse would convey a need for this medication?
   a. The client's level of agitation increases.
   b. The client complains of a sore throat.
   c. The client's skin has a yellowish cast.
   d. The client develops tremors and a shuffling gait.

5. Tony begins to tell the nurse about how the CIA is looking for him and will kill him if they find him. The most appropriate response by the nurse is:
   a. "That's ridiculous, Tony. No one is going to hurt you."
   b. "The CIA isn't interested in people like you, Tony."
   c. "Why do you think the CIA wants to kill you?"
   d. "I find that very hard to believe, Tony."

6. Tony's belief about the CIA is an example of a:
   a. Delusion of persecution.
   b. Delusion of reference.
   c. Delusion of control or influence.
   d. Delusion of grandeur.

7. Tony tilts his head to the side, stops talking in midsentence, and listens intently. The nurse recognizes from these signs that Tony is likely experiencing:

    a. Somatic delusions.
    b. Catatonic stupor.
    c. Auditory hallucinations.
    d. Pseudoparkinsonism.

8. The most appropriate nursing intervention for the symptom just described is to:

    a. Ask the client to describe his physical symptoms.
    b. Ask the client to describe what he is hearing.
    c. Administer a dose of benztropine.
    d. Call the physician for additional orders.

9. Should Tony suddenly become aggressive and violent on the unit, which of the following approaches would be *best* for the nurse to use *first?*

    a. Provide large motor activities to relieve Tony's pent-up tension.
    b. Administer a large dose of sedative to keep Tony calm.
    c. Call for sufficient help to control the situation safely.
    d. Convey to Tony that his behavior is unacceptable and will not be permitted.

10. Tony and his parents attend a weekly family therapy group. The primary focus of this type of group is:

    a. To discuss concrete problem solving and adaptive behaviors for coping with stress.
    b. To introduce the family to others with the same problem.
    c. To keep the client and family in touch with the health care system.
    d. To promote family interaction and increase understanding of the illness.

REFERENCES

American Psychiatric Association. (1987). *Diagnostic and statistical manual of mental disorders* (3rd ed., revised). Washington, DC: American Psychiatric Association.

American Psychiatric Association. (1994). *Diagnostic and statistical manual of mental disorders* (4th ed.). Washington, DC: American Psychiatric Association.

Anderson, C.M., et al. (1980). Family treatment of adult schizophrenic patients: A psychoeducational approach. *Schizophrenia Bulletin, 6,* 490–505.

Bateson, G., et al. (1956). Towards a theory of schizophrenia. *Behavioral Science, 1,* 251–264.

Bellack, A.S. (1984). *Schizophrenia: Treatment, management, and rehabilitation.* Orlando, FL: Grune & Stratton.

Birchwood, M.J., et al. (1989). *Schizophrenia: An integrated approach to research and treatment.* New York: New York University Press.

Black, D.W., & Andreasen, N.C. (1994). Schizophrenia, schizophreniform disorder, and delusional (paranoid) disorder. In R.E. Hales, S.C. Yudofsky, & J.A. Talbott (Eds.), *Textbook of psychiatry* (2nd ed.). Washington, D.C.: American Psychiatric Press.

Bowen, M. (1978). A family concept of schizophrenia. In M. Bowen (Ed.), *Family therapy in clinical practice.* New York: Aronson.

Brown, G.W., & Birley, J. (1968). Crises and life changes and the onset of schizophrenia. *Journal of Health and Social Behavior, 9,* 203–214.

Cutting, J. (1985). *The psychology of schizophrenia.* New York: Churchill Livingstone.

Erikson, E. (1963). *Childhood and society* (2nd ed.). New York: W.W. Norton.

Freud, S. (1961). The ego and the id. In *Standard edition of the complete psychological works of Freud* (Vol. XIX). London: The Hogarth Press.

Goldstein, M.J. (1987). Psychosocial issues. *Schizophrenia Bulletin, 13*(1), 157–172.

Gomes-Schwartz, B. (1984). Individual psychotherapy of schizophrenia. In A.S. Bellack (Ed.), *Schizophrenia: Treatment, management, and rehabilitation.* Orlando, FL: Grune & Stratton.

Haber, J., Hoskins, P.P., Leach, A.M., & Sideleau, B.F. (1987). *Comprehensive psychiatric nursing* (3rd ed.). New York: McGraw-Hill.

Hall, L.L. (1996). The best of times, the worst of times. Unpublished remarks at symposium on schizophrenia to U.S. Congress. National Alliance for the Mentally Ill. [on line]. Available: www.schizophrenia.nami.org./schizophrenia/schizophrenia.html

Hollandsworth, J.G. (1990). *The physiology of psychological disorders.* New York: Plenum Press.

Kaplan, H.I., & Sadock, B.J. (1985). *Modern synopsis of comprehensive textbook of psychiatry* (4th ed.). Baltimore: Williams & Wilkins.

Kaplan, H.I., & Sadock, B.J. (1998). *Synopsis of psychiatry: Behavioral sciences/clinical psychiatry* (8th ed.). Baltimore: Williams & Wilkins.

Kaplan, H.I., Sadock, B.J., & Grebb, J.A. (1994). *Synopsis of psychiatry* (7th ed.). Baltimore: Williams & Wilkins.

Keith, S.J., & Matthews, S. (1984). Group psychotherapy. In A.S. Bellack (Ed.), *Schizophrenia: Treatment, management, and rehabilitation.* Orlando, FL: Grune & Stratton.

Liberman, R.P. (1970). Behavior modification with chronic mental patients. *Journal of Chronic Diseases, 23,* 803–812.

Liberman, R.P., et al. (1984). The nature and problem of schizophrenia. In A.S. Bellack (Ed.), *Schizophrenia: Treatment, management, and rehabilitation.* Orlando, FL: Grune & Stratton.

Lickey, M.E., & Gordon, B. (1983). *Drugs for mental illness: A revolution in psychiatry.* New York: W.H. Freeman.

Mahler, M., Pine, F., & Bergman, A. (1975). *The psychological birth of the human infant.* New York: Basic Books.

Pfohl, B., & Winokur, G. (1983). The micropsychopathology of hebephrenic/catatonic schizophrenia. *Journal of Nervous and Mental Disorders, 171,* 296–300.

Safier, E. (1997). Our families, the context of our lives. *Menninger Perspective, 28*(1), 4–9.

Schatzberg, A.F., & Cole, J.O. (1986). *Manual of clinical psychopharmacology.* Washington, DC: American Psychiatric Press.

Scheibel, A.B. (1991, Summer). Schizophrenia: Cells in disarray. *Journal of the California Alliance for the Mentally Ill*, 2(4), 9–10.

Stevens, J.R. (1982). Neuropathology of schizophrenia. *Archives of General Psychiatry*, 39, 1131–1139.

Strauss, J.S. (1983). The evolution of psychotherapeutic approaches for affective and schizophrenic disorders. In M.R. Zales (Ed.), *Affective and schizophrenic disorders*. New York: Brunner/Mazel.

Sullivan, H.S. (1953). *The interpersonal theory of psychiatry*. New York: W.W. Norton.

Tsuang, M.T., & Faraone, S.V. (1994). Schizophrenia. In G. Winokur & P.J. Clayton (Eds.), *The medical basis of psychiatry* (2nd ed.). Philadelphia: W.B. Saunders.

Bibliography

Altshuler, L. (1991, Summer). Neuroanatomy in schizophrenia and affective disorder. *Journal of the California Alliance for the Mentally Ill*, 2(4), 27–30.

Bailey, K.P. (1996, October). Pharmacologic agents for the treatment of schizophrenia: Similarities and differences. *Journal of the American Psychiatric Nurses Association*, 2(5), 181–185.

Bleuler, E. (1966). *Dementia praecox or the group of schizophrenias* (1908). J. Zinkin (Trans.) New York: International University Press.

Chapman, T. (1991, June). The nurse's role in neuroleptic medications. *Journal of Psychosocial Nursing*, 29(6), 6–8.

Dzurec, L.C. (1990, August). How do they see themselves? Self-perception and functioning for people with chronic schizophrenia. *Journal of Psychosocial Nursing*, 28(8), 10–14.

Feinberg, I. (1991, Summer). Synaptic pruning and the adolescent brain. *Journal of the California Alliance for the Mentally Ill*, 2(4), 22–24.

Field, W.E. (1985, January). Hearing voices. *Journal of Psychosocial Nursing*, 23(1), 8–14.

Hall, B.A. (1997, February). Looking at chronic mental illness through new trifocal lenses. *Journal of the American Psychiatric Nurses Association*, 3(1), 27–30.

Jernigan, T.L. (1991, Summer). When and why does schizophrenia develop? *Journal of the California Alliance for the Mentally Ill*, 2(4), 25–26.

Kahn, E.M. (1984, July). Psychotherapy with chronic schizophrenics. *Journal of Psychosocial Nursing*, 22(7), 20–25.

Littrell, K.H., & Freeman, L.Y. (1995, December). Maximizing psychosocial interventions. *Journal of the American Psychiatric Nurses Association*, 1(6), 214–218.

Littrell, K.H., & Littrell, S.H. (1997, February). Therapeutic efficacy of olanzapine. *Journal of the American Psychiatric Nurses Association*, 3(1), S8–S13.

Littrell, K.H., & Littrell, S.H. (1997, February). Choosing an antipsychotic in the treatment of schizophrenia: Conversions to olanzapine. *Journal of the American Psychiatric Nurses Association*, 3(1), S18–S23.

Littrell, S.H., & Littrell, K.H. (1997, August). Recent advances in the understanding of negative symptoms in schizophrenia. *Journal of the American Psychiatric Nurses Association*, 3(4), 111–117.

Malone, J.A. (1990, August). Schizophrenia research update: Implications for nursing. *Journal of Psychosocial Nursing*, 28(8), 4–9.

Mednick, S.A. (1991, Summer). Fetal neural development and adult schizophrenia. *Journal of the California Alliance for the Mentally Ill*, 2, 6–8.

Nihart, M.A. (1996, October). The neurobiology of schizophrenia. *Journal of the American Psychiatric Nurses Association*, 2(5), 174–180.

Nihart, M.A. (1997, February). Atypical antipsychotics and the pharmacology of olanzapine. *Journal of the American Psychiatric Nurses Association*, 3(1), S2–S7.

Peschel, E., & Peschel, R. (1991, Summer). Neurobiological disorders. *Journal of the California Alliance for the Mentally Ill*, 2(4), 4.

Smith, S.F., Karasik, D.A., & Meyer, B.J. (1984). *Psychiatric and psychosocial nursing*. Los Altos, CA: National Nursing Review.

Spitzer, V.M. (1995, December). Biologic aspects of schizophrenia. *Journal of the American Psychiatric Nurses Association*, 1(6), 204–207.

Stevenson, S. (1991, September). Heading off violence with verbal de-escalation. *Journal of Psychosocial Nursing*, 29(9), 6–10.

Townsend, M.C. (1997). *Nursing diagnoses in psychiatric nursing: A pocket guide for care plan construction* (4th ed.). Philadelphia: F.A. Davis.

Tugrul, K.C. (1995, December). Pharmacologic treatment of schizophrenia: A review. *Journal of the American Psychiatric Nurses Association*, 1(6), 208–213.

Tugrul, K.C., & Bennett, J.A. (1997, February). Olanzapine: Safety profile and dosing strategies. *Journal of the American Psychiatric Nurses Association*, 3(1), S14–S17.

Wirshing, W.C. (1991, Summer). Searching the brain: Trying to see neurobiological disorders. *Journal of the California Alliance for the Mentally Ill*, 2(4), 2–3.

Wirshing, W.C. (1991, Summer). Schizophrenia, neuroleptics, and brain rust: Speculations from the research fringe. *Journal of the California Alliance for the Mentally Ill*, 2(4), 31–34.

MOOD DISORDERS

KEY TERMS

mood
mania
melancholia
bipolar disorder
mourning
grief
anticipatory grieving

delayed grief
prolonged grief
exaggerated grief
dysthymic disorder
premenstrual dysphoric
    disorder
hypomania

cyclothymic disorder
bereavement overload
postpartum depression
psychomotor retardation
delirious mania
cognitive therapy
tyramine

OBJECTIVES

After reading this chapter, the student will be able to:

1. Recount historical perspectives of mood disorders.
2. Discuss epidemiological statistics related to mood disorders.
3. Differentiate between normal and maladaptive responses to loss.
4. Describe various types of mood disorders.
5. Identify predisposing factors in the development of mood disorders.
6. Discuss implications of depression related to developmental stage.
7. Identify symptomatology associated with mood disorders and use this information in client assessment.
8. Formulate nursing diagnoses and outcome criteria for clients with mood disorders.
9. Identify topics for client and family teaching relevant to mood disorders.
10. Describe appropriate nursing interventions for behaviors associated with mood disorders.
11. Describe relevant criteria for evaluating nursing care of clients with mood disorders.
12. Discuss various modalities relevant to treatment of mood disorders.

epression is likely the oldest and still one of the most frequently diagnosed psychiatric illnesses. Symptoms of depression have been described almost as far back as there is evidence of written documentation.

An occasional bout with the "blues," a feeling of sadness or downheartedness, is common among healthy people and considered to be a normal response to everyday disappointments in life. These episodes are short-lived as the individual adapts to the loss, change, or failure (real or perceived) that has been experienced. Pathological depression occurs when adaptation is ineffective.

This chapter focuses on the consequences of dysfunctional grieving, as it is manifested by mood disorders. **Mood** describes an individual's sustained emotional tone, which significantly influences behavior, personality, and perception. Mood disorders are classified as depressive or bipolar.

A historical perspective and epidemiological statistics related to mood disorders are presented here. Predisposing factors that have been implicated in the etiology of mood disorders provide a framework for studying the dynamics of depression and bipolar disorder. A discussion of the normal grief process precedes an explanation of the maladaptive response.

The implications of depression relevant to individuals of various developmental stages are discussed. An explanation of the symptomatology is presented as background knowledge for assessing the client with a mood disorder. Nursing care is described in the context of the six steps of the nursing process, and critical pathways of care are included as guidelines for use in a case management approach. Various medical treatment modalities are explored.

HISTORICAL PERSPECTIVE

Many ancient cultures (e.g., Babylonian, Egyptian, Hebrew) have believed in the supernatural or divine origin of depression and mania (Georgotas & Cancro, 1988). The Old Testament states in the Book of Samuel that King Saul's depression was inflicted by an "evil spirit" sent from God to "torment" him.

A clearly nondivine point of view regarding depressive and manic states was held by the Greek medical community from the 5th century BC through the 3rd century AD. This represented the thinking of Hippocrates, Celsus, and Galen, among others. They strongly rejected the idea of divine origin, and considered the brain as the seat of all emotional states (Georgotas & Cancro, 1988). Hippocrates believed that melancholia was caused by an excess of black bile, a heavily toxic substance produced in the spleen or intestine, which affected the brain.

During the Renaissance, several new theories evolved. Depression was viewed by some as being the result of obstruction of vital air circulation, excessive brooding, or helpless situations beyond the client's control. These

strong emotions of depression and mania were reflected in major literary works of the time, including Shakespeare's *King Lear*, *Macbeth*, and *Hamlet*.

In the 19th century, the definition of **mania** was narrowed down from the concept of total madness to that of a disorder of affect and action (Berrios, 1988). The old notion of **melancholia** was refurnished with meaning, and emphasis was placed on the primary affective nature of the disorder. Finally, an introduction was made to the possibility of an alternating pattern of affective symptomatology associated with the disorders.

Contemporary thinking has been shaped a great deal by the works of Sigmund Freud, Emil Kraepelin, and Adolf Meyer. Having evolved from these early 20th-century models, current thinking about mood disorders generally encompasses the intrapsychic, behavioral, and biological perspectives. These various perspectives support the notion of multiple causation in the development of mood disorders.

EPIDEMIOLOGY

Current estimates suggest that 10 to 14 million Americans are afflicted with some form of major affective disorder. Approximately 20 percent of the population will suffer an episode of depressive illness at least once in their lifetime; some estimates put the risk at 30 percent (Quitkin & Endicott, 1992). This preponderance has led to the consideration of depression by some researchers as "the common cold of psychiatric disorders" and this generation as an "age of melancholia."

Gender

Studies indicate that the incidence of depressive disorder is higher in women than it is in men by about 2 to 1. The incidence of **bipolar disorder** is roughly equal, with a ratio of women to men of 1.2 to 1.

Age

Several studies have shown that the incidence of depression is higher in young women and has a tendency to decrease with age. The opposite has been found in men, with the prevalence of depressive symptoms being lower in younger men and increasing with age (Boyd & Weissman, 1982). Studies suggest that the median age at onset of bipolar disorder is 18 years in men and 20 years in women (Burke, Burke, & Regier, 1990).

Social Class

Results of studies have indicated an inverse relationship between social class and report of depressive symptoms.

Bipolar disorder appears to occur more frequently among the higher social classes, especially professionals and the highly educated. (Craig, 1994).

Race

Studies have shown no consistent relationship between race and affective disorder. One problem encountered in reviewing racial comparisons has to do with the socioeconomic class of the race being investigated. Sample populations of nonwhite clients are many times predominantly lower class and are often compared with white populations from middle and upper social classes. Other studies suggest a second problematic factor in the study of racial comparisons. Clinicians tend to underdiagnose mood disorders and to overdiagnose schizophrenia in clients who have racial or cultural backgrounds different from their own (Kaplan, Sadock, & Grebb, 1994). This misdiagnosis may result from language barriers between clients and physicians who are unfamiliar with cultural aspects of nonwhite clients' language and behavior.

Marital Status

The highest incidence of depressive symptoms has been indicated in single and divorced persons (Kaplan, Sadock, & Grebb, 1994). When gender and marital status are considered together, the differences reveal lowest rates of depressive symptoms among married men, the highest by married women and single men. Kaplan, Sadock, and Grebb (1994) state, "Bipolar I disorder may be more common in divorced and single persons than among married persons, but that difference may reflect the early onset and the resulting marital discord that are characteristic of the disorder."

Seasonality

A number of studies have examined seasonal patterns associated with mood disorders. These studies have revealed two prevalent periods of seasonal involvement: one in the spring (March, April, and May) and one in the fall (September, October, and November). This pattern tends to parallel the seasonal pattern for suicide, which shows a large peak in the spring and a smaller one in October (Goodwin & Jamison, 1990).

THE GRIEF RESPONSE

Loss can be defined as "an experience in which an individual relinquishes a connection to a valued object." The *object* may be animate or inanimate, a relationship or situation, or even a change or a failure (real or perceived). Following are examples of some notable forms of loss.

1. A significant other, through death, divorce, or separation for any reason.
2. Illness or hospitalization can represent a loss for an individual caused by the many changes that may be incurred, as well as the possible fears associated with threat to physiological integrity.
3. A decrease in self-esteem can be experienced as a loss, if one is unable to meet self-expectations or the expectations of others (or even if these expectations are only *perceived* by the individual as unfulfilled).
4. Personal possessions symbolize familiarity and security in a person's life. Separation from these familiar and personally valued external objects represents a loss of material extensions of the self.

Some texts differentiate the terms **mourning** and **grief** by describing mourning as "the psychological process (or stages) through which the individual passes on the way to successful adaptation to the loss of a valued object." *Grief* is defined as "the subjective states that accompany mourning, or the emotional work involved in the mourning process." For purposes of this text, grief work and the process of mourning are collectively referred to as the *grief response*.

Stages of Grief

Behavior patterns associated with the grief response include many individual variations. However, sufficient similarities have been observed to warrant characterization of grief as a syndrome that has a predictable course with an expected resolution (Kaplan & Sadock, 1985). A number of theorists, including Kübler-Ross (1969), Bowlby (1961), and Engel (1964), have described behavioral stages through which individuals advance in their progression toward resolution. A number of variables influence one's progression through the grief process. Some individuals may reach acceptance, only to revert back to an earlier stage; some may never complete the sequence; and indeed, some may never progress beyond the initial stage. A comparison of the similarities among these three models is presented in Table 26.1.

Elisabeth Kübler-Ross

These well-known stages of the grief process were identified by Kübler-Ross in her extensive work with dying patients. Behaviors associated with each of these stages can be observed in individuals experiencing the loss of any object of personal value.

Stage I: Denial. In this stage the individual does not acknowledge that the loss has occurred. He or she may say "No, it can't be true!" or "It's just not possible." This stage may protect the individual against the psychological pain of reality.

TABLE 26.1 STAGES OF THE NORMAL GRIEF RESPONSE

A COMPARISON OF MODELS BY ELISABETH KÜBLER-ROSS, JOHN BOWLBY, AND GEORGE ENGEL

| STAGES | | | POSSIBLE TIME | |
KÜBLER-ROSS	BOWLBY	ENGEL	DIMENSION	BEHAVIORS
I. Denial	I. Numbness/Protest	I. Shock/Disbelief	Occurs immediately upon experiencing the loss. Usually lasts no more than 2 wk.	Individual refuses to acknowledge that the loss has occurred.
II. Anger	II. Disequilibrium	II. Developing awareness	In most cases begins within hours of the loss. Peaks within 2 to 4 wk.	Anger is directed toward self or others. Ambivalence and guilt may be felt toward the lost object.
III. Bargaining				The individual fervently seeks alternatives to improve current situation.
		III. Restitution		Attends to various rituals associated with the culture in which the loss has occurred.
IV. Depression	III. Disorganization and despair	IV. Resolution of the loss	A year or more.	The actual work of grieving. Preoccupation with the lost object. Feelings of helplessness and loneliness occur in response to realization of the loss. Feelings associated with the loss are confronted.
V. Acceptance	IV. Reorganization	V. Recovery		Resolution is complete. The bereaved person experiences a reinvestment in new relationships and new goals. Terminally ill persons express a readiness to die.

Stage II: Anger. This is the stage when reality sets in. Feelings associated with this stage include sadness, guilt, shame, helplessness, and hopelessness. Self-blame or blaming of others may lead to feelings of anger toward self and others. The anxiety level may be elevated, and the individual may experience confusion and a decreased ability to function independently. He or she may be preoccupied with an idealized image of the lost object. Numerous somatic complaints are common.

Stage III: Bargaining. At this stage in the grief response, the individual attempts to strike a bargain with God for a second chance, or for more time. The person acknowledges the loss, or impending loss, but holds out hope for additional alternatives, as evidenced by statements such as, "If only I could. . . ." or "If only I had. . . ."

Stage IV: Depression. In this stage, the individual mourns for that which has been or will be lost. This is a very painful stage during which the individual must confront feelings associated with having lost an object of value (called *reactive* depression). An example might be the individual who is mourning a change in body image. Feelings associated with an impending loss (called *preparatory* depression) are also confronted. Examples include permanent lifestyle changes related to the altered body image or even an impending loss of life itself. Regression, withdrawal, and social isolation may be observed behaviors with this stage. Therapeutic intervention should be available, but not imposed, and with guidelines for implementation based on client readiness.

Stage V: Acceptance. At this time, the individual has worked through the behaviors associated with the other stages and either accepts or is resigned to the loss. Anxiety decreases, and methods for coping without the lost object have been established. The client is less preoccupied with what has been lost and increasingly interested in other aspects of the environment. If this is an impending death of self, the individual is ready to die. The person may become very quiet and withdrawn, seemingly devoid of feelings. These behaviors are an attempt to facilitate the passage by slowly disengaging from the environment.

John Bowlby

John Bowlby hypothesized four stages in the grief process. He implies that these behaviors can be observed in all individuals who have experienced the loss of a valued object, even in babies as young as 6 months of age (Bowlby, 1973).

Stage I: Numbness or Protest. This stage is characterized by a feeling of shock and disbelief that the loss has occurred. Reality of the loss is not acknowledged.

Stage II: Disequilibrium. During this stage, the individual has a profound urge to recover the lost object. Behaviors associated with this stage include a preoccupation with the lost object, intense weeping and expressions of anger toward self and others, and feelings of ambivalence and guilt toward the lost object.

Stage III: Disorganization and Despair. Feelings of despair occur in response to realization that the loss has occurred. Activities of daily living become increasingly disorganized, and behavior is characterized by restlessness and aimlessness. Efforts to regain productive patterns of behavior are ineffective and the individual experiences fear, helplessness, and hopelessness. Somatic complaints are common. Perceptions of visualizing or being in the presence of the lost object may occur. Social isolation is common and the individual may feel a great deal of loneliness.

Stage IV: Reorganization. The individual accepts or becomes resigned to the loss. New goals and patterns of organization are established. The individual begins a reinvestment in new relationships and indicates a readiness to move forward within the environment. Grief subsides and recedes into valued remembrances.

George Engel

Stage I: Shock and Disbelief. The initial reaction to a loss is a stunned, numb feeling and refusal by the individual to acknowledge the reality of the loss. Engel (1964) states that this stage is an attempt on the part of the individual to protect the self "against the effects of the overwhelming stress by raising the threshold against its recognition or against the painful feelings evoked thereby."

Stage II: Developing Awareness. This stage begins within minutes to hours of the loss. Behaviors associated with this stage include excessive crying and regression to a state of helplessness and a childlike manner. Awareness of the loss creates feelings of emptiness, frustration, anguish, and despair. Anger may be directed toward the self or toward others in the environment who are held accountable for the loss.

Stage II: Restitution. In this stage, the various rituals associated with loss within a culture are performed. Examples include funerals, wakes, special attire, a gathering of friends and family, and religious practices customary to the spiritual beliefs of the bereaved. Participation in these rituals is thought to assist the individual to accept the reality of the loss and to facilitate the recovery process.

Stage IV: Resolution of the Loss. This stage is characterized by a preoccupation with the lost object. The concept of the lost object is idealized, and the individual may even imitate admired qualities of that which has been lost. Preoccupation with the lost object gradually decreases over a year or more, and the individual eventually begins to reinvest feelings in others.

Stage V: Recovery. Obsession with the lost object has ended, and the individual is able to go on with his or her life.

Length of the Grief Process

Stages of grief allow bereaved persons an orderly approach to the resolution of mourning. Each stage presents tasks that must be overcome through a painful experiential process. Engel (1964) has stated that successful resolution of the grief response is thought to have occurred when a bereaved individual is able "to remember comfortably and realistically both the pleasures and disappointments of the lost [object]." Length of the grief process is exceedingly individual and can last for a number of years without being maladaptive. The acute phase of normal grieving usually lasts 6 to 8 weeks—longer in older adults—but complete resolution of the grief response may take much longer.

Kaplan, Sadock, and Grebb (1994) state:

> "Traditionally, grief lasts about six months to one year, as the grieving person experiences the calendar year at least once without the lost person. Some signs and symptoms of grief may persist much longer than one or two years, and a survivor may have various grief-related feelings, symptoms, and behavior throughout life. In general, the acute grief symptoms gradually lessen, and within one or two months the grieving person is able to eat, sleep, and return to functioning." (p. 82)

Smith, Karasik, and Meyer, (1984) have identified the following factors that influence the eventual outcome of the grief response:

1. The importance of the lost object as a source of support.
2. The degree of dependence on the relationship with the lost object. The greater the degree of dependency, the more difficult is the task of resolution.
3. The degree of ambivalence felt toward the lost object. A love-hate relationship may instill feelings of guilt that can interfere with the grief work.
4. The number and nature of other meaningful relationships the mourner has. Letting go of the attachment to the lost object is facilitated by support from significant others.

5. The number and nature of previous grief experiences. Grief is cumulative, and if previous losses have not been resolved, each succeeding grief response becomes more difficult.
6. The age of a lost person is influential. The loss of a child usually has a more profound effect on the survivor than that of an elderly parent.
7. Health of the mourner at the time of loss. The state of one's physical and psychological condition influences the capacity to cope with stress of the loss.
8. The degree of preparation for the loss. The experience of *anticipatory grieving* is thought to facilitate the grief response that occurs at the time of the actual loss.

Anticipatory Grief

Anticipatory grieving is the initiation and actual process of grieving that takes place when anticipating a significant loss, before it actually takes place (Thompson et al., 1986). In anticipatory grieving, the stages of grief and the feelings and behaviors associated with them are very similar to those experienced in normal grieving. One dissimilar aspect relates to the fact that conventional grief tends to diminish in intensity with the passage of time. Conversely, anticipatory grief may increase in intensity as the expected loss becomes more imminent.

Although anticipatory grief is thought to facilitate the actual mourning process following the loss, there may be some problems. In the case of a dying person, difficulties can arise when the family members complete the process of anticipatory grief and detachment from the dying person occurs prematurely. Feelings of loneliness and isolation are experienced by the dying person as the psychological pain of imminent death is faced without family support. Another example of difficulties associated with premature completion of the grief response is described by Kaplan, Sadock, and Grebb (1994):

> "Once anticipatory grief has been expended, the bereaved person may find it difficult to reestablish the prior relationship. That phenomenon is experienced with the return of persons long gone (for example, in combat or concentration camps) and of persons thought to have been dead." (p. 82)

Anticipatory grieving may serve as a defense for some individuals to ease the burden of loss when it actually occurs. It may prove to be less functional for others who, because of interpersonal, psychological, or sociocultural variables, are unable in advance of the actual loss to express the intense feelings that accompany the grief response.

MALADAPTIVE RESPONSES TO LOSS

When, then, is the grieving response considered to be maladaptive? Lindemann (1944) described two types of pathological grief reactions: the delayed reaction and the distorted (or exaggerated) reaction. Most theorists agree that resolution has failed to occur when the grief process has been delayed, inhibited, prolonged, or exaggerated.

Delayed or Inhibited Grief

Delayed or inhibited grief refers to the absence of evidence of grief when it ordinarily would be expected (Kaplan, Sadock, & Grebb, 1994). Many times, cultural influences, such as the expectation to keep a "stiff upper lip," cause the delayed response.

Delayed or inhibited grief is potentially pathological because the person is simply not dealing with the reality of the loss. He or she remains fixed in the denial stage of the grief process, sometimes for many years. When this occurs, the grief response may be triggered, sometimes many years later, when the individual experiences a subsequent loss. Sometimes the grief process is triggered spontaneously or in response to a seemingly insignificant event. Overreaction to another person's loss may be one manifestation of delayed grief.

The recognition of **delayed grief** is critical because, depending on the profoundness of the loss, the failure of the mourning process may prevent assimilation of the loss and thereby delay a return to satisfying living (Ruark & Gonda, 1988). Delayed grieving most commonly occurs because of ambivalent feelings toward the lost object, outside pressure to resume normal function, or perceived lack of internal and external resources to cope with a profound loss.

Prolonged Grief

The grief response is considered to be pathologically prolonged if there has been no resumption of normal activities of daily living within 4 to 8 weeks of a loss (Ruark & Gonda, 1988). The **prolonged grief** pattern has been associated with self-blame on the part of the bereaved, difficulty accepting the loss, sudden and untimely loss, and a history of a dependent relationship with the one who has died (Parkes, 1975).

Stories abound in the literature of bereaved individuals who establish shrines to their dead and conduct rituals that perpetuate the grieving process. Other evidences of prolonged grief may include an intensification, rather than diminishment, of the behaviors associated with normal grieving; development of physical symptoms similar to those experienced by the deceased person before death; progressive social isolation and interrupted interpersonal relationships with friends and relatives; and participation in activities that are detrimental to one's social or economic existence (Shives, 1990).

Exaggerated Grief Response

Lindemann (1944) described a distorted grief reaction in which all of the symptoms associated with normal grieving are exaggerated. Feelings of sadness, helplessness, hopelessness, powerlessness, anger, and guilt as well as numerous somatic complaints render the individual dysfunctional in terms of management of daily living. Horowitz and associates (1980) describe an **exaggerated grief** reaction as:

"... the intensification of grief to the level where the person is overwhelmed, resorts to maladaptive behavior, or remains interminably in the state of grief without progression of the mourning process toward completion."

When the exaggerated grief reaction occurs, the individual remains fixed in the anger stage of the grief response. This anger may be directed toward others in the environment to whom the individual may be attributing the loss. However, many times the anger is turned inward on the self. When this occurs, depression is the result. Depressive mood disorder is a type of exaggerated grief reaction.

Normal versus Maladaptive Grieving

Several authors have identified one crucial difference between normal and maladaptive grieving: the loss of self-esteem. Henderson and Nite (1978) state, "The loss of self-esteem that almost invariably occurs in depression is not present with normal grief." Eisendrath (1996) affirms, "Grief is usually accompanied by intact self-esteem, whereas depression is marked by a sense of guilt and worthlessness."

Becker (1964) also expounds on this major difference between normal grieving and a maladaptive response (depression): "It is the threat to self-esteem, or the threat of reduction in self-esteem, which ultimately precipitates the depression."

TYPES OF MOOD DISORDERS

The *DSM-IV* (American Psychiatric Association [APA], 1994) describes the essential feature of these disorders as a disturbance of mood, characterized by a full or partial manic or depressive syndrome, that cannot be attributed to another mental disorder. Mood disorders are classified under two major categories: depressive disorders and bipolar disorders.

Depressive Disorders

Major Depressive Disorder

This disorder is characterized by depressed mood or loss of interest or pleasure in usual activities. Evidence of im-

paired social and occupational functioning has existed for at least 2 weeks. There is no history of manic behavior and the symptoms cannot be attributed to use of substances or a general medical condition.

Major depressive disorder may be further classified as follows:

1. **Single Episode or Recurrent.** A *single episode* specifier is used for an individual's first diagnosis of depression. *Recurrent* is specified when the history reveals two or more episodes of depression.
2. **Mild, Moderate, or Severe.** These categories are identified by the number and severity of symptoms.
3. **With Psychotic Features.** The impairment of reality testing is evident. The individual experiences delusions or hallucinations.
4. **With Melancholic Features.** This is a typically severe form of major depressive episode. Symptoms are exaggerated. Even temporary reactivity to usually pleasurable stimuli is absent. History reveals a good response to antidepressant or other somatic therapy.
5. **Chronic.** This classification applies when the current episode of depressed mood has been evident continuously for at least the past 2 years.
6. **With Seasonal Pattern.** This diagnosis indicates the presence of depressive symptoms during the fall or winter months. This diagnosis is made when the number of seasonal depressive episodes substantially outnumber the nonseasonal depressive episodes that have occurred over the individual's lifetime (APA, 1994). This disorder has previously been identified in the literature as seasonal affective disorder (SAD).
7. **With Postpartum Onset.** This specifier is used when symptoms of major depression occur within 4 weeks postpartum.

The *DSM-IV* diagnostic criteria for major depressive disorder are presented in Table 26.2.

Dysthymic Disorder

Characteristics of this mood disturbance are similar to, if somewhat milder than, those ascribed to major depressive disorder. Individuals with **dysthymic disorder** describe their mood as sad or "down in the dumps" (APA, 1994). There is no evidence of psychotic symptoms. The essential feature is a chronically depressed mood (or possibly an irritable mood in children or adolescents) for most of the day, more days than not, for at least 2 years (1 year for children and adolescents).

Dysthymic disorder may be further classified as:

1. **Early Onset.** Identifies cases of dysthymic disorder when the onset occurs before age 21 years.

TABLE 26.2 DIAGNOSTIC CRITERIA FOR MAJOR DEPRESSIVE DISORDER

A. Five (or more) of the following symptoms have been present during the same 2-week period and represent a change from previous functioning; at least one of the symptoms is either (1) depressed mood, or (2) loss of interest or pleasure.

    1. Depressed mood most of the day, nearly every day, as indicated by either subjective report (e.g., feels sad or empty) or observation made by others (e.g., appears tearful). Note: In children and adolescents, can be irritable mood.

    2. Markedly diminished interest or pleasure in all, or almost all, activities most of the day, nearly every day (as indicated either by subjective account or observation made by others).

    3. Significant weight loss when not dieting or weight gain (e.g., a change of more than 5% of body weight in a month), or a decrease or increase in appetite nearly every day.

       NOTE: In children, consider failure to make expected weight gains.

    4. Insomnia or hypersomnia nearly every day.

    5. Psychomotor agitation or retardation nearly every day (observable by others, not merely subjective feelings of restlessness or being slowed down).

    6. Fatigue or loss of energy nearly every day.

    7. Feelings of worthlessness or excessive or inappropriate guilt (which may be delusional) nearly every day (not merely self-reproach or guilt about being sick).

    8. Diminished ability to think or concentrate, or indecisiveness, nearly every day (either by subjective account or as observed by others).

    9. Recurrent thoughts of death (not just fear of dying), recurrent suicidal ideation without a specific plan, or a suicide attempt or a specific plan for committing suicide.

B. There has never been a manic episode, a mixed episode, or a hypomanic episode that was not substance or treatment induced or due to the direct physiological effects of a general medical condition.

C. The symptoms cause clinically significant distress or impairment in social, occupational, or other important areas of functioning.

D. The symptoms are not due to the direct physiological effects of a substance (e.g., a drug of abuse, a medication) or a general medical condition (e.g., hypothyroidism).

E. The symptoms are not better accounted for by bereavement (i.e., after the loss of a loved one, the symptoms persist for longer than 2 months or are characterized by marked functional impairment, morbid preoccupation with worthlessness, suicidal ideation, psychotic symptoms, or psychomotor retardation).

SOURCE: APA (1994), with permission.

    2. **Late Onset.** Identifies cases of dysthymic disorder when the onset occurs at age 21 years or older.

The *DSM-IV* diagnostic criteria for dysthymic disorder are presented in Table 26.3.

Premenstrual Dysphoric Disorder

The *DSM-IV* (APA, 1994) does not include this disorder as an official diagnostic category but provides a set of research criteria to promote further study of the disorder. The essential features include markedly depressed mood, marked anxiety, mood swings, and decreased interest in activities during the week prior to menses and subsiding shortly after the onset of menstruation (APA, 1994). The *DSM-IV* research criteria for **premenstrual dysphoric disorder** are presented in Table 26.4.

Bipolar Disorders

Bipolar disorders are characterized by mood swings from profound depression to extreme euphoria (mania), with intervening periods of normalcy. Delusions or hallucinations may or may not be a part of the clinical picture, and onset of symptoms may reflect a seasonal pattern.

During a manic episode, the mood is elevated, expansive, or irritable. The disturbance is sufficiently severe to cause marked impairment in occupational functioning or in usual social activities or relationships with others, or to require hospitalization to prevent harm to self or others. Motor activity is excessive and frenzied. Psychotic features may be present. A somewhat milder degree of this clinical symptom picture is called **hypomania.** Hypomania is not severe enough to cause marked impairment in social or occupational functioning or to require hospitalization, and it does not include psychotic features. The DSM-IV diagnostic criteria for mania are presented in Table 26.5.

The diagnostic picture for depression associated with bipolar disorder is identical to that described for major depressive disorder, with one addition. The client must have a history of one or more manic episodes.

When the symptom presentation includes rapidly alternating moods (sadness, irritability, euphoria) accompanied by symptoms associated with both depression and mania, the individual is given a diagnosis of *bipolar disorder, mixed.* This disturbance is severe enough to cause marked impairment in social or occupational functioning or to require hospitalization. Psychotic features may be evident.

TABLE 26.3 DIAGNOSTIC CRITERIA FOR DYSTHYMIC DISORDER

A. Depressed mood for most of the day, more days than not, as indicated either by subjective account or observation by others, for at least 2 years. Note: In children and adolescents, mood can be irritable and duration must be at least 1 year.

B. Presence, while depressed, of two (or more) of the following:
 1. Poor appetite or overeating.
 2. Insomnia or hypersomnia.
 3. Low energy or fatigue.
 4. Low self-esteem.
 5. Poor concentration or difficulty making decisions.
 6. Feelings of hopelessness.

C. During the 2-year period (1 year for children or adolescents) of the disturbance, the person has never been without the symptoms in A and B for more than 2 months at a time.

D. No major depressive disorder has been present during the first 2 years of the disturbance (1 year for children and adolescents).

E. There has never been a manic, mixed or hypomanic episode, and criteria have never been met for cyclothymic disorder.

F. The disturbance does not occur exclusively during the course of a chronic psychotic disorder, such as schizophrenia or delusional disorder.

G. The symptoms are not due to the direct physiological effects of a substance (e.g., a drug of abuse, a medication) or a general medical condition (e.g., hypothyroidism).

H. The symptoms cause clinically significant distress or impairment in social, occupational, or other important areas of functioning.

Specify if:
 Early onset: Before age 21 years.
 Late onset: Age 21 years or older.

SOURCE: APA (1994), with permission.

Bipolar I Disorder

Bipolar I disorder is the diagnosis given to an individual who is experiencing, or has experienced, a full syndrome of manic or mixed symptoms. The client may also have experienced episodes of depression. This diagnosis is further specified by the current or most recent behavioral episode experienced. For example, the specifier might be single manic episode (to describe individuals having a first episode of mania) or current (or most recent) episode manic, hypomanic, mixed, or depressed (to describe individuals who have had recurrent mood episodes). This diagnosis is synonymous with what was called bipolar disorder in the *DSM-III-R*.

Bipolar II Disorder

This diagnostic category is characterized by recurrent bouts of major depression with the episodic occurrence of hypomania. The individual who is assigned this diagnosis may

TABLE 26.4 RESEARCH CRITERIA FOR PREMENSTRUAL DYSPHORIC DISORDER

A. In most menstrual cycles during the past year, five (or more) of the following symptoms were present for most of the time during the last week of the luteal phase, began to remit within a few days after the onset of the follicular phase, and were absent in the week postmenses, with at least one of the symptoms being 1, 2, 3, or 4:
 1. Markedly depressed mood, feelings of hopelessness, or self-deprecating thoughts.
 2. Marked anxiety, tension, feelings of being "keyed up," or "on edge."
 3. Marked affective lability (e.g., feeling suddenly sad or tearful or increased sensitivity to rejection).
 4. Persistent and marked anger or irritability or increased interpersonal conflicts.
 5. Decreased interest in usual activities (e.g., work, school, friends, hobbies).
 6. Subjective sense of difficulty in concentrating.
 7. Lethargy, easy fatigability, or marked lack of energy.
 8. Marked change in appetite, overeating, or specific food cravings.
 9. Hypersomnia or insomnia.
 10. A subjective sense of being overwhelmed or out of control.
 11. Other physical symptoms, such as breast tenderness or swelling, headaches, joint or muscle pain, a sensation of "bloating," weight gain.

B. The disturbance markedly interferes with work or school or with usual social activities and relationships with others (e.g., avoidance of social activities, decreased productivity and efficiency at work or school).

C. The disturbance is not merely an exacerbation of the symptoms of another disorder, such as major depressive disorder, panic disorder, dysthymic disorder, or a personality disorder (although it may be superimposed on any of these disorders).

D. Criteria A, B, and C must be confirmed by prospective daily ratings during at least two consecutive symptomatic cycles.

SOURCE: APA (1994), with permission.

TABLE 26.5　DIAGNOSTIC CRITERIA FOR MANIC EPISODE

A. A distinct period of abnormally and persistently elevated, expansive, or irritable mood, lasting 1 wk (or any duration if hospitalization is necessary).

B. During the period of mood disturbance, three (or more) of the following symptoms have persisted (four if the mood is only irritable) and have been present to a significant degree:
   1. Inflated self-esteem or grandiosity.
   2. Decreased need for sleep (e.g., feels rested after only 3 hours of sleep).
   3. More talkative than usual or pressure to keep talking.
   4. Flight of ideas or subjective experience that thoughts are racing.
   5. Distractibility (i.e., attention too easily drawn to unimportant or irrelevant external stimuli).
   6. Increase in goal-directed activity (either socially, at work or school, or sexually) or psychomotor agitation.
   7. Excessive involvement in pleasurable activities that have a high potential for painful consequences (e.g., engaging in unrestrained buying sprees, sexual indiscretions, or foolish business investments).

C. The mood disturbance is sufficiently severe to cause marked impairment in occupational functioning or in usual social activities or relationships with others, or to necessitate hospitalization to prevent harm to self or others, or there are psychotic features.

D. The symptoms are not due to the direct physiological effects of a substance (e.g., a drug of abuse, a medication, or other treatment) or a general medical condition (e.g., hyperthyroidism).

SOURCE: APA (1994), with permission.

present with symptoms (or history) of depression or hypomania. The client has never experienced an episode that meets the full criteria for mania or mixed symptomatology. Bipolar II disorder is a new diagnosis in the *DSM-IV*.

Cyclothymic Disorder

The essential feature of this disorder is a chronic mood disturbance of at least 2 years' duration, involving numerous episodes of hypomania and depressed mood of insufficient severity or duration to meet the criteria for either bipolar I or II disorder. The individual is never without hypomanic or depressive symptoms for more than 2 months. The *DSM-IV* criteria for **cyclothymic disorder** are presented in Table 26.6.

Other Mood Disorders

Mood Disorder Due to a General Medical Condition

This disorder is characterized by a prominent and persistent disturbance in mood that is judged to be the result of direct physiological effects of a general medical condition (APA, 1994). The mood disturbance may involve depression or elevated, expansive, or irritable mood, and causes clinically significant distress or impairment in social, occupational, or other important areas of functioning. Types of physiological influences are included in the discussion of predisposing factors to mood disorders.

Substance-Induced Mood Disorder

The disturbance of mood associated with this disorder is considered to be the direct result of physiological effects of a substance (e.g., a drug of abuse, a medication, or toxin exposure). The mood disturbance may involve depression or elevated, expansive, or irritable mood, and causes clinically significant distress or impairment in social, occupational, or other important areas of functioning.

Mood disturbances are associated with *intoxication* from substances such as alcohol, amphetamines, cocaine, hallucinogens, inhalants, opioids, phencyclidine, sedatives, hypnotics, and anxiolytics. Symptoms can occur with *withdrawal* from substances such as alcohol, amphetamines, cocaine, sedatives, hypnotics, and anxiolytics. Heavy met-

TABLE 26.6　DIAGNOSTIC CRITERIA FOR CYCLOTHYMIC DISORDER

A. For at least 2 years, the presence of numerous periods with hypomanic symptoms and numerous periods with depressive symptoms that do not meet the criteria for major depressive disorder.
   NOTE: In children and adolescents, the duration must be at least 1 year.

B. During the 2-year period (1 year in children and adolescents), the person has not been without the symptoms in criterion A for more than 2 months at a time.

C. No major depressive episode, manic episode, or mixed episode has been present during the first 2 years of the disturbance.

D. The symptoms in criterion A are not better accounted for by schizoaffective disorder and are not superimposed on schizophrenia, schizophreniform disorder, delusional disorder, or psychotic disorder not otherwise specified.

E. The symptoms are not due to the direct physiological effects of a substance (e.g., a drug of abuse, a medication) or a general medical condition (e.g., hyperthyroidism).

F. The symptoms cause clinically significant distress or impairment in social, occupational, or other important areas of functioning.

SOURCE: APA (1994), with permission.

als and toxins, such as gasoline, paint, organophosphate insecticides, nerve gases, carbon monoxide, and carbon dioxide, may also cause mood symptoms (APA, 1994).

A number of medications have been known to evoke mood symptoms. Classifications include anesthetics, analgesics, anticholinergics, anticonvulsants, antihypertensives, antiparkinsonian agents, antiulcer agents, cardiac medications, oral contraceptives, psychotropic medications, muscle relaxants, steroids, and sulfonamides. Some specific examples are included in the discussion of predisposing factors to mood disorders.

DEPRESSIVE DISORDERS

Predisposing Factors

Biological Theories

Genetics. Affective illness has been the subject of considerable research on the relevance of hereditary factors. A genetic link has been suggested in numerous studies; however, no definitive mode of genetic transmission has yet to be demonstrated.

Twin Studies. Twin studies suggest a genetic factor in the illness, as about 65 percent of monozygotic twins are concordant for the illness, concordant referring to twins who are both affected with the illness. Similar results were revealed in studies of monozygotic twins raised apart. The concordance rate in dizygotic twins is 10 to 25 percent. (Kaplan, Sadock, & Grebb, 1994).

Family Studies. Most family studies have shown that major depression is 1.5 to 3 times more common among first-degree biological relatives of people with the disorder than among the general population (APA, 1994). Indeed, the evidence to support an increased risk of depressive disorder in individuals with positive family history is quite compelling. It is unlikely that random environmental factors could cause the concentration of illness that is seen within families.

Adoption Studies. Further support for heritability as an etiological influence in depression comes from studies of the adopted offspring of affectively ill biological parents. Kaplan, Sadock, and Grebb (1994) state, "Studies have found that the biological children of affected parents remain at increased risk of a mood disorder, even if they are reared in nonaffected, adoptive families."

Biochemical Influences

Biogenic Amines. It has been hypothesized that depressive illness may be related to a deficiency of the neurotransmitters norepinepherine, serotonin, and dopamine at functionally important receptor sites in the brain (Janowsky et al., 1988). Historically, the biogenic amine hypothesis of mood disorders grew out of the observation that reserpine, which depletes the brain of amines, was associated with the development of a depressive syndrome (Winokur, 1994). The catecholamine norepinephrine has been identified as a key component in the mobilization of the body to deal with stressful situations. Neurons that contain serotonin are critically involved in the regulation of such diverse functions as sleep, temperature, pain sensitivity, appetite, locomotor activity, neuroendocrine secretions, and mood (Janowsky et al., 1988). Tryptophan, the amino acid precursor of serotonin, has been shown to enhance the efficacy of antidepressant medications and, on occasion, to be effective as an antidepressant itself. The level of dopamine in the mesolimbic system of the brain is thought to exert a strong influence over human mood and behavior. A diminished supply of these biogenic amines inhibits the transmission of impulses from one neuronal fiber to another, causing a failure of the cells to fire or become charged.

More recently, the biogenic amine hypothesis has been expanded to include another neurotransmitter, acetylcholine. Because cholinergic agents do have profound effects on mood, electroencephalogram (EEG), sleep, and neuroendocrine function, it has been suggested that the problem in depression and mania may be an imbalance between the biogenic amines and acetylcholine (Hollandsworth, 1990).

The precise role that any of the neurotransmitters plays in the etiology of depression is unknown. As the body of research grows, there is no doubt that increased knowledge regarding the biogenic amines will contribute to a greater capacity for understanding and treating affective illness.

Neuroendocrine Disturbances. Neuroendocrine disturbances may play a role in the pathogenesis or persistence of depressive illness. This notion has arisen in view of the marked disturbances in mood observed with the administration of certain hormones or in the presence of spontaneously occurring endocrine disease (Stokes, 1988).

Hypothalamic-Pituitary-Adrenocortical Axis. In clients who are depressed, the normal system of hormonal inhibition fails, resulting in a hypersecretion of cortisol. This elevated serum cortisol is the basis for the dexamethasone suppression test that is sometimes used to determine if an individual has somatically treatable depression.

Hypothalamic-Pituitary-Thyroid Axis. Thyrotropin-releasing factor (TRF) from the hypothalamus stimulates the release of thyroid-stimulating hormone (TSH) from the anterior pituitary gland. In turn, TSH stimulates the thyroid gland. Diminished TSH response to administered TRF is observed in approximately 25 percent of depressed persons. This laboratory test has future potential for identifying clients at high risk for affective illness.

Physiological Influences. Depressive symptoms that occur as a consequence of a nonmood disorder or as an adverse effect of certain medications are called a *secondary* depression. Secondary depression may be related to medication side effects, neurological disorders, electrolyte or hormonal disturbances, nutritional deficiencies, and other physiological or psychological conditions.

Medication Side Effects. A number of drugs, either alone or in combination with other medications, can produce a depressive syndrome. Most common among these drugs are those that have a direct effect on the central nervous system. Examples of these include the anxiolytics, antipsychotics, and sedative-hypnotics. Certain antihypertensive medications, such as propranolol and reserpine, have been known to produce depressive symptoms. Depressed mood may also occur with any of the following medications (Hollandsworth, 1990):

Antiparkinsonians: levodopa, amantadine
Hormones: estrogen, progesterone
Corticosteroids: cortisone
Antituberculars: cyloserine
Antineoplastics: vincristine, vinblastine
Antiulcers: cimetidine

Neurological Disorders. An individual who has suffered a cardiovascular accident (CVA) may experience a despondency unrelated to the severity of the CVA. These are true mood disorders, and antidepressant drug therapy may be indicated. Brain tumors, particularly in the area of the temporal lobe, often cause symptoms of depression. Agitated depression may be part of the clinical picture associated with Alzheimer's disease, Parkinson's disease, and Huntington's disease. Agitation and restlessness may also represent an underlying depression in the individual with multiple sclerosis.

Electrolyte Disturbances. Excessive levels of sodium bicarbonate or calcium can produce symptoms of depression, as can deficits in magnesium and sodium. Potassium is also implicated in the syndrome of depression. Symptoms have been observed with excesses of potassium in the body, as well as in instances of potassium depletion.

Hormonal Disturbances. Depression is associated with dysfunction of the adrenal cortex and is commonly observed in both Addison's disease and Cushing's syndrome. Other endocrine conditions that may result in symptoms of depression include hypoparathyroidism, hyperparathyroidism, hypothyroidism, and hyperthyroidism.

An imbalance of the hormones estrogen and progesterone has been implicated in the predisposition to premenstrual dysphoric disorder. It is postulated that excess estrogen or a high estrogen-to-progesterone ratio during the luteal phase causes water retention and that this hormonal imbalance has other effects as well, resulting in the symptoms associated with premenstrual syndrome (Kaplan, Sadock, & Grebb, 1994).

Nutritional Deficiencies. Deficiencies in vitamin B_1 (thiamine), vitamin B_6 (pyridoxine), vitamin B_{12}, niacin, vitamin C, iron, folic acid, zinc, and protein may produce symptoms of depression (Field, 1985; Hollandsworth, 1990).

A number of nutritional alterations have also been implicated in the etiology of premenstrual dysphoric disor-

der (Casey & Dwyer, 1987). They include vitamin B_6 deficiency, glucose tolerance fluctuations, abnormal fatty acid metabolism, magnesium deficiency, vitamin E deficiency, and caffeine sensitivity. No definitive evidence exists to support any specific nutritional alteration in the etiology of these symptoms.

Other Physiological Conditions. Other conditions that have been associated with secondary depression include collagen disorders, such as systemic lupus erythematosus (SLE) and polyarteritis nodosa; cardiovascular disease, such as cardiomyopathy, congestive heart failure, and myocardial infarction; infections, such as encephalitis, hepatitis, mononucleosis, pneumonia, and syphilis; and metabolic disorders, such as diabetes mellitus and porphyria.

Psychosocial Theories

Psychoanalytical Theories. Freud (1957) presented his classic paper "Mourning and Melancholia" in 1917. He defined the distinguishing features of melancholia as:

"... a profoundly painful dejection, cessation of interest in the outside world, loss of the capacity to love, inhibition of all activity, and a lowering of the self-regarding feelings to a degree that finds utterances in self-reproaches and self-revilings, and culminates in a delusional expectation of punishment."

He observed that melancholia occurs after the loss of a loved object, either actually by death or emotionally by rejection, or the loss of some other abstraction of value to the individual. Freud indicated that in melancholia, the depressed patient's rage is internally directed because of identification with the lost object (Kaplan, Sadock, & Grebb, 1994).

Freud believed that the individual predisposed to melancholia experienced ambivalence in love relationships. He postulated, therefore, that once the loss had been incorporated into the self (ego), the hostile part of the ambivalence that had been felt for the lost object is then turned inward against the ego.

Klein (1948) viewed the predisposition to depression as stemming from the quality of the mother-infant relationship. She postulated that the "depressive position" occurred as a normal stage in development when the child began to realize that whole love objects were composed of both "good" and "bad" parts. At this point the child is aware of his or her own ambivalence in relationships with others. However, until the child is able to integrate these feelings and become confident of the mother's love, each disappointment, each frustration, each separation is interpreted as the loss of a good object. These losses are related to the child's own destructive fantasies and are accompanied by feelings of sadness, guilt, and regret. Klein believed that children who never received sufficient love to achieve a sense of security from the mothering figure were always predisposed to return to the depressive position: to feelings of loss, sadness, guilt, and low self-esteem. In other words, they become particularly vulnerable to depressive episodes throughout their life.

Learning Theory. The model of "learned helplessness" arises out of Seligman's (1973) experiments with dogs. The animals were exposed to electrical stimulation from which they could not escape. Later, when they were given the opportunity to avoid the traumatic experience, they reacted with helplessness and made no attempt to escape. A similar state of helplessness exists in humans who have experienced numerous failures (either real or perceived). The individual abandons any further attempt to succeed. Seligman theorized that learned helplessness predisposes individuals to depression by imposing a feeling of lack of control over their life situation. McKinney and Moran (1982) state:

> "Negative expectations about the effectiveness of one's own efforts in bringing about the control of one's own environment leads to passivity and diminished initiation of responses."

Object Loss Theory. The theory of object loss (Bowlby, 1973) suggests that depressive illness occurs if the person is abandoned by, or otherwise separated from, a significant other during the first 6 months of life. Because during this period the mother represents the child's main source of security, she is the "object." This absence of attachment, which may be either physical or emotional, leads to feelings of helplessness and despair that contribute to lifelong patterns of depression in response to loss.

Spitz (1946) described behaviors that he observed in infants who were responding to maternal deprivation during the first year of life. He referred to the reaction as "anaclitic depression," which included behaviors such as excessive crying, anorexia, withdrawal, psychomotor retardation, stupor, and a generalized impairment in the normal process of growth and development. Some researchers suggest that loss in adult life afflicts people much more severely in the form of depression if the subjects have suffered early childhood loss.

Cognitive Theory. Beck and colleagues (1979) have proposed a theory suggesting that the primary disturbance in depression is cognitive rather than affective. The underlying cause of the depressive affect is seen as cognitive distortions that result in negative, defeated attitudes. Beck identifies three cognitive distortions that he believes serve as the basis for depression:

1. Negative expectations of the environment.
2. Negative expectations of the self.
3. Negative expectations of the future.

These cognitive distortions arise out of a defect in cognitive development, and the individual feels inadequate, worthless, and rejected by others. Outlook for the future is one of pessimism and hopelessness.

Cognitive theorists believe that depression is the product of negative thinking. This is in contrast to the other theorists, who suggest that negative thinking occurs when an individual is depressed. Cognitive therapy focuses on helping the individual to alter mood by changing the way he or she thinks. The individual is taught to control negative thought distortions that lead to pessimism, lethargy, procrastination, and low self-esteem.

The Transactional Model

The etiology of depression remains unclear. No single theory or hypothesis has been postulated that substantiates a clear-cut explanation for the disease. Evidence continues to mount in support of multiple causation. The transactional model recognizes the combined effects of genetic, biochemical, and psychosocial influences on an individual's susceptibility to depression. The dynamics of depression using the transactional model of stress/adaptation are presented in Figure 26.1.

Developmental Implications

Childhood

Only in recent years has a consensus developed among investigators identifying major depressive disorder as an entity in children and adolescents that can be identified using criteria similar to those used for adults (APA, 1994; Lewis & Volkmar, 1990). However, it is not uncommon for the symptoms of depression to be manifested differently in childhood. Herskowitz (1988) has stated:

> "A child doesn't have to be sad to be depressed. You have to look and see what is the child's prevailing mood. It could be anger or irritability. There don't have to be tears."

Herskowitz described the following symptoms specific to preschoolers:

1. Appearing bored, angry, or sad.
2. Crying for no apparent reason.
3. Needing to rest, or seeming tired or listless.
4. Being rejected by or rejecting others.
5. Seeming cranky or irritable.
6. Being moody, changeable.
7. Being restless, fidgety, constantly on the move.
8. Fighting with others.
9. Talking excessively.

Other symptoms of childhood depression may include hyperactivity, delinquency, school problems, psychosomatic complaints, sleeping and eating disturbances, social isolation, and suicidal thoughts or actions.

Children may become depressed for various reasons. In many depressed children, there is a genetic predisposition toward the condition, which is then precipitated by a stressful situation. Common precipitating factors include

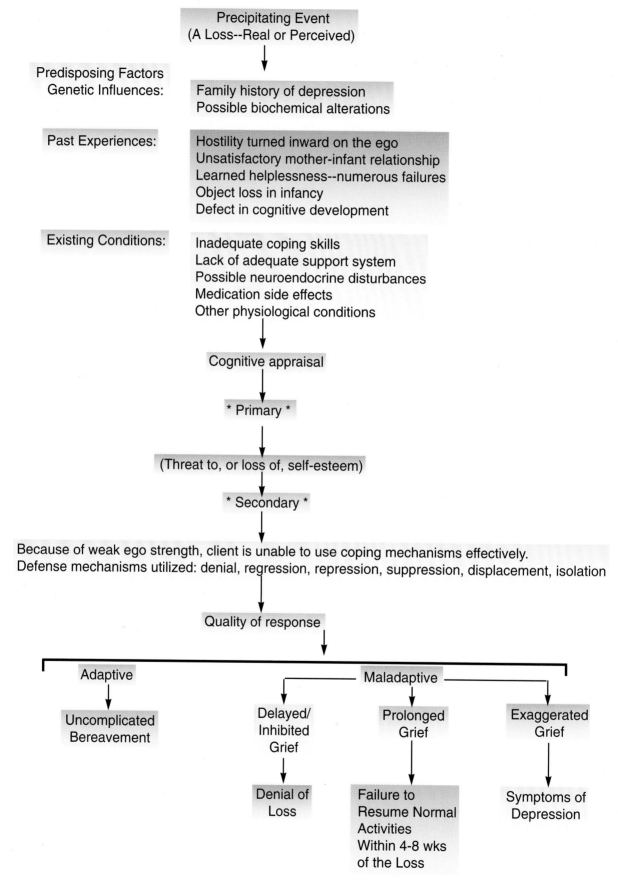

Figure 26.1 The dynamics of depression using the transactional model of stress/adaptation.

physical or emotional detachment from the primary care-giver, parental separation or divorce, death of a loved one (person or pet), a move, academic failure, or physical illness. In any event, the common denominator is loss.

The focus of therapy with depressed children is to alleviate the child's symptoms and strengthen the child's coping and adaptive skills, with the hope of possibly preventing future psychological problems. Some studies have shown that untreated childhood depression may lead to subsequent problems in adolescence and adult life (Sargent, 1989). Most children are treated on an outpatient basis. Hospitalization of the depressed child usually occurs only if he or she is actively suicidal, when the home environment precludes adherence to a treatment regimen, or if the child needs to be separated from the home because of psychosocial deprivation.

Parental and family therapy are commonly used to help the younger depressed child. Recovery is facilitated by emotional support and guidance to family members. Children older than age 8 usually participate in family therapy. In some situations, individual treatment may be appropriate for older children. Medications, such as antidepressants or lithium, can be important in the treatment of children, especially for the more serious and recurrent forms of depression.

Adolescence

Depression may be even harder to recognize in an adolescent than in a younger child. Feelings of sadness, loneliness, anxiety, and hopelessness associated with depression may be perceived as the normal emotional stresses of growing up. Therefore, many young people whose symptoms are attributed to the "normal adjustments" of adolescence do not get the help they need. Depression is a major cause of suicide among teens. During the past three decades, suicide among adolescents has almost tripled (Ghosh & Victor, 1994), and it is the third leading cause of death in this age group (Kestenbaum & Trautman, 1992).

Common symptoms of depression in the adolescent are inappropriately expressed anger, aggressiveness, running away, delinquency, social withdrawal, sexual acting out, substance abuse, restlessness, and apathy. Loss of self-esteem, sleeping and eating disturbances, and psychosomatic complaints are also common.

Bipolar disorder, which often emerges during adolescence, is manifested by episodes of impulsivity, irritability, and loss of control, sometimes alternating with periods of withdrawal. These behaviors are often confused with the emotional cycles of adolescence, delaying necessary treatment.

What, then, is the indicator that differentiates mood disorder from the typical stormy behavior of adolescence? The clue is revealed by a visible manifestation of *behavioral change that lasts for several weeks*. For example, the normally outgoing and extroverted adolescent who has become withdrawn and antisocial; the good student who previously received consistently high marks but is now failing and skipping classes; the usually self-confident teenager who is now inappropriately irritable and defensive with others.

Adolescents become depressed for all the same reasons that were discussed in childhood depression. Rosenn (1982) stated:

"It has been suggested that repeated childhood losses cause disturbances in early ego development. The biologic and psychosocial drive toward autonomy during adolescence overly taxes the teenager's defenses. When actual separation from the real or surrogate parents (e.g., girlfriend or boyfriend) is threatened, the usual defensive network may break down."

This threat of imminent abandonment by parents or closest peer relationship is thought to be the most frequent immediate precipitant to adolescent suicide.

Treatment of the depressed adolescent is often conducted on an outpatient basis. Geller and Carr (1988) suggest the following guidelines for hospitalization of depressed adolescents:

1. When the adolescent is suicidal and the family cannot set up the appropriate precautions at home.
2. When the psychosocial situation precludes adherence to a treatment regimen (i.e., the family is unable to keep therapy appointments or administer medications as required at home).
3. When the adolescent, because of depressive stupor or marked anorexia, is unable to sustain his or her own biological needs.
4. When the adolescent's anger is excessive and imposes a risk of harm to younger siblings in the home.

Antidepressant or lithium therapy, in addition to supportive psychosocial intervention, is the common modality for treatment of adolescent mood disorders. Various treatments may have to be attempted in order to determine the one that is most effective.

Senescence

Depression is the most common psychiatric disorder of the elderly, who make up 12.8 percent of the general population of the United States (Duncker & Greenberg, 1997). This is not surprising considering the disproportionate value our society places on youth, vigor, and uninterrupted productivity. These societal attitudes continually nurture the feelings of low self-esteem, helplessness, and hopelessness that become more pervasive and intensive with advanced age. Further, the aging individual's adaptive coping strategies may be seriously challenged by major stressors, such as financial problems, physical illness, changes in bodily functioning, and an increasing awareness of approaching death. The problem is often intensified by the numerous losses individuals experience during this period in life, such as spouse, friends, children, home, and independence. A phenomenon called **bereavement overload** occurs when individuals experience so many losses in their lives that they are not able to resolve one grief response before another one begins. Bereavement overload predisposes elderly individuals to depressive illness.

The elderly account for about 25 percent of the suicides in the United States, although they make up only 12.8 percent of the population. The rate of suicide for individuals 75 or older is more than three times the rate among the young (Kaplan, Sadock, & Grebb, 1994).

Symptoms of depression in the elderly are not very different from those in younger adults. However, depressive syndromes are often confused with other illnesses associated with the aging process. Symptoms of depression are often misdiagnosed as senile dementia, when in fact the memory loss, confused thinking, or apathy symptomatic of senility actually may be due to depression. The early awakening and reduced appetite typical of depression are common among many older persons who are not depressed. Compounding this situation is the fact that many medical conditions, such as endocrinological, neurological, nutritional, and metabolic disorders, often present with classic symptoms of depression. Many medications commonly used by the elderly, such as antihypertensives, corticosteroids, and analgesics, can also produce a depressant effect.

On the other hand, depression does accompany many of the illnesses that afflict older persons, such as Parkinson's disease, cancer, arthritis, and the early stages of Alzheimer's disease. Treating depression in these situations can reduce unnecessary suffering and help afflicted individuals cope with their medical problems (Sargent, 1989).

The most effective treatment of depression in the elderly individual is thought to be a combination of psychosocial and biological approaches (Blazer, 1994). Antidepressant medications are administered with consideration for age-related physiological changes in absorption, distribution, elimination, and brain receptor sensitivity. Because of these changes, plasma concentrations of these medications can reach very high levels despite moderate oral doses.

Electroconvulsive therapy (ECT) still remains one of the safest and most effective treatments for major depression in the elderly (Georgotas & Cancro, 1988). The response to ECT appears to be slower with advancing age, and the therapeutic effects are of limited duration. However, it may be considered the treatment of choice for the elderly individual who is an acute suicidal risk or is unable to tolerate antidepressant medications.

Other therapeutic approaches include interpersonal, behavioral, group, and family psychotherapies. Appropri-

ate treatment of the depressed elderly individual can bring relief from suffering and offer a new lease on life with a feeling of renewed productivity.

Postpartum Depression

The severity of depression in the postpartum period varies from a feeling of the "blues," to moderate depression, to psychotic depression or melancholia. Seventy to 80 percent of women who give birth experience the "blues" following delivery. The incidence of moderate depression is 10 to 20 percent. Severe, or psychotic, depression occurs rarely, in about 1 or 2 out of 1000 postpartum women (Person, 1992).

Symptoms of the "maternity blues" include tearfulness, despondency, anxiety, and subjectively impaired concentration appearing in the early puerperium. Typically, the condition appears between 1 and 10 days postpartum, and lasts no longer than 2 weeks (Ugarriza, 1992).

Symptoms of moderate **postpartum depression** have been described as depressed mood varying from day to day, with more bad days than good, tending to be worse toward evening and associated with fatigue, irritability, loss of appetite, sleep disturbances, and loss of libido. In addition, the new mother expresses a great deal of concern about her inability to care for her baby. These symptoms begin somewhat later than those described in the "maternity blues," and take from a few weeks to several months to abate.

Postpartum melancholia, or depressive psychosis, is characterized by depressed mood, agitation, indecision, lack of concentration, guilt, and an abnormal attitude toward bodily functions. There may be lack of interest in, or rejection of, the baby, or a morbid fear that the baby may be harmed. Risks of suicide and infanticide should not be overlooked. These symptoms generally develop within 3 weeks following delivery, and most women who are treated improve within 2 to 3 months (Ugarriza, 1992).

The etiology of postpartum depression remains unclear. "Maternity blues" may be associated with hormonal changes, tryptophan metabolism, or alterations in membrane transport during the early postpartum period. Besides being exposed to these same somatic changes, the woman who experiences moderate-to-severe symptoms probably possesses a vulnerability to depression related to heredity, upbringing, early life experiences, personality, or social circumstances. Pitt (1982) reported on the results of two studies, one of which found a close association between postpartum depression and loss of a parent before age 11. The second reported a relationship between postpartum depression and women who had had insufficient contact with their mothers during childhood. The etiology of postpartum depression may very likely be a combination of hormonal, metabolic, and psychosocial influences.

Treatment of postpartum depression varies with the

severity of the illness. Psychotic depression may be treated with antidepressant medication, along with supportive psychotherapy, group therapy, and possibly family therapy. Moderate depression may be relieved with supportive psychotherapy and continuing assistance with home management until the symptoms subside. "Maternity blues" usually need no treatment beyond a word of reassurance from the physician or nurse that these feelings are common and will soon pass, along with a bit of extra support and comfort from significant others.

APPLICATION OF THE NURSING PROCESS TO DEPRESSIVE DISORDERS

Background Assessment Data

Symptomatology of depression can be viewed on a continuum according to severity of the illness. All individuals become depressed from time to time. These are the transient symptoms that accompany the everyday disappointments of life. Examples of the disappointments include failing an examination or breaking up with a boyfriend or girlfriend. Transient symptoms of depression subside relatively quickly, as the individual advances toward other goals and achievements.

Mild depressive episodes occur when the grief process is triggered in response to the loss of a valued object. This can occur with the loss of a loved one, pet, friend, home, or significant other. As one is able to work through the stages of grief, the loss is accepted, symptoms subside, and activities of daily living are resumed within a few weeks. If this does not occur, grief is prolonged or exaggerated, and symptoms intensify.

Moderate depression occurs when grief is prolonged or exaggerated. The individual becomes fixed in the anger stage of the grief response, and the anger is turned inward on the self. All of the feelings associated with normal grieving are exaggerated out of proportion, and the individual is unable to function without assistance. Dysthymic disorder is an example of moderate depression.

Severe depression is an intensification of the symptoms associated with the moderate level. The individual who is severely depressed may also demonstrate a loss of contact with reality. This level is associated with a complete lack of pleasure in all activities, and ruminations about suicide are common. Major depressive disorder is an example of severe depression.

A continuum of depression is presented in Figure 26.2.

Symptoms of depression can be described as alterations in four spheres of human functioning: affective, behavioral, cognitive, and physiological. Alterations within these spheres differ according to degree of severity of symptomatology.

Transient Depression

Symptoms at this level of the continuum are not necessarily dysfunctional. Alterations include:

1. *Affective:* sadness, dejection, feeling downhearted, having the "blues."
2. *Behavioral:* some crying possible.
3. *Cognitive:* some difficulty getting mind off of one's disappointment.
4. *Physiological:* feeling tired and listless.

Mild Depression

Symptoms at the mild level of depression are identified by those associated with normal grieving. Alterations include:

1. *Affective:* denial of feelings, anger, anxiety, guilt, helplessness, hopelessness, sadness, despondency.
2. *Behavioral:* tearfulness, regression, restlessness, agitation, withdrawal.
3. *Cognitive:* preoccupation with the loss, self-blame, ambivalence, blaming others.
4. *Physiological:* anorexia or overeating, insomnia or hypersomnia, headache, backache, chest pain, or other symptoms associated with the loss of a significant other.

Moderate Depression

This level of depression represents a more problematic disturbance. Symptoms associated with dysthymic disorder include:

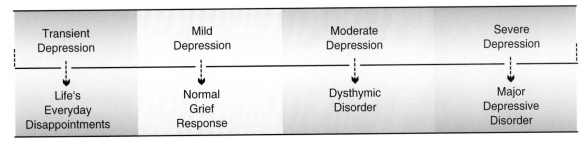

Transient Depression	Mild Depression	Moderate Depression	Severe Depression
↓	↓	↓	↓
Life's Everyday Disappointments	Normal Grief Response	Dysthymic Disorder	Major Depressive Disorder

Figure 26.2   A continuum of depression.

1. *Affective:* feelings of sadness, dejection, helplessness, powerlessness, hopelessness; gloomy and pessimistic outlook; low self-esteem; difficulty experiencing pleasure in activities.
2. *Behavioral:* slowed physical movements (i.e., **psychomotor retardation**); slumped posture; slowed speech; limited verbalizations, possibly consisting of ruminations about life's failures or regrets; social isolation with a focus on the self; increased use of substances possible; self-destructive behavior possible; decreased interest in personal hygiene and grooming.
3. *Cognitive:* retarded thinking processes; difficulty concentrating and directing attention; obsessive and repetitive thoughts, generally portraying pessimism and negativism; verbalizations and behavior reflecting suicidal ideation.
4. *Physiological:* anorexia or overeating; insomnia or hypersomnia; sleep disturbances; amenorrhea; decreased libido; headaches; backaches; chest pain; abdominal pain; low energy level; fatigue and listlessness; feeling best early in the morning and continually worse as the day progresses. This may be related to the diurnal variation in the level of neurotransmitters that affect mood and level of activity.

Severe Depression

Severe depression is characterized by an intensification of the symptoms described for moderate depression. Examples of severe depression include major depressive disorder and bipolar depression. Symptoms include:

1. *Affective:* feelings of total despair, hopelessness, and worthlessness; flat (unchanging) affect, appearing devoid of emotional tone; prevalent feelings of nothingness and emptiness; apathy; loneliness; sadness; inability to feel pleasure.
2. *Behavioral:* psychomotor retardation so severe that physical movement may literally come to a standstill, or psychomotor behavior manifested by rapid, agitated, purposeless movements; slumped posture; sitting in a curled-up position; walking slowly and rigidly; virtually nonexistent communication (when verbalizations do occur, they may reflect delusional thinking); no personal hygiene and grooming; social isolation common, with virtually no inclination toward interaction with others.
3. *Cognitive:* prevalent delusional thinking, with delusions of persecution and somatic delusions being most common; confusion, indecisiveness, and an inability to concentrate; hallucinations reflecting misinterpretations of the environment; excessive self-deprecation, self-blame, and thoughts of suicide.

NOTE: Because of the low energy level and retarded thought processes, the individual may be un-

able to follow through on suicidal ideas. However, the desire is strong at this level.

4. *Physiological:* a general slowdown of the entire body, reflected in sluggish digestion, constipation, and urinary retention; amenorrhea; impotence; diminished libido; anorexia; weight loss; difficulty falling asleep and awakening very early in the morning; feeling worse early in the morning and somewhat better as the day progresses. As with moderate depression, this may reflect the diurnal variation in the level of neurotransmitters that affect mood and activity.

Diagnosis/Outcome Identification

From the assessment data, the nurse formulates the appropriate nursing diagnoses for the depressed client. From these identified problems, care planning is executed, nursing actions are implemented, and relevant criteria for evaluation are established. Possible nursing diagnoses for depressed clients include:

Risk for self-directed violence related to depressed mood, feelings of worthlessness, anger turned inward on the self, misinterpretations of reality.

Dysfunctional grieving related to real or perceived loss, bereavement overload, evidenced by denial of loss, inappropriate expression of anger, idealization of or obsession with the lost object, inability to carry out activities of daily living.

Self-esteem disturbance related to learned helplessness, feelings of abandonment by significant other, impaired cognition fostering negative view of self, evidenced by expressions of worthlessness, hypersensitivity to a slight or criticism, and a negative, pessimistic outlook.

Powerlessness related to dysfunctional grieving process, lifestyle of helplessness, evidenced by feelings of lack of control over life situation, overdependence on others to fulfill needs.

Spiritual distress related to dysfunctional grieving over loss of valued object evidenced by anger toward God, questioning meaning of own existence, inability to participate in usual religious practices.

Social isolation/impaired social interaction related to developmental regression, egocentric behaviors, fear of rejection or failure of the interaction, evidenced by being uncommunicative and withdrawn, seeking to be alone, and dysfunctional interaction with peers, family, or others.

Altered thought processes related to withdrawal into the self, underdeveloped ego, punitive superego, impaired cognition fostering negative perception of self or environment, evidenced by delusional thinking, confusion, difficulty concentrating, impaired problem-solving ability.

Altered nutrition, less than body requirements related to depressed mood, loss of appetite, or lack of interest in food, evidenced by weight loss, poor muscle tone, pale conjunctiva and mucous membranes, poor skin turgor, weakness.

Sleep pattern disturbance related to depressed mood, anxiety, and fears, evidenced by difficulty falling asleep, awakening earlier or later than desired, verbal complaints of not feeling well rested.

Self-care deficit (hygiene, grooming) related to depressed mood, feelings of worthlessness, evidenced by uncombed hair, disheveled clothing, offensive body odor.

The following criteria may be used for measurement of outcomes in the care of the depressed client.

THE CLIENT:

1. Has experienced no physical harm to self.
2. Discusses the loss with staff and family members.
3. No longer idealizes or obsesses about the lost object.
4. Sets realistic goals for self.
5. Is no longer afraid to attempt new activities.
6. Is able to identify aspects of self-control over life situation.
7. Expresses personal satisfaction and support from spiritual practices.
8. Interacts willingly and appropriately with others.
9. Is able to maintain reality orientation.
10. Is able to concentrate, reason, and solve problems.
11. Eats a well-balanced diet with snacks, to prevent weight loss and maintain nutritional status.
12. Sleeps 6 to 8 hours per night and verbalizes feeling well rested.
13. Bathes, washes and combs hair, and dresses in clean clothing without assistance.

Planning/Implementation

Table 26.7 provides a plan of care for the depressed client. Selected nursing diagnoses are presented, along with outcome criteria, appropriate nursing interventions, and rationales for each.

Some institutions are using a case management model to coordinate care (see Chapter 7 for more detailed explanation). In case management models, the plan of care may take the form of a critical pathway. Table 26.8 depicts an example of a critical pathway of care for a depressed client.

Client/Family Education

The role of client teacher is important in the psychiatric area, as it is in all areas of nursing. A list of topics for client/family education relevant to depression is presented in Table 26.9.

Evaluation of Care for the Depressed Client

In the final step of the nursing process, a reassessment is conducted to determine if the nursing actions have been successful in achieving the objectives of care. Evaluation of the nursing actions for the depressed client may be facilitated by gathering information using the following types of questions:

1. Has self-harm to the individual been avoided?
2. Have suicidal ideations subsided?
3. Does the individual know where to seek assistance outside the hospital when suicidal thoughts occur?
4. Has the client discussed the recent loss with staff and family members?
5. Is he or she able to verbalize feelings and behaviors associated with each stage of the grieving process and recognize own position in the process?
6. Has obsession with and idealization of the lost object subsided?
7. Is anger toward the lost object expressed appropriately?
8. Does client set realistic goals for self?
9. Is he or she able to verbalize positive aspects about self, past accomplishments, and future prospects?
10. Can the client identify areas of life situation over which he or she has control?
11. Is the client able to participate in usual religious practices and feel satisfaction and support from them?
12. Is the client seeking out interaction with others in an appropriate manner?
13. Does the client maintain reality orientation with no evidence of delusional thinking?
14. Is he or she able to concentrate and make decisions concerning own self-care?
15. Is the client selecting and consuming foods sufficiently high in nutrients and calories to maintain weight and nutritional status?
16. Does the client sleep without difficulty and wake feeling rested?
17. Does the client show pride in appearance by attending to personal hygiene and grooming?
18. Have somatic complaints subsided?

BIPOLAR DISORDER (MANIA)

Predisposing Factors

Biological Theories

Genetics

Twin Studies. Twin studies have indicated that if one twin has bipolar disorder, the other twin is four to five times more likely to also have the disorder if the twins are

TABLE 26.7   CARE PLAN FOR THE DEPRESSED CLIENT

NURSING DIAGNOSIS: RISK FOR SELF-DIRECTED VIOLENCE

RELATED TO: Depressed mood, feelings of worthlessness, anger turned inward on the self, misinterpretations of reality

OUTCOME CRITERIA	NURSING INTERVENTIONS	RATIONALE
Client will not harm self.	1. Ask client directly: "Have you thought about harming yourself in any way? If so, what do you plan to do? Do you have the means to carry out this plan?"	1. The risk of suicide is greatly increased if the client has developed a plan and particularly if means exist for the client to execute the plan.
	2. Create a safe environment for the client. Remove all potentially harmful objects from client's access (sharp objects, straps, belts, ties, glass items, alcohol). Supervise closely during meals and medication administration. Perform room searches as deemed necessary.	2. Client safety is a nursing priority
	3. Formulate a short-term verbal or written contract that the client will not harm self. When time is up, make another, and so forth. Secure a promise that the client will seek out staff when feeling suicidal.	3. A degree of the responsibility for his or her safety is given to the client. Increased feelings of self-worth may be experienced when client feels accepted unconditionally regardless of thoughts or behavior.
	4. Encourage client to express honest feelings, including anger. Provide hostility release if needed.	4. Depression and suicidal behaviors may be viewed as anger turned inward on the self. If this anger can be verbalized in a nonthreatening environment, the client may be able to eventually resolve these feelings.

NURSING DIAGNOSIS: DYSFUNCTIONAL GRIEVING

RELATED TO: Real or perceived loss, bereavement overload

EVIDENCED BY: Denial of loss, inappropriate expression of anger, idealization of or obsession with lost object, inability to carry out activities of daily living

OUTCOME CRITERIA	NURSING INTERVENTIONS	RATIONALE
Client will be able to verbalize normal behaviors associated with grieving and begin progression toward resolution.	1. Assess stage of fixation in grief process.	1. Accurate baseline data is required in order to plan accurate care.
	2. Develop trust. Show empathy, caring, and unconditional positive regard.	2. Developing trust provides the basis for a therapeutic relationship.
	3. Explore feelings of anger and help client direct them toward the intended object or person. Promote the use of large motor activities for relieving pent-up tension.	3. Until client can recognize and accept personal feelings regarding the loss, grief work cannot progress. Physical exercise is a safe and effective way of relieving internalized anger.
	4. Teach normal behaviors associated with grieving.	4. Understanding of the grief process will help prevent feelings of guilt generated by these responses.
	5. Help client with honest review of relationship with lost object.	5. Only when the client is able to see both positive and negative aspects related to the lost object will the grieving process be complete.

NURSING DIAGNOSIS: SELF-ESTEEM DISTURBANCE

RELATED TO: Learned helplessness, feelings of abandonment by significant other, impaired cognition fostering negative view of self

EVIDENCED BY: Expressions of worthlessness, hypersensitivity to slights or criticism, negative, pessimistic outlook

OUTCOME CRITERIA	NURSING INTERVENTIONS	RATIONALE
Client will be able to attempt new activities without fear of failure. Client will be able to verbalize positive aspects about self.	1. Be accepting of client and spend time with him or her even though pessimism and negativism may seem objectionable. Focus on strengths and accomplishments and minimize failures. 2. Promote attendance in therapy groups that offer client simple methods of accomplishment. Encourage client to be as independent as possible. 3. Encourage client to recognize areas of change and provide assistance toward this effort. 4. Teach assertiveness and communication techniques.	1. Interventions that focus on the positive contribute toward feelings of self-worth. 2. Success and independence promote feelings of self-worth. 3. Client will need assistance with problem solving. 4. Effective communication and assertiveness techniques enhance self-esteem.

NURSING DIAGNOSIS: POWERLESSNESS

RELATED TO: Dysfunctional grieving process, lifestyle of helplessness

EVIDENCED BY: Feelings of lack of control over life situation, overdependence on others to fulfill needs

OUTCOME CRITERIA	NURSING INTERVENTIONS	RATIONALE
Client will be able to solve problems to take control of life situation.	1. Allow client to participate in goal setting and decision making regarding own care. 2. Ensure that goals are realistic and that client is able to identify areas of life situation that are realistically under his or her control. 3. Encourage client to verbalize feelings about areas that are not within his or her ability to control.	1. Providing client with choices will increase his or her feelings of control 2. Realistic goals will avoid setting client up for further failures. 3. Verbalization of unresolved issues may help client accept what cannot be changed.

NURSING DIAGNOSIS: SPIRITUAL DISTRESS

RELATED TO: Dysfunctional grieving over loss of valued object

EVIDENCED BY: Anger toward God, questioning meaning of own existence, inability to participate in usual religious practices

OUTCOME CRITERIA	NURSING INTERVENTIONS	RATIONALE
Client will express achievement of support and personal satisfaction from spiritual practices.	1. Be accepting and nonjudgmental when client expresses anger and bitterness toward God. Stay with client. 2. Encourage client to ventilate feelings related to meaning of own existence in the face of current loss.	1. The nurse's presence and nonjudgmental attitude increase the client's feelings of self-worth and promote trust in the relationship. 2. Client may believe he or she cannot go on living without lost object. Catharsis can provide relief and put life back into realistic perspective.

Continued on following page

TABLE 26.7 *(Continued)*

3. Encourage client as part of grief work to reach out to previously used religious practices for support. Encourage client to discuss these practices and how they provided support in the past.	3. Client may find comfort in religious rituals with which he or she is familiar.
4. Assure client that he or she is not alone when feeling inadequate in the search for life's answers.	4. Validations of client's feelings and assurance that they are shared by others offers reassurance and an affirmation of acceptability
5. Contact spiritual leader of client's choice, if he or she requests.	5. These individuals serve to provide relief from spiritual distress and often can do so when other support persons cannot.

identical than if they are fraternal (Kelsoe, 1991). Because identical twins have identical genes and fraternal twins share only approximately half their genes, this is strong evidence that genes play a major role in the etiology.

Family Studies. Family studies have shown that if one member of a family has bipolar disorder, then the other members are 7 to 10 times more likely to also have bipolar disorder than in the general population (Kelsoe, 1991). This has also been shown to be the case in studies of children born to parents with bipolar disorder who were adopted at birth and reared by adoptive parents without evidence of the disorder. These results strongly indicate that genes play a role separate from that of the environment. Kelsoe adds:

> "It is important to understand that if an individual inherits a gene for bipolar disorder, he or she has only about a 50% to 80% chance of ever having a mood disorder. Hence, it is a predisposition or susceptibility that is inherited." (p. 21)

Biochemical Influences

Biogenic Amines. Early studies have associated symptoms of depression with a functional deficiency of norepinephrine and dopamine, and mania with a functional excess of these amines. The neurotransmitter serotonin appears to remain low in both states (Goodwin & Jamison, 1990). These conclusions have been substantiated by the effects of neuroleptic drugs that influence the levels of these biogenic amines to produce the desired effect.

Electrolytes. Some studies have indicated that bipolar illness is accompanied by increased intracellular sodium and calcium. These electrolyte imbalances may be related to abnormalities in cellular membrane function in bipolar disorder. A possible deficiency in the membrane-bound sodium pump has been suggested as an explanation for the increased intracellular sodium. This link between increased intracellular calcium and symptoms of bipolar disorder may be indicated by calcium channel blockers, medications which inhibit the influx of calcium into the cell

and have been shown to have antimanic, and possibly antidepressant and anticycling, properties (Goodwin & Jamison, 1990).

Physiological Influences

Brain Lesions. Studies have shown that lesions in the left frontotemporal or right parieto-occipital quadrants tend to be associated with depression (Goodwin & Jamison, 1990). The most common affective sequelae of brain lesions involve poststroke depressions, the severity of which increases the closer the damage is to the left frontal pole. Secondary manic-like symptoms appear to be associated with right frontotemporal or left parieto-occipital lesions.

Medication Side Effects. Certain medications used to treat somatic illnesses have been known to trigger a manic response. The most common of these are the steroids, frequently used to treat chronic illnesses such as multiple sclerosis and SLE. Some clients whose first episode of mania occurred during steroid therapy have reported spontaneous recurrence of manic symptoms years later (Kaplan & Sadock, 1985). Amphetamines and tricyclic antidepressants also have the potential for initiating a manic episode.

Psychosocial Theories

The credibility of psychosocial theories has declined in recent years. Conditions such as schizophrenia and bipolar disorder are being viewed by many as diseases of the brain with biological etiologies. The etiology of these illnesses remains unclear, however, and it is possible that both biological and psychosocial factors could be influential. For this reason, a discussion of the psychosocial theories is included.

Psychoanalytical Theories. Freud (1957) believed that depression and mania were maladaptive responses to loss. He suggested that the lost object became merged

■ **TABLE 26.8   CRITICAL PATHWAY OF CARE FOR THE DEPRESSED CLIENT**

Estimated Length of Stay: 7 days—variations from designated pathway should be documented in progress notes

Nursing Diagnosis and Categories of Care	Time Dimension	Goals and/or Actions	Time Dimension	Goals and/or Actions	Time Dimension	Discharge Outcome
Risk for self-directed violence	Day 1	Environment is made safe for client.	Ongoing	Client does not harm self.	Day 7	Client is discharged without harm to self.
Referrals	Day 1	Psychiatrist: May give order to isolate if risk is great or may do ECT For relaxation therapy: Music therapist Clinical nurse specialist Stress management specialist			Day 7	Discharge with follow-up appointments as required.
Additional assessments	Day 1	Suicidal assessment: ● ideation ● gestures ● threats ● plan ● means ● anxiety level ● thought disorder	Day 2–7	Ongoing assessments.	Day 7	Client discharged. Denies suicidal ideations.
	Day 1	Secure no-suicide contract.				
Medications	Day 1	Antidepressant medication, as ordered. Antianxiety agents p.r.n.	Day 1–7	Assess for effectiveness and side effects of medications. Be alert for sudden lifts in mood.	Day 7	Discharged with antidepressant medications.
Client education	Day 3–6	Teach relaxation techniques. Discuss resources outside the hospital from whom client may seek assistance when feeling suicidal.	Day 6–7	Reinforce teaching.	Day 7	Discharge with understanding of instruction given.
Dysfunctional grieving	Day 1	Assess stage of fixation in grief process.			Day 7	Discharge with evidence of progression toward resolution of grief.
Referrals	Day 1	Psychiatrist Psychologist Social worker Clinical nurse specialist Music therapist Occupational therapist Recreational therapist, chaplain			Day 7	Discharge with follow-up appointments as required.

Continued on following page

TABLE 26.8 (*Continued*)

Estimated Length of Stay: 7 days—variations from designated pathway should be documented in progress notes

Nursing Diagnosis and Categories of Care	Time Dimension	Goals and/or Actions	Time Dimension	Goals and/or Actions	Time Dimension	Discharge Outcome
Diagnostic studies	Day 1 Day 2–3	Any of the following tests *may* be ordered: Drug screen Urine test for norepinephrine and serotonin Dexamethasone-suppression test A measure of TSH response to administered TRH. Serum and urine studies for nutritional deficiencies.				
Medications	Day 1	Antidepressant medication, as ordered. Antianxiety agent p.r.n.	Day 1–7	Assess for effectiveness and side effects of medications.	Day 7	Client is discharged with medications.
Diet	Day 1	If antidepressant medication is MAO inhibitor: Low tyramine			Day 7	Client has experienced no symptoms of hypertensive crisis.
Additional assessments	Day 1 Day 1	VS every shift Assess: ● mental status ● mood, affect ● thought disorder ● communication patterns ● level of interest in environment ● participation in activities ● weight	Day 2–7 Day 2–7	VS daily if stable. Ongoing assessments.	Day 7	Mood and affect appropriate. No evidence of thought disorder. Participates willingly and appropriately in activities.
Client education	Day 1	Orient to unit	Day 4 Day 5–6	Discuss importance of taking medications regularly, even when feeling well or if feeling medication is not helping. Discuss possible side effects of medication and when to see the physician. Teach which foods to eliminate from diet if taking MAO inhibitor. Reinforce teaching.	Day 7	Client is discharged. Verbalizes understanding of information presented prior to discharge.

TABLE 26.9 TOPICS FOR CLIENT/FAMILY EDUCATION RELATED TO DEPRESSION

Name of the Illness
1. Stages of grief and symptoms associated with each stage.
2. What is depression?
3. Why do people get depressed?
4. What are the symptoms of depression?

Management of the Illness
1. Medication management
   a. Nuisance side effects
   b. Side effects to report to physician
   c. Importance of taking regularly
   d. Length of time to take effect
   e. Diet (related to MAO inhibitors)
2. Assertiveness techniques
3. Stress-management techniques
4. Ways to increase self-esteem
5. Electroconvulsive therapy

Support Services
1. Suicide hotline
2. Support groups
3. Legal and financial assistance

---

with the ego, and the rage felt for having been rejected or abandoned was then directed inward against the self. In this way, the individual can remain unaware of the unacceptable anger against the love object. Freud assumed that in mania the lost object is rapidly relinquished (although he could not explain why), and a vast amount of psychic energy becomes free to be invested upon the self and the surrounding world (Aleksandrowicz, 1980). In this model, mania is viewed as a denial of depression.

Klein (1948) viewed depression as a developmental phase, occurring toward the end of the first year of life, caused by weaning and gradual weakening of the deep bond between the infant and the mothering figure. Mania is viewed as a denial of, or defense against, the depression, and represents a reactivation of the corresponding infantile state.

Theory of Family Dynamics. A study by Cohen and coworkers (1954) found that the individual with bipolar disorder most likely began life in a loving, nurturing environment. All physical and emotional needs were fulfilled by the primary caregiver, who assumed the image of "goodness" in the mind of the infant. As the child developed and became increasingly independent, some of the nurturing was withdrawn. The child, who had not yet achieved object constancy by this time, was unable to incorporate the concepts of both "good" and "bad" in the primary caregiver. A feeling of ambivalence developed toward the primary caregiver as the child learned the necessity of fulfilling expectations in order to gain affection, even at the expense of negating his or her own needs and desires.

As the child matured, he or she had a tendency to be particularly sensitive, and to crave approval, support, and affection from others. Gibson and colleagues (1959) found that the childhood family of the manic-depressive had been characterized by a striving for social prestige, and that as a child the client had borne the brunt of this, with heavy pressure from one or both parents to succeed in social life. The family showed little interest in the child in his or her own right, but only in the role as carrier of prestige. Parental approval depended not on "who you are" but on "what you do." Expectations were often unrealistic, and the child's social and psychological life became greatly restricted, resulting in the development of rigid behavior patterns. A love-hate relationship is established as resentment toward the parents continues to grow, even though the child strongly desires and continues to try to please them.

The child's ego development is disrupted in this dysfunctional family system, and the adult bipolar client's gratification and security are strongly tied to unfulfilled needs for approval. The depressive and manic episodes are precipitated by a loss in which the client feels rejected, rebuked, or not appreciated (Aleksandrowicz, 1980). The loss need not be a conspicuous and obviously stressful life event. Cohen and associates (1954) pointed out that even a change in the client's appraisal of existing relationships may be subjectively experienced as loss of love.

Because there is weak ego development, the response to loss is directed by influences from the id or superego component of the personality. If the superego becomes punitive, the individual turns anger inward on the self and experiences depression. When the depression subsides, the ego may still be too weak to control the impulsive, excessive behavior dominated by the id, and the symptoms of mania are manifested (Aleksandrowicz, 1980).

The Transactional Model

Bipolar disorder most likely results from an interaction between genetic, biological, and psychosocial determinants. Kaplan, Sadock, and Grebb (1994) state:

"The causative factors (of mood disorders) can artificially be divided into biological factors, genetic factors, and psychosocial factors. That division is artificial because of the likelihood that the three realms interact among themselves. For example, psychosocial factors and genetic factors can affect biological factors (for example, concentrations of a certain neurotransmitter). Biological and psychosocial factors can also affect gene expression. And biological and genetic factors can affect the response of a person to psychosocial factors." (p. 518)

The transactional model takes these various etiological influences, as well as those associated with past experiences, existing conditions, and the individual's perception of the event, into consideration. Figure 26.3 depicts the dynamics of bipolar disorder, mania, using the transactional model of stress/adaptation.

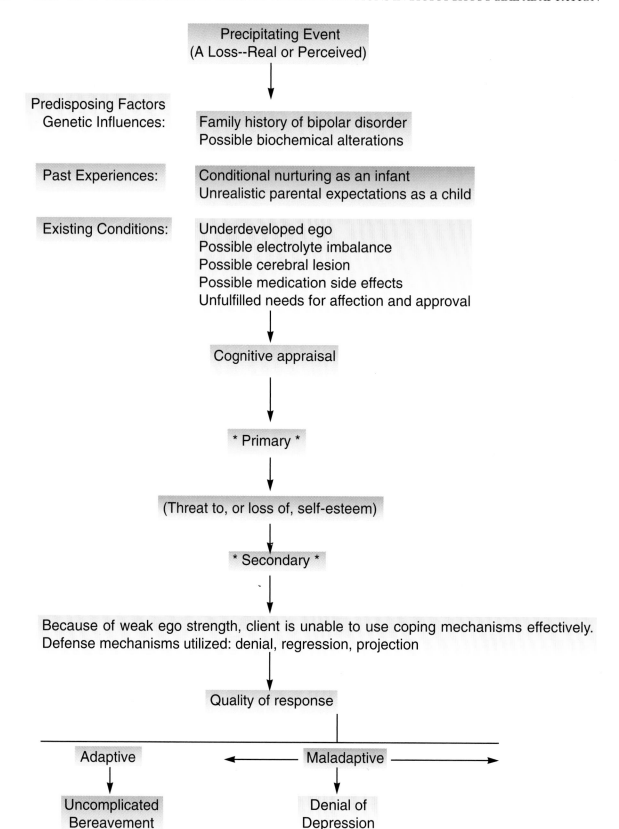

Figure 26.3 The dynamics of bipolar disorder, mania, using the transactional model of stress/adaptation.

APPLICATION OF THE NURSING PROCESS TO BIPOLAR DISORDER (MANIA)

Background Assessment Data

Goodwin and Jamison (1990) describe symptoms of manic states according to three stages: hypomania, acute mania, and **delirious mania.** Symptoms of mood, cognition and perception, and activity and behavior are presented for each stage.

Stage I: Hypomania

At this stage the disturbance is not sufficiently severe to cause marked impairment in social or occupational functioning or to require hospitalization (APA, 1994).

Mood. The mood of a hypomanic person is cheerful and expansive. However, there is an underlying irritability that surfaces rapidly when the person's wishes and desires go unfulfilled. The nature of the hypomanic person is very volatile and fluctuating.

Cognition and Perception. Perceptions of the self are exalted—ideas of great worth and ability. Thinking is flighty, with a rapid flow of ideas. Perception of the environment is heightened, but the individual is so easily distracted by irrelevant stimuli that goal-directed activities are difficult.

Activity and Behavior. Hypomanic individuals exhibit increased motor activity. They are perceived as being very extroverted and sociable, and because of this they attract numerous acquaintances. However, they lack the depth of personality and warmth to formulate close friendships. They talk and laugh a lot, usually very loudly and often inappropriately. Increased libido is common. Some individuals experience anorexia and weight loss. The exalted self-perception leads some hypomanics to engage in inappropriate behaviors, such as calling the president of the United States or buying huge amounts on a credit card without having the resources to pay.

Stage II: Acute Mania

Symptoms of acute mania may be a progression in intensification of those experienced in hypomania or may be manifested directly. Most individuals experience marked impairment in functioning and require hospitalization.

Mood. Acute mania is characterized by euphoria and elation. The person appears to be on a continuous "high." However, the mood is always subject to frequent variation, easily changing to irritability and anger or even to sadness and crying.

Cognition and Perception. Cognition and perception become fragmented and often psychotic in acute mania. Rapid thinking proceeds to racing and disjointed thinking (flight of ideas) and may be manifested by a continuous flow of accelerated, pressured speech (loquaciousness), with abrupt changes from topic to topic. When flight of ideas is severe, speech may be disorganized and incoherent. Distractibility becomes all-pervasive. Attention can be diverted by even the smallest of stimuli. Paranoid and grandiose delusions are common, as are illusions and hallucinations (Goodwin & Jamison, 1990).

Activity and Behavior. Psychomotor activity is excessive. Sexual interest is increased. There is poor impulse control, and the individual who is normally discreet may become socially and sexually uninhibited. Excessive spending is common. Individuals with acute mania have the ability to manipulate others to carry out their wishes, and if things go wrong, they can skillfully project responsibility for the failure onto others (Janowsky et al., 1974). Energy seems inexhaustible, and the need for sleep is diminished. They may go for many days without sleep and still not feel tired. Hygiene and grooming may be neglected. Dress may be disorganized, flamboyant, or bizarre, and the use of excessive makeup or jewelry is common.

Stage III: Delirious Mania

Delirious mania is a grave form of the disorder characterized by severe clouding of consciousness and representing an intensification of the symptoms associated with acute mania (Goodwin & Jamison, 1990). This condition has become relatively rare since the availability of antipsychotic medication.

Mood. The mood of the delirious person is very labile. He or she may exhibit feelings of despair, quickly converting to unrestrained merriment and ecstasy, or becoming irritable or totally indifferent to the environment. Panic anxiety may be evident.

Cognition and Perception. Cognition and perception are characterized by a clouding of consciousness, with accompanying confusion, disorientation, and sometimes stupor. Other common manifestations include religiosity, delusions of grandeur or persecution, and auditory or visual hallucinations. The individual is extremely distractible and incoherent.

Activity and Behavior. Psychomotor activity is frenzied and characterized by agitated, purposeless movements. The safety of these individuals is at stake unless this activity is curtailed. Exhaustion, injury to self or others, and eventually death could occur without intervention.

Diagnosis/Outcome Identification

From the assessment data, nursing diagnoses are formulated from which the plan of care is derived. Possible nursing diagnoses for the client with bipolar disorder (mania) include:

Risk for injury related to extreme hyperactivity, evidenced by increased agitation and lack of control over purposeless and potentially injurious movements.

Risk for violence: Self-directed or directed at others related to manic excitement, delusional thinking, hallucinations.

Altered nutrition: Less than body requirements related to refusal or inability to sit still long enough to eat, evidenced by loss of weight, amenorrhea.

Altered thought processes related to unresolved grief—denial of depression, evidenced by delusions of grandeur and persecution.

Sensory-perceptual alteration related to unresolved grief—denial of depression, possible sleep deprivation, evidenced by auditory and visual hallucinations.

Impaired social interaction related to egocentric and narcissistic behavior, evidenced by inability to develop satisfying relationships and manipulation of others for own desires.

Sleep pattern disturbance related to excessive hyperactivity and agitation, evidenced by difficulty falling asleep and sleeping only short periods.

The following criteria may be used for measuring outcomes in the care of the manic client.

THE CLIENT:

1. Exhibits no evidence of physical injury.
2. Has not harmed self or others.
3. Is no longer exhibiting signs of physical agitation.
4. Eats a well-balanced diet with snacks to prevent weight loss and maintain nutritional status.
5. Verbalizes an accurate interpretation of the environment.
6. Verbalizes that hallucinatory activity has ceased and demonstrates no outward behavior indicating hallucinations.
7. Accepts responsibility for own behaviors.
8. Does not manipulate others for gratification of own needs.
9. Interacts appropriately with others.
10. Is able to fall asleep within 30 minutes of retiring.
11. Is able to sleep 6 to 8 hours per night without medication.

Planning/Implementation

Table 26.10 provides a plan of care for the manic client. Selected nursing diagnoses are presented, along with outcome criteria, appropriate nursing interventions, and rationales for each.

Some institutions are using a case management model to coordinate care (see Chapter 7 for a more detailed explanation). In case management models, the plan of care may take the form of a critical pathway. Table 26.11 depicts an example of a critical pathway of care for a manic client.

Client/Family Education

The role of client teacher is important in the psychiatric area, as it is in all areas of nursing. A list of topics for client/family education relevant to bipolar disorder is presented in Table 26.12.

Evaluation of Care for the Manic Client

In the final step of the nursing process, a reassessment is conducted in order to determine if the nursing actions have been successful in achieving the objectives of care. Evaluation of the nursing actions for the manic client may be facilitated by gathering information using the following types of questions.

1. Has the individual avoided personal injury?
2. Has violence to client or others been prevented?
3. Has agitation subsided?
4. Have nutritional status and weight been stabilized? Is the client able to select foods to maintain adequate nutrition?
5. Have delusions and hallucinations ceased? Is the client able to interpret the environment correctly?
6. Is the client able to make decisions about own self-care? Have hygiene and grooming improved?
7. Is behavior socially acceptable? Is client able to interact with others in a satisfactory manner? Has the client stopped manipulating others to fulfill own desires?
8. Is the client able to sleep 6 to 8 hours per night and awaken feeling rested?
9. Does the client understand the importance of maintenance lithium therapy? Does he or she understand that symptoms may return if lithium is stopped?
10. Can the client verbalize early signs of lithium toxicity? Does he or she understand the necessity for monthly blood level checks?

TREATMENT MODALITIES FOR MOOD DISORDERS

Psychological Treatments

Individual Psychotherapy

For Depression. Research has documented both the importance of close and satisfactory attachments in the prevention of depression and the role of disrupted attachments in the development of depression (Klerman, 1988). With this concept in mind, interpersonal psychotherapy focuses on the client's current interpersonal relations. Interpersonal psychotherapy with the depressed person proceeds through the following phases and interventions (Klerman, 1988):

Phase I. During the first phase, the client is assessed to

TABLE 26.10 CARE PLAN FOR THE CLIENT EXPERIENCING A MANIC EPISODE

NURSING DIAGNOSIS: RISK OF INJURY
RELATED TO: Extreme hyperactivity
EVIDENCED BY: Increased agitation and lack of control over purposeless and potentially injurious movements

OUTCOME CRITERIA	NURSING INTERVENTIONS	RATIONALE
Client will not experience injury.	1. Reduce environmental stimuli. Assign private room with simple decor, on quiet unit if possible. Keep lighting and noise level low.	1. Client is extremely distractible and responses to even the slightest stimuli are exaggerated. A milieu unit may be too stimulating.
	2. Remove hazardous objects and substances (including smoking materials).	2. Rationality is impaired, and client may harm self inadvertently.
	3. Stay with the client who is hyperactive and agitated.	3. Nurse's presence may offer support and provide feeling of security for the client.
	4. Provide physical activities.	4. Physical activities help relieve pent-up tension.
	5. Administer tranquilizing medication as ordered by physician.	5. Antipsychotics are common and very effective for providing rapid relief from symptoms of hyperactivity.

NURSING DIAGNOSIS: RISK FOR VIOLENCE: SELF-DIRECTED OR DIRECTED AT OTHERS
RELATED TO: Manic excitement, delusional thinking, hallucinations

OUTCOME CRITERIA	NURSING INTERVENTIONS	RATIONALE
Client will not harm self or others	1. Maintain low level of stimuli in client's environment.	1. To minimize anxiety, agitation, and suspiciousness.
	2. Observe client's behavior at least every 15 minutes.	2. This is important so that intervention can occur if required to ensure client's (and others') safety.
	3. Ensure that all sharp objects, glass or mirrored items, belts, ties, smoking materials have been removed from client's environment.	3. These objects must be removed so that client cannot use them to harm self or others.
	4. Redirect violent behavior with physical outlets.	4. Physical activity is good for relieving pent-up tension and hostility.
	5. Maintain and convey a calm attitude to client. Respond matter-of-factly to verbal hostility.	5. Anxiety is contagious and can be transmitted from staff to client.
	6. Have sufficient staff to indicate a show of strength to client if necessary.	6. This conveys evidence of control over the situation and provides some physical security for staff.
	7. Offer tranquilizing medication. If client refuses, use of mechanical restraints may be necessary.	7. Client should be offered an avenue of the "least restrictive alternative."
	8. Medication may then be administered following application of mechanical restraints. Observe client every 15 minutes.	8. Ensure that needs for circulation, nutrition, hydration, and elimination are met. Client safety is a nursing priority.
	9. Remove restraints gradually, one at a time.	9. Removal of restraints gradually minimizes potential for injury to client and staff.

Continued on following page

TABLE 26.10 (Continued)

NURSING DIAGNOSIS: ALTERED NUTRITION: LESS THAN BODY REQUIREMENTS
RELATED TO: Refusal or inability to sit still long enough to eat
EVIDENCED BY: Weight loss, amenorrhea

OUTCOME CRITERIA	NURSING INTERVENTIONS	RATIONALE
Client will exhibit no signs or symptoms of malnutrition.	1. Provide high-protein, high-calorie, nutritious finger foods and drinks that can be consumed "on the run."	1. Client has difficulty sitting still long enough to eat a meal.
	2. Have juice and snacks on the unit at all times.	2. Nutritious intake is required on a regular basis to compensate for increased caloric requirement due to hyperactivity.
	3. Maintain accurate record of intake, output, calorie count, and weight. Monitor daily laboratory values.	3. Nutritional assessment data are important.
	4. Provide favorite foods.	4. Encourages eating.
	5. Supplement diet with vitamins and minerals.	5. Improves nutritional status.
	6. Walk or sit with client while he or she eats.	6. Nurse's presence offers support and encouragement to client to eat food that will maintain adequate nutrition.

NURSING DIAGNOSIS: IMPAIRED SOCIAL INTERACTION
RELATED TO: Egocentric and narcissistic behavior
EVIDENCED BY: Inability to develop satisfying relationships and manipulation of others for own desires

OUTCOME CRITERIA	NURSING INTERVENTIONS	RATIONALE
Client will interact appropriately with others.	1. Recognize that manipulative behaviors help to reduce feelings of insecurity by increasing feelings of power and control.	1. Understanding the motivation behind the behavior may facilitate greater acceptance of the individual.
	2. Set limits on manipulative behaviors. Explain what is expected and the consequences if limits are violated. Terms of the limitations must be agreed on by all staff who will be working with the client.	2. Consequences for violation of limits must be consistently administered, or behavior will not be eliminated.
	3. Ignore attempts by client to argue, bargain, or charm his or her way out of the limit setting.	3. Lack of feedback may decrease these manipulative behaviors.
	4. Give positive reinforcement for nonmanipulative behaviors.	4. Positive reinforcement enhances self-esteem and promotes repetition of desirable behaviors.
	5. Discuss consequences of client's behavior and how attempts are made to attribute them to others.	5. Client must accept responsibility for own behavior before adaptive change can occur.
	6. Help client identify positive aspects about self, recognize accomplishments, and feel good about them.	6. As self-esteem is increased, client will feel less need to manipulate others for own gratification.

determine the extent of the illness. Complete information is then given to the individual regarding the nature of depression, symptom pattern, frequency, clinical course, and alternative treatments. If the level of depression is severe, interpersonal psychotherapy has been shown to be more effective if conducted in combination with antidepressant medication. The client is encouraged to continue working and participating in regular activities during therapy. A mutually agreeable therapeutic contract is negotiated.

Phase II. Treatment at this phase focuses on helping the client resolve dysfunctional grief reactions. This may include resolving the ambivalence with the lost relationship, serving as a temporary substitute for the lost relationship, and assistance with establishing new relationships.

TABLE 26.11   CRITICAL PATHWAY OF CARE FOR THE CLIENT EXPERIENCING A MANIC EPISODE

Estimated Length of Stay: 7 days—variations from designated pathway should be documented in progress notes

Nursing Diagnosis and Categories of Care	Time Dimension	Goals and/or Actions	Time Dimension	Goals and/or Actions	Time Dimension	Discharge Outcome
Risk for injury/ violence	Day 1	Environment is made safe for client and others.	Ongoing	Client does not harm self or others.	Day 7	Client has not harmed self or others.
Referrals	Day 1	Psychiatrist Clinical nurse specialist Internist (may need to determine if symptoms are caused by other illness or medication side effects) Neurologist (may want to check for brain lesion) Alert hostility management team			Day 7	Discharge with follow-up appointments as required.
Diagnostic studies	Day 1	Drug screen Electrolytes Lithium level	Day 5	Lithium level	Day 7	Lithium level and discharge with instructions to return monthly to have level drawn.
Additional assessments	Day 1 Ongoing Ongoing	VS q4h Restraints p.r.n. Assess for signs of impending violent behavior: increase in psychomotor activity, angry affect, verbalized persecutory delusions or frightening hallucinations.	Day 2–7	Ongoing assessments		
Medications	Day 1	Antipsychotic medications, scheduled and p.r.n. Lithium carbonate 600 mg t.i.d. or q.i.d.	Day 2–7	Administer medications as ordered and observe for effectiveness and side effects.	Day 7	Client is discharged on maintenance dose lithium carbonate.
Client education			Day 4	Teach about lithium: Continue to take medication even when feeling okay. Teach symptoms of toxicity. Emphasize importance of monthly blood levels.	Day 7	Client is discharged with written instructions and verbalizes understanding of material presented.
			Day 6	Reinforce teaching.		

Continued on following page

TABLE 26.11 *(Continued)*

Estimated Length of Stay: 7 days—variations from designated pathway should be documented in progress notes

Nursing Diagnosis and Categories of Care	Time Dimension	Goals and/or Actions	Time Dimension	Goals and/or Actions	Time Dimension	Discharge Outcome
Altered nutrition: Less than body requirements					Day 7	Nutritional condition and weight have stabilized.
Referrals	Day 1	Consult dietitian.	Day 1–7	Fulfill nutritional needs.		
Diet	Day 1	High-protein, high-calorie nutritious finger foods. Juice and snacks as tolerated.	As mania subsides.	Regular diet with foods of client's choice.		
Diagnostic studies	Day 1	Chemistry profile Urinalysis	Day 2–7	Repeat of selected diagnostic studies as required.		
Additional assessments	Day 1–7	Weight I&O Skin turgor Color of mucous membranes				
Medications	Day 1–7	Multiple vitamin/mineral tab				
Client education			Day 4	Principles of nutrition; foods for maintenance of wellness; adequate sodium; 6–8 glasses of water/day. Contact dietitian if weight gain becomes a problem.	Day 5–7	Client demonstrates ability to select appropriate foods for healthy diet and verbalizes understanding of material presented.
			Day 6	Reinforce teaching.		

Other areas of treatment focus may include interpersonal disputes between the client and a significant other, difficult role transitions at various developmental life cycles, and correction of interpersonal deficits that may interfere with the client's ability to initiate or sustain interpersonal relationships.

Phase III. During the final phase of interpersonal psychotherapy, the therapeutic alliance is terminated. With emphasis on reassurance, clarification of emotional states, improvement of interpersonal communication, testing of perceptions, and performance in interpersonal settings, interpersonal psychotherapy has been successful in helping depressed persons recover enhanced social functioning.

For Mania. Manic clients traditionally have been difficult candidates for psychotherapy. They form a therapeutic relationship easily because they are eager to please and grateful for the therapist's interest. However, the relationship tends to remain shallow and rigid (Aleksandrowicz, 1980). Some reports have indicated that psychotherapy (in conjunction with lithium maintenance treatment) and counseling may indeed be useful with these individuals.

Lyness (1997) states:

"Individual or family psychotherapies are often crucial to forming and maintaining the treatment alliances within which compliance issues can be addressed. Psychotherapy also provides the framework for management of ongoing

TABLE 26.12 TOPICS FOR CLIENT/FAMILY EDUCATION RELATED TO BIPOLAR DISORDER

Nature of the Illness
1. Causes of bipolar disorder
2. Cyclic nature of the illness
3. Symptoms of depression
4. Symptoms of mania

Management of the Illness
1. Medication management
   a. Lithium
   b. Others: carbamazepine, valproic acid, clonazepam, verapamil
   c. Side effects
   d. Symptoms of lithium toxocity
   e. Importance of regular blood tests
   f. Adverse effects
   g. Importance of not stopping medication, even when feeling well
2. Assertive techniques
3. Anger management

Support Services
1. Crisis hotline
2. Support groups
3. Individual psychotherapy
4. Legal and financial assistance

stressors or dysfunctional behavioral patterns that might precipitate or exacerbate the bipolar disorder." (pp. 55–56)

Group Therapy for Depression and Mania

Group therapy forms an important dimension of multimodal treatment of the manic or depressed client (Spitz, 1988). Once an acute phase of the illness is passed, groups can provide an atmosphere in which individuals may discuss issues in their lives that cause, maintain, or arise out of having a serious affective disorder. The element of peer support provides a feeling of security, as troublesome or embarrassing issues are discussed and resolved. Some groups have other specific purposes, such as helping to monitor medication-related issues or serving as an avenue for promoting education related to the affective disorder and its treatment.

Support groups help members gain a sense of perspective on their condition and tangibly encourage them to link up with others who have common problems. A sense of hope is conveyed when the individual is able to see that he or she is not alone or unique in experiencing affective illness.

Self-help groups offer another avenue of support for the depressed or manic client. These groups are usually peer-led and are not meant to substitute for, or compete with, professional therapy. They offer supplementary support that frequently enhances compliance with the medical regimen. Examples of self-help groups are the National Depressive and Manic-Depressive Association (NDMDA), Depressives Anonymous, Families of Depressives, Manic and Depressive Support Group, Recovery Inc., and New Images for Widows. Although self-help groups are not psychotherapy groups, they do provide important adjunctive support experiences, which often have therapeutic benefit for participants (Spitz, 1988).

Family Therapy for Depression and Mania

The ultimate objective in working with families of clients with mood disorders is to synthesize the available data to formulate a therapeutic plan with two key goals: resolution of the symptoms and restoration or creation of adaptive family function (Spitz, 1988). As with group therapy, the most effective approach appears to be with a combination of psychotherapeutic and pharmacotherapeutic treatments. Some studies of bipolar disorder have shown that behavioral family treatment combined with lithium substantially reduces relapse rate compared with lithium therapy alone (Miklowitz, Goldstein, & Nuechterlein, 1988).

Kaplan, Sadock, & Grebb (1994) state:

"Family therapy is indicated if the disorder jeopardizes the patient's marriage or family functioning or if the mood disorder is promoted or maintained by the family situation. Family therapy examines the role of the mood-disordered member in the overall psychological well-being of the whole family; it also examines the role of the entire family in the maintenance of the patient's symptoms." (p. 545)

Cognitive Therapy for Depression and Mania

In **cognitive therapy,** the individual is taught to control thought distortions that are considered to be a factor in the development and maintenance of mood disorders. In the cognitive model, depression is characterized by a triad of negative distortions related to expectations of the environment, self, and future. The environment and activities within it are viewed as unsatisfying, the self is unrealistically devalued, and the future is perceived as hopeless. In the same model, mania is characterized by a positive cognitive triad—the self is seen as highly valued and powerful, experiences within the environment are viewed as overly positive, and the future is seen as one of unlimited opportunity (Leahy & Beck, 1988).

The general goals in cognitive therapy are to obtain symptom relief as quickly as possible, to assist the client in identifying dysfunctional patterns of thinking and behaving, and to guide the client to evidence and logic that effectively tests the validity of the dysfunctional thinking. Therapy focuses on changing "automatic thoughts" that occur spontaneously and contribute to the distorted affect. Examples of automatic thoughts in depression include:

1. Personalizing: "I'm the only one who failed."
2. All or nothing: "I'm a complete failure."
3. Mind reading: "He thinks I'm foolish."
4. Discounting positives: "The other questions were so easy. Any dummy could have gotten them right."

Examples of automatic thoughts in mania include:

1. Personalizing: "She's this happy only when she's with me."
2. All or nothing: "Everything I do is great."
3. Mind reading: "She thinks I'm wonderful."
4. Discounting negatives: "None of those mistakes are really important."

The client is asked to describe evidence that both supports and disputes the automatic thought. The logic underlying the inferences is then reviewed with the client. Another technique involves evaluating what would most likely happen if the client's automatic thoughts were true. Implications of the consequences are then discussed.

Clients should not become discouraged if one technique seems not to be working. No single technique works with all clients. He or she should be reassured that any of a number of techniques may be used, and both therapist and client may explore these possibilities (see Chapter 18).

Finally, the use of cognitive therapy does not preclude the value of administering medication (Leahy & Beck, 1988). Particularly in the treatment of mania, cognitive therapy should be considered a secondary treatment to pharmacological treatment. Cognitive therapy alone has offered encouraging results in the treatment of depression. In fact, the results of several studies with depressed clients show that in some cases cognitive therapy may be equally or even more effective than antidepressant medication (Wright & Thase, 1992; Hollon, DeRubeis, & Evans, 1992).

Organic Treatments

Psychopharmacology

For Depression. The tricyclic antidepressants (TCAs) have been the most widely prescribed drugs used to treat depression (Goodwin & Jamison, 1990). Since the initial discovery of their antidepressant properties, the tricyclic drugs have been subjected to hundreds of controlled trials, and their efficacy in treating depressive illness is now firmly established (see Chapter 19 for a detailed discussion of antidepressant medications).

A subsiding of symptoms may not occur for up to 4 weeks after beginning therapy with antidepressant medications. It is important, therefore, for clients to understand that even though it may seem the medication is not producing the desired effects, he or she must continue taking it for at least a month to determine efficacy. The greater effectiveness of one medication over another with any given client is not yet fully understood. Choice of drug may be based on symptoms. For example, anxious clients may be started on TCAs with the most sedative properties and clients with psychomotor retardation may be prescribed those antidepressants with the least sedative properties. When possible, selection of the appropriate drug is based on a history of previous responses to antidepressant therapy.

Common side effects of the TCAs include sedation, tachycardia, dry mouth, constipation, urinary retention, blurred vision, orthostatic hypotension, lowering of the seizure threshold, weight gain, and changes in sexual functioning. Elderly individuals may be particularly sensitive to these medications, and adjustments in dosage must be considered. TCAs are absolutely contraindicated in cases of severe heart disease and untreated narrow-angle glaucoma (Kragh-Sorensen, 1988).

Monoamine oxidase (MAO) inhibitors have a unique place in the history of antidepressant medications. They were originally used in the treatment of tuberculosis. Evidence that individuals who were treated with the medication experienced a sense of well-being, without bacteriological improvement, led to the discovery of their enzyme inhibition properties and the subsequent hypothesis that monoamines have a function in regulating mood (Schildkraut, 1965).

Following the initial enthusiasm about MAO inhibitors, they fell into relative disuse for nearly two decades because of a perceived poor risk-to-benefit ratio (Kurtz & Robinson, 1988). They have now regained widespread acceptance as a viable alternative to TCAs, as it has been shown that some individuals respond more beneficially to MAO inhibitors than to any other antidepressant medication.

The greatest concern with using MAO inhibitors is the potential for hypertensive crisis, which is considered a medical emergency. Hypertensive crisis occurs in clients receiving MAO inhibitor therapy who consume foods or drugs high in **tyramine** content (see Table 19.4). Typically, symptoms develop within 2 hours after ingestion of a food or drug high in tyramine, and include severe occipital and/or temporal pounding headaches with occasional photophobia. Sensations of choking, palpitations, and a feeling of "dread" are common. Marked systolic and diastolic hypertension occurs, sometimes with neck stiffness (Kurtz & Robinson, 1988). In addition to hypertensive crisis, side effects are similar to those associated with the TCAs.

A second generation of antidepressants has been marketed since the early 1970s. These include maprotiline (Ludiomil), amoxapine (Asendin), trazodone (Desyrel), bupropion (Wellbutrin), and most recently, mirtazapine (Remeron). Although some of these newer antidepressants were initially touted as being better than drugs used in the past, accumulated evidence and experience have dampened some of this initial enthusiasm (McCue & Georgotas, 1988).

Maprotiline, although as effective as the older antidepressants in treating depressive symptoms, carries an increased risk of seizures and greater toxicity in overdose.

Amoxapine, a derivative of the antipsychotic loxapine, is effective in treating psychotic depression but has a potential for causing neuroleptic malignant syndrome and tardive dyskinesia.

Trazodone is just as effective as the older antidepressants and has fewer side effects (the most common being sedation). A relatively rare adverse effect that has been observed with trazodone is priapism (prolonged, painful erection). This is a very problematic condition requiring surgical intervention in some clients.

Bupropion is as effective as the older antidepressants and has notably fewer anticholinergic and cardiovascular side effects. There have been some difficulties in the past, however, with increased risk of seizures, especially in emaciated clients.

Mirtazapine is the newest medication to be included with this group of antidepressants. A great deal is yet to be learned about the safety and efficacy of this drug, although in clinical trials it was associated with several cases of agranulocytosis. Clients should be closely monitored for signs and symptoms while on this medication.

The newest classifications of antidepressants include the selective serotonin reuptake inhibitors (SSRIs) and the nonselective reuptake inhibitors. The SSRIs include fluoxetine (Prozac), paroxetine (Paxil), sertraline (Zoloft), fluvoxamine (Luvox), and citalopram (Celexa). The nonselective reuptake inhibitors include venlafaxine (Effexor) and nefazodone (Serzone). These drugs have fewer anticholinergic and cardiovascular side effects than the TCAs and often work faster. Although long-term studies are not yet available, they appear to be just as effective in alleviating symptoms of depression as the older antidepressants.

For Mania. Lithium carbonate is the drug of choice for acute manic episodes, as well as for maintenance therapy to prevent or diminish the intensity of subsequent manic episodes. Its mode of action in the control of manic symptoms is unclear. It has also been indicated for treatment of bipolar depression (see Chapter 19 for a detailed discussion of lithium carbonate).

Common side effects of lithium therapy include drowsiness, dizziness, headache, dry mouth, thirst, gastrointestinal upset, fine hand tremors, pulse irregularities, polyuria, and weight gain. In initiating lithium therapy with an acutely manic individual, physicians commonly order an antipsychotic as well. Because normalization of symptoms with lithium may not be achieved for 1 to 3 weeks, the antipsychotic medication will calm the excessive hyperactivity of the manic client until the lithium reaches therapeutic level.

Therapeutic level of lithium carbonate is 1.0 to 1.5 mEq/L for acute mania and 0.6 to 1.2 mEq/L for maintenance therapy. There is a narrow margin between the therapeutic and toxic levels, and lithium levels should be drawn weekly until the therapeutic level is reached, and then monthly during maintenance therapy (Townsend, 1995). Because lithium toxicity is a life-threatening condition, monitoring of lithium levels is critical. The initial signs of lithium toxicity include ataxia, blurred vision, severe diarrhea, persistent nausea and vomiting, and tinnitis. Symptoms intensify as toxicity increases and include excessive output of dilute urine, psychomotor retardation, mental confusion, tremors and muscular irritability, seizures, impaired consciousness, oliguria or anuria, arrhythmias, coma, and eventually death.

Pretreatment assessments should include adequacy of renal functioning, as 95 percent of ingested lithium is eliminated via the kidneys (Johnson, 1988). Use of lithium during pregnancy is not recommended owing to results of studies that indicate a greater number of cardiac anomalies in babies born to mothers who consumed lithium, particularly in the first trimester.

A number of other medications have been tried on an investigational basis in the treatment of mania, with varying degrees of success. Examples include anticonvulsants

---

RESEARCH NOTE

Prevention of recurrent depression with cognitive behavioral therapy: Preliminary findings. *Archives of General Psychiatry* (1998, September), 55(9), 816–820. Fava, G.A., Rafanelli, C., Grandi, S., Conti, S., and Belluardo, P.

Description of the Study: This study was conducted to examine the effectiveness of cognitive behavioral therapy (CBT) in the reduction of recurrence of major depressive episodes in individuals with a history of recurrent major depression. Forty patients were treated on an outpatient basis for 3 to 5 months with usual doses of either tricyclic or SSRI antidepressant medication. Upon having achieved 10 weeks of remission of symptoms, the individuals were randomly assigned to receive either ten 30-minute sessions of CBT or unstructured clinical management (CM) as the medication was slowly tapered and discontinued. All patients were reassessed every 3 months for 2 years using the Paykel Clinical Interview for Depression.

Results of the Study: At the 2-year follow-up, the individuals who had received CBT had a significantly lower incidence (25 percent) of recurrence of depression than the CM patients (80 percent). The average length of time relapse in CBT patients was also significantly longer than in the CM patients (92 weeks versus 62 weeks).

Comments: The authors conclude that these results challenge the assumption that long-term drug treatment is the only tool to prevent relapse in patients with recurrent depression. Although maintenance pharmacotherapy may be necessary for some patients, adding a brief course of CBT may have an additive effect on patients who continue medications, as well as perhaps reducing the risk of symptom recurrence in patients who may be inclined to stop taking their antidepressants.

TEST YOUR CRITICAL THINKING SKILLS

Alice, age 29, had been working in the typing pool of a large corporation for 6 years. Her immediate supervisor recently retired and Alice was promoted to supervisor, in charge of 20 people in the department. Alice was flattered by the promotion but anxious about the additional responsibility of the position. Shortly after the promotion, she overheard two of her former coworkers saying, "Why in the world did they choose her? She's not the best one for the job. I know *I* certainly won't be able to respect her as a boss!" Hearing these comments added to Alice's anxiety and self-doubt.

Shortly after Alice began her new duties, her friends and coworkers noticed a change. She had a great deal of energy and worked long hours on her job. She began to speak very loudly and rapidly. Her roommate noticed that Alice slept very little, yet seldom appeared tired. Every night she would go out to bars and dances. Sometimes she brought men she had just met home to the apartment, something she had never done before. She bought lots of clothes and makeup and had her hair restyled in a more youthful look. She failed to pay her share of the rent and bills but came home with a brand new convertible. She lost her temper and screamed at her roommate to "Mind your own business!" when asked to pay her share.

She became irritable at work, and several of her subordinates reported her behavior to the corporate manager. When the manager confronted Alice about her behavior, she lost control, shouting, cursing, and striking out at anyone and anything that happened to be within her reach. The security officers restrained her and took her to the emergency department of the hospital, where she was admitted to the psychiatric unit. She had no previous history of psychiatric illness.

The psychiatrist assigned a diagnosis of bipolar I disorder and wrote orders for chlorpromazine (Thorazine) 50 mg IM STAT and p.r.n., chlorpromazine 25 mg PO q.i.d., and lithium carbonate 600 mg q.i.d.

Answer the following questions related to Alice:

1. What are the most important considerations with which the nurse who is taking care of Alice should be concerned?
2. Why was Alice given the diagnosis of bipolar I disorder?
3. The doctor should order a lithium level drawn after 4 to 6 days. For what symptoms should the nurse be on the alert?
4. Why did the physician order chlorpromazine in addition to the lithium carbonate?

(carbamazapine, clonazepam, valproic acid) and calcium channel blockers (verapamil). These drugs have been used as alternate or adjunctive approaches to management of clients with bipolar illness refractory to lithium.

Electroconvulsive Therapy for Depression and Mania

ECT is the induction of a grand mal (generalized) seizure through the application of electrical current to the brain.

ECT is effective with clients who are acutely suicidal and in the treatment of severe depression, particularly in those clients who are also experiencing psychotic symptoms and those with psychomotor retardation and neurovegetative changes, such as disturbances in sleep, appetite, and energy. It is often considered for treatment only after a trial of therapy with antidepressant medication has proved ineffective.

Episodes of acute mania are occasionally treated with ECT, particularly when the client does not tolerate or fails to respond to lithium or other drug treatment, or when life is threatened by dangerous behavior or exhaustion (see Chapter 20 for a detailed discussion of ECT).

SUMMARY

Depression is one of the oldest recognized psychiatric illnesses that is still prevalent today. It is so common, in fact, that it has been referred to as the "common cold of psychiatric disorders."

Everyone experiences transient feelings of depression from time to time, most commonly in response to a real or perceived loss. Several theorists have described the grief response as it progresses through stages over a predictable period. Grieving is considered to be maladaptive when the response is delayed, prolonged, or exaggerated. Pathological depression is an exaggerated grief response and occurs when an individual experiences a threat to the self-esteem.

The cause of depressive disorders is not entirely known. A number of factors, including genetics, biochemical influences, and psychosocial experiences likely enter into the development of the disorder. Secondary depression occurs in response to other physiological disorders. Symptoms occur along a continuum according to the degree of severity from transient to severe. The disorder occurs in all developmental levels, including childhood, adolescence, senescence, and during the puerperium.

Bipolar disorder, mania, is a maladaptive response to loss and has been referred to as the "mirror image of depression." Symptoms occur in response to a real or perceived

INTERNET REFERENCES

- Additional information about mood disorders, including psychosocial and pharmacological treatment of these disorders, may be located at the following websites:
  a. http://pw2.netcom.com/~shakey/bipolar.html
  b. http://www.pslgroup.com/DEPRESSION.HTM
  c. http://depression.miningco.com/
  d. http://www.snap.com
  e. http://www.ndmda.org
  f. http://www.fadavis.com
  g. http://www.laurus.com

loss, and are considered a denial of depression. Genetic influences have been strongly implicated in the development of the disorder. Various other physiological factors, such as biochemical and electrolyte alterations, as well as cerebral structural changes, have been implicated. Side effects of certain medications may also induce symptoms of mania. No single theory can explain the etiology of bipolar disorder, and it is likely that the illness is caused by a combination of biological and psychosocial factors. Symptoms of mania may be observed on a continuum of three phases, each identified by the degree of severity: phase I, hypomania; phase II, acute mania; and phase III, delirious mania.

Treatment of mood disorders includes individual, group, family, and cognitive therapies. Somatic therapies include psychopharmacology and ECT. Nursing care is accomplished using the six steps of the nursing process.

REVIEW QUESTIONS

SELF-EXAMINATION/LEARNING EXERCISE

Select the answer that is most appropriate for the questions that follow each section of the situation.

Situation: Margaret, age 68, was brought to the emergency department of a large regional medical center by her sister-in-law, who stated, "She does nothing but sit and stare into space. I can't get her to eat or anything!" Upon assessment, it was found that 6 months ago Margaret's husband of 45 years had died of a massive myocardial infarction. They had no children and had been inseparable. Since her husband's death, Margaret has visited the cemetery every day, changing the flowers often on his grave. She has not removed any of his clothes from the closet or chest of drawers. His shaving materials still occupy the same space in the bathroom. Over the months, Margaret has become more and more socially isolated. She refuses invitations from friends, preferring instead to make her daily trips to the cemetery. She has lost 15 lb and her sister-in-law reports that there is very little food in the house. Today she said to her sister-in-law, "I don't really want to live anymore. My life is nothing without Frank." Her sister-in-law became frightened and, with forceful persuasion, was able to convince Margaret she needed to see a doctor. Margaret is admitted to the psychiatric unit.

1. The *priority* nursing diagnosis for Margaret would be:

    a. Altered nutrition: less than body requirements.
    b. Dysfunctional grieving.
    c. Risk for self-directed violence.
    d. Social isolation.

2. The physician orders amitriptyline (Elavil) 20 mg q.i.d. for Margaret. After 3 days of taking the medication, Margaret says to the nurse, "I don't think this medicine is doing any good. I don't feel a bit better." What is the most appropriate response by the nurse?

    a. "Cheer up, Margaret. You have so much to be happy about."
    b. "Sometimes it takes a few weeks for the medicine to bring about an improvement in symptoms."
    c. "I'll report that to the physician, Margaret. Maybe he will order something different."
    d. "Try not to dwell on your symptoms, Margaret. Why don't you join the others down in the dayroom?"

After being stabilized on her medication, Margaret was released from the hospital with directions to continue taking the amitriptyline as ordered. A week later her sister-in-law found Margaret in bed and was unable to awaken her. An empty prescription bottle was by her side. She was revived in the emergency department and transferred to the psychiatric unit in a state of severe depression. The physician determines that ECT may help Margaret. Consent is obtained.

3. About 30 minutes prior to the first treatment the nurse administers atropine sulfate 0.4 mg IM. Rationale for this order is:

    a. To decrease secretions and increase heart rate.
    b. To relax muscles.
    c. To produce a calming effect.
    d. To induce anesthesia.

4. When Margaret is in the treatment room, the anesthesiologist administers thiopental sodium (Pentothal) followed by IV succinylcholine (Anectine). The purposes of these medications are to:

    a. Decrease secretions and increase heart rate.
    b. Prevent nausea and induce a calming effect.
    c. Minimize memory loss and stabilize mood.
    d. Induce anesthesia and relax muscles.

5. After three ECTs, Margaret's mood begins to lift and she tells the nurse, "I feel so much better, but I'm having trouble remembering some things that happened this last week." The nurse's best response would be:

   a. "Don't worry about that. Nothing important happened."
   b. "Memory loss is just something you have to put up with in order to feel better."
   c. "Memory loss is a side effect of ECT, but it is only temporary. Your memory should return within a few weeks."
   d. "Forget about last week, Margaret. You need to look forward from here."

A year later, Margaret presents in the emergency department, once again accompanied by her sister-in-law. This time Margaret is agitated, pacing, demanding, and speaking very loudly. "I didn't want to come here! My sister-in-law is just jealous, and she's trying to make it look like I'm insane!" Upon assessment, the sister-in-law reports that Margaret has become engaged to a 25-year-old construction worker to whom she has willed her sizable inheritance and her home. Margaret loudly praises her fiance's physique and sexual abilities. She has been spending large sums of money on herself and giving her fiance $500 a week. The sister-in-law tells the physician, "I know it is Margaret's business what she does with her life, but I'm really worried about her. She is losing weight again. She eats very little and almost never sleeps. I'm afraid she's going to just collapse!" Margaret is once again admitted to the psychiatric unit.

6. The *priority* nursing diagnosis for Margaret is:

   a. Altered nutrition: less than body requirements related to not eating.
   b. Risk for injury related to hyperactivity.
   c. Sleep pattern disturbance related to agitation.
   d. Ineffective individual coping related to denial of depression.

7. One way to promote adequate nutritional intake for Margaret is to:

   a. Sit with her during meals to ensure that she eats everything on her tray.
   b. Have her sister-in-law bring all her food from home, as she knows Margaret's likes and dislikes.
   c. Provide high-calorie, nutritious finger foods and snacks that Margaret can eat "on the run."
   d. Tell Margaret that she will be on room restriction until she starts gaining weight.

8. The physician orders lithium carbonate 600 mg t.i.d. for Margaret. There is a narrow margin between the therapeutic and toxic levels of lithium. Therapeutic range for acute mania is:

   a. 1.0 to 1.5 mEq/L.
   b. 10 to 15 mEq/L.
   c. 0.5 to 1.0 mEq/L.
   d. 5 to 10 mEq/L.

9. After an appropriate length of time, the physician determines that Margaret does not respond satisfactorily to lithium therapy. He changes her medication to another drug that has been found to be effective in the treatment of bipolar mania. This drug is:

   a. Molindone (Moban).
   b. Paroxetine (Paxil).
   c. Carbamazepine (Tegretol).
   d. Tranylcypromine (Parnate).

10. Margaret's statement, "My sister-in-law is just jealous, and she's trying to make it look like I'm insane!" is an example of:

    a. A delusion of grandeur.
    b. A delusion of persecution.
    c. A delusion of reference.
    d. A delusion of control or influence.

REFERENCES

Aleksandrowicz, D.R. (1980). Psychoanalytic studies of mania. In R.H. Belmaker & H.M. vanPraag (Eds.), *Mania: An evolving concept.* Jamaica, NY: Spectrum Publications.

American Psychiatric Association. (1994). *Diagnostic and statistical manual of mental disorders* (4th ed.). Washington, DC: American Psychiatric Association.

Beck, A.T., Rush, A.J., Shaw, B.F., & Emery, G. (1979). *Cognitive theory of depression.* New York: Guilford Press.

Becker, E. (1964). *The revolution in psychiatry: The new understanding of man.* Glencoe, IL: Free Press.

Berrios, G.E. (1988). Depressive and manic states during the nineteenth century. In A. Georgotas & R. Cancro (Eds.), *Depression and mania.* New York: Elsevier Science Publishing.

Blazer, D. (1994). Geriatric psychiatry. In R.E. Hales, S.C. Yudofsky, & J.A. Talbott (Eds.), *The American Psychiatric Press textbook of psychiatry* (2nd ed.). Washington, DC: American Psychiatric Press.

Bowlby, J. (1961). Processes of mourning. *International Journal of Psychoanalysis, 42,* 22.

Bowlby, J. (1973). *Attachment and loss: Separation, anxiety, and anger.* New York: Basic Books.

Boyd, J.H., & Weissman, M.M. (1982). Epidemiology. In E.S. Paykel (Ed.), *Handbook of affective disorders.* New York: Guilford Press.

Burke, K.C., Burke, J.D., & Regier, D.A. (1990). Age at onset of selected mental disorders in five community populations. *Archives of General Psychiatry, 47,* 511–518.

Casey, V., & Dwyer, J.T. (1987, Nov/Dec). Premenstrual syndrome: Theories and evidence. *Nutrition Today,* 4–12.

Cohen, M.B., et al. (1954). An intensive study of twelve cases of manic-depressive psychosis. *Psychiatry, 17,* 103–138.

Craig, T.J. (1994). Epidemiology of psychiatric illness. In G. Winokur & P.J. Clayton (Eds.), *The medical basis of psychiatry.* Philadelphia: W.B. Saunders.

Duncker, A.P., & Greenberg, S.R. (1997). *A profile of older Americans.* Washington, DC: American Association of Retired Persons and Administration on Aging. U.S. Department of Health and Human Services.

Eisendrath, S.J. (1996). Psychiatric disorders. In L.M. Tierney, S.J. McPhee, & M.A. Papadakis (Eds.), *Current medical diagnosis and treatment* (35th ed.). Norwalk, CT: Appleton & Lange.

Engel, G. (1964). Grief and grieving. *American Journal of Nursing, 64,* 93.

Field, W.E. (1985). Physical causes of depression. *Journal of Psychosocial Nursing and Mental Health Services, 23*(10), 6–11.

Freedman, A.M., et al. (1976). *Modern synopsis of psychiatry II.* Baltimore: Williams & Wilkins.

Freud, S. (1957). *Mourning and melancholia,* Vol. 14 (standard ed.). London: Hogarth Press. (Original work published 1917.)

Geller, B., & Carr, L.G. (1988). Similarities and differences between adult and pediatric major depressive disorders. In A. Georgotas & R. Cancro (Eds.), *Depression and mania.* New York: Elsevier Science Publishing.

Georgotas, A., & Cancro, R. (Eds.) (1988). *Depression and mania.* New York: Elsevier Science Publishing.

Ghosh, T.B., & Victor, B.S. (1994). Suicide. In R.E. Hales, S.C. Yudofsky, & J.A. Talbott (Eds.), *The American Psychiatric Press textbook of psychiatry* (2nd ed.). Washington, DC: American Psychiatric Press.

Gibson, R.W., et al. (1959). On the dynamics of the manic-depressive personality. *American Journal of Psychiatry, 115,* 1101–1107.

Goodwin, F.K., & Jamison, K.R. (1990). *Manic-depressive illness.* New York: Oxford University Press.

Henderson, V., & Nite, G. (1978). *Principles and practice of nursing* (6th ed.). New York: Macmillan.

Herskowitz, J. (1988). *Is your child depressed?* New York: Pharos Books.

Hollandsworth, J.G. (1990). *The physiology of psychological disorders.* New York: Plenum Press.

Hollon, S.D., DeRubeis, R.J., & Evans, M.D. (1992). Cognitive therapy and pharmacotherapy for depression: Singly and in combination. *Archives of General Psychiatry, 49,* 774–781.

Horowitz, M.J., et al. (1980). Pathological grief and the activation of latent self-images. *American Journal of Psychiatry, 137*(10), 1157–1162.

Janowsky, D.S., et al. (1974). Interpersonal maneuvers of manic patients. *American Journal of Psychiatry, 131,* 250–255.

Janowsky, D.S., et al. (1988). Neurochemistry of depression and mania.

In A. Georgotas & R. Cancro (Eds.), *Depression and mania.* New York: Elsevier Science Publishing.

Johnson, G.F.S. (1988). Highlights on the main pharmacological treatments for mania. In A. Georgotas & R. Cancro (Eds.), *Depression and mania.* New York: Elsevier Science Publishing.

Kaplan, H.I., & Sadock, B.J. (1985). *Modern synopsis of comprehensive textbook of psychiatry* (4th ed.). Baltimore: Williams & Wilkins.

Kaplan, H.I., Sadock, B.J., & Grebb, J.A. (1994). *Synopsis of psychiatry: Behavioral sciences, clinical psychiatry* (7th ed.). Baltimore: Williams & Wilkins.

Kelsoe, J.R. (1991, Summer). Molecular genetics of mood disorders. *Journal of California Alliance for the Mentally Ill, 2*(4), 20–22.

Kestenbaum, C.J., & Trautman, P.D. (1992). Normal development and major problems of adolescents. In F.I. Kass, J.M. Oldham, & H. Pardes (Eds.), *The Columbia University College of Physicians and Surgeons complete home guide to mental health.* New York: Henry Holt and Company.

Klein, M. (1948). Mourning and its relation to manic-depressive states. In M. Klein (Ed.), *Contributions to psychoanalysis, 1921–1945.* London: Hogarth Press.

Klerman, G.L. (1988). Principles of interpersonal psychotherapy for depression. In A. Georgotas & R. Cancro (Eds.), *Depression and mania.* New York: Elsevier Science Publishing.

Kragh-Sorensen, P. (1988). Tricyclic antidepressants. In A. Georgotas & R. Cancro (Eds.), *Depression and mania.* New York: Elsevier Science Publishing.

Kübler-Ross, E. (1969). *On death and dying.* New York: Macmillan.

Kurtz, N.M., & Robinson, D.S. (1988). Monoamine oxidase inhibitors. In A. Georgotas & R. Cancro (Eds.), *Depression and mania.* New York: Elsevier Science Publishing.

Leahy, R.L., & Beck, A.T. (1988). Cognitive therapy of depression and mania. In A. Georgotas & R. Cancro (Eds.), *Depression and mania.* New York: Elsevier Science Publishing.

Lewis, M., & Volkmar, F. (1990). *Clinical aspects of child and adolescent development.* Philadelphia: Lea & Febiger.

Lindemann, E. (1944). Symptomatology and management of acute grief. *American Journal of Psychiatry, 101,* 141–148.

Lyness, J.M. (1997). *Psychiatric pearls.* Philadelphia: F.A. Davis.

McCue, R.E., & Georgotas, A. (1988). Newer generation antidepressants and lithium. In A. Georgotas & R. Cancro (Eds.), *Depression and mania.* New York: Elsevier Science Publishing.

McKinney, W.T., & Moran, E.C. (1982). Animal models. In E.S. Paykel (Ed.), *Handbook of affective disorders.* New York: Guilford Press.

Miklowitz, D.J., Goldstein, M.J., & Nuechterlein, K.H. (1988). Family factors and the course of bipolar affective disorder. *Archives of General Psychiatry, 45,* 225–231.

Parkes, C.M. (1975). Determinants of outcome following bereavement. *Omega, 6*(4), 303–323.

Person, E.S. (1992). Women's issues at a time of social change. In F.I. Kass, J.M. Oldham, & H. Pardes (Eds.), *The Columbia University College of Physicians and Surgeons complete home guide to mental health.* New York: Henry Holt and Company.

Pitt, B. (1982). Depression and childbirth. In E.S. Paykel (Ed.), *Handbook of affective disorders.* New York: Guilford Press.

Quitkin, F.M., & Endicott, J. (1992). Depression and other mood disorders. In F.I. Kass, J.M. Oldham, & H. Pardes (Eds.), *The Columbia University College of Physicians and Surgeons complete home guide to mental health.* New York: Henry Holt and Company.

Rosenn, D.W. (1982). Suicidal behavior in children and adolescents. In Bassuk et al. (Eds.), *Lifelines: Clinical perspectives on suicide.* New York: Plenum Press.

Ruark, J.E., & Gonda, T.A. (1988). Grief and mourning. In A. Georgotas & R. Cancro (Eds.), *Depression and mania.* New York: Elsevier Science Publishing.

Sargent, M. (1989). *Depressive illnesses: Treatments bring new hope.* Rockville, MD: National Institute of Mental Health.

Schildkraut, J.J. (1965). The catecholamine hypothesis of affective disorder: A review of supportive evidence. *American Journal of Psychiatry, 122,* 505–518.

Seligman, M.E.P. (1973). Fall into helplessness. *Psychology Today, 7,* 43–48.

Shives, L.R. (1990). *Basic concepts of psychiatric-mental health nursing* (2nd ed.). Philadelphia: J.B. Lippincott.

Smith, S.F., Karasik, D.A., & Meyer, B.J. (1984). *Psychiatric and psychosocial nursing*. Los Altos, CA: National Nursing Review.

Spitz, H.I. (1988). Principles of group and family therapy for depression and mania. In A. Georgotas & R. Cancro (Eds.), *Depression and mania*. New York: Elsevier Science Publishing.

Spitz, R.A. (1946). Anaclitic depression: An inquiry into the genesis of psychiatric conditions in early childhood, II. *Psychoanalytic Study of the Child, 2*, 313–347.

Stokes, P.E. (1988). Psychoendocrinology of depression and mania. In A. Georgotas & R. Cancro (Eds.), *Depression and mania*. New York: Elsevier Science Publishing.

Thompson, J.M., McFarland, G.K., Hirsch, J.E., Tucker, S.M., & Bowers, A.C. (1986). *Clinical nursing*. St. Louis: C.V. Mosby.

Townsend, M.C. (1995). *Drug guide for psychiatric nursing* (2nd ed.). Philadelphia: F.A. Davis.

Ugarriza, D.N. (1992). Postpartum affective disorders: Incidence and treatment. *Journal of Psychosocial Nursing, 30*(5), 29–32.

Winokur, G. (1994). Unipolar depression. In G. Winokur & P.J. Clayton (Eds.), *The medical basis of psychiatry* (2nd ed.). Philadelphia: W.B. Saunders.

Wright, J.H., & Thase, M.E. (1992). Cognitive and biological therapies: A synthesis. *Psychiatric Annals, 22*, 451–458.

Bibliography

Anonymous. A positive note . . . on being depressed. (1997). *Journal of Psychosocial Nursing and Mental Health Services, 35*(2), 44.

Chuong, C.J., Pearsall-Otey, L.R., & Rosenfeld, B.L. (1995, May/June). A practical guide to relieving PMS. *Contemporary Nurse Practitioner, 1*(3), 31–37.

Davis, K.M., & Mathew, E. (1998). Pharmacologic management of depression in the elderly. *The Nurse Practitioner, 23*(6), 16–47.

Doenges, M.E., Townsend, M.C., & Moorhouse, M.F. (1998). *Psychiatric care plans: Guidelines for client care* (3rd ed.). Philadelphia: F.A. Davis.

Egan, M.P., Rivera, S.G., Robillard, R.R., & Hanson, A. (1997). The no suicide contract: Helpful or harmful? *Journal of Psychosocial Nursing and Mental Health Services, 35*(3), 31–33.

Fagan-Pryor, E.C., Gonzalez, A, & Richardson, D. (1997). Effects of venlafaxine on blood pressure: A case report. *Journal of the American Psychiatric Nurses Association, 3*(6), 198–202.

Flowers, E.M. (1997). Recognition and psychopharmacologic treatment of geriatric depression. *Journal of the American Psychiatric Nurses Association, 3*(2), 32–41.

Isaacs, A. (1998). Depression and your patient. *American Journal of Nursing, 98*(7), 26–32.

Knop, D.S., Bergman-Evans, B., & McCabe, B.W. (1998). In sickness and in health: An exploration of the perceived quality of the marital relationship, coping, and depression in caregivers of spouses with Alzheimer's disease. *Journal of Psychosocial Nursing and Mental Health Services, 36*(1), 16–21.

McEnany, G. (1996). Rhythm & blues revisited: Biological rhythm disturbances in depression, Part I. *Journal of the American Psychiatric Nurses Association, 2*(1), 15–22.

McEnany, G. (1996). Rhythm & blues revisited: Biological rhythm disturbances in depression, Part II. *Journal of the American Psychiatric Nurses Association, 2*(2), 54–57.

McEnany, G. (1996). Phototherapy and sleep manipulations: An examination of two nondrug biologic interventions for depression. *Journal of the American Psychiatric Nurses Association, 2*(3), 86–93.

Mohr, W.K. (1998). Updating what we know about depression in adolescents. *Journal of Psychosocial Nursing and Mental Health Services, 36*(9), 12–19.

Shea, N.M., McBride, L., Gavin, C., & Bauer, M.S. (1997). The effects of an ambulatory collaborative practice model on process and outcome of care for bipolar disorder. *Journal of the American Psychiatric Nurses Association, 3*(2), 49–57.

Townsend, M.C. (1997). *Nursing diagnoses in psychiatric nursing: A pocket guide for care plan construction* (4th ed.). Philadelphia: F.A. Davis.

Zerhusen, J.D., Boyle, K., & Wilson, W. (1991). Out of the darkness: Group cognitive therapy for depressed elderly. *Journal of Psychosocial Nursing and Mental Health Services, 29*(9), 16–21.

the other hand, a fear of elevators may very well interfere with this individual's daily functioning.

Specific phobias have been classified according to the phobic stimulus. A list of some of the more common ones appears in Table 27.4. This list is by no means all-inclusive. People can become phobic about almost any object or situation, and anyone with a little knowledge of Greek or Latin can produce a phobia classification, thereby making possibilities for the list almost infinite.

The *DSM-IV* identifies subtypes of the most common specific phobias. They include the following:

1. **Animal Type.** This subtype would be identified as part of the diagnosis if the fear is of animals or insects.
2. **Natural Environment Type.** Examples of this subtype include objects or situations that occur within the natural environment, such as heights, storms, or water.
3. **Blood-Injection–Injury Type.** This diagnosis should be specified if the fear is of seeing blood or an injury or of receiving an injection or other invasive medical or dental procedure.
4. **Situational Type.** This subtype is designated if the fear is of a specific situation, such as public transportation, tunnels, bridges, elevators, flying, driving, or enclosed places.
5. **Other Type.** This category covers all other excessive or irrational fears. It may include fear of contracting a serious illness, fear of situations that might lead to vomiting or choking, fear of loud noises, or fear of driving.

The *DSM-IV* diagnostic criteria for specific phobia are presented in Table 27.5.

Predisposing Factors to Phobias

The cause of phobias is unknown; however, various theories exist that may offer insight into the etiology.

TABLE 27.4 CLASSIFICATIONS OF SPECIFIC PHOBIAS

CLASSIFICATION	FEAR
Acrophobia	Height
Ailurophobia	Cats
Algophobia	Pain
Anthophobia	Flowers
Anthropophobia	People
Aquaphobia	Water
Arachnophobia	Spiders
Astraphobia	Lightning
Belonophobia	Needles
Brontophobia	Thunder
Claustrophobia	Closed spaces
Cynophobia	Dogs
Dementophobia	Insanity
Equinophobia	Horses
Herpetophobia	Lizards, reptiles
Mikrophobia	Germs
Murophobia	Mice
Mysophobia	Dirt, germs, contamination
Numerophobia	Numbers
Nyctophobia	Darkness
Ophidiophobia	Snakes
Pyrophobia	Fire
Siderodromophobia	Railways
Taphaphobia	Being buried alive
Thanatophobia	Death
Trichophobia	Hair
Triskaidekaphobia	Concerning the number 13
Xenophobia	Strangers
Zoophobia	Animals

SOURCE: From Goodwin (1983), with permission.

TABLE 27.5 DIAGNOSTIC CRITERIA FOR SPECIFIC PHOBIA

A. Marked and persistent fear that is excessive or unreasonable, cued by the presence or anticipation of a specific object or situation (e.g., flying, heights, animals, receiving an injection, seeing blood).

B. Exposure to the phobic stimulus almost invariably provokes an immediate anxiety response, which may take the form of a situationally bound or situationally predisposed panic attack.
   NOTE: In children, the anxiety may be expressed by crying, tantrums, freezing, or clinging.

C. The person recognizes that the fear is excessive or unreasonable.
   NOTE: In children, this feature may be absent.

D. The phobic situation(s) is avoided or else is endured with intense anxiety or distress.

E. The avoidance, anxious anticipation, or distress in the feared situation(s) interferes significantly with the person's normal routine, occupational (academic) functioning, or social activities or relationships, or there is marked distress about having the phobia.

F. In individuals under 18 years, the duration is at least 6 months.

G. The anxiety, panic attacks, or phobic avoidance associated with the specific object or situation are not better accounted for by another mental disorder.

The diagnosis may be further specified as:
   Animal type
   Natural environment type (e.g., heights, storms, water)
   Blood-injection–injury type
   Situational type (e.g., airplanes, elevators, enclosed places)
   Other type

SOURCE: From APA (1994), with permission.

Psychoanalytical Theory. Freud believed that phobias developed when a child, feeling normal incestual feelings toward the opposite-sex parent (Oedipal complex), becomes frightened of the aggression he fears the same-sex parent feels for him (castration anxiety). To protect themselves, these children *repress* this fear of hostility from the father and *displace* it onto something safer and more neutral, which becomes the phobic stimulus. The phobic stimulus becomes the symbol for the father, but the child does not realize this.

Modern-day psychoanalysts believe in the same concept of phobic development but that castration anxiety is not the sole source of phobias. They believe that other unconscious fears may also be expressed in a symbolic manner as phobias. For example, a female child who was sexually abused by an adult male family friend while he was taking her for a ride in his boat grew up with an intense, irrational fear of all water vessels. Psychoanalytical theory postulates that fear of the man was repressed and displaced onto boats. Boats became an unconscious symbol for the feared person, but one that the young girl viewed as safer since her fear of boats prevented her from having to confront the real fear.

Learning Theory. Classic conditioning in the case of phobias may be explained as follows—a stressful stimulus produces an "unconditioned" response: fear. When the stressful stimulus is repeatedly paired with a harmless object, eventually the harmless object alone produces a "conditioned" response: fear. If, to avoid fear, the person avoids the harmless object, the fear becomes a phobia (Goodwin, 1983).

Some learning theorists hold that fears are conditioned responses and thus learned by imposing rewards for appropriate behaviors. What then is the reward if a phobia is learned? Goodwin (1983) states:

"The reward is powerful indeed. Every time a person avoids a phobic situation, he escapes fear. Avoidance may be a nuisance, but it is clearly preferable to panic."

Phobias may also be acquired by direct learning or imitation (modeling) (e.g., a mother who exhibits fear toward an object will provide a model for the child, who may also develop a phobia toward the same object).

Cognitive Theory. Cognitive theorists espouse that anxiety is the product of faulty cognitions or anxiety-inducing self-instructions (Emmelkamp, 1982). Two types of faulty thinking have been investigated: negative self-statements and irrational beliefs. Cognitive theorists believe that some individuals engage in negative and irrational thinking that produces anxiety reactions. The individual begins to seek out avoidance behaviors to prevent the anxiety reactions, and phobias result.

Somewhat related to the cognitive theory is the involvement of locus of control. Johnson and Sarason (1978) suggested that individuals with internal locus of control and those with external locus of control might respond differently to life change. These researchers propose that locus of control orientation may be an important variable in the development of phobias. Emmelkamp (1982) proposed that individuals with an external control orientation experiencing anxiety attacks in a stressful period are likely to mislabel the anxiety and attribute it to external sources (e.g., crowded areas) or to a disease (e.g., heart attack). They may perceive the experienced anxiety as being outside of their control. Figure 27.2 depicts a graphic model of the relationship between locus of control and the development of phobias.

Biological Aspects

Temperament. Goodwin (1983) suggests that some fears are innate. He states:

"These fears even follow a kind of biological timetable. At six months, the infant is frightened by loud noises and sudden movements. At age three he is frightened by strangers; at five by animals. Fear of open spaces and social situations occur (if they occur) much later: in adolescence or early adulthood."

Innate does not necessarily mean *genetic*. Innate fears represent a part of the overall characteristics or tendencies with which one is born that influence how one responds throughout life to specific situations. Innate fears usually do not reach phobic intensity but may have the capacity for such development if reinforced by events in later life. For example, a 4-year-old girl is afraid of dogs. By age 5, however, she has overcome her fear and plays with her own dog and the neighbors' dogs without fear. Then, when she is 19, she is bitten by a stray dog and develops a dog phobia.

Life Experiences. Certain early experiences may set the stage for phobic reactions later in life. Some researchers believe that phobias, particularly specific phobias, are symbolic of original anxiety-producing objects or situations that have been repressed. Examples include:

1. A child who is punished by being locked in a closet develops a phobia for elevators or other closed places.
2. A child who falls down a flight of stairs develops a phobia for high places.
3. A young woman who, as a child, survived a plane crash in which both her parents were killed has a phobia of airplanes.

Transactional Model of Stress/Adaptation. The etiology of phobic disorders is most likely influenced by multiple factors. In Figure 27.3, a graphic depiction of this theory of multiple causation is presented in the transactional model of stress/adaptation.

Diagnosis/Outcome Identification

Nursing diagnoses are formulated from the data gathered during the assessment phase and with background knowl-

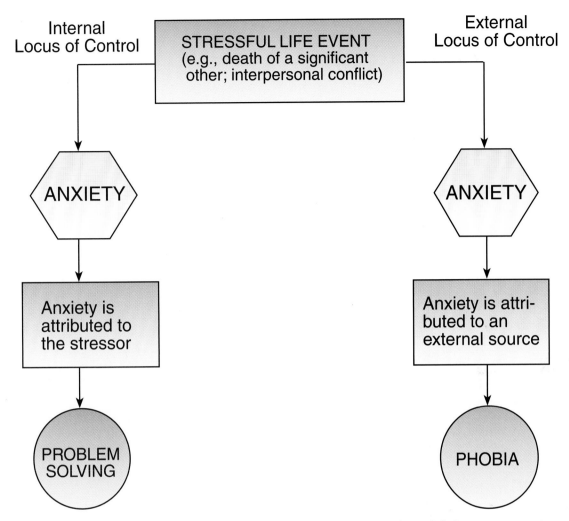

**Internal
Locus of Control**

**External
Locus of Control**

STRESSFUL LIFE EVENT
(e.g., death of a significant
other; interpersonal conflict)

ANXIETY

ANXIETY

Anxiety is
attributed to
the stressor

Anxiety is attri-
buted to an
external source

PROBLEM
SOLVING

PHOBIA

Figure 27.2   Locus of control as a variable in the etiology of phobias.

edge regarding predisposing factors to the disorder. Some common nursing diagnoses for clients with phobias include:

> Fear related to causing embarrassment to self in front of others; to being in a place from which one is unable to escape; or to a specific stimulus, evidenced by behavior directed toward avoidance of the feared object or situation.

> Social isolation related to fears of being in a place from which one is unable to escape, evidenced by staying alone, refusing to leave room or home.

The following criteria may be used for measurement of outcomes in the care of the client with phobic disorders.

THE CLIENT:

1. Functions adaptively in the presence of the phobic object or situation without experiencing panic anxiety.
2. Demonstrates techniques that can be used to maintain anxiety at a manageable level.

3. Voluntarily attends group activities and interacts with peers.
4. Discusses feelings that may have contributed to irrational fears.
5. Verbalizes a future plan of action for responding in the presence of the phobic object or situation without developing panic anxiety.

Planning/Implementation

Table 27.6 provides a plan of care for the client with phobic disorder. Nursing diagnoses are presented, along with outcome criteria, appropriate nursing interventions, and rationales for each.

Evaluation

Reassessment is conducted to determine if the nursing actions have been successful in achieving the objectives of care. Evaluation of the nursing actions for the client with

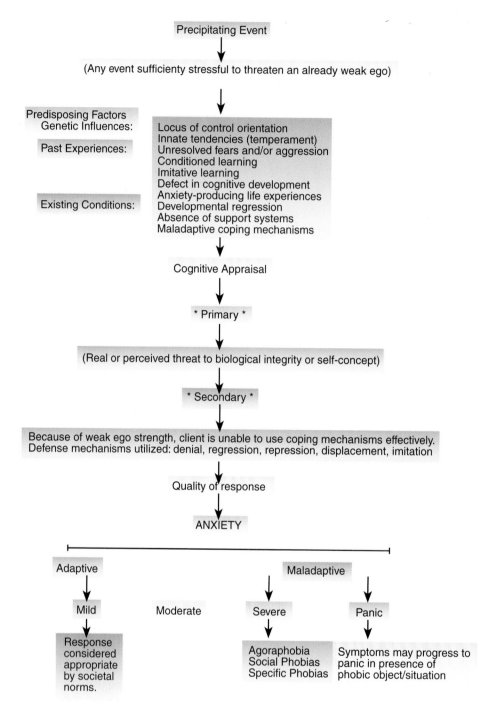

Figure 27.3 The dynamics of phobic disorder using the transactional model of stress/adaptation.

a phobic disorder may be facilitated by gathering information using the following types of questions:

1. Can the client discuss the phobic object or situation without becoming anxious?
2. Can the client function in the presence of the phobic object or situation without experiencing panic anxiety?
3. Does the client voluntarily leave the room or home to attend group activities?
4. Is the client able to verbalize the signs and symptoms of escalating anxiety?
5. Is the client able to demonstrate techniques that he or she may use to prevent the anxiety from escalating to the panic level?
6. Can the client verbalize the thinking process that promoted the irrational fears?
7. Is the client capable of creating change in his or her life to confront (or eliminate, or avoid) the phobic situation?

TABLE 27.6 CARE PLAN FOR CLIENTS WITH PHOBIC DISORDERS

NURSING DIAGNOSIS: FEAR

RELATED TO: Causing embarrassment to self in front of others; being in a place from which one is unable to escape; or a specific stimulus

EVIDENCED BY: Behavior directed toward avoidance of the feared object or situation

OUTCOME CRITERIA	NURSING INTERVENTIONS	RATIONALE
Client will be able to function in presence of phobic object or situation without experiencing panic anxiety.	1. Reassure client that he or she is safe.	1. At the panic level of anxiety, client may fear for his or her own life.
	2. Explore client's perception of the threat to physical integrity or threat to self-concept.	2. It is important to understand client's perception of the phobic object or situation to assist with the desensitization process.
	3. Discuss reality of the situation with client to recognize aspects that can be changed and those that cannot.	3. Client must accept the reality of the situation (aspects that cannot change) before the work of reducing the fear can progress.
	4. Include client in making decisions related to selection of alternative coping strategies. (Example: Client may choose either to avoid the phobic stimulus or to attempt to eliminate the fear associated with it.)	4. Allowing the client choices provides a measure of control and serves to increase feelings of self-worth.
	5. If client elects to work on elimination of the fear, techniques of desensitization or implosion therapy may be employed. (See explanation of these techniques under "Treatment Modalities" at the end of this chapter.	5. Fear is decreased as the physical and psychological sensations diminish in response to repeated exposure to the phobic stimulus under nonthreatening conditions.
	6. Encourage client to explore underlying feelings that may be contributing to irrational fears and to face them rather than suppress them.	6. Exploring underlying feelings may help the client to confront unresolved conflicts and develop more adaptive coping abilities.

NURSING DIAGNOSIS: SOCIAL ISOLATION

RELATED TO: Fears of being in a place from which one is unable to escape

EVIDENCED BY: Staying alone; refusing to leave room or home

OUTCOME CRITERIA	NURSING INTERVENTIONS	RATIONALE
Client will voluntarily participate in group activities with peers.	1. Convey an accepting attitude and unconditional positive regard. Make brief, frequent contacts. Be honest and keep all promises.	1. These interventions increase feelings of self-worth and facilitate a trusting relationship.
	2. Attend group activities with client if it may be frightening for him or her.	2. The presence of a trusted individual provides emotional security.
	3. Be cautious with touch. Allow client extra space and an avenue for exit if anxiety becomes overwhelming.	3. A person in panic anxiety may perceive touch as threatening.
	4. Administer tranquilizing medications as ordered by physician. Monitor for effectiveness and adverse side effects.	4. Antianxiety medications, such as diazepam, chlordiazepoxide, or alprazolam, help to reduce level of anxiety in most individuals, thereby facilitating interactions with others.

Continued on following page

TABLE 22.6 *(Continued)*

5. Discuss with client signs and symptoms of increasing anxiety and techniques to interrupt the response (e.g., relaxation exercises, "thought stopping").	5. Maladaptive behaviors, such as withdrawal and suspiciousness, are manifested during times of increased anxiety.
6. Give recognition and positive reinforcement for voluntary interactions with others.	6. Recognition enhances self-esteem and encourages repetition of acceptable behaviors.

8. Is the client able to verbalize resources outside the hospital from whom he or she can seek assistance during times of extreme stress?

Obsessive-Compulsive Disorder

Background Assessment Data

The *DSM-IV* describes this disorder as recurrent obsessions or compulsions that are severe enough to be time consuming or to cause marked distress or significant impairment (APA, 1994).

Obsessions are defined as unwanted, intrusive, persistent ideas, thoughts, impulses, or images that cause marked anxiety or distress. The most common ones include repeated thoughts about contamination, repeated doubts, a need to have things in a particular order, aggressive or horrific impulses, and sexual imagery (APA, 1994).

Compulsions denote unwanted repetitive behavior patterns or mental acts (e.g., praying, counting, repeating words silently) that are intended to reduce anxiety, not to provide pleasure or gratification (APA, 1994). They may be performed in response to an obsession or in a stereotyped fashion. The individual recognizes that the behavior is excessive or unreasonable but, because of the feeling of relief from discomfort that it promotes, is compelled to continue the act. The most common compulsions involve washing and cleaning, counting, checking, requesting or demanding assurances, repeating actions, and ordering (APA, 1994). The *DSM-IV* diagnostic criteria for obsessive-compulsive disorder (OCD) are presented in Table 27.7.

The disorder is equally common among men and women. It may begin in childhood, but more often begins in adolescence or early adulthood. The course is usually chronic, and may be complicated by depression or substance abuse. Single people are affected by OCD more often than are married people (Kaplan & Sadock, 1998).

Predisposing Factors to Obsessive-Compulsive Disorder

Psychoanalytical Theory. Psychoanalytical theorists propose that individuals with obsessive-compulsive disorder have weak, underdeveloped egos (for any of a variety of reasons: unsatisfactory parent-child relationship, conditional love, or provisional gratification). The psychoanalytical concept views clients with obsessive-compulsive disorder as having regressed to developmentally earlier stages of the infantile superego, the harsh, exacting, punitive characteristics of which now reappear as part of the psychopathology (Kaplan & Sadock, 1989). Regression to the pre-Oedipal anal-sadistic phase, combined with use of specific ego defense mechanisms (isolation, undoing, displacement, reaction formation), produces the clinical symptoms of obsessions and compulsions. Aggressive impulses (common during the anal-sadistic developmental phase) are channeled into thoughts and behaviors that prevent the feelings of aggression from surfacing and producing intense anxiety fraught with guilt (generated by the punitive superego).

Learning Theory. Learning theorists explain obsessive-compulsive behavior as a conditioned response to a traumatic event. The traumatic event produces anxiety and discomfort, and the individual learns to prevent the anxiety and discomfort by avoiding the situation with which it is associated. This type of learning is called *passive avoidance* (staying away from the source). When passive avoidance is not possible, the individual learns to engage in behaviors that provide relief from the anxiety and discomfort associated with the traumatic situation. This type of learning is called *active avoidance* and describes the behavior pattern of the individual with obsessive-compulsive disorder (Kaplan, Sadock, & Grebb, 1994).

According to this classic conditioning interpretation, a traumatic event should mark the beginning of the obsessive-compulsive behaviors. However, in a significant number of cases, the onset of the behavior is gradual and the clients relate the onset of their problems to life stress in general rather than to one or more traumatic events (Emmelkamp, 1982).

Biological Aspects. Recent findings suggest that neurobiological disturbances may play a role in the pathogenesis and maintenance of obsessive-compulsive disorder (Kaplan & Sadock, 1989).

Neuroanatomy. Abnormalities in various regions of the brain have been implicated in the neurobiology of obsessive-compulsive disorder. Functional neuroimaging techniques have shown abnormal metabolic rates in the basal ganglia and orbitalfrontal cortex of individuals with OCD (MacKenzie, 1994).

TABLE 27.7   DIAGNOSTIC CRITERIA FOR OBSESSIVE-COMPULSIVE DISORDER

A. Either obsessions or compulsions:

Obsessions as defined by 1, 2, 3, and 4:
1. Recurrent and persistent thoughts, impulses, or images that are experienced at some time during the disturbance as intrusive and inappropriate and that cause marked anxiety or distress.
2. The thoughts, impulses, or images are not simply excessive worries about real-life problems.
3. The person attempts to ignore or suppress such thoughts, impulses, or images, or to neutralize them with some other thought or action.
4. The person recognizes that the obsessional thoughts, impulses, or images are a product of his or her own mind (not imposed from without as in thought insertion).

Compulsions as defined by 1 and 2:
1. Repetitive behaviors (e.g., hand washing, ordering, checking) or mental acts (e.g., praying, counting, repeating words silently) that the person feels driven to perform in response to an obsession, or according to rules that must be applied rigidly.
2. The behaviors or mental acts are aimed at preventing or reducing distress or preventing some dreaded event or situation; however, these behaviors or mental acts either are not connected in a realistic way with what they are designed to neutralize or prevent or are clearly excessive.

B. At some point during the course of the disorder, the person has recognized that the obsessions or compulsions are excessive or unreasonable.
   NOTE: This does not apply to children.

C. The obsessions or compulsions cause marked distress, are time consuming (take more than 1 hr a day), or significantly interfere with the person's normal routine, occupational (or academic) functioning, or usual social activities or relationships.

D. If another axis I disorder is present, the content of the obsessions or compulsions is not restricted to it (e.g., preoccupation with food in the presence of an eating disorder; hair pulling in the presence of trichotillomania; concern with appearance in the presence of body dysmorphic disorder; preoccupation with having a serious illness in the presence of hypochondriasis; preoccupation with sexual urges or fantasies in the presence of a paraphilia; or guilty ruminations in the presence of major depressive disorder).

E. This disturbance is not due to the direct physiological effects of a substance (e.g., drug of abuse, a medication) or a general medical condition.

SOURCE: From APA (1994), with permission.

Physiology. Some individuals with obsessive-compulsive disorder exhibit nonspecific electroencephalogram (EEG) changes. Some researchers have hypothesized that obsessive-compulsive disorder may represent a nonconvulsive epileptiform disorder (e.g., abnormal discharges in selective brain regions) or an abnormality in left-frontal brain functions (Kaplan & Sadock, 1989).

Biochemical. A number of studies have implicated the neurotransmitter serotonin as influential in the etiology of obsessive-compulsive behaviors. Drugs that have been used successfully in alleviating the symptoms of obsessive-compulsive disorder are clomipramine and the selective serotonin reuptake inhibitors (SSRIs), all of which are believed to block the neuronal reuptake of serotonin, thereby potentiating serotoninergic activity in the central nervous system.

Transactional Model of Stress Adaptation. The etiology of obsessive-compulsive disorder is most likely influenced by multiple factors. In Figure 27.4 a graphic depiction of this theory of multiple causation is presented in the transactional model of stress/adaptation.

Diagnosis/Outcome Identification

Nursing diagnoses are formulated from the data gathered during the assessment phase and with background knowledge regarding predisposing factors to the disorder. Some common nursing diagnoses for clients with obsessive-compulsive disorder include:

Ineffective individual coping related to underdeveloped ego, punitive superego; avoidance learning; possible biochemical changes; evidenced by ritualistic behavior and/or obsessive thoughts.

Altered role performance related to need to perform rituals, evidenced by inability to fulfill usual patterns of responsibility.

The following criteria may be used to measure outcomes in the care of the client with obsessive-compulsive disorder.

THE CLIENT:
1. Is able to maintain anxiety at a manageable level without resorting to the use of ritualistic behavior.
2. Is able to perform activities of daily living independently.
3. Verbalizes understanding of relationship between anxiety and **ritualistic behavior.**
4. Verbalizes specific situations that in the past have provoked anxiety and resulted in seeking relief through rituals.
5. Demonstrates more adaptive coping strategies to deal with stress, such as thought stopping, relaxation techniques, and physical exercise.
6. Is able to resume role-related responsibilities because of decreased need for ritualistic behaviors.

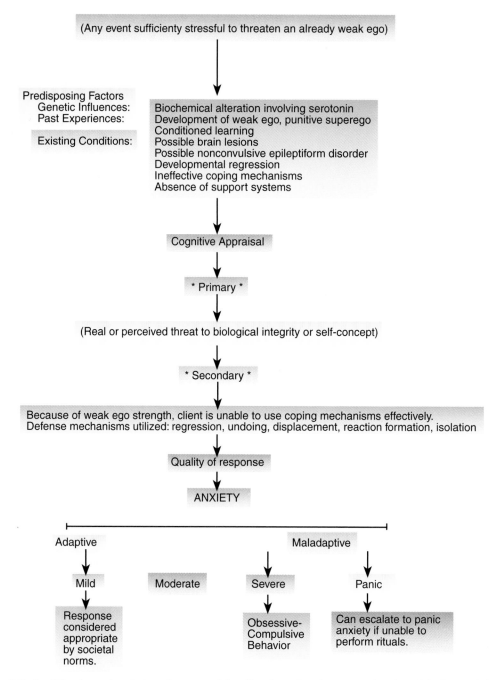

Figure 27.4 The dynamics of obsessive-compulsive disorder using the transactional model of stress/adaptation.

Planning/Implementation

Table 27.8 provides a plan of care for the client with obsessive-compulsive disorder. Nursing diagnoses are presented, along with outcome criteria, appropriate nursing interventions, and rationales for each.

Evaluation

Reassessment is conducted in order to determine if the nursing actions have been successful in achieving the objectives of care. Evaluation of the nursing actions for the client with

obsessive-compulsive disorder may be facilitated by gathering information using the following types of questions:

1. Can the client refrain from performing rituals when anxiety level rises?
2. Can the client demonstrate substitute behaviors to maintain anxiety at a manageable level?
3. Does the client recognize the relationship between escalating anxiety and the dependence on ritualistic behaviors for relief?
4. Can the client verbalize situations that occurred in the past during which this strategy was used?

TABLE 27.8   CARE PLAN FOR THE CLIENT WITH OBSESSIVE-COMPULSIVE DISORDER

NURSING DIAGNOSIS: INEFFECTIVE INDIVIDUAL COPING

RELATED TO: Underdeveloped ego, punitive superego; avoidance learning; possible biochemical changes

EVIDENCED BY: Ritualistic behavior or obsessive thoughts

OUTCOME CRITERIA	NURSING INTERVENTIONS	RATIONALE
Client will demonstrate ability to cope effectively without resorting to obsessive-compulsive behaviors or increased dependency.	1. Work with client to determine types of situations that increase anxiety and result in ritualistic behaviors. 2. Initially meet the client's dependency needs as required. Encourage independence and give positive reinforcement for independent behaviors. 3. In the beginning of treatment, allow plenty of time for rituals. Do not be judgmental or verbalize disapproval of the behavior. 4. Support client's efforts to explore the meaning and purpose of the behavior. 5. Provide structured schedule of activities for client, including adequate time for completion of rituals. 6. Gradually begin to limit amount of time allotted for ritualistic behavior as client becomes more involved in unit activities. 7. Give positive reinforcement for nonritualistic behaviors. 8. Help client learn ways of interrupting obsessive thoughts and ritualistic behavior with techniques such as thought stopping, relaxation, and exercise.	1. Recognition of precipitating factors is the first step in teaching the client to interrupt the escalating anxiety. 2. Sudden and complete elimination of all avenues for dependency would create intense anxiety on the part of the client. Positive reinforcement enhances self-esteem and encourages repetition of desired behaviors. 3. To deny client this activity may precipitate panic anxiety. 4. Client may be unaware of the relationship between emotional problems and compulsive behaviors. Recognition is important before change can occur. 5. Structure provides a feeling of security for the anxious client. 6. Anxiety is minimized when client is able to replace ritualistic behaviors with more adaptive ones. 7. Positive reinforcement enhances self-esteem and encourages repetition of desired behaviors. 8. Knowledge and practice of coping techniques that are more adaptive will help client change and let go of maladaptive responses to anxiety.

NURSING DIAGNOSIS: ALTERED ROLE PERFORMANCE

RELATED TO: Need to perform rituals

EVIDENCED BY: Inability to fulfill usual patterns of responsibility

OUTCOME CRITERIA	NURSING INTERVENTIONS	RATIONALE
Client will be able to resume role-related responsibilities.	1. Determine client's previous role within the family and extent to which this role is altered by the illness. Identify roles of other family members. 2. Discuss client's perception of role expectations. 3. Encourage client to discuss conflicts evident within the family system. Identify how client and other family members have responded to this conflict.	1. Determining family roles is important in formulating an appropriate plan of care. 2. Determine if client's perception of his or her role expectations are realistic. 3. Identifying specific stressors, as well as adaptive and maladaptive responses within the system, is necessary before assistance can be provided in an effort to create change.

Continued on following page

TABLE 27.8 *(Continued)*

4. Explore available options for changes or adjustments in role. Practice through role-play.	4. Planning and rehearsal of potential role transitions can reduce anxiety.
5. Encourage family participation in the development of plans to effect positive change, and work to resolve the cause of the anxiety from which the client seeks relief through use of ritualistic behaviors.	5. Input from the individuals who will be directly involved in the change will increase the likelihood of a positive outcome.
6. Give client lots of positive reinforcement for ability to resume role responsibilities by decreasing need for ritualistic behaviors.	6. Positive reinforcement enhances self-esteem and promotes repetition of desired behaviors.

5. Can the client verbalize a plan of action for dealing with these stressful situations in the future?

6. Can client perform self-care activities independently?

7. Can the client demonstrate an ability to fulfill role-related responsibilities?

8. Can the client verbalize resources from whom he or she can seek assistance during times of extreme stress?

Posttraumatic Stress Disorder

Background Assessment Data

This disorder is described by the *DSM-IV* as the development of characteristic symptoms following exposure to an extreme traumatic stressor involving a personal threat to physical integrity or to the physical integrity of others. The symptoms may occur after learning about unexpected or violent death, serious harm, or threat of death or injury to a family member or other close associate (APA, 1994). These symptoms are not related to common experiences such as uncomplicated bereavement, marital conflict, or chronic illness but are associated with events that would be markedly distressing to almost anyone. The individual may experience the trauma alone or in the presence of others. Examples of some experiences that may produce this type of response include military combat, violent personal assault, being kidnapped or taken hostage, being tortured, being incarcerated as a prisoner of war, natural or manmade disasters, severe automobile accidents, or being diagnosed with a life-threatening illness (APA, 1994).

Characteristic symptoms include reexperiencing the traumatic event, a sustained high level of anxiety or arousal, or a general numbing of responsiveness. Intrusive recollections or nightmares of the event are common. Some individuals may be unable to remember certain aspects of the trauma.

Symptoms of depression are common with this disorder and may be severe enough to warrant a diagnosis of a depressive disorder. In the case of a life-threatening trauma shared with others, survivors often describe painful guilt feelings about surviving when others did not, or about the things they had to do to survive (APA, 1994). Substance abuse is common.

The full symptom picture must be present for more than 1 month and cause significant interference with social, occupational, and other areas of functioning. If the symptoms have not been present for more than 1 month, the diagnosis assigned is acute stress disorder (APA, 1994).

The disorder can occur at any age. Symptoms may begin within the first 3 months after the trauma, or there may be a delay of several months or even years. The *DSM-IV* diagnostic criteria for posttraumatic stress disorder (PTSD) are presented in Table 27.9.

Studies reveal a lifetime prevalence for PTSD ranging from 1 to 4 percent (APA, 1994). In a separate study investigating the incidence of combat-related posttraumatic stress disorder in Vietnam War veterans, the rate was found to be 15 percent (Kulka, Schlenger, & Fairbank, 1988).

Predisposing Factors to Posttraumatic Stress Disorder

Reports of symptoms and syndromes with PTSD-like features have existed in writing throughout the centuries. In the early part of the 20th century, traumatic neurosis was viewed as the ego's inability to master the degree of trauma that resulted in the disorganization of ego functioning (Kardiner, 1941). Very little was written about posttraumatic neurosis during the years between 1950 and 1970. This absence was followed in the 1970s and 1980s with an explosion in the amount of research and writing on the subject. Peterson, Prout, and Schwarz (1991) have stated:

TABLE 27.9 DIAGNOSTIC CRITERIA FOR POSTTRAUMATIC STRESS DISORDER

A. The person has been exposed to a traumatic event in which both of the following were present:
   1. The person experienced, witnessed, or was confronted with an event or events that involved actual or threatened death or serious injury, or a threat to the physical integrity of self or others.
   2. The person's response involved intense fear, helplessness, or horror.
      NOTE: In children, this may be expressed instead by disorganized or agitated behavior.
B. The traumatic event is persistently reexperienced in one (or more) of the following ways:
   1. Recurrent and intrusive distressing recollections of the event, including images, thoughts, or perceptions.
      NOTE: In young children, repetitive play may occur in which themes or aspects of the trauma are expressed.
   2. Recurrent distressing dreams of the event.
      NOTE: In children, there may be frightening dreams without recognizable content.
   3. Acting or feeling as if the traumatic event were recurring (includes a sense of reliving the experience, illusions, hallucinations, and dissociative flashback episodes, including those that occur on awakening or when intoxicated).
      NOTE: In young children, trauma-specific reenactment may occur.
   4. Intense psychological distress at exposure to internal or external cues that symbolize or resemble an aspect of the traumatic event.
   5. Physiological reactivity on exposure to internal or external cues that symbolize or resemble an aspect of the traumatic event.
C. Persistent avoidance of stimuli associated with the trauma and numbing of general responsiveness (not present before the trauma), as indicated by three (or more) of the following:
   1. Efforts to avoid thoughts or feelings associated with the trauma.
   2. Efforts to avoid activities, places, or people that arouse recollections of the trauma.
   3. Inability to recall an important aspect of the trauma.
   4. Markedly diminished interest or participation in significant activities.
   5. Feeling of detachment or estrangement from others.
   6. Restricted range of affect (e.g., unable to have loving feelings).
   7. Sense of a foreshortened future (e.g., does not expect to have a career, marriage, children, or a normal lifespan).
D. Persistent symptoms of increased arousal (not present before the trauma), as indicated by two (or more) of the following:
   1. Difficulty falling or staying asleep.
   2. Irritability or outbursts of anger.
   3. Difficulty concentrating.
   4. Hypervigilance.
   5. Exaggerated startle response.
E. Duration of the disturbance more than 1 month
F. Disturbance that causes clinically significant distress or impairment in social, occupational, or other important areas of functioning

Specify if acute (symptoms less than 3 months), chronic (symptoms 3 months or more), or delayed onset (onset of symptoms at least 6 months after the stressor).

SOURCE: From APA (1994), with permission.

"Clearly, the psychological casualties of the Vietnam War were largely responsible for the renewed interest in posttraumatic neurosis. Most of the early papers on posttraumatic neurosis were about Vietnam veterans."

Indeed, the category of PTSD did not appear until the third edition of the *Diagnostic and Statistical Manual of Mental Disorders* (*DSM-III*) in 1980. The increasingly obvious problems of Vietnam veterans plus clinical work with victims of multiple disasters made clear a need for this posttraumatic stress category in the *DSM-III* (Kaplan & Sadock, 1989).

Psychosocial Theory. Green, Wilson, and Lindy (1985) have proposed an etiological model of PTSD that has become widely accepted. This theory seeks to explain why certain persons exposed to massive trauma develop PTSD and others do not. Variables include characteristics that relate to (1) the traumatic experience, (2) the individual, and (3) the recovery environment.

The Traumatic Experience. Specific characteristics relating to the trauma have been identified as crucial elements in the determination of an individual's long-term response to stress. They include:

1. Severity and duration of the stressor.
2. Degree of anticipatory preparation prior to the onset.
3. Exposure to death.
4. Numbers affected by life threat.
5. Degree of control over recurrence.
6. Location of where the trauma was experienced (e.g., familiar surroundings, at home, in a foreign country).

Individual Characteristics. Variables that are considered important in determining an individual's response to trauma include:

1. Degree of ego-strength.
2. Effectiveness of coping resources.

3. Presence of preexisting psychopathology.
4. Outcomes of previous experiences with stress/trauma.
5. Behavioral tendencies (temperament).
6. Current psychosocial developmental stage (Erikson, 1968).
7. Demographic factors (e.g., age, socioeconomic status, education).

The Recovery Environment. Green, Wilson, and Lindy (1985) suggest that the quality of the environment in which the individual attempts to work through the traumatic experience is correlated with outcome. Environmental variables include:

1. Availability of social supports.
2. The cohesiveness and protectiveness of family and friends.
3. The attitudes of society regarding the experience.
4. Cultural and subcultural influences.

Peterson, Prout, and Schwarz (1991) suggest that the recovery environment for Vietnam veterans and rape victims has often been less supportive than that for disaster victims or the victims of assault or other crimes. In research conducted by Wilson and Krauss (1985) using this model with Vietnam combat veterans, the best predictors of PTSD were the severity of the stressor and the degree of psychosocial isolation in the recovery environment.

Learning Theory. Learning theorists view negative reinforcement as behavior that leads to a reduction in an aversive experience. This reduction is the reinforcement that enhances the repetition of the behavior. The avoidance behaviors and psychic numbing in response to a trauma are mediated by negative reinforcement (behaviors that decrease the emotional pain of the trauma). Behavioral disturbances such as anger and aggression, and drug and alcohol abuse, "are conceptualized as behavioral patterns that are functionally reinforced by their capacity to reduce aversive feelings" (Keane et al., 1985).

Cognitive Theory. These models take into consideration the cognitive appraisal of an event and focus on assumptions that an individual makes about the world. Epstein (1990) outlines three fundamental beliefs that most people construct within a personal theory of reality. They include:

1. The world is benevolent and a source of joy.
2. The world is meaningful and controllable.
3. The self is worthy (e.g., lovable, good, and competent).

As life situations occur, some disequilibrium is expected to occur until accommodation for the change has been made and it has become assimilated into one's personal theory of reality. An individual is vulnerable to PTSD when the fundamental beliefs are invalidated by a trauma that cannot be comprehended, and a sense of helplessness and hopelessness prevails. One's appraisal of the environment can be drastically altered.

Biological Aspects. Kaplan and Sadock (1989) explain a biological hypothesis for chronic PTSD that suggests reactivation of symptoms stimulated by a situation that resembles the original trauma. This arousal state, which is mediated by the sympathetic nervous system, is central in promoting the return of the traumatic images.

Van der Kolk (1988) has suggested that an endogenous opioid peptide response may assist in the maintenance of chronic PTSD. The hypothesis supports a type of "addiction to the trauma," which is explained in the following manner.

Opioids, including endogenous opioid peptides, have the following psychoactive properties:

1. Tranquilizing action.
2. Reduction of rage/aggression.
3. Reduction of paranoia.
4. Reduction of feelings of inadequacy.
5. Antidepressant action.

Van der Kolk suggests that physiological arousal initiated by reexposure to trauma-like situations enhances production of endogenous opioid peptides and results in increased feelings of comfort and control. When the stressor terminates, the individual may experience opioid withdrawal, the symptoms of which bear strong resemblance to those of PTSD.

Transactional Model of Stress/Adaptation. The etiology of PTSD is most likely influenced by multiple factors. In Figure 27.5, a graphic depiction of this theory of multiple causation is presented in the transactional model of stress/adaptation.

Diagnosis/Outcome Identification

Nursing diagnoses are formulated from the data gathered during the assessment phase and with background knowledge regarding predisposing factors to the disorder. Some common nursing diagnoses for clients with PTSD include:

Posttrauma response related to distressing event considered to be outside the range of usual human experience, evidenced by flashbacks, intrusive recollections, nightmares, psychological numbness related to the event, dissociation, or amnesia.

Dysfunctional grieving related to loss of self as perceived before the trauma or other actual or perceived losses incurred during or after the event, evidenced by irritability and explosiveness, self-destructiveness, substance abuse, verbalization of survival guilt or guilt about behavior required for survival.

The following criteria may be used for measurement of outcomes in the care of the client with PTSD.

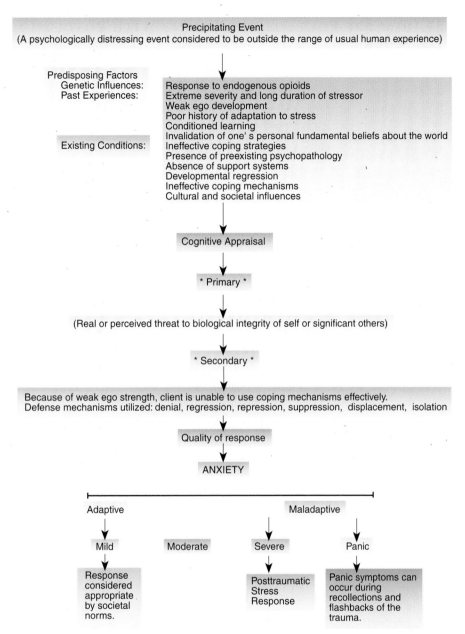

Figure 27.5 The dynamics of posttraumatic stress disorder using the transactional model of stress/adaptation.

THE CLIENT:

1. Can acknowledge the traumatic event and the impact it has had on his or her life.
2. Is experiencing fewer flashbacks, intrusive recollections, and nightmares than he or she was on admission (or at the beginning of therapy).
3. Can demonstrate adaptive coping strategies (e.g., relaxation techniques, mental imagery, music, art).
4. Can concentrate and has set realistic goals for the future.
5. Includes significant others in the recovery process and willingly accepts their support.
6. Verbalizes no ideas or intent of self-harm.
7. Has worked through feelings of survivor's guilt.
8. Gets enough sleep to avoid risk of injury.
9. Verbalizes community resources from whom he or she may seek assistance in times of stress.
10. Attends support group of individuals who have recovered or are recovering from similar traumatic experiences.
11. Verbalizes desire to put the trauma in the past and progress with his or her life.

Planning/Implementation

Table 27.10 provides a plan of care for the client with PTSD. Nursing diagnoses are presented, along with outcome criteria, appropriate nursing interventions, and rationales for each.

TABLE 27.10 CARE PLAN FOR THE CLIENT WITH POSTTRAUMATIC STRESS DISORDER

NURSING DIAGNOSIS: POSTTRAUMA RESPONSE

RELATED TO: Distressing event considered to be outside the range of usual human experience

EVIDENCED BY: Flashbacks, intrusive recollections, nightmares, psychological numbness related to the event, dissociation, or amnesia

OUTCOME CRITERIA	NURSING INTERVENTIONS	RATIONALE
The client will integrate the traumatic experience into his or her persona, renew significant relationships, and establish meaningful goals for the future.	1. a. Assign the same staff as often as possible. b. Use a nonthreatening, matter-of-fact, but friendly approach. c. Respect client's wishes regarding interaction with individuals of opposite sex at this time (especially important if the trauma was rape). d. Be consistent; keep all promises; convey acceptance; spend time with client.	1. All of these interventions serve to facilitate a trusting relationship.
	2. Stay with client during periods of flashbacks and nightmares. Offer reassurance of safety and security and that these symptoms are not uncommon following a trauma of the magnitude he or she has experienced.	2. Presence of a trusted individual may calm fears for personal safety and reassure client that he or she is not "going crazy."
	3. Obtain accurate history from significant others about the trauma and the client's specific response.	3. Various types of traumas elicit different responses in clients (e.g., human-engendered traumas often generate a greater degree of humiliation and guilt in victims than trauma associated with natural disasters).
	4. Encourage the client to talk about the trauma at his or her own pace. Provide a nonthreatening, private environment, and include a significant other if the client wishes. Acknowledge and validate client's feelings as they are expressed.	4. This debriefing process is the first step in the progression toward resolution.
	5. Discuss coping strategies used in response to the trauma, as well as those used during stressful situations in the past. Determine those that have been most helpful, and discuss alternative strategies for the future. Include available support systems, including religious and cultural influences. Identify maladaptive coping strategies (e.g., substance use, psychosomatic responses), and practice more adaptive coping strategies for possible future posttrauma responses.	5. Resolution of the posttrauma response is largely dependent on the effectiveness of the coping strategies employed.
	6. Assist the individual to try to comprehend the trauma if possible. Discuss feelings of vulnerability and the individual's "place" in the world following the trauma.	6. Posttrauma response is largely a function of the shattering of basic beliefs the victim holds about self and world. Assimilation of the event into one's persona requires that some degree of meaning associated with the event be incorporated into the basic beliefs, which will affect how the individual eventually comes to reappraise self and world (Epstein, 1990).

NURSING DIAGNOSIS: DYSFUNCTIONAL GRIEVING

RELATED TO: Loss of self as perceived prior to the trauma or other actual/perceived losses incurred during/following the event

EVIDENCED BY: Irritability and explosiveness, self-destructiveness, substance abuse, verbalization of survival guilt or guilt about behavior required for survival

OUTCOME CRITERIA	NURSING INTERVENTIONS	RATIONALE
Client will demonstrate progress in dealing with stages of grief and will verbalize a sense of optimism and hope for the future.	1. Acknowledge feelings of guilt or self-blame that client may express.	1. Guilt at having survived a trauma in which others died is common. The client needs to discuss these feelings and recognize that he or she is not responsible for what happened but must take responsibility for own recovery.
	2. Assess stage of grief in which the client is fixed. Discuss normalcy of feelings and behaviors related to stages of grief	2. Knowledge of grief stage is necessary for accurate intervention. Guilt may be generated if client believes it is unacceptable to have these feelings. Knowing they are normal can provide a sense of relief.
	3. Assess impact of the trauma on client's ability to resume regular activities of daily living. Consider employment, marital relationship, sleep patterns.	3. Following a trauma, individuals are at high risk for physical injury because of disruption in ability to concentrate and problem solve and because of lack of sufficient sleep. Isolation and avoidance behaviors may interfere with interpersonal relatedness.
	4. Assess for self-destructive ideas and behavior.	4. The trauma may result in feelings of hopelessness and worthlessness, leading to high risk for suicide.
	5. Assess for maladaptive coping strategies, such as substance abuse.	5. These behaviors interfere with and delay the recovery process.
	6. Identify available community resources from which the individual may seek assistance if problems with dysfunctional grieving persist.	6. Support groups for victims of various types of traumas exist within most communities. Presence of support systems in the recovery environment has been identified as a major predictor in the successful recovery from trauma (Wilson & Krauss, 1985).

Some institutions are using a case management model to coordinate care (see Chapter 7 for a more detailed explanation). In case management models, the plan of care may take the form of a critical pathway. Table 27.11 depicts an example of a critical pathway of care for a client with PTSD.

Evaluation

Reassessment is conducted in order to determine if the nursing actions have been successful in achieving the objectives of care. Evaluation of the nursing actions for the client with PTSD may be facilitated by gathering information using the following types of questions:

1. Can the client discuss the traumatic event without experiencing panic anxiety?
2. Does the client voluntarily discuss the traumatic event?
3. Can the client discuss changes that have occurred in his or her life because of the traumatic event?
4. Does the client have "flashbacks"?
5. Can the client sleep without medication?
6. Does the client have nightmares?
7. Has the client learned new, adaptive coping strategies for assistance with recovery?
8. Can the client demonstrate successful use of these new coping strategies in times of stress?
9. Can the client verbalize stages of grief and the normal behaviors associated with each?
10. Can he or she recognize own position in the grieving process?
11. Is guilt being alleviated?
12. Has the client maintained or regained satisfactory relationships with significant others?
13. Can the client look to the future with optimism?

TABLE 27.11   CRITICAL PATHWAY OF CARE FOR THE POSTTRAUMA CLIENT

Estimated length of stay: 7 days—Variations from designated pathway should be documented in progress notes

Nursing Diagnosis and Categories of Care	Time Dimension	Goals and/or Actions	Time Dimension	Goals and/or Actions	Time Dimension	Discharge Outcome
Posttrauma response	Day 1	Reassurance of client safety.	Ongoing	Environment is made safe for client.	Day 7	Client is able to carry out activities of daily living. Fewer flashbacks, nightmares.
Referrals	Day 1	Psychiatrist Psychologist Social worker Clinical nurse specialist Music therapist Occupational therapist Recreational therapist Chaplain			Day 7	Discharge with follow-up appointments as required.
Diagnostic studies	Day 1 Day 2–5	Drug screen EKG; EEG MMPI Impact of event scale (IES)				
Medications	Day 1	Antidepressant medication, as ordered (SSRIs, tricyclics, or MAO inhibitors). Antianxiety medication, as ordered (benzodiaze-pines); may be given p.r.n. because of addictive quality. Clonidine or propranolol (for intrusive thoughts and hyperarousal). Sedative-hypnotics for sleep distur-bances, may be given p.r.n.	Day 1–7	Assess for effectiveness and side effects of medications. Administer addictive medications judiciously and taper dosage.	Day 7	Discharged with scripts as ordered by physician (e.g., antidepressants; clonidine; propranolol).
Additional assessments	Day 1 Day 1	VS every shift Assess: ● Mental status ● Mood swings ● Anxiety level ● Social interaction ● Ability to carry out activities of daily living ● Suicide ideation ● Sleep disturbances	Day 2–7 Day 2–7	VS daily if stable Ongoing assessments	Day 7	Anxiety is maintained at manageable level. Mood is appropriate. Interacts with others. Carries out activities of daily living independently. Denies suicide ideation. Sleeps without medication.

		● "Flashbacks" ● Presence of guilt feelings				Is able to interrupt flashbacks with adaptive, coping stragegies. Has worked through feelings of guilt.
Diet	Day 1	Client's choice or low-tyramine if taking monoamine oxidase inhibitors (MAOIs)	Day 2–7	Same	Day 7	Client eats well-balanced diet.
Client education	Day 1	Orient to unit	Day 3–4 Day 6	Stages of grief Side effects of medications Coping strategies Low-tyramine diet Community resources Support group Importance of not mixing drugs and alcohol Reinforce teaching	Day 7	Client is discharged. Verbalizes understanding of information presented before discharge.

14. Does the client attend a regular support group for victims of similar traumatic experiences?
15. Does the client have a plan of action for dealing with symptoms, if they return?

Anxiety Disorder Due to a General Medical Condition

Background Assessment Data

The symptoms of this disorder are judged to be the direct physiological consequence of a general medical condition. Symptoms may include prominent generalized anxiety symptoms, panic attacks, or obsessions or compulsions (APA, 1994). History, physical examination, or laboratory findings must be evident to substantiate the diagnosis.

The *DSM-IV* (APA, 1994) lists the following types and examples of medical conditions that may cause anxiety symptoms:

Endocrine conditions:	Hyperthyroidism and hypothyroidism, pheochromocytoma, hypoglycemia, hyperadrenocorticism.
Cardiovascular conditions:	Congestive heart failure, pulmonary embolism, arrhythmia.
Respiratory conditions:	Chronic obstructive pulmonary disease, pneumonia, hyperventilation.
Metabolic conditions:	Vitamin B_{12} deficiency, porphyria.
Neurological conditions:	Neoplasms, vestibular dysfunction, encephalitis.

Care of clients with this disorder must take into consideration the underlying cause of the anxiety. Holistic nursing care is essential to ensure that the client's physiological and psychosocial needs are met. Nursing actions appropriate for the specific medical condition must be considered. Actions for dealing with the symptoms of anxiety were discussed previously.

Substance-Induced Anxiety Disorder

Background Assessment Data

The *DSM-IV* (APA, 1994) describes the essential features of this disorder as prominent anxiety symptoms that are judged to be due to the direct physiological effects of a substance (i.e., a drug of abuse, a medication, or toxin exposure). The symptoms may occur during substance intoxication or withdrawal, and may involve prominent anxiety, panic attacks, phobias, or obsessions or compulsions. Diagnosis of this disorder is made only if the anxiety symptoms are in excess of those usually associated with the intoxication or withdrawal syndrome and warrant independent clinical attention. Evidence of intoxication or withdrawal must be available from history, physical examination, or laboratory findings to substantiate the diagnosis. See Chapter 24 for a discussion of the types of substances that may produce these symptoms.

Nursing care of the client with substance-induced anxiety disorder must take into consideration the nature of

TABLE 27.12 TOPICS FOR CLIENT/FAMILY EDUCATION RELATED TO ANXIETY DISORDERS

Nature of the Illness
1. What is anxiety?
2. What might it be related to?
3. What is obsessive-compulsive disorder?
4. What is posttraumatic stress disorder?
5. Symptoms of anxiety disorders.

Management of the Illness
1. Medication Management: possible adverse effects; length of time to take effect; what to expect from the medication
   a. For panic disorder and generalized anxiety disorder: benzodiazepines, buspirone, tricyclics, SSRIs, propranolol, clonidine
   b. For phobic disorders: benzodiazepines, tricyclics, propranolol, SSRIs
   c. For obsessive-compulsive disorder: SSRIs, clomipramine
   d. For posttraumatic stress disorder: tricyclics, SSRIs, MAOIs, trazodone, propranolol, carbamazepine, valproic acid, lithium carbonate
2. Stress Management: Teach ways to interrupt escalating anxiety through relaxation techniques (see Chapter 12)
   a. Progressive muscle relaxation
   b. Imagery
   c. Music
   d. Meditation
   e. Yoga
   f. Physical exercise

Support Services
1. Crisis hotline
2. Support groups
3. Individual psychotherapy

the substance and the context in which the symptoms occur, that is, intoxication or withdrawal (see Chapter 24). Nursing actions for dealing with anxiety symptoms were discussed previously.

TREATMENT MODALITIES

Individual Psychotherapy

Most clients experience a marked lessening of anxiety when given the opportunity to discuss their difficulties with a concerned and sympathetic therapist (Kaplan & Sadock, 1989). Gray (1978) states that the ultimate goal of individual psychotherapy with clients who have anxiety disorders is "to help the client make responsible choices and to attain personal freedom." This is accomplished through four aspects of psychotherapy that are of particular importance:

1. **The Therapeutic Relationship.** An effective relationship ideally is based on mutual respect, confidence, and trust. Both therapist and client should participate in the process with feelings of openness and frankness. Dependence on the therapist must be prevented, and treatment should be terminated when optimal benefit has been attained for the client.
2. **Communication.** The ability of the client to talk to the therapist and unburden himself or herself of guilt, conflict, anxiety, shame, and so forth gives the client a feeling of relief and communion with another human being. The opportunity to reveal inner secrets that are a source of pain and suffering can free the individual to see and understand his or her behavior as never before. These shared insights open pathways for change.
3. **Education and Reeducation.** Uncertainties and doubts are relieved from the mind through education. Knowledge dissolves the fear that is fostered by ignorance. The therapist can use logical and rational explanations to increase the client's understanding about various situations that create anxiety in his or her life. Topics are presented in Table 27.12.
4. **Change or Transformation.** Gray (1978) suggests that this change in the client's total being leads to his or her personal freedom to make conscious choices, to act according to these choices, and to accept responsibility for the consequences of the action. The client is able to choose the degree to which others can influence him or her. The anxiety response diminishes with this achievement of personal control.

Cognitive Therapy

The cognitive model relates how individuals respond in stressful situations to their subjective cognitive appraisal of the event (Beck & Emery, 1985). Anxiety is experienced when the cognitive appraisal is one of danger with which the individual perceives that he or she is unable to cope. Impaired cognition can contribute to anxiety disorders when the individual's appraisals are chronically negative. Automatic negative appraisals provoke self-doubts, negative evaluations, and negative predictions. Anxiety is maintained by this dysfunctional appraisal of a situation.

Cognitive therapy strives to assist the individual to reduce anxiety responses by altering cognitive distortions. Anxiety is described as being the result of exaggerated, *automatic* thinking.

Cognitive therapy for anxiety is brief and time-limited, usually lasting from 5 to 20 sessions. Brief therapy discourages the client's dependency on the therapist, which is prevalent in anxiety disorders, and encourages the client's self-sufficiency.

A sound therapeutic relationship is a necessary condition for effective cognitive therapy. The client must be able to talk openly about fears and feelings for the therapeutic process to occur. A major part of treatment consists of encouraging the client to face frightening situations to be able to view them realistically, and talking about them is one way of achieving this. Treatment is a collaborative effort between client and therapist.

Rather than offering suggestions and explanations, the therapist uses questions to encourage the client to correct his or her anxiety-producing thoughts. The client is encouraged to become aware of the thoughts, examine them for cognitive distortions, substitute more balanced thoughts, and eventually develop new patterns of thinking.

Cognitive therapy is very structured and orderly, which is important for the anxious client who is often confused and lacks self-assurance. The focus is on solving current problems. Together, the client and therapist work to identify and correct maladaptive thoughts and behaviors that maintain a problem and block its solution.

Cognitive therapy is based on education. The premise is that one develops anxiety because he or she has learned inappropriate ways of handling life experiences. The belief is that with practice individuals can learn more effective ways of responding to these experiences. Homework assignments, a central feature of cognitive therapy, provide an experimental, problem-solving approach to overcoming long-held anxieties. Through fulfillment of these personal "experiments," the effectiveness of specific strategies and techniques is determined.

Behavior Therapy

Two common forms of behavior therapy include **systematic desensitization** and **implosion therapy (flooding)**. They are commonly used to treat clients with phobic disorders and to modify stereotyped behavior of clients with PTSD (Embry, 1990). They have also been shown to be effective in a variety of other anxiety-producing situations.

Systematic Desensitization

In systematic desensitization, the client is gradually exposed to the phobic stimulus, in either a real or imagined

situation. The concept was introduced by Joseph Wolpe in 1958 and is based on behavioral conditioning principles. Emphasis is placed on *reciprocal inhibition* or counterconditioning.

Reciprocal inhibition is described as the restriction of anxiety prior to the effort of reducing avoidance behavior. The rationale behind this concept is that because relaxation is antagonistic to anxiety, individuals cannot be anxious and relaxed at the same time.

Systematic desensitization with reciprocal inhibition involves two main elements:

1. Training in relaxation techniques.
2. Progressive exposure to a hierarchy of fear stimuli while in the relaxed state.

The individual is instructed in the art of relaxation, using techniques most effective for him or her (e.g., progressive relaxation, mental imagery, tense and relax, meditation). When the individual has mastered the relaxation technique, exposure to the phobic stimulus is initiated. He or she is asked to present a hierarchal arrangement of situations pertaining to the phobic stimulus in order from most disturbing to least disturbing. While in a state of maximum relaxation, the client may be asked to imagine the phobic stimulus. Initial exposure is focused on a concept of the phobic stimulus that produces the least amount of fear or anxiety. In subsequent sessions, the individual is gradually exposed to more fearful stimuli. Sessions may be executed in fantasy, in real-life (in vivo) situations, or sometimes in a combination of both.

CASE STUDY

John was afraid to ride on elevators. He had been known to climb 24 flights of stairs in an office building to avoid riding the elevator. John's own insurance office had plans for moving the company to a high-rise building soon, with offices on the 32nd floor. John sought assistance from a therapist for this problem. He was taught to achieve a sense of calmness and well-being, using a combination of mental imagery and progressive relaxation techniques. In the relaxed state, John was initially instructed to imagine the entry level of his office building, with a clear image of the bank of elevators. In subsequent sessions, and always in the relaxed state, John progressed to images of walking onto an elevator, having the elevator door close after he had entered, riding the elevator to the 32nd floor, and emerging from the elevator once the doors were opened. The progression included being accompanied in the activities by the therapist and eventually accomplishing them alone.

Therapy for John also included in vivo sessions, in which he was exposed to the phobic stimulus in real-life situations (always after achieving a state of relaxation). This technique, combining imagined and in vivo procedures, proved very successful for John, and his employment in the high-rise complex was no longer in jeopardy because of claustrophobia.

Implosion Therapy (Flooding)

Flooding is a therapeutic process in which the client must imagine situations or participate in real-life situations that he or she finds extremely frightening, for a prolonged period of time. Relaxation training is not a part of this technique. Plenty of time must be allowed for these sessions because brief periods may be ineffective or even harmful. A session is terminated when the client responds with considerably less anxiety than at the beginning of the session. Chambless and Goldstein (1979) describe flooding techniques in the following manner:

"The flooding technique requires that the therapist get as much information as possible concerning situations that trigger inappropriate anxiety. In a case of agoraphobia, a client reports that going out of the house leads to anxiety and that the anxiety is worse in public conveyances, elevators, and crowds. She fears she might be sent to an asylum and that no one will take care of her children, and so on. The client is asked to close her eyes and to imagine as vividly as possible what will be described without reflecting on it or evaluating its appropriateness. The therapist begins describing an anxiety-evoking situation in vivid detail starting with the client's preparing to go out alone. The flooding therapist is guided by the client's reactions: the more anxiety, the more appropriate the narrative. Modifications are made on the basis of new clues given by the client's reactions or statement. The same theme is repeated if it continues to arouse anxiety; it will be repeated as frequently as possible over as many sessions as necessary. Criteria for continuing are reports that anxiety is decreasing between sessions and that the client is instead entering formerly avoided situations." (p. 250)

Group/Family Therapy

Group therapy has been strongly advocated for clients with PTSD. It has proved especially effective with Vietnam veterans (Kaplan, Sadock, & Grebb, 1994). Kolb (1986) emphasized the importance of being able to share their experiences with empathetic fellow veterans, to talk about problems in social adaptation, and to discuss options for managing their aggression toward others. Some groups are informal and leaderless, such as veterans' "rap" groups, and some are led by experienced group therapists who may have had some firsthand experience with the trauma. Some groups involve family members, thereby recognizing that the symptoms of PTSD may also severely affect them (Kaplan & Sadock, 1989). Hollander, Simeon, and Gorman (1994) state:

"Because of past experiences, clients with PTSD are often mistrustful and reluctant to depend on authority figures, whereas the identification, support, and hopefulness of peer settings can facilitate therapeutic change."

Psychopharmacology

For Panic and Generalized Anxiety Disorders

Anxiolytics. The benzodiazepines have been the drug of choice in the treatment of generalized anxiety disorder (Kaplan & Sadock, 1998). They can be prescribed on an as-needed basis when the client is feeling particularly anxious. Recent investigations indicate that alprazolam, lorazepam, and clonazepam are particularly effective in the treatment of panic disorder. The major risks with benzodiazepine therapy are physical dependence and tolerance, which may encourage abuse. Because withdrawal symptoms can be life-threatening, clients must be warned against abrupt discontinuation of the drug and should be tapered off the medication at the end of therapy.

The antianxiety agent buspirone (Buspar) is effective in about 60 to 80 percent of clients with generalized anxiety disorder (Kaplan & Sadock, 1998). One disadvantage of buspirone is its 10- to 14-day delay in alleviating symptoms. However, the benefit of lack of physical dependence and tolerance with buspirone may make it the drug of choice in the treatment of generalized anxiety disorder.

Antidepressants. Several antidepressants are effective as major antianxiety agents. The tricyclics clomipramine and imipramine have been used with success in clients experiencing panic disorder. Since the advent of SSRIs, the tricyclics are less widely used because of their tendency to produce severe side effects at the high doses required to relieve symptoms of panic disorder (Kaplan & Sadock, 1998).

The SSRIs fluoxetine, sertraline, and paroxetine have been shown to be effective in the treatment of panic disorder. Paroxetine has been approved by the Food and Drug Administration (FDA) for this purpose. The dosage of these drugs must be titrated slowly, as clients with panic disorder appear to be sensitive to the overstimulation caused by SSRIs.

The use of antidepressants in the treatment of generalized anxiety disorder is still being investigated (Silver, Yudofsky, & Hurowitz, 1994). Some success has been reported with imipramine (Noyes & Holt, 1994), but the effectiveness of other antidepressants has yet to be determined.

Antihypertensive Agents. Recently several studies have called attention to the effectiveness of beta blockers (e.g., propranolol) and alpha₂-receptor agonists (e.g., clonidine) in the amelioration of anxiety symptoms (Perry, Alexander, & Garrey, 1994). Propranolol has potent effects on the somatic manifestations of anxiety (e.g., palpitations, tremors), with less dramatic effects on the psychic component of anxiety. It appears to be most effective in the treatment of acute situational anxiety (e.g., performance anxiety, test anxiety), but it is not the first-line drug of choice in the treatment of panic disorder and generalized anxiety disorder (Perry, Alexander, & Garvey, 1994).

Clonidine is effective in blocking the acute anxiety effects in conditions such as opioid and nicotine withdrawal. However, it has had limited usefulness in the long-term treatment of panic and generalized anxiety disorders, particularly because of the development of tolerance to its antianxiety effects (Kaplan & Sadock, 1989).

For Phobic Disorders

Anxiolytics. The benzodiazepines have been the most widely prescribed drugs for the relief of phobic disorders, with mixed results. Alprazolam and clonazepam appear to be successful in reducing the symptoms of agoraphobia associated with panic disorder (Kaplan & Sadock, 1989).

Antidepressants. The tricyclic imipramine and the MAOI phenelzine have been shown to be effective in diminishing symptoms of agoraphobia and social phobias. Evidence of the effectiveness of the SSRIs in treating social phobia is also accruing. Specific phobias are generally not treated with medication unless panic attacks accompany the phobia. In such case, the panic attacks may be treated with medication (Kaplan & Sadock, 1998).

Antihypertensives. The beta blocker propranolol has been tried with success in clients experiencing anticipatory performance anxiety, or "stage fright" (Silver, Yudofsky, & Hurowitz, 1994). This type of phobic response produces symptoms such as sweaty palms, racing pulse, trembling hands, dry mouth, labored breathing, nausea, and memory loss. Propranolol appears to be quite effective in reducing these symptoms in some individuals.

For Obsessive-Compulsive Disorder

Antidepressants. All of the SSRIs—fluoxetine, paroxetine, sertraline, and fluvoxamine—have been approved by the FDA for the treatment of obsessive-compulsive disorder. Side effects include sleep disturbances, headache, and restlessness. These effects are often transient and are less troublesome than those of the tricyclics.

The tricyclic antidepressant clomipramine was the first drug approved by the FDA in the treatment of obsessive-compulsive disorder. Clomipramine is more selective for serotonin reuptake than any of the other tricyclics. Its efficacy in the treatment of OCD is well established, although the adverse effects, such as those associated with all the tricyclics, may make it less desirable than the SSRIs.

For Posttraumatic Stress Disorder

Antidepressants. Studies have shown that tricyclic antidepressants, and in particular amitriptyline and imipraimine, have been effective in alleviating the depression, intrusive thoughts, sleep disorders and nightmares associated with PTSD. Other antidepressants that have been shown effective in the treatment of PTSD include the SSRIs, the MAOIs, and trazadone (Desyrel) (Kaplan & Sadock, 1998).

Anxiolytics. Alprazolam has been prescribed for PTSD clients for its antidepressant and antipanic effects. Other benzodiazepines have also been widely used, despite the absence of controlled studies demonstrating their efficacy in PTSD (Friedman, 1990). Kaplan, Sadock, and Grebb (1994) state:

> "Although some anecdotal reports point to the effectiveness of alprazolam in posttraumatic stress disorder, the use of that drug is complicated by the high association of substance-related disorders in patients with the disorder and by the emergence of withdrawal symptoms on discontinuation of the drug."

Antihypertensives. The beta blocker propranolol and alpha$_2$-receptor agonist clonidine have been successful in alleviating some of the symptoms associated with PTSD. In clinical trials, Kolb, Burris, and Griffiths, (1984) reported marked reductions in nightmares, intrusive recol-

---

TEST YOUR CRITICAL THINKING SKILLS

Sarah, age 25, was taken to the emergency room by her friends. They were at a dinner party when Sarah suddenly clasped her chest and started having difficulty breathing. She complained of nausea and was perspiring profusely. She had calmed down some by the time they reached the hospital. She denied any pain, and electrocardiogram and laboratory results were unremarkable.

Sarah told the admitting nurse that she had a history of these "attacks." She began having them in her sophomore year of college. She knew her parents had expectations that she should follow in their footsteps and become an attorney. They also expected her to earn grades that would promote acceptance by a top Ivy League university. Sarah experienced her first attack when she made a "B" in English during her third semester of college. Since that time, she has experienced these symptoms sporadically, often in conjunction with her perception of the need to excel. She graduated with top honors from Harvard.

Last week Sarah was promoted within her law firm. She was assigned her first solo case of representing a couple whose baby had died at birth and who were suing the physician for malpractice. She has experienced these panic symptoms daily for the past week, stating, "I feel like I'm going crazy!"

Sarah is transferred to the psychiatric unit. The psychiatrist diagnoses panic disorder without agoraphobia.

Answer the following questions related to Sarah:

1. What would be the priority nursing diagnosis for Sarah?
2. What is the priority nursing intervention with Sarah?
3. What medical treatment might you expect the physician to prescribe?

R E S E A R C H   N O T E

Outcomes of group cognitive behavioral training in the treatment of panic disorder and agoraphobia. *Journal of the American Psychiatric Nurses Association* (1995, June), 1(3), 83–91.
Schweitzer, P.B., Nesse, R.M., Fantone, R.F., & Curtis, G.C.

Description of the Study: The purpose of this study was to examine the effects of a 6-week, nurse-led, cognitive-behavioral training (CBT) program on severity of symptoms in clients with panic disorder and agoraphobia. Subjects included 40 individuals being treated in an outpatient facility for panic disorder with agoraphobia (38) and agoraphobia without history of panic disorder (2). The subjects completed a symptom check list and weekly ratings scale before and after participation in the training program. The comprehensive anxiety management program (CAMP) consisted of six 2-hour sessions. The objective for the group sessions included educating members to become proficient at self-exposure (to the phobia) in vivo and cognitive restructuring.

Results of the Study: Significant reduction in mean baseline scores for impairment, phobic anxiety, panic attacks, general anxiety, avoidance, and depression resulted by the end of the study. No significant differences were found between baseline and endpoints ratings in subjects who were taking medication and those who were not.

Comments: The authors suggest that knowledge of the following benefits were derived from this study: (1) Brief, nurse-facilitated group training in CBT can reduce symptoms of panic disorder and agoraphobia. (2) Format of the approach is an efficient use of the nurse-clinician time. (3) Teaching clients to help themselves may increase their self-esteem. (4) Effective, brief, outpatient treatment is cost-effective.

INTERNET REFERENCES

- Additional information about anxiety disorders and medications to treat these disorders may be located at the following websites:
  - a. http://www.adaa.org
  - b. http://www.mentalhealth.com
  - c. http://www.psychweb.com/obsessiv.htm
  - d. http://www.cmhc.com/articles/grohol/ocd.htm
  - e. http://www.wvhealth.wvu.edu/mentalhealth/ansocial.htm
  - f. http://www.nimh.nih.gov/events/socifact.htm
  - g. http://www.anxietynetwork.com/pdhome.html
  - h. http://www.uams.edu/department_of_psychiatry/syllabus/anxiolytics/anxiolytics.htm

The psychological implications for the symptoms were not recognized until the early 1900s.

Anxiety is considered a normal reaction to a realistic danger or threat to biological integrity or self-concept. Normality of the anxiety experienced in response to a stressor is defined by societal and cultural standards.

Anxiety disorders are more common in women than in men by at least two to one. Studies of familial patterns suggest that a familial predisposition to anxiety disorders probably exists.

The *DSM-IV* identifies several broad categories of anxiety disorders. They include panic and generalized anxiety disorders, phobic disorders, obsessive-compulsive disorder, posttraumatic stress disorder, anxiety disorder due to a general medical condition, and substance-induced anxiety disorder. A number of elements, including psychosocial factors, biological influences, and learning experiences most likely contribute to the development of these disorders.

Treatment of anxiety disorders include individual psychotherapy, cognitive therapy, behavior therapy, group and family therapy, and psychopharmacology. Common behavior therapies include systematic desensitization and implosion therapy (flooding). Nursing care is accomplished using the six steps of the nursing process.

Nurses encounter clients experiencing anxiety in virtually all types of health care settings. Nurses should be able to recognize the symptoms of anxiety and assist clients to understand that these symptoms are normal and acceptable.

Clients with anxiety disorders are usually seen in emergency departments or psychiatric facilities. Here nurses help clients to gain insight and increase self-awareness in relation to their illness. Intervention focuses on assisting clients to learn techniques with which they may interrupt the escalation of anxiety before it reaches unmanageable proportions. Maladaptive behavior patterns are replaced by new, more adaptive, coping skills.

lections, hypervigilance, insomnia, startle responses, and angry outbursts with the use of these drugs.

Other Drugs. Carbamazepine and lithium carbonate alleviate symptoms of intrusive recollections, flashbacks, nightmares, impulsivity, irritability, and violent behavior in PTSD clients (Lipper, Davidson, & Grady, 1986; van der Kolk, 1988; Szymanski & Olympia, 1991). Antipsychotics have been used with success in the treatment of refractory PTSD marked by paranoid behavior, aggressive psychotic symptoms, uncontrollable anger, self-destructive behavior, and frequent flashback episodes marked by frank auditory and visual hallucinations of traumatic episodes (Friedman, 1990). Further controlled trials with these drugs are needed to validate their efficacy in treating PTSD.

SUMMARY

Anxiety is a necessary force for survival and has been experienced by humanity throughout the ages. It was first described as a physiological disorder and identified by its physical symptoms, particularly the cardiac symptoms.

REVIEW QUESTIONS

SELF-EXAMINATION/LEARNING EXERCISE

For each situation select the answer that is most appropriate for the questions that follow.

Situation: Ms. T has been diagnosed with agoraphobia.

1. Which behavior would be most characteristic of this disorder?

   a. Ms. T experiences panic anxiety when she encounters snakes.
   b. Ms. T refuses to fly in an airplane.
   c. Ms. T will not eat in a public place.
   d. Ms. T stays in her home for fear of being in a place from which she cannot escape.

2. The therapist who works with Ms. T would likely choose which of the following therapies for her?

   a. 10 mg Valium q.i.d.
   b. Group therapy with other agoraphobics
   c. Facing her fear in gradual step progression
   d. Hypnosis

3. Should the therapist choose to use implosion therapy, Ms. T would be:

   a. taught relaxation exercises.
   b. subjected to graded intensities of the fear.
   c. instructed to stop the therapeutic session as soon as anxiety is experienced.
   d. presented with massive exposure to a variety of stimuli associated with the phobic object/situation.

Situation: Sandy is a 29-year-old woman who has been admitted to the psychiatric unit with a diagnosis of obsessive-compulsive disorder. She spends many hours during the day and night washing her hands.

4. The most likely reason Sandy washes her hands so much is that it

   a. relieves her anxiety.
   b. reduces the probability of infection.
   c. gives her a feeling of control over her life.
   d. increases her self-concept.

5. The initial care plan for Sandy would include which of the following nursing interventions?

   a. Keep Sandy's bathroom locked so she cannot wash her hands all the time.
   b. Structure Sandy's schedule so that she has plenty of time for washing her hands.
   c. Put Sandy in isolation until she promises to stop washing her hands so much.
   d. Explain Sandy's behavior to her, since she is probably unaware that it is maladaptive.

6. On Sandy's fourth hospital day, she says to the nurse, "I'm feeling better now. I feel comfortable on this unit, and I'm not ill-at-ease with the staff or other patients anymore." In light of this change, which nursing intervention is most appropriate?

   a. Give attention to the ritualistic behaviors each time they occur and point out their inappropriateness.
   b. Ignore the ritualistic behaviors, and they will be eliminated for lack of reinforcement.
   c. Set limits on the amount of time Sandy may engage in the ritualistic behavior.
   d. Continue to allow Sandy all the time she wants to carry out the ritualistic behavior.

Situation: John is a 28-year-old high school science teacher whose Army Reserve unit was called to fight in Operation Desert Storm. John did not want to fight. He admits that he joined the reserves to help pay off his college loans. In Saudi Arabia, he participated in combat and witnessed the wounding of several from his unit, as well as the death of his best friend. He has been experiencing flashbacks, intrusive recollections, and nightmares. His wife reports he is afraid to go to sleep, and his work is suffering. Sometimes he just sits as though he is in a trance. John is diagnosed with PTSD.

7. John says to the nurse, "I can't figure out why God took my buddy instead of me." From this statement, the nurse assesses which of the following in John?

    a. Repressed anger.
    b. Survivor's guilt.
    c. Intrusive thoughts.
    d. Spiritual distress.

8. John experiences a nightmare during his first night in the hospital. He explains to the nurse that he was dreaming about gunfire all around and people being killed. The nurse's most appropriate initial intervention is:

    a. administer alprazolam as ordered p.r.n. for anxiety.
    b. call the physician and report the incident.
    c. stay with John and reassure him of his safety.
    d. have John listen to a tape of relaxation exercises.

9. Which of the following therapy regimens would most appropriately be ordered for John?

    a. Imipramine and group therapy.
    b. Diazepam and implosion therapy.
    c. Alprazolam and behavior therapy.
    d. Carbamazepine and cognitive therapy.

10. Which of the following may be influential in the predisposition to PTSD?

    a. Unsatisfactory parent-child relationship.
    b. Excess of the neurotransmitter serotonin.
    c. Distorted, negative cognitions.
    d. Severity of the stressor and availability of support systems.

REFERENCES

American Psychiatric Association. (1994). *Diagnostic and statistical manual of mental disorders* (4th ed.). Washington DC: American Psychiatric Association.

Beck, A.T., & Emery, G. (1985). *Anxiety disorders and phobias.* New York: Basic Books.

Chambless, D.L., & Goldstein, A.J. (1979). Behavioral psychotherapy. In R.J. Corsini (Ed.), *Current psychotherapies* (2nd ed.). Itasca, IL: F.E. Peacock.

Charney, D.S., Woods, S.W., & Nagg, L.M. (1990). Noradrenergic function in panic disorder. *Journal of Clinical Psychiatry, 51*(suppl), 5–11.

Embry, C.K. (1990). Psychotherapeutic interventions in chronic posttraumatic stress disorder. In M.E. Wolf & A.D. Mosnaim (Eds.), *Posttraumatic stress disorder: Etiology, phenomenology, and treatment.* Washington, DC: American Psychiatric Press.

Emmelkamp, P.M.G. (1982). *Phobic and obsessive-compulsive disorders: Theory, research, and practice.* New York: Plenum Press.

Epstein, S. (1990). Beliefs and symptoms in maladaptive resolutions of the traumatic neurosis. In Ozer et al. (Eds.), *Perspectives on personality* (Vol. 3). London: Jessica Kingsley.

Erikson, E. (1968). *Youth, identity, and crisis.* New York: Norton.

Freud, S. (1959). On the grounds for detaching a particular syndrome from neurasthenia under the description 'anxiety neurosis.' In *The standard edition of the complete psychological works of Sigmund Freud* (Vol. 3). London: Hogarth Press.

Friedman, M.J. (1990). Interrelationships between biological mechanisms and pharmacotherapy of posttraumatic stress disorder. In M.E. Wolf & A.D. Mosnaim (Eds.), *Posttraumatic stress disorder: Etiology, phenomenology, and treatment.* Washington, DC: American Psychiatric Press.

Goodwin, D.W. (1983). *Phobia: The facts.* New York: Oxford University Press.

Gray, M. (1978). *Neuroses: A comprehensive and critical view.* New York: Van Nostrand Reinhold.

Green, B.L., Wilson, J.P., & Lindy, J.D. (1985). Conceptualizing posttraumatic stress disorder: A psychosocial framework. In C.R. Figley (Ed.), *Trauma and its wake: The study and treatment of posttraumatic stress disorder.* New York: Brunner/Mazel.

Halpern, R. (1990). Poverty and early childhood parenting: Toward a framework for intervention. *American Journal of Orthopsychiatry, 60*(1), 6–8.

Hollander, E., Simeon, D., & Gorman, J.M. (1994). Anxiety disorders. In R.E. Hales, S.C. Yudofsky, & J.A. Talbott (Eds.), *Textbook of psychiatry* (2nd ed.). Washington, DC: American Psychiatric Press.

Johnson, B.S. (1995). Mental health of children, adolescents, and families. In B.S. Johnson (Ed.), *Child, adolescent & family psychiatric nursing.* Philadelphia: J.B. Lippincott.

Johnson, J.H., & Sarason, I.G. (1978). Life stress, depression and anxiety: Internal-external control as a moderator variable. *Journal of Psychosomatic Research, 22,* 205–208.

Kaplan, H.I., and Sadock, B.J. (1989). *Comprehensive textbook of psychiatry* (Vol. 1) (5th ed.). Baltimore: Williams & Wilkins.

Kaplan, H.I., and Sadock, B.J. (1998). *Synopsis of psychiatry: Behavioral sciences/clinical psychiatry* (8th ed.). Baltimore: Williams & Wilkins.

Kaplan, H.I., Sadock, B.J., & Grebb, J.A. (1994). *Kaplan and Sadock's synopsis of psychiatry* (7th ed.). Baltimore: Williams & Wilkins.

Kardiner, A. (1941). *The traumatic neuroses of war.* New York: Hoeber.

Keable, D. (1989). *The management of anxiety: A manual for therapists.* New York: Churchill Livingstone.

Keane, T.M., et al. (1985). A behavioral approach to assessing and treating PTSD in Vietnam veterans. In C.R. Figley (Ed.), *Trauma and its wake.* New York: Brunner/Mazel.

Kolb, L.C. (1986). Treatment of chronic posttraumatic stress disorder. *Current Psychiatric Therapies, 23,* 119–126.

Kolb, L.C., Burris, B.C., & Griffiths, S. (1984). Propranolol and clonidine in the treatment of the chronic posttraumatic stress disorders of war. In B.A. van der Kolk (Ed.), *Posttraumatic stress disorder: Psychological and biological sequelae.* Washington, DC: American Psychiatric Press.

Kulka, R., Schlenger, W., & Fairbank, J. (1988). *National Vietnam veterans readjustment study (NVVRS) report: Description, current status, and initial PTSD prevalence estimates.* Washington, DC: Veterans Administration.

Lipper, S., Davidson, J.R.T., & Grady. T.A. (1986). Preliminary study of carbamazepine in posttraumatic stress disorder. *Psychosomatics, 27,* 849–854.

MacKenzie, T.B. (1994). Obsessive-compulsive neurosis. In G. Winokur & P.J. Clayton (Eds.), *The medical basis of psychiatry* (2nd ed.). Philadelphia: W.B. Saunders.

Noyes, R., & Holt, C.S. (1994). Anxiety disorders. In G. Winokur & P.J. Clayton (Eds.), *The medical basis of psychiatry* (2nd ed.). Philadelphia: W.B. Saunders.

Perry, P.J., Alexander, B., & Garvey, M.J. (1994). In G. Winokur & P.J. Clayton (Eds.), *The medical basis of psychiatry* (2nd ed.). Philadelphia: W.B. Saunders.

Peterson, K.C., Prout, M.F., & Schwarz, R.A. (1991). *Posttraumatic stress disorder: A clinician's guide.* New York: Plenum Press.

Silver, J.M., Yudofsky, S.C., & Hurowitz, G.I. (1994). Psychopharmacology and electroconvulsive therapy. In R.E. Hales, S.C. Yudofsky, & J.A. Talbott (Eds.), *Textbook of psychiatry* (2nd ed.). Washington, DC: American Psychiatric Press.

Szymanski, H.V., & Olympia, J. (1991). Divalproex in posttraumatic stress disorder. *American Journal of Psychiatry, 148,* 1086–1087.

Uhde, T.W., & Nemiah, J.C. (1989). Anxiety disorders. In H.I. Kaplan & B.J. Sadock (Eds.), *Comprehensive textbook of psychiatry* (Vol. 1) (5th ed.). Baltimore: Williams & Wilkins.

van der Kolk, B.A. (1988). The biological response to trauma. In F. Ochberg (Ed.), *Posttraumatic therapy and victims of violence.* New York: Brunner/Mazel.

Wilson, J.P., & Krauss, G.E. (1985). Predicting posttraumatic stress disorders among Vietnam veterans. In W.E. Kelly (Ed.), *Posttraumatic stress disorder and the war veteran patient.* New York: Brunner/Mazel.

Wolpe, J. (1958). *Psychotherapy and reciprocal inhibition.* Stanford: Stanford University Press.

Bibliograpy

Beeber, L.S. (1989). Treatment of anxiety. *Journal of Psychosocial Nursing, 27,* 42.

Blair, D.T., & Hildreth, N.A. (1991). PTSD and the Vietnam veteran: The battle for treatment. *Journal of Psychosocial Nursing, 29*(10), 15–20.

Gerlock, A.A. (1991). Vietnam: Returning to the scene of the trauma. *Journal of Psychosocial Nursing, 29*(2), 4–8.

Glod, C.A., & Cawley, D. (1997, August). The neurobiology of obsessive-compulsive disorder. *Journal of the American Psychiatric Nurses Association, 3*(4), 120–122.

Harvard Medical School (1998, November). Obsessive-Compulsive Disorder—Part II. *The Harvard Mental Health Letter, 15*(5), 1–4.

Harvard Medical School (1998, October). Obsessive-Compulsive Disorder—Part I. *The Harvard Mental Health Letter, 15*(4), 1–4.

Harvard Medical School (1996, July). Posttraumatic Stress Disorder—Part II. *The Harvard Mental Health Letter, 13*(1), 1–5.

Harvard Medical School (1996, June). Posttraumatic Stress Disorder—Part I. *The Harvard Mental Health Letter, 12*(12), 1–4.

Mowrer, O.H. (1960). *Learning theory and behavior.* New York: Wiley.

Nymberg, J.H., & Van Noppen, B. (1994, April). Obsessive-compulsive disorder: A concealed diagnosis. *American Family Physician, 49*(5), 1129–1137.

Roy-Byrne, P.P., & Katon, W. (1987, August). An update on treatment of the anxiety disorders. *Hospital and Community Psychiatry, 38,* 835–843.

Simoni, P.S. (1991). Obsessive-compulsive disorder: The effect of research on nursing care. *Journal of Psychosocial Nursing, 29*(4), 19–23.

Snell, F.I., & Padin-Rivera, E. (1997, February). Group treatment for older veterans with posttraumatic stress disorder. *Journal of Psychosocial Nursing, 35*(2), 10–16.

Townsend, M.C. (1995). *Drug guide for psychiatric nursing* (2nd ed.). Philadelphia: F.A. Davis.

Townsend, M.C. (1997). *Nursing diagnoses in psychiatric nursing: A pocket guide for care plan construction* (4th ed.). Philadelphia: F.A. Davis.

Tuma, A.H., & Maser, J. (Eds.). *Anxiety and the anxiety disorders.* Hillsdale, NJ: Lawrence Erlbaum Associates.

Whitley, G.G. (1991). Ritualistic behavior: Breaking the cycle. *Journal of Psychosocial Nursing, 29*(10), 31–35.

Wolf, M.E., & Mosnaim, A.D. (Eds.). (1990). *Posttraumatic stress disorder: Etiology, phenomenology, and treatment.* Washington, DC: American Psychiatric Press.

SOMATOFORM AND SLEEP DISORDERS

KEY TERMS

hysteria
hypochondriasis
somatization
tertiary gain
aphonia

anosmia
pseudocyesis
primary gain
secondary gain
la belle indifference

insomnia
hypersomnia
parasomnias
narcolepsy

OBJECTIVES

After reading this chapter, the student will be able to:

1. Define the term *hysteria.*
2. Discuss historical aspects and epidemiological statistics related to somatoform and sleep disorders.
3. Describe various types of somatoform and sleep disorders and identify symptomatology associated with each; use this information in client assessment.
4. Identify predisposing factors in the development of somatoform and sleep disorders.
5. Formulate nursing diagnoses and goals of care for clients with somatoform and sleep disorders.
6. Describe appropriate nursing interventions for behaviors associated with somatoform and sleep disorders.
7. Identify topics for client and family teaching relevant to somatoform and sleep disorders.
8. Evaluate the nursing care of clients with somatoform and sleep disorders.
9. Discuss various modalities relevant to treatment of somatoform and sleep disorders.

omatoform disorders are characterized by physical symptoms suggesting medical disease, but without demonstrable organic pathology or known pathophysiological mechanism to account for them (Barsky, 1989). They are classified as mental disorders because pathophysiological processes are not demonstrable or understandable by existing laboratory procedures, and there is either evidence or strong presumption that psychological factors are the major cause of the symptoms. Somatization refers to all those mechanisms by which anxiety is translated into physical illness or bodily complaints.

It is now well documented that a large proportion of clients in general medical outpatient clinics and private medical offices do not have organic disease requiring medical treatment. It is likely that many of these clients have somatoform disorders, but they do not perceive themselves as having a psychiatric problem and thus do not seek treatment from psychiatrists.

Disordered sleep is a problem for a great many individuals. For some, the problem may be a temporary one related to stress or anxiety; for others, the cause could be physiological. The study of sleep physiology in psychiatric disorders remains a powerful tool in the research of brain function (Neyland, Reynolds, & Kupfer, 1994).

This chapter focuses on the process of nursing clients exhibiting symptoms of disordered sleep and those who are characterized by repressed anxiety that is being expressed in the form of physiological symptoms. Historical and epidemiological statistics are presented. Predisposing factors that have been implicated in the etiology of somatoform and sleep disorders provide a framework for studying the dynamics of somatization disorder, pain disorder, hypochondriasis, conversion disorder, body dysmorphic disorder, and sleep disorders.

An explanation of the symptomatology is presented as background knowledge for assessing clients with these disorders. Nursing care is described in the context of the nursing process. Various medical treatment modalities are explored.

SOMATOFORM DISORDERS

Historical Aspects

The term **hysteria** describes a polysymptomatic disorder that usually begins in adolescence, rarely after the 20s, chiefly affects women, and is characterized by recurrent, multiple somatic complaints often described dramatically (Goodwin & Guze, 1989). The concept of hysteria is at least 4000 years old and probably originated in Egypt. The name has been in use since the time of Hippocrates.

In the Middle Ages, hysteria was associated with witchcraft, demonology, and sorcery. Mysterious symptoms and unusual behavior were frequently considered manifestations of supernatural, evil influences, with the client being considered as either the evil spirit itself or the victim of the evil force.

In the 19th century, the French physician Paul Briquet attributed the disorder to dysfunction in the nervous system (Stoudemire, 1988). He believed that the disorder resulted from stressful events that acted on the affective part of the brain in vulnerable individuals. Another French physician, Jean Martin Charcot, proposed an essentially physical theory for the disorder, attributing the symptoms to a hereditary degenerative process of the nervous system. Despite his feelings about a physical basis for hysteria, he became famous for his use of hypnosis in the treatment of the disorder (Goodwin & Guze, 1989).

Freud, whose interest in hysterical disorders had developed while he was working in Paris with Charcot, observed that under hypnosis, clients could recall past memories and emotional experiences that would relieve their symptoms. This led to his proposal that unexpressed emotion can be "converted" into physical symptoms (Jones, 1980).

In the 1960s a series of studies originated with a subgroup of hysteria clients who presented with multiple somatic symptoms, a chronic course, and excessive amounts of medical and surgical care. The disorder that delineated this homogeneous group came to be known as Briquet's syndrome and is occasionally designated by this terminology even today (Barsky, 1989). Somatization disorder, as it is described in the *DSM-IV*, is a simplified version of Briquet's syndrome.

Epidemiological Statistics

The lifetime prevalence rate for somatoform disorders in women is 1 or 2 percent (Kaplan & Sadock, 1998). Women are 5 to 20 times more likely to be diagnosed with the disorder than men. Tendencies toward somatization are apparently more common in those who are poorly educated and from the lower socioeconomic classes.

Lifetime prevalence rates of conversion disorder vary widely. Statistics within the general population have been reported from 5 to 30 percent. The disorder occurs more frequently in women than in men and more frequently in adolescents and young adults than in other age groups. A higher prevalence exists in lower socioeconomic groups, rural populations, and among those with less education (Kaplan & Sadock, 1998).

Hypochondriasis is present in 4 percent to 9 percent of clients in general medical practice (APA, 1994). The disorder is equally common among men and women, and the most common age at onset is in early adulthood (APA, 1994).

Pain is likely the most frequent presenting complaint in medical practice today. Pain disorder (previously called somatoform pain disorder) is diagnosed more frequently in women than in men by about 2 to 1. Its onset can occur at any age, with the peak ages of onset in the 40s and

50s. It is more common among people in so-called blue-collar occupations, perhaps because of increased likelihood of job-related injuries (Kaplan & Sadock, 1998).

Body dysmorphic disorder is rare, although it may be more common than once believed (APA, 1994). As many as 2 percent of plastic surgery consultations have been reported from clients with this disorder (Stoudemire, 1988). Psychiatrists see only a small fraction of the cases. A profile of these clients reveals that they are usually in the late teens or 20s and unmarried. Comorbidity with another psychiatric disorder, such as major depression, anxiety disorder, or even a psychotic disorder, is not uncommon with body dysmorphic disorder (Kaplan & Sadock, 1998).

APPLICATION OF THE NURSING PROCESS TO SOMATOFORM DISORDERS

Background Assessment Data

Somatization disorder is a syndrome of multiple somatic symptoms that cannot be explained medically and are associated with psychosocial distress and long-term seeking of assistance from health care professionals (Barsky, 1989). The disorder is chronic, with symptoms beginning before age 30. The symptoms are identified as pain (in as least four different sites), gastrointestinal symptoms (e.g., nausea, vomiting, diarrhea), sexual symtoms (e.g., irregular menses, erectile or ejaculatory dysfunction), and pseudoneurological symptoms (e.g., paralysis, blindness, deafness) (APA, 1994). Anxiety and depression are frequently manifested, and suicidal threats and attempts are not uncommon.

The disorder usually runs a fluctuating course, with periods of remission and exacerbation. Clients often receive medical care from several physicians, sometimes concurrently, leading to the possibility of dangerous combinations of treatments (APA, 1994). They have a tendency to seek relief through overmedicating with prescribed analgesics or antianxiety agents. Drug abuse and dependence are not uncommon complications of somatization disorder. When suicide results, it is usually in association with substance abuse (Purcell, 1988).

McCracken (1985) described personality characteristics common to clients with somatization disorder. He has suggested that there may be some overlapping of features associated with histrionic personality disorder, such as heightened emotionality, vague impressionistic thought, seductiveness, strong dependency needs, and a preoccupation with symptoms and oneself.

The *DSM-IV* diagnostic criteria for somatization disorder are presented in Table 28.1.

Predisposing Factors to Somatization Disorder

Psychodynamic Theory. This theory emphasizes a disturbance in the early mother-child relationship. McCracken (1985) describes the mother as one who, because of her own conflicts regarding sexuality and dependency, alternately clings to and rejects the child. From this conditional nurturing by the mother, the child fails to develop feelings of self-security. These children defend themselves against this insecurity by learning to gain affection and care through illness.

Theory of Family Dynamics. In some families, the

TABLE 28.1 DIAGNOSTIC CRITERIA FOR SOMATIZATION DISORDER

A. A history of physical complaints beginning before age 30 yr that occur over a period of several years and result in treatment being sought or significant impairment in social, occupational, or other important areas of functioning.

B. Each of the following criteria must have been met, with individual symptoms occurring at any time during the course of the disturbance:
1. Four Pain Symptoms: A history of pain related to at least four different sites or functions (e.g., head, abdomen, back, joints, extremities, chest, rectum, during menstruation, during sexual intercourse, or during urination).
2. Two Gastrointestinal Symptoms: A history of at least two gastrointestinal symptoms other than pain (e.g., nausea, bloating, vomiting other than during pregnancy, diarrhea, or intolerance of several different foods).
3. One Sexual Symptom: A history of at least one sexual or reproductive symptom other than pain (e.g., sexual indifference, erectile or ejaculatory dysfunction, irregular menses, excessive menstrual bleeding, vomiting throughout pregnancy).
4. One Pseudoneurological Symptom: A history of at least one symptom of deficit suggesting a neurological condition not limited to pain (e.g., conversion symptoms such as impaired coordination or balance, paralysis or localized weakness, difficulty swallowing or lump in throat, aphonia, urinary retention, hallucinations, loss of touch or pain sensation, double vision, blindness, deafness, seizures; dissociative symptoms such as amnesia; or loss of consciousness other than fainting).

C. Either 1 or 2:
1. After appropriate investigation, each of the symptoms in criterion B cannot be fully explained by a known general medical condition or the direct effects of a substance (e.g., a drug of abuse, a medication).
2. When there is a related general medical condition, the physical complaints or resulting social or occupational impairment are in excess of what would be expected from the history, physical examination, or laboratory findings.

D. The symptoms are not intentionally produced or feigned (as in factitious disorder or malingering).

SOURCE: From APA (1994), with permission.

family members are unable to express emotions openly and resolve conflicts verbally. They tend to deny psychological problems in general. In these "psychosomatic families," when the child becomes ill, the focus shifts from the open conflict to the child's illness, leaving unresolved the underlying issues that the family cannot confront openly. Thus, somatization by the child brings some stability to the family, as harmony replaces discord and the child's welfare becomes the common concern. The child in turn receives positive reinforcement for the illness (Minuchin et al., 1975).

Somatization may also have its roots in the family system due to parental teaching and parental example. The effectiveness of learning through role modeling has been well established and may be instrumental in teaching children to respond to anxious situations with somatization.

Cultural and Environmental Factors. Some cultures and religions carry implicit sanctions against verbalizing or directly expressing emotional states (Stoudemire, 1988). Cross-cultural studies have shown that the somatization symptoms associated with depression are relatively similar, but the "cognitive" or emotional symptoms such as guilt are predominantly seen in Western societies (Kleinman & Mechanic, 1980). In Middle Eastern and Asian cultures, depression is almost exclusively manifested by somatic or vegetative symptoms. This unacceptability of emotional expression is reinforced in various cultures by the absence of vocabulary within the language to express psychological and emotional states (Leff, 1973).

Environmental influences may be significant in the predisposition to somatization disorder. Some studies have suggested that a tendency toward somatization appears to be more common in the poorly educated, rural, and lower socioeconomic classes (Stoudemire, 1988). It is thought that this may be related to a lack of language sophistication required to express oneself psychologically or social restrictions against conceptualizing life difficulties in psychological terminology (Barsky, 1979; Mechanic, 1972).

Genetic Factors. Studies have shown a ten- to twentyfold increased incidence in female first-degree relatives of persons with the disorder (Kaplan & Sadock, 1998). These statistics may imply a possible inheritable predisposition. Studies with monozygotic and dizygotic twins have also provided information that suggests a possible genetic influence.

Transactional Model of Stress/Adaptation. The etiology of somatization disorder is most likely influenced by multiple factors. In Figure 28.1 a graphic depiction of this theory of multiple causation is presented in the transactional model of stress/adaptation.

Diagnosis/Outcome Identification

Nursing diagnoses are formulated from the data gathered during the assessment phase and with background knowledge regarding predisposing factors to the disorder. Some common nursing diagnoses for clients with somatization disorder include:

Ineffective individual coping related to repressed anxiety and unmet dependency needs, evidenced by verbalization of numerous physical complaints in the absence of any pathophysiological evidence; focus on the self and physical symptoms.

Knowledge deficit (psychological causes for physical symptoms) related to strong denial defense system evidenced by history of "doctor shopping" for evidence of organic pathology to substantiate physical symptoms and by statements such as, "I don't know why the doctor put me on the psychiatric unit. I have a physical problem."

The following criteria may be used for measurement of outcomes in the care of the client with somatization disorder.

THE CLIENT:

1. Demonstrates adaptive coping strategies.
2. Effectively uses adaptive coping strategies during stressful situations without resorting to physical symptoms.
3. Identifies stressors that cause anxiety level to rise.
4. Verbalizes understanding of correlation between times of increased anxiety and onset of physical symptoms.
5. Demonstrates control over life situation by meeting needs in an assertive manner.

Planning/Implementation

Table 28.2 provides a plan of care for the client with somatization disorder. Nursing diagnoses are presented, along with outcome criteria, appropriate nursing interventions, and rationales for each.

Evaluation

Reassessment is conducted to determine if the nursing actions have been successful in achieving the objectives of care. Evaluation of the nursing actions for the client with somatization disorder may be facilitated by gathering information using the following types of questions:

1. Can the client recognize signs and symptoms of escalating anxiety?
2. Can the client intervene with adaptive coping strategies to interrupt the escalating anxiety before physical symptoms are exacerbated?
3. Can the client verbalize an understanding of the correlation between physical symptoms and times of escalating anxiety?

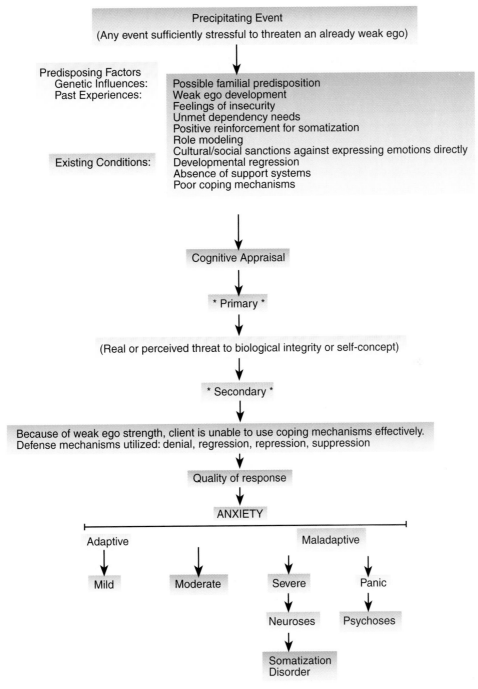

Figure 28.1   The dynamics of somatization disorder using the transactional model of stress/adaptation.

4. Does the client have a plan for dealing with increased stress to prevent exacerbation of physical symptoms?
5. Can the client demonstrate assertiveness skills?
6. Does the client exercise control over life situation by participating in the decision-making process?
7. Can the client verbalize resources outside the hospital from whom he or she may seek assistance during times of extreme stress?

Pain Disorder

Background Assessment Data

The essential feature of pain disorder is severe and prolonged pain that causes clinically significant distress or impairment in social, occupational, or other important areas of functioning (APA, 1994). This diagnosis is made when psychological factors have been judged to have a major role in the onset, severity, exacerbation, or maintenance of the

TABLE 28.2 CARE PLAN FOR THE CLIENT WITH SOMATIZATION DISORDER

NURSING DIAGNOSIS: INEFFECTIVE INDIVIDUAL COPING

RELATED TO: Repressed anxiety and unmet dependency needs

EVIDENCED BY: Verbalization of numerous physical complaints in the absence of any pathophysiological evidence; total focus on the self and physical symptoms

OUTCOME CRITERIA	NURSING INTERVENTIONS	RATIONALE
Client will demonstrate ability to cope with stress by means other than preoccupation with physical symptoms.	1. Monitor physician's ongoing assessments, laboratory reports, and other data to maintain assurance that possibility of organic pathology is clearly ruled out. Review findings with client.	1. Accurate medical assessment is vital for the provision of adequate and appropriate care. Honest explanation may help client understand psychological implications.
	2. Recognize and accept that the physical complaint is real to the client, even though no organic etiology can be identified.	2. Denial of the client's feelings is nontherapeutic and interferes with establishment of a trusting relationship.
	3. Identify gains that the physical symptoms are providing for the client: increased dependency, attention, distraction from other problems.	3. Identification of underlying motivation is important in assisting the client with problem resolution.
	4. Initially, fulfill the client's most urgent dependency needs, but gradually withdraw attention to physical symptoms. Minimize time given in response to physical complaints.	4. Anxiety and maladaptive behaviors will increase if dependency needs are ignored initially. Gradual lack of positive reinforcement will discourage repetition of maladaptive behaviors.
	5. Explain to client that any new physical complaints will be referred to the physician and give no further attention to them. Ensure physician's assessment of the complaint.	5. The possibility of organic pathology must always be considered. Failure to do so could jeopardize client safety.
	6. Encourage client to verbalize fears and anxieties. Explain that attention will be withdrawn if rumination about physical complaints begins. Follow through.	6. Without consistency of limit-setting, change will not occur.
	7. Discuss possible alternative coping strategies client may use in response to stress (e.g., relaxation exercises, physical activities, assertiveness skills). Give positive reinforcement for use of these alternatives.	7. Client may need help with problem solving. Positive reinforcement encourages repetition.
	8. Help client identify ways to achieve recognition from others without resorting to physical symptoms.	8. Positive recognition from others enhances self-esteem and minimizes the need for attention through maladaptive behaviors.

NURSING DIAGNOSIS: KNOWLEDGE DEFICIT (PSYCHOLOGICAL CAUSES FOR PHYSICAL SYMPTOMS)

RELATED TO: Strong denial defense system

EVIDENCED BY: History of doctor shopping for evidence of organic pathology to substantiate physical symptoms and statements such as, "I don't know why the doctor put me on the psychiatric unit. I have a physical problem."

OUTCOME CRITERIA	NURSING INTERVENTIONS	RATIONALE
Client will verbalize psychological implications for physical symptoms.	1. Assess client's level of knowledge regarding effects of psychological problems on the body. Assess level of anxiety and readiness to learn.	1. An adequate database is necessary for the development of an effective teaching plan. Learning does not occur beyond the moderate level of anxiety.

2. Discuss results of laboratory tests and physical examinations with client.
3. Have client keep a diary of appearance, duration, and intensity of physical symptoms. A separate record of situations that the client finds especially stressful should also be kept.
4. Help client identify needs that are being met through the sick role. Formulate a more adaptive means for fulfilling these needs. Practice by role-playing.

5. Have client demonstrate adaptive methods of stress management, such as relaxation exercises, meditation, deep-breathing exercises, autogenics, mental imagery, and assertiveness techniques.

2. Objective information about physical condition may help to break through the strong denial defense.
3. Comparison of these records may provide objective data from which to observe the relationship between physical symptoms and stress.

4. Change cannot occur until the client realizes that physical symptoms are used to fulfill unmet needs. Anxiety is relieved by role-playing, as the client is able to anticipate responses to stressful situations.
5. Demonstration by the client provides a measurable means of evaluating the effectiveness of what has been taught.

---

pain, even when the physical examination reveals pathology that is associated with the pain. Psychological implications in the etiology of the pain complaint may be evidenced by the correlation of a stressful situation with the onset of the symptom. Additional psychological implications may be supported by the facts that (1) appearance of the pain enables the client to avoid some unpleasant activity and (2) the pain promotes emotional support or attention that the client might not otherwise receive (Stoudemire, 1988).

Characteristic behaviors include frequent visits to physicians in an effort to obtain relief, excessive use of analgesics, and requests for surgery (Kaplan, Sadock, & Grebb, 1994). Symptoms of depression are common and often severe enough to warrant a diagnosis of major depression. Dependence on addictive substances is not an uncommon complication of pain disorder. *DSM-IV* diagnostic criteria for this disorder are presented in Table 28.3.

Predisposing Factors to Pain Disorder

Psychoanalytical Theory. Engel (1959) associated psychogenic pain with unconscious guilt and masochism. He theorized that pain in these clients could often serve the purposes of punishment and atonement for unconscious guilt. He found that life histories of these clients were characterized by repeated episodes of real or perceived failures. Childhood was marked by physical abuse, the use of pain as punishment, and emotional distance from parents, resulting in repressed anger and feelings of helplessness. Children who have been severely punished feel guilty and unconsciously come to believe that they must indeed be bad. Such children may grow up with an unconscious need for suffering and pain to assuage this guilt (Barsky, 1989).

Behavioral Theory. In behavioral terminology, psychogenic pain is explained as a response that is learned through operant and classical conditioning. In classical conditioning, a previously neutral stimulus may become a trigger for pain-related behaviors when it becomes associated in the mind of the individual with a painful stimulus. For example, the room where a painful event occurred may itself alone evoke pain-related behaviors because it has become associated with the painful event.

In operant conditioning, learning occurs when pain behaviors are positively or negatively reinforced. When pain behavior elicits attention, sympathy, and nurturing, this positive reinforcement increases the probability of the pain behavior continuing. Negative reinforcement results when the pain behavior prevents an undesirable response from occurring (e.g., provides relief from responsibilities for the client).

Theory of Family Dynamics. "Pain games" may be played in families burdened by conflict. Pain may be used by a family member to control and coerce others and for manipulating and gaining the advantage in interpersonal relationships. Pain may also serve as a **tertiary gain** for a family that maintains the identified client in such a position that the real issue is disregarded and remains unresolved, even though some of the conflict is relieved.

Neurophysiological Theory. This theory postulates that the cerebral cortex and medulla are involved in inhibiting the firing of afferent pain fibers (Cloninger, 1994). Serotonin and the endorphins probably play a role in the central modulation of pain. The levels of serotonin and endorphins are believed to be decreased in clients with chronic, intractable pain. This deficiency seems to correlate with the augmentation of incoming sensory (pain) stimuli.

TABLE 28.3 DIAGNOSTIC CRITERIA FOR PAIN DISORDER

A. Pain in one or more anatomical sites is the predominant focus of the clinical presentation and is of sufficient severity to warrant clinical attention.

B. The pain causes clinically significant distress or impairment in social, occupational, or other important areas of functioning.

C. Psychological factors are judged to have an important role in the onset, severity, exacerbation, or maintenance of the pain.

D. The symptom or deficit is not intentionally produced or feigned (as in factitious disorder or malingering).

E. The pain is not better accounted for by a mood, anxiety, or psychotic disorder and does not meet criteria for dyspareunia.

May be coded as:

- **Acute:** Duration of fewer than 6 months.
- **Chronic:** Duration of 6 months or longer.
- **Associated with Psychological Factors:** Psychological factors are judged to have the major role in the onset, severity, exacerbation, or maintenance of the pain.
- **Associated with Both Psychological Factors and a General Medical Condition:** Both psychological factors and a general medical condition are judged to have important roles in the onset, severity, exacerbation, or maintenance of the pain.

SOURCE: From APA (1994), with permission.

Transactional Model of Stress/Adaptation. The etiology of pain disorder is most likely influenced by multiple factors. Figure 28.2 presents a graphic depiction of this theory of multiple causation in the transactional model of stress/adaptation.

Diagnosis/Outcome Identification

Nursing diagnoses are formulated from the data gathered during the assessment phase and with background knowledge regarding predisposing factors to the disorder. Some common nursing diagnoses for clients with pain disorder include:

Chronic pain related to repressed anxiety and learned maladaptive coping skills, evidenced by verbal complaints of pain, with evidence of psychological contributing factors and excessive use of analgesics.

Social isolation related to preoccupation with self and pain, evidenced by seeking to be alone; refusal to participate in therapeutic activities.

The following criteria may be used for measurement of outcomes in the care of the client with pain disorder:

THE CLIENT:

1. Demonstrates adaptive coping strategies.
2. Verbalizes relief from pain.
3. Effectively uses adaptive coping strategies during stressful situations to prevent the onset of pain.
4. Has identified stressors that raise the anxiety level.
5. Verbalizes understanding of correlation between times of increased anxiety and onset of pain.
6. Demonstrates control over life situation by meeting needs assertively.
7. Interacts with others appropriately.
8. Demonstrates the ability to focus on the needs of others rather than focusing on the self and pain.

Planning/Implementation

Table 28.4 provides a plan of care for the client with pain disorder. Nursing diagnoses are presented, along with outcome criteria, appropriate nursing interventions, and rationales.

Evaluation

Reassessment is conducted to determine if the nursing actions have been successful in achieving the objectives of care. Evaluation of the nursing actions for the client with pain disorder may be facilitated by gathering information using the following types of questions:

1. Can the client recognize signs and symptoms of escalating anxiety?
2. Can the client intervene with adaptive coping strategies to interrupt the escalating anxiety before pain becomes unmanageable?
3. Can the client verbalize an understanding of the correlation between onset of pain and times of escalating anxiety?
4. Does the client have a plan for dealing with increased stress so that the pain response can be diminished?
5. Can the client demonstrate assertiveness skills?
6. Does the client exercise control over life situation by participating in decision-making process?
7. Is the client willingly and voluntarily interacting with others in an appropriate manner?
8. Does the client verbalize understanding of how pain behaviors interfere with the development of satisfactory interpersonal relationships?
9. Does the client show concern for the needs of others and focus less on self and pain?
10. Can the client verbalize resources outside the hospital from whom he or she may seek assistance during times of extreme stress?

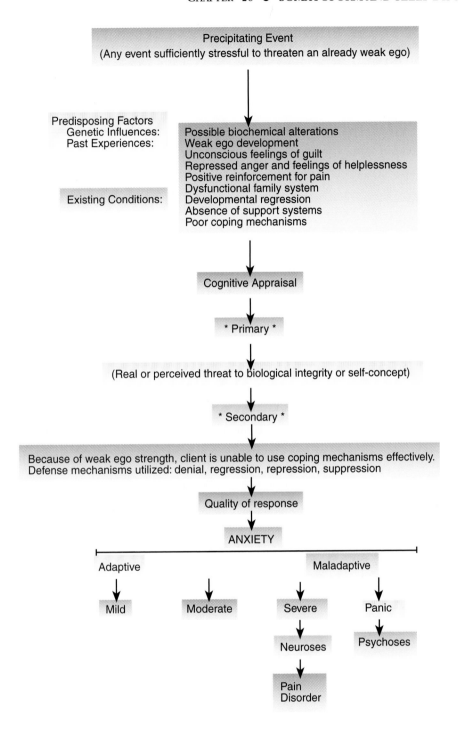

Figure 28.2 The dynamics of pain disorder using the transactional model of stress/adaptation.

Hypochondriasis

Background Assessment Data

Hypochondriasis may be defined as an unrealistic or inaccurate interpretation of physical symptoms or sensations, leading to preoccupation and fear of having a serious disease (Kaplan, Sadock, & Grebb, 1994). The fear becomes disabling and persists despite appropriate reassurance that no organic pathology can be detected. Occasionally medical disease may be present, but in the hypochondriacal individual, the symptoms are grossly disproportionate to the degree of pathology (Barsky, 1989).

The preoccupation may be with a specific organ or disease (e.g., cardiac disease), with bodily functions, such as

TABLE 28.4 CARE PLAN FOR THE CLIENT WITH PAIN DISORDER

NURSING DIAGNOSIS: CHRONIC PAIN

RELATED TO: Repressed anxiety and learned maladaptive coping skills

EVIDENCED BY: Verbal complaints of pain, with evidence of psychological contributing factors, and excessive use of analgesics

OUTCOME CRITERIA	NURSING INTERVENTIONS	RATIONALE
Client will verbalize relief from pain while demonstrating more adaptive coping strategies for dealing with life situation.	1. Monitor physician's ongoing assessments and laboratory reports. 2. Recognize and accept that the pain is indeed real to the client even though no organic etiology can be identified. 3. Observe and record the duration and intensity of the pain. Note factors that precipitate the onset of pain. 4. Provide pain medication as prescribed by physician. 5. Provide nursing comfort measures (e.g., backrub, warm bath, heating pad) with a matter-of-fact approach that does not reinforce the pain behavior. 6. Offer attention at times when client is not focusing on pain. 7. Identify activities that serve to distract client from focus on self and pain. 8. Encourage verbalization of feelings. Explore meaning that pain holds for client. Help client connect symptoms of pain to times of increased anxiety and to identify specific situations that cause anxiety to rise. 9. Encourage client to identify alternative methods of coping with stress. 10. Explore ways to intervene as symptoms begin to intensify (e.g., visual or auditory distractions, mental imagery, deep-breathing exercises, application of hot or cold compresses, relaxation exercises). 11. Provide positive reinforcement for times when client is not focusing on pain.	1. Organic pathology must be clearly ruled out. 2. Denying the client's feelings is nontherapeutic and hinders the development of a trusting relationship. 3. Identification of the precipitating stressor is important for assessment and care planning. 4. Client comfort and safety are nursing priorities. 5. Comfort measures may provide some relief from pain. Secondary gains from physical symptoms may prolong maladaptive behaviors. 6. Positive reinforcement encourages repetition of adaptive behaviors. 7. These distracters serve in a therapeutic manner as a transition from focus on self and pain to focus on unresolved psychological issues. 8. Verbalization of feelings in a nonthreatening environment facilitates expression and resolution of disturbing emotional issues. 9. Alternative stress management techniques may avert the use of pain as a maladaptive response to stress. 10. Adaptive ways of preventing the pain from becoming disabling should be explored. 11. Positive reinforcement, in the form of the nurse's presence and attention, may encourage a continuation of more adaptive behaviors.

NURSING DIAGNOSIS: SOCIAL ISOLATION

RELATED TO: Preoccupation with self and pain

EVIDENCED BY: Seeking to be alone; refusal to participate in therapeutic activities

OUTCOME CRITERIA	NURSING INTERVENTIONS	RATIONALE
Client will voluntarily spend time with other clients and staff members in group activities.	1. Spend more time with the client after setting limits on attention-seeking behaviors. Withdraw presence if ruminations about pain begin.	1. The nurse's presence conveys a sense of worthiness to the client. Lack of reinforcement of maladaptive behaviors may help to decrease their repetition.

2. Increase amount of attention given during times when client is not focusing on pain.

2. This separates the person from the behavior. The client experiences unconditional acceptance without a need for the pain behavior.

3. Describe to the client how the focus on pain and self discourages others from wanting to spend time with him or her.

3. Client may not realize how own behavior is perceived and may result in alienation from others.

4. Teach client to recognize the differences among passive, assertive, and aggressive behaviors and the importance of respecting the human rights of others while protecting one's own basic human rights.

4. These assertive techniques enhance self-esteem and facilitate communication and mutual acceptance in interpersonal relationships.

5. Provide positive feedback for any attempts at social interaction in which the client's focus is on others rather than on self or pain

5. Positive feedback enhances self-esteem and encourages repetition of desirable behaviors.

peristalsis or heartbeat, or even with minor physical alterations, such as a small sore or an occasional cough (APA, 1994). Individuals with hypochondriasis may become convinced that a rapid heart rate indicates they have heart disease or that the small sore is skin cancer. They are profoundly preoccupied with their bodies and are totally aware of even the slightest change in feeling or sensation. However, their response to these small changes is usually unrealistic and exaggerated.

Individuals with hypochondriasis often have a long history of "doctor shopping" and are convinced that they are not receiving the proper care. Anxiety and depression are common, and obsessive-compulsive traits frequently accompany the disorder.

Preoccupation with the fear of serious disease may interfere with social or occupational functioning. However, some individuals are able to function appropriately on the job, while limiting their physical complaints to nonwork time.

Individuals with hypochondriasis are so totally convinced that their symptoms are related to organic pathology that they adamantly reject, and are often irritated by, any implication that stress or psychosocial factors play any role in their condition (Barsky, 1989). They are so apprehensive and fearful that they become alarmed at the slightest intimation of serious illness. Even reading about a disease or hearing that someone they know has been diagnosed with an illness precipitates alarm on their part.

The *DSM-IV* diagnostic criteria for hypochondriasis are presented in Table 28.5.

Predisposing Factors to Hypochondriasis

Psychodynamic Theory. Some psychodynamicists view hypochondriasis as an ego defense mechanism. Physical complaints are the expression of low self-esteem and feelings of worthlessness, as it is easier to feel something is wrong with the body than to feel something is wrong with the self (Barsky, 1989).

Another psychodynamic view explains hypochondriasis as the transformation of aggressive and hostile wishes toward others into physical complaints to others. Repressed anger, originating from past disappointments and unfulfilled needs for nurturing and caring, is expressed in the present by soliciting other people's help and concern and then thwarting and rejecting them as ineffective.

Still other psychodynamicists have viewed hypochon-

TABLE 28.5 DIAGNOSTIC CRITERIA FOR HYPOCHONDRIASIS

A. Preoccupation with fears of having, or the idea that one has, a serious disease, based on the person's misinterpretation of bodily symptoms.

B. The preoccupation persists despite appropriate medical evaluation and reassurance.

C. The belief in criterion A is not of delusional intensity (as in delusional disorder, somatic type) and is not restricted to a circumscribed concern about appearance (as in body dysmorphic disorder).

D. The preoccupation causes clinically significant distress or impairment in social, occupational, or other important areas of functioning.

E. The duration of the disturbance is at least 6 months.

F. The preoccupation is not better accounted for by generalized anxiety disorder, obsessive-compulsive disorder, panic disorder, a major depressive episode, separation anxiety, or another somatoform disorder.

SOURCE: From APA (1994), with permission.

driasis as a defense against guilt (Kenyon, 1976). The individual views the self as "bad," based on real or imagined past misconduct, and views physical suffering as the deserved punishment required for atonement.

Cognitive Theory. Studies show that noxious sensory input undergoes a cognitive screening process involving assessment and clarification, which may amplify or reduce the sensations (Chapman, 1978). Cognitive theorists view hypochondriasis as arising out of perceptual and cognitive abnormalities. Barsky and Klerman (1983) cite three components of this theory:

1. These clients amplify normal bodily sensory input.
2. They incorrectly assess and misinterpret somatic symptoms of emotional arousal.
3. They are innately predisposed to thinking and perceiving in concrete rather than emotional or subjective terms.

Benign bodily sensations are misinterpreted and negative cognitive meanings are attached to them. Barsky and Klerman (1983) have stated:

"Once formed, the incorrect attribution tends to persist because all future perceptions are interpreted to fit the cognitive set that the individual has a disease."

Sociocultural/Familial Factors. Somatic complaints are often reinforced when the sick role relieves the individual from the need to deal with a stressful situation, whether it be within society or within the family. When the sick person is allowed to avoid stressful obligations and postpone unwelcome challenges, is excused from troublesome duties, or becomes the prominent focus of attention because of the illness, positive reinforcement virtually guarantees repetition of the response. Barsky (1989) stated:

"Sick clients have special powers within their families—sickness and suffering allow them to avoid intimacy ('Not tonight, dear, I have a headache'), to control and manipulate others, and to express their hostility, since temper tantrums and irritability are excusable if one is sick."

Past Experiences With Physical Illness. Individuals with hypochondriasis seem to have an increased incidence of childhood medical illness and more extensive past medical histories (Barksy, 1989). This early exposure instills a knowledge of the terminology required to translate psychological distress into physical expression.

Personal experience, or the experience of close family members, with serious or life-threatening illness can predispose an individual to hypochondriasis. Once an individual has experienced a threat to biological integrity, he or she may develop a fear of recurrence. Increased bodily sensitivity develops, and the individual becomes strongly in tune to changes that may occur. The fear of recurring illness generates an exaggerated response leading to hypochondriacal behaviors.

Genetic Influences. Although little is known about the inheritance of hypochondriasis, some evidence indicates an increased prevalence of hypochondriasis among identical twins and other first-degree relatives (Barsky, 1989).

Transactional Model of Stress/Adaptation. The etiology of hypochondriasis is most likely influenced by multiple factors. In Figure 28.3 a graphic depiction of this theory of multiple causation is presented in the transactional model of stress/adaptation.

Diagnosis/Outcome Identification

Nursing diagnoses are formulated from the data gathered during the assessment phase and with background knowledge regarding predisposing factors to the disorder. Common nursing diagnoses for clients with hypochondriasis include:

Fear (of having serious disease) related to past experience with life-threatening illness (of self or significant others), evidenced by preoccupation with and unrealistic interpretation of bodily signs and sensations.

Self-esteem disturbance related to unfulfilled childhood needs for nurturing and caring, evidenced by transformation of internalized anger into physical complaints and hostility toward others.

The following criteria may be used to measure outcomes in the care of the client with hypochondriasis:

THE CLIENT:
1. Interprets bodily sensations rationally.
2. Verbalizes significance that the irrational fear held for him or her.
3. Has decreased the number and frequency of physical complaints.
4. Has identified the correlation between increased anxiety and the exacerbation of physical symptoms.
5. Has identified life situations that precipitate anxiety.
6. Demonstrates more adaptive ways of coping with stress than with physical symptoms.
7. Demonstrates acceptance of self as a worthwhile person.
8. Expresses self-confidence in dealing with stressful life situations.
9. Makes life changes for improvement and accepts situations that cannot be changed.
10. Sets realistic goals for the future.

Planning/Implementation

Table 28.6 provides a plan of care for the client with hypochondriasis. Nursing diagnoses are presented, along with outcome criteria, appropriate nursing interventions, and rationales.

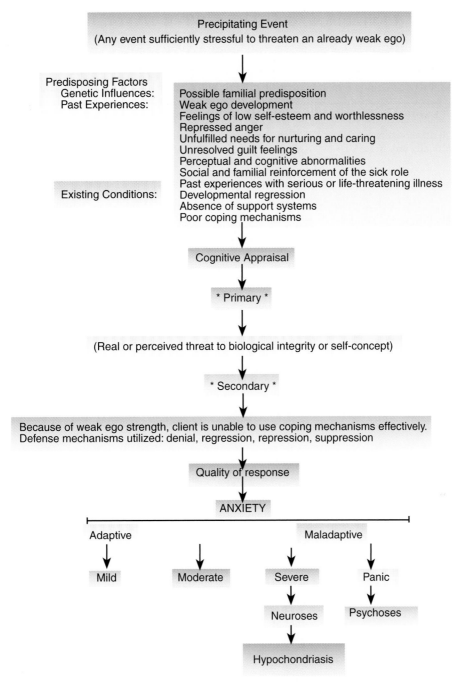

Figure 28.3 The dynamics of hypochondriasis using the transactional model of stress/adaptation.

Evaluation

Reassessment is conducted to determine if the nursing actions have been successful in achieving the objectives of care. Evaluation of the nursing actions for the client with hypochondriasis may be facilitated by gathering information using the following types of questions:

1. Does the client demonstrate a decrease in ruminations about physical symptoms?
2. Have fears of serious illness diminished?

3. Can the client correlate the exacerbation of physical symptoms to times of escalating anxiety?
4. Can the client use more adaptive coping mechanisms to interrupt the anxiety response?
5. Can the client demonstrate assertiveness and effective communication skills?
6. Does the client exercise control over life situation by participating in the decision-making process?
7. Does the client set realistic goals for the future?
8. Can the client maximize his or her potential by making the most of personal strengths?

TABLE 28.6 CARE PLAN FOR CLIENT WITH HYPOCHONDRIASIS

NURSING DIAGNOSIS: FEAR (OF HAVING A SERIOUS DISEASE)
RELATED TO: Past experience with life-threatening illness of self or significant others
EVIDENCED BY: Preoccupation with and unrealistic interpretation of bodily signs and sensations

OUTCOME CRITERIA	NURSING INTERVENTIONS	RATIONALE
Client will verbalize irrationality of fear and interpret bodily sensations correctly.	1. Monitor physician's ongoing assessments and laboratory reports.	1. Organic pathology must be clearly ruled out.
	2. Refer all new physical complaints to physician.	2. To assume that all physical complaints are hypochondriacal would place client's safety in jeopardy.
	3. Assess function client's illness is fulfilling for him or her (e.g., unfulfilled needs for dependency, nurturing, caring, attention, or control).	3. This information may provide insight into reasons for maladaptive behavior and provide direction for planning client care.
	4. Identify times during which preoccupation with physical symptoms is worse. Determine extent of correlation of physical complaints with times of increased anxiety.	4. Client is unaware of the psychosocial implications of the physical complaints. Knowledge of the relationship is the first step in the process for creating change.
	5. Convey empathy. Let client know that you understand how a specific symptom may conjure up fears of previous life-threatening illness.	5. Unconditional acceptance and empathy promote a therapeutic nurse-client relationship.
	6. Initially allow client a limited amount of time (e.g., 10 minutes each hour) to discuss physical symptoms.	6. Because this has been his or her primary method of coping for so long, complete prohibition of this activity would likely raise client's anxiety level significantly, further exacerbating the hypochondriacal behavior.
	7. Help client determine what techniques may be most useful for him or her to implement when fear and anxiety are exacerbated (e.g., relaxation techniques, mental imagery, thought-stopping techniques, physical exercise).	7. All of these techniques are effective in reducing anxiety and may assist client in the transition from focusing on fear of physical illness to the discussion of honest feelings.
	8. Gradually increase the limit on amount of time spent each hour in discussing physical symptoms. If client violates the limits, withdraw attention.	8. Lack of positive reinforcement may help to extinguish maladaptive behavior.
	9. Encourage client to discuss feelings associated with fear of serious illness.	9. Verbalization of feelings in a nonthreatening environment facilitates expression and resolution of disturbing emotional issues. When the client can express feelings directly, there is less need to express them through physical symptoms.
	10. Role play the client's plan for dealing with the fear the next time it assumes control and before it becomes disabling through the exacerbation of physical symptoms.	10. Anxiety and fears are minimized when client has achieved a degree of comfort through practicing a plan for dealing with stressful situations in the future.

NURSING DIAGNOSIS: SELF-ESTEEM DISTURBANCE
RELATED TO: Unfulfilled childhood needs for nurturing and caring
EVIDENCED BY: Transformation of internalized anger into physical complaints and hostility toward others

OUTCOME CRITERIA	NURSING INTERVENTIONS	RATIONALE
Client will demonstrate acceptance of self as a person of worth, as evidenced by setting realistic goals, limiting physical complaints and hostility toward others, and verbalizing positive prospects for the future.	1. Convey acceptance, unconditional positive regard, and remain nonjudgmental at all times.	1. Offering the client respect and dignity adds to feelings of self-worth.
	2. Encourage client to participate in decision making regarding care as well as life situations.	2. Feelings of personal control decreases feelings of powerlessness.
	3. Help client to recognize and focus on strengths and accomplishments. Minimize attention given to past (real or perceived) failures.	3. Lack of attention may help to eliminate negative ruminations.
	4. Encourage participation in group activities.	4. Through participation in group activities, client may receive positive feedback and support from peers.
	5. Ensure that client is not becoming increasingly dependent. Withdraw attention at times when client is focusing on physical symptoms.	5. Independent functioning increases feelings of self-worth. Lack of reinforcement may help to extinguish maladaptive behaviors.
	6. Ensure that therapy groups offer client simple methods of achievement. Offer recognition and positive feedback for actual accomplishments.	6. Successes and recognition increase self-esteem.
	7. Teach assertiveness techniques and effective communication techniques.	7. Self-esteem is enhanced by the ability to interact with others in an effective manner.
	8. Offer positive feedback when client responds to stressful situation with coping strategies other then physical complaints.	8. Positive feedback enhances self-esteem and encourages repetition of desirable behaviors.

9. Can the client verbalize resources outside the hospital from whom he or she may seek assistance during times of extreme stress?

Conversion Disorder

Background Assessment Data

Conversion disorder is a loss of or change in body function resulting from a psychological conflict, the physical symptoms of which cannot be explained by any known medical disorder or pathophysiological mechanism (Barsky, 1989). Clients are unaware of the psychological basis and are therefore unable to control their symptoms.

Conversion symptoms affect voluntary motor or sensory functioning suggestive of neurological disease and are therefore sometimes called "pseudoneurological" (APA, 1994). Examples include paralysis, **aphonia,** seizures, coordination disturbance, difficulty swallowing, urinary retention, akinesia, blindness, deafness, double vision, **anosmia,** loss of pain sensation, and hallucinations. **Pseudocyesis** (false pregnancy) is a conversion symptom and may represent a strong desire to be pregnant (Cloninger, 1994).

Precipitation of conversion symptoms must be explained by psychological factors, and this may be evidenced by the presence of primary or secondary gain. When an individual achieves **"primary gain,"** the conversion symptoms serve to prevent internal conflicts or painful issues or events from attaining awareness. Conversion symptoms promote **"secondary gain"** for the individual by enabling him or her to avoid difficult situations or to obtain support that might not otherwise be forthcoming.

The symptom usually occurs after a situation that produces extreme psychological stress for the individual. The symptom appears suddenly, and often the person expresses a relative lack of concern that is out of keeping with the severity of the impairment (APA, 1994). This lack of concern is identified as **la belle indifference** and is often a clue to the physician that the problem may be psychological rather than physical. Other individuals, however, may present symptoms in a dramatic or histrionic fashion (APA, 1994).

The prognosis of conversion disorder seems to be highly variable. Some conversion symptoms resolve themselves over a period of days to months without treatment, whereas some may persist for years in spite of intense efforts at treatment (Purcell, 1988). The prognosis seems to have little to do with the specific symptom involved and seemingly depends on the interplay of the individual's psychological makeup, the social environment, and the response to the symptom by people who are important to the client. Symptoms of blindness, aphonia, and paralysis are associated with good prognosis, whereas seizures and tremor are associated with poorer prognosis (Martin & Yutzy, 1994). The *DSM-IV* diagnostic criteria for conversion disorder are presented in Table 28.7.

Predisposing Factors to Conversion Disorder

Psychoanalytical Theory. This theory proposes that emotions associated with a traumatic event that the individual cannot express because of moral or ethical unacceptability are "converted" into physical symptoms. The unacceptable emotions are repressed and converted to a somatic hysterical symptom that is symbolic in some way of the original emotional trauma. An example might be the young soldier who, knowing that at daybreak he will be sent to the front lines to participate in battle, develops a paralysis of his arms and is unable to pick up his rifle.

Theory of Interpersonal Communication. In this conceptual model, conversion symptoms are viewed as a type of nonverbal communication. When direct verbal communication becomes blocked in an interpersonal relationship, a message is conveyed through the use of "somatic" language (Ford & Folks, 1985). With physical symptoms, the individual communicates that he or she (or the relationship) needs special treatment or consideration. Physical symptoms also may function as a nonverbal means of controlling or manipulating others (Barsky, 1989).

Neurophysiological Theory. This theory suggests that some clients with conversion disorder have a distur-

bance in central nervous system (CNS) arousal. Symptoms are thought to be derived from an excessive cortical arousal, creating a negative feedback loop between the cerebral cortex and the brainstem reticular formation (Kaplan & Sadock, 1998). This activity diminishes the awareness of bodily sensation and would explain the observed sensory deficits in some conversion disorder clients and their apparently low levels of anxiety and relative indifference to their impairment.

Behavioral Theory. Behavioral theorists believe that conversion symptoms are learned through positive reinforcement from cultural, social, and interpersonal influences (Stoudemire, 1988). The individual uses physical symptoms to communicate helplessness and, in return, gains attention and support from the environment. These secondary gains reinforce the perpetuation of symptoms during times of stress or conflict.

Transactional Model of Stress/Adaptation. The etiology of conversion disorder is most likely influenced by multiple factors. In Figure 28.4, a graphic depiction of this theory of multiple causation is presented in the transactional model of stress/adaptation.

Diagnosis/Outcome Identification

Nursing diagnoses are formulated from the data gathered during the assessment phase and with background knowledge regarding predisposing factors to the disorder. Common nursing diagnoses for clients with conversion disorder include:

Sensory-perceptual alteration related to repressed severe anxiety, evidenced by loss or alteration in physical functioning without evidence of organic pathology; and "la belle indifference."

Self-care deficit related to loss or alteration in physical functioning, evidenced by the need for assistance to

---

> ![icon] **TABLE 28.7 DIAGNOSTIC CRITERIA FOR CONVERSION DISORDER**

A. One or more symptoms or deficits affecting voluntary motor or sensory function that suggest a neurological or other general medical condition.

B. Psychological factors are judged to be associated with the symptom or deficit because the initiation or exacerbation of the symptom or deficit is preceded by conflicts or other stressors.

C. The symptom or deficit is not intentionally produced or feigned (as in factitious disorder or malingering).

D. The symptom or deficit cannot, after appropriate investigation, be fully explained by a general medical condition, by the direct effects of a substance, or as a culturally sanctioned behavior or experience.

E. The symptom or deficit causes clinically significant distress or impairment in social, occupational, or other important ideas of functioning or warrants medical evaluation.

F. The symptom or deficit is not limited to pain or sexual dysfunction, does not occur exclusively during the course of somatization disorder, and is not better accounted for by another mental disorder.

Specify type of symptom or deficit:

With motor symptom or deficit.

With sensory symptom or deficit.

With seizures or convulsions.

With mixed presentation.

SOURCE: From APA (1994), with permission.

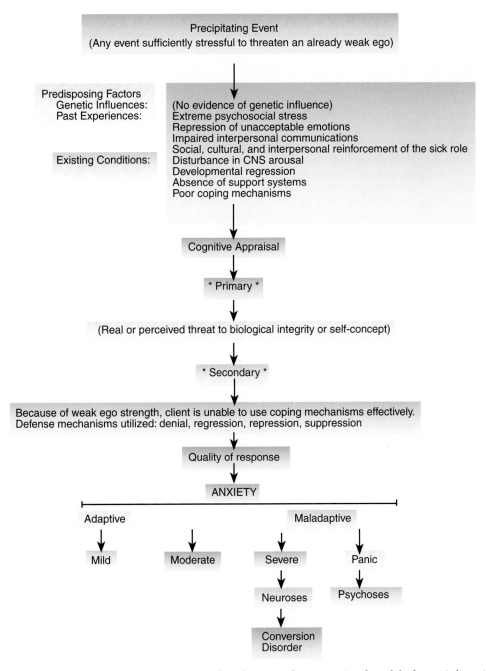

Figure 28.4   The dynamics of conversion disorder using the transactional model of stress/adaptation.

carry out self-care activities such as eating, dressing, maintaining hygiene, and toileting.

The following criteria may be used for measurement of outcomes in the care of the client with conversion disorder.

THE CLIENT:

1. Is free of physical disability.
2. Verbalizes the correlation between the loss of or alteration in function and extreme emotional stress.
3. Is able to identify the stressful situation that precipitated the physical disability.
4. Verbalizes the purpose the disability serves for him or her.
5. Demonstrates more adaptive coping strategies for dealing with stress in the future.
6. Performs all self-care activities without assistance.

Planning/Implementation

Table 28.8 provides a plan of care for the client with conversion disorder. Nursing diagnoses are presented, along with outcome criteria, appropriate nursing interventions, and rationales.

TABLE 28.8 CARE PLAN FOR THE CLIENT WITH CONVERSION DISORDER

NURSING DIAGNOSIS: SENSORY-PERCEPTUAL ALTERATION

RELATED TO: Repressed severe anxiety

EVIDENCED BY: Loss or alteration in physical functioning, without evidence of organic pathology; "la belle indifference"

OUTCOME CRITERIA	NURSING INTERVENTIONS	RATIONALE
Client will demonstrate recovery of lost or altered function.	1. Monitor physician's ongoing assessments, laboratory reports, and other data to ensure that possibility of organic pathology is clearly ruled out.	1. Failure to do so may jeopardize client safety.
	2. Identify primary or secondary gains that the physical symptom is providing for the client (e.g., increased dependency, attention, protection from experiencing a stressful event).	2. Primary and secondary gains are etiological factors and will be used to assist in problem resolution.
	3. Do not focus on the disability, and encourage client to be as independent as possible. Intervene only when client requires assistance.	3. Positive reinforcement would encourage continual use of the maladaptive response for secondary gains, such as dependency.
	4. Do not allow the client to use the disability as a manipulative tool to avoid participation in therapeutic activities. Withdraw attention if client continues to focus on physical limitation.	4. Lack of reinforcement may help to extinguish the maladaptive response.
	5. Encourage client to verbalize fears and anxieties. Help identify physical symptoms as a coping mechanism that is used in times of extreme stress.	5. Clients with conversion disorder are usually unaware of the psychological implications of their illness.
	6. Help client identify coping mechanisms that he or she could use when faced with stressful situations, rather than retreating from reality with a physical disability.	6. Client needs assistance with problem solving at this severe level of anxiety.
	7. Give positive reinforcement for identification or demonstration of alternative, more adaptive coping strategies.	7. Positive reinforcement enhances self-esteem and encourages repetition of desirable behaviors.

NURSING DIAGNOSIS: SELF-CARE DEFICIT

RELATED TO: Loss or alteration in physical functioning

EVIDENCED BY: Need for assistance to carry out self-care activities, such as eating, dressing, hygiene, and toileting

OUTCOME CRITERIA	NURSING INTERVENTIONS	RATIONALE
Client will be able to perform self-care activities independently.	1. Assess client's level of disability. Note areas of strength and impairment.	1. Information about strengths and impairments will be used to plan care for the client.
	2. Encourage client to perform self-care to his or her level of ability. Intervene when client is unable to perform.	2. Successful performance of independent activities enhances self-esteem.
	3. Maintain nonjudgmental attitude when providing assistance to the client. The physical symptom is not within the client's conscious control and is very real to him or her.	3. A judgmental attitude interferes with the nurse's ability to provide therapeutic care for the client.

4. a. Feed client, if necessary, or provide assistance with containers, positioning, and so forth.
   b. Bathe client, or assist with bath, as required.
   c. Assist with dressing, oral hygiene, combing hair, applying makeup.
   d. Provide bedpan, commode, or assistance to bathroom, as required.
5. Avoid fostering dependency by intervening when client is capable of performing independently. Allow ample time to complete these activities to the best of client's ability without assistance. Provide positive reinforcement for independent accomplishments.
6. Help client understand the purpose this disability is serving for him or her. Discuss honest feelings.

4. Client comfort and safety are nursing priorities.

5. Success and positive reinforcement enhance self-esteem and encourage repetition of desirable behaviors.

6. Self-disclosure and exploration of feelings with a trusted individual may help client fulfill unmet needs and confront unresolved issues.

Evaluation

Reassessment is conducted to determine if the nursing actions have been successful in achieving the objectives of care. Evaluation of the nursing actions for the client with conversion disorder may be facilitated by gathering information using the following types of questions:

1. Does the client demonstrate full recovery from previous physical disability?
2. Can the client perform all self-care activities independently?
3. Can the client verbalize why the disability occurred?
4. Can the client verbalize the relationship between loss of function and the stressful event?
5. Does the client recognize what unfulfilled need the loss of function was serving?
6. Can the client openly discuss feelings associated with the stressful event?
7. Can the client directly confront the conflict that was previously repressed and somaticized?
8. Can the client demonstrate more adaptive coping skills for dealing with stress or conflict?
9. Does he or she have a plan for coping with future stressful situations?
10. Can the client verbalize resources outside the hospital to whom he or she may turn when feeling the need for assistance?

Body Dysmorphic Disorder
Background Assessment Data

This disorder, formerly called dysmorphophobia, is characterized by the exaggerated belief that the body is deformed or defective in some specific way. The most common complaints involve imagined or slight flaws of the face or head, such as thinning hair, acne, wrinkles, scars, vascular markings, facial swelling or asymmetry, or excessive facial hair (APA, 1994). Other complaints may have to do with some aspect of the nose, ears, eyes, mouth, lips, or teeth. Some clients may present with complaints involving other parts of the body, and in some instances a true defect is present. However, the significance of the defect is unrealistically exaggerated and the person's concern is grossly excessive.

Symptoms of depression and characteristics associated with obsessive-compulsive personality are common in individuals with body dysmorphic disorder. Social and occupational impairment may occur because of the excessive anxiety experienced by the individual in relation to the imagined defect. The person's medical history may reflect numerous visits to plastic surgeons and dermatologists in an unrelenting drive to correct the imagined defect. He or she may undergo unnecessary surgical procedures toward this effort.

This disorder has been closely associated with delusional thinking, and the *DSM-IV* suggests that if the perceived body defect is in fact of delusional intensity, the appropriate diagnosis would be delusional disorder, somatic type (APA, 1994). Traits associated with schizoid and narcissistic personality disorders are not uncommon (Kaplan & Sadock, 1998). In Europe, where the syndrome has been more widely studied, it is considered to be a psychosis (Barsky, 1989).

The *DSM-IV* diagnostic criteria for body dysmorphic disorder are presented in Table 28.9.

■ **Table 28.9 Diagnostic Criteria for Body Dysmorphic Disorder**

A. Preoccupation with an imagined defect in appearance. If a slight physical anomaly is present, the person's concern is markedly excessive.
B. The preoccupation causes clinically significant distress or impairment in social, occupational, or other important areas of functioning.
C. The preoccupation is not better accounted for by another mental disorder (e.g., dissatisfaction with body shape and size in anorexia nervosa).

SOURCE: From APA (1994), with permission.

Predisposing Factors to Body Dysmorphic Disorder

The etiology of body dysmorphic disorder is unknown. In some clients the belief is due to another more pervasive psychiatric disorder, such as schizophrenia, major mood disorder, or anxiety disorder. This has been supported by the responsiveness of the condition to the serotonin-specific drugs (Kaplan & Sadock, 1998).

Body dysmorphic disorder has been classified as one of several *monosymptomatic hypochondriacal syndromes.* Each of these syndromes is characterized by a single hypochondriacal belief about one's body. Body dysmorphic disorder is one of the most common such syndromes. Others include delusions of parasitosis (i.e., false belief that one is infested with some parasite or vermin) and of bromosis (i.e., false belief that one is emitting an offensive body odor).

Body dysmorphic disorder has also been defined as the fear of some physical defect thought to be noticeable to others although the client appears normal. These interpretations suggest that the disorder may be related to predisposing factors similar to those associated with hypochondriasis or phobias. The psychodynamic view suggests that unresolved emotional conflict is displaced onto a body part through symbolization and projection (Kaplan & Sadock, 1998). Repression of morbid anxiety is undoubtedly an underlying factor, and it is very likely that multiple factors are involved in the predisposition to body dysmorphic disorder.

Diagnosis/Outcome Identification

Nursing diagnoses are formulated from the data gathered during the assessment phase and with background knowledge regarding predisposing factors to the disorder. Nursing diagnoses for clients with body dysmorphic disorder may include:

Body image disturbance related to repressed severe anxiety, evidenced by preoccupation with imagined defect; verbalizations that are out of proportion to any actual physical abnormality that may exist; and numerous visits to plastic surgeons or dermatologists seeking relief.

The following criteria may be used for measurement of outcomes in the care of the client with body dysmorphic disorder:

The Client:

1. Verbalizes a realistic perception of his or her appearance.
2. Expresses feelings of self-worth that reflect a positive body image and acceptance of personal appearance.
3. Verbalizes fears and anxieties that may contribute to altered body image.
4. Verbalizes adaptive strategies for dealing with fears and anxieties more effectively.
5. Expresses satisfaction with accomplishments unrelated to physical appearance.
6. Verbalizes intent to participate in a support group.

Planning/Implementation

Table 28.10 provides a plan of care for the client with body dysmorphic disorder. The nursing diagnosis is presented, along with the outcome criterion, appropriate nursing interventions, and rationales.

Evaluation

Reassessment is conducted in order to determine if the nursing actions have been successful in achieving the objectives of care. Evaluation of the nursing actions for the client with body dysmorphic disorder may be facilitated by gathering information using the following types of questions:

1. Does the client demonstrate a decrease in ruminations about the imagined defect?
2. Can the client maximize his or her potential by making the most of personal strengths?
3. Has the client verbalized a realistic perception of personal appearance?
4. Does he or she demonstrate satisfactory acceptance of personal appearance?
5. Does the client interact with others comfortably?
6. Does the client focus attention on activities or personal accomplishments rather than personal appearance?
7. Does the client demonstrate a positive self-worth not based on appearance?
8. Has he or she expressed fears and anxieties that may have provided the foundation for preoccupation with the imagined defect?

TABLE 28.10   CARE PLAN FOR THE CLIENT WITH BODY DYSMORPHIC DISORDER

NURSING DIAGNOSIS: BODY IMAGE DISTURBANCE

RELATED TO: Repressed severe anxiety

EVIDENCED BY: Preoccupation with imagined defect; verbalizations that are out of proportion to any actual physical abnormality that may exist; and numerous visits to plastic surgeons or dermatologists seeking relief

OUTCOME CRITERIA	NURSING INTERVENTIONS	RATIONALE
Client will verbalize realistic perception of body appearance.	1. Assess client's perception of his or her body image. Keep in mind that this image is real to the client.	1. Assessment information is necessary in developing an accurate plan of care. Denial of the client's feelings impedes the development of a trusting, therapeutic relationship.
	2. Help client to see that his or her body image is distorted or that it is out of proportion in relation to the significance of an actual physical anomaly.	2. Recognition that a misperception exists is necessary before the client can accept reality and reduce the significance of the imagined defect.
	3. Encourage verbalization of fears and anxieties associated with identified stressful life situations. Discuss alternative adaptive coping strategies.	3. Verbalization of feelings with a trusted individual may help the client come to terms with unresolved issues. Knowledge of alternative coping strategies may help the client respond to stress more adaptively in the future.
	4. Involve client in activities that reinforce a positive sense of self not based on appearance.	4. When the client is able to develop self-satisfaction based on accomplishments and unconditional acceptance, significance of the imagined defect or minor physical anomaly will diminish.
	5. Make referrals to support groups of individuals with similar histories (e.g., Adult Children of Alcoholics [ACOA], Victims of Incest, Survivors of Suicide [SOS], Adults Abused as Children).	5. Having a support group of understanding, empathic peers can help the client accept the reality of the situation, correct distorted perceptions, and make adaptive life changes.

9. Can the client demonstrate strategies for coping more adaptively with stress in the future?

10. Can the client verbalize resources from whom he or she may seek assistance during times of extreme stress (including regular attendance in a support group)?

SLEEP DISORDERS

The main purposes of sleep are to restore homeostatic function, maintain normal thermoregulation, and conserve energy (Kaplan, Sadock, & Grebb, 1994). Some individuals require fewer than 6 hours, whereas others need more than 9 hours of sleep per night to function adequately. Individuals who require less sleep are generally efficient, ambitious, socially adept, and content. The longer sleepers tend to be mildly depressed, anxious, and socially withdrawn (Kaplan, Sadock, & Grebb, 1994). The need for sleep increases with physical activity, illness, pregnancy, emotional stress, and increased mental activity.

Each year, approximately 10 million Americans seek treatment from physicians for sleep-related disturbances (Neyland, Reynolds, & Kupfer, 1994). Kaplan, Sadock, and Grebb (1994) identify four major symptomatic manifestations that characterize most sleep disorders: **insomnia, hypersomnia, parasomnias,** and sleep-wake schedule disturbances.

APPLICATION OF THE NURSING PROCESS TO SLEEP DISORDERS

Background Assessment Data

Insomnia. Insomnia is defined as difficulty with initiating or maintaining sleep (American Sleep Disorders Association [ASDA], 1990). The *DSM-IV* identifies this disorder as primary insomnia, to differentiate it from insomnia that is secondary to physical or mental conditions. The *DSM-IV* specifies that the symptom must be of at least 1 month's duration; must cause significant impairment in social, occupational, or other important areas of functioning;

and must not be due to the direct effects of a substance, a general medical condition, or a mental disorder (APA, 1994).

Primary insomnia may be manifested by a combination of difficulty falling asleep and intermittent wakefulness during sleep. The disorder often becomes a vicious cycle when the individual becomes more and more distressed by the inability to achieve sleep, and the additional stress in turn contributes to the insomnia.

Individuals with this disorder often have an anxious overconcern with their general health. Depression and anxiety are not uncommon. Lack of sleep results in daytime irritability and problems with attention and concentration. Inappropriate use of substances, both hypnotics for sleep and stimulants to counteract fatigue, often occurs.

Primary insomnia typically begins in early to middle adulthood and increases with age. It is more common in women than in men.

Hypersomnia. Hypersomnia, or *somnolence*, can be defined as excessive sleepiness or seeking excessive amounts of sleep. Primary hypersomnia refers to the condition when no other cause for the symptom can be found. The term should be used for individuals who have difficulty staying awake during what should be considered the waking hours of the sleep-wake cycle; it should not be used for those who are simply physically tired or weary (Kaplan, Sadock, & Grebb, 1994). The *DSM-IV* specifies that the symptom must be of at least 1 month's duration; must be severe enough to interfere with social, occupational, or other important areas of functioning; and must not be due to the direct physiological effects of a substance or a general medical condition (APA, 1994).

Excessive sleepiness interferes with attention, concentration, memory, and productivity. It can also lead to disruption in social and family relationships. Depression is a common side effect of hypersomnia, as are substance-related disorders, particularly those related to self-medication with stimulants (APA, 1994).

Approximately 5 percent to 10 percent of individuals who present to sleep disorders clinics with complaints of daytime sleepiness are diagnosed as having primary hypersomnia (APA, 1994). The disorder usually begins in late adolescence or early adulthood and is more common in men than in women.

Narcolepsy is a disorder similar to hypersomnia. They both produce excessive sleepiness, have similar age at onset, and run the same stable course over time. The characteristic manifestation of narcolepsy is sleep attacks. The individual cannot prevent falling asleep. He or she may be in the middle of a task or even in the middle of a sentence when the attack occurs. Associated with the attack in 50 percent to 70 percent of the cases is cataplexy, a sudden loss of muscle tone, such as jaw drop, head drop, weakness of the knees, or paralysis of all skeletal muscles with collapse (Kaplan, Sadock, & Grebb, 1994). The episode is followed by full return of muscle strength. Individuals

with narcolepsy are at risk for injury to self or others if they participate in dangerous activities, such as driving an automobile or operating dangerous machinery.

The onset of narcolepsy occurs most frequently in late adolescence or early adulthood. Clinical history may reveal, however, that excessive sleepiness may have been present in childhood. The disorder is equally common in men and women.

Parasomnias. Parasomnias are unusual to undesirable behaviors that occur during sleep. Examples of parasomnias include nightmares, sleep terrors, and sleepwalking.

Nightmare Disorder. Nightmares are frightening dreams that lead to awakenings from sleep (APA, 1994). Nightmare disorder is diagnosed when there is a repeated occurrence of the frightening dreams, which interferes with social or occupational functioning.

Content of the nightmares usually relates to imminent physical danger to the individual, personal failure or embarrassment, or the replication of a traumatic experience. They occur during rapid-eye-movement (REM) sleep and can occur at any time during that sleep episode. The individual is usually fully alert upon awakening from the nightmare and, because of lingering fear or anxiety, may have difficulty returning to sleep.

Nightmares are not uncommon between the ages of 3 and 6 years, and most children outgrow the phenomenon. Many adults report an occasional nightmare, but the incidence of nightmare disorder is not known.

Sleep Terror Disorder. The manifestations of sleep terrors include abrupt arousal from sleep with a piercing scream or cry. The individual is difficult to awaken or comfort, and if wakefulness does occur, the individual is usually disoriented, expresses a sense of intense fear, but cannot recall the dream episode. Upon awakening in the morning, the individual has amnesia for the whole experience.

Sleep terrors are closely associated with sleepwalking, and often a night terror episode progresses into a sleepwalking episode (Kaplan, Sadock, & Grebb, 1994). Approximately 1 percent to 6 percent of children experience sleep terrors, the incidence appears to be more common in boys than in girls. Resolution usually occurs spontaneously during adolescence (APA, 1994). If the disorder begins in adulthood, it usually runs a chronic course.

Sleepwalking. The disorder of sleepwalking is characterized by the performance of motor activity initiated during sleep in which the individual may leave the bed and walk about, dress, go to the bathroom, talk, scream, or even drive (Kaplan, Sadock, & Grebb, 1994). Episodes may last from a few minutes to a half hour. Most often the person returns to bed and has no memory of the event upon awakening. Occasionally, the individual may awaken during the episode, experiencing several minutes of confusion and disorientation. Individuals with sleepwalking disorder are at risk of injuring themselves or others.

The incidence of sleepwalking disorder among children ranges from 1 percent to 5 percent. Onset most commonly occurs between ages 4 and 8 years and usually subsides spontaneously during adolescence. The disorder is equally common in boys and girls. Sleepwalking episodes can occur as isolated behaviors at any age.

Sleep-Wake Schedule Disturbances. Sleep-wake schedule disturbances can be described as a misalignment between sleep and wake behaviors (Kaplan, Sadock, & Grebb, 1994). The normal sleep-wake schedule is disrupted from its usual circadian rhythm. The individual is unable to sleep (or be awake) when he or she wants to sleep (or be awake), but can do so at other times. The *DSM-IV* calls this condition *circadian rhythm sleep disorder.* Sleep-wake schedule disturbances are common among shift workers and airplane travelers.

The disorder is common in shift workers who experience rapid and repeated changes in their work schedules. Many rotating-shift workers sleep fewer hours and have more disturbances in their sleep patterns than those shift workers who maintain a night or evening routine. Social and family demands, as well as environmental disturbances (e.g., telephone, traffic noise) during intended sleep times, also interfere with these individuals' ability to achieve adequate sleep (APA, 1994).

Airplane travel contributes to sleep-wake schedule disturbances when individuals travel through a number of time zones in a short period of time. This phenomenon is commonly called *jet lag*, which arises from conflict between the pattern of sleep and wakefulness generated by the circadian system and the pattern of sleep and wakefulness required by a new time zone (APA, 1994). Advancing the sleep-wake cycle (travel from west to east) appears to be more difficult for most people than delaying the sleep-wake cycle (travel from east to west).

Predisposing Factors to Sleep Disorders

Various factors have been shown to predispose individuals to sleep disorders. Genetic or familial patterns are thought to play a contributing role in primary insomnia, primary hypersomnia, narcolepsy, sleep terror disorder, and sleepwalking.

A number of medical conditions, as well as aging, have been implicated in the etiology of insomnia. They include pain; sleep apnea syndrome; restless leg syndrome; the use of, or withdrawal from, substances (including alcohol); endocrine or metabolic disorders; infectious, neoplastic, or other diseases; and CNS lesions (Kaplan, Sadock, & Grebb, 1994).

Medical conditions associated with hypersomnia include metabolic and encephalitic conditions, the use of alcohol or other CNS depressants, withdrawal from stimulants, sleep apneas, and hypoventilation syndromes (Kaplan, Sadock, & Grebb, 1994).

Psychiatric or environmental conditions that can contribute to insomnia or hypersomnia include anxiety, depression, environmental changes, circadian rhythm sleep disturbances, posttraumatic stress disorder, and schizophrenia (Kaplan, Sadock, & Grebb, 1994).

Night terrors may be related to minor neurological abnormalities, particularly in the temporal lobe. Onset of sleep terror episodes in adolescence or early adulthood often prove to be the initial symptoms of temporal lobe epilepsy (Kaplan, Sadock, & Grebb, 1994). The use of alcohol or other CNS depressants, sleep deprivation, sleep-wake disruptions, fatigue, and physical or emotional stress increase the incidence of episodes of night terrors (APA, 1994). Episodes of sleepwalking are exacerbated by extreme fatigue and sleep deprivation.

Activities that interfere with the 24-hour circadian rhythm of hormonal and neurotransmitter functioning within the body predispose individuals to sleep-wake schedule disturbances. See Chapter 4 for a more detailed explanation of the relationship between circadian rhythm and sleep.

Diagnosis/Outcome Identification

Nursing diagnoses are formulated from the data gathered during the assessment phase and with background knowledge regarding predisposing factors to the disorder. Common nursing diagnoses for clients with sleep disorders include:

Sleep pattern disturbance related to (specific medical condition); use of, or withdrawal from, substances; anxiety or depression; circadian rhythm disruption; familial patterns; evidenced by insomnia, hypersomnia, nightmares, sleep terrors, or sleepwalking.

Risk for injury related to excessive sleepiness, sleep terrors, or sleepwalking.

The following criteria may be used to measure outcomes in the care of the client with sleep disorders:

THE CLIENT:
1. Has not experienced injury.
2. Verbalizes understanding of the sleep disorder.
3. Demonstrates individually appropriate interventions that promote sleep.
4. Adjusts lifestyle to accommodate alteration in biological rhythms.
5. Demonstrates improvement in sleep patterns.
6. Reports increased sense of well-being and feeling rested.

Planning/Implementation

Table 28.11 provides a plan of care for the client with a sleep disorder. Nursing diagnoses are presented, along with outcome criteria, appropriate nursing interventions, and rationales.

TABLE 28.11   CARE PLAN FOR THE CLIENT WITH A SLEEP DISORDER

NURSING DIAGNOSIS: SLEEP PATTERN DISTURBANCE

RELATED TO: Use of, or withdrawal from, substances; anxiety or depression; circadian rhythm disruption; familial patterns; or specific medical condition

EVIDENCED BY: Insomnia, hypersomnia, nightmares, sleep terrors, or sleepwalking

OUTCOME CRITERIA	NURSING INTERVENTIONS	RATIONALE

Client will be able to achieve adequate, uninterrupted sleep.
Client will report feeling rested and demonstrate a sensation of well-being.
	1. To promote sleep:
	  a. Encourage activities that prepare one for sleep: soft music, relaxation exercises, warm bath.
	  b. Discourage strenuous exercise within 1 hr of bedtime.
	  c. Control intake of caffeine-containing substances within 4 hr of bedtime (e.g., coffee, tea, colas, chocolate, and certain analgesic medications).
	  d. Provide a high-carbohydrate snack before bedtime.
	
	  e. Keep the temperature of the room between 68° and 72°F.
	  f. Instruct the client not to use alcoholic beverages to relax.
	
	  g. Discourage smoking and use of other tobacco products near sleep time.
	  h. Discourage daytime napping. Increase program of activities to keep the person busy.
	  i. Individuals with chronic insomnia should use sleeping medications judiciously.
	
	2. To prevent "jet lag" circadian rhythm disruption:
	  a. If time permits, use a preventive strategy of altering mealtimes and sleep times in the appropriate direction.
	  b. If preventive measures are impossible, increase the amount of sleep upon arrival.
	  c. Provide short-term use of sleep medication by physician's order.
		a. These activities promote relaxation.
		
		b. Strenuous exercise can be stimulating and keep one awake.
		c. Caffeine is a CNS stimulant and can interfere with the promotion of sleep.
		
		d. Carbohydrates increase the levels of the amino acid tryptophan, a precursor to the neurotransmitter serotonin. Serotonin is thought to play a role in the promotion of sleep.
		e. This range provides the temperature most conducive to sleep.
		f. Although alcohol may initially induce drowsiness and promote falling asleep, a rebound stimulation occurs in the CNS within several hours after drinking alcohol. The individual may fall asleep, only to be wide awake a few hours later.
		g. Tobacco produces a stimulant effect on the CNS.
		
		h. Sleeping during the day can interfere with the ability to achieve sleep at night.
		i. Sedatives and hypnotics have serious side effects and are highly addicting. Life-threatening symptoms can occur with abrupt withdrawal and discontinuation should be tapered under a physician's supervision. Long-term use can result in rebound insomnia.
		
		a. This strategy will prepare the body for the oncoming change.
		
		b. This may help to reduce fatigue and restore the rested feeling.
		
		c. May provide restful sleep when other measures are unsuccessful.

NURSING DIAGNOSIS: RISK FOR INJURY

RELATED TO: Excessive sleepiness, sleep tremors, or sleepwalking

OUTCOME CRITERIA	NURSING INTERVENTIONS	RATIONALE
Client will not experience injury.	1. Ensure that siderails are up on the bed.	1. An individual who experiences serious nightmares or night terrors can fall from the bed during an episode.
	2. Keep the bed in a low position.	2. To diminish the risk of injury by the person who gets out of bed during a sleepwalking episode.
	3. Equip the bed with a bell (or other audible device) that is activated when the bed is exited.	3. This may alert the caretaker so that supervision to prevent accidental injury can be instituted.
	4. Keep a night light on and arrange the furniture in the bedroom in a manner that promotes safety.	4. To provide a safe environment for the individual who awakens (fully or partially) during the night.
	5. Administer drug therapy as ordered (see "Treatment Modalities"). For the child who experiences nightmares, encourage him or her to talk about the dream. Tell the child that all people have dreams. Validate his or her feeling of fearfulness while ensuring safety. Keep a light on in the room or give the child a flashlight.	5. Talking about the dream helps to promote the unreality of the dream and to differentiate between what is real and what is not real. Light gives the child a feeling of control over the darkness within the room.

Evaluation

Reassessment is conducted in order to determine if the nursing actions have been successful in achieving the objectives of care. Evaluation of the nursing actions for the client with a sleep disorder may be facilitated by gathering information using the following types of questions.

1. Is the client free from injury?
2. Have appropriate measures been taken to ensure that the environment has been made as risk-free from injury as possible?
3. Can the client verbalize knowledge about his or her sleep disorder and understand about possible causes?
4. Does the client demonstrate appropriate interventions that promote sleep? Can he or she verbalize activities and behaviors that may interfere with the promotion of sleep?
5. Does the pattern of sleep indicate improvement since the beginning of treatment?
6. Does the client report feeling rested and demonstrate a noticeable sense of well-being?

Table 28.12 presents topics for client/family education related to somatoform and sleep disorders.

TREATMENT MODALITIES

Somatoform Disorders

Clients with somatoform disorders are difficult to treat. The typical clinical picture of recurrent, multiple, vague symptoms combined with "doctor-shopping" and frequent requests for time and attention may generate frustration and anger in the physician. Many clients with these disorders ignore referrals to psychiatrists, and those who do follow through rarely persist with the treatment. Thus, the majority of care for these clients continues to rest with other physicians, even though studies show that psychiatric consultation can reduce both the extent and cost of medical care (Smith et al., 1986).

Individual Psychotherapy

The goal of psychotherapy is to help clients develop healthy and adaptive behaviors, encourage them to move beyond their somatization, and manage their lives more effectively (Barsky, 1989). The focus is on personal and social difficulties that the client is experiencing in daily life and the achievement of practical solutions for these difficulties.

Treatment is initiated with a complete physical examination to rule out organic pathology. Once this has been ensured, the physician turns his or her attention to the client's social and personal problems and away from the somatic complaints.

In the case of conversion disorder, the therapist will attempt to identify precipitating stressors and conflicts. He or she may be assisted in this effort by the use of hypnosis and narcoanalysis (amytal interview). These techniques

TABLE 28.12 TOPICS FOR CLIENT/FAMILY EDUCATION RELATED TO SOMATOFORM AND SLEEP DISORDERS

Nature of the Illness
1. Define and describe symptoms of
   a. Somatization disorder
   b. Pain disorder
   c. Hypochondriasis
   d. Conversion disorder
   e. Body dysmorphic disorder
   f. Primary insomnia or hypersomnia
   g. Parasomnias
   h. Sleep-wake schedule disturbances
2. Discuss etiologies of above disorders

Management of the Illness
1. Discuss ways to identify onset of escalating anxiety
2. Ways to intervene to prevent exacerbation of physical symptom
3. Assertive techniques
4. Relaxation techniques
5. Physical activities
6. Ways to increase feelings of control and decrease feelings of powerlessness
7. Pain management
8. Family: How to prevent reinforcing the illness
9. Ways to minimize sleep-wake circadian rhythm cycle
10. Activities to promote sleep
    a. Soft music
    b. Relaxation exercises
    c. Warm bath
    d. Control caffeine intake
    e. High carbohydrate snack before bedtime
    f. Control temperature of bedroom
    g. Discourage use of alcohol and tobacco
    h. Discourage daytime napping
11. Family with member who sleepwalks: Ways to prevent injury.
12. Pharmacology:
    a. For pain: aspirin, nonsteroidal antiinflammatory agents (NSAIDs), some antidepressants
    b. For insomnia: benzodiazepines, chloral hydrate, zolpidem
    c. For hypersomnia/narcolepsy: CNS stimulants, selective serotonin reuptake inhibitors (SSRIs)

Support Services
1. Support groups
2. Individual psychotherapy
3. Biofeedback
4. Behavior therapy

consist of placing the client in a relaxed state and, through questioning and suggestion, allowing him or her to reexperience the precipitating stress, fully reliving the repressed emotions, thereby freeing the client of the psychological need for the symptom (McCracken, 1985).

Psychotherapy appears to be useful with very few hypochondriacal clients. Treatment consists of a complete medical examination by the primary physician to rule out organic pathology. Because most people with hypochondriasis are opposed to psychiatric treatment, the best approach seems to be a supportive and accepting relationship with a general medical practitioner who tolerates the client's behavior without judgment and who is available during periods of distress and increased symptoms. This type of support can help to minimize incapacitating anxiety, "doctor-shopping," and further regression (McCracken, 1985).

Group Psychotherapy

Group therapy may be helpful for somatoform disorders because it provides a setting where clients can share their experiences of illness, learn to verbalize thoughts and feelings, and be confronted by group members and leaders when they reject responsibility for maladaptive behaviors (McCracken, 1985). It has been reported to be the treatment of choice for both somatization disorder and hypochondriasis, in part because it provides the social support and social interaction that these clients need (Barsky, 1989).

Behavior Therapy

Behavior therapy is more likely to be successful in instances when secondary gain is prominent. This may involve working with the client's family or other significant others who may be perpetuating the physical symptoms by rewarding passivity and dependency and by being overly solicitous and helpful (Barsky, 1989). Behavioral therapy focuses on teaching these individuals to reward the client's autonomy, self-sufficiency, and independence. This process becomes more difficult when the client is very regressed and the sick role well established.

Psychopharmacology

With somatoform pain disorder, the drugs of choice are aspirin and the nonsteroidal anti-inflammatory agents. They are most effective if used on a regularly scheduled basis rather than as needed. Opiates have a high addiction potential and should be reserved for clients suffering from pain that is clearly pathogenic (Barsky, 1989).

Some clinicians believe that antianxiety agents and antidepressants are helpful in these clients, when anxiety or depression is prominent. Careful monitoring of the use of antianxiety agents is important because of the high addiction potential.

Antidepressants are also used to treat chronic pain. Amitriptyline (Elavil), imipramine (Tofranil), doxepin (Sinequan), and phenelzine (Nardil) have been used, often providing pain relief at a dosage below that used to treat depression. The analgesic action of antidepressant medications is not known.

Anticonvulsants such as phenytoin (Dilantin), carbamazepine (Tegretol), and clonazepam (Klonopin) have been reported to be effective in treating neuropathic and neuralgic pain, at least for short periods. Their efficacy in other somatoform pain disorders is less clear.

Sleep Disorders

Primary Insomnia

Relaxation Therapy. Relaxation therapies can be helpful in the treatment of chronic insomnia. Hypnosis, meditation, deep breathing, and progressive muscle relaxation are effective. Success with these interventions requires a great deal of practice and motivation on the part of the client (McClusky, Milby, & Switzer, 1991).

Biofeedback. Biofeedback has been used with success in some clients (Neyland, Reynolds, & Kupfer, 1994). The use of a biological variable, such as electromyography or electroencephalography, helps these clients increase sensitivity to their internal state of arousal.

Drug Therapy. The efficacy of drug therapy in the treatment of insomnia cannot be disputed. When used judiciously, sedatives and hypnotics produce the calming effect needed for many individuals to achieve much needed sleep. These drugs are CNS depressants that, with long-term use, have the capacity for psychological and physiological dependence. The most commonly used group are the benzodiazepines. Some of those most frequently used include flurazepam (Dalmane), temazepam (Restoril), and triazolam (Halcion). Nonbenzodiazepines frequently used include chloral hydrate (Noctec) and zolpidem (Ambien). Common side effects of these medications include dizziness, confusion, impairment of cognitive and psychomotor skills, and nausea. Caution is required in using these drugs with elderly clients, as they have reduced clearance of hypnotics and hence experience more sedation and cognitive side effects than younger clients (Greenblatt, Harmatz, & Sharpiro, 1991). Gradual discontinuation and tapering of the dosage is required with all long-term users to diminish the risk of withdrawal symptoms and rebound insomnia.

Primary Hypersomnia/Narcolepsy

Drug Therapy. The usual treatment for hypersomnolence is with CNS stimulants such as amphetamines (Kaplan, Sadock, & Grebb, 1994). In some instances, the nonsedating serotonin-specific reuptake inhibitor antidepressants (fluoxetine, sertraline, and paroxetine) may be helpful with this problem.

Narcolepsy is also treated with CNS stimulants, such as amphetamine, methylphenidate, or pemoline. Tricyclic antidepressants have been effective in the treatment of symptoms of cataplexy.

Parasomnias

Treatment of parasomnias usually centers around measures to relieve obvious stress within the family. Individual or family therapy is sometimes useful. Interventions to prevent injury are required. In severe cases, pharmacological intervention may be instituted with tricyclic antidepressants or low-dose benzodiazepines.

Sleep-Wake Schedule Disturbances

Disturbances of the sleep-wake cycle are usually treated with behavior modification; that is, the individual trains himself or herself to adapt to the change in schedule. Phototherapy (also called "bright light" therapy) has been shown to be effective in treating delayed sleep-phase disorder and jet lag. Typically, individuals require 30 minutes to 2 hours of daily exposure to bright light to achieve a therapeutic response (Terman, 1989).

SUMMARY

Somatoform disorders, known historically as hysteria, affect about 1 or 2 percent of the female population. There is a higher prevalence rate among the lower socioeconomic groups and the less educated. Somatoform disorders include somatization disorder, pain disorder, hypochondriasis, conversion disorder, and body dysmorphic disorder.

TEST YOUR CRITICAL THINKING SKILLS

Ricky, age 11, was recently hospitalized on the psychiatric unit for evaluation. His parents stated to the nurse, "We are beside ourselves about what to do with him." They explained that Ricky has been sleepwalking almost nightly for the last 2 months. Before that, he had experienced an occasional episode (perhaps three per year at the most) beginning at about age 7. During sleepwalking, Ricky seldom awakens, and when he does, he appears confused and just returns to bed and sleep. In the morning he has no memory of the episode. Several times his parents have found him wandering around the front yard. They called the physician today after finding him riding his bicycle down the middle of the street in the middle of the night last night. Ricky says he cannot remember the incident. His parents are afraid for Ricky's safety.

Answer the following questions related to Ricky:

1. What is the *priority* nursing consideration when caring for Ricky?
2. Describe some nursing interventions that may be implemented for the consideration in question number 1.
3. What treatment might you expect the physician to prescribe for Ricky?

RESEARCH NOTE

A prospective 4- to 5-year study of DSM-III-R hypochondriasis. *Archives of General Psychiatry* (1998, August), 55, 737–744.
Barsky, A.J., Fama, J.M., Bailey, E.D., and Ahern, D.K.

Description of Study: This study consisted of a sample of 250 clients from a medical outpatient setting. One hundred twenty of the subjects met the *DSM-III-R* criteria for hypochondriasis, and the control group consisted of 133 nonhypochondriacal clients. Both groups completed an extensive research battery assessing hypochondriacal symptoms, medical and psychiatric comorbidity, functional status and role impairment, and medical care. Four to five years later, 74 percent of the subjects underwent reassessment.

Results of the Study: Average scores for hypochondriacal symptoms and functional status improved significantly for the study group at follow-up, while control group scores showed minimal change. However, 64 percent of the study group still met the *DSM-III-R* criteria for hypochondriasis. Interestingly, 3 percent of the control group also met the criteria at the 5-year reassessment. Changes in medical and psychiatric comorbidity did not differ between the two groups.

Comments: The authors concluded that, although hypochondriacal symptoms improved on average over 5 years, a majority of clients continued to meet the standard diagnostic criteria. They noted that many who showed improvement described positive changes that had occurred in their lives, and some had replaced traditional medical treatment with "alternative" strategies, such as acupuncture, yoga, and massage. The authors do suggest that the high percentage of clients who continued to meet the *DSM-III-R* criteria at follow-up may indicate that hypochondriasis carries with it a substantial, long-term burden of morbidity, functional impairment, and personal distress.

The person with somatization disorder has physical symptoms that may be vague, dramatized, or exaggerated in their presentation. No evidence of organic pathology can be identified. In pain disorder, the predominant symptom is pain, for which there is either no medical explanation or for which the symptom is exaggerated out of proportion to what would be the expected reaction. Psychological factors can be identified as contributing to the symptom. Individuals with these disorders commonly have long histories of "doctor shopping" in search of validation of their symptoms.

Hypochondriasis is an unrealistic preoccupation with fear of having a serious illness. This disorder may follow a personal experience, or the experience of a close family member, with serious or life-threatening illness.

The individual with conversion disorder experiences a loss of or alteration in bodily functioning, unsubstantiated by medical or pathophysiological explanation. Psychological factors are evident by the primary or secondary gains the individual achieves from experiencing the physiological manifestation. A relative lack of con-

INTERNET REFERENCES

- Additional information about somatoform disorders may be located at the following websites:
  a. http://www.psyweb.com/Mdisord.somatd.html
  b. http://www.delmarnursing.com/frisch/web2.html#psychosomatic
  c. http://www.mc.vanderbilt.edu/peds/pidl/adolesc/convreac.htm
  d. http://www.emedicine.com/EMERG/topic112.Htm
  e. http://www.lifewell.com/educenter/294.cfm
  f. http://www.yahoo.com/Health/Mental_Health/Diseases_and_Conditions/Hypochondria/

cern regarding the symptom is identified as "la belle indifference."

Body dysmorphic disorder, formerly called dysmorphophobia, is the exaggerated belief that the body is deformed or defective in some way. It may be related to more serious psychiatric illness.

RESEARCH NOTE

Association of physical activity and human sleep disorders. *Archives of Internal Medicine* (1998, September 28), 158, 1894–1898.
Sherrill, D.L., Kotochou, K., and Quan, S.F.

Description of the Study: This was a study of 319 men and 403 women who were taking part in the Tucson epidemiological study of obstructive airways disease. Part of the study included completing health questionnaires related to physical exercises and sleep disorders. Sleep disorders were classified as disorders in maintaining sleep, excessive daily sleepiness, nightmares, and any other symptoms indicative of sleep disorders.

Results of the Study: More women than men reported participating in a regular program of exercise, while more men than women reported participating in vigorous activity and walking at a brisk pace for more than 6 blocks per day. More women than men reported having symptoms of sleep disorders in maintaining sleep and nightmares. A significantly reduced risk of disorders in maintaining sleep, as well as symptoms of any sleep disorder, was positively correlated with a regular exercise program for both men and women, and walking at a brisk pace for more than 6 blocks for men. A risk for nightmares was inversely related to age in women.

Comments: The authors suggest that most studies related to this topic have correlated the benefits of physical exercise on the efficiency of sleep. They conclude that the data from this study provide evidence that a program of regular exercise may be a useful therapeutic modality for clients with sleep disorders.

INTERNET REFERENCES

- Additional information about sleep disorders may be located at the following websites:
  a. http://www.sleepnet.com/disorder.htm
  b. http://sleepcpmc.groupwork.com/
  c. http://www.asda.org/
  d. http://www.sleepmedservices.com/
  e. http://sleepdisorderscenter.com/
- Information about medications for sleep disorders may be located at the following websites:
  a. http://www.rxmed.com/prescribe.html
  b. http://www.mentalhealth.com/drug/

Sleep disorders include primary insomnia, primary hypersomnia, parasomnias, and sleep-wake schedule disturbances. Clients with primary insomnia have difficulty initiating or maintaining sleep. Primary hypersomnia manifests as excessive amounts of sleep and excessive daytime sleepiness.

Parasomnias include nightmare disorder, sleep terror disorder, and sleepwalking. These disorders primarily begin in childhood but can also affect adults.

Sleep-wake schedule disturbances occur when there is a disruption in an individual's regular pattern of fluctuation in physiology that is linked to the 24-hour light-dark cycle. This commonly occurs in individuals whose jobs require rotating shifts and in those who frequently travel long distances over a short period of time (commonly called "jet lag").

Various modalities have been implemented in the treatment of somatoform and sleep disorders, including individual psychotherapy, group psychotherapy, behavior therapy, and psychopharmacology. Nursing care is accomplished using the steps of the nursing process. Nurses can assist clients with these disorders by helping them to understand their problem and identify and establish new, more adaptive behavior patterns.

REVIEW QUESTIONS

SELF-EXAMINATION/LEARNING EXERCISE

For each situation select the answer that is most appropriate for the questions that follow.

Situation: Amy, age 24, was selected to represent the local children's home in the upcoming 26-mile marathon. If she wins, the children's home gets the new playground equipment they want so badly. If she loses, they will have to wait until another financial source can be located. Amy wants desperately to win for them. The morning of the race, she falls when she tries to get out of bed. She discovers her right leg is paralyzed.

1. Amy's mother takes her to the emergency department. Her physician is notified. It is likely that his initial intervention will be to:
   a. Prescribe an antianxiety medication.
   b. Rule out organic pathology.
   c. Refer her to the rehabilitation clinic.
   d. Refer her to a psychiatrist.

2. Amy shows a relative lack of concern for her sudden paralysis, even though her athletic abilities have always been a source of pride to her. This manifestation is known as:
   a. Tardive dyskinesia.
   b. Secondary gain.
   c. Malingering.
   d. "La belle indifference."

3. Amy is admitted to the psychiatric unit with a diagnosis of conversion disorder. The primary nursing diagnosis for Amy would be:
   a. Self-care deficit related to inability to walk without assistance.
   b. Severe anxiety related to fear of losing the race.
   c. Ineffective individual coping related to severe anxiety.
   d. Fear related to lack of confidence in her athletic ability.

4. Which of the following nursing interventions would be most appropriate for Amy?
   a. Promote Amy's dependence, so that unfulfilled dependency needs can be met.
   b. Encourage her to discuss her feelings about the paralysis.
   c. Explain to her that the paralysis is not "real."
   d. Promote independence and withdraw attention when she continues to focus on the paralysis.

5. Conversion symptoms provide primary and secondary gains for the individuals experiencing them. Which of the following is an example of a primary gain for Amy?
   a. Allows her to receive additional personal attention.
   b. Allows her to be totally dependent on others.
   c. Allows her an acceptable excuse for not running in the race.
   d. Allows her to feel more accepted and cared for by others.

Situation: Lorraine is a frequent visitor to the outpatient clinic. She has been diagnosed with somatization disorder.

6. Which of the following symptom profiles would you expect when assessing Lorraine?
   a. Multiple somatic symptoms in several body systems.
   b. Fear of having a serious disease.
   c. Loss or alteration in sensorimotor functioning.
   d. Belief that the body is deformed or defective in some way.

7. Which of the following ego defense mechanisms describes the underlying dynamics of somatization disorder?

   a. Denial of depression.
   b. Repression of anxiety.
   c. Suppression of grief.
   d. Displacement of anger.

8. Nursing care for Lorraine would focus on helping her to:

   a. Eliminate the stress in her life.
   b. Discontinue her numerous physical complaints.
   c. Take her medication only as prescribed.
   d. Learn more adaptive coping strategies.

9. Lorraine states, "My doctor thinks I should see a psychiatrist. I can't imagine why he would make such a suggestion!" What is the basis for Lorraine's statement?

   a. She thinks her doctor wants to get rid of her as a client.
   b. She does not understand the correlation of symptoms and stress.
   c. She thinks psychiatrists are only for "crazy" people.
   d. She thinks her doctor has made an error in diagnosis.

10. Lorraine tells the nurse about a pain in her side. She says she has not experienced it before. Which is the most appropriate response by the nurse?

   a. "I don't want to hear about another physical complaint. You know they are all in your head. It's time for group therapy now."
   b. "Let's sit down here together and you can tell me about this new pain you are experiencing. You'll just have to miss group therapy today."
   c. "I will report this pain to your physician. In the meantime, group therapy starts in 5 minutes. You must leave now to be on time."
   d. "I will call your physician and see if he will order a new pain medication for your side. The one you have now doesn't seem to provide relief. Why don't you get some rest for now?"

REFERENCES

American Psychiatric Association. (1994). *Diagnostic and statistical manual of mental disorders* (4th ed.). Washington, DC: American Psychiatric Association.

American Sleep Disorders Association. (1990). *International classification of sleep disorders: Diagnostic and coding manual.* Rochester, MN: American Sleep Disorders Association.

Barsky, A.J. (1979). Patients who amplify bodily sensations. *Annals of Internal Medicine, 91,* 63–70.

Barsky, A.J. (1989). Somatoform disorders. In H.I. Kaplan & B.J. Sadock (Eds.), *Comprehensive textbook of psychiatry* (Vol. 1) (5th ed.). Baltimore: Williams & Wilkins.

Barsky, A.J., & Klerman, G.L. (1983). Overview: Hypochondriasis, bodily complaints, and somatic styles. *American Journal of Psychiatry, 140,* 273–283.

Chapman, C.R. (1978). Pain: The perception of noxious events. In R.A. Sternbach (Ed.), *The psychology of pain.* New York: Raven Press.

Cloniger, C.R. (1994). Somatoform and dissociative disorders. In G. Winokur & P.J. Clayton (Eds.), *The medical basis of psychiatry* (2nd ed.). Philadelphia: W.B. Saunders.

Engel, G.E. (1959). Psychogenic pain and the pain-prone patient. *American Journal of Medicine, 16,* 899–918.

Ford, C.V., & Folks, D.G. (1985). Conversion disorders: An overview. *Psychosomatics, 26,* 371–383.

Goodwin, D.W., & Guze, S.B. (1989). *Psychiatric diagnosis* (4th ed.). New York: Oxford University Press.

Greenblatt, D.J., Harmatz, J.S., & Shapiro, L. (1991). Sensitivity to triazolam in the elderly. *New England Journal of Medicine, 324,* 1691–1698.

Jones, M.M. (1980). Conversion reaction: Anachronism or evolutionary form? A review of the neurologic, behavioral, and psychoanalytic literature. *Psychology Bulletin, 87,* 427–441.

Kaplan, H.I., & Sadock, B.J. (1998). *Synopsis of psychiatry: Behavioral sciences/clinical psychiatry* (8th ed.). Baltimore: Williams & Wilkins.

Kaplan, H.I., Sadock, B.J., & Grebb, J.A.: (1994). *Kaplan and Sadock's synopsis of psychiatry* (7th ed.). Baltimore: Williams & Wilkins.

Kenyon, F.E. (1976). Hypochondriacal states. *British Journal of Psychiatry, 129,* 1–14.

Kleinman, A., & Mechanic, D. (1980). Mental illness and psychosocial aspects of medical problems in China. In Kleinman et al. (Eds.), *Normal and abnormal behavior in Chinese culture.* Boston: Reidel Publishing.

Leff, J. (1973). Culture and the differentiation of emotional states. *British Journal of Psychiatry, 123,* 299–306.

Ludwig, A.M. (1972). Hysteria: A neurobiological theory. *Archives of General Psychiatry, 27,* 771–777.

Martin, R.L., & Yutzy, S.H. (1994). Somatoform disorders. In R.E. Hales, S.C. Yudofsky, & J.A. Talbott (Eds.), *The American Psychiatric Press textbook of psychiatry* (2nd ed.). Washington, DC: American Psychiatric Press.

McClusky, H.Y., Milby, J.B., & Switzer, P.K. (1991). Efficacy of behavioral versus triazolam treatment in persistent sleep-onset insomnia. *American Journal of Psychiatry, 148,* 121–126.

McCracken, J.T. (1985). Somatoform disorders. In J.I. Walker (Ed.), *Essentials of clinical psychiatry.* Philadelphia: J.B. Lippincott.

Mechanic, D. (1972). Social psychological factors affecting the presentation of bodily complaints. *New England Journal of Medicine, 286,* 1132–1139.

Minuchin, S., et al. (1975). Family organization and family therapy. *Archives of General Psychiatry, 32,* 1031–1038.

Neyland, T.C., Reynolds, C.F., & Kupfer, D.J. (1994). Sleep disorders. In R.E. Hales, S.C. Yudofsky, & J.A. Talbott (Eds.). *Textbook of psychiatry* (2nd ed.). Washington, DC: American Psychiatric Press.

Purcell, S.D. (1988). Somatoform disorders. In H.H. Goldman (Ed.), *Review of general psychiatry* (2nd ed.). Norwalk, CT: Appleton & Lange.

Smith, G.R., et al. (1986). Psychiatric consultation in somatization disorder: A randomized controlled study. *New England Journal of Medicine, 314*, 1407–1413.

Stoudemire, G.A. (1988). Somatoform disorders, factitious disorders, and malingering. In J.A. Talbott, R.E. Hales, & S.C. Yudofsky (Eds.), *Textbook of psychiatry*. Washington, DC: American Psychiatric Press.

Terman, J. (1989). Light therapy. In M.H. Kryger, T. Roth, & W.C. Dement (Eds.), *Principles and practices of sleep medicine*. Philadelphia: W.B. Saunders.

Bibliography

Barbee, J.G., et al. (1997, September). Explained and unexplained medical symptoms in generalized anxiety and panic disorder: Relationship to the somatoform disorders. *Annals of Clinical Psychiatry, 9*, 149–155.

Fritz, G.K., Fritsch, S., and Hagino, O. (1997, October). Somatoform disorders in children and adolescents: A review of the past 10 years. *Journal of the American Academy of Child and Adolescent Psychiatry, 36*, 1329–1338.

Hiller, W., Janca, A., & Burke, K.C. (1997, December). Association between tinnitus and somatoform disorders. *Journal of Psychosomatic Research 43*, 613–624.

Hiller, W., Rief, W., & Fichter M.M. (1997, November). How disabled are patients with somatoform disorders? *General Hospital Psychiatry, 19*, 432–438.

Kroenke, K., Spitzer, R.L., deGruy, F.V., & Swindle, R. (1998, May–June). A symptom checklist to screen for somatoform disorders in primary care. *Pychosomatics, 39*, 263–272.

Rogers, M.P., et al. (1996, January–February). Prevalence of somatoform disorders in a large sample of patients with anxiety disorders. *Psychosomatics, 37*, 17–22.

Singh, B.S. (1998, June 1). Managing somatoform disorders. *Medical Journal of Australia, 168*, 572–577.

Townsend, M.C. (1995). *Drug guide for psychiatric nursing* (2nd ed.). Philadelphia: F.A. Davis.

Townsend, M.C. (1997). *Nursing diagnoses in psychiatric nursing: A pocket guide for care plan construction* (4th ed.). Philadelphia: F.A. Davis.

Yamadera, H., Takahashi, K., & Okawa, M. (1996, August). A multicenter study of sleep-wake rhythm disorders: Clinical features of sleep-wake rhythm disorders. *Psychiatry and Clinical Neurosciences, 50*, 195–201.

DISSOCIATIVE DISORDERS

CHAPTER OUTLINE

OBJECTIVES

INTRODUCTION

HISTORICAL ASPECTS

EPIDEMIOLOGICAL STATISTICS

APPLICATION OF THE NURSING PROCESS

TREATMENT MODALITIES

SUMMARY

REVIEW QUESTIONS

KEY TERMS

amnesia
fugue
depersonalization

integration
derealization
free association

directed association
hypnosis
abreaction

OBJECTIVES

After reading this chapter, the student will be able to:

1. Discuss historical aspects and epidemiological statistics related to dissociative disorders.
2. Describe various types of dissociative disorders and identify symptomatology associated with each; use this information in client assessment.
3. Identify predisposing factors in the development of dissociative disorders.
4. Formulate nursing diagnoses and goals of care for clients with dissociative disorders.
5. Describe appropriate nursing interventions for clients with dissociative disorders.
6. Identify topics for client and family teaching relevant to dissociative disorders.
7. Evaluate nursing care of clients with dissociative disorders.
8. Discuss various modalities relevant to treatment of dissociative disorders.

he *DSM-IV* describes the essential feature of dissociative disorders as a disruption in the usually integrated functions of consciousness, memory, identity, or perception of the environment (American Psychiatric Association [APA], 1994). Dissociative responses occur when anxiety becomes overwhelming and the personality becomes disorganized. Defense mechanisms that normally govern consciousness, identity, and memory break down, and behavior occurs with little or no participation on the part of the conscious personality (Kolb & Brodie, 1982). Four types of dissociative disorders are described by the *DSM-IV*: dissociative **amnesia**, dissociative **fugue**, dissociative identity disorder, and **depersonalization** disorder.

This chapter focuses on disorders characterized by severe anxiety that has been repressed and is being expressed in the form of dissociative behavior. In these clients, certain mental contents are removed from consciousness to protect the ego from experiencing the painful anxiety. Historical and epidemiological statistics are presented. Predisposing factors that have been implicated in the etiology of dissociative disorders provide a framework for studying the dynamics of dissociative amnesia, dissociative fugue, dissociative identity disorder, and depersonalization disorder.

An explanation of the symptomatology is presented as background knowledge for assessing the client with a dissociative disorder. Nursing care is described in the context of the nursing process. Various medical treatment modalities are explored.

HISTORICAL ASPECTS

There was a great deal of interest in the phenomena of dissociative processes during the 19th century, when the concept of dissociation was first formulated by the French physician and psychologist, Pierre Janet. He used it to explain the myriad bizarre symptoms of hysteria, which he characterized as "a form of mental disintegration characterized by a tendency toward the permanent and complete undoubling of consciousness" (Janet, 1907).

Freud (1962) viewed dissociation as a type of repression, an active defense mechanism used to remove threatening or unacceptable mental contents from conscious awareness. He also described the defense of splitting of the ego in the management of incompatible mental contents.

Professional interest in the dissociative disorders waned after the turn of the century but has recently been revived, with the study of dissociative identity disorder in particular achieving a level surpassing such study in all previous periods. Despite the fact that Janet pioneered the study of dissociative processes in the 1890s, scientists still know remarkably little about the phenomena. Are dissociative disorders psychopathological processes or ego-

protective devices? Are dissociative processes under voluntary control, or are they a totally unconscious effort? The wide scope of current studies concerning the dissociative syndromes promises to lead to a more accurate picture of their scope, etiology, and underlying mechanisms.

EPIDEMIOLOGICAL STATISTICS

Dissociative syndromes are statistically quite rare, but when they do occur they may present very dramatic clinical pictures of severe disturbances in normal personality functioning (Purcell, 1988). Dissociative amnesia is relatively rare, occurring most frequently under conditions of war or during natural disasters. However, in recent years, there has been an increase in the number of reported cases, possibly attributed to increased awareness of the phenomenon, and identification of cases that were previously undiagnosed (APA, 1994). It appears to be more common in women than in men and in young adults than in older adults (Kaplan & Sadock, 1998). Dissociative amnesia can occur at any age, but it is difficult to diagnose in children because it is easily confused with inattention or oppositional behavior.

Dissociative fugue is also rare and occurs most often under conditions of war, natural disasters, or intense psychosocial stress. Information regarding gender distribution and familial patterns of occurrence is not available.

Estimates of the prevalence of dissociative identity disorder (DID) vary widely. Kaplan and Sadock (1998) report that perhaps as many as 5 percent of all patients with psychiatric disorders meet the criteria for DID. The disorder occurs from three to nine times more frequently in women than in men, and onset likely occurs in childhood, although manifestations of the disorder may not be recognized until much later (APA, 1994). Clinical symptoms usually are not recognized until late adolescence or early adulthood, although they have probably existed for a number of years prior to diagnosis (Kaplan & Sadock, 1998). There appears to be some evidence that the disorder is more common in first-degree biological relatives of people with the disorder than in the general population.

The prevalence of severe episodes of depersonalization disorder is unknown, although single brief episodes of depersonalization may occur at some time in as many as half of all adults, particularly in the event of severe psychosocial stress (APA, 1994). Symptoms usually begin in adolescence or early adulthood. The disorder is chronic, with periods of remission and exacerbation. The incidence of depersonalization disorder is high under conditions of sustained traumatization, such as in military combat or prisoner-of-war camps. It has also been reported in many individuals who endure near-death experiences (Kluft, 1988).

APPLICATION OF THE NURSING PROCESS

Dissociative Amnesia

Background Assessment Data

Dissociative amnesia is an inability to recall important personal information, usually of a traumatic or stressful nature, that is too extensive to be explained by ordinary forgetfulness and is not due to the direct effects of substance use or a general medical condition (APA, 1994). Five types of disturbance in recall have been described. In the following examples, the individual is involved in a traumatic automobile accident in which a loved one is killed.

1. **Localized Amnesia.** The inability to recall all incidents associated with the traumatic event for a specific time period following the event (usually a few hours to a few days).

EXAMPLE:

The individual cannot recall events of the automobile accident and events occurring during a period after the accident (a few hours to a few days).

2. **Selective Amnesia.** The inability to recall only certain incidents associated with a traumatic event for a specific period after the event.

EXAMPLE:

The individual may not remember events leading to the impact of the accident but may remember being taken away in the ambulance.

3. **Generalized Amnesia.** The rare phenomenon of not being able to recall anything that has happened during the individual's entire lifetime, including his or her personal identity.

4. **Continuous Amnesia.** The inability to recall events occurring after a specific time up to and including the present.

EXAMPLE:

The individual cannot remember events associated with the automobile accident and anything that has occurred since. That is, the individual cannot form new memories, even though apparently alert and aware (Purcell, 1988).

5. **Systematized Amnesia.** With this type of amnesia, the individual cannot remember events that relate to a specific category of information, such as one's family, or to one particular person or event.

The individual with amnesia usually appears alert and may give no indication to observers that anything is wrong, although at the onset of the episode there may be a brief period of disorganization or clouding of consciousness (Kaplan & Sadock, 1998). Clients suffering from amnesia are often brought to general hospital emergency departments by police who have found them wandering confusedly around the streets (Nemiah, 1989).

Onset of an amnestic episode usually follows severe psychosocial stress. Termination is typically abrupt and followed by complete recovery. Recurrences are unusual. *DSM-IV* diagnostic criteria for dissociative amnesia are presented in Table 29.1.

Predisposing Factors to Dissociative Amnesia

Psychodynamic Theory. Freud (1962) described amnesia as the result of repression of distressing mental contents from conscious awareness. He believed the unconscious was a dynamic entity in which repressed mental contents were stored and unavailable to conscious recall. Current psychodynamic explanations of dissociation are based on Freud's concepts. The repression of mental contents is perceived as a mechanism for protecting the client from emotional pain that has arisen either from disturbing external circumstances or from anxiety-provoking internal sources (Nemiah, 1989).

Behavioral Theory. Dissociative amnesia may also be explained by potential gains derived from the response. Reinforcement, in the form of primary and secondary gains for the individual, may contribute to the maladaptive

---

TABLE 29.1   DIAGNOSTIC CRITERIA FOR DISSOCIATIVE AMNESIA

A. The predominant disturbance is one or more episodes of inability to recall important personal information, usually of a traumatic or stressful nature, that is too extensive to be explained by ordinary forgetfulness.

B. The disturbance does not occur exclusively during the course of dissociative identity disorder, dissociative fugue, posttraumatic stress disorder, acute stress disorder, or somatization disorder and is not due to the direct physiological effect of a substance (e.g., a drug of abuse, a medication) or a neurological or other general medical condition (e.g., amnestic disorder due to head trauma).

C. The symptoms cause clinically significant distress or impairment in social, occupational, or other important areas of functioning.

SOURCE: From APA (1994), with permission.

functioning associated with this disorder. Primary gain from the amnesia would be protection from a painful emotional experience. Secondary gains may be derived from the gratifying responses of others that fulfill certain psychological needs and thus serve to maintain the amnesia after it is established (Purcell, 1988).

Biological Theory. Some efforts have been made to explain dissociative amnesia on the basis of neurophysiological dysfunction, particularly in the ascending reticular activating system, thalamocortical projections, and other neurological pathways (Nemiah, 1989).

Cloninger (1994) cites studies from which he reports the following:

> "Dissociative reactions may be precipitated by excessive cortical arousal, which in turn triggers reactive inhibition of signals at synapses in sensorimotor pathways by way of negative feedback relationships between the cerebral cortex and the brainstem reticualr formation." (p. 182)

Transactional Model of Stress/Adaptation. The etiology of dissociative amnesia is most likely influenced by multiple factors. In Figure 29.1 a graphic depiction of

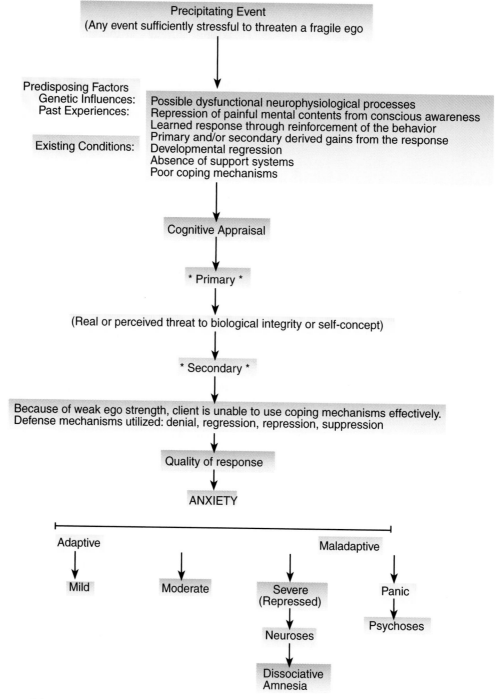

Figure 29.1 The dynamics of dissociative amnesia using the transactional model of stress/adaptation.

this theory of multiple causation is presented in the transactional model of stress/adaptation.

Diagnosis/Outcome Identification

Nursing diagnoses are formulated from the data gathered during the assessment phase and with background knowledge regarding predisposing factors to the disorder. The following nursing diagnoses may be used for the client with dissociative amnesia:

Altered thought processes related to severe psychological stress and repression of anxiety, evidenced by loss of memory.

Powerlessness related to inability to cope effectively with severe anxiety, evidenced by verbalizations of frustration over lack of control and dependence on others.

The following criteria may be used for measurement of outcomes in the care of the client with dissociative amnesia:

THE CLIENT:

1. Can recall events associated with a traumatic or stressful situation.
2. Can recall all events of past life.
3. Can demonstrate more adaptive coping strategies to avert amnestic behaviors in the face of severe anxiety.
4. Verbalizes control over certain life situations.
5. Verbalizes acceptance of certain life situations over which he or she has no control.
6. Sets realistic goals and expresses a sense of control over outcomes for the future.

Planning/Implementation

Table 29.2 provides a plan of care for the client with dissociative amnesia. Nursing diagnoses are presented, along with outcome criteria, appropriate nursing interventions, and rationales.

Evaluation

Reassessment is conducted to determine if the nursing actions have been successful in achieving the objectives of care. Evaluation of the nursing actions for the client with dissociative amnesia may be facilitated by gathering information using the following types of questions:

1. Has the client's memory been restored?
2. Can the client connect occurrence of psychological stress to loss of memory?
3. Can the client verbalize more adaptive methods of coping with stress?
4. Can the client demonstrate use of these more adaptive coping strategies?
5. Can the client carry out activities of daily living independently?
6. Can the client identify aspects of life situation over which control can be achieved?

7. Does he or she verbalize acceptance of aspects of life situation over which control is not possible?
8. Does the client set realistic goals for the future?
9. Does he or she express positive outcomes for the future?
10. Can the client verbalize the names of support groups of which he or she may become a member in an effort to deal successfully with stressful life situations?
11. Does he or she express an intention to become affiliated with one of these self-help groups?

Dissociative Fugue

Background Assessment Data

The characteristic feature of dissociative fugue is sudden, unexpected travel away from home or customary place of daily activities, with inability to recall some or all of one's past (APA, 1994). An individual in a fugue state cannot recall personal identity and often assumes a new identity. Nemiah (1989) states:

"During the fugue they completely forget their past lives and associations. But unlike the clients with amnesia, they are unaware that they have forgotten anything. It is only when they suddenly come back to their former selves that they recall the time preceding the onset of the fugue, but now they are amnesic for the period covered by the fugue itself."

Individuals in a fugue state do not appear to be behaving in any way out of the ordinary. Contacts with other people are minimal. The assumed identity may be simple and incomplete or complex and elaborate. If a complex identity is established, the individual engages in intricate interpersonal and occupational activities and is often more socially gregarious and uninhibited than was his or her previous style (Purcell, 1988).

Clients with dissociative fugue often are picked up by the police when they are found wandering in a somewhat confused and frightened condition after emerging from the fugue in unfamiliar surroundings. They are usually presented to emergency departments of general hospitals. Upon assessment, they are able to provide details of their earlier life situation but have no recall from the beginning of the fugue state. Information from other sources usually reveals that the occurrence of severe psychological stress or excessive alcohol use precipitated the fugue behavior.

Duration is usually brief—that is, hours to days or, more rarely, months—and recovery is rapid and complete. Recurrences are not common. *DSM-IV* diagnostic criteria for dissociative fugue are presented in Table 29.3.

Predisposing Factors to Dissociative Fugue

The theoretical models described as predisposing factors to dissociative amnesia also have relevance for dissociative fugue. Psychodynamic features, behavioral aspects, and possible biological factors have etiological

TABLE 29.2 CARE PLAN FOR THE CLIENT WITH DISSOCIATIVE AMNESIA

NURSING DIAGNOSIS: ALTERED THOUGHT PROCESSES
RELATED TO: Severe psychological stress and repression of anxiety
EVIDENCED BY: Loss of memory

OUTCOME CRITERIA	NURSING INTERVENTIONS	RATIONALE
Client will recover deficits in memory and develop more adaptive coping mechanisms to deal with stress.	1. Obtain as much information as possible about the client from family and significant others if possible. Consider likes, dislikes, important people, activities, music, pets. 2. Do not flood client with data regarding his or her past life. 3. Instead, expose client to stimuli that represent pleasant experiences from the past such as smells associated with enjoyable activities, beloved pets, and music known to have been pleasurable to the client. As memory begins to return, engage client in activities that may provide additional stimulation. 4. Encourage client to discuss situations that have been especially stressful and to explore the feelings associated with those times. 5. Identify specific conflicts that remain unresolved, and assist client to identify possible solutions. Provide instruction regarding more adaptive ways to respond to anxiety.	1. A comprehensive baseline assessment is important for the development of an effective plan of care. 2. Individuals who are exposed to painful information from which the amnesia is providing protection may decompensate even further into a psychotic state. 3. Recall may occur during activities that simulate life experiences. 4. Verbalization of feelings in a non-threatening environment may help client come to terms with unresolved issues that may be contributing to the dissociative process. 5. Unless these underlying conflicts are resolved, any improvement in coping behaviors must be viewed as only temporary.

NURSING DIAGNOSIS: POWERLESSNESS
RELATED TO: Inability to cope effectively with severe anxiety
EVIDENCED BY: Verbalizations of frustration over lack of control and dependence on others

OUTCOME CRITERIA	NURSING INTERVENTIONS	RATIONALE
Client will be able to effectively problem solve ways to take control of life situation.	1. Allow client to take as much responsibility as possible for own self-care practices. 2. Provide positive feedback for decisions made. Respect client's right to make those decisions independently, and refrain from attempting to influence him or her toward those that may seem more logical. 3. Assist client to set realistic goals for the future. 4. Help client identify areas of life situation that he or she can control.	1. Providing client with choices will increase feelings of control. 2. Positive feedback encourages repetition of desirable behaviors. 3. Unrealistic goals set client up for failure and reinforce feelings of powerlessness. 4. Client's memory deficits may interfere with his or her ability to solve problems. Assistance is required to perceive the benefits and consequences of available alternatives accurately.

5. Help client identify areas of life situation that are not within his or her ability to control. Encourage verbalization of feelings related to this inability.
6. Identify ways in which client can achieve. Encourage participation in these activities, and provide positive reinforcement for participation, as well as for achievement.
7. Encourage client's participation in supportive self-help groups.

5. Client learns to deal with unresolved issues and accept what cannot be changed.

6. Positive reinforcement enhances self-esteem and encourages repetition of desirable behaviors.

7. In support groups, client can learn ways to achieve greater control over life situation through direct feedback and by hearing about the experiences of others.

---

implications for both disorders. In addition, dysfunctional family dynamics may be implicated in the predisposition to dissociative fugue. The theory of family dynamics is described here. Other theoretical models may be reviewed under the section on dissociative amnesia.

Theory of Family Dynamics. In the theory of family dynamics, fugue is thought to be related to a person's search for a lost parent (Berger, 1985). The unsatisfactory parent-child relationship, with subsequent internalization of loss, results in episodes of depression and suicidal ideation, common in clients who experience fugues. Unfulfilled separation anxiety, a defect in personality development, and unmet dependency needs are other associated features of dissociative fugue that are related to dysfunctional family dynamics.

Transactional Model of Stress/Adaptation. The etiology of dissociative fugue is most likely influenced by multiple factors. In Figure 29.2, a graphic depiction of this theory of multiple causation is presented in the transactional model of stress/adaptation.

Diagnosis/Outcome Identification

Nursing diagnoses are formulated from the data gathered during the assessment phase and with background knowledge regarding predisposing factors to the disorder. Some common nursing diagnoses for clients with dissociative fugue include:

Risk for violence directed toward others related to fear of unknown circumstances surrounding emergence from fugue state.

Ineffective individual coping related to dysfunctional family system and repressed severe anxiety, evidenced by sudden travel away from home with inability to recall previous identity.

The following criteria may be used for measurement of outcomes in the care of the client with dissociative fugue:

THE CLIENT:

1. Has not harmed self or others.
2. Can maintain anxiety at a level at which he or she feels no need for aggression.
3. Can discuss fears and anxieties with staff.
4. Can verbalize the extreme anxiety that precipitated the fugue state.
5. Can demonstrate more adaptive coping strategies in the face of extreme anxiety.
6. Can verbalize resources from whom he or she may seek assistance in times of extreme anxiety.

Planning/Implementation

Table 29.4 provides a plan of care for the client with dissociative fugue. Nursing diagnosis are presented, along with outcome criteria, appropriate nursing interventions, and rationales.

▄▄ TABLE 29.3 DIAGNOSTIC CRITERIA FOR DISSOCIATIVE FUGUE

A. The predominant disturbance is sudden, unexpected travel away from home or one's customary place of work, with inability to recall one's past.

B. Confusion about personal identity or assumption of a new identity (partial or complete).

C. The disturbance does not occur exclusively during the course of DID and is not due to the direct physiological effects of a substance (e.g., a drug of abuse, a medication) or a general medical condition (e.g., temporal lobe epilepsy).

D. The symptoms cause clinically significant distress or impairment in social, occupational, or other important areas of functioning.

SOURCE: From APA (1994), with permission.

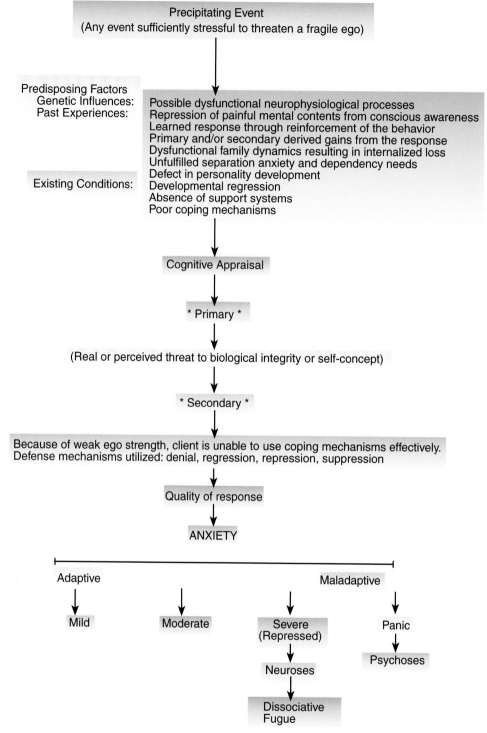

Figure 29.2   The dynamics of dissociative fugue using the transactional model of stress/adaptation.

Evaluation

Reassessment is conducted in order to determine if the nursing actions have been successful in achieving the objectives of care. Evaluation of the nursing actions for the client with dissociative fugue may be facilitated by gathering information using the following types of questions:

1. Can the client control anxiety without using violence?
2. Can he or she demonstrate strategies for relieving anxiety without resorting to aggression?
3. Does the client discuss fears and anxieties with members of the staff?

TABLE 29.4   CARE PLAN FOR THE CLIENT WITH DISSOCIATIVE FUGUE

NURSING DIAGNOSIS: RISK FOR VIOLENCE DIRECTED TOWARD OTHERS

RELATED TO: Fear of unknown circumstances surrounding emergence from fugue state

OUTCOME CRITERIA	NURSING INTERVENTIONS	RATIONALE
Client will not harm self or others.	1. Maintain low level of stimuli in client's environment (low lighting, few people, simple decor, low noise level). 2. Observe client's behavior frequently. 3. Remove all dangerous objects from client's environment. 4. Try to redirect violent behavior with physical outlets for the client's anxiety (e.g., punching bag). 5. Staff should maintain and convey a calm attitude to client. 6. Have sufficient staff available to indicate a show of strength to client if it becomes necessary. 7. Administer tranquilizing medications as ordered by physician. Monitor medication for its effectiveness and for any adverse side effects. 8. If the client is not calmed by "talking down" or by medication, use of mechanical restraints may be necessary. Be sure to have sufficient staff available to assist. Follow protocol established by the institution. Most states require that the physician reevaluate and issue a new order for restraints every 3 hr, except between midnight and 8:00 AM. If the client has previously refused medication, administer after restraints have been applied. Most states consider this intervention appropriate in emergency situations or in the event that a client would likely harm self or others. Observe client in restraints every 15 minutes (or according to institutional policy). Ensure that circulation is not compromised (check temperature, color, pulse). Assist client with needs related to nutrition, hydration, and elimination. Position client so that comfort is facilitated and aspiration can be prevented. 9. As agitation decreases, assess client's readiness for restraint removal or reduction. Remove one restraint at a time, while assessing client's response.	1. Anxiety level rises in stimulating environment. Individuals may be perceived as threatening by a fearful and agitated client. 2. Close observation is necessary so that intervention can occur if required to ensure client's (and others') safety. 3. This will prevent the confused and agitated client from using them to harm self or others. 4. Physical exercise is a safe and effective way of relieving pent-up tension. 5. Anxiety is contagious and can be transmitted from staff to client. 6. This shows the client evidence of control over the situation and provides some physical security for staff. 7. The avenue of the "least restrictive alternative" (see Chap. 40) must be selected when planning intervention for a psychiatric client. 8. Client safety is a nursing priority. 9. This minimizes risk of injury to client and staff.

Continued on following page

TABLE 29.4 *(Continued)*

NURSING DIAGNOSIS: INEFFECTIVE INDIVIDUAL COPING
RELATED TO: Dysfunctional family system and repressed severe anxiety
EVIDENCED BY: Sudden travel away from home with inability to recall previous identity

OUTCOME CRITERIA	NURSING INTERVENTIONS	RATIONALE
Client will demonstrate more adaptive ways of coping in stressful situations than resorting to dissociation.	1. Reassure client of safety and security through your presence. Dissociative behaviors may be frightening to the client. 2. Identify stressor that precipitated severe anxiety. 3. Explore feelings that client experienced in response to the stressor. Help client understand that the disequilibrium felt is acceptable in times of severe stress. 4. As anxiety level decreases and memory returns, use exploration and an accepting, nonthreatening environment to encourage client to identify repressed traumatic experiences that contribute to chronic anxiety. 5. Have client identify methods of coping with stress in the past and determine whether the response was adaptive or maladaptive. 6. Help client define more adaptive coping strategies. Make suggestions of alternatives that might be tried. Examine benefits and consequences of each alternative. Assist client in the selection of those that are most appropriate for him or her. 7. Provide positive reinforcement for client's attempts to change. 8. Identify community resources to which the individual may go for support if past maladaptive coping patterns return.	1. Presence of a trusted individual provides feeling of security and assurance of freedom from harm. 2. This information is necessary to the development of an effective plan of client care and problem resolution. 3. Client's self-esteem is preserved by the knowledge that others may experience these behaviors under similar circumstances. 4. Client must confront and deal with painful issues to achieve resolution. 5. In times of extreme anxiety, client is unable to evaluate appropriateness of response. This information is necessary for client to develop a plan of action for the future. 6. Depending on current level of anxiety, client may require assistance with problem solving and decision making. 7. Positive reinforcement enhances self-esteem and encourages repetition of desired behaviors. 8. Knowledge alone that this type of support exists may provide the client with a feeling of security. Use of the resources may help the client from decompensating.

4. Has he or she confronted these fears and anxieties and dealt with them in an effort toward resolution?
5. Can the client verbalize and demonstrate adaptive coping strategies for dealing with extreme stress without resorting to dissociation?
6. Does the client recall the extreme stressor that precipitated the fugue state?
7. Does he or she have a plan for dealing with the stressor should it recur in the future?
8. Can he or she verbalize resources for seeking assistance in the face of extreme stress?

Dissociative Identity Disorder

Background Assessment Data

Dissociative identity disorder was formerly called multiple personality disorder. This disorder is characterized by the existence of two or more personalities within a single individual. Only one of the personalities is evident at any given moment, and one of them is dominant most of the time over the course of the disorder. Each personality is unique and composed of a complex set of memories, behavior patterns, and social relationships that surface during the dominant interval. The transition from one personality to another is usually sudden, often dramatic, and usually precipitated by stress. O'Regan and Hurley (1985) state:

> "Transition may be voluntary or involuntary, initiated either through conscious willing, in response to an unconscious emotion or a situation which triggers 'automatic' switching, or as a result of biochemical changes in the body." (p. 4)

Before therapy, the original personality usually has no knowledge of the other personalities, but when there are two or more subpersonalities, they are usually aware of each other's existence. Most often, the various subpersonalities have different names, but they may be unnamed and may be of a different sex, race, and age (Purcell, 1988). The various personalities are almost always quite disparate and may even appear to be the exact opposite of the original personality. For example, a normally shy, socially withdrawn, faithful husband may become a gregarious womanizer and heavy drinker with the emergence of another personality.

Various personalities may respond to a stressful situation in different ways. An example cited by the *DSM-III-R* suggests that a person may have one personality that responds to aggression with childlike fright and flight, another that responds with masochistic submission, and yet another that responds with counterattack (APA, 1987).

Generally, there is amnesia for the events that took place when another personality was in the dominant position. Often, however, one personality state is not bound by such amnesia and retains complete awareness of the existence, qualities, and activities of the other personalities (Nemiah, 1989). Subpersonalities that are amnestic for the other subpersonalities experience the periods when others are dominant as "lost time" or blackouts. They may "wake up" in unfamiliar situations with no idea where they are, how they got there, or who the people around them are. They may frequently be accused of lying when they deny remembering or being responsible for events or actions that occurred while another personality controlled the body.

Dissociative identity disorder is not always incapacitating. Some individuals with DID maintain responsible positions, complete graduate degrees, and are successful spouses and parents before diagnosis and while in treatment. Many individuals are misdiagnosed with depression, borderline and antisocial personality disorders, schizophrenia, epilepsy, or bipolar disorder before being diagnosed with DID.

The *DSM-IV* diagnostic criteria for dissociative identity disorder are presented in Table 29.5.

Predisposing Factors to Dissociative Identity Disorder

Kluft (1984, 1987) developed the "four-factor" theory of the etiology of DID. The four factors he considers necessary for the development of this disorder are:

1. A biological capacity for dissociation.
2. A history of trauma or abuse.
3. Specific psychological factors that influence the shaping of the various personalities as they take form at the time of the traumatic mobilization of the dissociative defense. These would be factors such as developmental state, cultural, societal, and family influences.
4. A lack of adequate nurturing or opportunities to recover from the abuse.

These four factors may be explained by the following theories.

Biological Theories

Genetics. Several studies have indicated that DID is more common in first-degree biological relatives of people with the disorder than in the general population (APA, 1994). Braun (1986) concludes from his studies that at least one early caretaker of the individual who will develop DID has exhibited severe psychopathology. The disorder is often seen in more than one generation of a family. Although some psychiatrists believe this may reflect a genetic component of DID, perhaps linked to the psychobiological capacity for dissociation, others correlate this dissociation process to the effects of the violent personalities of adult caregivers (O'Regan & Hurley, 1985).

Organic. The role of organic influences in the development of DID remains unclear. Studies (Horton & Miller, 1972; Schenk & Bear, 1981) have suggested a possible link between certain neurological alterations and DID. These neurological conditions include temporal lobe epilepsy, severe migraine headaches, cerebral cortical damage, and visual alterations. Electroencephalographic abnormalities were observed in some clients with DID (Kaplan & Sadock, 1998).

TABLE 29.5 DIAGNOSTIC CRITERIA FOR DISSOCIATIVE IDENTITY DISORDER

A. The presence of two or more distinct personality states (each with its own relatively enduring pattern of perceiving, relating to, and thinking about the environment and self).

B. At least two of these identities or personality states recurrently take control of the person's behavior.

C. Inability to recall important personal information that is too extensive to be explained by ordinary forgetfulness.

D. The disturbance is not due to the direct physiological effects of a substance (e.g., blackouts or chaotic behavior during alcohol intoxication) or a general medical condition (e.g., complex partial seizures). Note: In children, the symptoms are not attributable to imaginary playmates or other fantasy play.

SOURCE: From APA (1994), with permission.

The majority of individuals with these organic alterations show no signs of DID. Based on the body of present knowledge, the hypothesis of organic dysfunction as a determinant of DID should be approached with caution.

Psychological Influences. A growing body of evidence points to the etiology of DID as a set of traumatic experiences that overwhelms the individual's capacity to cope by any means other than dissociation. These experiences usually take the form of severe physical, sexual, or psychological abuse by a parent or significant other in the child's life (O'Regan & Hurley, 1985). Benjamin (1990) has stated, "DID develops when people have been so overcome by early traumas that they have to put up mental partitions in order to function in everyday life." The most widely accepted etiological explanation for DID is that it begins as a survival strategy that serves to help children cope with horrendous sexual, physical, or psychological abuse. In this traumatic environment, the child is reduced to experiencing the self as a passive victim unable to ward off cruel and unwanted stimuli (Confer & Ables, 1983). He or she creates a new being who is able to experience the overwhelming pain of the cruel reality, while the primary self can then escape awareness of the pain. Each new personality has as its nucleus a means of responding without anxiety and distress to various painful or dangerous stimuli.

Studies have revealed a great diversity in the nature and scope of the trauma that individuals with DID have suffered (O'Regan & Hurley, 1985). *Sexual* abuse has included rape, incest, sodomy, and heterosexual and homosexual fellatio. Some individuals report being forced to witness the physical or sexual abuse of other children. Individuals with the disorder have given such examples of *psychological* abuse as being compelled to participate in murders, including cult activities involving ritual murders. *Physical* abuse has included being buried, tortured, beaten, given excessive enemas and massive doses of cathartics, as well as enduring total neglect. Kluft (1984) has suggested that the number of an individual's alternate personalities may be related to the number of different types of abuse he or she suffered as a child. Individuals with many personalities have usually been severely abused well into adolescence.

Theory of Family Dynamics. Studies by Braun (1986) indicate that individuals with DID do not find the necessary healing support in their environment. Research has revealed a profile of the family of origin of the individual with DID. Characteristics include:

1. Upholding rigid religious or mystical beliefs.
2. Presenting a united front to the community, while internally riddled with conflict.
3. Isolation from the community and lack of cooperation regarding intervention or assistance.
4. At least one caretaker who exhibits severe psychopathology.

5. Subjecting the child to contradictory communications.
6. Polarization by one overadequate parent (the abuser) and one underadequate parent (the enabler).

The individual who is not given the opportunity to heal following abuse and dissociation adopts this defense as a routine strategy for dealing with life problems.

Transactional Model of Stress/Adaptation. The etiology of DID is most likely influenced by multiple factors. In Figure 29.3, a graphic depiction of this theory of multiple causation is presented in the transactional model of stress/adaptation.

Diagnosis/Outcome Identification

Nursing diagnoses are formulated from the data gathered during the assessment phase and with background knowledge regarding predisposing factors to the disorder. Some common nursing diagnoses for clients with dissociative identity disorder include:

Risk for self-directed violence related to unresolved grief and self-blame associated with childhood abuse.
Personal identity disturbance related to childhood trauma/abuse, evidenced by the presence of more than one personality within the individual.

The following criteria may be used for measurement of outcomes in the care of the client with dissociative identity disorder:

THE CLIENT:

1. Has not harmed self or others.
2. Seeks out staff when aggressive feelings emerge.
3. Verbalizes understanding of the existence of multiple personalities.
4. Verbalizes understanding of the purpose the various personalities serve.
5. Verbalizes understanding that transition from one personality to another occurs in times of stress.
6. Verbalizes knowledge of various situations that precipitate stress.
7. Verbalizes understanding of and willingness to participate in integration therapy.

Planning/Implementation

Table 29.6 provides a plan of care for the client with DID. Nursing diagnoses are presented, along with outcome criteria, appropriate nursing interventions, and rationales.

Evaluation

Hospitalization of the client with DID usually occurs only in an acute situation (e.g., an attempted suicide, or

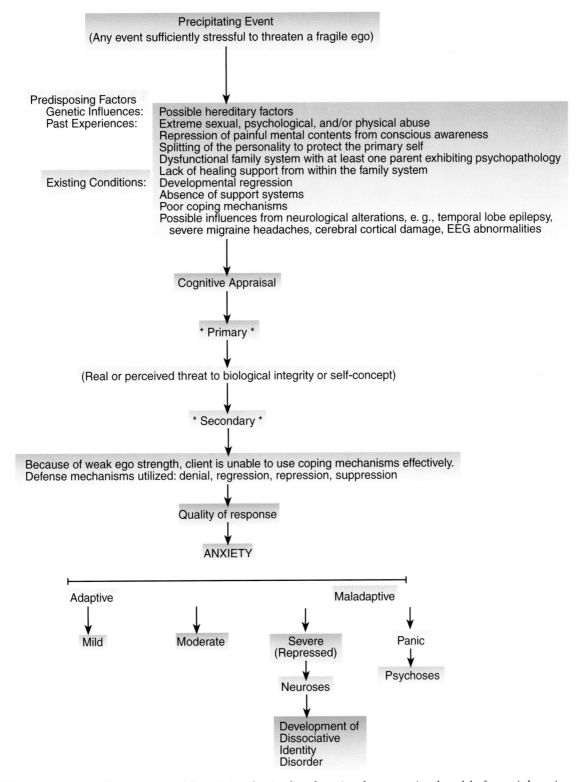

Figure 29.3   The dynamics of dissociative identity disorder using the transactional model of stress/adaptation.

an attempt to integrate a personality that the therapist is anticipating may precipitate violence and requires a more structured setting). In these cases, the nursing interventions would be directed toward the most critical issues.

Reassessment is ongoing, to determine if the nursing actions have been successful in achieving the stated objectives of care. Evaluation of the nursing actions for the client with DID may be facilitated by gathering information using the following types of questions:

TABLE 29.6 CARE PLAN FOR THE CLIENT WITH DISSOCIATIVE IDENTITY DISORDER

NURSING DIAGNOSIS: RISK FOR SELF-DIRECTED VIOLENCE
RELATED TO: Unresolved grief and self-blame associated with childhood abuse

OUTCOME CRITERIA	NURSING INTERVENTIONS	RATIONALE
Client will not harm self.	1. Assess suicidal or harmful intent. Discuss consideration of a plan and availability of means. Assess sudden changes in behavior.	1. Impulse control may be impaired. Sudden changes may signal a switch to the "suicidal" personality.
	2. Help client identify stressful precipitating factors that initiate emergence of the "suicidal" personality.	2. Early detection allows time to manipulate the environment to reduce the possibility of injury.
	3. Establish trust and secure a promise that client seek out support when self-destructive impulses are present.	3. This allows the client to assume some of the responsibility for his or her behavior, while still offering assistance if self-control is lacking.
	4. Seek assistance from another, strong-willed personality.	4. A strong-willed personality may help to control the behavior of the "suicidal" personality.
	5. Assist the client in identifying alternative behaviors to self-destructive behaviors (e.g., verbal or written expression, physical activity).	5. These activities may provide a nondestructive alternative in the face of overwhelming aggressive impulses.
	6. If necessary, place in isolation or provide physical restraint in a nonpunitive manner.	6. Physical restraints will ensure client safety when internal controls fail.
	7. Assess physical and emotional status every 15 minutes while in restraints.	7. Client safety and security are nursing priorities.
	8. Administer antidepressant and antianxiety medications as ordered by physician.	8. Depression is common and the client may become frustrated with the long-term treatment (sometimes in excess of 10 yr). Anxiolytics may be required to reduce anxiety until internal controls are achieved.

NURSING DIAGNOSIS: PERSONAL IDENTITY DISTURBANCE
RELATED TO: Childhood trauma/abuse
EVIDENCED BY: The presence of more than one personality within the individual

OUTCOME CRITERIA	NURSING INTERVENTIONS	RATIONALE
Client will verbalize understanding about the existence of multiple personalities within the self, the reason for their existence, and the importance of eventual integration of the personalities into one.	1. The nurse must develop a trusting relationship with the original personality and with each of the subpersonalities.	1. Trust is the basis of a therapeutic relationship. Each of the personalities views itself as a separate entity and must initially be treated as such.
	2. Help client understand the existence of the subpersonalities and the need each serves in the personal identity of the individual.	2. Client may initially be unaware of the dissociative response. Knowledge of the needs each personality fulfills is the first step in the integration process.
	3. Help client identify stressful situations that precipitate transition from one personality to another. Carefully observe and record these transitions.	3. Identification of stressors is required to assist client in responding more adaptively and to eliminate the need for transition to another personality.
	4. Use nursing interventions necessary to deal with maladaptive behaviors associated with individual subpersonalities. For example, if one personality is suicidal, precau-	4. The safety of client and others is a nursing priority.

5. Help subpersonalities to understand that their "being" will not be destroyed but rather integrated into a unified identity within the individual.

6. Provide support during disclosure of painful experiences and reassurance when client becomes discouraged with lengthy treatment.

5. Because subpersonalities function as separate entities, the idea of total elimination generates fear and defensiveness.

6. Positive reinforcement may encourage repetition of desirable behaviors.

tions must be taken to guard against the client's self-harm. If another personality has a tendency toward physical hostility, precautions must be taken to protect others.

---

1. Can the client maintain control over hostile impulses?
2. Has injury to client and others been avoided?
3. Does the client seek support from staff when aggressive feelings emerge?
4. Can the client discuss the presence of various personalities within the self?
5. Can he or she verbalize why these personalities exist?
6. Can the client verbalize situations that precipitate transition from one personality to another?
7. Does he or she ever switch from one personality to another voluntarily?
8. Can the client demonstrate alternative, more adaptive coping strategies?
9. Does the client verbalize understanding of the process of **integration?**
10. Is he or she willing to undergo the lengthy therapy required for integration?
11. Do the alternate personalities resist integration?
12. Do the alternate personalities understand that integration means not extinction, but rather instead a "coming together," of all the personalities into one identity?
13. Does the client have a plan for dealing with stress outside the therapy setting, particularly those situations that provoke feelings of violence to self or others? If so, has the plan been demonstrated (e.g., through role-play)?
14. Can the client verbalize resources outside the hospital from whom he or she may seek assistance during times of extreme stress?

Depersonalization Disorder

Background Assessment Data

Depersonalization disorder is characterized by a temporary change in the quality of self-awareness, which often takes the form of feelings of unreality, changes in body image, feelings of detachment from the environment, or a sense of observing oneself from outside the body

(Marciniak, 1985). Depersonalization (a disturbance in the perception of oneself) is differentiated from **derealization,** which describes an alteration in the perception of the external environment. Both of these phenomena also occur in a variety of psychiatric illnesses such as schizophrenia, depression, anxiety states, and organic mental disorders. As stated earlier, the symptom of depersonalization is very common. It is estimated that approximately half of all adults experience transient episodes of depersonalization (APA, 1994). The diagnosis of depersonalization disorder is not made, even if episodes are recurrent, unless the symptom causes social or occupational dysfunction (Purcell, 1988).

The *DSM-IV* describes this disorder as the persistence or recurrence of episodes of depersonalization characterized by a feeling of detachment or estrangement from one's self (APA, 1994). There may be a mechanical or dreamlike feeling, or belief that the body's physical characteristics have changed. If derealization is present, objects in the environment are perceived as altered in size or shape. Other people in the environment may seem automated or mechanical.

These altered perceptions are experienced as disturbing and are often accompanied by anxiety, depression, fear of going insane, obsessive thoughts, somatic complaints, and a disturbance in the subjective sense of time (APA, 1994). The disorder has been found to occur at least twice as often in women as in men and is a disorder of younger people, rarely occurring in individuals older than 40 years of age (Nemiah, 1989). The diagnostic criteria for depersonalization disorder are presented in Table 29.7.

Predisposing Factors to Depersonalization Disorder

Physiological Theories. A variety of empirical observations have led some investigators to suggest that the phenomenon of depersonalization has a neurophysiological basis (Purcell, 1988). Clients with diseases of the central nervous system, such as brain tumors and epilepsy, have reported depersonalization episodes in association

Table 29.7 Diagnostic Criteria for Depersonalized Disorder

A. Persistent or recurrent experiences of feeling detached from, and as if one is an outside observer of, one's mental processes or body (e.g., feeling like one is in a dream).

B. During the depersonalization experience, reality testing remains intact.

C. The depersonalization causes clinically significant distress or impairment in social, occupational, or other important areas of functioning.

D. The depersonalization experience does not occur exclusively during the course of another mental disorder, such as schizophrenia, panic disorder, acute stress disorder, or another dissociative disorder, and is not due to the direct physiological effects of a substance (e.g., a drug of abuse, a medication) or a general medical condition (e.g., temporal lobe epilepsy).

SOURCE: From APA (1994), with permission.

with their neurological impairment. Electrical stimulation of the cortex of the temporal lobes has produced the same effect. Some psychotomimetic drugs, such as lysergic acid diethylamide (LSD) and mescaline, create distortions of perception and alterations in the sense of reality. A number of researchers have reported that individuals subjected to severe sensory deprivation sometimes experience depersonalization.

Psychodynamic Theories. Psychodynamic explanations emphasize psychological conflict and disturbances of ego structure in the predisposition to depersonalization disorder.

Perceiving the self as "not real" would serve as a defense mechanism and offer protection or escape from anxiety or some other unpleasant emotion resulting from internal psychological conflict (Purcell, 1988). For example, an individual who experiences extreme anxiety after a severe automobile accident perceives himself or herself (or the situation) as "not real" and therefore escapes the emotional pain associated with the incident.

Theories related to disturbances in ego structure focus on problems with personal identity and ego boundaries. Depersonalization occurs in response to psychological conflicts within the ego itself. The conflict results in a split in the ego between an observing self and an acting self, or a split between conflicting identifications (Nemiah, 1989). Proponents of this theory believe that explanation of depersonalization lies primarily in understanding the pathology of the structure and function of the ego.

Transactional Model of Stress/Adaptation. The etiology of depersonalization disorder is most likely influenced by multiple factors. In Figure 29.4, a graphic depiction of this theory of multiple causation is presented in the transactional model of stress/adaptation.

Diagnosis/Outcome Identification

Nursing diagnoses are formulated from the data gathered during the assessment phase and with background knowledge regarding predisposing factors to the disorder. Some common nursing diagnoses for clients with depersonalization disorder include:

Sensory-perceptual alteration (visual and kinesthetic) related to repressed severe anxiety and underdeveloped ego, evidenced by alteration in the perception or experience of the self or the environment.

Anxiety (severe to panic) related to fears of losing control or going insane, evidenced by somatic complaints, obsessive thoughts, and disturbances in the sense of time.

The following criteria may be used for measurement of outcomes in the care of the client with depersonalization disorder:

The client:

1. Maintains a sense of reality during stressful situations.
2. Perceives self and environment accurately.
3. Verbalizes correlation between severe anxiety and symptoms of depersonalization.
4. Can maintain anxiety at a manageable level.
5. Verbalizes an understanding of the role depersonalization behaviors play in the management of anxiety.
6. Can verbalize more adaptive strategies for coping with stress.

Planning/Implementation

Table 29.8 provides a plan of care for the client with depersonalization disorder. Nursing diagnoses are presented, along with outcome criteria, appropriate nursing interventions, and rationales.

Evaluation

Reassessment is conducted in order to determine if the nursing actions have been successful in achieving the objectives of care. Evaluation of the nursing actions for the client with depersonalization disorder may be facilitated by gathering information using the following types of questions:

1. Does the client demonstrate the ability to perceive stimuli correctly?

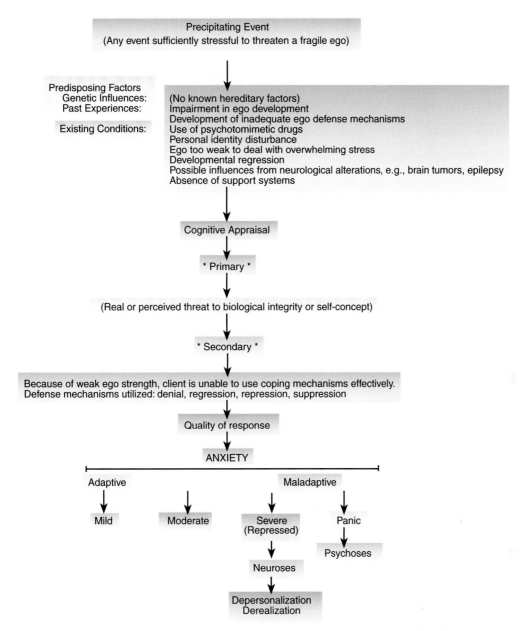

Figure 29.4   The dynamics of depersonalization disorder using the transactional model of stress/adaptation.

2. Does he or she maintain a sense of reality during stressful situations?
3. Can the client verbalize the purpose depersonalization behaviors serve?
4. Can the client verbalize a correlation between stressful situations and the onset of depersonalization behaviors?
5. Can the client demonstrate more adaptive coping strategies for dealing with stress without resorting to dissociation?
6. Has the client role played these strategies in preparation for their use in real-life situations?
7. Can the client verbalize types of situations that precipitate extreme stress?
8. Can the client discuss more adaptive ways that he or she plans to deal with these times of extreme stress in the future?
9. Can the client verbalize resources outside the hospital to whom he or she may turn when feeling the need for assistance?

Table 29.9 presents topics for client/family education related to dissociative disorders.

TREATMENT MODALITIES

Dissociative Amnesia

Many cases of dissociative amnesia resolve spontaneously when the individual is removed from the stressful situation (Purcell, 1988). For other, more refractory conditions,

TABLE 29.8 CARE PLAN FOR THE CLIENT WITH DEPERSONALIZATION DISORDER

NURSING DIAGNOSIS: SENSORY-PERCEPTUAL ALTERATION (VISUAL/KINESTHETIC)
RELATED TO: Repressed severe anxiety and underdeveloped ego
EVIDENCED BY: Alteration in the perception or experience of the self or the environment

OUTCOME CRITERIA	NURSING INTERVENTIONS	RATIONALE
Client will demonstrate the ability to perceive stimuli correctly and maintain a sense of reality during stressful situations.	1. Provide support and encouragement during times of depersonalization. Clients manifesting these symptoms may express fear and anxiety at experiencing such behaviors. They do not understand the response and may express a fear of going insane.	1. Support and encouragement from a trusted individual provide a feeling of security when fears and anxieties are manifested.
	2. Explain the depersonalization behaviors and the purpose they usually serve for the client.	2. Client learning may help to minimize fears and anxieties associated with their occurrence.
	3. Explain the relationship between severe anxiety and depersonalization behaviors. Help relate these behaviors to times of severe psychological stress that client has experienced.	3. The client may be unaware that the occurrence of depersonalization behaviors is related to severe anxiety.
	4. Explore past experiences and possibly repressed painful situations, such as trauma or abuse.	4. Traumatic experiences may predispose individuals to dissociative disorders.
	5. Discuss these painful experiences with client, and encourage him or her to deal with the feelings associated with these situations. Work to resolve the conflicts these repressed feelings have nurtured.	5. Conflict resolution will serve to decrease the need for the dissociative response to anxiety.
	6. Discuss ways the client may more adaptively respond to stress, and use role-play to practice these new methods.	6. Having practiced through role-play helps to prepare client to face stressful situations by using these new behaviors when they occur in real life.

NURSING DIAGNOSIS: ANXIETY (SEVERE TO PANIC)
RELATED TO: Fears of losing control or going insane
EVIDENCED BY: Somatic complaints, obsessive thoughts, and disturbances in the sense of time

OUTCOME CRITERIA	NURSING INTERVENTIONS	RATIONALE
Client will verbalize understanding of purpose depersonalization behaviors fulfill, thereby decreasing fears and anxieties associated with experiencing them.	1. Maintain a calm, nonthreatening manner while working with the client.	1. Anxiety is contagious and may be transferred from staff to a client or vice versa. Client develops feeling of security in presence of calm staff person.
	2. Reassure the client of his or her safety and security. This can be conveyed by the physical presence of the nurse. Do not leave the client alone at this time.	2. The client may fear for his or her life. The presence of a trusted individual provides client with a feeling of security and assurance of personal safety.
	3. Use simple words and brief messages, spoken calmly and clearly.	3. In an intensely anxious situation, the client is unable to comprehend anything but the most elemental communication.
	4. Explain to the client what is happening. Assure the client that the experiencing of depersonalization behaviors does not mean that he or she is going crazy.	4. The feeling of a lack of control over behavior he or she does not understand will contribute to anxiety. Explanations should offer some relief.

5. When depersonalization behaviors have diminished and anxiety has been reduced, explore with the client the stressful situation that may have precipitated the response.
6. Discuss with the client ways in which he or she might respond to stressful situations that would be less likely to result in depersonalization behaviors.
7. Use role-play to practice new, more adaptive coping strategies.

5. The client may be unaware that the occurrence of depersonalization behaviors is related to severe anxiety.
6. This may have been the client's way of dealing with stress for a long time. He or she may need help to identify alternative coping strategies.
7. Role-play allows the client to practice and be better prepared to deal with the stressful situation should it recur. Being prepared provides a feeling of security and offers a sense of control to the client.

---

intravenous administration of amobarbital is useful in the retrieval of lost memories. Most clinicians recommend supportive psychotherapy also to reinforce adjustment to the psychological impact of the retrieved memories and the emotions associated with them (Kaplan & Sadock, 1998).

In some instances, psychotherapy is used as the primary treatment. Techniques of persuasion and **free** or **directed association** are used to help the client remember. In other cases, **hypnosis** may be required to mobilize the memories. Once the memories are obtained, the suggestion is made to clients that they will retain them in consciousness after awakening (Nemiah, 1989).

Dissociative Fugue

Recovery from dissociative fugue is usually rapid, spontaneous, and complete. Treatment is similar to that of dissociative amnesia (Kaplan & Sadock, 1998). In some instances, manipulation of the environment or psychotherapeutic support may help to diminish stress or help the client adapt to stress in the future.

When the fugue is prolonged, techniques of gentle encouragement, persuasion, or directed association may be helpful, either alone or in combination with hypnosis or amobarbital interviews, which are also aimed at facilitating recall of the previous identity (Purcell, 1988).

Dissociative Identity Disorder

The goal of therapy for the client with DID is to optimize the client's function and potential. The achievement of integration (a blending of all the personalties into one) is usually considered desirable, but in some cases resolution, or a smooth collaboration among the subpersonalities, may be all that is realistic. (Kluft, 1991).

Some success has been achieved with intensive, long-term psychotherapy directed toward uncovering the underlying psychological conflicts, providing the client with

insight into these conflicts, and striving to synthesize the various identities into one integrated personality (Purcell, 1988). Clients are assisted to recall past traumas in detail. They must mentally reexperience the abuse that caused their illness. This process, called **abreaction,** or "remembering with feeling," is so painful that clients sometimes scream, sob, and flail about, just as they did during the actual event (Gupta, 1990).

During therapy, each personality is actively explored and encouraged to become aware of the others across previously amnestic barriers. Traumatic memories associated with the different personality manifestations, especially those related to childhood abuse, are examined.

Braun (1986) and Kluft (1988) have identified the following principles of therapy for the person with DID:

1. Use hypnosis to access personalities that do not emerge spontaneously.
2. Identify the relationships among subpersonalities and work with each personality equally.
3. Provide each personality with information about its role in the dissociated system.
4. Encourage awareness, communication, empathy, and cooperation among personalities.
5. Use medications sparingly. Almost any medicine is fraught with "switch potential"—idiosyncratic responses to medication that vary across personalities.
6. Expect some degree of relapse following initial integration.
7. Do not assume that the course of treatment will be smooth. The course of treatment is often difficult and anxiety provoking to client and therapist alike, especially when aggressive or suicidal personalities are in the dominant role. In these instances, brief periods of hospitalization may be necessary as an interim supportive measure (Nemiah, 1989).

When integration is achieved, the individual becomes a total of all the feelings, experiences, memories, skills, and talents that were previously in the command of the various per-

TABLE 29.9 TOPICS FOR CLIENT/FAMILY EDUCATION RELATED TO DISSOCIATIVE DISORDERS

Nature of the Illness
1. Define and describe symptoms of:
   a. Dissociative amnesia
   b. Dissociative fugue
   c. Dissociative identity disorder (DID)
   d. Depersonalization disorder
2. Discuss etiologies of above disorders.
3. Discuss possibility of long-term course, particularly in the case of DID.

Management of the Illness
1. Discuss ways to identify onset of escalating anxiety.
2. Discuss ways to intervene to prevent exacerbation of symptoms.
3. Teach relaxation techniques.
4. Teach assertiveness techniques.
5. Pharmacology: Teach about any medications that may be used to treat symptoms associated with dissociative disorders or disorders of comorbidity. (For example, anxiolytics, antipsychotics, antidepressants)

Support Services
1. Support groups
2. Individual psychotherapy

---

sonalities. He or she learns how to function effectively without the necessity for creating new personalities to cope with life. This is possible only after years of intense psychotherapy, and even then, recovery is very often incomplete.

Depersonalization Disorder

Information about the treatment of depersonalization disorder is sparse and inconclusive. Various regimens have been tried, although none have proven widely successful. Pharmacotherapy with dextroamphetamines or amobarbital (Amytal) has been tried with inconclusive results (Purcell, 1988). Benzodiazepines provide symptomatic relief if anxiety is an important element of the clinical condition (Kaplan & Sadock, 1998). If other psychiatric disorders, such as schizophrenia, are evident, they too may be treated pharmacologically. For clients with evident intrapsychic conflict, analytically oriented insight psychotherapy may be useful, although many clinicians believe that a successful outcome requires a minimum of 5 years of therapy (Nemiah, 1989). Specific recommendations for the management of depersonalization disorder must await more extensive clinical investigation.

SUMMARY

A dissociative response has been described as a defense mechanism to protect the ego in the face of overwhelming anxiety. Dissociative responses result in an alteration in the normally integrative functions of identity, memory, or consciousness. Classification of dissociative disorders includes dissociative amnesia, dissociative fugue, dissociative identity disorder, and depersonalization disorder.

TEST YOUR CRITICAL THINKING SKILLS

Sam[1] was admitted to the psychiatric unit from the emergency department of a general hospital in the Midwest. The owner of a local bar called the police when Sam suddenly seemed to "lose control. He just went ballistic." The police reported that Sam did not know where he was or how he got there. He kept saying, "My name is John Brown, and I live in Philadelphia." When the police ran an identity check on Sam, they found that he was indeed John Brown from Philadelphia and his wife had reported him missing a month ago. Mrs. Brown explained that about 18 months before his disappearance, her husband, who was a middle-level manager at a large manufacturing company, had been having considerable difficulty at work. He had been passed over for a promotion, and his supervisor had been very critical of his work. Several of his staff had left the company for other jobs, and Sam found it impossible to meet production goals. Work stress made him very difficult to live with at home. Previously an easygoing, gregarious person, he became withdrawn and critical of his wife and children. Immediately preceding his disappearance, he had had a violent argument with his 18-year-old son. The son had called him a "failure" and stormed out of the house to live with some friends who had an apartment. It was the day after this argument that Sam disappeared. The psychiatrist assigns a diagnosis of dissociative fugue.

Answer the following questions related to Sam:

1. Describe the priority nursing intervention with Sam as he is admitted to the psychiatric unit.
2. What approach should be taken to help Sam with his problem?
3. What is the long-term goal of therapy for Sam?

[1]Adapted from Spitzer et al. (1994).

In comparison to other primary psychiatric disorders, dissociative disorders are relatively rare. However, dissociative behaviors are not uncommonly observed in clients with other disorders.

The individual with dissociative amnesia is unable to recall important personal information that is too extensive to be explained by ordinary forgetfulness. The memory deficit may be described as *localized, selective, generalized, continuous,* or *systematized.* Dissociative fugue is character-

---

R E S E A R C H N O T E

Outpatient group therapy for dissociative trauma survivors. *Journal of the American Psychiatric Nurses Association* **(1996, April), 2(2), 37–43.**
Applegate, M.

Description of the Study: This article reviews a clinical experience of three long-standing (3-year) groups of female survivors with posttraumatic stress disorder (PTSD), dissociative disorder not otherwise specified (DDNOS), and dissociative identity disorder (DID). Three group experiences were offered to adult female trauma survivors who exhibited dissociative symptoms.

Results of the Study: Group placement was correlated to the degree of frequency and the severity of dissociative symptoms based on scores obtained on the Dissociative Experiences Scale (DES). The low-score group (scores of 7–20) reflected normal dissociative experiences to those suggestive of PTSD. The middle group (scores of 20–35) was composed of those women with symptoms indicative of PTSD, DDNOS, or DID. The third group consisted of the women who scored 35 or greater, which indicated either clinically documented personality states or a strong indication of undiagnosed DID. Interventions within the groups were focused on promotion of safety and trust, personal validation, social support, and patient education.

Comments: The author describes the DES as a cost-effective assessment tool that may be used in practice to objectively measure dissociative phenomena exhibited by clients who are survivors of trauma. She identifies group therapy in the outpatient setting as an effective treatment for these clients with PTSD, DDNOS, and DID. Group experiences for female trauma survivors can "enhance validation and promote a heightened sense of personal well-being and psychological wellness."

INTERNET REFERENCES

● Additional information about dissociative disorders may be located at the following websites:
  a. http://www.human-nature.com/odmh/
     dissociative.html
  b. http://www.nami.org/helpline/
     whatdiss.htm
  c. http://www.voiceofwomen.com/
     VOW2_11950/center.html
  d. http://www.shakey.net/dissoc.html
  e. http://www.webcrawler.com/health/
     mental_health/dissociative_disorders
  f. http://www.issd.org/isdabout.htm
  g. http://www.lifewell.com/InfoSprings/
     spring14.cfm

---

ized by a sudden, unexpected travel away from home with an inability to recall the past, including personal identity. Duration of the fugue is usually brief, and once it is over the individual recovers memory of the past life but is amnestic for the time period covered by the fugue. The prominent feature of DID is the existence of two or more personalities within a single individual. An individual may have many personalities, each of which serves a purpose for that individual of enduring painful stimuli that the original personality is too weak to face. Depersonalization disorder is characterized by an alteration in the perception of oneself (sometimes described as a feeling of having separated from the body and watching the activities of the self from a distance).

Nursing care of individuals with dissociative disorders is accomplished using the steps of the nursing process. Background assessment data were presented, along with nursing diagnoses common to each disorder. Interventions appropriate to each nursing diagnosis and relevant outcome criteria for each were included. An overview of current medical treatment modalities was discussed.

Nurses in all areas of clinical practice should be aware of client potential for dissociative responses and be able to recognize these behaviors should they occur. Clients exhibiting dissociative behaviors often receive health care initially in areas other than psychiatry.

REVIEW QUESTIONS

SELF-EXAMINATION/LEARNING EXERCISE

Select the answer that is most appropriate for the questions that follow the situation.

Situation: Ellen, age 32, was diagnosed as having DID at age 28. Since that time she has been in therapy with a psychiatrist, who has detected the presence of 12 personalities and identified a history of childhood abuse. Yesterday, Beth, the personality with suicidal ideations, swallowed a bottle of 20 diazepam (Valium) tablets. Ellen's roommate found her when she returned from work and called the emergency medical service. She was stabilized in the emergency department and 48 hours later transferred to the psychiatric unit.

1. The primary nursing diagnosis for Ellen would be:

   a. Personal identity disturbance related to childhood abuse.
   b. Sensory-perceptual alteration related to repressed anxiety.
   c. Altered thought processes related to memory deficit.
   d. Risk for self-directed violence related to unresolved grief.

2. In establishing trust with Ellen, the nurse must:

   a. Try to relate to Ellen as though she did not have multiple personalities.
   b. Establish a relationship with each of the personalities separately.
   c. Ignore behaviors that Ellen attributes to Beth.
   d. Explain to Ellen that he or she will work with her only if she maintains the status of the primary personality.

3. The ultimate goal of therapy for Ellen is:

   a. Integration of the personalities into one.
   b. For her to have the ability to switch from one personality to another voluntarily.
   c. For her to select which personality she wants to be her dominant self.
   d. For her to recognize that the various personalities exist.

4. The ultimate goal of therapy will most likely be achieved through:

   a. Crisis intervention and directed association.
   b. Psychotherapy and hypnosis.
   c. Psychoanalysis and free association.
   d. Insight psychotherapy and dextroamphetamines.

5. Which of the following is an appropriate nursing intervention for controlling the behavior of the "suicidal personality," Beth?

   a. When Beth emerges, put the client in restraints.
   b. Keep Ellen in isolation during her hospitalization.
   c. Make a verbal contract with Ellen that Beth will do no harm.
   d. Elicit the help of another, strong-willed personality to help control Beth's behavior.

The following are general questions related to dissociative disorders:

6. Which of the following nursing interventions is most appropriate for the nurse working with the client experiencing dissociative amnesia?

   a. Use the technique of implosion therapy (flooding) to help the client remember.
   b. Use hypnosis to help the client remember.
   c. Expose the client to stimuli that represent pleasant memories from the past.
   d. Expose the client to stimuli that represent the painful stimuli for which the amnesia is providing the protection.

7. It is important for the nurse to understand that, when an individual awakens from a fugue state, he or she:
    a. Will have no memory for what occurred during the fugue.
    b. Will remember everything that occurred during the fugue.
    c. Will have no memory for life before the fugue occurred.
    d. Will have total recall of the time before and during the fugue.

8. Bob was driving his automobile when it was involved in an accident in which his wife and child were killed. Unable to carry on with his life, he has sought emotional help. He says to the nurse, "I don't know how I managed to make all the funeral arrangements. At times it seemed as though I was an outside observer of everything that was happening." What is this phenomenon called?
    a. Derealization.
    b. Abreaction.
    c. Depersonalization.
    d. Psychosis.

9. Bob continues, "At other times, when I was with a group of people, it would appear as though everyone was moving in slow motion." What is this phenomenon called?
    a. Derealization.
    b. Abreaction.
    c. Depersonalization.
    d. Psychosis.

10. Which of the following examples of Bob's situation describes selective amnesia?
    a. Bob was unable to remember anything having to do with the accident until 3 days following the accident.
    b. Bob could not remember the accident, but remembered hearing the ambulance siren and being admitted to the emergency room.
    c. Bob is unable to remember anything that has happened during his entire lifetime.
    d. Bob can remember nothing since the time of the accident.

REFERENCES

American Psychiatric Association. (1994). *Diagnostic and statistical manual of mental disorders* (4th ed.). Washington, DC: American Psychiatric Association.

American Psychiatric Association. (1987). *Diagnostic and statistical manual of mental disorders* (3rd ed., rev.). Washington, DC: American Psychiatric Association.

Benjamin, R. (1990, March). In N.E. Gupta, Who am I? *Ladies Home Journal, CVII* (3), 233.

Berger, D.M. (1985). Dissociative disorders. In S.E. Greben, V.M. Rakoff, & G. Voineskos (Eds.), *A method of psychiatry* (2nd ed.). Philadelphia: Lea & Febiger.

Braun, B.G. (1986). *Treatment of multiple personality disorder.* Washington, DC: American Psychiatric Press.

Braun, B.G. (1989). The transgenerational incidence of dissociation and multiple personality disorder: A preliminary report. In R.P. Kluft (Ed.), *Childhood antecedents of multiple personality.* Washington, DC: American Psychiatric Press.

Cloninger, C.R. (1994). Somatoform and dissociative disorders. In G. Winokur & P.J. Clayton (Eds.), *The medical basis of psychiatry* (2nd ed.). Philadelphia: W.B. Saunders.

Confer, W.N., & Ables, B.S. (1983). *Multiple personality: Etiology, diagnosis, and treatment.* New York: Human Sciences Press.

Freud, S. (1962). The neuro-psychoses of defense (1894). In J. Strachey (Ed.), *Standard edition of the complete psychological works of Sigmund Freud,* Vol. 3. London: Hogarth Press. (Original work published 1894).

Gupta, N.E. (1990, March). Who am I? *Ladies Home Journal, CVII* (3): 161, 233–237.

Horton, P.C., & Miller, D.H. (1972). The etiology of multiple personality. *Comprehensive Psychiatry, 13*(2), 151–159.

Janet, P. (1907). *The major symptoms of hysteria.* New York: Macmillan.

Kaplan, H.I., & Sadock, B.J. (1998). Synopsis of psychiatry: *Behavioral sciences/clinical psychiatry* (8th ed.). Baltimore: Williams & Wilkins.

Kluft, R.P. (1984). Multiple personality in childhood. *Psychiatric Clinics of North America, 7,* 121–134.

Kluft, R.P. (1987). Multiple personality disorder: An update. *Hospital and Community Psychiatry, 38,* 363–373.

Kluft, R.P. (1988). The dissociative disorders. In J.A. Talbott, R.E. Hales, & S.C. Yodofsky (Eds.), *Textbook of psychiatry.* Washington, D.C.: American Psychiatric Press.

Kluft, R.P. (1991). Multiple personality disorder. In A. Tasman & S.M. Goldfinger (Eds.), *American Psychiatric Press review of psychiatry,* Vol. 10. Washington, DC: American Psychiatric Press.

Kolb, L.C., & Brodie, H.K.H. (1982). *Modern clinical psychiatry* (10th ed.). Philadelphia: W.B. Saunders.

Marciniak, R.D. (1985). Other psychiatric disorders. In J.I. Walker (Ed.), *Essentials of clinical psychiatry.* Philadelphia: J.B. Lippincott.

Nemiah, J.C. (1989). Dissociative disorders (hysterical neuroses, dissociative type). In H.I. Kaplan & B.J. Sadock (Eds.), *Comprehensive textbook of psychiatry* (5th Ed., Vol. I). Baltimore: Williams & Wilkins.

O'Regan, B., & Hurley, T.J. (1985). Multiple personality—Mirrors of a new model of mind? *Investigations, 1* (3/4), 1–23. Sausalito, CA: The Institute of Noetic Sciences.

Purcell, S.D. (1988). Dissociative disorders. In H.H. Goldman (Ed.), *Review of general psychiatry* (2nd ed.) Norwalk, CT: Appleton & Lange.

Schenk, L., & Bear, D. (1981). Multiple personality and related dissociative phenomena in patients with temporal lobe epilepsy. *American Journal of Psychiatry, 138,* 1311–1316.

Spitzer, R.L., Gibbon, M., Skodol, A.E., Williams, J.B., & First, M.B. (1994). *DSM-IV casebook: A learning companion to the diagnostic and statistical manual of mental disorders, 4th edition.* Washington, DC: American Psychiatric Press.

Bibliography

Appelbaum, S.A. (1996). Multiple personality disorder and the choice of self: Change factors in a brief therapy case. *Journal of Contemporary Psychotherapy, 26,* 103–116.

Applegate, M. (1997). Multiphasic short-term therapy for dissociative identity disorder. *Journal of the American Psychiatric Nurses Association, 3*(1), 1–9.

Curtin, S.L. (1993). Recognizing multiple personality disorder. *Journal of Psychosocial Nursing, 31*(2), 29–33.

Dallam, S., & Manderino, M.A. (1997). Free to be peer group supports patients with MPD/DD. *Journal of Psychosocial Nursing, 35*(5), 22–27.

Egeland, B., & Susman-Stillman, A. (1996). Dissociation as a mediator of child abuse across generations. *Child Abuse and Neglect, 20,* 1123–1132.

Ellason, J.W., & Ross, C.A. (1996). Lifetime Axis I and II comorbidity and childhood trauma history in dissociative identity disorder. *Psychiatry, 59,* 255–266.

O'Reilly-Knapp, M. (1996). From fragmentation to wholeness: An integrative approach with clients who dissociate. *Perspectives in Psychiatric Care, 32*(4), 5–11.

Stafford, L.L. (1993). Dissociation and multiple personality disorder: A challenge for psychosocial nurses. *Journal of Psychosocial Nursing, 31*(1), 15–20.

Townsend, M.C. (1997). *Nursing diagnoses in psychiatric nursing: A pocket guide for care plan construction* (4th ed.). Philadelphia: F.A. Davis.

SEXUAL AND GENDER IDENTITY DISORDERS

CHAPTER OUTLINE

OBJECTIVES

INTRODUCTION

DEVELOPMENT OF HUMAN SEXUALITY

SEXUAL DISORDERS

GENDER IDENTITY DISORDERS

VARIATIONS IN SEXUAL ORIENTATION

SEXUALLY TRANSMITTED DISEASES

SUMMARY

REVIEW QUESTIONS

KEY TERMS

orgasm
paraphilia
pedophilia
exhibitionism
voyeurism
fetishism
transvestic fetishism

frotteurism
masochism
sadism
anorgasmia
retarded ejaculation
premature ejaculation
vaginismus

dyspareunia
sensate focus
homosexuality
lesbianism
transsexualism
gonorrhea
syphilis

OBJECTIVES

After reading this chapter, the student will be able to:

1. Describe developmental processes associated with human sexuality.
2. Discuss historical and epidemiological aspects of paraphilias and sexual dysfunction disorders.
3. Identify various types of paraphilias, sexual dysfunction disorders, and gender identity disorders.
4. Discuss predisposing factors associated with the etiology of paraphilias, sexual dysfunction disorders, and gender identity disorders.
5. Describe the physiology of the human sexual response.
6. Conduct a sexual history.
7. Formulate nursing diagnoses and goals of care for clients with sexual and gender identity disorders.
8. Identify appropriate nursing interventions for clients with sexual and gender identity disorders.
9. Identify topics for client and family education relevant to sexual disorders.
10. Evaluate care of clients with sexual and gender identity disorders.
11. Describe various treatment modalities for clients with sexual and gender identity disorders.
12. Discuss variations in sexual orientation.
13. Identify various types of sexually transmitted diseases and discuss the consequences of each.

uman beings are sexual beings. Sexuality is a basic human need and an innate part of the total personality. It influences our thoughts, actions, and interactions and is involved in aspects of physical and mental health.

Society's attitude toward sexuality is changing. Clients are more open to seeking assistance in matters that pertain to sexuality. Although not all nurses need to be educated as sex therapists, they can readily integrate information on sexuality into the care they give by focusing on preventive, therapeutic, and educational interventions to assist individuals to attain, regain, or maintain sexual wellness.

This chapter focuses on disorders associated with sexual function and gender identity. Primary consideration is given to the categories of paraphilias, sexual dysfunction, and gender identity disorders as classified in the *DSM-IV* (American Psychiatric Association [APA], 1994). An overview of human sexual development throughout the life span is presented. Historical and epidemiological information associated with sexual disorders is included. Predisposing factors that have been implicated in the etiology of sexual and gender identity disorders provide a framework for studying the dynamics of these disorders. Various medical treatment modalities are explored. A discussion of variations in sexual orientation is included. Various types of sexually transmitted diseases are described, and an explanation of the consequences of each is presented.

Symptomatology of each disorder is presented as background knowledge for assessing clients with sexual and gender identity disorders. A tool for acquiring a sexual history is included. Nursing care is described in the context of the nursing process.

DEVELOPMENT OF HUMAN SEXUALITY

Birth Through Age 12

Although the sexual identity of an infant is determined before birth by chromosomal factors and physical appearance of the genitals, postnatal factors can greatly influence the way developing children perceive themselves sexually. Masculinity and femininity, as well as sex roles, are for the most part culturally defined. For example, differentiation of roles may be initiated at birth by painting a child's room pink or blue and by clothing the child in frilly, delicate dresses or tough, sturdy rompers.

It is not uncommon for infants to touch and explore their genitals. In fact, research on infantile sexuality indicates that both male and female infants are capable of sexual arousal and **orgasm** (Reinisch, 1990).

By age 2 or 2½, children know what gender they are (Hyde, 1986). They know that they are like the parent of the same gender and different from the parent of the opposite gender and from other children of the opposite

gender. They become acutely aware of anatomical sex differences during this time period (Clunn, 1991).

By age 4 or 5, children engage in heterosexual play. "Playing doctor" can be a popular game at this age. In this way, children form a concept of marriage to a member of the opposite gender.

Children increasingly gain experience with masturbation during childhood, although certainly not all children masturbate during this period. In a study of college students, 15 percent of the men and 20 percent of the women recalled that their first masturbation experiences occurred between ages 5 and 8 (Arafat & Cotton, 1974).

Late childhood and preadolescence may be characterized by homosexual play (Reinisch, 1990). Generally the activity involves no more than touching the other's genitals. Girls at this age become interested in menstruation, and both sexes are interested in learning about fertility, pregnancy, and birth. Interest in the opposite sex increases. Children of this age become self-conscious about their bodies and are concerned with physical attractiveness.

Children ages 10 to 12 are preoccupied with pubertal changes and the beginnings of romantic interest in the opposite gender. Prepubescent boys may engage in group sexual activities such as genital exhibition or group masturbation. Homosexual sex play is not uncommon. Prepubescent girls may engage in some genital exhibition but are usually not as preoccupied with the genitalia as are boys of this age (Reinisch, 1990).

Adolescence

Adolescence represents an acceleration in terms of biological changes and psychosocial and sexual development. This time of turmoil is nurtured by awakening endocrine forces and a new set of psychosocial tasks to undertake (Bell, 1998). Included in these tasks are issues relating to sexuality, such as how to deal with new or more powerful sexual feelings, whether to participate in various types of sexual behavior, how to recognize love, how to prevent unwanted pregnancy, and how to define age-appropriate sex roles.

Biologically, puberty begins for the female adolescent with breast enlargement, widening of the hips, and growth of pubic and ancillary hair. The onset of menstruation usually occurs between the ages of 11 and 13 years. In the male adolescent, growth of pubic hair and enlargement of the testicles begin at 12 to 16 years of age. Penile growth and the ability to ejaculate usually occur from the ages of 13 to 17. There is a marked growth of the body between ages 11 and 17, accompanied by the growth of body and facial hair, increased muscle mass, and a deeper voice.

Sexuality is slower to develop in the female than in the male adolescent. Women show steady increases in sexual responsiveness that peak in their middle 20s or early 30s. Men reach the sexual acme of their lives during adolescence (Hogan, 1980). Masturbation is a common sexual activity among male adolescents. Studies have indicated that nearly all males and almost two thirds of females have masturbated to orgasm by the time they complete adolescence (Kinsey, Pomeroy, & Martin, 1948).

Many individuals have their first experience with sexual intercourse during the adolescent years. Although studies indicate a variety of statistics related to incidence of adolescent coitus, three notable trends have become evident during the past two decades. They are:

1. More adolescents are engaging in premarital intercourse.
2. The incidence of premarital intercourse for girls has increased.
3. The average age of first intercourse is decreasing (Kaplan, Sadock, & Grebb, 1994).

The American culture has ambivalent feelings toward adolescent sexuality. Psychosexual development is desired, but most parents want to avoid anything that may encourage teenage sex. The rise in the number of cases of sexually transmitted diseases, some of which are considered life-threatening, also contributes to fears associated with unprotected sexual activity in all age groups.

Adulthood

This period of the life cycle begins at approximately 20 years of age and continues to age 65. Sexuality associated with ages 65 and older will be discussed in Chapter 35.

Marital Sex

Choosing a marital partner or developing a sexual relationship with another individual is one of the major tasks in the early years of this life-cycle stage. Current cultural perspective reflects that the institution of marriage has survived. About 80 percent to 90 percent of all people in the United States marry, and of those who divorce, a high percentage remarry. Intimacy in marriage is one of the most common forms of sexual expressions for adults. The average American couple has coitus about two or three times per week when they are in their 20s, with the frequency gradually declining to about once per week for those aged 45 and over (Hyde, 1986). Many adults continue to masturbate even though they are married and have ready access to heterosexual sex. This behavior is perfectly normal, although it often evokes feelings of guilt and may be done secretly.

Extramarital Sex

Approximately 20 to 30 percent of men have extramarital sex at some time during their marriages compared with

about 15 to 20 percent of women (McCarthy & McCarthy, 1998). Although the incidence of extramarital sex for men seems to be holding constant, some evidence exists to suggest that the incidence for women may be increasing.

Although attitudes toward premarital sex have changed substantially during the last several decades, attitudes toward extramarital sex have remained relatively stable. The majority of women and men say they believe sexual exclusivity should be a goal in marriage, although they were less certain about what would happen if their partner did not live up to that ideal. Some studies place the incidence of divorce caused by infidelity or adultery at around 20 percent of all divorce cases (Reinisch, 1990).

Sex and the Single Person

Attitudes about sexual intimacy among singles—never married, divorced, or widowed—vary from individual to individual. Some single people will settle for any kind of relationship, casual or committed, that they believe will enrich their lives. Others deny any desire for marriage or sexual intimacy, cherishing instead the independence they retain by being "unattached." Still others may desperately search for a spouse, with the desperation increasing as the years wear on.

Most divorced women, but fewer widowed women, return to having an active sex life following separation from, or loss of, their spouse. Virtually all divorced and widowed men return to an active sex life (Hyde, 1986).

The "Middle" Years—46 to 65

With the advent of the middle years, a decrease in hormonal production initiates a number of changes in the sex organs, as well as the rest of the body. The average age of onset of menopause for the woman is around 50, although changes can be noted from about age 46 to 60 (Sands, 1995). This decrease in the amount of estrogen can result in loss of vaginal lubrication, making intercourse painful. Other symptoms may include insomnia, "hot flashes," headaches, heart palpitations, and depression. Hormonal supplements may alleviate some of these symptoms.

With the decrease of androgen production during these years, men also experience sexual changes. The amount of ejaculate may decrease, and ejaculation may be less forceful. The testes decrease in size, and erections may be less frequent and less rigid. By age 50, the refractory period increases, and men may require 8 to 24 hours after orgasm before another erection can be achieved (Becker, 1992).

Biological drives decrease, and interest in sexual activity may decrease during these "middle" years. Although men need longer stimulation to reach orgasm and intensity of pleasure may decrease, women stabilize at the same level of sexual activity as at the previous stage in the life cycle and often have a greater capacity for orgasm in middle adulthood than in young adulthood (Kaplan, Sadock, & Grebb, 1994). Both sexes should continue sexual activity because long sexual abstinence decreases sexual functioning (Masters & Johnson, 1966).

SEXUAL DISORDERS

Paraphilias

The term **paraphilia** is used to identify repetitive or preferred sexual fantasies or behaviors that involve any of the following:

1. The preference for use of a nonhuman object.
2. Repetitive sexual activity with humans that involves real or simulated suffering or humiliation.
3. Repetitive sexual activity with nonconsenting partners (Abel, 1989).

The *DSM-IV* specifies that these sexual fantasies or behaviors must persist for at least 6 months and cause the individual clinically significant distress or impairment in social, occupational, or other important areas of functioning (APA, 1994).

Historical Aspects

Historically, it seems, some restrictions on human sexual expression have always existed. Sexual prohibitions provide possible containment for sexuality's potentially disruptive power (Abel, 1989). Under the code of Orthodox Judaism, masturbation was punishable by death. In ancient Catholicism it was considered a carnal sin. In the late 19th century this activity was viewed as a major cause of insanity.

Pedophilia, the sexual exploitation of children, was condemned in ancient cultures, as it continues to be today. Incest remains the one taboo that crosses cultural barriers. It was punishable by death in Babylonia, Judea, and ancient China, and offenders were given the death penalty as late as 1650 in England (Abel, 1989).

Oral-genital, anal, homosexual, and animal sexual contacts were viewed by the early Christian church as unnatural and, in fact, as greater transgressions than extramarital sexual activity because they did not lead to biological reproduction (Abel, 1989). Today, of these church-condemned, nonprocreative behaviors, only sex with animals (zoophilia) retains its classification as a paraphilia in the *DSM-IV.*

Epidemiological Statistics

Relatively limited data exist on the prevalence or course of the paraphilias. Most information that is available has been obtained from studies of incarcerated sex offenders.

Another source of information has been from outpatient psychiatric services for paraphiliacs outside the criminal justice system.

Because few paraphiliacs experience personal distress from their behavior, most individuals come for treatment because of pressure from their partners or the authorities (Becker & Kavoussi, 1988). Data suggest that the majority of paraphiliacs seeking outpatient treatment do so for pedophilia (45 percent), **exhibitionism** (25 percent), or **voyeurism** (12 percent).

The majority of individuals with paraphilias are men, and more than 50 percent of these individuals develop the onset of their paraphilic arousal before age 18 (Abel, Rouleau, & Osborn, 1994). The behavior peaks between ages 15 and 25 and gradually declines so that, by age 50, the occurrence of paraphilic acts is very low, except for those paraphilic behaviors that occur in isolation or with a cooperative partner. Some individuals with these disorders experience multiple paraphilias (Kaplan, Sadock, & Grebb, 1994).

Types of Paraphilias

The following types of paraphilias are identified by the *DSM-IV:*

Exhibitionism. Exhibitionism is characterized by recurrent, intense sexual urges, behaviors, or sexually arousing fantasies, of at least 6 months' duration, involving the exposure of one's genitals to an unsuspecting stranger (APA, 1994). Masturbation may occur during the exhibitionism. In almost 100 percent of cases of exhibitionism, the perpetrators are men and the victims are women (Kaplan, Sadock, & Grebb, 1994).

The exhibitionist's urges to expose himself intensify when he has excessive free time or is under significant stress (Abel, 1989). Most exhibitionists have rewarding sexual relationships with adult partners but concomitantly expose themselves to other women.

Fetishism. **Fetishism** involves recurrent, intense sexual urges or behaviors, or sexually arousing fantasies, of at least 6 months' duration, involving the use of nonliving objects (APA, 1994). The sexual focus is commonly on objects intimately associated with the human body (e.g., shoes, gloves, stockings) (Kaplan, Sadock, & Grebb, 1994). The fetish object is usually used during masturbation or incorporated into sexual activity with another person in order to produce sexual excitation.

When the fetish involves cross-dressing, the disorder is called **transvestic fetishism.** The individual is a heterosexual man who keeps a collection of women's clothing that he intermittently uses to dress in when alone. While cross-dressed, he usually masturbates and imagines himself to be both the male subject and the female object of his sexual fantasy (APA, 1994).

Requirement of the fetish object for sexual arousal may become so intense in some individuals that to be without it may result in impotence. Onset of the disorder usually occurs during adolescence.

The disorder is chronic, and the complication arises when the individual becomes progressively more intensely aroused by sexual behaviors that exclude a sexual partner. The paraphiliac and his partner may become so distant that the partner eventually terminates the relationship.

In addition to their fetishism, significant numbers of fetishists are concomitantly or have previously been involved in exhibitionism, **frotteurism,** pedophilia, rape, or voyeurism (Abel, 1989).

Frotteurism. Frotteurism is the recurrent preoccupation with intense sexual urges, behaviors, or fantasies of at least 6 months' duration involving touching and rubbing against a nonconsenting person (APA, 1994). Sexual excitement is derived from the actual touching or rubbing, not from the coercive nature of the act. Almost without exception, the gender of the frotteur is male.

The individual usually chooses to commit the act in crowded places, such as on buses or subways during rush hour. In this way, he can provide rationalization for his behavior should someone complain and more easily escape arrest. The frotteur waits in a crowd until he identifies a victim, then he follows her and allows the rush of the crowd to push him against her. He fantasizes a relationship with his victim while rubbing his genitals against her thighs and buttocks or touching her genitalia or breasts with his hands. He often escapes detection owing to the victim's initial shock and denial that such an act has been committed in this public place.

Significant numbers of frotteurs are concomitantly or have previously been involved in exhibitionsim, pedophilia, sadism, rape, or voyeurism (Abel, 1989).

Pedophilia. The *DSM-IV* describes the essential feature of this disorder as recurrent sexual urges, behaviors, or sexually arousing fantasies, of at least 6 months' duration, involving sexual activity with a prepubescent child. The age of the molester is at least 16 and at least 5 years older than the child. This category of paraphilia is the most common of sexual assaults (Abel, 1989).

The majority of child molestations involve genital fondling or oral sex. Vaginal or anal penetration of the child is most common in cases of incest (Abel, 1989). Others may limit their activity to undressing the child and looking, exposing themselves, masturbating in the presence of the child, or gentle touching and fondling of the child (APA, 1994).

Onset usually occurs during adolescence, and the disorder often runs a chronic course, particularly with male pedophiles who demonstrate a preference for little boys. A significant number of pedophiles are concomitantly or have previously been involved in exhibitionism, voyeurism, or rape (Able, 1989).

Sexual Masochism. The identifying feature of sexual **masochism** is recurrent, intense sexual urges, behaviors, or sexually arousing fantasies of at least 6 months' dura-

tion, involving the act (real, not simulated) of being humiliated, beaten, bound, or otherwise made to suffer (APA, 1994). These masochistic activities may be fantasized (e.g., being raped), solitary (e.g., self-inflicted pain), or with a partner (e.g., being restrained, spanked, or beaten by the partner). Some masochistic activities have resulted in death, in particular those that involve sexual arousal by oxygen deprivation.

The disorder is usually chronic and can progress to the point at which the individual cannot achieve sexual satisfaction without masochistic fantasies or activities. A significant number of masochists are concomitantly or have previously been involved in exhibitionism, pedophilia, rape, or transvestism (Abel, 1989).

Sexual Sadism. The *DSM-IV* identifies the essential feature of sexual **sadism** as recurrent, intense sexual urges, behaviors, or sexually arousing fantasies, of at least 6 months' duration, involving acts (real, not simulated) in which the psychological or physical suffering (including humiliation) of the victim is sexually exciting (APA, 1994). The sadistic activities may be fantasized or acted on with a consenting or nonconsenting partner. In all instances, sexual excitation occurs in response to the suffering of the victim. Examples of sadistic acts include restraint, beating, burning, rape, cutting, torture, and even killing.

The course of the disorder is usually chronic, with the severity of the sadistic acts often increasing over time. Activities with nonconsenting partners are usually terminated by legal apprehension. A significant number of sadists are concomitantly or have previously been involved in exhibitionism, frotteurism, pedophilia, rape, or voyeurism (Abel, 1989).

Voyeurism. This disorder is identified by recurrent, intense sexual urges, behaviors, or sexually arousing fantasies, of at least 6 months' duration, involving the act of observing an unsuspecting person who is naked, in the process of disrobing, or engaging in sexual activity (APA, 1994). Sexual excitement is achieved through the act of looking, and no contact with the person is attempted. Masturbation usually accompanies the "window peeping" but may occur later as the individual fantasizes about the voyeuristic act.

Onset of voyeuristic behavior is usually before age 15, and the disorder is often chronic. Most voyeurs enjoy satisfying sexual relationships with an adult partner. Few apprehensions occur because most targets of voyeurism are unaware that they are being observed. In addition to their voyeurism, a significant number of voyeurs are concomitantly or have previously been involved in exhibitionism, frotteurism, pedophilia, rape, or sadism (Abel, 1989).

Predisposing Factors to Paraphilias

Biological Factors. Various studies have implicated several organic factors in the etiology of paraphilias. Destruction of parts of the limbic system in animals has been shown to cause hypersexual behavior (Becker & Kavoussi, 1988). Temporal lobe diseases, such as psychomotor seizures or temporal lobe tumors, have been implicated in some paraphiliacs. Abnormal levels of androgens also may contribute to inappropriate sexual arousal. The results of these studies are inconclusive at this time. The majority of studies involved violent sex offenders and the results cannot accurately be generalized to specific paraphiliacs (Bradford & McLean, 1984).

Psychoanalytical Theory. The psychoanalytical approach defines a paraphiliac as one who has failed the normal developmental process toward heterosexual adjustment (Abel, 1989). This occurs when the individual fails to resolve the oedipal crisis and either identifies with the parent of the opposite gender or selects an inappropriate object for libido cathexis. Becker and Kavoussi (1988) offer the following explanation:

> "Severe castration anxiety during the oedipal phase of development leads to the substitution of a symbolic object (inanimate or an anatomic part) for the mother, as in fetishism and transvestism. Similarly, anxiety over arousal to the mother can lead to the choice of 'safe,' inappropriate sexual partners, as in pedophilia and zoophilia, or 'safe' sexual behaviors in which there is no sexual contact, as in exhibitionism and voyeurism."

Behavioral Theory. The behavioral model hypothesizes that whether or not an individual engages in paraphiliac behavior depends on the type of reinforcement he or she receives following the behavior. Abel (1989) suggests that the initial act may be committed for various reasons. Some examples include recalling memories of experiences from an individual's early life (especially the first shared sexual experience), modeling behavior of others who have carried out paraphilic acts, mimicking sexual behavior depicted in the media, and recalling past trauma such as one's own molestation.

Once the initial act has been committed, the paraphiliac consciously evaluates the behavior and decides whether or not to repeat it. Fear of punishment or perceived harm or injury to the victim, or a lack of pleasure derived from the experience, may lead to nonrecurrence of the paraphilic act. However, when negative consequences do not occur, when the act itself is highly pleasurable, or when the paraphilic person immediately escapes and thereby avoids seeing any negative consequences experienced by the victim, the activity is more likely to be repeated (Abel, 1989).

Transactional Model of Stress/Adaptation. Marshall and Barbaree (1990) contend that one model alone is not sufficient to explain the etiology of paraphilias. They suggest that an integration of learning experiences, sociocultural factors, and biological processes must occur to account for these deviant sexual behaviors. A combination of biological inheritance, hormonal variations, poor parenting, sociocultural attitudes, and aspects of the learning paradigm previous described probably provides the most comprehensive etiological explanation for paraphilias to date (Abel, Rouleau, & Osborn, 1994). In Figure 30.1, a graphic depiction of the theory of multiple causation is presented in the transactional model of stress/adaptation.

Treatment Modalities

Biological Treatment. Biological treatment of individuals with paraphilias has focused on blocking or decreasing the level of circulating androgens. The most extensively used of the antiandrogenic medications are the progestin derivatives that block testosterone synthesis (Becker & Kavoussi, 1988). They do not influence the direction of sexual drive toward appropriate adult partners. Instead they act to decrease libido and thus break the individual's pattern of compulsive deviant sexual behavior (Becker & Kavoussi, 1988). They are not meant to be the sole source of treatment and work best when given in conjunction with the paraphiliac's participation in individual or group psychotherapy.

Psychoanalytical Therapy. Psychoanalytical approaches have been tried in the treatment of paraphilias. In this type of therapy, the therapist assists the client to identify unresolved conflicts and traumas from early childhood. The therapy focuses on helping the individual resolve these early conflicts, thus relieving the anxiety that prevents him or her from forming appropriate sexual relationships. In turn, the individual has no further need for paraphilic fantasies.

Behavioral Therapy. Aversion techniques have been used to modify undesirable behavior. Aversion therapy methods in the treatment of paraphilias include noxious stimuli, such as electric shocks and bad odors, that are paired with the impulse, which then diminishes. The stimuli can be self-administered and used by clients whenever they feel the urge to act on the impulse (Kaplan, Sadock, & Grebb, 1994).

Other behavioral approaches to decreasing inappropriate sexual arousal have included covert sensitization and satiation. With covert sensitization, the individual combines inappropriate sexual fantasies with aversive, anxiety-provoking scenes under the guidance of the therapist (Becker & Kavoussi, 1988). Satiation is a technique in which the postorgasmic individual repeatedly fantasizes deviant behaviors to the point of saturation with the deviant stimuli, consequently making the fantasies and behavior boring (Marshall & Barbaree, 1978).

Role of the Nurse

Treatment of the paraphiliac is often very frustrating for both the client and the therapist. Most paraphiliacs deny that they have a problem and seek psychiatric care only after their inappropriate behavior comes to the attention of

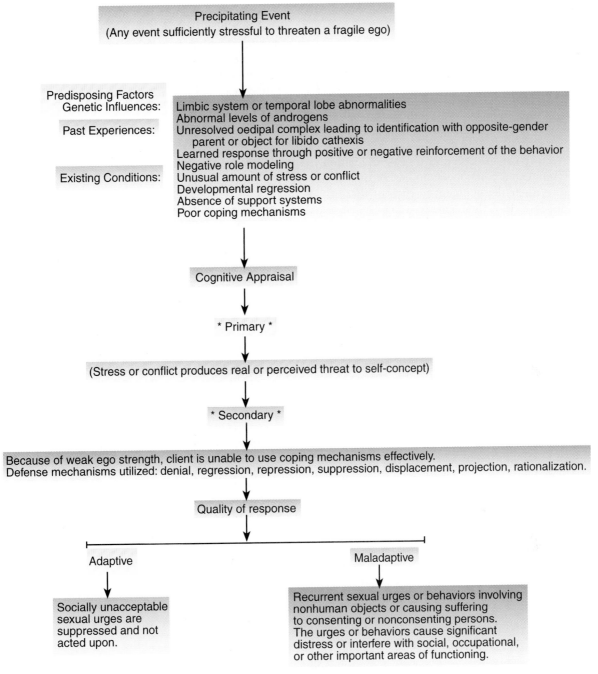

Figure 30.1 The dynamics of paraphilia using the transactional model of stress/adaptation.

others. In secondary prevention, the focus is to diagnose and treat the problem as early as possible, to minimize difficulties. These individuals should be referred to specialists who are accustomed to working with this very special population.

Nursing may best become involved in the primary prevention process. The focus of primary prevention in sexual disorders is to intervene in home life or other facets of childhood in an effort to prevent problems from developing. An additional concern of primary prevention is to as-

sist in the development of adaptive coping strategies to deal with stressful life situations.

Bancroft (1978) has suggested that there are three components of sexual development. A disturbance in one or more of these components in development might lead to a variety of sexual deviations. These three components include:

1. Gender identity—the sense of maleness or femaleness developed in early childhood.

2. Sexual responsiveness—arousal to appropriate stimuli.
3. Formation of relationships with others.

Different developmental components seem to be disturbed in the various sexual deviations. For example, gender identity may be disturbed in transvestism or transsexualism. The second component, sexual responsiveness to appropriate stimuli, is disturbed in the case of the fetishist. In the case of the exhibitionist or the frotteur, the ability to form relationships may be disturbed.

Nurses can participate in the regular evaluation of these developmental components to ensure that as children mature, their development in each of these three components is healthy, thereby preventing deviant sexual behaviors. Nurses who work in pediatrics, psychiatry, public health, ambulatory clinics, schools, and any other facility requiring contact with children must be knowledgeable about human sexual development. Accurate assessment and early intervention by these nurses can contribute a great deal toward primary prevention of sexual disorders.

Sexual Dysfunctions

The Sexual Response Cycle

Because sexual dysfunctions occur as disturbances in any of the phases of the sexual response cycle, an understanding of anatomy and physiology is a prerequisite to considerations of pathology and treatment.

Phase I: Desire. During this phase, the desire to have sexual activity occurs in response to verbal, physical, and/or visual stimulation. Sexual fantasies can also bring about this desire.

Phase II: Excitement. This is the phase of sexual arousal and erotic pleasure. Physiological changes occur. The male responds with penile tumescence and erection. Female changes include vasocongestion in the pelvis, vaginal lubrication and expansion, and swelling of the external genitalia (APA, 1994).

Phase III: Orgasm. Orgasm is identified as a peaking of sexual pleasure, with release of sexual tension and rhythmic contraction of the perineal muscles and reproductive organs (APA, 1994). Orgasm in women is marked by simultaneous rhythmic contractions of the uterus, the orgasmic platform, and the anal sphincter. In the man, a forceful emission of semen occurs in response to rhythmic spasms of the prostate, seminal vesicles, vas, and urethra (APA, 1994; Kaplan, Sadock, & Grebb, 1994).

Phase IV: Resolution. If orgasm has occurred, this phase is characterized by disgorgement of blood from the genitalia (detumescence), creating a sense of general relaxation, well-being, and muscular relaxation. If orgasm does not occur, resolution may take 2 to 6 hours and be associated with irritability and discomfort (Kaplan, Sadock, & Grebb, 1994).

After the resolution period, men have a refractory period that may last from several minutes to many hours, during which time they cannot be stimulated to further orgasm (Kaplan, Sadock, & Grebb, 1994). For most men, this interval lengthens with age. Women experience no refractory period and may be able to respond to additional stimulation almost immediately (APA, 1994).

Historical and Epidemiological Aspects Related to Sexual Dysfunction

Concurrent with the cultural changes occurring during the sexual revolution of the 1960s and 1970s came an increase in scientific research into sexual physiology and sexual dysfunctions. Masters and Johnson (1966, 1970) pioneered this work with their studies on human sexual response and the treatment of sexual dysfunctions. Sadock (1989) states:

> "Historically, problems of sexual conflict and sexual dysfunction have always been the province of psychiatry. Problems of dysfunction are particularly distressing to clients and have often been resistant to treatment. The current approach to sexual dysfunctions reflects the cultural and scientific developments of recent years, the development of specific techniques for the treatment of these problems, the historical interest of psychiatry in this area, and the recognition of its importance in psychiatric practice."

Sexual dysfunction consists of an impairment or disturbance in any of the phases of the sexual response cycle. No one knows exactly how many people experience sexual dysfunctions. Knowledge exists only about those who seek some kind of treatment for the problem, and they may be few in number compared with those who have a dysfunction but suffer quietly and never seek therapy (Hyde, 1986).

Masters and Johnson (1970) reported that 50 percent of all American couples suffer from some type of sexual dysfunction. A study by Robins and coworkers (1984) estimated that 24 percent of the U.S. population will experience a sexual dysfunction at some time in their lives. In 1990, Spector and Carey reviewed 23 studies conducted over the past 50 years in an effort to evaluate the incidence and prevalence of the sexual dysfunctions. The results of this study are presented in Table 30.1.

Types of Sexual Dysfunction

Sexual Desire Disorders

Hypoactive Sexual Desire Disorder. This disorder is defined by the *DSM-IV* (APA, 1994) as a persistent or recurrent deficiency or absence of sexual fantasies and desire for sexual activity. The judgment of deficiency or absence is made by the clinician, taking into account factors

TABLE 30.1   ESTIMATES OF PREVALENCE RATES FOR SEXUAL DYSFUNCTIONS*

DISORDER	MEN	WOMEN
Orgasm disorders		
Inhibited female orgasm		5%–10%
Inhibited male orgasm	4%–10%	
Premature ejaculation	36%–38%	
Sexual arousal disorders		
Male erectile disorder	4%–9%	
Female arousal disorders		NA

*Prevalence rate refers to an estimate of the number of people who have a disorder at any given time.
SOURCE: Adapted from Spector & Carey (1990).

that affect sexual functioning, such as age and the context of the person's life.

An individual's absolute level of sexual desire may not be the problem; rather, the problem may be a discrepancy between the partners' levels (Hyde, 1986). The conflict may occur if one partner wants to have sexual relations more often than the other. Care must be taken not to label one partner as pathological when the problem actually lies in the discrepancy of sexual desire between the partners.

An estimated 20 percent of the total population have hypoactive sexual desire disorder (Sadock, 1989). The complaint is more common in women then in men.

Sexual Aversion Disorder. This disorder is characterized by a persistent or recurrent extreme aversion to, and avoidance of, all (or almost all) genital sexual contact with a sexual partner (APA, 1994). Whereas individuals displaying hypoactive desire are often neutral or indifferent toward sexual interaction, sexual aversion implies disgust, anxiety, or even panic responses to genital contact (Leiblum & Rosen, 1988).

Sexual Arousal Disorders

Female Sexual Arousal Disorder. This disorder is identified in the *DSM-IV* as a persistent or recurrent inability to attain, or to maintain until completion of the sexual activity, an adequate lubrication/swelling response of sexual excitement.

Male Erectile Disorder. This disorder is characterized by persistent or recurrent inability to attain, or to maintain until completion of the sexual activity, an adequate erection (APA, 1994). *Primary erectile dysfunction* refers to cases in which the man has never been able to have intercourse; *secondary erectile dysfunction* refers to cases in which the man has difficulty getting or maintaining an erection but has been able to have vaginal or anal intercourse at least once (Hyde, 1986).

Orgasmic Disorders

Female Orgasmic Disorder. This disorder is defined by the *DSM-IV* as persistent or recurrent delay in, or ab-

sence of, orgasm following a normal sexual excitement phase. This condition is sometimes referred to as **anorgasmia.** Women who can achieve orgasm through noncoital clitoral stimulation but are not able to experience it during coitus in the absence of manual clitoral stimulation are not necessarily categorized as anorgasmic (Sadock, 1989).

A woman is considered to have *primary orgasmic dysfunction* when she has never experienced orgasm by any kind of stimulation. *Secondary orgasmic dysfunction* exists if the woman has experienced at least one orgasm, regardless of the means of stimulation, but no longer does so.

Male Orgasmic Disorder. This disorder, sometimes referred to as **retarded ejaculation,** is characterized by persistent or recurrent delay in, or absence of, orgasm following a normal sexual excitement phase during sexual activity that the clinician, taking into account the person's age, judges to be adequate in focus, intensity, and duration (APA, 1994). With this disorder, the man is unable to ejaculate, even though he has a firm erection and has had more than adequate stimulation (Hyde, 1986). The severity of the problem may range from only occasional problems ejaculating (secondary disorder) to a history of never having experienced an orgasm (primary disorder). In the most common version, the man cannot ejaculate during coitus but may be able to ejaculate as a result of other types of stimulation.

Premature Ejaculation. The *DSM-IV* describes **premature ejaculation** as persistent or recurrent ejaculation with minimal sexual stimulation before, on, or shortly after penetration and before the person wishes it. Diagnosis should take into account factors that affect duration of the excitement phase, such as age, novelty of the sexual partner or situation, and recent frequency of sexual activity (APA, 1994).

An estimated 30 percent of the male population have this dysfunction, and about 40 percent of men treated for sexual disorders have premature ejaculation as the chief complaint (Sadock, 1989). It is particularly common among young men who have a very high sex drive and have not yet learned to control ejaculation (Hyde, 1986).

Sexual Pain Disorders

Dyspareunia. This disorder is recurrent or persistent genital pain associated with sexual intercourse in either a man or a woman (APA, 1994). It is not caused by **vaginismus,** lack of lubrication, other general medical condition, or physiological effects of substance use. In women, the pain may be felt in the vagina, around the vaginal entrance and clitoris, or deep in the pelvis. In men, the pain is felt in the penis. **Dyspareunia** makes intercourse very unpleasant and may even lead to abstention from sexual activity (Hyde, 1986).

Prevalence studies of dyspareunia have provided estimates ranging from 8 to 33 percent in women and 1 percent in men (Wincze & Carey, 1991). Dyspareunia in men is often associated with urinary tract infection, with pain being experienced during urination as well as during ejaculation.

Vaginismus. Vaginismus is an involuntary constriction of the outer one third of the vagina that prevents penile insertion and intercourse (Sadock, 1989). Vaginismus is less prevalent than female orgasmic disorder, and most often afflicts highly educated women and those in the high socioeconomic groups (Kaplan, Sadock, & Grebb, 1994). On the basis of data obtained from infertility studies, Barnes (1981) found that vaginismus occurred in 5 out of every 1000 women, a rate of 0.5 percent.

Sexual Dysfunction Due to a General Medical Condition and Substance-Induced Sexual Dysfunction. With these disorders, the sexual dysfunction is judged to be caused by the direct physiological effects of a general medical condition or use of a substance. The dysfunction may involve pain, impaired desire, impaired arousal, or impaired orgasm. Types of medical conditions that are associated with sexual dysfunction include neurological, such as multiple sclerosis and neuropathy; endocrine, such as diabetes mellitus and thyroid dysfunctions; vascular, such as atherosclerosis; and genitourinary, such as testicular disease and urethral or vaginal infections. Substances that can interfere with sexual functioning include alcohol, amphetamines, cocaine, opioids, sedatives, hypnotics, anxiolytics, and others.

Predisposing Factors to Sexual Dysfunctions

Biological Factors

Sexual Desire Disorders. Studies have correlated decreased levels of serum testosterone with hypoactive sexual desire disorder in men (Sadock, 1989). Evidence also exists that suggests a relationship between serum testosterone and increased female libido (Segraves, 1988). Diminished libido has been observed in both men and women with elevated levels of serum prolactin (Segraves, 1988). Various medications have also been implicated in the etiology of hypoactive sexual desire disorder. Some examples include antihypertensives, antipsychotics, antidepressants, anxiolytics, and anticonvulsants. Alcohol and cocaine have also been associated with impaired desire, especially after chronic use (Abel, 1985).

Sexual Arousal Disorders. Postmenopausal women require a longer period of stimulation for lubrication to occur, and there is generally less vaginal transudate after menopause (Sadock, 1989). Various medications, particularly those with antihistaminic and anticholinergic properties, may also contribute to decreased ability for arousal in women. Arteriosclerosis is a common cause of male erectile disorder as a result of arterial insufficiency (Goldberg, 1998). Various neurological disorders can contribute to erectile dysfunctions as well. The most com-

mon neurologically based cause may be diabetes, which places men at high risk for neuropathy (Wincze & Carey, 1991). Others include temporal lobe epilepsy and multiple sclerosis. Trauma (e.g., spinal cord injury or pelvic cancer surgery) can also result in erectile dysfunction. Several medications have been implicated in the etiology of this disorder, including antihypertensives, antipsychotics, antidepressants, and anxiolytics. Chronic use of alcohol has also been shown to be a contributing factor.

Orgasmic Disorders. Results of research on the increased ability to achieve orgasm in posthysterectomy women by administering an estrogen-androgen hormone combination have been mixed (Wincze & Carey, 1991). Although the hormone replacement did influence sexual desire and arousal, effects on orgasmic response remain unclear. In a study on female orgasmic response by Malatesta and associates (1982), acute alcohol intoxication was found to be associated with difficulty achieving orgasm, as well as a decreased subjective intensity of orgasm. Some medical conditions (e.g., hypothyroidism, diabetes mellitus, and hyperprolactinemia) and some medications (e.g., antihypertensives, antidepressants) can affect a woman's ability to have orgasms (Sadock, 1989).

Biological factors associated with inhibited male orgasm include surgery of the genitourinary tract (e.g., prostatectomy), various neurological disorders (e.g., Parkinson's disease), and other diseases (e.g., diabetes mellitus). Medications that have been implicated include antihypertensives, anticholinergics, and antipsychotics. Transient cases of the disorder may occur with excessive alcohol intake (Sadock, 1989).

Although premature ejaculation is commonly caused by psychological factors, general medical conditions or substance use may also be contributing influences. Particularly in cases of secondary dysfunction, in which a man at one time had ejaculatory control but later lost it, physical factors may be involved (Hyde, 1986). Examples include a local infection such as prostatitis or a degenerative neural disorder such as multiple sclerosis.

Sexual Pain Disorders. A number of organic factors can contribute to painful intercourse in women, including intact hymen, episiotomy scar, vaginal or urinary tract infection, ligament injuries, endometriosis, or ovarian cysts or tumors.

Painful intercourse in men may also be caused by various organic factors. For example, infection caused by poor hygiene under the foreskin of an uncircumsized man can cause pain. Phimosis, a condition in which the foreskin cannot be pulled back, can also cause painful intercourse (Hyde, 1986). An allergic reaction to various vaginal spermicides or irritation caused by vaginal infections may be a contributing factor. Finally, various prostate problems may cause pain on ejaculation (Hyde, 1986).

Psychosocial Factors

Sexual Desire Disorders. LoPiccolo and Friedman (1988) have identified a number of individual and relationship causes of hypoactive sexual desire disorder. Individual causes include religious orthodoxy, obsessive-compulsive personality, conflicts with gender identity or sexual preference, sexual phobias, fear of losing control over sexual urges, secret sexual deviations, fear of pregnancy, "widower's syndrome" (inadequate grieving following the death of a spouse), depression, and aging-related concerns (e.g., changes in physical appearance). Among the relationship causes are lack of physical attraction to one's partner, poor sexual skills in the partner, conflict in the marriage, and fear of closeness (for fear of personal vulnerability or rejection).

Sadock (1989) describes the possible etiology of sexual aversion disorder as follows:

"The disorder may result from a traumatic sexual assault, such as rape or childhood abuse, from repeated painful experiences with coitus, and from early developmental conflicts that have left the client with unconscious connections between the sexual impulse and overwhelming feelings of shame and guilt. The disorder may also be a reaction to a perceived psychological assault by one's partner and to relationship difficulties."

Sexual Arousal Disorders. A number of psychological factors have been cited as possible impediments to female arousal. They include doubt, guilt, fear, anxiety, shame, conflict, embarrassment, tension, disgust, irritation, resentment, grief, hostility toward partner, and a puritanical or moralistic upbringing. Clinical experience suggests that history of sexual abuse may also be an important etiological factor (Becker, 1989).

The etiology of male erectile disorder may be related to an inability to express the sexual impulse because of fear, anxiety, anger, or moral prohibition (Sadock, 1989). Developmental factors that hinder the ability to be intimate, that lead to a feeling of inadequacy or distrust, or that develop a sense of being unloving or unlovable may also result in impotence. Relationship factors that may affect erectile functioning include lack of attraction to one's partner, anger toward one's partner, or being in a relationship that is not characterized by trust (Wincze & Carey, 1991). Unfortunately, regardless of the etiology of the impotence, once it occurs, the man may become increasingly anxious about his next sexual encounter. This anticipatory anxiety about achieving and maintaining an erection may then perpetuate the problem.

Orgasmic Disorders. Numerous psychological factors are associated with inhibited female orgasm. They include fears of becoming pregnant or rejection by the sexual partner, hostility toward men, and feelings of guilt regarding sexual impulses (Sadock, 1989). Negative cultural conditioning ("nice girls don't enjoy sex") may also influence the adult female's sexual response. Various developmental factors also have relevance to orgasmic dysfunction. Examples include childhood exposure to rigid religious orthodoxy, negative family attitudes toward nudity and sex, and traumatic sexual experiences during childhood or adolescence,

such as incest or rape (Kolodny, Masters, & Johnson, 1979; Kaplan, & Sadock, 1998).

Psychological factors are also associated with inhibited male orgasm. In the primary disorder (never experienced prior orgasm), the man often comes from a rigid, puritanical background. He perceives sex as sinful and the genitals as dirty, and he may have conscious or unconscious incest wishes and guilt (Sadock, 1989). In the case of secondary disorder (previously experienced orgasms that have now stopped), interpersonal difficulties are usually implicated. There may be some ambivalence about commitment, fear of pregnancy, or unexpressed hostility.

Kaplan (1974) focused on the main cause of premature ejaculation as being the man's lack of awareness of the premonitory sensations before ejaculation. The ability to control ejaculation occurs as a gradual maturing process with a sexual partner in which foreplay becomes more give-and-take "pleasuring," rather than strictly goal-oriented. The man becomes aware of the sensations and learns to delay the point of ejaculatory inevitability. Relationship problems such as a stressful marriage, unexpressed anger, anxiety over intimacy, and lack of comfort in the sexual relationship may also contribute to this disorder (McCarthy, 1989).

Sexual Pain Disorders. Vaginismus may occur in response to having experienced dyspareunia (painful intercourse) for various organic reasons stated in the "Biological Factors" section. This previous experience results in involuntary constriction within the vagina in response to anticipatory pain, making intercourse impossible. No organic process can be implicated as the cause of vaginismus itself (Kaplan & Sadock, 1998). A variety of psychosocial factors have been implicated, including negative childhood conditioning of sex as dirty, sinful, and shameful. Early traumatic sexual experiences (e.g., rape or incest) may also cause vaginismus. Other factors that may be important in the etiology of vaginismus include homosexual orientation, traumatic experience with an early pelvic examination, pregnancy phobia, venereal disease phobia, or cancer phobia (Kolodny, Masters, & Johnson, 1979; Kaplan & Sadock, 1998).

Transactional Model of Stress/Adaptation. The etiology of sexual dysfunction is most likely influenced by multiple factors. In Figure 30.2, a graphic depiction of the theory of multiple causation is presented in the transactional model of stress/adaptation.

Application of the Nursing Process to Sexual Disorders

Assessment. Most assessment tools for taking a general nursing history contain some questions devoted to sexuality. It is a subject about which many nurses feel uncomfortable obtaining information. However, accurate data must be collected if problems are to be identified and resolutions attempted. Sexual health is an integral part of

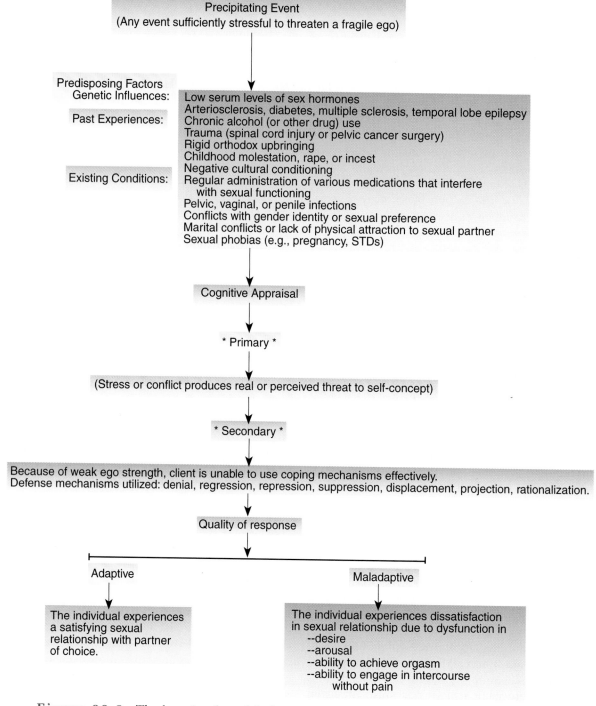

Figure 30.2   The dynamics of sexual dysfunction using the transactional model of stress/adaptation.

physical and emotional well-being. The nursing history is incomplete if items directed toward sexuality are not included.

Indeed, most nurses are not required to obtain a sexual history as in-depth as the one presented in this chapter. However, certain clients require a more extensive sexual history than that which is included in the general nursing history. These include clients who have medical or surgical conditions that may affect their sexuality; clients with infertility problems, sexually transmitted disease, or complaints of sexual inadequacy; clients who are pregnant or present with gynecological problems; those seeking information on abortion or family planning; and individuals in premarital, marital, and psychiatric counseling (Hogan, 1980).

The best approach for taking a sexual history is a nondirective one; that is, it is best to use the sexual history

TABLE 30.2   SEXUAL HISTORY: CONTENT OUTLINE

I. Identify data
  A. Client
    1. Age.
    2. Gender.
    3. Marital status.
  B. Parents
    1. Ages.
    2. Dates of death and ages at death.
    3. Birthplace.
    4. Marital status.
    5. Religion.
    6. Education.
    7. Occupation.
    8. Congeniality.
    9. Demonstration of affection.
    10. Feelings toward parents.
  C. Siblings (same information as above)
  D. Marital partner (same information as above)
  E. Children
    1. Ages.
    2. Gender.
    3. Strengths.
    4. Identified problems.

II. Childhood sexuality
  A. Family attitudes about sex
    1. Parents' openness about sex.
    2. Parents' attitudes about nudity.
  B. Learning about sex
    1. Asking parents about sex.
    2. Information volunteered by parents.
    3. At what age and how did client learn about: pregnancy, birth, intercourse, masturbation, nocturnal emissions, menstruation, homosexuality, STDs.
  C. Childhood sex activity
    1. First sight of nude body:
      a. Same gender.
      b. Opposite gender.
    2. First genital self-stimulation:
      a. Age.
      b. Feelings
      c. Consequences.
    3. First sexual exploration at play with another child:
      a. Age (of self and other child).
      b. Gender of other child.
      c. Nature of the activity.
      d. Feelings and consequences.
    4. Sexual activity with older persons:
      a. Age (of self and other person).
      b. Gender of other person.
      c. Nature of the activity.
      d. Client willingness to participate.
      e. Feelings and consequences.
  D. Did you ever see your parents (or others) having intercourse? Describe your feelings.
  E. Childhood sexual theories or myths:
    1. Thoughts about conception and birth.
    2. Roles of male/female genitals and other body parts in sexuality.

III. Onset of adolescence
  A. In girls:
    1. Information about menstruation:
      a. How received; from whom.
      b. Age received.
      c. Feelings.
    2. Age:
      a. Of first period.
      b. When breasts began to develop.
      c. At appearance of ancillary and pubic hair.
    3. Menstruation:
      a. Regularity; discomfort; duration.
      b. Feelings about first period.
  B. In boys:
    1. Information about puberty:
      a. How received; from whom.
      b. Age received.
      c. Feelings.
    2. Age:
      a. Of appearance of ancillary and public hair.
      b. Change of voice.
      c. First orgasm (with or without ejaculation); emotional reaction.

IV. Orgastic experiences
  A. Nocturnal emissions (male) or orgasms (female) during sleep
    1. Frequency.
  B. Masturbation
    1. Age begun; ever punished?
    2. Frequency; methods used.
    3. Marital partner's knowledge.
    4. Practiced with others? Spouse?
    5. Emotional reactions.
    6. Accompanying fantasies.
  C. Necking and petting ("making out")
    1. Age when begun.
    2. Frequency.
    3. Number of partners.
    4. Types of activity.
  D. Premarital intercourse
    1. Frequency.
    2. Relationship with and number of partners.
    3. Contraceptives used.
    4. Feelings.
  E. Orgasmic frequency
    1. Past.
    2. Present.

V. Feelings about self as masculine/feminine
  A. The male client:
    1. Does he feel masculine?
    2. Accepted by peers?
    3. Sexually adequate?
    4. Feelings/concerns about body:
      a. Size.
      b. Appearance.
      c. Function.
  B. The female client:
    1. Does she feel feminine?
    2. Accepted by peers?
    3. Sexually adequate?

Continued on following page

TABLE 30.2   SEXUAL HISTORY: CONTENT OUTLINE *(Continued)*

4. Feelings/concerns about body:
   a. Size.
   b. Appearance.
   c. Function.

VI. Sexual fantasies and dreams
   A. Nature of sex dreams
   B. Nature of fantasies
      1. During masturbation.
      2. During intercourse.

VII. Dating
   A. Age and feelings about:
      1. First date.
      2. First kissing.
      3. First petting or "making out."
      4. First going steady.

VIII. Engagement
   A. Age
   B. Sex activity during engagement period:
      1. With fiancee.
      2. With others.

IX. Marriage
   A. Date of marriage.
   B. Age at marriage: Spouse:
   C. Spouse's occupation.
   D. Previous marriages: Spouse:
   E. Reason for termination of previous marriages:
      Client: Spouse:
   F. Children from previous marriages:
      Client: Spouse:
   G. Wedding trip (honeymoon):
      1. Where? How long?
      2. Pleasant or unpleasant?
      3. Sexual considerations?
   H. Sex in marriage:
      1. General satisfaction/dissatisfaction.
      2. Thoughts about spouse's general
         satisfaction/dissatisfaction.
   I. Pregnancies
      1. Number: Ages of couple:
      2. Results (normal birth, cesarean delivery,
         miscarriage, abortion).
      3. Planned or unplanned.
      4. Effects on sexual adjustment.
      5. Sex of child wanted or
         unwanted.

X. Extramarital sex
   A. Emotional attachments
      1. Number; frequency; feelings.
   B. Sexual intercourse
      1. Number; frequency; feelings.
   C. Postmarital masturbation
      1. Frequency; feelings.
   D. Postmarital homosexuality
      1. Frequency; feelings.
   E. Multiple sex ("swinging")
      1. Frequency; feelings.

XI. Sex after widowhood, separation, or divorce:
   A. Outlet
      1. Orgasms in sleep.
      2. Masturbation.
      3. Petting.
      4. Intercourse.
      5. Homosexuality.
      6. Other.
   B. Frequency; feelings

XII. Sexual variations and disorders:
   A. Homosexuality
      1. First experience; describe circumstances.
      2. Frequency since adolescence.
   B. Sexual contact with animals
      1. First experience; describe nature of
         contact.
      2. Frequency and recent contact.
      3. Feelings.
   C. Voyeurism
      1. Describe types of observation experienced.
      2. Feelings.
   D. Exhibitionism
      1. To whom? When?
      2. Feelings.
   E. Fetishes; transvestism
      1. Nature of fetish.
      2. Nature of transvestite activity.
      3. Feelings.
   F. Sadomasochism
      1. Nature of activity.
      2. Sexual response.
      3. Frequency; recency.
      4. Consequences.
   G. Seduction and rape
      1. Has client seduced/raped another?
      2. Has client ever been seduced/raped?
   H. Incest
      1. Nature of the sexual activity.
      2. With whom?
      3. When occurred? Frequency; recency.
      4. Consequences.
   I. Prostitution
      1. Has client ever accepted/paid money for sex?
      2. Type of sexual activity engaged in.
      3. Feelings about prostitution.

XIII. Certain effects of sex activities
   A. STDs
      1. Age at learning about STDs.
      2. Type of STD contracted.
      3. Age and treatment received.
   B. Illegitimate pregnancy
      1. At what age(s).
      2. Outcome of the pregnancy(ies).
      3. Feelings.
   C. Abortion
      1. Why performed?
      2. At what age(s)?
      3. How often?
      4. Before or after marriage?

◼ TABLE 30.2 SEXUAL HISTORY: CONTENT OUTLINE

5. Circumstances: who, where, how?	2. Mild pleasure.
6. Feelings about abortion: at the time; in retrospect; anniversary reaction.	3. Disinterest; disgust.
	B. Use in connection with sexual activity
XIV. Use of erotic material	1. Type and frequency of use.
A. Personal response to erotic material	2. To accompany what type of sexual activity.
1. Sexual pleasure—arousal.	

SOURCE: Adapted from an outline prepared by the Group for Advancement of Psychiatry, based on the Sexual Performance Evaluation Questionnaire of the Marriage Council of Philadelphia. Used with permission.

outline as a guideline but allow the interview to progress in a less restrictive manner than the outline permits (with one question immediately following the other). The order of the questions should be adjusted according to the client's needs as they are identified during the interview. A nondirective approach allows time for the client to interject information related to feelings or concerns about his or her sexuality.

The language used should be understandable to the client. If he or she uses terminology that is unfamiliar, ask for clarification. Take level of education and cultural influences into consideration.

The nurse's attitude must convey warmth, openness, honesty, and objectivity. Personal feelings, attitudes, and values should be clarified and should not interfere with acceptance of the client. The nurse must remain nonjudgmental. This is conveyed by listening in an interested, but matter-of-fact, manner without overreacting or underreacting to any information the client may present.

The content outline for a sexual history presented in Table 30.2 is not intended to be used as a rigid questionnaire but as guidelines from which the nurse may select appropriate topics for gathering information about the client's sexuality. The outline should be individualized according to client needs.

Diagnosis/Outcome Identification. Nursing diagnoses are formulated from the data gathered during the assessment phase and with background knowledge regarding predisposing factors to the disorder. The following nursing diagnoses may be used for the client with sexual disorders:

Sexual dysfunction related to depression and conflict in relationship or to certain biological or psychological contributing factors, evidenced by loss of sexual desire.

Altered sexuality patterns related to conflicts with sexual orientation or variant preferences, evidenced by expressed dissatisfaction with sexual behaviors (e.g., voyeurism, transvestism).

The following criteria may be used for measurement of outcomes in the care of the client with sexual disorders.

THE CLIENT:

1. Can correlate stressful situations that decrease sexual desire.
2. Can communicate with partner about sexual situation without discomfort.
3. Can verbalize ways to enhance sexual desire.
4. Verbalizes resumption of sexual activity at level satisfactory to self and partner.
5. Can correlate variant behaviors with times of stress.
6. Can verbalize fears about abnormality and inappropriateness of sexual behaviors.
7. Expresses desire to change variant sexual behavior.
8. Participates and cooperates with extended plan of behavior modification.
9. Expresses satisfaction with own sexuality pattern.

Planning/Implementation. Table 30.3 provides a plan of care for the client with sexual disorders. Nursing diagnoses are presented, along with outcome criteria, appropriate nursing interventions, and rationales.

Client/Family Education. The role of client teacher is important in the psychiatric area, as it is in all areas of nursing. A list of topics for client and family education relevant to sexual disorders is presented in Table 30.4.

Evaluation. Reassessment is necessary to determine if selected interventions have been successful in assisting the client to overcome problems with sexual functioning. Evaluation may be facilitated by gathering information using the following types of questions.

For the client with sexual dysfunction:

1. Has the client identified life situations that promote feelings of depression and decreased sexual desire?
2. Can he or she verbalize ways to deal with this stress?
3. Can the client satisfactorily communicate with sexual partner about the problem?
4. Have the client and sexual partner identified ways to enhance sexual desire and the achievement of sexual satisfaction for both?
5. Are client and partner seeking assistance with relationship conflict?
6. Do both partners agree on what the major problem is? Do they have the motivation to attempt change?

TABLE 30.3 CARE PLAN FOR THE CLIENT WITH A SEXUAL DISORDER

NURSING DIAGNOSIS: SEXUAL DYSFUNCTION

RELATED TO: Depression and conflict in relationship; biological or psychological factors contributing to the disorder

EVIDENCED BY: Loss of sexual desire

OUTCOME CRITERIA	NURSING INTERVENTIONS	RATIONALE
Client identifies stressors that contribute to loss of sexual desire. Client resumes sexual activity at level satisfactory to self and partner.	1. Assess client's sexual history and previous level of satisfaction in sexual relationship. 2. Assess client's perception of the problem. 3. Help client determine time dimension associated with the onset of the problem and discuss what was happening in life situation at that time. 4. Assess client's level of energy. 5. Review medication regimen; observe for side effects. 6. Provide information regarding sexuality and sexual functioning. 7. Refer for additional counseling or sex therapy if required.	1. Client history establishes a database from which to work and provides a foundation for goal setting. 2. Client's idea of what constitutes a problem may differ from the nurse's. It is the client's perception on which the goals of care must be established. 3. Stress in all areas of life will affect sexual functioning. Client may be unaware of correlation between stress and sexual dysfunction. 4. Fatigue decreases client's desire and enthusiasm for participation in sexual activity. 5. Many medications can affect sexual functioning. Evaluation of drug and individual response is important to ascertain whether drug is responsible for the problem. 6. Increasing knowledge and correcting misconceptions can decrease feelings of powerlessness and anxiety and facilitate problem resolution. 7. Client and partner may need additional or more in-depth assistance if problems in sexual relationship are severe or remain unresolved.

NURSING DIAGNOSIS: ALTERED SEXUALITY PATTERNS

RELATED TO: Conflicts with sexual orientation or variant preferences

EVIDENCED BY: Expressed dissatisfaction with sexual behaviors (e.g., voyeurism, transvestism)

OUTCOME CRITERIA	NURSING INTERVENTIONS	RATIONALE
Client will express satisfaction with own sexuality pattern.	1. Take sexual history, noting client's expression of areas of dissatisfaction with sexual pattern. 2. Assess areas of stress in client's life and examine relationship with sexual partner. 3. Note cultural, social, ethnic, racial, and religious factors that may contribute to conflicts regarding variant sexual practices. 4. Be accepting and nonjudgmental. 5. Assist therapist in plan of behavior modification to help client decrease variant behaviors.	1. Knowledge of what client perceives as the problem is essential for providing the type of assistance he or she may need. 2. Variant sexual behaviors are often associated with added stress in the client's life. 3. Client may be unaware of the influence these factors exert in creating feelings of shame and guilt. 4. Sexuality is a very personal and sensitive subject. The client is more likely to share this information if he or she does not fear being judged by the nurse. 5. Individuals with paraphilias are treated by specialists who have experience in modifying variant sexual behaviors. Nurses can intervene by providing assistance with implementation of the plan for behavior modification.

6. Teach client that sexuality is a normal human response and is not synonymous with any one sexual act; that it involves complex interrelationships among one's self-concept, body image, personal history, family and cultural influences; and all interactions with others (Vande-Vusse & Simandl, 1992).

6. If client feels abnormal or very unlike everyone else, the self-concept is likely to be very low—even worthless. Helping him or her to see that even though the behavior is variant, feelings and motivations are common may help to increase feelings of self-worth and desire to change behavior.

7. Do client and partner verbalize an increase in sexual satisfaction?

For the client with variant sexual behaviors:

1. Can the client correlate an increase in variant sexual behavior to times of severe stress?
2. Has the client been able to identify those stressful situations and verbalize alternative ways to deal with them?
3. Does the client express a desire to change variant sexual behavior and a willingness to cooperate with extended therapy to do so?
4. Does the client express an understanding about the normality of sexual feelings, aside from the inappropriateness of his or her behavior?
5. Are expressions of increased self-worth evident?

Treatment Modalities For Sexual Dysfunctions

Sexual Desire Disorders

Hypoactive Sexual Desire Disorder. This disorder has been treated in the past in both men and women with the administration of testosterone. The masculinizing side effects makes this approach unacceptable to women, and there is no conclusive evidence that it increases libido in men, even when normal levels are low (Bancroft, 1984).

Becker and Kavoussi (1994) describe the most effective treatment as a combination of cognitive therapy to deal with maladaptive beliefs; psychodynamic therapy to explore intrapsychic conflicts; behavioral treatment, such as exercises to enhance sexual pleasuring and communication; and relationship therapy to deal with the individual's use of sex as a method of control.

Low sexual desire is not uncommonly the result of partner incompatibility. If this is the case, the therapist may choose to shift from the sexual issue to helping a couple identify and deal with their incompatibility (Wincze & Carey, 1991).

Sexual Aversion Disorder. Systematic desensitization (see Chapter 27) is often the treatment of choice for this disorder, to reduce the client's fear and avoidance of sex (Becker & Kavoussi, 1994). Gradual exposure, under relaxed conditions, to imagined and actual sexual situations decreases the amount of anxiety generated by these experiences. Successful treatment of sexual phobias has also been reported by Kaplan (1979) using tricyclic or monoamine oxidase inhibitor medications and psychosexual therapy aimed at developing insight into unconscious conflicts.

Sexual Arousal Disorders

Female Sexual Arousal Disorder. The goal of treatment is to reduce the anxiety associated with sexual activity. Masters and Johnson (1970) reported successful results using their behaviorally oriented **sensate focus** exercises to treat this disorder. The objective is to reduce the goal-

> ▰ **TABLE 30.4 TOPICS FOR CLIENT/FAMILY EDUCATION RELATED TO SEXUAL DISORDERS**
>
> **Nature of the Illness**
> 1. The human sexual response cycle
> 2. What is "normal" and "abnormal"?
> 3. Types of sexual dysfunctions
> 4. Cause of sexual dysfunctions
> 5. Types of paraphilias
> 6. Causes of paraphilias
> 7. Symptoms associated with sexual dysfunctions and paraphilias
>
> **Management of the Disorder**
> 1. Teach practices and ways of sexual expression.
> 2. Teach relaxation techniques.
> 3. Teach side effects of medications that may be contributing to sexual dysfunction.
> 4. Teach effects of alcohol consumption on sexual functioning.
> 5. Teach about sexually transmitted diseases (see Table 30.6).
>
> **Support Services**
> 1. Provide appropriate referral for assistance from sex therapist
> 2. One national association to which many qualified sex therapists belong is:
>   American Association of Sex Educators, Counselors and Therapists
>   435 N. Michigan Avenue, Suite 1717
>   Chicago, IL 60611–4067
>   (312) 644-0828

oriented demands of intercourse on both the man and the woman, thus reducing performance pressures and anxiety associated with possible failure. Kolodny and colleagues (1979) describe sensate focus exercises in the following manner:

"The couple are instructed to take turns touching one another's bodies—avoiding the breasts and genitals—to establish a sense of tactile awareness by noticing textures, contours, temperatures, and contrasts (while doing the touching) or to be aware of the sensations of being touched by their partner. They are carefully instructed that sexual excitation is not the purpose of this exercise (although it may occur); instead, their attention should focus on their own physical sensations and should minimize cognitive processes. The couple gradually moves through various levels of sensate focus that progress from nongenital touching to touching that includes the breasts and genitals; touching that is done in a simultaneous, mutual format rather than by one person at a time; and touching that extends to and allows eventually for the possibility of intercourse."

Male Erectile Disorder. Sensate focus has been used effectively for male erectile disorder as well. Clinicians widely agree that even when significant organic factors have been identified, psychological factors may also be present and must be considered in treatment (Wincze & Carey, 1991).

Group therapy, hypnotherapy, and systematic desensitization have also been used successfully in reducing the anxiety that may contribute to erectile difficulties. Psychodynamic interventions may help alleviate intrapsychic conflicts contributing to performance anxiety (Becker & Kavoussi, 1994).

Various medications, including testosterone and yohimbine, have been used to treat male erectile dysfunction. Penile injections of papaverine or prostaglandin have been used to produce an erection lasting from 1 to 4 hours (Abel, Rouleau, & Osborn, 1994).

The most recent medication to be approved by the Federal Drug Administration in the treatment of erectile dysfunction is sildenafil (Viagra). Sildenafil blocks the action of phosphodiesterase (PDE5), an enzyme that breaks down cyclic guanosine monophosphate (cGMP), a compound that is required to produce an erection. This action only occurs, however, in the presence of nitric oxide (NO), which is released during sexual arousal. Sildenafil does not result in sexual arousal. It works to achieve penile erection in the presence of sexual arousal. In research trials, sildenafil was effective in improving erections for 63 to 82 percent of men who took from 25- to 100-mg dosages. Adverse effects include headache, facial flushing, indigestion, nasal congestion, dizziness, and visual changes (color tinges and blurred vision that was mild and temporary in nature) (Goldberg, 1998).

Goldberg (1998) also reports that two other oral medications for erectile dysfunction, apomorphine and phentolamine, are being investigated at this time. Also being investigated are a variety of topical creams, intraurethral agents, and new injection agents for men who do not respond to the current available treatments.

For erectile dysfunction refractory to current medication therapy, penile prostheses may be implanted. Two basic types are currently available: a bendable silicone implant and an inflatable device. The bendable variety requires a relatively simple surgical technique for insertion of silicone rods into the erectile areas of the penis. This results in a perpetual state of semierection for the client. The inflatable penile prosthesis produces an erection only when it is desired, and the appearance of the penis in both the flaccid and erect states is completely normal. Potential candidates for penile implantation should undergo careful psychological and physical screening. Although penile implants do not enable the client to recover the ability to ejaculate or to have an orgasm, men with prosthetic devices have generally reported satisfaction with their subsequent sexual functioning (Kaplan, Sadock, & Grebb, 1994).

Female Orgasmic Disorder. Because anxiety may contribute to the lack of orgasmic ability in women, sensate focus is often advised to reduce anxiety, increase awareness of physical sensations, and transfer communication skills from the verbal to the nonverbal domain (Kolodny, Masters, & Johnson, 1979). LoPiccolo and Stock (1986) describe a program of directed masturbation training for the individual with primary anorgasmia (never having had an orgasm). The systematic program involves discussion of feelings, special exercises, and gradual self-exploration of the body, and moves toward focused genital stimulation in combination with sexual fantasies. Treatment for secondary anorgasmia (had orgasms, then stopped) focuses on the couple and their relationship. Therapy with both partners is essential to the success of this disorder.

Male Orgasmic Disorder. Treatment for this disorder is very similar to that described for the anorgasmic woman. A combination of sensate focus and masturbatory training has been used with a high degree of success in the Masters and Johnson (1970) clinic. Treatment for male orgasmic disorder almost always includes the sexual partner.

Premature Ejaculation. Masters and Johnson (1970) developed a highly successful technique for the treatment of premature ejaculation. Sensate focus is used, with progression to genital stimulation. When the man reaches the point of imminent ejaculation, the woman is instructed to apply the "squeeze" technique—applying pressure at the base of the glans penis with her thumb and first two fingers. Pressure is held for 5 seconds and then released. This technique is continued until the man is no longer on the verge of ejaculating. This technique is practiced during subsequent periods of sexual stimulation. Kolodny and associates (1979) state, "For unknown neurophysiological reasons, this maneuver reduces the urgency of ejaculatory tension and, used with consistency, reconditions the pattern of ejaculatory timing to improve control surprisingly well."

Sexual Pain Disorders

Dyspareunia. Treatment for the pain of intercourse begins with a thorough physical and gynecological examination. When organic pathology has been eliminated, the client's fears and anxieties underlying sexual functioning are investigated (Becker & Kavoussi, 1994). Systematic desensitization has been used successfully to decrease fears and anxieties associated with painful intercourse.

Vaginismus. Treatment of this disorder begins with education of the woman and her sexual partner regarding the anatomy and physiology of the disorder (i.e., what exactly is occurring during the vaginismus reflex and possible etiologies). The involuntary nature of the disorder is stressed in an effort to alleviate the perception on the part of the sexual partner that this occurrence is an act of willful withholding by the woman (Kolodny, Masters, & Johnson, 1979).

The second phase of treatment involves systematic desensitization. The client is taught a series of tensing and relaxing exercises aimed at relaxation of the pelvic musculature. Relaxation of the pelvic muscles is followed by a procedure involving the systematic insertion of dilators of graduated sizes until the woman is able to accept the penis into the vagina without discomfort. This physical therapy, combined with treatment of any identified relationship problems, has been used by the Masters and Johnson (1970) clinic with a high degree of success.

GENDER IDENTITY DISORDERS

Gender identity is the sense of knowing to which sex one belongs—that is, the awareness of one's masculinity or femininity. Gender identity disorders occur when there is an incongruence between anatomical sex and gender identity. The *DSM-IV* categorizes diagnosis of the disorder according to the client's current age: gender identity disorder in children and gender identity disorder in adolescents or adults. Although most cases of the disorder begin in childhood, persons who present clinically with gender identity problems may be of any age (Kaplan, Sadock, & Grebb, 1994). It is for this reason that they are categorized together.

For purposes of this text, differentiation between the age groups will be discussed, but the major focus will be on the disorder as it emerges in childhood. Nurses who work in areas of primary prevention with children can make the greatest impact in terms of treating this disorder. Treatment aimed at reversal in behavior is considered cautiously optimistic if initiated in childhood. After one has established a clear-cut core gender identity, it is difficult later in life to instill attributes of an opposite identity (Kaplan & Sadock, 1985).

Predisposing Factors

Biological Influences. Abel, Rouleau, and Osborn (1994) report the results of a study with girls and women diagnosed with congenital adrenal hyperplasia (CAH). The data are interesting but inconclusive. They state:

"In this condition, the adrenal gland does not produce normal amounts of corticosteroids, which causes an increase in testosterone production and the subsequent masculinization of the external genitalia. Although the girls with CAH are more masculine in gender role behavior, the evidence of frank identity disorder is not clear."

Because the incidence of gender identity disorder is relatively low, genetic studies have been difficult to conduct. Becker and Kavoussi (1994) state, "To date, no clear increase in familial incidence has been demonstrated."

Family Dynamics. It appears that family dynamics plays the most influential role in the etiology of gender disorders. In Green's (1976) classic study with feminine boys, he concluded that the requisite variable was that, as any feminine behavior began to emerge, there was no discouragement of that behavior by the child's principal caretaker. He found this to be the case in nearly every family. This type of family influence may include strong interests in opposite-gender activities and weak reinforcement of normative gender-role behavior by the parents. In boys, there may also be an absence or unavailability of a father and encouragement of extreme physical and psychological closeness with her son by the mother.

Psychoanalytical Theory. The psychoanalytical theory suggests that gender identity problems begin during the struggle of the oedipal conflict. Problems may reflect both real family events and those created in the imagination of the child. These conflicts, whether real or imagined, interfere with the child's loving of the opposite-gender parent and identifying with the same-gender parent, and ultimately with normal gender identity.

Application of the Nursing Process to Gender Identity Disorders

Background Assessment Data (Symptomatology)

Gender Identity Disorder in Children. The *DSM-IV* describes the manifestations of this disorder as the presence of four (or more) of the following:

1. Repeatedly stated desire to be, or insistence that he or she is, the other sex.
2. In boys, preference for cross-dressing or simulating female attire; in girls, insistence on wearing only stereotypical masculine clothing.
3. Strong and persistent preferences for cross-sex roles in make-believe play or persistent fantasies of being the other sex.
4. Intense desire to participate in the stereotypical games and pastimes of the other sex.
5. Strong preference for playmates of the other sex.

They may be subjected to teasing and rejection by their peers and disapproval from family members. This occurs early in childhood for boys, but often does not occur before adolescence in girls. Because of this rejection, interpersonal relationships are hampered. The disorder is not common but occurs more frequently in boys than in girls.

Gender Identity Disorder in Adolescents and Adults. The *DSM-IV* describes this disorder as one in which there is a strong and persistent cross-gender identification (not merely a desire for any perceived cultural advantages of being the other sex) (APA, 1994). Symptomatic manifestations include a stated desire to be of the opposite gender, frequently passing as the opposite gender, a desire to live or be treated as the opposite gender, or the conviction that he or she has the typical feelings and reactions of the opposite gender (APA, 1994). These symptoms are accompanied by a persistent discomfort with or sense of inappropriateness in the assigned gender role. Some individuals are so convinced they were born the wrong gender that they become preoccupied with methods to eliminate the sex characteristics of the assigned gender, such as requesting opposite gender hormones or surgery to alter sexual characteristics.

Diagnosis/Outcome Identification

Kaplan, Sadock, and Grebb (1994) report that intervention with adolescents and adults with gender identity disorder is difficult. Adolescents commonly act out and rarely have the motivation required to alter their cross-gender roles. Adults generally seek therapy to learn how to cope with their altered sexual identity, not to correct it. Becker and Kavoussi (1994) state,

> "Treatment of the child with gender identity disorder is offered in an attempt to help the child avoid peer ostracism and humiliation, be comfortable with his or her own sex, and avoid the possible development of adult gender dissatisfaction."

Most of the treatment conducted with children with this disorder has been in outpatient clinics. Nurses working in these settings may encounter these clients from time to time, although the disorder is not common. One-to-one nursing intervention may be provided by a master's-prepared psychiatric clinical nurse specialist.

Based on the data collected during the nursing assessment, possible nursing diagnoses for the client with gender identity disorder in children may include:

Personal identity disturbance related to parenting patterns that encourage culturally unacceptable behaviors for assigned gender.

Impaired social interaction related to socially and culturally unacceptable behaviors.

Self-esteem disturbance related to rejection by peers.

The following criteria may be used for measurement of outcomes in the care of the client with gender identity disorder in children.

THE CLIENT:

1. Demonstrates trust in a therapist of the same gender.
2. Demonstrates development of a close relationship with the parent of the same gender.
3. Demonstrates interruption in the excessively close relationship with the parent of the opposite gender.
4. Demonstrates behaviors that are culturally appropriate for assigned gender.
5. Verbalizes and demonstrates comfort in, and satisfaction with, assigned gender role.
6. Interacts appropriately with others demonstrating culturally acceptable behaviors.
7. Verbalizes and demonstrates self-satisfaction with assigned gender role.

Planning/Implementation

Table 30.5 provides a plan of care for the client with gender identity disorder in children. Nursing diagnoses are presented, along with outcome criteria, appropriate nursing interventions, and rationales.

Evaluation

The final step of the nursing process is to determine if the nursing interventions have been effective in achieving the intended goals of care. This evaluation process requires that the nurse reassess the client's behaviors and determine if the changes at which the interventions had been directed have occurred. For the child with gender identity disorder, this may be accomplished by using the following types of questions:

1. Does the client demonstrate use of behaviors that are culturally accepted for his or her assigned gender?
2. Does the client perceive that a problem existed that requires a change in behavior for resolution?
3. Can the client use these culturally accepted behaviors in interactions with others?
4. Is the client accepted by peers when same-sex behaviors are used?
5. If the client is refusing to change behaviors, what is peer reaction?
6. What is the client's response to negative peer reaction?
7. Can the client verbalize positive statements about self?

TABLE 30.5 CARE PLAN FOR THE CLIENT WITH GENDER IDENTITY DISORDER IN CHILDREN

NURSING DIAGNOSIS: PERSONAL IDENTITY DISTURBANCE

RELATED TO: Parenting patterns that encourage culturally unacceptable behaviors for assigned gender

EVIDENCED BY: Statements of desiring to be of the opposite gender; exhibiting behaviors culturally associated with the opposite gender

OUTCOME CRITERIA	NURSING INTERVENTIONS	RATIONALE
Client will verbalize knowledge of and demonstrate behaviors that are appropriate and culturally acceptable for assigned gender.	1. Spend time with client and show positive regard. 2. Be aware of own feelings and attitudes toward this client and his or her behavior. 3. Allow client to describe his or her perception of the problem. 4. Discuss with client the types of behaviors that are more culturally acceptable. Practice these behaviors through role-playing or with play therapy strategies (e.g., male and female dolls). Positive reinforcement or social attention may be given for use of appropriate behaviors. No response is given for opposite-sex-stereotype behaviors.	1. Trust and unconditional acceptance are essential to the establishment of a therapeutic nurse-client relationship. 2. Attitudes influence behavior. The nurse must not allow negative attitudes to interfere with the effectiveness of interventions. 3. It is important to know how the client perceives the problem before attempting to correct misperceptions. 4. The goal is to enhance culturally appropriate same-sex behaviors, but not necessarily to extinguish all coexisting opposite-sex behaviors (Rosen, Rekers, & Bentler, 1978).

NURSING DIAGNOSIS: IMPAIRED SOCIAL INTERACTION

RELATED TO: Social and culturally unacceptable behaviors

EVIDENCED BY: Peer rejection and identification with members of the opposite gender

OUTCOME CRITERIA	NURSING INTERVENTIONS	RATIONALE
Client will interact with others using culturally acceptable behaviors.	1. Once client feels comfortable with the new behaviors in role-playing or one-to-one nurse-client interactions, they may be tried in group situations. If possible, remain with client during interactions with others. Observe client behaviors and the responses he or she elicits from others. Give social attention (e.g., smile, nod) to desired behaviors. Follow up these "practice" sessions with one-to-one processing of the interaction. Give positive reinforcement for efforts. Offer support if client is feeling hurt from peer ridicule. Matter-of-factly discuss the behaviors that elicited the ridicule. Offer no personal reaction to the behavior.	1. The goal is to create a trusting, nonthreatening atmosphere for the client in an attempt to change behavior and improve social interactions. Long-term studies have not yet revealed the significance of therapy with these children on psychosexual relationship development in adolescence or adulthood. One variable that must be considered is the evidence of psychopathology within the families of many of these children (Zucker, 1985).

Continued on following page

TABLE 30.5 *(Continued)*

NURSING DIAGNOSIS: SELF-ESTEEM DISTURBURANCE
RELATED TO: Rejection by peers
EVIDENCED BY: Difficulty accepting positive reinforcement; self-negating verbalizations; inability to form close, personal relationships

OUTCOME CRITERIA	NURSING INTERVENTIONS	RATIONALE
Client will verbalize positive statements about self, including past accomplishments and future prospects.	1. Encourage child to engage in activities in which he or she is likely to achieve success. Help the child to focus on aspects of his or her life for which positive feelings exist. Discourage rumination about situations that are perceived as failures or over which client has no control. Give positive reinforcement for these behaviors. 2. Help client identify behaviors or aspects of life he or she would like to change. If realistic, assist child in problem solving to find ways to bring about the change. 3. Offer to be available for support to the child when he or she is feeling rejected by peers.	1. Success and positive feedback enhance self-esteem. 2. Having some control over his or her life may decrease feelings of powerlessness and increase feelings of self-worth. 3. Having an available support person who does not judge the child's behavior and who provides unconditional acceptance assists the child to progress toward acceptance of self as a worthwhile person.

8. Can the client discuss past accomplishments without dwelling on the perceived failures?

9. Has the client shown progress toward accepting self as a worthwhile person regardless of others' responses to his or her behavior?

VARIATIONS IN SEXUAL ORIENTATION

Homosexuality

Homosexual activity occurs under some circumstances in probably all known human cultures and all mammalian species in which it has been studied (Gadpaille, 1989). The term **homosexuality** is derived from the Greek root *homo* meaning "same" and refers to sexual preference for individuals of the same gender. It may be applied in a general way to homosexuals of both genders but is often used to specifically denote male homosexuality. The term **lesbianism,** used to identify female homosexuality, is traced to the Greek poet Sappho, who lived on the island of Lesbos and is famous for the love poems she wrote to other women. Most homosexuals prefer the term "gay," as it is less derogatory in its lack of emphasis on the sexual aspects of the orientation (Hyde, 1986). A heterosexual is then referred to as "straight."

The psychiatric community in general does not consider consensual homosexuality to be a mental disturbance (Kaplan & Sadock, 1998). The concept of homosexuality as a disturbance in sexual orientation no longer appears in the *DSM*. Instead, the *DSM-IV* (APA, 1994) is concerned only with the individual who experiences "persistent and marked distress about his or her sexual orientation."

Many members of the American culture disapprove of homosexuality. In a survey by the *Washington Post*, Harvard University, and the Henry J. Kaiser Family Foundation (1998), 53 percent of those surveyed responded that they believed sexual relations between two adults of the same sex was always wrong. Some experts believe that many Americans' attitudes toward homosexuals can best be described as homophobic. *Homophobia* is defined as a negative attitude toward or fear of homosexuality or homosexuals (Kaplan & Sadock, 1998). It may be indicative of a deep-seated insecurity about one's own gender identity. Homophobic behaviors include extreme prejudice against, abhorrence of, and discomfort around homosexuals. These behaviors are usually rationalized by religious, moral, or legal considerations.

Relationship patterns are as varied among homosexuals as they are among heterosexuals (Gadpaille, 1989). Some homosexuals may remain with one partner for an extended period of time, even for a lifetime, whereas others prefer not to make a commitment, and "play the field" instead.

No one knows for sure why people become homosexual or heterosexual. Various theories have been proposed regarding the issue, but no single etiological factor has consistently emerged. Many contributing factors likely influence the development of sexual orientation.

Predisposing Factors

Biological Theories. As early as 1952, Kallman (1952) argued that there is a genetic predisposition to homosexuality. He based this theory on a study in which he found 100 percent concordance for homosexuality among all the identical-twin pairs he studied. Subsequent investigators have failed to duplicate his findings. A more recent study by Bailey and Pillard (1991) has provided some concurrence, however. This study showed 52 percent concordance for homosexual orientation in monozygotic twins and 22 percent in dizygotic twins. These data were significant enough to suggest a possible heritable trait.

A number of studies have been conducted to determine whether or not there is a hormonal influence in the etiology of homosexuality. It has been hypothesized that levels of testosterone may be lower and levels of estrogen higher in homosexual men than in heterosexual men. Results have been inconsistent. Some studies did find higher testosterone levels and lower estrogen levels among lesbians than among a control group of heterosexual women (Hyde, 1986). It has also been suggested that exposure to inappropriate levels of androgens during the critical fetal period of sexual differentiation may contribute to homosexual orientation (Kaplan & Sadock, 1998). This hypothesis lacks definitive evidence, and conclusions regarding its validity remain tentative.

Psychosocial Theories. Freud (1930) believed that all humans are inherently bisexual, with the capacity for both heterosexual and homosexual behavior. He theorized that all individuals go through a homoerotic phase as children. Thus, if homosexuality occurs later in life it is due to arrest of normal psychosexual development. He also believed homosexuality could occur as a result of pathological family relationships in which the child adopts a negative oedipal position, that is, there is sexualized attachment to the parent of the same gender and identification with the parent of the opposite gender.

Bieber and coworkers (1962) found a dysfunctional family pattern as an etiological influence in the development of male homosexuality. The mother was described as dominant, overprotective, possessive, and seductive in her interactions with her son. The father was found to be passive, distant, and covertly or overtly hostile, and was openly devalued and dominated by the mother. Her behavior succeeds in undermining the father's availability as an acceptable object of gender identification for the boy, while hindering the child's capacity for trust in members of the opposite sex.

A study by Wolff (1971) revealed characteristics about the families of lesbians. Mothers of lesbians were found to be rejecting or indifferent and the fathers distant or absent. Wolff concluded from these findings that because the girl does not receive adequate love from her mother, she continues throughout her life to search for that missing love in other women. Having a distant or absent father results in her lack of ability to form satisfactory relationships with men.

These theories of family dynamics have been disputed by some clinicians who believe that parents have very little influence on the outcome of their children's sexual-partner orientation (Reinisch, 1990).

Special Concerns

People with homosexual preferences have problems that are similar to those of their heterosexual counterparts. Considerations of attractiveness, finding a partner, and concerns about sexual adequacy are common to both. Sexually transmitted diseases are epidemic among sexually active individuals of all sexual persuasions. Of particular concern is acquired immunodeficiency syndrome (AIDS), which was considered a "gay disease" for the first few years of the epidemic (see Chapter 36). AIDS is a fatal viral illness that in the Western world initially was indeed mainly transmitted during male homosexual activity (Bancroft, 1989). Although it is now well known that AIDS is also spread through contaminated blood products, the sharing of needles by intravenous drug users, and heterosexual contact, some individuals still believe AIDS is God's way of punishing homosexuals. These types of societal attitudes are described by many homosexuals as being their greatest burden.

Some homosexual individuals live in fear of the discovery of their sexual orientation—fear of being rejected by parents and significant others. They experience a great deal of cognitive dissonance related to the disparity between their overt behavior and their inner feelings. Social sanctions still exist in some areas for homosexuals in regard to employment, housing, and public accommodations. Gay rights are protected by the Human Rights Commission; however, discrimination is still widespread.

Nurses must examine their personal attitudes and feelings about homosexuality. They must be able to recognize when negative feelings are compromising the care they give. Increasing numbers of homosexuals are being honest about their lifestyles. Health care workers must ensure that these individuals receive the care with dignity that is the right of all human beings. Nurses who have come to terms with their own feelings about homosexuality are better able to separate the person from the behavior. Acceptance of the alternative sexual orientation is not an essential component of nursing; unconditional acceptance of the individual is.

Transsexualism

Transsexualism is a disorder of gender identity or gender dysphoria (unhappiness or dissatisfaction with one's gender) of the most extreme variety. An individual, despite having the anatomical characteristics of a given gender, has the self-perception of being of the opposite gender (Becker & Kavoussi, 1988). The disorder is rare, with an estimated prevalence of 1 in 30,000 for men and 1 in 100,000 for women (Kaplan, Sadock, & Grebb, 1994).

The *DSM-IV* does not identify transsexualism as a specific disorder, choosing instead to discuss the broader category of *gender identity disorder*; however, transsexualism is included in the 10th revision of the *International Classification of Diseases* (*ICD-10*).

Individuals with this disorder do not feel comfortable wearing the clothes of their assigned gender and often engage in cross-dressing. They may find their own genitals repugnant and may repeatedly submit requests to the health care system for hormonal and surgical gender reassignment. Depression and anxiety are common and are often attributed by the individual to his or her inability to live in the desired gender role.

Predisposing Factors

Biological Theories. Several studies have been conducted to determine if sex hormone levels are abnormal in individuals with gender dysphoria. Some researchers did find decreased levels of testosterone in male transsexuals and abnormally high levels of testosterone in female transsexuals, but the results have been inconsistent (Becker & Kavoussi, 1994).

As with homosexuality, there has been some speculation that gender-disordered individuals may be exposed to inappropriate hormones during the prenatal period, which can result in a genetic woman having male genitals, or a genetic man having female genitals (Ehrhardt et al., 1985). Evidence that prenatal exposure to these hormones predisposes to transsexualism, however, remains inconclusive.

Psychosocial Theories. Much emphasis has been placed on the importance of social learning in gender identity development. The *DSM-III-R* states, "Extensive, pervasive childhood femininity in a boy or childhood masculinity in a girl increases the likelihood of transsexualism" (APA, 1987). Green (1976, 1985) found a number of factors believed to influence femininity in boys:

1. Parental indifference to feminine behavior in a boy.
2. Parental encouragement of feminine behavior in a boy.
3. Repeated cross-dressing of a young boy by a female.
4. Maternal overprotection of a son and prohibition of "rough, boyish" play.
5. Excessive maternal attention and physical contact, resulting in lack of separation and individuation of the boy from his mother.
6. Absence of or rejection by the father.
7. Physical beauty of a boy, influencing adults to treat him in a feminine manner.
8. Lack of male playmates during early years of socialization.

Factors that influence masculinity in girls are not as clear cut. These characteristics are considerably more common and are also regarded as more socially acceptable; hence, less attention is given to their significance. In a study of "tomboy" girls, Green and associates (1982) found a preference for male gender–typed toys, male-gender peer group, participation in sports, male roles taken in playing house, as well as the stated wish to be a boy. Pauly (1974) found that a disturbed parental relationship was also commonly reported by a substantial majority of adult female transsexuals. The dynamics often included a weak or depressive mother or an aggressive, excessively masculine and often alcoholic father. Encouragement by both parents of masculinity in the daughter appears to be common.

Special Concerns

Treatment of the transsexual is a complex process. The true transsexual intensely desires to have the genitalia and physical appearance of the assigned gender changed to conform with his or her gender identity. This change requires a great deal more than surgical alteration of physical features. In most cases, the individual must undergo extensive psychological testing and counseling, as well as live in the role of the desired gender for up to 2 years before surgery.

Hormonal treatment is initiated during this period. Male clients receive estrogen, which results in a redistribution of body fat in a more "feminine" pattern, enlargement of the breasts, a softening of the skin, and reduction in body hair. Females receive testosterone, which also causes a redistribution of body fat, growth of facial and body hair, enlargement of the clitoris, and deepening of the voice (Becker & Kavoussi, 1988). Amenorrhea usually occurs within 4 months (Levine, 1989).

Surgical treatment for the male-to-female transsexual involves removal of the penis and testes and creation of an artificial vagina. Care is taken to preserve sensory nerves in the area so that the individual may continue to experience sexual stimulation.

Surgical treatment for the female-to-male transsexual is more complex and usually less successful (Reinisch, 1990). A mastectomy and sometimes a hysterectomy are preformed. A penis and scrotum are constructed from tissues in the genital and abdominal area, and the vaginal orifice is closed. A penile implant is used to attain erection.

Both men and women continue to receive maintenance

hormone therapy following surgery. Satisfaction with the results is high, and most consider the pain and discomfort worthwhile. Kaplan and Sadock (1998) state:

> "Outcome studies are highly variable in terms of how success is defined and measured (for example, successful intercourse and body image satisfaction). About 70 percent of male-to-female and 80 percent of female-to-male reassignment surgery patients report satisfactory results." (p. 718)

Nursing care of the post–sex-reassignment surgical client is similar to that of most other postsurgical clients. Particular attention is given to maintaining comfort, preventing infection, preserving integrity of the surgical site, maintaining elimination, and meeting nutritional needs. Psychosocial needs may have to do with body image, fears and insecurities about relating to others, and being accepted in the new gender role. Meeting these needs can begin with nursing in a nonthreatening, nonjudgmental healing atmosphere.

Bisexuality

A bisexual person is not exclusively heterosexual or homosexual but engages in sexual activity with members of both genders. Bisexuals are also sometimes referred to as ambisexual.

Bisexuality is more common than exclusive homosexuality. Statistics suggest that approximately 75 percent of all men are exclusively heterosexual and only 2 percent are exclusively homosexual, leaving a relatively large percentage who have engaged in sexual activity with both men and women (Hyde, 1986).

MacDonald (1982) describes a diversity of sexual preferences among bisexuals. Some prefer men and women equally, whereas others have a preference for one gender but also accept sexual activity with the other gender. Some bisexuals may alternate between homosexual and heterosexual activity for long periods; others may have both a male and a female lover at the same time. Whereas some individuals maintain their bisexual orientation throughout their lives, others may become exclusively homosexual or heterosexual.

Predisposing Factors

Little research exists on the etiology of bisexuality. Freud (1930) believed that all humans are inherently bisexual; that is, he believed that all individuals have the capacity for both heterosexual and homosexual interactions.

Much research on the development of homosexuality rests on the assumption that it is somehow determined by pathological conditions in childhood. Many heterosexual individuals, however, have their first homosexual encounter later in life. It is unlikely that an initial homosexual encounter that occurs in the 30s or 40s was deter-mined by a pathological condition that occurred when the individual was 3 or 4 years old. Some encounters, too, are based solely on the situation, such as the heterosexual man who engages in homosexual behavior while in prison, then returns to heterosexuality following his release. This behavior most likely was determined by the circumstances rather than some pathological process that occurred in childhood.

Riddle (1978) suggests that gender identity (determining whether one is male or female) is established during the preschool years. Sexual identity (determining whether one is heterosexual or homosexual or both), however, most likely continues to evolve throughout one's lifetime.

SEXUALLY TRANSMITTED DISEASES

Phipps (1995) defines *sexually transmitted diseases* (*STDs*) as diseases that usually are or can be transmitted from one person to another through intimate contact with the genitalia, mouth, or rectum. They may be transmitted from one person to another through heterosexual or homosexual contact, and external genital evidence of pathology may or may not be manifested.

Sexually transmitted diseases are at epidemic levels in the United States. Individuals are beginning an active sex life at an earlier age. More women are sexually active than ever before. The social changes that may have contributed to the increase in STDs are sometimes referred to as the three Ps: permissiveness, promiscuity, and the pill. The widespread knowledge that antibiotics were available to cure infections and the availability of the pill to prevent pregnancy resulted in significant increases in promiscuity and the subsequent exposure to and spread of STDs.

A primary nursing responsibility in STD control is education that is aimed at prevention of the diseases. Nurses must know which diseases are most prevalent, how they are transmitted, their signs and symptoms, available treatment, and consequences of avoiding treatment (Table 30.6). They must teach this information to clients in hospitals and clinics and take an active role in programs of education in the community. Early education is important in order to decrease the spread of STDs.

Sexually transmitted diseases have a particularly emotive significance because they can be transmitted between sexual partners. Consequently, STDs carry strong connotations of illicit or immoral sex and considerable social stigma, as well as potentially horrifying medical consequences (Bancroft, 1989). Feelings of guilt in clients with STDs can be overwhelming. These individuals need strong support to overcome not only the physical difficulties but also the social and emotional ones associated with having this type of illness.

Prevention of STDs is the ideal goal, but early detection and appropriate treatment continue to be considered a realistic objective. Nurses are in an excellent position to

TABLE 30.6 SEXUALLY TRANSMITTED DISEASES

DISEASE	ORGANISM OF TRANSMISSION	METHOD OF TRANSMISSION	SIGNS AND SYMPTOMS	AVAILABLE TREATMENT	POTENTIAL COMPLICATIONS
Gonorrhea	*Neisseria gonorrhoeae* (bacterium)	Vaginal sex; anal sex; genital-oral sex; via hand moistened with infected secretions and placed in contact with mucous membranes such as the eyes.	Males: urethritis; dysuria, purulent discharge from urethra; proctitis; pharyngitis. Females: initially asymptomatic. Progress to infection of cervix, urethra, and fallopian tubes.	Tetracycline; penicillin G; amoxicillin; ampicillin; spectinomycin	Men: sterility from orchitis or epididymitis. Women: chronic pelvic inflammatory disease; infertility; ectopic pregnancy; blindness from gonococcal conjunctivitis.
Syphilis	*Treponema pallidum* (spirochete)	Vaginal sex; anal sex; genital-oral sex; via contact of infected secretions with intact mucous membranes or abraded skin.	Primary stage: painless chancre on penis, vulva, vagina, mouth, anus, or other point of contact with mucous membranes or abraded skin. Secondary stage: rash, headache, anorexia, weight loss, fever, sore throat, body aches, anemia.	Long-acting penicillin G; tetracycline; erythromycin	Latent stage: lasts many years; no symptoms but can be passed on to fetus. Tertiary stage: blindness, heart disease, insanity, ulcerated lesions on skin, mucous membranes, or internal organs.
Chlamydial infection	*Chlamydia trachomatis* (intracellular bacterium)	Vaginal sex; anal sex; via hand moistened with infected secretions and placed in contact with mucous membranes.	Women: cervicitis (either asymptomatic or may have discharge, dysuria, soreness, bleeding). Men: urethral discharge and dysuria.	Tetracycline; erythromycin	Scarring in the fallopian tubes; ectopic pregnancy; infertility.
Genital herpes	Herpes simplex virus, type 1 or type 2	Vaginal sex; anal sex; genital-oral sex; skin-to-skin contact with infected areas; to newborn through vaginal delivery.	Blistery lesions in the genital area causing pain, itching, burning. Also vaginal or urethral discharge, fever, headache, malaise, and myalgias.	Acyclovir applied directly to the area provides symptomatic relief. No cure.	Recurrences are possible. Potential complications include: meningitis, encephalitis, urethral strictures. Possible risk of cervical cancer.
Genital warts	Condyloma acuminatum (human papilloma virus)	Vaginal sex; anal sex; skin-to-skin contact with infected areas.	Cauliflowerlike warts that appear on penis or scrotum in men, labia, vaginal walls or cervix in women. Mild itching may occur.	Application of fluorouracil (5-FU); cryotherapy; electrocautery; surgical removal.	Recurrences are possible. Possible increased risk of cervical cancer.

TABLE 30.6 SEXUALLY TRANSMITTED DISEASES

DISEASE	ORGANISM OF TRANSMISSION	METHOD OF TRANSMISSION	SIGNS AND SYMPTOMS	AVAILABLE TREATMENT	POTENTIAL COMPLICATIONS
Hepatitis B	NHepatitis B virus	Vaginal sex; anal sex; genital-oral sex; contact with infectious blood or blood products; contact of infectious secretions with mucous membranes or abrased skin.	Malaise, anorexia, nausea/vomiting, fever, headache, mild pain in right upper quadrant of abdomen, jaundice.	No cure. Treatment involves supportive care; bedrest for extended period. Medications have not generally been found to be useful.	Complications include chronic hepatitis; cirrhosis; liver cancer.
AIDS	Human immunodeficiency virus (HIV)	Exchange of body fluids via: Anal sex; vaginal sex; genital-oral sex; shared use of needles during drug use. Skin-to-skin contact when there are open sores on the skin. Transfusion with contaminated blood.	May be asymptomatic for as long as 10 years following infection with HIV. Early signs of AIDS include severe weight loss, diarrhea, fever, night sweats or the presence of a persistent opportunistic infection (e.g., herpes or candidiasis).	No cure. Antiretroviral used to slow growth of the virus. Other medications given for symptomatic relief.	Regardless of treatment, AIDS is eventually fatal.

provide the education required for prevention, as well as the physical treatment and social and emotional support to assist clients with STDs regain and maintain optimal wellness.

SUMMARY

This chapter has provided information related to the development of sexuality throughout the life cycle. Normal sexual response patterns were described in an effort to provide background information for the recognition and treatment of sexual and gender identity disorders.

The *DSM-IV* identifies two major categories of sexual disorders (paraphilias and sexual dysfunctions) and two categories of gender identity disorders (those occurring in children and those occurring in adolescents and adults).

Paraphilias are a group of behaviors involving sexual activity with nonhuman objects or with nonconsenting partners or that involve suffering to others. Types of paraphilias include exhibitionism, fetishism, frotteurism, pedophilia, sexual masochism or sadism, and voyeurism.

Sexual dysfunctions are disturbances that occur in any of the phases of the normal human sexual response cycle. They include sexual desire disorders, sexual arousal disorders, orgasmic disorders, and sexual pain disorders.

TEST YOUR CRITICAL THINKING SKILLS

Sarah was hospitalized on the psychiatric unit for depression. During her nursing assessment interview, she stated, "According to my husband, I can't do anything right—not even have sex." When asked to explain further, Sarah said she and her husband had been married for 17 years. She said that in the beginning, they had experienced a mutually satisfying sexual relationship and "made love" two or three times a week. Their daughter was born after they had been married 2 years, followed 2 years later by the birth of their son. They now have two teenagers (ages 15 and 13) who, by Sarah's admission, require a great deal of her time and energy. She says, "I'm too tired for sex. And, besides, the kids might hear. I would be so embarrassed if they did. I walked in on my parents having sex once when I was a teenager, and I thought I would die! And my parents never mentioned it. It was just like it never happened! It was so awful! But sex is just so important to my husband, though, and we haven't had sex in months. We argue all the time about it. I'm afraid it's going to break us up."

Answer the following questions related to Sarah:

1. What would be the primary nursing diagnosis for Sarah?
2. What interventions might the nurse include in the treatment plan for Sarah?
3. What would be a realistic goal for which Sarah might strive?

RESEARCH NOTE

Adolescents' views of sexual decision-making. *IMAGE: Journal of Nursing Scholarship* **(1996, Summer), 28(2), 125–130.**
Keller, M.L., Duerst, B.L., and Zimmerman, J.

Description of the Study: Because large numbers of adolescents continue, despite intensive educational efforts, to engage in behaviors that place them at high risk for sexually transmitted diseases (STDs), this study was undertaken in an attempt to determine reasons adolescents give for abstinence, engaging in safer sex (intercourse with a condom), or unprotected intercourse. The sample included 62 male and 53 female students enrolled in the health or social science classes of six rural school districts in Wisconsin. Average age was 17.5 years. Respondents completed a study questionnaire in which they responded to a vignette in which a teenage couple became sexually aroused. They were to choose an ending to the vignette in one of three ways: the couple abstains from intercourse, the couple has sexual intercourse using a condom, or the couple has intercourse without using a condom. The subjects were then asked to give reasons why they chose the particular ending, and possible feelings associated with all three choices from the perspective of the couple in the vignette.

Results of the Study: By a large margin, most of the subjects chose an ending in which the couple had sexual intercourse.

Forty-three percent chose the outcome of intercourse with a condom; 33 percent chose the ending of unprotected sexual intercourse; and 23 percent chose the abstinence ending. Reasons given for response of intercourse with a condom included responsibility, safety, and "People expect to use condoms these days." Reasons given for the outcome of unprotected sexual intercourse included, "It's what usually happens," no condom available, and loss of control. The most frequent reason given for choosing the abstinence ending was that "The couple did not know each other well enough to have sexual intercourse."

Comments: The authors suggest that data from this study imply the importance of helping adolescents know that they have control over a situation. Unprotected sex was attributed to loss of control and being "swept away by desire." A second aspect might be to use fear-inducing strategies. Reasons given for abstinence and use of condoms included fear about pregnancy and STDs. Reinforcement of the legitimacy of these fears can be part of an educational intervention to motivate teens to engage in desirable behaviors. The ability to help adolescents think about the *positive* consequences of safer sex was also a consideration for nursing intervention. The authors cited limitations of the study as the difficulty to generalize the results because of homogeneous nature of the sample (rural, white, middle class) and the use of open-ended questions, which were often difficult to interpret.

Gender identity disorders occur when there is an incongruence between anatomical sex and the assigned gender role. Individuals experience extreme discomfort in the assigned gender and desire to be, or insist that they are, the opposite gender. Cross-dressing is common, and some individuals pursue hormonal therapy or surgery to alter physical characteristics to match cognitive self-perception.

Predisposing factors and symptomatology for each of these disorders were presented as background assessment data. A content outline for obtaining a sexual history was included. The delivery of nursing care was described in the context of the nursing process.

A description of current medical treatment modalities for each of the disorders was presented. Alternative sexual orientations, including homosexuality, transsexualism, and bisexuality, were discussed. Finally, information on the transmission, signs and symptoms, treatment, and potential complications of the most prevalent STDs was suggested as material for use in programs of education targeted at decreasing the spread of sexually transmitted diseases.

Human sexuality influences all aspects of physical and mental health. Clients are becoming more open to discussing matters pertaining to sexuality, and it is therefore important for nurses to integrate information on sexuality into the care they give. This can be done by focusing on preventive, therapeutic, and educational interventions to assist individuals to attain, regain, or maintain sexual wellness.

INTERNET REFERENCES

- Additional information about sexual disorders may be located at the following websites:
  a. http://www.sexualhealth.com/
  b. http://www.hscsyr.edu/~icm/Sexuality.htm
  c. http://www.sexualhealthinstitute.com/
  d. http://www-hsl.mcmaster.ca/tomflem/sexual.html
- Additional information about gender identity disorders may be located at the following websites:
  a. http://www.avitale.com/
  b. http://english-www.hss.cmu.edu/gender/
- Additional information about sexually transmitted diseases may be located at the following websites:
  a. http://www.nau.edu/~fronske/stdintro.html
  b. http://www.shamino.quincy.edu/counseling/STD.htm

REVIEW QUESTIONS

SELF-EXAMINATION/LEARNING EXERCISE

Select the answer that is most appropriate for each of the following questions.

1. Janice, age 24, and her husband are seeking treatment at the sex therapy clinic. They have been married for 3 weeks and have never had sexual intercourse together. Pain and vaginal tightness prevent penile entry. Sexual history reveals Janice was raped when she was 15 years old. The physician would most likely assign which of the following diagnoses to Janice?

   a. Dyspareunia
   b. Vaginismus
   c. Anorgasmia
   d. Sexual aversion disorder

2. The most appropriate nursing diagnosis for Janice would be:

   a. Pain related to vaginal constriction.
   b. Altered sexuality patterns related to inability to have vaginal intercourse.
   c. Sexual dysfunction related to history of sexual trauma.
   d. Dysfunctional grieving related to loss of self-esteem because of rape.

3. The first phase of treatment may be initiated by the nurse. It would include which of the following?

   a. Sensate focus exercises
   b. Tense and relaxation exercises
   c. Systematic desensitization
   d. Education about the disorder

4. The second phase of treatment includes which of the following?

   a. Gradual dilation of the vagina
   b. Sensate focus exercises
   c. Hypnotherapy
   d. Administration of minor tranquilizers

5. Statistically, the outcome of therapy for Janice and her husband is likely to:

   a. be unsuccessful.
   b. be very successful.
   c. be of very long duration.
   d. result in their getting a divorce.

Match each of the paraphilias listed on the left with its correct behavioral description from the column on the right.

_____ 6. Exhibitionism

_____ 7. Transvestic fetishism

_____ 8. Voyeurism

_____ 9. Frotteurism

_____ 10. Pedophilia

a. Tom watches his neighbor through her window each night as she undresses for bed. Later he fantasizes about having sex with her.

b. Frank drives his car up to a strange woman, stops, and asks her for directions. As she is explaining, he reveals his erect penis to her.

c. Tim, age 17, babysits for his 11-year-old neighbor, Jeff. Six months ago, Tim began fondling Jeff's genitals. They now engage in mutual masturbation each time they are together.

d. John is 32 years old. He buys women's clothing at the thrift shop. Sometimes he dresses as a woman and goes to a singles' bar. He becomes sexually excited as he fantasizes about men being attracted to him as a woman.

e. Fred rides a crowded subway every day. He stands beside a woman he views as very attractive. Just as the subway is about to stop, he places his hand on her breast and rubs his genitals against her buttock. As the door opens, he dashes out and away. Later he fantasizes she is in love with him.

REFERENCES

Abel, E.L. (1985). *Psychoactive drugs and sex.* New York: Plenum.

Abel, G.G. (1989). Paraphilias. In H.I. Kaplan & B.J. Sadock (Eds.), *Comprehensive textbook of psychiatry* (Vol. I) (5th ed.). Baltimore: Williams & Wilkins.

Abel, G.G., Rouleau, J.L., & Osborn, C.A. (1994). Sexual disorders. In G. Winokur & P.J. Clayton (Eds.), *The medical basis of psychiatry* (2nd ed.). Philadelphia: W.B. Saunders.

American Psychiatric Association (APA). (1994). *Diagnostic and Statistical Manual of Mental Disorders* (4th ed.). Washington, DC: American Psychiatric Association.

American Psychiatric Association (APA). (1987). *Diagnostic and statistical manual of mental disorders* (3rd ed., rev). Washington, DC: American Psychiatric Association.

Arafat, I.S., & Cotton, W.L. (1974). Masturbation practices of males and females. *Journal of Sex Research, 10,* 293–307.

Bailey, J.M., & Pillard, R.C. (1991). A genetic study of male sexual orientation. *Archives of General Psychiatry, 48,* 1089–1096.

Bancroft, J. (1978). The prevention of sexual offenses. In C.B. Qualls et al. (Eds.), *The prevention of sexual disorders.* New York: Plenum.

Bancroft, J. (1984). Testosterone therapy for low sexual interest and erectile dysfunctions in men. *British Journal of Psychiatry, 144,* 146–151.

Bancroft, J. (1989). *Human sexuality and its problems* (2nd ed.). New York: Churchill-Livingstone.

Barnes, J. (1981). Non-consummation of marriage. *Irish Medical Journal, 74,* 19–21.

Becker, J.V. (1989). Impact of sexual abuse on sexual functioning. In S.R. Leiblum & R.C. Rosen (Eds.), *Principles and practice of sex therapy: Update for the 1990s* (2nd ed.). New York: Guilford Press.

Becker, J.V., & Kavoussi, R.J. (1988). Sexual disorders. In J.A. Talbott, R.E. Hales, & S.C. Yudofsky (Eds.), *Textbook of psychiatry.* Washington, DC: American Psychiatric Press.

Becker, J.V., & Kavoussi, R.J. (1994). Sexual and gender identity disorders. In R.E. Hales, S.C. Yudofsky, & J.A. Talbott (Eds.), *Textbook of psychiatry* (2nd ed.) Washington, DC: American Psychiatric Press.

Bell, R. (1998). *Changing bodies, changing lives* (3rd ed.). New York: Random House.

Bieber, I., et al. (1962). *Homosexuality.* New York: Basic Books.

Bradford, J.M., & McLean, D. (1984). Sexual offenders, violence, and testosterone: A clinical study. *Canadian Journal of Psychiatry, 29,* 335–343.

Clunn, P. (1991). *Child psychiatric nursing.* St. Louis: Mosby Year Book.

Ehrhardt, A.A., et al. (1985). Sexual orientation after prenatal exposure to exogenous estrogen. *Archives of Sexual Behavior, 14,* 57–78.

Freud, S. (1930). *Three contributions to the theory of sex* (4th ed.). New York: Nervous and Mental Disease Publishing.

Gadpaille, W.J. (1989). Homosexuality. In H.I. Kaplan & B.J. Sadock (Eds.), *Comprehensive textbook of psychiatry* (Vol. I) (5th ed.). Baltimore: Williams & Wilkins.

Goldberg, K.A. (1998). *Viagra: The potency pill.* Lincolnwood, IL: Publications International.

Green, R. (1976). One hundred and ten feminine and masculine boys: Behavioral contrasts and demographic similarities. *Archives of Sexual Behavior, 5,* 425–446.

Green, R. (1985). Gender identity in childhood and later sexual orientation: Follow up of 78 males. *American Journal of Psychiatry, 142,* 339–341.

Green, R., et al. (1982). Ninety-nine 'tomboys' and 'non-tomboys': Behavioral contrasts and demographic similarities. *Archives of Sexual Behavior, 11,* 247–266.

Hogan, R.M (1980). *Human sexuality: A nursing perspective.* New York: Appleton-Century-Crofts.

Hyde, J.S. (1986). *Understanding human sexuality* (3rd ed.). New York: McGraw-Hill.

Kallman, F.J. (1952). Comparative twin study on the genetic aspects of male homosexuality. *Journal of Nervous and Mental Disorders, 115,* 283.

Kaplan, H.I., & Sadock, B.J. (1985). *Modern synopsis of comprehensive textbook of psychiatry* (4th ed.). Baltimore: Williams & Wilkins.

Kaplan, H.I., & Sadock, B.J. (1998). *Synopsis of psychiatry: Behavioral sciences/clinical psychiatry* (8th ed.). Baltimore: Williams & Wilkins.

Kaplan, H.I., Sadock, B.J., & Grebb, J.A. (1994). *Kaplan and Sadock's synopsis of psychiatry* (7th ed.). Baltimore: Williams & Wilkins.

Kaplan, H.S. (1974). *The new sex therapy.* New York: Brunner/Mazel.

Kaplan, H.S. (1979). *Disorders of sexual desire and other new concepts and techniques in sex therapy.* New York: Brunner/Mazel.

Kinsey, A.C., Pomeroy, W.B., & Martin, C.E. (1948). *Sexual behavior in the human male.* Philadelphia: W.B. Saunders.

Leiblum, S.R., & Rosen, R.C. (Eds.). (1988). *Sexual desire disorders.* New York: Guilford.

Levine, S.B. (1989). Gender identity disorders of childhood, adolescence, and adulthood. In H.I. Kaplan & B.J. Sadock (Eds.). *Comprehensive textbook of psychiatry* (Vol. I) (5th ed.). Baltimore: Williams & Wilkins.

LoPiccolo, J., & Friedman, J.M. (1988). Broad-spectrum treatment of low sexual desire: Integration of cognitive, behavioral, and systemic therapy. In S.R. Leiblum & R.C. Rosen (Eds.), *Sexual desire disorders.* New York: Guilford Press.

LoPiccolo, J., & Stock, W.E. (1986). Treatment of sexual dysfunction. *Journal of Consulting Clinical Psychology, 54,* 158–167.

MacDonald, A.P. (1982). Research on sexual orientation: A bridge that touches both shores but doesn't meet in the middle. *Journal of Sex Education and Therapy, 8,* 9–13.

Malatesta, V.J., et al. (1982). Acute alcohol intoxication and female orgasmic response. *Journal of Sex Research, 18,* 1–17.

Marshall, W.L., & Barbaree, H.E. (1978). The reduction of deviant arousal: Satiation treatment for sexual aggressors. *Criminal Justice and Behavior 5,* 294–303.

Marshall, W.L., & Barbaree, H.E. (1990). An integrated theory of the etiology of sexual offending. In W.L. Marshall, D.R. Laws, & H.E. Barbaree (Eds.), *Handbook of sexual assault: Issues, theories, and treatment of the offender.* New York: Plenum Press.

Masters, W.H., & Johnson, V.E. (1966). *Human sexual response.* Boston: Little, Brown.

Masters, W.H., & Johnson, V.E. (1970). *Human sexual inadequacy.* Boston: Little, Brown.

McCarthy, B.W. (1989). Cognitive-behavioral strategies and techniques in the treatment of early ejaculation. In S.R. Leiblum & R.C. Rosen (Eds.), *Principles and practice of sex therapy: Update for the 1990s* (2nd ed.). New York: Guilford Press.

McCarthy, B., & McCarthy, E. (1998). *Couple sexual awareness.* New York: Carroll & Graf Publishers.

Pauly, I.B. (1974). Female transsexualism. *Archives of Sexual Behaviors, 3,* 487–526.

Phipps, W.J. (1995). Management of persons with sexually transmitted diseases. In W.J. Phipps, V.L. Cassmeyer, J.K. Sands, & M.K. Lehman (Eds.), *Medical-surgical nursing: Concepts and clinical practice* (5th ed.). St. Louis: Mosby.

Reinisch, J.M. (1990). *The Kinsey Institute new report on sex.* New York: St. Martin's Press.

Riddle, D.I. (1978). Relating to children: Gays as role models. *Journal of Social Issues, 34,* 38–58.

Robins, L.N., et al. (1984). Lifetime prevalence of specific psychiatric disorders in three sites. *Archives of General Psychiatry, 41,* 949–958.

Rosen, A.C., Rekers, G.A., & Bentler, P.M. (1978). Ethical issues in the treatment of children. *Journal of Social Issues, 32,*84.

Sadock, V.A. (1989). Normal human sexuality and sexual disorders. In H.I. Kaplan & B.J. Sadock (Eds.), *Comprehensive textbook of psychiatry* (Vol. I) (5th ed.). Baltimore: Williams & Wilkins.

Sands, J.K. (1995). Human sexuality. In W.J. Phipps, V.L. Cassmeyer, J.K. Sands, & M.K. Lehman (Eds.), *Medical-surgical nursing: Concepts and clinical practice* (5th ed.). St. Louis: Mosby.

Segraves, R.T. (1988). Hormones and libido. In S.R. Leiblum & R.C. Rosen. *Sexual desire disorders.* New York: The Guilford Press.

Spector, I.P., & Carey, M.P. (1990) Incidence and prevalence of the sexual dysfunctions: A critical review of the empirical literature. *Archives of Sexual Behavior, 19,* 374–389.

VandeVusse, L., & Simandl, G. (1992). Sexuality patterns, altered. In K.V. Gettrust & P.D. Brabec (Eds.), *Nursing diagnosis in clinical practice: Guides for care planning.* Albany, NY: Delmar.

The Washington Post, Harvard University, and the Henry J. Kaiser Family Foundation. (1998). *A sense of moral decline.* Washington, DC: The Washington Post.

Wincze, J.P., & Carey, M.P. (1991). *Sexual dysfunction: A guide for assessment and treatment.* New York: The Guilford Press.

Wolff, C. (1971). *Love between women.* New York: Harper & Row.

Zucker, K.J. (1985). Cross-gender-identified children. In B.W. Steiner (Ed.), *Gender dysphoria: Development, research, management.* New York: Plenum.

Bibliography

Carver, C. (1998, December). Premature ejaculation: A common and treatable concern. *Journal of the American Psychiatric Nurses Association, 4*(6), 199–204.

Doenges, M.E., Townsend, M.C., & Moorhouse, M.F. (1998). *Psychiatric care plans: Guidelines for individualizing care* (3rd ed.). Philadelphia: F.A. Davis.

Leifer, C., & Young, E.W. (1997, October). Homeless lesbians: Psychology of the hidden, the disenfranchised, and the forgotten. *Journal of Psychosocial Nursing, 35*(10), 28–33.

LeMone, P., & Jones, D. (1997, July–Sept). Nursing assessment of altered sexuality: A review of salient factors and objective measures. *Nursing Diagnosis, 8*(3), 120–128.

LeMone, P., & Weber, J. (1995, April–June). Validating gender-specific defining characteristics of altered sexuality. *Nursing Diagnosis, 6*(2), 64–69.

McEnany, G. (1998, February). Sexual dysfunction in the pharmacologic treatment of depression: When "don't ask, don't tell" is an unsuitable approach to care. *Journal of the American Psychiatric Nurses Association, 4*(1), 24–29.

Patel, S., Long, T.E., McCammon, S.L., & Wuensch, K.L. (1995). Personality and emotional correlates of self-reported antigay behaviors. *Journal of Interpersonal Violence, 10,* 354–366.

Townsend, M.C. (1997). *Nursing diagnoses in psychiatric nursing: A pocket guide for care plan construction* (4th ed.). Philadelphia: F.A. Davis.

EATING DISORDERS

KEY TERMS

obesity
anorexia
body image

emaciated
amenorrhea
binging

purging
anorexigenics

OBJECTIVES

After reading this chapter, the student will be able to:

1. Identify and differentiate among the various eating disorders.
2. Discuss epidemiological statistics related to eating disorders.
3. Describe symptomatology associated with anorexia nervosa, bulimia nervosa, and obesity, and use the information in client assessment.
4. Identify predisposing factors in the development of eating disorders.

5. Formulate nursing diagnoses and goals of care for clients with eating disorders.
6. Describe appropriate interventions for behaviors associated with eating disorders.
7. Identify topics for client and family teaching relevant to eating disorders.
8. Evaluate the nursing care of clients with eating disorders.
9. Discuss various modalities relevant to treatment of eating disorders.

utrition is required to sustain life, and most individuals acquire nutrients from eating food; however, nutrition and life sustenance are not the only reasons most people eat food. Indeed, in an affluent culture, life sustenance may not even be a consideration. It is sometimes difficult to remember that many people within this affluent American culture, as well as all over the world, are starving from lack of food.

The hypothalamus contains the appetite regulation center within the brain. This complex neural system regulates the body's ability to recognize when it is hungry and when it has been sated. Halmi (1994) states:

"Eating behavior is now known to reflect an interaction between an organism's physiological state and environmental conditions. Salient physiological variables include the balance of various neuropeptides and neurotransmitters, metabolic state, metabolic rate, condition of the gastrointestinal tract, amount of storage tissue, and sensory receptors for taste and smell. Environmental conditions include features of the food such as taste, texture, novelty, accessibility, and nutritional composition, and other external conditions such as ambient temperature, presence of other people, and stress." (p. 857)

Society and culture have a great deal of influence on eating behaviors. Eating is a social activity; seldom does an event of any social significance occur without the presence of food. Yet society and culture also influence how people (and in particular, women) must look. History reveals a regularity of fluctuation in what society has considered desirable in the human female body. Archives and historical paintings reveal the fashionableness and desirability of the plump, full-figured women of the 16th and 17th centuries. Beauty in the Victorian era was characterized by a slender, wan appearance that continued through the flapper era of the 1920s. During the depression era and World War II, the full-bodied woman was again admired, only to be superseded in the late 1960s by the image of the superthin models propagated by the media, which remains the ideal of today. As it has been said, "A woman can't be too rich or too thin." Eating disorders as we know them can dispute this quote.

This chapter explores the disorders associated with undereating and overeating. Because psychological or behavioral factors play a potential role in the presentation of these disorders, they fall well within the realm of psychiatry and psychiatric nursing. Epidemiological statistics are presented along with predisposing factors that have been implicated in the etiology of anorexia nervosa, bulimia nervosa, and obesity. An explanation of the symptomatology is presented as background knowledge for assessing the client with an eating disorder. Nursing care is described in the context of the nursing process. Various treatment modalities are explored.

EPIDEMIOLOGICAL FACTORS

The incidence of anorexia nervosa has increased in the past 30 years both in the United States and in Western Europe (Halmi, 1994). One study indicated that incidence of the disorder nearly doubled from 1960 to 1976 (Jones et al., 1980). Recent studies indicate an incidence rate among young women in the United States of approximately 14 per 100,000 population (Eckert & Mitchell, 1994). Anorexia nervosa occurs predominantly in females aged 12 to 30 years. Only 4 percent to 10 percent of the cases are males (Eckert & Mitchell, 1994). Anorexia nervosa was once believed to be more prevalent in the higher socioeconomic classes, but evidence is lacking to support this hypothesis.

Bulimia nervosa is more prevalent than anorexia nervosa. Estimates of the disorder range from 1 percent to 3 percent of young women. Onset of bulimia nervosa occurs in late adolescence or early adulthood, with a mean age of onset of 18 years (Eckert & Mitchell, 1994). Cross-cultural research suggests that bulimia nervosa occurs primarily in societies that place emphasis on thinness as the model of attractiveness for women and where an abundance of food is available (Eckert & Mitchell, 1994).

Obesity has been defined as a body mass index (weight/height^2) of 30 or greater. Estimates show that 24 percent of adult males and 27 percent of adult females in the United States today suffer from obesity (Schmidt, 1998). Obesity is more common in black women than in white women and more common in white men than in black men. The prevalence among lower socioeconomic classes is six times that in upper socioeconomic classes, and there is a somewhat greater prevalence of obesity among Jews, followed by Roman Catholics, and then Protestants (Lomax, 1989). Approximately 0.1 percent of the population are categorized as "morbidly" obese, which is defined by the National Institutes of Health as a body mass index (BMI) greater than 40 kg/m^2 (Long, 1995).

APPLICATION OF THE NURSING PROCESS

Background Assessment Data (Symptomatology)

Anorexia Nervosa

This disorder is characterized by a morbid fear of obesity. Symptoms include gross distortion of body image, preoccupation with food, and refusal to eat. The term **anorexia** is actually a misnomer. It was initially believed that anorexics did not experience sensations of hunger. However, research indicates that they do indeed suffer from pangs of hunger, and it is only with food intake of less than

200 calories per day that hunger sensations actually cease (Leon & Dinklage, 1989).

The distortion in **body image** is manifested by the individual's perception of being "fat" when he or she is obviously underweight or even **emaciated.** Weight loss is usually accomplished by reduction in food intake and often extensive exercising. Self-induced vomiting may also occur, along with the abuse of laxatives or diuretics.

Weight loss is marked. For example, the individual may present for health care services weighing less than 85 percent of expected weight. Other symptoms include hypothermia, bradycardia, hypotension, edema, lanugo, and a variety of metabolic changes. **Amenorrhea** usually follows weight loss but in some instances may precede it (APA, 1994).

There may be an obsession with food. For example, these individuals may hoard or conceal food, talk about food and recipes at great length, or prepare elaborate meals for others, only to restrict themselves to a limited amount of low-calorie food intake. Compulsive behaviors, such as hand-washing, may also be present.

Age at onset is usually early to late adolescence. It is estimated to occur in approximately 0.5 to 1 percent of adolescent females, and is 10 to 20 times more common in females than in males (Kaplan & Sadock, 1998). Psychosexual development is generally delayed.

Feelings of depression and anxiety often accompany this disorder. In fact, several studies have suggested a possible interrelationship between eating disorders and affective disorders (Leon & Dinklage, 1989). Table 31.1 outlines the *DSM-IV* (APA, 1994) diagnostic criteria for anorexia nervosa.

Bulimia Nervosa

Bulimia is an episodic, uncontrolled, compulsive, rapid ingestion of large quantities of food over a short period of time (**binging**), followed by inappropriate compensatory behaviors to rid the body of the excess calories. The food consumed during a binge often has a high caloric content, a sweet taste, and a soft or smooth texture that can be eaten rapidly, sometimes even without being chewed (Kaplan, Sadock, & Grebb, 1994). The binging episodes often occur in secret and are usually only terminated by abdominal discomfort, sleep, social interruption, or self-induced vomiting. Although the eating binges may bring pleasure while they are occurring, self-degradation and depressed mood commonly follow.

In order to rid the body of the excessive calories, the individual may engage in **purging** behaviors (self-induced vomiting, or the misuse of laxatives, diuretics, or enemas) or other inappropriate compensatory behaviors, such as fasting or excessive exercise. There is a persistent overconcern with personal appearance, particularly regarding how they believe others perceive them. Weight fluctuations are common because of the alternating binges and fasts. However, most bulimics are within a normal weight range, some slightly underweight, some slightly overweight.

Excessive vomiting and laxative/diuretic abuse may lead to problems with dehydration and electrolyte imbalance. Gastric acid in the vomitus also contributes to the erosion of tooth enamel. In rare instances, the individual may experience tears in the gastric or esophageal mucosa.

Some people with this disorder are subject to mood disorders, anxiety disorders, substance abuse or dependence, most frequently involving amphetamines or alcohol (APA, 1994). Diagnostic criteria for bulimia nervosa are presented in Table 31.2.

Predisposing Factors to Anorexia Nervosa and Bulimia Nervosa

Biological Influences

Genetics. A hereditary predisposition to eating disorders has been hypothesized on the basis of family histories

---

■ **TABLE 31.1   DIAGNOSTIC CRITERIA FOR ANOREXIA NERVOSA**

A. Refusal to maintain body weight at or above a minimally normal weight for age and height (e.g., weight loss leading to maintenance of body weight less than 85% of that expected; or failure to make expected weight gain during period of growth, leading to body weight less than 85% of that expected).

B. Intense fear of gaining weight or becoming fat, even though underweight.

C. Disturbance in the way one's body weight or shape is experienced, undue influence of body weight or shape on self-evaluation, or denial of the seriousness of the current low body weight.

D. In postmenarcheal females, amenorrhea; that is, the absence of at least three consecutive menstrual cycles. (A woman is considered to have amenorrhea if her periods occur only following hormone, such as estrogen, administration.)

Specify type:
   Restricting Type: During the current episode of anorexia nervosa, the person has not regularly engaged in binge-eating or purging behavior (i.e., self-induced vomiting or the misuse of laxatives, diuretics, or enemas).
   Binge-Eating/Purging Type: During the current episode of anorexia nervosa, the person has regularly engaged in binge-eating or purging behavior (i.e., self-induced vomiting or the misuse of laxatives, diuretics, or enemas).

SOURCE: From APA (1994), with permission.

TABLE 31.2   DIAGNOSTIC CRITERIA FOR BULIMIA NERVOSA

A. Recurrent episodes of binge eating. An episode of binge eating is characterized by both of the following:
   1. Eating, in a discrete period of time (e.g., within any 2-hour period) an amount of food that is definitely larger than most people would eat during a similar period of time and under similar circumstances.
   2. A sense of lack of control over eating during the episode (e.g., a feeling that one cannot stop eating or control what or how much one is eating).
B. Recurrent inappropriate compensatory behavior in order to prevent weight gain, such as self-induced vomiting; misuse of laxatives, diuretics, enemas, or other medications; fasting; or excessive exercise.
C. The binge eating and inappropriate compensatory behaviors both occur, on average, at least twice a week for 3 months.
D. Self-evaluation is unduly influenced by body shape and weight.
E. The disturbance does not occur exclusively during episodes of anorexia nervosa.
Specify type:
   Purging Type: During the current episode of bulimia nervosa, the person has regularly engaged in self-induced vomiting or the misuse of laxatives, diuretics, or enemas.
   Nonpurging Type: During the current episode of bulimia nervosa, the person has used other inappropriate compensatory behaviors, such as fasting or excessive exercise, but has not regularly engaged in self-induced vomiting or the misuse of laxatives, diuretics, or enemas.

SOURCE: From APA (1994), with permission.

and an apparent association with other disorders for which the likelihood of genetic influences exist. Anorexia nervosa is more common among sisters and mothers of those with the disorder than among the general population. Several studies have reported a higher than expected frequency of mood disorders among first-degree biological relatives of people with anorexia nervosa and bulimia nervosa, and of substance abuse and dependence in relatives of individuals with bulimia nervosa (APA, 1994).

Neuroendocrine Abnormalities. Some speculation has occurred regarding a primary hypothalamic dysfunction in anorexia nervosa. Studies consistent with this theory have revealed elevated cerebral-spinal-fluid cortisol levels and a possible impairment of dopaminergic regulation in anorexics (Eckert & Mitchell, 1994). Additional evidence in the etiological implication of hypothalamic dysfunction is gathered from the fact that many anorexics experience amenorrhea before the onset of starvation and significant weight loss.

Biological influences in bulimia may be associated with the neurotransmitters serotonin and norepinephrine (Kaplan & Sadock, 1998). This hypothesis has been supported by the positive response these individuals have shown to therapy with the selective serotonin reuptake inhibitors (SSRIs). Some studies have found high levels of endogenous opioids in the spinal fluid of anorectic clients, promoting the speculation that these chemicals may contribute to denial of hunger (Kaplan & Sadock, 1998; Harvard Medical School, 1997). Some of these individuals have been shown to gain weight when given naloxone, an opioid antagonist.

Psychodynamic Influences

Psychodynamic theories suggest that eating disorders result from very early and profound disturbances in mother-infant interactions. The result is retarded ego development in the child and an unfulfilled sense of separation-individuation. This problem is compounded when the mother responds to the child's physical and emotional needs with food. Manifestations include a disturbance in body identity and a distortion in body image. When events occur that threaten the vulnerable ego, feelings emerge of lack of control over one's body (self). Behaviors associated with food and eating serve to provide feelings of control over one's life.

Family Influences

Conflict Avoidance. In the theory of the family as a system, psychosomatic symptoms, including anorexia nervosa, are reinforced in an effort to avoid spousal conflict. Parents are able to deny marital conflict by defining the sick child as the family problem. In these families, there is an unhealthy involvement between the members (enmeshment); the members strive at all costs to maintain "appearances"; and the parents endeavor to retain the child in the dependent position. Conflict avoidance may be a strong factor in the interpersonal dynamics of some families in which children develop eating disorders.

Elements of Power and Control. The issue of control may become the overriding factor in the family of the client with an eating disorder. These families often consist of a passive father, a domineering mother, and an overly dependent child. A high value is placed on perfectionism in this family, and the child feels he or she must satisfy these standards. Parental criticism promotes an increase in obsessive and perfectionistic behavior on the part of the child, who continues to seek love, approval, and recognition. The child eventually begins to feel helpless and ambivalent toward the parents. In adolescence, these distorted eating patterns may represent a rebellion against the parents, viewed by the child as a means of gaining, and remaining in, control. The symptoms are often triggered by a stressor that the adolescent perceives as a loss of control in some aspect of his or her life.

Obesity

Obesity is not classified as a psychiatric disorder in the *DSM-IV* but because of the strong emotional factors associated with the condition, it may be considered under *Psychological Factors Affecting Medical Condition*. A third category of eating disorder is also being considered by the American Psychiatric Association. Research criteria for binge-eating disorder (BED) is presented in the *DSM-IV* (see Table 31.3). Obesity is a factor in BED because the individual binges on large amounts of food but does not engage in behaviors to rid the body of the excess calories. The following formula is used to determine degree of obesity in an individual:

$$\text{Body mass index} = \frac{\text{Weight}}{\text{Height}^2}$$

The BMI range for normal weight is 20 to 24.9. Studies by the National Center for Health Statistics indicate that *overweight* is defined as a BMI of 25.0–29.9 (based on U.S. Dietary Guidelines for Americans) and *obesity* is defined as a BMI of 30.0 or greater (based on criteria of the World Health Organization; American Heart Association, 1998). These guidelines, which were released by the National Heart, Lung, and Blood Institute in June 1998, have been received by the medical community with a great deal of controversy. This change in guidelines increased the number of individuals in the United States considered to be obese from one third to approximately one half. The average American woman has a BMI of 26, and fashion models typically have BMIs of 18 (America's Health Network, 1998). Table 31.4 presents an example of some BMIs based on weight (in pounds) and height (in inches).

Obese people often present with hyperlipidemia, particularly elevated triglyceride and cholesterol levels. They commonly have hyperglycemia and are at risk for developing diabetes mellitus. Osteoarthritis may be evident owing to trauma to weight-bearing joints. Work load on the heart and lungs is increased, often leading to symptoms of angina or respiratory insufficiency (Long, 1995).

Predisposing Factors to Obesity
Biological Influences

Genetics. Genetics have been implicated in the development of obesity in that 80 percent of offspring of two obese parents are obese (Halmi, 1994). Studies of twins and adoptees reared by normal and overweight parents have also supported this implication of heredity as a predisposing factor to obesity.

Physiological Factors. Lesions in the appetite and satiety centers in the hypothalamus may contribute to overeating and lead to obesity. Hypothyroidism is a problem that interferes with basal metabolism and may lead to weight gain. Weight gain can also occur in response to the decreased insulin production of diabetes mellitus and the increased cortisone production of Cushing's disease.

Lifestyle Factors. On an elementary level, obesity can be viewed as an ingestion of a greater number of calories than are expended. Weight gain occurs when caloric intake exceeds caloric output in terms of basal metabolism and physical activity. Many overweight individuals lead sedentary lifestyles, making it very difficult to burn off calories.

■ **TABLE 31.3   RESEARCH CRITERIA FOR BINGE-EATING DISORDER**

A. Recurrent episodes of binge eating. An episode of binge eating is characterized by both of the following:
   1. Eating, in a discrete period of time (e.g., within any 2-hour period), an amount of food that is definitely larger than most people would eat in a similar period of time under similar circumstances.
   2. A sense of lack of control over eating during the episode (e.g., a feeling that one cannot stop eating or control what or how much one is eating).
B. The binge-eating episodes are associated with three (or more) of the following:
   1. Eating much more rapidly than normal.
   2. Eating until feeling uncomfortably full.
   3. Eating large amounts of food when not feeling physically hungry.
   4. Eating alone because of being embarrassed by how much one is eating.
   5. Feeling disgusted with oneself, depressed, or very guilty after overeating.
C. Marked distress regarding binge eating is present.
D. The binge eating occurs, on average, at least 2 days a week for 6 months.
   Note: The method of determining frequency differs from that used for bulimia nervosa; future research should address whether the preferred method of setting a frequency threshold is counting the number of days on which binges occur or counting the number of episodes of binge eating.
E. The binge eating is not associated with the regular use of inappropriate compensatory behaviors (e.g., purging, fasting, excessive exercise) and does not occur exclusively during the course of anorexia nervosa or bulimia nervosa.

SOURCE: From APA (1994), with permission.

TABLE 31.4   BODY MASS INDEX (BMI) CHART

To use this table, find the appropriate height in the left-hand column. Move across to a given weight. The number at the top of the column is the BMI at that height and weight. Pounds have been rounded off.

BMI Height (inches)	19	20	21	22	23	24	25	26	27	28	29	30	31	32	33	34	35	36	37	38	39	40
								Body Weight (pounds)														
58	91	96	100	105	110	115	119	124	129	134	138	143	148	153	158	162	167	172	177	181	186	191
59	94	99	104	109	114	119	124	128	133	138	143	148	153	158	163	168	173	178	183	188	193	198
60	97	102	107	112	118	123	128	133	138	143	148	153	158	163	168	174	179	184	189	194	199	204
61	100	106	111	116	122	127	132	137	143	148	153	158	164	169	174	180	185	190	195	201	206	211
62	104	109	115	120	126	131	136	142	147	153	158	164	169	175	180	186	191	196	202	207	213	218
63	107	113	118	124	130	135	141	146	152	158	163	169	175	180	186	191	197	203	208	214	220	225
64	110	116	122	128	134	140	145	151	157	163	169	174	180	186	192	197	204	209	215	221	227	232
65	114	120	126	132	138	144	150	156	162	168	174	180	186	192	198	204	210	216	222	228	234	240
66	118	124	130	136	142	148	155	161	167	173	179	186	192	198	204	210	216	223	229	235	241	247
67	121	127	134	140	146	153	159	166	172	178	185	191	198	204	211	217	223	230	236	242	249	255
68	125	131	138	144	151	158	164	171	177	184	190	197	203	210	216	223	230	236	243	249	256	262
69	128	135	142	149	155	162	169	176	182	189	196	203	209	216	223	230	236	243	250	257	263	270
70	132	139	146	153	160	167	174	181	188	195	202	209	216	222	229	236	243	250	257	264	271	278
71	136	143	150	157	165	172	179	186	193	200	208	215	222	229	236	243	250	257	265	272	279	286
72	140	147	154	162	169	177	184	191	199	206	213	221	228	235	242	250	258	265	272	279	287	294
73	144	151	159	166	174	182	189	197	204	212	219	227	235	242	250	257	265	272	280	288	295	302
74	148	155	163	171	179	186	194	202	210	218	225	233	241	249	256	264	272	280	287	295	303	311
75	152	160	168	176	184	192	200	208	216	224	232	240	248	256	264	272	279	287	295	303	311	319
76	156	164	172	180	189	197	205	213	221	230	238	246	254	263	271	279	287	295	304	312	320	328

SOURCE: National Heart, Lung, & Blood Institute, a division of the National Institutes of Health (1998).

Psychosocial Influences

The psychoanalytical view of obesity proposes that obese individuals have unresolved dependency needs and are fixed in the oral stage of psychosexual development (Norman, 1984). The symptoms of obesity are viewed as depressive equivalents, attempts to regain "lost" or frustrated nurturance and care.

Lomax (1989) describes an oral character structure, the traits of which include excessive optimism or pessimism, greed, demandingness, dependency, and impatience. Together, these traits form a characteristic personality configuration that is etiologically significant and is found in strong association with obesity.

Kaplan, Sadock, and Grebb (1994) suggest that psychodynamic factors related to obesity include oral fixation, oral regression, and the overvaluation of food. These characteristics are thought to be especially important in the case of binge eating.

Transactional Model of Stress/Adaptation

The etiology of eating disorders is most likely influenced by multiple factors. In Figure 31.1, a graphic depiction of this theory of multiple causation is presented in the transactional model of stress/adaptation.

Diagnosis/Outcome Identification

Based on the data collected during the nursing assessment, possible nursing diagnoses for the client with eating disorders include:

Altered nutrition: Less than body requirements related to refusal to eat.

Fluid volume deficit (risk for or actual) related to decreased fluid intake; self-induced vomiting; laxative and/or diuretic abuse.

Ineffective denial related to retarded ego development and fear of losing the only aspect of life over which he or she perceives some control (eating).

Altered nutrition: More than body requirements related to compulsive overeating.

Body image/self-esteem disturbance related to retarded ego development, dysfunctional family system, or feelings of dissatisfaction with body appearance.

Anxiety (moderate to severe) related to feelings of helplessness and lack of control over life events.

The following criteria may be used for measurement of outcomes in the care of clients with eating disorders:

THE CLIENT(S):

1. Has achieved and maintained at least 85 percent of expected body weight.

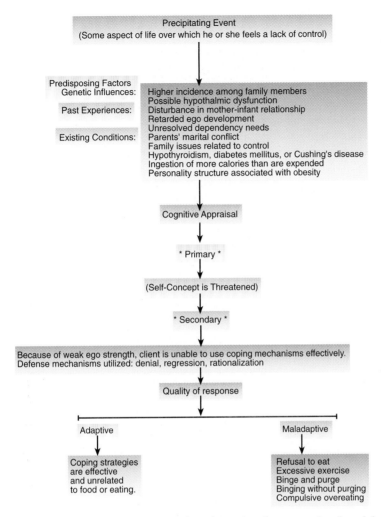

Figure 31.1   The dynamics of eating disorders using the transactional model of stress/adaptation.

2. Vital signs, blood pressure, and laboratory serum studies are within normal limits.

3. Verbalizes importance of adequate nutrition.

4. Verbalizes knowledge regarding consequences of fluid loss caused by self-induced vomiting (or laxative/diuretic abuse) and importance of adequate fluid intake.

5. Verbalizes events that precipitate anxiety and demonstrates techniques for its reduction.

6. Verbalizes ways in which he or she may gain more control of the environment and thereby reduce feelings of helplessness.

7. Expresses interest in welfare of others and less preoccupation with own appearance.

8. Verbalizes that image of body as "fat" was misperception and demonstrates ability to take control of own life without resorting to maladaptive eating behaviors (anorexia nervosa).

9. Has established a healthy pattern of eating for weight control with weight loss toward a desired goal progressing.

10. Verbalizes plans for future maintenance of weight control.

Planning/Implementation

Tables 31.5 and 31.6 provide plans of care for clients with eating disorders. Nursing diagnoses are presented, along with outcome criteria, appropriate nursing interventions, and rationales.

Some institutions are using a case management model to coordinate care (see Chapter 7 for more detailed explanation). In case management models, the plan of care may take the form of a critical pathway. Table 31.7 depicts an example of a critical pathway of care for a client with anorexia nervosa.

Client/Family Education

The role of client teacher is important in the psychiatric area, as it is in all areas of nursing. A list of topics for client

TABLE 31.5   CARE PLAN FOR CLIENT WITH EATING DISORDERS: ANOREXIA NERVOSA AND BULIMIA NERVOSA

NURSING DIAGNOSES: ALTERED NUTRITION: LESS THAN BODY REQUIREMENTS/ FLUID VOLUME DEFICIT (RISK FOR OR ACTUAL)

RELATED TO: Refusal to eat/drink; self-induced vomiting; abuse of laxatives/diuretics

EVIDENCED BY: Loss of weight; poor muscle tone and skin turgor; lanugo; bradycardia; hypotension; cardiac arrhythmias; pale, dry mucous membranes

OUTCOME CRITERIA	NURSING INTERVENTIONS	RATIONALE
Client will achieve 80%–85% of body weight and be free of signs and symptoms of malnutrition/dehydration.	1. Dietitian will determine number of calories required to provide adequate nutrition and realistic weight gain.	1. Adequate calories are required to allow a weight gain of 2–3 lb per week.
	2. Explain to the client that privileges and restrictions will be based on compliance with treatment and direct weight gain. Do not focus on food and eating.	2. The real issues have little to do with food or eating patterns. Focus on the control issues that have precipitated these behaviors.
	3. Weigh client daily, immediately upon arising and following first voiding. Always use same scale, if possible. Keep strict record of intake and output. Assess skin turgor and integrity regularly. Assess moistness and color of oral mucous membranes.	3. These assessments are important measurements of nutritional status and provide guidelines for treatment.
	4. Stay with client during established time for meals (usually 30 min) and for at least 1 hr following meals.	4. Lengthy mealtimes put excessive focus on food and eating and provide client with attention and reinforcement. The hour following meals may be used to discard food stashed from tray or to engage in self-induced vomiting.
	5. If weight loss occurs, employ restrictions. Client must understand that if nutritional status deteriorates, tube feedings will be initiated. This is implemented in a matter-of-fact, nonpunitive way.	5. Restrictions and limits must be established and carried out consistently to avoid power struggles, to encourage client compliance with therapy, and to ensure client safety.

NURSING DIAGNOSIS: INEFFECTIVE DENIAL

RELATED TO: Retarded ego development and fear of losing the only aspect of life over which client perceives some control (eating)

EVIDENCED BY: Inability to admit the impact of maladaptive eating behaviors on life pattern

OUTCOME CRITERIA	NURSING INTERVENTIONS	RATIONALE
Client will verbalize understanding that eating behaviors are maladaptive and demonstrate the ability to cope with issues of control in a more adaptive manner.	1. Develop a trusting relationship. Convey positive regard.	1. Trust and unconditional acceptance promote dignity and self-worth and provide a strong foundation for a therapeutic relationship.
	2. Avoid arguing or bargaining with the client who is resistant to treatment. State matter-of-factly which behaviors are unacceptable and how privileges will be restricted for noncompliance.	2. The person who is denying a problem and who also has a weak ego will use manipulation to achieve control. Consistency and firmness by staff will decrease use of these behaviors.
	3. Encourage client to verbalize feelings regarding role within the family and issues related to dependence/ independence, the intense need for achievement, and sexuality. Help client recognize ways in which he or she can gain control over these problematic areas of life.	3. When client feels control over major life issues, the need to gain control through maladaptive eating behaviors will diminish.

NURSING DIAGNOSIS: BODY IMAGE/SELF-ESTEEM DISTURBANCE
RELATED TO: Retarded ego development and dysfunctional family system
EVIDENCED BY: Distorted body image; difficulty accepting positive reinforcement; depressed mood and self-deprecating thoughts

OUTCOME CRITERIA	NURSING INTERVENTIONS	RATIONALE
Client will acknowledge misperception of body image as "fat" and verbalize positive self-attributes.	1. Help client to develop a realistic perception of body image and relationship with food. Compare specific measurement of the client's body with the client's perceived calculations. 2. Promote feelings of control within the environment through participation and independent decision making. Through positive feedback, help client learn to accept self as is, including weaknesses as well as strengths. 3. Help client realize that perfection is unrealistic, and explore this need with him or her.	1. There may be a large discrepancy between the actual body size and the client's perception of his or her body size. Client needs to recognize that the misperception of body image is unhealthy and that maintaining control through maladaptive eating behaviors is dangerous—even life threatening. 2. Client must come to understand that he or she is a capable, autonomous individual who can perform outside the family unit and who is not expected to be perfect. Control of his or her life must be achieved in other ways besides dieting and weight loss. 3. As client begins to feel better about self and identifies positive self-attributes, as well as develops the ability to accept certain personal inadequacies, the need for unrealistic achievement should diminish.

and family education relevant to eating disorders is presented in Table 31.8.

Evaluation

Evaluation of the client with an eating disorder requires a reassessment of the behaviors for which the client sought treatment. Behavioral change will be required on the part of both the client and family members. The following types of questions may provide assistance in gathering data required for evaluating whether the nursing interventions have been effective in achieving the goals of therapy.

FOR ANOREXIA OR BULIMIA:

1. Has the client steadily gained 2 to 3 lb per week to at least 80 percent of body weight for age and size?
2. Is the client free of signs and symptoms of malnutrition and dehydration?
3. Does the client consume adequate calories as determined by the dietitian?
4. Have there been any attempts to stash food from tray to discard later?
5. Have there been any attempts to self-induce vomiting?
6. Has the client admitted that a problem exists and that eating behaviors are maladaptive?

7. Have behaviors aimed at manipulating the environment been discontinued?
8. Is the client willing to discuss the real issues concerning family roles, sexuality, dependence/independence, and the need for achievement?
9. Does the client understand how he or she has used maladaptive eating behaviors in an effort to achieve a feeling of some control over life events?
10. Has the client acknowledged that perception of body image as "fat" is incorrect?

FOR OBESITY:

1. Has the client shown a steady weight loss since starting the new eating plan?
2. Does he or she verbalize a plan to help stay on the new eating plan?
3. Does the client verbalize positive self-attributes not associated with body size or appearance?

FOR ANOREXIA, BULIMIA, AND OBESITY:

1. Has the client been able to develop a more realistic perception of body image?
2. Has the client acknowledged that past self-expectations may have been unrealistic?
3. Does client accept self as less than perfect?
4. Has the client developed adaptive coping strategies to deal with stress without resorting to maladaptive eating behaviors?

TABLE 31.6   CARE PLAN FOR THE CLIENT WITH AN EATING DISORDER: OBESITY

NURSING DIAGNOSIS: ALTERED NUTRITION: MORE THAN BODY REQUIREMENTS
RELATED TO: Compulsive overeating
EVIDENCED BY: Weight of more than 20% over expected body weight for age and height; BMI > 30

OUTCOME CRITERIA	NURSING INTERVENTIONS	RATIONALE
Client will demonstrate change in eating patterns resulting in a steady weight loss.	1. Encourage the client to keep a diary of food intake.	1. A food diary provides the opportunity for client to gain a realistic picture of the amount of food ingested and provides a database on which to tailor the dietary program.
	2. Discuss feelings and emotions associated with eating.	2. This helps to identify when client is eating to satisfy an emotional need rather than a physiological one.
	3. With input from the client, formulate an eating plan that includes food from the basic food groups with emphasis on low-fat intake. It is helpful to keep the plan as similar to client's usual eating pattern as possible.	3. Diet must eliminate calories while maintaining adequate nutrition. Client is more likely to stay on the eating plan if he or she is able to participate in its creation and it deviates as little as possible from usual types of foods.
	4. Identify realistic increment goals for weekly weight loss.	4. Reasonable weight loss (1–2 lb/wk) results in more lasting effects. Excessive, rapid weight loss may result in fatigue and irritability and ultimately lead to failure in meeting goals for weight loss. Motivation is more easily sustained by meeting "stair-step goals."
	5. Plan progressive exercise program tailored to individual goals and choice.	5. Exercise may enhance weight loss by burning calories and reducing appetite, increasing energy, toning muscles, and enhancing sense of well-being and accomplishment. Walking is an excellent choice for overweight individuals.
	6. Discuss the probability of reaching plateaus when weight remains stable for extended periods.	6. Client should know this is likely to happen as changes in metabolism occur. Plateaus cause frustration, and client may need additional support during these times to remain on the weight-loss program.
	7. Administer medications to assist with weight loss if ordered by physician.	7. Appetite-suppressant drugs (e.g., diethylproprion) and drugs that have weight loss as a side effect (e.g., fluoxetine) may be helpful to someone who is morbidly obese. They should be used for this purpose for only a short period while the individual attempts to adjust to the new pattern of eating.

NURSING DIAGNOSIS: BODY IMAGE/SELF-ESTEEM DISTURBANCE
RELATED TO: Dissatisfaction with appearance
EVIDENCED BY: Verbalization of negative feelings about the way he or she looks and desire to lose weight

OUTCOME CRITERIA	NURSING INTERVENTIONS	RATIONALE
Client will begin to accept self based on self-attributes rather than on appearance, while actively pursuing weight loss as desired.	1. Assess client's feelings and attitudes about being obese.	1. Obesity and compulsive eating behaviors may have deep-rooted psychological implications, such as compensation for lack of love and nurturing or a defense against intimacy.

2. Ensure that the client has privacy during self-care activities.

3. Have client recall coping patterns related to food in family of origin and explore how these may affect current situation.

4. Determine client's motivation for weight loss and set goals.

5. Help client identify positive self-attributes. Focus on strengths and past accomplishments unrelated to physical appearance.

6. Refer client to support or therapy group.

2. The obese individual may be sensitive or self-conscious about his or her body.

3. Parents are role models for their children. Maladaptive eating behaviors are learned within the family system and are supported through positive reinforcement. Food may be substituted by the parent for affection and love, and eating is associated with a feeling of satisfaction, becoming the primary defense.

4. The individual may harbor repressed feelings of hostility, which may be expressed inward on the self. Because of a poor self-concept, the person often has difficulty with relationships. When the motivation is to lose weight for someone else, successful weight loss is less likely to occur.

5. It is important that self-esteem not be tied solely to size of the body. Client needs to recognize that obesity need not interfere with positive feelings regarding self-concept and self-worth.

6. Support groups can provide companionship, increase motivation, decrease loneliness and social ostracism, and give practical solutions to common problems. Group therapy can be helpful in dealing with underlying psychological concerns.

TREATMENT MODALITIES

The immediate aim of treatment in eating disorders is to restore the client's nutritional status. Complications of emaciation, dehydration, and electrolyte imbalance can lead to death. Once the physical condition is no longer life-threatening, other treatment modalities may be initiated.

Behavior Modification

Efforts to change the maladaptive eating behaviors of clients with anorexia and bulimia have become the widely accepted treatment. The importance of instituting a behavior modification program with these clients is to ensure that the program does not "control" them. Issues of control are central to the etiology of these disorders, and in order for the program to be successful, the client must perceive that he or she is in control of the treatment.

Successes have been observed when the client is allowed to contract for privileges based on weight gain (Sanger & Cassino, 1984). The client has input into the care plan and can clearly see what the treatment choices are. The client has control over eating, over the amount

of exercise pursued, and even over whether or not to induce vomiting. Goals of therapy are agreed on by client and staff, along with the responsibilities of each for goal achievement.

Staff and client also agree on a system of rewards and privileges that can be earned by the client, who is given ultimate control. He or she has a choice of whether or not to abide by the contract—a choice of whether or not to gain weight—a choice of whether or not to earn the desired privilege.

Individual Therapy

Although individual psychotherapy is not the therapy of choice for eating disorders, it can be helpful when underlying psychological problems are contributing to the maladaptive behaviors. In supportive psychotherapy, the therapist encourages the client to explore unresolved conflicts and to recognize the maladaptive eating behaviors as defense mechanisms used to ease the emotional pain. The goals are to resolve the personal issues and establish more adaptive coping strategies for dealing with stressful situations.

TABLE 31.7 CRITICAL PATHWAY OF CARE FOR CLIENT WITH ANOREXIA NERVOSA ON A BEHAVIORAL UNIT

Estimated Length of Stay: 28 days—Variations from designated pathway should be documented in progress notes

Nursing Diagnoses and Categories of Care	Time Dimension	Goals and/or Actions	Time Dimension	Goals and/or Actions	Time Dimension	Discharge Outcome
Altered nutrition: Less than body requirements. Fluid volume deficit, risk for	Ongoing	Client will gain 3 lb/wk and maintain adequate state of hydration			Day 28	Client will exhibit no signs/symptoms of malnutrition or dehydration.
Referrals	Day 1 and ongoing	Consult dietitian	Day 2–28	Fulfill nutritional needs. Client consumes 75% of food provided and at least 1000 ml fluid/day.		
Diagnostic studies	Day 1	Electrolytes Electrocardiogram Blood urea nitrogen/ creatinine Urinalysis Complete blood count Thyroid function	Day 14	Repeat of selected diagnostic studies.	Day 28	All laboratory values are within normal limits.
Additional assessments	Daily; q shift Daily; q shift Day 1 Day 1	Vital signs Input and output Weight Monitor for purging following meals.	Day 7–28 Day 7–28 Day 2–28 Day 1–21	Vital signs within normal limits. Appropriate balance is achieved. Client gains approximately ½ lb/day. Client bathroom is locked for 1 hr following meals.	Day 22–28	Client is able to refrain from self-induced vomiting.
Patient education	Day 1	Unit orientation; behavior modification plan	Day 7–14	Principles of nutrition; foods for maintenance of wellness.	Day 15–28	Client demonstrates ability to select appropriate foods for healthy diet.
Ineffective denial	Day 1	Client will cooperate with orientation to unit and explanation of behavior modification plan.	Day 2–28	Client cooperates with therapy to restore nutritional status.	Day 18–28	Client accepts that eating behaviors are maladaptive and demonstrates ability to cope more adaptively.
Referrals	Day 7 (or when physical condition is stable)	Psychologist; social worker; psycho- dramatist	Day 8–28	Client attends group psychotherapies daily.	Day 28	Client verbalizes ways to gain control in life situation.
Additional assessments	Day 1–17	Assess client's ability to trust; use of manipulation to achieve control.	Day 14	Client has developed trust- ing relationship with at least one staff member on each shift.	Day 28	Client no longer manipulates others to achieve control.

Nursing Diagnoses and Categories of Care	Time Dimension	Goals and/or Actions	Time Dimension	Goals and/or Actions	Time Dimension	Discharge Outcome
Patient education	Day 1 and ongoing as required.	Describe privileges and responsibilities of behavior modification program. Explain consequences of noncompliance.	Day 21	Discuss role of support groups for individuals with eating disorders.	Day 28	Client and family verbalize intention to attend community support group.
Body image/self-esteem disturbance	Day 7	Client acknowledges that attention will not be given to the discussion of body image and food.	Day 21	Client acknowledges misperception of body image as fat and verbalizes positive self-attributes.	Day 28	Client perceives body image correctly, is not obsessed with food, and has given up the need for perfection.
Referrals	Day 1 (or when condition is stable)	Occupational therapy; recreational therapy; music therapy; art therapy.	Day 2–28	Client attends therapy sessions on a daily basis.	Day 28	Through self-expression, client has gained self-awareness and and verbalizes positive attributes of self.
Additional assessments	Day 7	Compare specific measurements of client's body with client's perceived calculations. Clarify discrepancies.	Day 8–28	Discuss strengths and weaknesses. Client should strive to achieve self-acceptance.	Day 28	Client verbalizes acceptance of self, including "imperfections."
Client education	Day 14–28	Discuss alternative coping strategies for dealing with feelings. Have client keep diary of feelings, particularly when thinking about food.			Day 28	Client demonstrates adaptive coping strategies unrelated to eating behaviors for dealing with feelings.

Family Therapy

Eckert and Mitchell (1994) state:

"Counseling of family members is a necessary component of an effective treatment program. This involves educating the family about the disorder, assessing the family's impact on maintaining the disorder, and assisting in methods to promote normal functioning of the patient." (p. 199)

In many instances, eating disorders may be considered *family* disorders, and resolution cannot be achieved until dynamics within the family have improved.

Family therapy deals with education of the members about the disorder's manifestations, possible etiology, and prescribed treatment. Support is given to family members as they deal with feelings of guilt associated with the perception that they may have contributed to the onset of the disorder. Support is also given as they deal with the social stigma of having a family member with emotional problems.

In some instances when the dysfunctional family dynamics are related to conflict avoidance, the family may be noncompliant with therapy, as they attempt to maintain equilibrium by keeping a member in the sick role. When this occurs, it is essential to focus on the functional operations within the family and to help them manage conflict and create change.

Referrals are made to local support groups for families of individuals with eating disorders. Resolution and growth can sometimes be achieved through interaction

TABLE 31.8   TOPICS FOR CLIENT/FAMILY EDUCATION RELATED TO EATING DISORDERS

Nature of the Illness
1. Symptoms of anorexia nervosa
2. Symptoms of bulimia nervosa
3. What constitutes obesity
4. Causes of eating disorders
4. Effects of the illness or condition on the body

Management of the Illness
1. Principles of nutrition (foods for maintenance of wellness)
2. Ways client may feel in control of life (aside from eating)
3. Importance of expressing fears and feelings, rather than holding them inside
4. Alternative coping strategies (to maladaptive eating behaviors)
5. For the obese client:
   a. How to plan a reduced-calorie, nutritious diet
   b. How to read food content labels
   c. How to establish a realistic weight-loss plan
   d. How to establish a planned program of physical activity
6. Correct administration of prescribed medications (e.g., antidepressants, anorexigenics)
7. Indication for and side effects of prescribed medications
8. Relaxation techniques
9. Problem-solving skills

Support Services
1. Weight Watchers International
2. Overeaters Anonymous
3. National Association of Anorexia Nervosa and Associated Disorders (ANAD)
   P.O. Box 7
   Highland Park, IL 60035
   (847) 831-3438
4. The American Anorexia/Bulimia Association, Inc.
   165 W. 46th St., Suite 1108
   New York, NY 10036
   (212) 575-6200

with others who are experiencing, or have experienced, the numerous problems of living with a family member with an eating disorder.

Psychopharmacology

There are no medications specifically indicated for eating disorders. Various medications have been prescribed for associated symptoms, such as anxiety and depression. Halmi, Mitchell, and Rigotti (1995) report on the use of fluoxetine (Prozac), sertraline (Zoloft), and clomipramine (Anafranil) in clients with anorexia nervosa. Cyproheptadine (Periactin), in its unlabeled use as an appetite stimulant, antipsychotics such as chlorpromazine (Thorazine), and lithium carbonate have also been used to treat this disorder in selected clients.

Fluoxetine (Prozac) is the drug of choice for treating bulimia nervosa. (Halmi, Mitchell, & Rigotti, 1995). A dosage of 60 mg/day (triple the usual antidepressant dosage) was found to be most effective with bulimic clients. It is possible

that fluoxetine, a selective serotonin reuptake inhibitor, may decrease the craving for carbohydrates, thereby decreasing the incidence of binge eating, which is often associated with consumption of large amounts of carbohydrates. Other antidepressants, such as imipramine (Tofranil), desipramine (Norpramine), trazodone (Desyrel), and phenelzine (Nardil), also have been shown to be effective in controlled treatment studies (Halmi, 1994; Halmi, Mitchell, & Rigotti, 1995). Fluoxetine has also been successful in treating overweight clients, possibly for the same reason that was explained for bulimic clients. The effective dosage for promoting weight loss is 60 mg/day.

Kaplan, Sadock, and Grebb (1994) state:

"Sympathomimetics were previously used in the treatment of obesity because of their anorexia-inducing effects. Because tolerance develops for the anorectic effects and because of the drugs' high abuse potential, that indication is no longer considered justified." (p. 982)

Withdrawal from **anorexigenics** may result in a rebound weight gain and, in some clients, a concomitant lethargy and depression. Two once widely used anorexigenics, fenfluramine and dexfenfluramine, have been removed from the market because of their association with serious heart and lung disease.

A new medication for treating obesity became available in March 1998. Sibutramine (Meridia) has been suggested only for individuals who have a significant amount of weight to lose. The mechanism of action in the control of appetite appears to occur by inhibiting the neurotransmitters serotonin and norepinephrine. Common side effects include headache, dry mouth, constipation, and insomnia. More troublesome side effects include increased blood

---

TEST YOUR CRITICAL THINKING SKILLS

Cathy,[1] a high school sophomore, saw herself as an aspiring actress. When she was not chosen for the lead part in the school play, she believed it was because she was too fat. She was 5′3″ tall and weighed 110 lb. She decided to skip lunches to try and lose weight. When the pounds did not come off as quickly as she wanted, she began to skip breakfast also. She tried to keep her daily consumption to no more than 300 calories.

After weeks of starving herself, Cathy fainted in gym class. She was rushed to the emergency department. She weighed 90 lb. The physician saw how emaciated she was and admitted her immediately. Her diagnosis was anorexia nervosa.

Answer the following questions about Cathy:

1. What will be the primary consideration in her care?
2. How will treatment be directed toward helping her gain weight?
3. How will the nurse know if Cathy is using self-induced vomiting to rid herself of food consumed at meals?

[1]Adapted from Arnold (1996).

R E S E A R C H   N O T E

Guided self-change for bulimia nervosa incorporating use of a self-care manual. *American Journal of Psychiatry* (1998, July), 155, 947–953.
Thiels, C., Schmidt, U., Treasure, J., Garthe, R., and Troop, N.

Description of the Study: This was a study of 62 patients with the diagnosis of bulimia nervosa, who were randomly assigned to either: (1) 16 weekly sessions of conventional individual cognitive behavioral therapy (CBT) or (2) use of a self-help manual, plus eight sessions of CBT scheduled every other week to review and provide reinforcement for use of the self-help manual (guided self-change). The manual encouraged keeping a food diary, and it provided information about eating disorders and strategies for dealing with symptoms as well as skills associated with CBT. Outcomes were measured according to the following:

1. Eating Disorder Examination (experts' ratings on overeating, vomiting, dietary restraint, and shape and weight concerns)
2. Bulimic Investigatory Test Edinburgh (Subjects' self-reports)
3. Beck Depression Inventory
4. Self-Concept Questionnaire
5. Knowledge of nutrition, weight, and shape

Results of the Study: Measures were taken at the end of treatment and at follow-up an average of 43 weeks after treatment. Results at follow-up showed that 71 percent of the CBT group had not binged or vomited during the preceding week, while 70 percent of the guided self-help group had not binged and 61 percent had not vomited during the week before follow-up. Improvements in depression were also similar between the two groups.

Comments: On the basis of this study, the authors suggest that guided self-help may be an alternative to conventional CBT for treating certain ambulatory patients with eating disorders. Amount of therapist contact is about one half, cost of treatment is significantly reduced, and outcomes are comparably effective.

pressure and pulse rate. Although it has not been associated with the serious cardiopulmonary diseases for which the previously mentioned medications were recalled, precautions should be taken when considering this medication for an individual with a history of cardiac disease.

SUMMARY

The incidence of eating disorders has continued to increase over the past 30 years. Individuals with anorexia nervosa, a disorder that is characterized by a morbid fear of obesity and a gross distortion of body image, can literally starve themselves to death. The individual believes he or she is fat even when emaciated. The disorder is commonly accompanied by depression and anxiety.

Bulimia nervosa is an eating disorder characterized by the consumption of huge amounts of food, usually in a short period of time, and often in secret. Tension is relieved and pleasure felt during the time of the "binge" but is soon followed by feelings of guilt and depression. Individuals with this disorder "purge" themselves of the excessive intake with self-induced vomiting or the misuse of laxatives, diuretics, or enemas. They, too, are subject to mood and anxiety disorders.

Compulsive eating can result in obesity, which is defined by the National Institutes of Health as a BMI of 30. Obesity predisposes the individual to many health concerns, and at the morbid level (a BMI of 40.0), the weight alone can contribute to increases in morbidity and mortality.

This chapter explored the predisposing factors to these three eating disorders. Symptomatology was identified as background assessment data. Nursing care was presented in the context of the six steps of the nursing process. Care plans for anorexia/bulimia and obesity and a critical pathway of care for the anorexic client were included. The treatment modalities of behavior modification, individual psychotherapy, family therapy, and psychopharmacology were discussed.

INTERNET REFERENCES

- Additional information about anorexia nervosa and bulimia nervosa may be located at the following websites:
  a. http://members.aol.com/amanbu/
  b. http://www.psych.org/public_info/eating.html
  c. http://www.mentalhealth.com/dis/p20-et01.html
  d. http://www.anred.com/
  e. http://www.mentalhealth.com/dis/p20-et02.html
  f. http://www.nimh.nih.gov/publicat/eatdis.htm
  g. http://www.medlineplus.nlm.nih.gov/medlineplus/eatingdisorders.html

- Additional information about obesity may be located at the following websites:
  a. http://www.shapeup.org/bmi/index.html
  b. http://www.obesity.org/
  c. http://medlineplus.nlm.nih.gov/medlineplus/obesity.html
  d. http://www.asbp.org/bariatrics/obesity.htm
  e. http://www.niddk.nih.gov/health/nutrit/pubs/binge.htm

REVIEW QUESTIONS

SELF-EXAMINATION/LEARNING EXERCISE

Select the answer that is most appropriate for each of the following questions.

1. Some obese individuals take amphetamines to suppress appetite and help them lose weight. Which of the following is an adverse effect associated with use of amphetamines that makes this practice undesirable?

   a. Bradycardia.
   b. Amenorrhea.
   c. Tolerance.
   d. Convulsions.

2. Psychoanalytically, the theory of obesity relates to the individual's unconscious equation of food with:

   a. Love and affection.
   b. Power and control.
   c. Autonomy and emotional growth.
   d. Strength and endurance.

3. From a physiological point of view, the *most common* cause of obesity is probably:

   a. Lack of nutritional education.
   b. More calories consumed than expended.
   c. Impaired endocrine functioning.
   d. Low basal metabolic rate.

4. Nancy, age 14, has just been admitted to the psychiatric unit for anorexia nervosa. She is emaciated and refusing to eat. What is the primary nursing diagnosis for Nancy?

   a. Dysfunctional grieving.
   b. Altered nutrition: Less than body requirements.
   c. Alteration in family process.
   d. Anxiety (severe).

5. Which of the following physical manifestations would you expect to assess in Nancy?

   a. Tachycardia, hypertension, hyperthermia.
   b. Bradycardia, hypertension, hyperthermia.
   c. Bradycardia, hypotension, hypothermia.
   d. Tachycardia, hypotension, hypothermia.

6. Nancy continues to refuse to eat. What is the most appropriate response by the nurse?

   a. "You know that if you don't eat, you will die."
   b. "If you continue to refuse to take food orally, you will be fed through a nasogastric tube."
   c. "You might as well leave if you are not going to follow your therapy regimen."
   d. "You don't have to eat if you don't want to. It is your choice."

7. Which medication might you expect the physician to prescribe for Nancy?

   a. Chlorpromazine (Thorazine).
   b. Diazepam (Valium).
   c. Fluoxetine (Prozac).
   d. Carbamazepine (Tegretol).

8. Jane is hospitalized on the psychiatric unit. She has a history and current diagnosis of bulimia nervosa. Which of the following symptoms would be congruent with Jane's diagnosis?

   a. Binging, purging, obesity, hyperkalemia.
   b. Binging, purging, normal weight, hypokalemia.

c. Binging, laxative abuse, amenorrhea, severe weight loss.

d. Binging, purging, severe weight loss, hyperkalemia.

9. Jane has stopped vomiting in the hospital and tells the nurse she is afraid she is going to gain weight. Which is the most appropriate response by the nurse?

   a. "Don't worry. The dietitian will ensure you don't get too many calories in your diet."

   b. "Don't worry about your weight. We are going to work on other problems while you are in the hospital."

   c. "I understand that you are concerned about your weight, but I want you to tell me about your recent invitation to join the National Honor Society. That's quite an accomplishment."

   d. "You are not fat, and the staff will ensure that you do not gain weight while you are in the hospital, because we know that is important to you."

10. The binging episode is thought to involve:

    a. A release of tension, followed by feelings of depression.

    b. Feelings of fear, followed by feelings of relief.

    c. Unmet dependency needs and a way to gain attention.

    d. Feelings of euphoria, excitement, and self-gratification.

REFERENCES

American Psychiatric Association. (1994). *Diagnostic and statistical manual of mental disorders* (4th ed.). Washington, DC: American Psychiatric Association.

America's Health Network. (1998). Easy answer to weight-loss in America? Fat Chance! [On-line]. Available: http://www.ahn.com/ community/wellness/authors/twinkle/fatchance/HTM

Arnold, M.K. (1996). Get the help you need to recover from an eating disorder. *Psychopharmacology update*. Providence, RI: Manisses Communications Group.

Eckert, E.D., & Mitchell, J.E. (1994). Anorexia nervosa and bulimia nervosa. In G. Winokur & P.J. Clayton (Eds.), *The medical basis of psychiatry* (2nd ed.). Philadelphia: WB Saunders.

Halmi, K.A. (1994). Eating disorders: Anorexia nervosa, bulimia nervosa, and obesity. In R.E. Hales, S.C. Yudofsky, & J.A. Talbott (Eds.), *Textbook of psychiatry* (2nd ed.). Washington, DC: American Psychiatric Press.

Halmi, K.A., Mitchell, J.E., & Rigotti, N.A. (1995). Recognizing and treating eating disorders. *Contemporary Nurse Practitioner*, 1(1), 26–39.

Harvard Medical School. (1997, October). Eating disorders—Part I. *Harvard Mental Health Letter*, 14(4), 1–5.

Jones, D.J., Fox, M.M., Babigian, H.M., & Hutton, H.E. (1980). Epidemiology of anorexia nervosa in Monroe County, New York: 1960–1976. *Psychosomatic Medicine*, 42, 551.

Kaplan, H.I., & Sadock, B.J. (1998). *Synopsis of psychiatry: Behavioral sciences/clinical psychiatry* (8th ed.). Baltimore: Williams & Wilkins.

Kaplan, H.I., Sadock, B.J., & Grebb, J.A. (1994). *Synopsis of psychiatry* (7th ed.). Baltimore: Williams & Wilkins.

Leon, G.R., & Dinklage, D. (1989). Obesity and anorexia nervosa. In T.H. Ollendick & M. Hersen (Eds.), *Handbook of child psychopathology* (2nd ed.). New York: Plenum Press.

Lomax, J.W. (1989). Obesity. In H.I. Kaplan & B.J. Sadock (Eds.), *Comprehensive textbook of psychiatry* (5th ed.). Baltimore: Williams & Wilkins.

Long, B.C. (1995). Healthy life-styles: Nutrition, exercise, rest, and sleep. In W.J. Phipps, V.L. Cassmoyer, J.K. Sands, & M.K. Lehman (Eds.), *Medical-surgical nursing: Concepts and clinical practice* (5th ed.). St. Louis: C.V. Mosby.

Long, B.C., & Neville, J. (1987). Interventions for persons with problems of ingestion. In W.J. Phipps, B.C. Long, & N.F. Woods (Eds.), *Medical-surgical nursing: Concepts and clinical practice* (3rd ed.). St. Louis: C.V. Mosby.

National Heart, Lung, & Blood Institute. (1998). Body mass index (BMI) chart. Bethesda, MD: National Institute of Health.

Norman, K. (1984). Eating disorders. In H.H. Goldman (Ed.), *Review of general psychiatry*. Los Altos, CA: Lange Medical Publications.

Sanger, E., & Cassino, T. (1984, January). Eating disorders: Avoiding the power struggle. *American Journal of Nursing*, 84 (1), 31–33.

Schmidt, N.J. (1998). Obesity [On-line]. Available: http://www.pitt.edu/~nasst25/obesity.html

Bibliography

Anderson, A.E., & Holman, J.E. (1997). Males with eating disorders: Challenges for treatment and research. *Psychopharmacology Bulletin*, 33, 391–397.

Bulik, C.M., Sullivan, P.F., Joyce, P.R., Carter, F.A., & McIntosh, V.V. (1998, July–August). Predictors of 1-year treatment outcome in bulimia nervosa. *Comprehensive Psychiatry*, 39, 206–214.

Carlat, D.J., Camargo, C.A., & Herzog, D.B. (1997, August). Eating disorders in males: A report on 135 patients. *American Journal of Psychiatry*, 154, 1127–1132.

Coren, S., & Hewitt, P.L. (1998, August). Is anorexia nervosa associated with elevated rates of suicide? *American Journal of Public Health*, 88, 1206–1207.

Harvard Medical School. (1997, November). Eating disorders—Part II. *Harvard Mental Health Letter*, 14(5), 1–5.

Hofland, S.L., & Dardis, P.O. (1992). Bulimia nervosa: Associated physical problems. *Journal of Psychosocial Nursing*, 30(2), 23–27.

Mcgilley, B.M., & Pryor, T.L. (1998, June). Assessment and treatment of bulimia nervosa. *American Family Physician*, 57, 2743–2750.

McGowan, A., & Whitbread, J. (1996). Out of control! The most effective way to help the binge-eating patient. *Journal of Psychosocial Nursing*, 34(1), 30–37.

O'Meara, S., & Glenny, A.M. (1997 May 28–June 3). What are the best ways of tackling obesity? *Nursing Times*, 93, 50–51.

Owen, S.V., & Fullerton, M.L. (1995). Would it make a difference? A discussion group in a behaviorally oriented inpatient eating disorder program. *Journal of Psychosocial Nursing*, 33(11), 35–40.

Pike, K.M. (1998, June). Long-term course of anorexia nervosa: Response, relapse, remission, and recovery. *Clinical Psychology Review*, 18, 447–475.

Roselin, J.M. (1997). Eating disorders: Not just a young women's problem. *Seasons*, 7, 18–20.

Sobal, J., & Bursztyn, M. (1998). Dating people with anorexia nervosa and bulimia nervosa: Attitudes and beliefs of university students. *Women and Health, 27,* 73–88.

Staples, N.R., & Schwartz, M. (1990). Anorexia nervosa support group: Providing transitional support. *Journal of Psychosocial Nursing, 28(2),* 6–10.

Steiner, H., & Lock, J. (1998, April). Anorexia nervosa and bulimia nervosa in children and adolescents: A review of the past 10 years. *Journal of the American Academy of Child and Adolescent Psychiatry, 37,* 352–359.

Sullivan, P.F., Bulik, C.M., Fear, J.L., & Pickering, A. (1998, July). Outcome of anorexia nervosa: A case-control study. *American Journal of Psychiatry, 155,* 939–946.

Whitaker, R.C., et al. (1997, September 25). Predicting obesity in young adulthood from childhood and parental obesity. *New England Journal of Medicine, 337,* 869–873.

Wilfley, D.E., & Cohen, L.R. (1997). Psychological treatment of bulimia nervosa and binge eating disorder. *Psychopharmacology Bulletin, 33,* 437–454.

ADJUSTMENT AND IMPULSE CONTROL DISORDERS

KEY TERMS

adjustment disorder
kleptomania

pathological gambling
pyromania

trichotillomania
Gamblers Anonymous

OBJECTIVES

After reading this chapter, the student will be able to:

1. Discuss historical aspects and epidemiological statistics related to adjustment and impulse control disorders.
2. Describe various types of adjustment and impulse control disorders and identify symptomatology associated with each; use this information in client assessment.
3. Identify predisposing factors in the development of adjustment and impulse control disorders.
4. Formulate nursing diagnoses and goals of care for clients with adjustment and impulse control disorders.

5. Describe appropriate nursing interventions for behaviors associated with adjustment and impulse control disorders.
6. Identity topics for client and family teaching relevant to adjustment and impulse control disorders.
7. Evaluate nursing care of clients with adjustment and impulse control disorders.
8. Discuss various modalities relevant to treatment of adjustment and impulse control disorders.

lthough **adjustment disorder** and impulse control disorders are two separate diagnostic categories in the *DSM-IV* (American Psychiatric Association [APA], 1994), they do share some common characteristics. It is likely that they are precipitated by a type of psychosocial stress, the severity of which may or may not directly affect the individual response. Conversely, adjustment disorders are quite common, and impulse control disorders are relatively rare.

This chapter focuses on disorders that occur in response to stressful situations with which the individual cannot cope. The behavior may include:

1. Impairment in an individual's usual social and occupational functioning.
2. Compulsive acts that may be harmful to the person or others.

Historical and epidemiological statistics are presented. Predisposing factors that have been implicated in the etiology of adjustment and impulse control disorders provide a framework for studying the dynamics of these pathological conditions.

An explanation of the symptomatology is presented as background knowledge for assessing the client with an adjustment or impulse control disorder. Nursing care is described in the context of the nursing process. Various medical treatment modalities are explored.

HISTORICAL AND EPIDEMIOLOGICAL FACTORS

Historically, clients with symptoms identified by adjustment or impulse control disorders were classified as having personality disturbances. Problems with these diagnostic categories began after World War II, when, as a result of the lack of a standardized diagnostic system, psychiatrists began to experience difficulties formulating diagnoses for behaviors attributed to combat stress.

The concept of impulse disorders dates back to the 19th century and was identified by the term *instinctive monomania* (Wise & Tierney, 1994). The original monomanias included alcoholism, firesetting, homicide, and kleptomania.

A number of studies have indicated that adjustment disorders are probably quite common (Yates, 1994). In one study by Andreasen and Wasek (1980), 5 percent of inpatients received this diagnosis, and they also reported, "the percentage of new outpatients receiving this diagnosis was almost certainly substantially higher." A 1986 study by Hales and associates, who reviewed the records of more than 1000 medical and surgical inpatients who had subsequently been referred to the psychiatric service of a large general hospital, found that adjustment disorder composed the most frequent diagnosis given (almost 19 percent). It is more common in women than in men by about 2 to 1 (Kaplan & Sadock, 1998).

The *DSM-IV* (APA, 1994) identifies five specific categories of impulse control disorders: intermittent explosive disorder, **kleptomania, pathological gambling, pyromania,** and **trichotillomania.** Apparently these disorders are quite rare. Various sources place the prevalence range at from less than 1 percent to 5 percent of the adult population, with kleptomania being at the higher end of the range. Intermittent explosive disorder, pathological gambling, and pyromania are more common among men whereas kleptomania and trichotillomania are diagnosed more often in women (APA, 1994).

APPLICATION OF THE NURSING PROCESS

Adjustment Disorders

Classifications of Adjustment Disorder: Background Assessment Data

An adjustment disorder is characterized by a maladaptive reaction to an identifiable psychosocial stressor or stressors that occurs within 3 months after onset of the stressor and has persisted for no longer than 6 months (APA, 1994). An exception to the 6 months' criterion is if the symptoms occur in response to a chronic stressor, such as a chronic, disabling physical illness.

The individual shows impairment in social and occupational functioning or exhibits symptoms that are in excess of an expected reaction to the stressor. The symptoms are expected to remit soon after the stressor is relieved, or if the stressor persists, when a new level of adaptation is achieved. The *DSM-IV* diagnostic criteria for adjustment disorders are presented in Table 32.1.

The stressor itself can be almost anything, but an individual's response to any particular stressor cannot be predicted. If an individual is highly predisposed or vulnerable to maladaptive response, a severe form of the disorder may follow what most people would consider only a mild or moderate stressor. On the other hand, a less vulnerable individual may develop only a mild form of the disorder in response to what others might consider a severe stressor.

A number of clinical presentations are associated with adjustment disorders. The following categories, identified by the *DSM-IV*, are distinguished by the predominant features of the maladaptive response.

Adjustment Disorder With Anxiety. This category denotes a maladaptive response to a psychosocial stressor in which the predominant manifestation is anxiety. For example, the symptoms may reveal nervousness, worry, and jitteriness. The pervasiveness of anxiety as a symptom in psychiatric illness may contribute to the vagueness and subsequent infrequent use of this category of adjustment disorder (Popkin, 1989). The clinician must differentiate this diagnosis from those of anxiety disorders.

Adjustment Disorder With Depressed Mood. This

TABLE 32.1 DIAGNOSTIC CRITERIA FOR ADJUSTMENT DISORDERS

A. The development of emotional or behavioral symptoms in response to an identifiable stressor(s) occurring within 3 months of the onset of the stressor(s).

B. These symptoms or behaviors are clinically significant as evidenced by either of the following:
 1. Marked distress that is in excess of what would be expected from exposure to the stressor.
 2. Significant impairment in social or occupational (academic) functioning.

C. The stress-related disturbance does not meet the criteria for another specific axis I disorder and is not merely an exacerbation of a preexisting axis I or axis II disorder.

D. The symptoms do not represent bereavement.

E. Once the stressor (or its consequences) has terminated, the symptoms do not persist for more than an additional 6 months.

Specify if:
 Acute: If the disturbance lasts less than 6 months.
 Chronic: If the disturbance lasts for 6 months or longer.

SOURCE: From APA (1994), with permission.

category is the most commonly diagnosed adjustment disorder. The clinical presentation is one of predominant mood disturbance, although less pronounced than that of major depression. The symptoms, such as depressed mood, tearfulness, and feelings of hopelessness, exceed what is an expected or normative response to an identified psychosocial stressor.

Adjustment Disorder With Disturbance of Conduct. This category is characterized by conduct in which there is violation of the rights of others or of major age-appropriate societal norms and rules. Examples include truancy, vandalism, reckless driving, fighting, and defaulting on legal responsibilities. Differential diagnosis must be made from conduct disorder or antisocial personality disorder.

Adjustment Disorder With Mixed Disturbance of Emotions and Conduct. The predominant features of this category include emotional disturbances (e.g., anxiety or depression) as well as disturbances of conduct in which there is violation of the rights of others or of major age-appropriate societal norms and rules (e.g., truancy, vandalism, fighting).

Adjustment Disorder Unspecified. This subtype is used when the maladaptive reaction is not consistent with any of the other categories. Manifestations may include physical complaints, social withdrawal, or work or academic inhibition, without significant depressed or anxious mood (APA, 1994; Kaplan & Sadock, 1998).

Predisposing Factors to Adjustment Disorders

Biological Theory. Chronic disorders, such as cognitive disorders or mental retardation, are thought to impair the ability of an individual to adapt to stress, causing increased vulnerability to adjustment disorders. Yates (1994) suggests that genetic factors also may influence individual risks for maladaptive response to stress.

Psychosocial Theories. Some proponents of psycho-analytical theory view adjustment disorder as a maladaptive response to stress that is caused by early childhood trauma, increased dependency, and retarded ego development. Other psychoanalysts put considerable weight on the constitutional factor, or birth characteristics that contribute to the manner in which individuals respond to stress. In many instances, adjustment disorder is precipitated by a specific meaningful stressor having found a point of vulnerability in an individual of otherwise adequate ego strength.

DeWitt (1984) describes the predisposition to adjustment disorder as an inability to complete the grieving process in response to a painful life change. She describes the presumed cause of this inability to adapt as *psychic overload,* "a level of intrapsychic strain that exceeds the individual's ability to cope and may therefore disrupt normal functioning and cause psychological or somatic symptoms." Some individuals remain in denial, acting as though the event never occurred. In others, intrusive symptoms may predominate. In all instances, however, it is the persistence of unwanted emotions and images, and the feeling of being powerless to stop them, that precludes the dysfunctional response.

Transactional Model of Stress/Adaptation. Why are some individuals able to confront stressful situations adaptively and even gain strength from the experience, whereas others not only fail to cope adaptively, but may even encounter psychopathological dysfunction? The transactional model of stress/adaptation takes into consideration the interaction between the individual and the environment.

The type of stressor that one experiences may influence one's adaptation. Sudden-shock stressors occur without warning, and continuous stressors are those that an individual is exposed to over an extended period. Although many studies have been directed to individuals' responses to sudden-shock stressors, it has been found that continuous stressors are more commonly cited than sudden-shock stressors as precipitants to maladaptive functioning.

DeWitt (1984) cites situational context as a contributing factor to an individual's stress response. Situational factors include personal and general economic conditions; occupational and recreational opportunities; the availability of social supports such as family, friends, neighbors, and cultural or religious support groups.

Intrapersonal factors such as constitutional vulnerability have also been implicated in the predisposition to adjustment disorder. Chess and Thomas (1984) have suggested that a child with a difficult temperament (defined as one who cries loudly and often; adapts to changes slowly; and has irregular patterns of hunger, sleep, and elimination) is at greater risk of developing a behavior disorder. Freud (1964) theorized that traumatic childhood experiences created points of fixation to which the individual, during times of stress, would be likely to regress. This might also apply to other unresolved conflicts or developmental issues. Other intrapersonal factors that might influence one's ability to adjust to a painful life change include social skills, coping strategies, the presence of psychiatric illness, degree of flexibility, and level of intelligence.

The etiology of adjustment disorder is most likely influenced by multiple factors. A graphic depiction of this theory of multiple causation is presented in Figure 32.1.

Diagnosis/Outcome Identification

Nursing diagnoses are formulated from the data gathered during the assessment phase and with background knowledge regarding predisposing factors to the disorder. The following nursing diagnoses may be used for the client with an adjustment disorder:

Dysfunctional grieving related to real or perceived loss of any concept of value to the individual, evidenced by interference with life functioning, developmental regression, or somatic complaints.

Impaired adjustment related to change in health status requiring modification in lifestyle (e.g., chronic illness, physical disability), evidenced by inability to problem solve or set realistic goals for the future.

NOTE: According to the North American Nursing Diagnosis Association (NANDA) definition, this diagnosis would only be appropriate for the person with adjustment disorder if the precipitating stressor was a change in health status.

The following criteria may be used for measurement of outcomes in the care of the client with an adjustment disorder.

THE CLIENT:

1. Verbalizes acceptable behaviors associated with each stage of the grief process.
2. Demonstrates a reinvestment in the environment.
3. Accomplishes activities of daily living independently.
4. Demonstrates ability for adequate occupational and social functioning.

5. Verbalizes awareness of change in health status and the effect it will have on lifestyle.
6. Solves problems and sets realistic goals for the future.
7. Demonstrates ability to cope effectively with change in lifestyle.

Planning/Implementation

Table 32.2 provides a plan of care for the client with adjustment disorder. Nursing diagnoses are presented, along with outcome criteria, appropriate nursing interventions, and rationales.

Evaluation

Reassessment is conducted to determine if the nursing actions have been successful in achieving the objectives of care. Evaluation of the nursing actions for the client with adjustment disorder may be facilitated by gathering information using the following types of questions.

1. Does the client verbalize understanding of the grief process and his or her position in the process?
2. Does the client recognize his or her adaptive and maladaptive behaviors associated with the grief response?
3. Can the client accomplish activities of daily living independently?
4. If assistance is required, can he or she verbalize resources from whom help may be sought?
5. Does the client demonstrate evidence of progression along the grief response?
6. Does the client demonstrate the ability to perform occupational and social activities adequately?
7. Does the client discuss the change in health status and modification of lifestyle it will effect?
8. Does the client demonstrate acceptance of the modification?
9. Can the client participate in decision making and problem solving for his or her future?
10. Does the client set realistic goals for the future?
11. Does the client demonstrate new adaptive coping strategies for dealing with the change in lifestyle?
12. Can the client verbalize available resources to whom he or she may go for support or assistance should it be necessary?

Impulse Control Disorders

Classifications of Impulse Control Disorders: Background Assessment Data

The *DSM-IV* (APA, 1994) describes the essential features of impulse control disorders as follows:

1. Failure to resist an impulse, drive, or temptation to perform an act that is harmful to the person or others.

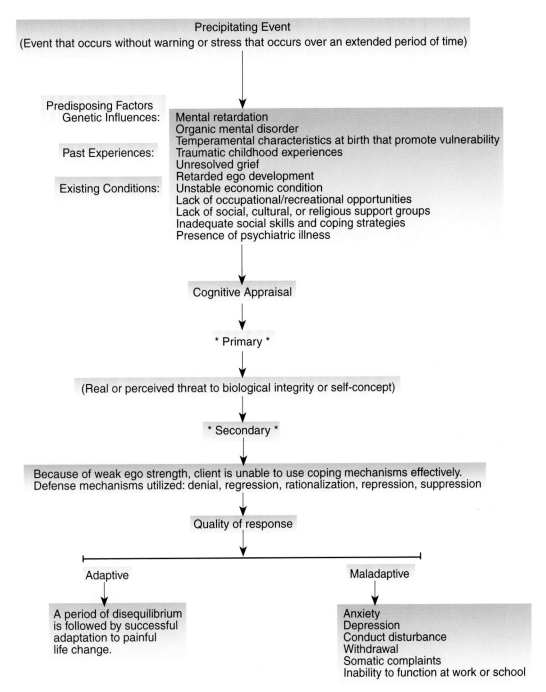

Precipitating Event
(Event that occurs without warning or stress that occurs over an extended period of time)

Predisposing Factors
Genetic Influences: Mental retardation
                       Organic mental disorder
                       Temperamental characteristics at birth that promote vulnerability
Past Experiences: Traumatic childhood experiences
                       Unresolved grief
                       Retarded ego development
Existing Conditions: Unstable economic condition
                       Lack of occupational/recreational opportunities
                       Lack of social, cultural, or religious support groups
                       Inadequate social skills and coping strategies
                       Presence of psychiatric illness

Cognitive Appraisal

* Primary *

(Real or perceived threat to biological integrity or self-concept)

* Secondary *

Because of weak ego strength, client is unable to use coping mechanisms effectively.
Defense mechanisms utilized: denial, regression, rationalization, repression, suppression

Quality of response

Adaptive

A period of disequilibrium
is followed by successful
adaptation to painful
life change.

Maladaptive

Anxiety
Depression
Conduct disturbance
Withdrawal
Somatic complaints
Inability to function at work or school

Figure 32.1   The dynamics of adjustment disorder using the transactional model of stress/adaptation.

2. An increasing sense of tension or arousal before committing the act.
3. An experience of pleasure, gratification, or relief at the time of committing the act. Following the act there may or may not be regret, self-reproach, or guilt.

Individuals who suffer from impulse control disorders follow their impulses to behave in a certain manner without regard to the consequences of their behavior. They seldom know why they do what they do or why it is plea-

surable. These behaviors have been likened to sexual excitement and orgasmic release; some authors have noted that many of the behaviors have adverse or even destructive consequences for the person.

Booth (1984) has stated:

"People with impulse control disorders usually function well enough in other areas of their lives. Many are stable individuals with no serious disorders of thought or cognition. Although other behavior disorders are occasionally associated with some impulse control disorders, the problem for many

Table 32.2 Care Plan for Client With Adjustment Disorder

NURSING DIAGNOSIS: DYSFUNCTIONAL GRIEVING

RELATED TO: Real or perceived loss of any concept of value to the individual

EVIDENCED BY: Interference with life functioning, developmental regression, or somatic complaints

OUTCOME CRITERIA	NURSING INTERVENTIONS	RATIONALE
Client will be able to function adequately at age-appropriate level with evidence of progression toward resolution of grief.	1. Determine stage of grief in which client is fixed. Identify behaviors associated with this stage.	1. Accurate baseline assessment data are necessary to plan effective care for the grieving client.
	2. Develop trusting relationship with the client. Show empathy and caring. Be honest and keep all promises.	2. Trust is the basis for a therapeutic relationship.
	3. Convey an accepting attitude so that the client is not afraid to express feelings openly.	3. An accepting attitude conveys to the client that you believe he or she is a worthwhile person. Trust is enhanced.
	4. Allow client to express anger. Do not become defensive if initial expression of anger is displaced on the nurse. Assist client to explore angry feelings so that they may be directed toward the intended object or person.	4. Verbalization of feelings in a non-threatening environment may help client come to terms with unresolved issues.
	5. Assist client to discharge pent-up anger through participation in large motor activities (e.g., brisk walks, jogging, volleyball, punching bag, exercise bike).	5. Physical exercise provides a safe and effective method for discharging pent-up tension.
	6. Explain to the client the normal stages of grief and the behaviors associated with each stage. Help client to understand that feelings such as guilt and anger toward the lost concept are appropriate and acceptable during the grief process.	6. Knowledge of the feelings and behaviors associated with normal grieving may help to relieve some of the guilt that these responses generate.
	7. Encourage client to review personal perception of the loss or change. With support and sensitivity, point out reality of the situation in areas where misrepresentations are expressed.	7. Client must give up idealized perception and be able to accept both positive and negative aspects about the painful life change before the grief process is complete.
	8. Communicate to client that crying is acceptable. Use of touch is generally therapeutic, although specific knowledge about the client is important before using it.	8. Use of touch is considered inappropriate in some cultures.
	9. Assist client in solving problems as he or she attempts to determine methods for more adaptive coping with the stressor. Provide positive feedback for strategies identified and decisions made.	9. Positive reinforcement enhances self-esteem and encourages repetition of desirable behaviors.
	10. Encourage client to reach out for spiritual support during this time in whatever form is desirable. Assess client's spiritual needs and assist as necessary in their fulfillment.	10. Spiritual support can enhance successful adaptation to painful life experiences.

NURSING DIAGNOSIS: IMPAIRED ADJUSTMENT
RELATED TO: Change in health status requiring modification in lifestyle
EVIDENCED BY: Inability to problem solve or set realistic goals for the future.

OUTCOME CRITERIA	NURSING INTERVENTIONS	RATIONALE
Client will willingly demonstrate competence to function independently to his or her optimal level of ability, considering change in health status.	1. Encourage client to talk about lifestyle prior to the change in health status. Discuss coping mechanisms that were used at stressful times in the past. 2. Encourage client to discuss the health change and particularly to express anger associated with it. 3. Encourage client to express fears associated with the change or alteration in lifestyle that the change has created. 4. Provide assistance with activities of daily living as required, but encourage independence to the limit that client's ability will allow. Give positive feedback for activities accomplished independently. 5. Help client with decision making regarding incorporation of change into lifestyle. Identify problems the change is likely to create. Discuss alternate solutions, weighing potential benefits and consequences of each alternative. Support client's decision in the selection of an alternative. 6. Use role-play to practice stressful situations that might occur in relation to the health status change. 7. Ensure that client and family are fully knowledgeable regarding the physiology of the change in health status and the necessity for optimal wellness. Encourage them to ask questions, and provide printed material about the health status change to which they may refer following discharge. Ensure that client can identify resources within the community from which he or she may seek assistance in adapting to the change in health status.	1. Identify the client's strengths so that they may be used to facilitate adaptation to the change in health status. 2. Anger is a normal stage in the grieving process and, if not released in an appropriate manner, may be turned inward on the self, leading to pathological depression. 3. Change often creates a feeling of disequilibrium, and the individual may respond with fears that are irrational or unfounded. He or she may benefit from feedback that corrects misperceptions about how life will be with the change in health status. 4. Independent accomplishments and positive feedback enhance self-esteem and encourage repetition of desired behaviors. Successes also provide hope that adaptive functioning is possible and decrease feelings of powerlessness. 5. The high degree of anxiety that usually accompanies a major lifestyle change often interferes with an individual's ability to solve problems and to make appropriate decisions. Client may need assistance with this process in an effort to progress toward successful adaptation. 6. This type of anticipatory guidance arms the client with a measure of security and serves to decrease anxiety. 7. Increased knowledge enhances successful adaptation.

of these individuals consists solely in a socially unacceptable discharge of tension that is momentarily gratifying but which causes misery and remorse later."

A description of the five categories of impulse control disorders identified by the *DSM-IV* (APA, 1994) follows.

Intermittent Explosive Disorder

This disorder is characterized by discrete episodes of failure to resist aggressive impulses resulting in serious assaults or destruction of property (APA, 1994). The individual is not normally an aggressive person between episodes, and the degree of aggressiveness expressed during the episodes is grossly out of proportion to any precipitating psychosocial stressor.

The symptoms appear suddenly, without any apparent provocation, and the violence is usually the result of an irresistible impulse to lash out. Some clients report sensorium changes, such as confusion during episodes or amnesia for events that occurred during episodes (Kaplan & Sadock, 1998). Symptoms terminate abruptly, commonly lasting only minutes or at most a few hours, and are followed by feelings of genuine remorse and self-reproach about the inability to control, and the consequences of, the aggressive behavior.

Symptoms of the disorder most often begin in adolescence or young adulthood and gradually disappear as the individual approaches middle age. Clients often have histories of learning disabilities, hyperkinesis, and proneness to accidents in childhood (Kaplan & Sadock, 1998; Wise & Tierney, 1994). The disorder, which is relatively rare, occurs more often in males than in females (APA, 1994). The *DSM-IV* diagnostic criteria for intermittent explosive disorder are presented in Table 32.3.

Predisposing Factors to Intermittent Explosive Disorder

Biological Influences

1. *Genetic.* The disorder is apparently more common in first-degree biological relatives of people with the disorder than in the general population (Kaplan, Sadock, & Grebb, 1994).
2. *Physiological.* Any central nervous system insult may predispose an individual to the syndrome. Predisposing factors in childhood are thought to include perinatal trauma, infantile seizures, head trauma, encephalitis, minimal brain dysfunction, and hyperactivity (Kaplan, Sadock, & Grebb, 1994). Individuals who show high-amplitude, paroxysmal, slow activation on the electroencephalogram (EEG) are more likely to have aggressive outbursts than are those with either classic "seizure disorder" or normal patterns on EEGs (Booth, 1984).

Psychosocial Influences.

1. *Family Dynamics.* Individuals with intermittent explosive disorder often have strong identifications with assaultive parental figures. The typical history includes a chaotic and violent early family milieu with heavy drinking by one or both parents, parental hostility, child abuse, threats to life, and the emotional or physical unavailability of a father figure. The individual often has childhood memories of parental inconsistencies and unpredictability.

Kleptomania

The *DSM-IV* describes kleptomania as "the recurrent failure to resist impulses to steal items even though the items are not needed for personal use or for their monetary value." The stolen items are either given away, discarded, returned surreptitiously, or kept and hidden. The individual usually has enough money to pay for the stolen objects (Kaplan, Sadock, & Grebb, 1994).

The individual with kleptomania steals purely for the sake of stealing and for the sense of relief and gratification that follows an episode. The impulsive stealing is in response to increasing tension, and even though the individual almost always knows that the act is wrong, he or she cannot resist the force of mounting tension and the pursuit of pleasure and relief that follows. Seldom is attention given to the possibility or consequences of being apprehended.

The individual, who usually steals without assistance or collaboration from others, may feel shame or remorse following the incident. Others never experience guilt or regret for their behavior. Symptoms of depression and anxiety have been associated with the disorder.

Onset of the disorder is usually in adolescence. It tends to be chronic, with periods of waxing and waning throughout the course of the disorder. The condition is rare but is thought to be more common among women than men. Fewer than 5 percent of arrested shoplifters give a history that is consistent with kleptomania (APA, 1994).

The *DSM-IV* diagnostic criteria for kleptomania are presented in Table 32.4.

TABLE 32.3 DIAGNOSTIC CRITERIA FOR INTERMITTENT EXPLOSIVE DISORDER

A. Several discrete episodes of failure to resist aggressive impulses that result in serious assaultive acts or destruction of property.

B. The degree of aggressiveness expressed during the episodes is grossly out of proportion to any precipitating psychosocial stressors.

C. The aggressive episodes are not better accounted for by another mental disorder (e.g., antisocial personality disorder, borderline personality disorder, a psychotic disorder, a manic episode, conduct disorder, or attention-deficit/hyperactivity disorder) and are not due to the direct physiological effects of a substance (e.g., a drug of abuse, a medication) or a general medical condition (e.g., head trauma, Alzheimer's disease).

SOURCE: From APA (1994), with permission.

TABLE 32.4 DIAGNOSTIC CRITERIA FOR KLEPTOMANIA

A. Recurrent failure to resist impulses to steal objects not needed for personal use or for their monetary value.

B. Increasing sense of tension immediately before committing the theft.

C. Pleasure, gratification, or relief at the time of committing the theft.

D. The stealing is not committed to express anger or vengeance and is not in response to a delusion or a hallucination.

E. The stealing is not better accounted for by conduct disorder, a manic episode, or antisocial personality disorder.

SOURCE: From APA (1994), with permission.

Predisposing Factors to Kleptomania

Biological Influences. As with other disorders of impulse control, brain disease and mental retardation have been associated with kleptomania (Kaplan, Sadock, & Grebb, 1994). Disinhibition and poor impulse control have been linked with cortical atrophy in the frontal region and enlargement of the lateral ventricles of the brain.

Psychosocial Influences. Abraham (1953) observed that many kleptomaniacs experienced feelings of being neglected, injured, or unwanted. They reported childhood memories of abandonment (real or imagined) and a sense of lovelessness and deprivation. Booth (1984) has stated:

> "Most dynamic theories of the causes of kleptomania center either on stealing as an attempt to obtain nourishment, esteem, and love or as a sexual equivalent—a quest for a penis in a woman or as a defense against castration anxiety in men. Some theories have been developed in which both mechanisms play a role."

Pathological Gambling

This disorder is defined by the *DSM-IV* as persistent and recurrent maladaptive gambling behavior (APA, 1994). The preoccupation with and impulse to gamble intensify when the individual is under stress. Many impulsive gamblers describe a physical sensation of restlessness and anticipation that can only be relieved by placing a bet. Booth (1984) stated:

> "During a game or a race, the tension is amplified. Whether the pathologic gambler wins or loses, there is typically an immediate urge to place another bet until all the money is gone or until the impulse is temporarily quelled by a run of winning chances, which confers a heightened sense of self-esteem or security."

As the need to gamble increases, the individual is forced to obtain money by any means available. This may include borrowing money from illegal sources or pawning personal items (or items that belong to others). As gambling debts accrue, or out of a need to continue gambling, the individual may desperately resort to forgery, theft, or even embezzlement. Family relationships are disrupted, and impairment in occupational functioning may occur because of absences from work in order to gamble.

Gambling behavior usually begins in adolescence; however, compulsive behaviors rarely occur before young adulthood. The disorder generally runs a chronic course, with periods of waxing and waning, largely dependent on periods of psychosocial stress.

The prevalence of pathological gambling in the United States is estimated at 1 percent to 3 percent of the adult population (APA, 1994). It is more common among men than women.

Various personality traits have been attributed to pathological gamblers. These individuals have been described as "fiercely competitive, highly independent, individualistic, overconfident, and profoundly optimistic" (Wise & Tierney, 1994). Many gamblers exhibit characteristics associated with narcissism and grandiosity and often have difficulties with intimacy, empathy, and trust.

The *DSM-IV* diagnostic criteria for pathological gambling are presented in Table 32.5.

Predisposing Factors to Pathological Gambling

Biological Influences

1. *Genetic.* The fathers of men with the disorder and the mothers of women with the disorder are more likely to have the disorder than is the population at large (Kaplan, Sadock, & Grebb, 1994). The *DSM-IV* reports that both pathological gambling and alcohol dependence are more common among the parents of individuals who display pathological gambling than in the general population (APA, 1994).

2. *Physiological.* Various neurophysiological dysfunctions have been associated with pathological gambling behaviors. They include epilepsy, subcortical lesions, and minimal brain dysfunction (Booth, 1984). Kaplan and Sadock (1998) suggest that a possible link may exist between pathological gambling and abnormalities in the catecholamine norepinephrine, the activation of which may accompany the tension that precedes the gambling. Other researchers have hypothesized that the problem may be associated with abnormalities in the serotonergic system.

Psychosocial Influences. Kaplan, Sadock, and Grebb (1994) report that the following may be predisposing factors to the development of pathological gambling: loss of a parent by death, separation, divorce, or desertion before

TABLE 32.5 DIAGNOSTIC CRITERIA FOR PATHOLOGICAL GAMBLING

A. Persistent and recurrent maladaptive gambling behavior as indicated by five (or more) of the following:
   1. Is preoccupied with gambling (e.g., preoccupied with reliving past gambling experiences, handicapping or planning the next venture, or thinking of ways to get money with which to gamble).
   2. Needs to gamble with increasing amounts of money in order to achieve the desired excitement.
   3. Has repeated unsuccessful efforts to control, cut back, or stop gambling.
   4. Is restless or irritable when attempting to cut down or stop gambling.
   5. Gambles to escape problems or relieve a dysphoric mood (e.g., feelings of helplessness, guilt, anxiety, depression).
   6. After losing money gambling, often returns another day to get even ("chasing" one's losses).
   7. Lies to family members, therapist, or others to conceal the extent of involvement with gambling.
   8. Has committed illegal acts such as forgery, fraud, theft, or embezzlement to finance gambling.
   9. Has jeopardized or lost a significant relationship, job, or educational or career opportunity because of gambling.
   10. Relies on others to provide money to relieve a desperate financial situation caused by gambling.
B. The gambling behavior is not better accounted for by a manic episode.

SOURCE: From APA (1994), with permission.

the child is 15 years of age; inappropriate parental discipline (absence, inconsistency, or harshness); exposure to and availability of gambling activities for the adolescent; a family emphasis on material and financial symbols; and a lack of family emphasis on saving, planning, and budgeting.

The early psychoanalytical view attempted to explain compulsive gambling in terms of psychosexual maturation. In this theory, the gambling is compared to masturbation; both of these activities derive motive force from a build-up of tension that is released through repetitive actions or the anticipation of them. A punitive superego fosters the gambler's inherent need for punishment, which is then achieved through losing, and is required for psychic equilibrium (Wise & Tierney, 1994).

Pyromania

Pyromania is the inability to resist the impulse to set fires. The act of starting the fire is preceded by tension or affective arousal. The individual experiences intense pleasure, gratification, or relief when setting the fires, witnessing their effects, or participating in their aftermath (APA, 1994). The sole motive for setting the fire is self-gratification, not revenge, insurance collection, or sabotage. They may take precautions to avoid apprehension; however, many pyromaniacs are totally indifferent to the consequences of their behavior.

The onset of symptoms is usually in childhood. Many pyromaniacs report early fascination with fire and excitement associated with firefighting equipment and activities. The disorder is relatively rare and is much more common in men than in women. Characteristics associated with pyromaniacs include low intelligence, learning disabilities, hyperkinesis and enuresis in childhood, explosive temper, recklessness, and fascination with high speed (Booth, 1984). Individuals with pyromania are often alcoholics and have fathers who are alcoholics (Linnoila, DeJong, & Virkkunen, 1989).

The *DSM-IV* diagnostic criteria for pyromania are presented in Table 32.6.

Predisposing Factors to Pyromania

Biological Influences. Various physiological influences have been associated with firesetting. They include mental retardation, dementia, epilepsy, minimal brain dysfunction, and learning disabilities (Booth, 1984; Popkin, 1989). A biochemical influence has been suggested based on evidence of significantly low cerebrospinal fluid

TABLE 32.6 DIAGNOSTIC CRITERIA FOR PYROMANIA

A. Deliberate and purposeful fire setting on more than one occasion.
B. Tension or affective arousal before the act.
C. Fascination with, interest in, curiosity about, or attraction to fire and its situational contexts (e.g., paraphernalia, uses, consequences).
D. Pleasure, gratification, or relief when setting fires, or when witnessing or participating in their aftermath.
E. The fire setting is not done for monetary gain, as an expression of sociopolitical ideology, to conceal criminal activity, to express anger or vengeance, to improve one's living circumstances, in response to a delusion or hallucination, or as a result of impaired judgment (e.g., in dementia, mental retardation, substance intoxication).
F. The fire setting is not better accounted for by conduct disorder, a manic episode, or antisocial personality disorder.

SOURCE: From APA (1994), with permission.

monoamine metabolite levels in a study of male arsonists (Virkkunen et al., 1987). The same study showed a possible hypoglycemic tendency in these individuals.

Psychosocial Influences. Booth (1984) describes three major psychoanalytical issues that have been associated with impulsive firesetting: (1) an association between firesetting and sexual gratification; (2) concerns about inferiority, impotence, and annihilation; and (3) unconscious anger toward a parent figure. This is consistent with Freud's (1964) view of fire as a symbol of sexuality. He suggested that the warmth radiated by fire can be compared to the sensation that accompanies a state of sexual excitation. Several authors have described clients who have masturbated after setting fires and describe the gratification they experience as "orgasmic." Other psychoanalytical writers have suggested that fire may symbolize activities deriving from various levels of libidinal and aggressive development. They view the act of firesetting as a means of relieving accumulated rage over the frustration caused by a sense of social, physical, and sexual inferiority (Kaplan, Sadock, & Grebb, 1994).

Trichotillomania

The *DSM-IV* defines this disorder as the recurrent pulling out of one's own hair that results in noticeable hair loss (APA, 1994). The impulse is preceded by an increasing sense of tension and results in a sense of release or gratification from pulling out the hair. The most common sites for hair pulling are the scalp, eyebrows, and eyelashes but may occur in any area of the body on which hair grows. These areas of hair loss are more likely found on the opposite side of the body from the dominant hand (Wise & Tierney, 1994). Pain is seldom reported to accompany the hairpulling, although tingling and pruritus in the area are not uncommon.

The disorder usually begins in childhood and may be accompanied by nail biting, head banging, scratching, biting, or other acts of self-mutilation (Kaplan, Sadock, & Grebb, 1994). This relatively rare phenomenon occurs more often in women than in men.

The *DSM-IV* diagnostic criteria for trichotillomania are presented in Table 32.7.

Predisposing Factors to Trichotillomania

Biological Influences. Krishnan, Davidson, and Guajardo (1985) report that trichotillomania may be present as a major symptom in mental retardation, obsessive-compulsive disorder, schizophrenia, borderline personality disorder, and depression. Kaplan, Sadock, and Grebb (1994) state:

> "Trichotillomania is increasingly being viewed as having a biologically determined substrate that may reflect inappropriately released motor activity or excessive grooming behaviors."

Psychosocial Influences. The onset of trichotillomania can be related to stressful situations in more than one quarter of cases. Other factors include disturbances in mother-child relationships, fear of abandonment, and recent object loss (Kaplan, Sadock, & Grebb, 1994).

The psychodynamic view associates trichotillomania with early emotional deprivation (Popkin, 1989). In this view, the mother is described as rejecting, sadistic, and condemning; the father as weak and passive. In some rudimentary and distorted way, hairpulling satisfies the need for tenderness and physical contact, and the fear of abandonment subsides.

Transactional Model of Stress/Adaptation. The etiology of impulse control disorders is most likely influenced by multiple factors. In Figure 32.2 a graphic depiction of this theory of multiple causation is presented in the transactional model of stress/adaptation.

Diagnosis/Outcome Identification

Nursing diagnoses are formulated from the data gathered during the assessment phase and with background knowledge regarding predisposing factors to the disorder. The following nursing diagnoses may be used for the client with impulse control disorder:

Risk for violence directed toward others related to dysfunctional family system; possible genetic or physiological influences evidenced by episodes of violent, aggressive, or assaultive behavior.

Ineffective individual coping related to possible hereditary factors, physiological alterations, dysfunctional family, or unresolved developmental issues, evidenced by inability to control impulse to gamble, steal, set fires, or pull out own hair.

◼ TABLE 32.7 DIAGNOSTIC CRITERIA FOR TRICHOTILLOMANIA

A. Recurrent pulling out of one's hair resulting in noticeable hair loss.

B. An increasing sense of tension immediately before pulling out the hair or when attempting to resist the behavior.

C. Pleasure, gratification, or relief when pulling out the hair.

D. The disturbance is not better accounted for by another mental disorder and is not due to a general medical condition (e.g., a dermatological condition).

E. The disturbance causes clinically significant distress or impairment in social, occupational, or other important areas of functioning.

SOURCE: From APA (1994), with permission.

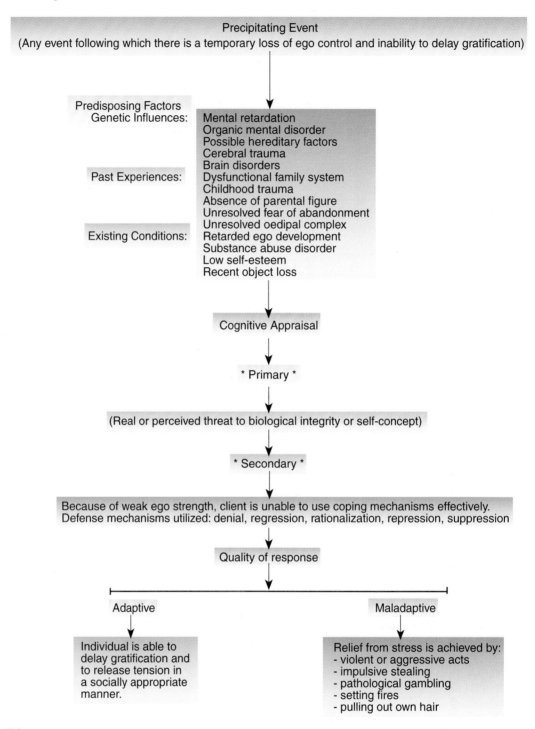

Figure 32.2   The dynamics of impulse control using the transactional model of stress/adaptation.

The following criteria may be used for measurement of outcomes in the care of the client with impulse control disorder.

THE CLIENT:

1. Has not caused harm to self or others.
2. Is able to inhibit the impulse for violence and aggression.
3. Verbalizes the symptoms of increasing tension.
4. Verbalizes strategies to avoid becoming violent.
5. Verbalizes actual object at which anger is directed.
6. Continues to work on increasing frustration tolerance.
7. Verbalizes more adaptive strategies for coping with stressful situations.
8. Demonstrates the ability to delay gratification.
9. Verbalizes understanding that behavior is unacceptable and accepts responsibility for own behavior.

Planning/Implementation

Table 32.8 provides a plan of care for the client with an impulse control disorder. Nursing diagnoses are presented, along with outcome criteria and appropriate nursing interventions and rationales.

Evaluation

Reassessment is conducted in order to determine if the nursing actions have been successful in achieving the objectives of care. Evaluation of the nursing actions for the client with an impulse control disorder may be facilitated by gathering information using the following types of questions:

1. Has violence, aggression, or assaultive behavior been avoided?
2. Have the client and others escaped harm?
3. Does the client verbalize understanding of the unacceptability of his or her behavior?
4. Can the client verbalize and demonstrate more adaptive strategies for coping with stress?
5. Can the client demonstrate the ability to delay gratification?
6. Can the client verbalize the symptoms of tension that precede unacceptable behavior?
7. Can the client demonstrate ways to intervene when tension rises that inhibit the compulsion for maladaptive behavior?
8. Can the client verbalize the types of stress that create the tension?
9. Can the client verbalize a plan to deal with the stress in the future without resorting to behaviors that are socially unacceptable?

Table 32.9 provides topics for client and family education related to adjustment and impulse control disorders.

TREATMENT MODALITIES

Adjustment Disorders

Various treatments are used for clients with adjustment disorder. The major goals of therapy for these individuals are:

1. To relieve symptoms associated with a stressor
2. To enhance coping with stressors that cannot be reduced or removed
3. To establish support systems that maximize adaptation (Strain et al., 1994)

Individual Psychotherapy

Individual psychotherapy is the most common treatment for adjustment disorder. Individual psychotherapy allows the client to examine the stressor that is causing the problem, possibly assign personal meaning to the stressor, and confront unresolved issues that may be exacerbating this crisis. Treatment works to remove these blocks to adaptation so that normal developmental progression can resume. Techniques are used to clarify links between the current stressor and past experiences, and to assist with the development of more adaptive coping strategies.

Family Therapy

Focus of treatment is shifted from the individual to the system of relationships in which the individual is involved. The maladaptive response of the identified client is viewed as symptomatic of a dysfunctional family system. All family members are included in the therapy, and treatment serves to improve the functioning within the family network. Emphasis is placed on communication, family rules, and interaction patterns among the family members.

Behavioral Therapy

The goal of behavioral therapy is to replace ineffective response patterns with more adaptive ones. The situations that promote ineffective responses are identified, and carefully designed reinforcement schedules, along with role modeling, coaching, and didactic presentations, are used to alter the maladaptive response patterns (DeWitt, 1984). This type of treatment is very effective when implemented in an inpatient setting where the client's behavior and its consequences may be more readily controlled.

Self-Help Groups

Group experiences with or without a professional facilitator provide an arena in which members may consider and compare their responses to those of individuals with similar life experiences. Members benefit from learning that they are not alone in their painful experiences. Hope is derived from knowing that others have survived and even grown from similar experiences. Members of the group exchange advice, share coping strategies, and provide support and encouragement for each other.

Crisis Intervention

In crisis intervention the therapist, or other intervener, becomes a part of the individual's life situation. Because of the individual's emotional state, he or she is unable to problem solve and requires guidance and support from another to help mobilize the resources needed to resolve the crisis. Crisis intervention is short-term and relies heavily on orderly problem-solving techniques and structured activities that are focused on change. The ultimate goal of crisis intervention in the treatment of adjustment disorder

TABLE 32.8 CARE PLAN FOR THE CLIENT WITH IMPULSE CONTROL DISORDER

NURSING DIAGNOSIS: HIGH RISK FOR VIOLENCE DIRECTED TOWARD OTHERS

RELATED TO: Dysfunctional family system; possible genetic or physiological influences

EVIDENCED BY: Episodes of violent, aggressive, or assaultive behavior

OUTCOME CRITERIA	NURSING INTERVENTIONS	RATIONALE
Client will not harm others or the property of others.	1. Convey an accepting attitude toward this client. Feelings of rejection are undoubtedly familiar to him or her. Work on development of trust. Be honest, keep all promises, and convey the message that it is not him or her but the behavior that is unacceptable.	1. An attitude of acceptance promotes feelings of self-worth. Trust is the basis of a therapeutic relationship.
	2. Maintain low level of stimuli in client's environment (low lighting, few people, simple decor, low noise level).	2. A stimulating environment may increase agitation and promote aggressive behavior.
	3. Remove all potentially dangerous objects from the client's environment. Help client identify the true object of his or her hostility.	3. Client safety is a nursing priority. Because of weak ego development, client may be unable to use ego defense mechanisms correctly. Helping him or her recognize this in a nonthreatening manner may help reveal unresolved issues so that they may be confronted.
	4. Staff should maintain and covey a calm attitude.	4. Anxiety is contagious and can be transferred from staff to client. A calm attitude provides client with a feeling of safety and security.
	5. Help client recognize the signs that tension is increasing and ways in which violence can be averted.	5. Activities that require physical exertion are helpful in relieving pent-up tension.
	6. Explain to client that should explosive behavior occur, staff will intervene in whatever way is required (e.g., tranquilizing medication, restraints, isolation) to protect client and others.	6. This conveys to the client evidence of control over the situation and provides a feeling of safety and security.

NURSING DIAGNOSIS: INEFFECTIVE INDIVIDUAL COPING

RELATED TO: Possible hereditary factors, physiological alterations, dysfunctional family, or unresolved developmental issues

EVIDENCED BY: Inability to control impulse to gamble, steal, set fires, or pull out own hair

OUTCOME CRITERIA	NURSING INTERVENTIONS	RATIONALE
Client will be able to delay gratification and use adaptive coping strategies in response to stress.	1. Help client gain insight into his or her own behaviors. Often these individuals rationalize to such an extent that they deny that what they have done is wrong.	1. Client must come to understand that certain behaviors will not be tolerated within the society and that severe consequences will be imposed upon those individuals who refuse to comply. Client must *want* to become a productive member of society before he or she can be helped.
	2. Talk about past behaviors with client. Discuss behaviors that are acceptable by societal norms and those that are not. Help client identify ways in which he or she has exploited others. Encourage client to explore how he or she would feel if the circumstances were reversed.	2. An attempt may be made to enlighten the client to the sensitivity of others by promoting self-awareness in an effort to gain insight into his or her own behavior.

3. Throughout relationship with client, maintain attitude of "It is not you, but your behavior, that is unacceptable."	3. An attitude of acceptance promotes feelings of dignity and self-worth.
4. Work with client to increase the ability to delay gratification. Reward desirable behaviors and provide immediate positive feedback.	4. Rewards and positive feedback enhance self-esteem and encourage repetition of desirable behaviors.
5. Help client identify and practice more adaptive strategies for coping with stressful life situations.	5. The impulse to perform the maladaptive behavior may be so great that the client is unable to see any other alternatives to relieve stress.

is to resolve the immediate crisis, restore adaptive functioning, and promote personal growth.

Psychopharmacology

Adjustment disorder is not commonly treated with medications. Reasons for this include: (1) their effect may be temporary and only mask the real problem, interfering with the possibility of finding a more permanent solution; and (2) psychoactive drugs carry the potential for physiological and psychological dependence.

When the client with adjustment disorder has symptoms of anxiety or depression, the physician may prescribe antianxiety or antidepressant medication. These medications are considered only adjuncts to psychotherapy and should not be given as the primary therapy. In these instances they are given to alleviate symptoms so that the individual may more effectively cope while attempting to adapt to the stressful situation.

Impulse Control Disorders

Intermittent Explosive Disorder

Individual psychotherapy for intermittent explosive disorder has not been successful. Group therapy, with its elements of group loyalty, peer pressure, expectation, and confrontation, may be more useful. Family therapy may be helpful when the client is an adolescent or young adult (Kaplan & Sadock, 1998).

Largely, clients with intermittent explosive disorder have been treated with psychopharmacological agents. A variety of agents have been tried, including lithium, carbamazepine, phenytoin, benzodiazepines, trazodoze, buspirone, phenothiazines, and propranolol (Kaplan & Sadock, 1998; Wise & Tierney, 1994). Recent data suggest a relationship between aggressive behavior and abnormal serotonin metabolism. Clinical management of the disorder with medications that block reuptake of serotonin, such as fluoxetine and other selective serotonin reuptake inhibihitors (SSRIs), have shown to be beneficial in some clients (Kaplan & Sadock, 1998).

Neurosurgical procedures have been used in the treatment of intractable explosive behavior. Evidence of the effectiveness of this type of treatment is lacking.

Kleptomania

Insight-oriented psychodynamic psychotherapy has been successful in the treatment of kleptomania. It has been most helpful with those individuals who experience guilt and shame and are thus motivated to change their behavior.

Various methods of behavior therapy have also been reported as useful (Popkin, 1989). Systematic desensitization, aversive conditioning, and alteration of interactional strategies have been helpful in some instances.

Several case reports cite success in the treatment of kleptomania using various medications (Kaplan & Sadock, 1998; Wise & Tierney, 1994). These have included the SSRIs, tricyclic antidepressants, trazodone, lithium, and valproate. Electroconvulsive therapy has also shown to be effective in some cases.

Pathological Gambling

Because most pathological gamblers deny that they have a problem, treatment is difficult. In fact, most gamblers only seek treatment due to legal difficulties, family pressures, or other psychiatric complaints (Kaplan, Sadock, & Grebb, 1994).

Behavioral therapy, cognitive therapy, psychoanalysis, and electroconvulsive therapy have been used with pathological gamblers, most with disappointing results (Wise & Tierney, 1994).

Some successes have been seen in pathological gamblers with various medications. Fluvoxamine, lithium carbonate, and clomipramine have provided a degree of efficacy for compulsive gambling. Other medications, such as antidepressants and antianxiety medications, have been useful in the relief of associated symptoms of depression and anxiety (Kaplan & Sadock, 1998).

Possibly the most effective treatment of pathological gambling is participation by the individual in **Gamblers**

TABLE 32.9 TOPICS FOR CLIENT/FAMILY EDUCATION RELATED TO ADJUSTMENT AND IMPULSE CONTROL DISORDERS

Nature of the Illness
1. Define adjustment disorder.
2. Describe types and symptoms of adjustment disorder.
3. Describe types and symptoms of impulse control disorder.
4. Discuss possible causes of the disorders.

Management of the Illness
1. Adjustment disorder
   a. Discuss possible need for lifestyle changes.
   b. Discuss ways to identify onset of escalating anxiety.
   c. Discuss problem-solving techniques.
   d. Teach assertive and relaxation techniques.
   e. Teach ways to increase feelings of control and decrease feelings of powerlessness.
   f. Pharmacology: Antianxiety agents and antidepressants. If these medications are given for associated symptoms, teach client about what to expect and possible adverse effects that may occur.
2. Impulse control disorder
   a. Discuss ways to identify onset of escalating anxiety and methods to prevent maladaptive responses.
   b. Discuss alternative adaptive coping strategies.
   c. Teach assertive and relaxation techniques.
   d. Teach ways to increase feelings of control and decrease feelings of powerlessness.
   e. Pharmacology: The following drugs may be prescribed for impulse control disorders. Ensure that client and family have sufficient knowledge about the medication prior to its administration.
      (1) Intermittent explosive disorder: lithium carbonate, phenothiazines, carbamazepine, benzodiazepines, propranolol, SSRIs
      (2) Kleptomania: SSRIs, tricyclic antidepressants, trazodone, lithium carbonate, valproate
      (3) Pathological gambling: fluvoxamine, lithium carbonate, clomipramine
      (4) Trichotillomania: chlorpromazine, amitriptyline, lithium carbonate, SSRIs/pimozide

Support Services
1. Support groups
   Gamblers Anonymous   National Council on Problem Gambling
   P. O. Box 17173   445 West 59th St., Room 1521
   Los Angeles, CA 90017   New York, NY 18019
   (213) 386-8789   1-800-522-4700
2. Individual psychotherapy
3. Crisis intervention
4. Behavior therapy
5. Family therapy

Anonymous (GA). This organization of inspirational group therapy is modeled after Alcoholics Anonymous. The only requirement for GA membership is an expressed desire to stop gambling (Wise & Tierney, 1994). Treatment is based on peer pressure, public confession, and the availability of other reformed gamblers to help individuals resist the urge to gamble. Gam-Anon (for family and spouses of compulsive gamblers) and Gam-a-Teen (for adolescent children of compulsive gamblers) are also important sources for treatment.

Pyromania

Treatment of individuals with pyromania has been difficult owing to the lack of motivation for change. Denial of problems, refusal to take responsibility for their behavior, and often the existence of alcoholism interfere with improvement in this disorder. Kaplan and Sadock (1998) state, "Incarceration may be the only method of prevent-

ing a recurrence. Behavior therapy can then be administered in the institution."

Trichotillomania

Behavior modification has been used to treat trichotillomania. Various techniques have been tried, including covert desensitization and habit-reversal practices. When the techniques are managed by a therapist, a system of rewards and punishment is applied in an effort to modify the hairpulling behaviors.

Psychodynamic intervention has been used in children with trichotillomania. Inquiry is made into areas of parent-child relationships or other areas of potential conflict that may provide some enlightenment about the problem (Wise & Tierney, 1994).

Various psychopharmacological agents, including chlorpromazine, amitriptyline, and lithium carbonate, have been tried in the treatment of trichotillomania, with

1. Impairment in an individual's usual social and occupational functioning.
2. Compulsive acts that may be harmful to the person or others.

Adjustment disorders are relatively common. In fact, some studies indicate it is the most commonly ascribed psychiatric diagnosis. Clinical symptoms include inability to function socially or occupationally in response to a psychosocial stressor. The disorder is distinguished by the predominant features of the maladaptive response. These include anxiety, depression, disturbance of conduct, disturbance of emotions and conduct, mixed emotional features, physical complaints, withdrawal, and inhibition of work or academics.

moderate results. Recent success with SSRIs augmented with pimozide has been reported (Kaplan & Sadock, 1998; Wise & Tierney, 1994).

SUMMARY

This chapter has focused on disorders that occur in response to stressful situations with which the individual cannot cope. The behavior may include:

RESEARCH NOTE

DSM-IV intermittent explosive disorder: A report of 27 cases. Journal of Clinical Psychiatry (1998, April), 59, 203–210
McElroy, S.L., Soutullo C.A., Beckman, D.A., Taylor, P., Jr., and Keck, P.E., Jr.

Description of the Study: The objective of this study was to obtain data regarding the demographic, phenomenological, course of illness, associated psychiatric and medical comorbidity, family history, and psychiatric treatment response characteristics in subjects meeting diagnostic criteria for intermittent explosive disorder in the *DSM-IV.* Twenty-seven subjects were given structured diagnostic interviews. Their and their families' medical and psychiatric histories were assessed along with the subjects' responses to psychiatric treatments.

Results of the Study: The following information was gathered from the assessments:

1. All 27 described aggressive impulses prior to their aggressive actions.
2. Twenty-one reported tension with the impulses.
3. Eighteen reported relief with the aggressive acts.
4. Eleven reported pleasure with the aggressive acts.
5. Most reported that their aggressive acts were associated with changes in mood.
6. Comorbidity reports were as follows:
   a. 93% had experienced mood disorders.
   b. 48% had experienced substance-use disorders.
   c. 48% had experienced anxiety disorders.
   d. 22% had experienced eating disorders.
   e. 44% had experienced an impulse control disorder other than intermittent explosive disorder.
   f. High rates of migraine headaches were reported.
   g. Family histories revealed high rates of mood disorders, substance-use disorders, and impulse control disorders.
7. Twelve of 20 subjects who received an antidepressant or mood stabilizer demonstrated a reduction in aggressive impulses and/or episodes.

Comments: The authors suggest that, although intermittent explosive disorder may correctly be regarded as an impulse control disorder, it may very well represent another form on the spectrum of affective disorders.

Of the two types of stressors discussed (i.e., sudden-shock and continuous), more individuals respond with maladaptive behaviors to long-term continuous stressors. Treatment modalities for adjustment disorders include individual psychotherapy, family therapy, behavior therapy, self-help groups, and psychopharmacology.

Impulse control disorders are quite rare but involve compulsive acts that may be harmful to the individual or to others. Individuals with impulse control disorders experience increased tension, followed by the inability to resist committing a specific act, after which the individual feels a sense of release and gratification.

Impulse control disorders include:

1. *Intermittent explosive disorder:* violent or aggressive behavior that culminates in serious assaultive acts or the destruction of property.

2. *Kleptomania:* inability to resist the impulse to steal.
3. *Pathological gambling:* inability to resist the impulse to gamble.
4. *Pyromania:* inability to resist the impulse to set fires.
5. *Trichotillomania:* inability to resist the impulse to pull out one's own hair.

Nursing care of individuals with adjustment and impulse control disorders is accomplished using the steps of the nursing process. Background assessment data were presented, along with nursing diagnoses common to each disorder. Interventions appropriate to each nursing diagnosis and relevant outcome criteria for each were included. An overview of current medical treatment modalities was discussed.

REVIEW QUESTIONS

SELF-EXAMINATION/LEARNING EXERCISE

Select the answer that is most appropriate for the questions that follow the situation.

Situation: Linda has been admitted to the psychiatric unit with a diagnosis of adjustment disorder with depressed mood. She recently left her husband after 10 years of a very stormy marriage. She did not want to leave but decided that the move was best for herself and her two children (who are living with her). Linda was very dependent on her husband and is having difficulty living an independent lifestyle.

1. The primary nursing diagnosis for Linda would be:
   a. Impaired adjustment related to breakup of marriage.
   b. Dysfunctional grieving related to breakup of marriage.
   c. High risk for self-directed violence related to depressed mood.
   d. Social isolation related to depressed mood.

2. Linda says to the nurse, "I feel so bad. I thought I would feel better once I left, but I feel worse!" Which is the *best* response by the nurse?
   a. "Cheer up, Linda. You have a lot to be happy about."
   b. "You are grieving for the marriage you did not have. It's natural for you to feel badly."
   c. "Try not to dwell on how you feel. If you don't think about it, you'll feel better."
   d. "You did the right thing, Linda. Knowing that should make you feel better."

3. The physician orders amitriptyline (Elavil) for Linda. This medication is intended to:
   a. Increase energy and elevate mood.
   b. Stimulate the central nervous system.
   c. Prevent psychotic symptoms.
   d. Produce a calming effect.

4. Which of the following is true regarding adjustment disorder?
   a. Linda will require long-term psychotherapy to achieve relief.
   b. Linda likely inherited a genetic tendency for the disorder.
   c. Linda's symptoms will likely remit once she has accepted the change in her life.
   d. Linda probably would not have experienced adjustment disorder if she had a higher level of intelligence.

5. The category of adjustment disorder with depressed mood identifies the individual who:
   a. Violates the rights of others to feel better.
   b. Expresses symptoms that reveal a high level of anxiety.
   c. Exhibits severe social isolation and withdrawal.
   d. Is experiencing a dysfunctional grieving process.

Match the behavior on the right to the appropriate diagnosis on the left.

_____   6. Kleptomania

_____   7. Intermittent explosive disorder

_____   8. Pathological gambling

_____   9. Pyromania

_____   10. Trichotillomania

a. Tony has been fascinated by fire for as long as he can remember. He played with matches as a child. As an adult, he has set numerous fires, always feeling exhilarated and even sexually stimulated afterward.

b. Janet received a great deal of money and property in a divorce settlement. Shortly after the divorce, she experienced an impulse to enter a large department store and steal some inexpensive costume jewelry. Although she had been apprehended twice for shoplifting, she was indifferent to being discovered at this time.

c. Frankie, a 16-year-old boy, had had temper tantrums since age 2. As he matured, the "tantrums" intensified, with explosions of rage, usually without identifiable provocation. He had attempted to molest his 12-year-old sister and went after his father with a butcher knife. He has an abnormal electroencephalogram.

d. Callie, a 10-year-old girl, has been pulling her hair out of the crown of her head for several years. She has been referred to psychiatry from the dermatology clinic. Her mother reports the hair pulling usually occurs at night when Callie is tired. Further history reveals Callie's father left her mother when Callie was 4 years old and has never been heard from since. Callie tells the psychiatrist he left because she was a bad girl.

e. Harold has borrowed a great deal of money from an illegal source in an effort to pay back a gambling debt. He has continued to gamble so that he can pay back the loan with his winnings. Last night, the loan sharks threatened harm if he did not pay soon. He withdraws all the money from his joint account with his wife and heads for the race track.

REFERENCES

Abraham, K. (1953). Manifestations of the female castration complex. In D. Bryan & A. Strachey (Eds.), *Selected papers on psychoanalysis.* New York: Basic Books.

American Psychiatric Association. (1994). *Diagnostic and statistical manual of mental disorders* (4th ed.). Washington, DC: American Psychiatric Association.

Andreasen, N.C., & Wasek, P. (1980). Adjustment disorders in adolescents and adults. *Archives of General Psychiatry, 37,* 1166–1170.

Booth, G.K. (1984). Disorders of impulse control. In H.H. Goldman (Ed.), *Review of general psychiatry.* Los Altos, CA: Lange Medical Publications.

Chess, S., & Thomas, A. (1984). *Origins and evolution of behavior disorders.* New York: Brunner/Mazel.

DeWitt, K.N. (1984). Adjustment disorder. In H.H. Goldman (Ed.), *Review of general psychiatry.* Los Altos, CA: Lange Medical Publications.

Freud, S. (1964). New introductory lectures on psychoanalysis and other works. In *The standard edition of the complete psychological works of Sigmund Freud* (Vol. 22). London: Hogarth Press.

Gibbens, T.C.N., & Prince, J. (1962). *Shoplifting.* London: Institute for the Study and Treatment of Delinquency.

Hales, R.E., et al. (1986). Psychiatric consultation in a military general hospital. *General Hospital Psychiatry, 8,* 173–182.

Kaplan, H.I., & Sadock, B.J. (1998). *Synopsis of psychiatry: Behavioral sciences/clinical psychiatry* (8th ed). Baltimore: Williams & Wilkins.

Kaplan, H.I., Sadock, B.J., & Grebb, J.A. (1994). *Synopsis of psychiatry* (7th ed.). Baltimore: Williams & Wilkins.

Krishnan, K.R.R., Davidson, J.R.T., & Guajardo, C. (1985). Trichotillomania—A review. *Comprehensive Psychiatry, 26,* 123–138.

Linnoila, M., DeJong, J., & Virkkunen, M. (1989). Family history of alcoholism in violent offenders and impulsive fire setters. *Archives of General Psychiatry, 46,* 613–616.

McConaghy, N., et al. (1983). Controlled comparison of aversive therapy and imaginal desensitization in compulsive gambling. *British Journal of Psychiatry, 142,* 366–372.

Moskowitz, J.A. (1980). Lithium and lady luck. *NY State Journal of Medicine, 80,* 785–788.

Popkin, M.K. (1989). Adjustment disorder and impulse control disorder. In H.I. Kaplan & B.J. Sadock (Eds.), *Comprehensive textbook of psychiatry* (Vol. 2) (5th ed.). Baltimore: Williams & Wilkins.

Strain, J.J., Newcorn, J., Wolf, D., & Fulop, G. (1994). Adjustment disorder. In R.E. Hales, S.C. Yudofsky, & J.A. Talbott (Eds.), *The American Psychiatric Press textbook of psychiatry* (2nd ed.). Washington, DC: American Psychiatric Press.

Virkkunen, M., et al. (1987). Cerebrospinal fluid monoamine metabolite levels in male arsonists. *Archives of General Psychiatry, 44,* 241–247.

Wise, M.G., & Tierney, J.G. (1994). Impulse control disorders not elsewhere classified. In R.E. Hales, S.C. Yudofsky, & J.A. Talbott (Eds.), *The American Psychiatric Press textbook of psychiatry* (2nd ed.). Washington, DC: American Psychiatric Press.

Yates, W.R. (1994). Other psychiatric syndromes: Adjustment disorder, factitious disorder, illicit steroid abuse. In G. Winokur & P.J. Clayton (Eds.), *The medical basis of psychiatry* (2nd ed.). Philadelphia: W.B. Saunders.

Bibliography

Bourin, M., Bougerol, T., Guitton, B., & Broutin, E. (1997). A combination of plant extracts in the treatment of outpatients with adjustment disorder with anxious mood: Controlled study versus placebo. *Fundamental and Clinical Pharmacology, 11,* 127–132.

Crockford, D.N., & el-Guebaly, N. (1998, February). Psychiatric co-morbidity in pathological gambling: A critical review. *Canadian Journal of Psychiatry, 43,* 43–50.

Daghestani, A.N., Elenz, E., & Crayton, J.W. (1996, August). Pathological gambling in hospitalized substance abusing veterans. *Journal of Clinical Psychiatry, 57,* 360–363.

Deater-Deckard, K., Reiss, D., Hetherington, E.M., & Plomin, R. (1997, July). Dimensions and disorders of adolescent adjustment: A quantitative genetic analysis of unselected samples and selected extremes. *Journal of Child Psychology and Psychiatry and Allied Disciplines, 38,* 515–525.

DeCaria, C.M., et al. (1996). Diagnosis, neurobiology, and treatment of pathological gambling. *Journal of Clinical Psychiatry, 57* (Suppl 8), 80–84.

Griffiths, M. (1996, December). Pathological gambling: A review of the literature. *Journal of Psychiatric and Mental Health Nursing, 3,* 347–353.

Kindler, S., Dannon, P.N., Iancu, I., Sasson, Y., & Zohar, J. (1997, April). Emergence of kleptomania during treatment for depression with serotonin selective reuptake inhibitors. *Clinical Neuropharmacology, 20,* 126–129.

McElroy, S.L., Pope, H.G., & Hudson, J.I. (1991, May). Kleptomania: A report of 20 cases. *American Journal of Psychiatry, 148,* 652–657.

McNeilly, D.P., & Burke, W.J. (1998, February). Stealing lately: A case of late-onset kleptomania. *International Journal of Geriatric Psychiatry, 13,* 116–121.

Shell, D., & Ferrante, A.P. (1996, January). Recognition of adjustment disorder in college athletes: A case study. *Clinical Journal of Sport Medicine, 6,* 60–62.

Steel, Z., & Blaszczynski, A. (1998, June). Impulsivity, personality disorders and pathological gambling severity. *Addiction 93,* 895–905.

Stilling, L. (1992). The pros and cons of physical restraints and behavior controls. *Journal of Psychosocial Nursing, 30*(3), 18–20.

Strain, J.J., et al. (1998, May). Adjustment disorder: A multisite study of its utilization and interventions in the consultation-liaison psychiatry setting. *General Hospital Psychiatry, 20,* 139–149.

Townsend, M.C. (1997). *Nursing diagnoses in psychiatric nursing: A pocket guide for care plan construction* (4th ed.). Philadelphia: F.A. Davis.

PSYCHOLOGICAL FACTORS AFFECTING MEDICAL CONDITIONS

CHAPTER OUTLINE

OBJECTIVES

INTRODUCTION

HISTORICAL ASPECTS

APPLICATION OF THE NURSING PROCESS

TREATMENT MODALITIES

SUMMARY

REVIEW QUESTIONS

KEY TERMS

psychophysiological
cachexia
carcinogens

type C personality
type A personality
type B personality

essential hypertension
migraine personality
autoimmune

OBJECTIVES

After reading this chapter, the student will be able to:

1. Differentiate between somatoform and psychophysiological disorders.
2. Identify various types of psychophysiological disorders.
3. Discuss historical and epidemiological statistics related to various psychophysiological disorders.
4. Describe symptomatology associated with various psychophysiological disorders and use this data in client assessment.
5. Identify various predisposing factors to psychophysiological disorders.
6. Formulate nursing diagnoses and goals of care for clients with various psychophysiological disorders.
7. Describe appropriate nursing interventions for behaviors associated with various psychophysiological disorders.
8. Identify topics for client and family teaching relevant to psychophysiological disorders.
9. Evaluate the nursing care of clients with psychophysiological disorders.
10. Discuss various modalities relevant to treatment of psychophysiological disorders.

sychophysiological responses are those in which it has been determined that psychological factors contribute to the initiation or exacerbation of the physical condition. They differ from somatoform disorders in that there is evidence of either demonstrable organic pathology or a known pathophysiological process involved. No such organic involvement can be identified in somatoform disorders.

The *DSM-IV* (American Psychiatric Association [APA], 1994) states:

"Psychological factors can influence the course of the general medical condition which can be inferred by a close temporal association between the factors and the development or exacerbation of, or delayed recovery from, the medical condition."

Several types of psychological factors are implicated by the *DSM-IV* as those which can affect the general medical condition. They include:

1. Mental disorders (e.g., axis I disorders, such as major depression).
2. Psychological symptoms (e.g., depressed mood or anxiety).
3. Personality traits or coping style (e.g., denial of the need for medical care).
4. Maladaptive health behaviors (e.g., smoking or overeating).
5. Stress-related physiological responses (e.g., tension headaches).
6. Other unspecified psychological factors (e.g., interpersonal or cultural factors).

The *DSM-IV* diagnostic criteria for psychological factors affecting medical condition are presented in Table 33.1.

Virtually any organic disorder can be considered psychophysiological. Kaplan (1989) states, ". . . all disease is influenced by psychological factors." A list of some (although certainly not all) psychophysiological disorders is presented in Table 33.2.

The following psychophysiological disorders are discussed in this chapter:

asthma
cancer
coronary heart disease
peptic ulcer
migraine headache
hypertension
rheumatoid arthritis
ulcerative colitis

Historical and epidemiological statistics are presented. Predisposing factors that have been implicated in the etiology of each psychophysiological disorder provide a framework for study. An explanation of the symptomatology is presented as background knowledge for assessing the client with a psychophysiological disorder. Nursing care is described in the context of the nursing process. Various medical treatment modalities are explored.

HISTORICAL ASPECTS

For more than a century, physicians have agreed that in some disorders there is an interaction between emotional and physical factors. Kaplan and Sadock (1985) describe four general types of reaction to stress:

1. *The normal reaction*, in which there is increased alertness and a mobilization of defenses for action.
2. *The psychophysiological reaction*, in which the defenses fail and the response is translated into somatic symptoms.
3. *The neurotic reaction*, in which the anxiety is so great

▬ TABLE 33.1   PSYCHOLOGICAL FACTORS (SPECIFY) AFFECTING MEDICAL CONDITION

A. A general medical condition is present.
B. Psychological factors adversely affect the general medical condition in one of the following ways:
 1. The factors have influenced the course of the general medical condition as shown by a close temporal association between the psychological factors and the development or exacerbation of, or delayed recovery from, the general medical condition.
 2. The factors interfere with the treatment of the general medical condition.
 3. The factors constitute additional health risks for the individual.
 4. Stress-related physiological responses precipitate or exacerbate symptoms of the general medical condition.
Specify type of psychological factor:
 Mental disorder (e.g., axis I disorder such as major depressive disorder delaying recovery from a myocardial infarction).
 Psychological symptoms (e.g., depressive symptoms delaying recovery from surgery, anxiety exacerbating asthma).
 Personality traits or coping style (e.g, pathological denial of the need for surgery in a patient with cancer; hostile, pressured behavior contributing to cardiovascular disease).
 Maladaptive health behaviors (e.g., overeating, lack of exercise, unsafe sex).
 Stress-related physiological response (e.g., stress-related exacerbations of ulcer, hypertension, arrhythmia, or tension headache).
 Other or unspecified psychological factors (e.g., interpersonal, cultural, or religious factors).

SOURCE: From APA (1994), with permission.

TABLE 33.2 EXAMPLES OF PSYCHOPHYSIOLOGICAL DISORDERS

Acne	Immune disease (e.g., multiple
Amenorrhea	sclerosis, systemic lupus
Angina pectoris	erythematosus)
Asthma	Impotence
Cancer	Irritable bowel syndrome
Cardiospasm	Migraine headache
Coronary heart disease	Nausea and vomiting
Duodenal ulcer	Neurodermatitis
Dysmenorrhea	Obesity
Enuresis	Pylorospasm
Essential hypertension	Regional enteritis
Gastric ulcer	Rheumatoid arthritis
Herpes	Sacroiliac pain
Hyperglycemia	Skin disease (e.g., psoriasis)
Hyperthyroidism	Tension headache
Hypoglycemia	Tuberculosis
	Ulcerative colitis

SOURCES: Modified from APA (1994), Kaplan (1989), and Pelletier (1992).

that the defense becomes ineffective and neurotic symptoms develop.

4. *The psychotic reaction,* in which loss of control results in misperception of the environment.

This explanation of stress response corresponds to the concept of anxiety described by Peplau (1963) and the type of responses associated with each level (see Chapter 2). Along the continuum of anxiety, psychophysiological disorders occur at the moderate-to-severe level.

Hans Selye (1976) studied the physiological response of a biological system to change imposed on it. He found that regardless of the stressor, the biological entity responded with a syndrome of symptoms that he called the *general adaptation syndrome.* (This syndrome of symptoms is described in Chapter 1.) In this aroused state, the individual garners the strength to face the stress and mobilize the defenses to resolve it. However, if the defenses fail and the stressor is not quickly resolved, the body remains in this aroused state indefinitely, becoming susceptible to psychophysiological illness.

Historically, mind and body have been viewed as two distinct entities, each subject to different laws of causality. Indeed, in many instances—particularly in highly specialized areas of medicine—the biological and psychological components of disease remain separate. However, medical research shows that a change is occurring. Research associated with biological functioning is being expanded to include also the psychological and social determinants of health and disease. This psychobiological approach to illness reflects a more holistic perspective and one that

promotes concern for helping clients achieve optimal functioning.

APPLICATION OF THE NURSING PROCESS

Background Assessment Data: Types of Psychophysiological Disorders

Asthma

Definition and Epidemiological Statistics. Asthma is a syndrome of airflow limitation characterized by increased responsiveness of the tracheobronchial tree to various stimuli and manifested by airway smooth muscle contraction, hypersecretion of mucus, and inflammation (Anderson, 1991). It affects approximately 10 million adults and children in the United States (Phipps & Brucia, 1995). The onset is commonly in childhood and the incidence is higher in boys until the teen years. During adolescence and thereafter, the incidence is higher in women than in men (Vachon, 1989).

Signs and Symptoms. Asthma is characterized by episodes of bronchial constriction resulting in dyspnea, wheezing, productive cough, restlessness, and eosinophilia. Expiration is prolonged and breathing reflects use of accessory muscles. Tachypnea and nasal flaring are common. The individual is usually diaphoretic and quite apprehensive, with total attention focused on his or her breathing.

Predisposing Factors

Biological Influences. Hereditary factors may play a role in the etiology of asthma. When both parents have the disease, it is known to occur in more than half the offspring, dropping to around 20 percent when only one parent is affected (Vachon, 1989). Twin studies show a concordance of about 50 percent.

Allergies play a major role in precipitating the attacks associated with asthma. Anderson (1991) lists the following specific agents known to stimulate bronchoconstriction: aspirin and all nonsteroidal anti-inflammatory drugs, chemicals, dust, grains, food additives, and beta blocking agents (e.g., propranolol). Other nonspecific factors known to stimulate bronchoconstriction include exercise, cold air, environmental pollutants and irritants (e.g., infection, cigarette smoke), pharmacological agents (e.g., histamine, cholinergic agonists), and reflux esophagitis.

Psychosocial Influences. Asthma has long been recognized as a "typical" psychophysiological response with evidence of symptoms being induced by emotional stress. Individuals with asthma are characterized as having excessive dependence needs, often with a strong unconscious wish for protection and for envelopment by the mother or surrogate mother. Kaplan and Sadock (1998) describe the mother figure as overprotective, oversolicitous, perfectionistic, dominating, and helpful. An asthmatic attack is thought to be precipitated when the child seeks but is denied protection from the mother.

Cancer

Definition and Epidemiological Statistics. Cancer is a malignant neoplasm in which the basic structure and activity of the cells have become deranged, usually because of changes in the DNA. These mutated cells grow wildly and rapidly and lose their similarity to the original cells. The malignant cells spread to other areas by invading surrounding tissues and by entering the blood and lymphatic system. If left untreated, the malignant neoplasms usually result in death.

Cancer is the second leading cause of death in the United States. However, 5-year survival rates have increased as a result of early diagnosis and treatment and the improvement of treatment modalities for most cancers. The largest number of deaths from cancer in both men and women is attributed to cancer of the lung (National Cancer Institute, 1999a).

The incidence and mortality rates for cancer are higher for blacks than for whites, and lower in Latino Americans than for both blacks and white (Deters, 1995). Cancer has been called a "disease of the aging," as the likelihood of developing cancer increases with age.

Signs and Symptoms. The American Cancer Society has identified seven significant changes that may occur as early warning signs of cancer (National Cancer Institute, 1999b). They include

1. A change in bowel or bladder habits.
2. A sore that does not heal.
3. Unusual bleeding or discharge.
4. A thickening or lump in the breast or elsewhere.
5. Indigestion or difficulty in swallowing.
6. An obvious change in a wart or mole.
7. A nagging cough or hoarseness.

Specific effects are determined by site. Malignant tumors can also create effects at sites distant to the primary site. Late-stage cancer symptoms may include anemias, infections, thrombocytopenia, **cachexia,** weakness, weight loss, dyspnea, ascites, and pleural effusion (Deters, 1995).

Predisposing Factors

Biological Influences. Certain cancers, such as those of the stomach, breast, colon, kidney, uterus, and lung, tend to occur in a familial pattern. Whether this indicates an inherited susceptibility or common exposure to an etiological factor is unknown.

Continuous irritation also may predispose individuals to certain types of cancer. For example, chronic exposure to the sun is thought to predispose to melanoma, and prolonged alcohol consumption may be related to the development of esophageal cancer.

Exposure to occupational or environmental **carcinogens** may lead to specific cancers. Examples include cigarette smoke, aniline dye, radium, asphalt, arsenic, chromate, uranium, and asbestos. Various drugs have been implicated in the onset of cancer. They include immunosuppressive agents, diethylstilbestrol, oral contraceptives, cytotoxic agents, and radioisotopes.

Certain viruses have been isolated and identified as the causative factor of cancer in some animals. However, the role that viruses play in the etiology of cancer in humans has not been definitely established.

Psychosocial Influences. Hafen and associates (1996) report on a number of research studies dealing with personality characteristics that have been associated with individuals who develop cancer. The term **type C personality** has been coined to describe these characteristics. Cancer has sometimes been called the "nice guy's disease." Common characteristics that were found to be associated with type C personality include repression of negative emotions, passivity, and being apologetic and overly cooperative.

Other researchers who have studied these characteristics identify the following profile for the type C personality:

● Extreme suppression of anger and hostility (experiences these emotions but does not express them).
● Exhibits a calm, placid exterior.
● Commonly feels depressed and in despair.
● Low self-esteem; low self-worth.
● Puts others' needs before their own.
● Has a tendency toward self-pity (acts as the martyr).
● Sets unrealistic standards and is inflexible in the enforcement of these standards.
● Resents others for perceived "wrongs," although others are never aware of these feelings.

LeShan (1977), who conducted psychotherapy for more than 30 years with cancer clients, says:

"The single most significant factor in the weakening of the cancer defense mechanism is the loss of hope in ever achieving any meaning, zest, or validity in life. It's the feeling that we can't ever really be ourselves—fully and richly as human beings—in being, relating or creating."

LeShan calls this the "loss of self." In his studies, he found that as children, cancer clients were not allowed to express themselves honestly but were forced to yield to the roles and expectations placed upon them by others. They come to believe that they can either be themselves (and therefore unloved and alone), or they can be what others want and thus be loved and accepted. It is viewed as a hopeless situation from which the individual can never achieve any real self-gratification. LeShan (1966) described the profile of the family of origin of cancer clients as follows:

● Lack of close relationship with one or both parents.
● Loss of parent through death in a large number of cases.

● Childhood characterized by feeling neglected, physically or emotionally.

● Childhood in which child feels loneliness and despair, and blames self for situation.

● Believing that one's life situation is hopeless, with little or no opportunity for self-gratification.

● Continual efforts to conform to others' expectations in order to win their love and approval.

Some studies have been conducted in an effort to determine if there is a link between psychosocial stress and the onset of cancer symptoms. Results suggest a positive correlation between the effects of stress and the induction and growth of neoplastic tumors in extensive work with experimental animals and in more limited studies with humans. Biopsychosocial events appear to reduce immunological competence at a critical time and may allow a mutant cell to thrive and grow (Pelletier, 1992).

Coronary Heart Disease

Definition and Epidemiological Statistics. Coronary heart disease (CHD) is defined as myocardial impairment caused by an imbalance between coronary blood flow and myocardial oxygen requirements resulting from changes in the coronary circulation (Woods, Underhill, & Cowan, 1991). It is the leading cause of death in the United States. Five million people have CHD. It is more prevalent in men than in women, although the number of women with CHD is increasing, probably as a result of greater social and economic pressures on women and changes in their lifestyles. The incidence of CHD is higher in older individuals and in the affluent (Abraham, 1995).

Signs and Symptoms. Atherosclerosis, or changes in the lining of the coronary arteries that affect lumen size, is the basic underlying problem associated with coronary heart disease. Size of the lumen is decreased because of an accumulation of cells, lipids, and connective tissue that adheres to the intima of the artery. This results in decreased oxygenated blood flow to the myocardium and possible myocardial ischemia. Myocardial ischemia may be asymptomatic or may cause discomfort in the chest.

Angina pectoris can occur spontaneously or in relation to increased myocardial oxygen demand. Common descriptions of pain associated with angina include sensations of strangling, aching, squeezing, pressing, expanding, choking, burning, constriction, indigestion, tightness, and heaviness (Woods, Underhill, & Cowan, 1991). The discomfort of angina usually lasts from 2 to 5 minutes, sometimes as long as 15 minutes, and rarely as long as 30 minutes.

Pain associated with myocardial infarction (MI) is similar to that experienced in angina but lasts longer than 15 to 30 minutes. Symptoms may also include indigestion, nausea and vomiting, diaphoresis, syncope, palpitations, or dyspnea. In approximately 15 percent to 20 percent of cases, clients experiencing MI will not experience chest discomfort (Abraham, 1995).

Predisposing Factors

Biological Influences. A number of risk factors have been identified as predisposing factors to the development of CHD. A family history of CHD increases an individual's risk of developing atherosclerosis. Other possible hereditary risk factors for CHD include high serum lipoprotein levels, particularly cholesterol and triglycerides, hypertension, and diabetes mellitus. It is not known whether there is a direct genetic link or if the risk is related more to environmental lifestyle patterns.

Various lifestyle habits have been implicated. The association between cigarette smoking and CHD has now been clearly established. Three compounds in cigarette smoke (tar, nicotine, and carbon monoxide) have been implicated as causative agents in CHD (Woods, Underhill, & Cowan, 1991).

Obesity, defined as body mass index (weight/height^2) of 30 or greater has been associated with increased risk of developing CHD. It is unclear whether the increased risk is associated with the obesity itself or to other factors that frequently accompany obesity, such as high blood pressure or diabetes.

Sedentary lifestyle has also been implicated. Physical exercise may reduce the risk of CHD and stroke, may help to maintain blood pressure at a lower level, help with weight maintenance, and increase levels of high-density lipoproteins (HDL) (Sobel & Ornstein, 1996).

Psychosocial Influences. Friedman and Rosenman (1974) have completed the most comprehensive work to date in the area of personality and CHD. They developed a detailed profile of the CHD-prone individual, which they identified as **type A personality.** They also studied personality characteristics of individuals who experienced stress in a different manner and seemed less prone to CHD. This personality profile was entitled **type B personality.**

Friedman and Rosenman identified two character traits that when occurring together automatically classify an individual as type A personality. These two traits are excessive competitive drive and a chronic, continual sense of time urgency. Additional type A characteristics include:

● Easily aroused hostility; usually kept under control but flaring up unexpectedly, often when others would consider it unwarranted.

● Very aggressive, very ambitious, concentrating almost exclusively on his or her career.

● Having no time for hobbies, and during any leisure time, feeling guilty just relaxing, as if wasting time.

● Seldom feeling satisfied with accomplishments; always feeling must do *more*.

● Measuring achievements in numbers produced and dollars earned.

- Continually struggling to achieve and feeling there is never enough time, time becoming the enemy of the person with type A personality.
- Appearing to be very extroverted and social; often dominating conversation; outgoing personality often concealing a deep-seated insecurity about own worth.
- Driving ambition and need to win leading the person with type A personality to undertake all activities with the same competitive drive, with even recreational activities becoming aggressive when the individual puts undue pressure on himself or herself to compete.

People with type B personalities are not the opposite of those with type A, only different. Those with type B personality are no less successful than those with type A. They may perform every bit as well on their jobs—maybe better. Those with type B do not feel the constant sense of time urgency that those with type A feel. They can function under time pressure when it is required, but it is not a pervasive part of their lives as it is with those type A individuals. Type B individuals' ambition is probably based on goals that have been well thought out. There is not the constant need for competition and comparison with peers. Self-worth often comes from goals other than material and social success. Type B personality individuals recognize and accept both strengths and limitations. They view leisure time as a time to relax, and they do so without feeling guilty. They take the time to consider alternatives and to think things through before deciding or acting. These characteristics often result in more creative output by persons with type B personality. Those with type A are prone to making more errors owing to their impulsivity (i.e., acting before thinking things through).

A study by Rosenman and colleagues (1975) reported the results of an 8½-year follow-up study for predicting CHD in men between the ages of 39 and 59. In this study, the incidence of CHD was significantly associated with parental history, diabetes, education, smoking, blood pressure, and serum cholesterol levels. The study also concluded that type A behavior was a strong factor and that "this association could not be explained by association of behavior pattern with any single predictive risk factor or any combination of them" (Rosenman et al., 1975). Type A behavior risk factor was clearly a contributing factor in itself.

Peptic Ulcer

Definition and Epidemiological Statistics. Peptic ulcers are an erosion of the mucosal wall in the esophagus, stomach, duodenum, or jejunum. Deeper lesions may penetrate the mucosal layer and extend into the muscular layers of the intestinal wall (Simmons & Heitkemper, 1991).

Peptic ulcers occur four times more frequently in men than in women. Peak ages have traditionally been identified as 40 to 50 years, although these ages are increasing. Within these vulnerable age groups, peptic ulcers are estimated to affect up to 10 percent of the general population (Sands, 1995a). Hospitalization, surgery, and mortality related to peptic ulcer disease place an economic burden on this country in the billions of dollars annually.

Signs and Symptoms. Pain is the characteristic clinical manifestation of peptic ulcer disease. It is usually experienced in the upper abdomen near the midline, and may radiate to the back, sternum, or lower abdomen. Pain is usually worse when the stomach is empty and gastric secretions are high. Food or antacid medication often relieves the pain.

Predisposing Factors

Biological Influences. There appears to be a hereditary predisposition to peptic ulcer disease, in that a person with a family member with ulcer disease has three times the risk of developing an ulcer compared with the general population (Simmons & Heitkemper, 1991). The ulcer itself occurs as a result of an imbalance in the secretion of hydrochloric acid and the mucosal resistance factors. Any factor that stimulates higher-than-normal hydrochloric acid secretion can promote the development of peptic ulcers.

Several environmental factors have been associated with peptic ulcer disease. Cigarette smoking and regular use of aspirin have been strongly implicated. Other agents such as alcohol, steroids, and nonsteroidal anti-inflammatory drugs are also ulcerogenic in that they can cause damage to the gastric mucosal barrier.

Most recently, gastric ulcers have been associated with infection by the bacterium *Helicobacter pylori*. It is not yet known if stress in a susceptible person increases the likelihood of infection with this bacterium.

Psychosocial Influences. Studies have observed increased gastric secretion and motility in the presence of hostility, resentment, guilt, and frustration (Hafen et al., 1996). The link between ulcers and stress has been related by some psychodynamic investigators to an unfulfilled dependency need in ulcer-prone individuals. These individuals tend to have an unhealthy attachment to others, and although they are dependent by nature, they perceive that they have few people on whom they can depend in time of crisis. They are excessive worriers and seem to have more times of crises than most people, possibly because they are such pessimists and always seem to expect the worst from a situation (Hafen et al., 1996). Anxiety and depression are common among ulcer-prone individuals.

Essential Hypertension

Definition and Epidemiological Statistics. Essential hypertension is the persistent elevation of blood pressure for which there is no apparent cause or associated underlying disease (Cunningham, 1991). It is a major cause of cerebrovascular accident (stroke), cardiac disease, and renal failure.

Twenty-five percent of the adult population in the United States are hypertensive, a condition characterized by a blood pressure of 140/90 mm Hg or higher (American Heart Association, 1999). Because hypertension is often asymptomatic, it is estimated that 50 percent of persons with hypertension do not know they have it (Walsh, 1995). The disorder is more common in men than in women and is twice as prevalent in the black population as it is in the white population.

Signs and Symptoms. Most commonly, hypertension produces no symptoms, particularly in the early stages. When symptoms do occur, they may include headache, vertigo, flushed face, spontaneous nosebleed, or blurred vision. Chronic, progressive hypertension may reveal signs and symptoms associated with specific organ system damage. For example, dyspnea, chest pain, or cardiac hypertrophy may indicate cardiovascular damage, confusion and parasthesia may suggest cerebrovascular damage, and elevated serum creatinine or blood urea nitrogen may signal kidney damage.

Predisposing Factors

Biological Influences. Individuals who have a positive family history of hypertension are at greater risk of developing the disorder than those who do not. Other environmental conditions that may contribute to hypertension are obesity and cigarette smoking.

Various physiological influences have been hypothesized. These include an imbalance of circulating vasoconstrictors (e.g., angiotensin) and vasodilators (e.g., prostaglandins), increased sympathetic nervous system activity resulting in increased vasoconstriction, and impairment of sodium and water excretion (Cunningham, 1991).

Psychosocial Influences. Hackett, Rosenbaum, and Cassem (1989) offer the following psychodynamic explanation of the individual with essential hypertension:

> "The person at risk for hypertension appears compliant and congenial, longing for approval. Although superficially easygoing, that person is inwardly suppressing anger and suspicion. This dilemma derives from childhood experiences with parents toward whom anger could not be expressed without real or imagined loss of love and security. The desire to please, in tandem with an antagonistic battle-ready stance, is felt to be characteristic of essential hypertensive persons."

Migraine Headache

Definition and Epidemiological Statistics. Migraine headache is a vascular event in which pain arises from the scalp, its blood vessels, and muscles; from the dura mater and its venous sinuses; and from the blood vessels at the base of the brain (Schenk, 1995). Pain most commonly originates in the muscles of the face, neck, and head; the blood vessels; and the dura mater. The blood vessels dilate and become congested with blood. Pain results from the exertion of pressure on nerves that lie in or around these congested blood vessels.

Migraine headaches can occur at any age but commonly begin in persons between ages 16 and 30 years. They are more common in women than in men and often are associated with various phases of the menstrual cycle. Approximately 5 percent of the general population suffer from migraine headaches.

Signs and Symptoms. The "classic" migraine headache occurs in two distinctive phases. In the prodromal phase, which may begin from minutes to days before the actual pain of the headache, the individual may experience visual disturbances, weakness and numbness on one side of the body, mental confusion, irritability, fatigue, sweating, and dizziness. The headache phase usually consists of pain on one side of the head. As it intensifies, the pain may spread to the other side as well. The ache is frequently dull, deep, and throbbing, and often begins in the forehead, ear, jaw, or in or around an eye or temple. Nausea, vomiting, mental cloudiness, total body achiness, abdominal pain, chills, and cold hands and feet commonly accompany the headache. The actual attack usually lasts from 1 hour to more than a day, after which sore muscles, total body exhaustion, and a continued mild mental cloudiness may persist for days.

The most common form of migraine headache is a variation of the classic version. Many of the symptoms are similar, but in common migraine the distinctive phases of the classic migraine do not occur. Photophobia (sensitivity to light) and hyperacusis (sensitivity to sound) may be present in both types.

Predisposing Factors

Biological Influences. A number of biological influences have been identified as triggers for headache-prone individuals. Periods of hormonal change have been implicated, such as during menstruation, during ovulation, during menopause, and at the beginning of or just following pregnancy.

Heredity appears to play an important role in the etiology of migraine headaches. It is common for individuals from several generations within the same family to experience the disorder. Occasionally members of one or two generations are spared, but it is not uncommon to track a history of headaches in aunts, uncles, cousins, or grandparents.

Some foods, beverages, and drugs can precipitate migraine in certain individuals. These substances include caffeine, chocolate, aged cheese, vinegar, organ meats, alcoholic beverages, sour cream, yogurt, aspartame, citrus fruits, bananas, raisins, avocados, onions, smoked meats, monosodium glutamate, and products preserved with nitrites. Drugs that lower blood pressure, in particular reserpine and hydralazine, have also been known to trigger migraine headaches.

Some people experience attacks only during or after physical exertion. This may be caused either by the chemical or blood vessel changes that occur during physical exertion or by the depletion of certain biological substances that may occur after exercise.

Various other factors that have been implicated in the development of migraine headaches include cigarette smoking, bright lights, changes in the weather, high elevations, oral contraceptives, altered sleep patterns, and skipping meals.

Psychosocial Influences. Certain characteristics have been identified as "the **migraine personality.**" Migraine sufferers have been described as perfectionistic, overly conscientious, and somewhat inflexible. They may be meticulously neat and tidy, compulsive, and often very hard workers. They are usually quite intelligent, exacting, and place a very high premium on success, setting high (sometimes unrealistic) expectations on themselves and others. Delegation of responsibility is difficult, as they feel no one can perform the task as well as they can. Classically, there is repressed or suppressed anger. The individual experiences hostility and anger but cannot express these feelings openly. Some researchers have identified the migraine personality as a clone of the type A personality (Hafen et al., 1996).

Emotions play a critical role in the precipitation of migraine headaches. An individual experiencing emotional stress may develop a migraine headache in response to the secondary gains one receives from assuming the sick role. Migraine headaches therefore may provide a means of escape from dealing with the stressful situation. Other individuals experience migraine attacks only *after* the emotionally distressing event has passed or lessened. This has been called "let-down" headache and can be one of the influential factors in provoking the weekend or holiday migraine, when the anxiety has been relieved and the individual finally relaxes (Robbins & Lang, 1995).

Rheumatoid Arthritis

Definition and Epidemiological Statistics. Rheumatoid arthritis is a disease characterized by chronic musculoskeletal pain caused by inflammatory disease of the joints (Kaplan & Sadock, 1998). It is a *systemic* disease, and may also be manifested by lesions of the major organs of the body. Rheumatoid arthritis is more prevalent in women than men by a ratio of 2:1 or 3:1. It affects 1 to 3 percent of the population of the United States, with an estimated 200,000 cases diagnosed annually (Marek, Buergin, & Paskert, 1995). The disease is characterized by periods of remission and exacerbation.

Signs and Symptoms. Onset of the disease is usually insidious, with joint inflammation preceding the systemic symptoms of fatigue, malaise, anorexia, weight loss, low-grade fever, myalgias, and parasthesias (Cicero, 1991). Some individuals recover from a first attack of the disorder and never suffer a recurrence, while others tend to suffer chronic and progressive systemic symptoms. Joint involvement is usually characterized by swelling, pain, redness, warmth, and tenderness. Joints of the hands and feet are often affected early. As the disease progresses, any freely movable joint may be involved.

About one out of every five rheumatoid arthritis clients develop systemic manifestations, which can occur in virtually any body system. Cardiac, pulmonary, and renal involvement are the most serious consequences of rheumatoid arthritis (Cicero, 1991).

Predisposing Factors

Biological Influences. Heredity appears to be influential in the predisposition to rheumatoid arthritis. The serum protein rheumatoid factor is found in at least half of rheumatoid arthritics and frequently in their close relatives (Pelletier, 1992). It is an inherited characteristic that increases one's vulnerability to the disease. Although the rheumatoid factor is present in clients with other diseases, it is rare in the population at large.

An additional theory postulates that rheumatoid arthritis may be the result of a dysfunctional immune mechanism initiated by an infectious process, although the causative agent is yet to be identified. In such an instance, antibodies that form in keeping with a normal reaction to infection become directed instead against the self in an **autoimmune** response that results in tissue damage.

Psychosocial Influences. Rheumatoid arthritis clients are postulated to be self-sacrificing, masochistic, conforming, self-conscious, inhibited, and perfectionistic, with an inherent inability to express anger (Hafen et al., 1996). Female rheumatoid clients are described as nervous, tense, worried, moody, and depressed, and typically had mothers whom they felt rejected them and fathers who were unduly strict (Pelletier, 1992).

Evidence has accumulated over the past four decades suggesting that emotionally traumatic life events, such as the loss of a key person by death or separation, often precede the first symptoms of rheumatoid arthritis and precipitate its onset in between 22 percent and 100 percent of clients (Ananth, 1989). Thus, emotional decompensation in predisposed individuals may result in the onset or exacerbation of rheumatoid arthritis.

Ulcerative Colitis

Definition and Epidemiological Statistics. Ulcerative colitis is a chronic inflammatory ulcerative disease of the colon, usually associated with bloody diarrhea (Kaplan & Sadock, 1998). The incidence of the disease in the

United States is approximately 5 to 7 per 100,000 population (Heitkemper & Martin, 1991). It can occur at any age but is most prevalent between the ages of 15 and 30 years. The disease is prevalent in Caucasians, rare in African Americans and Native Americans. There is a high incidence of ulcerative colitis among American and European Jews (Sands, 1995b).

Signs and Symptoms. The mucosa of the colon and rectum become inflamed, with diffuse areas of bleeding. Diarrhea is the predominant symptom of ulcerative colitis. There may be as many as 15 to 20 liquid stools a day containing blood, mucus, and pus (Sands, 1995b). Abdominal cramping may or may not precede the bowel movement. Generalized manifestations include fever, anorexia, weight loss, nausea, and vomiting. During exacerbation of the illness, anemia and elevated white cell count are common.

As the disease progresses, the inflammation advances up the colon and the bleeding points enlarge and become ulcerated. The ulcers may bleed or perforate, forming scar tissue as it heals. The scar tissue causes the colon to thicken and become rigid, and normal elasticity and absorptive capability are diminished. Changes in the mucosa may cause the formation of pseudopolyps that can become cancerous.

Predisposing Factors

Biological Influences. A genetic factor may be involved in the development, as individuals who have a family member with ulcerative colitis are at greater risk than the general population. This theory is supported by sibling and twin studies, although no genetic marker has been identified.

The possibility that ulcerative colitis may be an autoimmune disease has generated a great deal of research interest. High rates of anticolon antibodies are found in relatives of ulcerative colitis clients. This autoimmune precondition for inflammatory bowel disease may support Engel's (1955) statement that the disease may be caused by "unidentified changes which alter relationships in the colon so that it responds to its own flora as pathogens."

Psychosocial Influences. Lipsitt (1989) states:

"The precise role of psychosomatic factors in the pathogenesis of inflammatory bowel disease remains uncertain, although descriptions of clients as obsessive-compulsive, dependent, emotionally immature, and especially vulnerable to separations and loss have borne the test of time and clinical observation."

Engel (1955) described colitis clients as having an obsessive-compulsive behavior pattern involving excessive neatness, indecision, conformity, overintellectualism, rigid morality, anxiety, and depression. He found similarities between the personality profiles of colitis clients and those of rheumatoid arthritis clients. Both could not express hostility or anger directly and seemed immature and dependent. Colitis clients generally had mothers who were controlling and had a propensity to assume the role of martyr, much like the mothers of rheumatoid arthritis clients.

Kaplan and Sadock (1998) state, "Most studies show a predominance of compulsive personality traits. Clients with ulcerative colitis are neat, orderly, clean, punctual, hyperintellectual, timid, and inhibited in expressing their anger."

Onset or exacerbation of ulcerative colitis has been associated with stressful life events or psychological trauma. The altered immune status that accompanies psychological stress may be an influencing factor in predisposed individuals.

Transactional Model of Stress/Adaptation

The etiology of psychophysiological disorders is most likely influenced by multiple factors. In Figure 33.1, a graphic depiction of this theory of multiple causation is presented in the transactional model of stress/adaptation.

Diagnosis/Outcome Identification

Nursing diagnoses are formulated from the data gathered during the assessment phase and with background knowledge regarding predisposing factors to the disorder. Some common nursing diagnoses for clients with specific psychophysiological disorders include:

ASTHMA

Ineffective airway clearance
Activity intolerance
Anxiety (severe)

CANCER

Fear
Anticipatory grieving
Body image disturbance

CORONARY HEART DISEASE

Pain
Fear
Activity intolerance

PEPTIC ULCER DISEASE

Pain
Impaired tissue integrity

HYPERTENSION

Risk for altered tissue perfusion
Risk for sexual dysfunction

MIGRAINE HEADACHE

Pain
Altered role performance

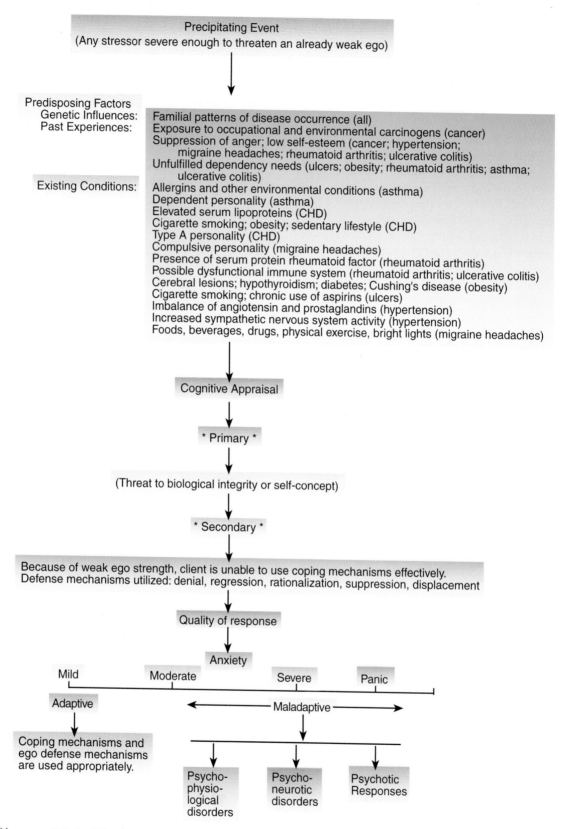

Figure 33.1 The dynamics of psychophysiological disorders using the transactional model of stress/adaptation.

RHEUMATOID ARTHRITIS

Pain

Self-care deficit

Activity intolerance

ULCERATIVE COLITIS

Pain

Diarrhea

Risk for altered nutrition: Less than body requirements

Some nursing diagnoses common to the general category of psychological factors affecting medical condition include:

Ineffective individual coping related to repressed anxiety and inadequate coping methods, evidenced by initiation or exacerbation of physical illness.

Knowledge deficit related to psychological factors affecting medical condition, evidenced by statements such as "I don't know why the doctor put me on the psychiatric unit. I have a physical problem."

Self-esteem disturbance related to unmet dependency needs, evidenced by self-negating verbalizations and demanding sick-role behaviors.

Altered role performance related to physical illness accompanied by real or perceived disabling symptoms, evidenced by changes in usual patterns of responsibility.

The following criteria may be used for measurement of outcomes in the care of the client with a psychophysiological disorder:

THE CLIENT:

1. Denies pain or other physical complaint.
2. Demonstrates the ability to perform more adaptive coping strategies in the face of stressful situations.
3. Verbalizes stressful situations that have led to or worsened physical symptoms in the past.
4. Verbalizes a plan to cope with stressful situations in an effort to prevent exacerbation of physical symptoms.
5. Performs activities of daily living independently.

Planning/Implementation

In Table 33.3, selected nursing diagnoses common to the general category are presented in a plan of care. Nursing diagnoses are included, along with outcome criteria, appropriate nursing interventions, and rationales.

Client/Family Education

The role of client teacher is important in the psychiatric area, as it is in all areas of nursing. A list of topics for client and family education relevant to psychological factors that affect the medical condition is presented in Table 33.4.

Evaluation

Reassessment is conducted to determine if the nursing actions have been successful in achieving the objectives of care. Evaluation of the nursing actions for the client with a psychophysiological disorder may be facilitated by gathering information using the following types of questions.

1. Does the client complain of pain or other physical symptoms?
2. Are the physical symptoms interfering with role responsibilities?
3. Does the client verbalize that physical symptoms have been relieved?
4. Can the client carry out activities of daily living independently?
5. Can the client verbalize alternative coping strategies for dealing with stress?
6. Can the client demonstrate the ability to utilize these more adaptive coping strategies in the face of stress?
7. Does client recognize which types of stressful situations or maladaptive health behaviors exacerbate physical symptoms?
8. Can the client correlate the appearance of the physical symptoms with a stressful situation or maladaptive health behavior?
9. Can the client verbalize unfulfilled needs for which the sick role may be compensating?
10. Can the client verbalize alternative ways to fulfill these needs?
11. Can the client verbalize resources to whom he or she may go when feeling the need for assistance in times of stress?

TREATMENT MODALITIES

Asthma

The goals of medical treatment for clients with asthma are prevention of acute attacks and promotion of normal functioning (Phipps & Brucia, 1995). The most commonly prescribed medications for asthma are bronchodilators and corticosteroids, usually from a metered-dose inhaler. Bronchodilators increase the airway diameter and corticosteroids reduce the inflammatory response.

The most commonly used bronchodilators are the beta-adrenergic agonists (e.g., metaproterenol, albuterol). Theophylline and other methylxanthines are also used, but, because they are usually given orally, they may produce greater side effects than those administered by inhaler.

Corticosteroids, such as prednisone and beclomethasone, may be given by inhaler in doses less than 15 mg/day; higher doses usually require oral administration (Anderson, 1991). Other medications prescribed for asthma include anticholinergics, which inhibit neural

TABLE 33.3 CARE PLAN FOR THE CLIENT WITH A PSYCHOPHYSIOLOGICAL DISORDER

NURSING DIAGNOSIS: INEFFECTIVE INDIVIDUAL COPING
RELATED TO: Repressed anxiety and inadequate coping methods
EVIDENCED BY: Initiation or exacerbation of physical illness

OUTCOME CRITERIA	NURSING INTERVENTIONS	RATIONALE
Client will achieve physical wellness and demonstrate the ability to prevent exacerbation of physical symptoms as a coping mechanism in response to stress.	1. Perform thorough physical assessment.	1. Physical assessment is necessary to determine specific care required for client's physical condition.
	2. Monitor laboratory values, vital signs, intake and output, and other assessments.	2. It is necessary to maintain an accurate ongoing appraisal.
	3. Together with the client, identify goals of care and ways in which client believes he or she can best achieve those goals. Client may need assistance with problem solving.	3. Personal involvement in his or her own care provides a feeling of control and increases chances for positive outcomes.
	4. Encourage client to discuss current life situations that he or she perceives as stressful and the feelings associated with each.	4. Verbalization of true feelings in a nonthreatening environment may help client come to terms with unresolved issues.
	5. During client's discussion, note times during which a sense of powerlessness or loss of control over life situations emerges. Focus on these times and discuss ways in which the client may maintain a feeling of control.	5. A sense of self-worth develops and is maintained when an individual feels power over his or her own life situations.
	6. As client becomes able to discuss feelings more openly, assist him or her in a nonthreatening manner to relate certain feelings to the appearance of physical symptoms.	6. Client may be unaware of the relationship between physical symptoms and emotional problems.
	7. Discuss stressful times when physical symptoms did not appear and the adaptive coping strategies that were used during those situations. Therapy is facilitated by considering areas of strength and using them to the client's benefit. Provide positive reinforcement for adaptive coping mechanisms identified or used. Suggest alternative coping strategies but allow client to determine which can most appropriately be incorporated into his or her lifestyle.	7. Positive reinforcement enhances self-esteem and encourages repetition of desired behaviors. Client may require assistance with problem solving but must be allowed and encouraged to make decisions independently.
	8. Help client to identify a resource within the community (friend, significant other, group) to use as a support system for the expression of feelings.	8. A positive support system may help to prevent maladaptive coping through physical illness.

NURSING DIAGNOSIS: KNOWLEDGE DEFICIT
RELATED TO: Psychological factors affecting medical condition
EVIDENCED BY: Statements such as "I don't know why the doctor put me on the psychiatric unit. I have a physical problem."

OUTCOME CRITERIA	NURSING INTERVENTIONS	RATIONALE
Client will be able to verbalize psychological factors affecting his or her physical condition.	1. Assess client's level of knowledge regarding effects of psychological problems on the body.	1. An adequate database is necessary for the development of an effective teaching plan.

2. Assess client's level of anxiety and readiness to learn.
3. Discuss physical examinations and laboratory tests that have been conducted. Explain purpose and results of each.
4. Explore feelings and fears held by client. Go slowly. These feelings may have been suppressed or repressed for so long that their disclosure may be a very painful experience. Be supportive.
5. Have client keep a diary of appearance, duration, and intensity of physical symptoms. A separate record of situations that the client finds especially stressful should also be kept.
6. Help client identify needs that are being met through the sick role. Together, formulate more adaptive means for fulfilling these needs. Practice by role-playing.
7. Provide instruction in assertiveness techniques, especially the ability to recognize the differences among passive, assertive, and aggressive behaviors and the importance of respecting the rights of others while protecting one's own basic rights.
8. Discuss adaptive methods of stress management, such as relaxation techniques, physical exercise, meditation, breathing exercises, and autogenics.

2. Learning does not occur beyond the moderate level of anxiety.
3. Client has the right to know about and accept or refuse any medical treatment.
4. Expression of feelings in the presence of a trusted individual and in a nonthreatening environment may encourage the individual to confront unresolved feelings.
5. Comparison of these records may provide objective data from which to observe the relationship between physical symptoms and stress.
6. Repetition through practice serves to reduce discomfort in the actual situation.
7. These skills will preserve client's self-esteem while also improving his or her ability to form satisfactory interpersonal relationships.
8. Use of these adaptive techniques may decrease appearance of physical symptoms in response to stress.

reflex effects that contribute to bronchoconstriction, and cromolyn sodium, which occupies a position on the mast cell and prevents release of the chemicals that stimulate bronchospasm and promote inflammation.

Some clients with asthma may be candidates for short-term or long-term psychotherapy. The internist or family physician maintains care of the physical component of the client's illness, whereas the psychotherapist focuses on attitudes and emotions, fears of confiding and rejection, and struggles between attachment and independence (Vachon, 1989). The psychological aspects are kept separate from the physical aspects of the illness so that the therapeutic relationship is not destroyed if the client suffers an asthmatic attack during psychotherapy. Exacerbations during the treatment offer both the therapist and the client an opportunity to become aware of the psychological context in which they occur. They then may be able to understand the emotional factors involved and, hopefully, to modify them.

Cancer

Surgery is perhaps the oldest method used to control or cure cancer. Surgical procedures can be used to diagnose

malignancy (e.g., biopsy), to cure malignancies (e.g., mastectomy, hysterectomy), for rehabilitation measures (e.g., breast reconstruction), and for various other purposes of improving quality of life for cancer clients when a cure is impossible (e.g., palliative and supportive measures).

Radiation therapy is the use of high-energy ionizing emissions from a radioactive source to eradicate malignant tumors with as little damage to normal tissues as possible (Wheeler, 1991). It can be used singly or in combination with other forms of treatment to achieve maximum tumor control. It is also used as a palliative measure to control the pain of bone metastasis in clients with advanced neoplastic disease.

Chemotherapy is the administration of antineoplastic drugs, in a systemic or regional manner, to cure or control a malignancy (Wheeler, 1991). These drugs can cure certain cancers. When a cure is not possible, they may be given for palliative measures, to control symptoms, or to extend the client's useful life. They are often given in combination with other therapies, such as surgery or radiation therapy. Most chemotherapeutic agents have significant adverse effects (e.g., bone marrow depression, severe nausea and vomiting, alopecia), which should be measured against the potential benefits when outlining a course of treatment for a cancer client.

Table 33.4 Topics for Client/Family Education Related to Psychological Factors Affecting Medical Condition

Nature of the Illness
1. Provide information to the client about specific disease process:
   a. Asthma
   b. Cancer
   c. Coronary heart disease
   d. Peptic ulcer
   e. Essential hypertension
   f. Migraine headache
   g. Rheumatoid arthritis
   h. Ulcerative colitis
   i. Other
2. Discuss psychological implications of exacerbation or delayed healing.

Management of the Illness
1. Discuss ways to identify onset of escalating anxiety.
2. Discuss ways to interrupt escalating anxiety.
   a. Assertive techniques
   b. Relaxation techniques
   c. Physical activities
   d. Talking with trusted individual
   e. Meditation
3. Discuss pain management.
4. Discuss how family can prevent reinforcing the illness.
5. Pharmacology
   a. Discuss why physician has prescribed certain medications.
   b. Discuss possible side effects of medications.
   c. Provide printed information about what symptoms to report to physician.
6. Discuss medical treatment modalities of the illness.
7. Discuss possible lifestyle changes related to the illness.

Support Services
1. Support groups
2. Individual psychotherapy
3. Biofeedback

In consideration of the psychosomatic dimensions of cancer, Simonton and Simonton (1975) reported positive results with autogenic relaxation and mental imagery in the role of adjunct therapy for clients with malignant disease. Once relaxation has been achieved, the individual is taught to visualize the malignancy within his or her body. Then the person visualizes a killer attack (from his or her own fantasy) on the malignant cells, followed by a visualization of the army of white cells transporting the dead cancer cells out of the body. The Simontons have had convincing results with this technique, particularly in clients who maintain a positive attitude about therapy. They strongly emphasize a high correlation between positive response to treatment and positive attitudes, both to the disease and to life in a more general sense. They also emphasize that the application of relaxation and visualization techniques is an *adjunct* to traditional treatment, not an *alternative*.

Psychotherapy may help those possibly cancer-prone individuals with type C personality characteristics. The individual must begin by searching for and finding the "lost self." He or she must learn to express the feelings and emotions that have been suppressed. Overcoming some of the characteristics associated with type C personality may have the potential of diminishing the risk of developing cancer, as well as facilitating recovery from the disease. It is thought that immune responses are enhanced when the individual perceives a greater feeling of well-being through the attainment of a more positive sense of self-control (Hafen et al., 1996).

Coronary Heart Disease

Abraham (1995) discusses several therapies in the treatment of CHD. Surgical intervention with coronary artery bypass grafting (CABG) is indicated for clients with significant obstruction of the major coronary arteries. It provides symptomatic relief in 85 to 90 percent of cases (Massie, 1996).

Percutaneous transluminal coronary angioplasty (PTCA) is a technique that does not alter the general disease process but is an alternative approach to CABG. PTCA attempts to restore patency of the arterial lumen by compressing atheromatous plaques.

Chemotherapeutic agents used in the treatment of CHD include:

1. Vasodilators: to increase coronary tissue perfusion (e.g., nitroglycerin, isosorbide).
2. Beta-adrenergic blocking agents: to treat angina and hypertension (e.g., propranolol, atenolol).
3. Calcium antagonists: to treat angina and hypertension (e.g., verapamil, nifedipine, diltiazem).
4. Antihyperlipidemic agents: to lower serum cholesterol and triglyceride levels (e.g., clofibrate, gemfibrozil, pravachol).

Various techniques, such as progressive relaxation, autohypnosis, meditation, biofeedback, and group therapy, have been tried in an attempt to modify the type A behavior pattern associated with CHD. Vaughn (1987) reports on a study by Friedman and Rosenman that began in 1978 at San Francisco's Mt. Zion Hospital and Medical Center. From this research project, they have devised a therapeutic program designed to reduce type A behavior. Combining education of the client with individualized counseling and behavior modification therapy, they were able to reduce type A behavior in a significant number of the experimental subjects. The recurrence rate of nonfatal MI was half that of the control subjects who received the educational program but did not participate in the behavior modification therapy. Hafen and associates, (1996) report that eighteen controlled studies have now shown that the toxic, hostile parts of type A (and even the excessive busyness) can indeed be transformed into safer behaviors.

Peptic Ulcer

The focus of treatment for peptic ulcer disease is to alleviate symptoms, promote healing, and prevent complications and recurrence (Simmons & Heitkemper, 1991).

Pharmacological interventions include:

1. Antacids: to neutralize gastric acid (e.g., calcium carbonate, magnesium/aluminum salts).
2. Antisecretory agents: to inhibit secretion of hydrochloric acid (HCl) in the stomach.
   a. Histamine H_2 antagonists (e.g., cimetidine, ranitidine).
   b. Anticholinergics (e.g., atropine, belladona, propantheline).
3. Cytoprotective agents: to coat ulcerated mucosal tissue and inhibit pepsin activity (e.g., sucralfate).
4. Gastric acid-pump inhibitor: decreases gastric acidity by interrupting the flow of hydrogen ions (e.g., omeprazole).
5. Antibiotics and anti-infectives: treatment of *H. pylori* infection (e.g., amoxicillin; tetracycline; metronidazole).

The selection of foods in dietary intervention is determined by client tolerance. The traditional bland diet with emphasis on dairy products has become controversial. Spicy foods do, however, cause dyspepsia in some individuals. A reduction or elimination of caffeine and alcohol is recommended. Smoking and the intake of aspirin should be avoided.

Surgical intervention may be necessary if medical management does not result in symptomatic relief, when serious, life-threatening complications occur, or when there is possible malignancy (Simmons & Heitkemper, 1991). The most common types of surgical intervention include gastrectomy (removal of a portion of the stomach), vagotomy (severing the vagus nerve to reduce vagally stimulated HCl), and pyloroplasty (repairing or reopening of the pylorus to enhance gastric emptying).

Psychotherapy with ulcer clients whose personality characteristics, ego strength, and coping mechanisms favor increased vulnerability to stress has been described as beneficial (Lipsitt, 1989). Troublesome conflicts that have been associated with peptic ulcer disease, such as passivity, dependency, aggression, anger, and frustration, need to be evaluated and properly addressed in treatment, respecting the client's defensive structure and need for support and reassurance. Various studies have been conducted with peptic ulcer clients (Lipsitt, 1989). The experimental groups received medication along with psychotherapy, whereas the control groups received medication alone. Results were significant for the experimental groups, who showed consistent and continuing improvement, while recurrence and complications were common among members of the control groups. Lipsitt (1989) states:

> "Cumulative evidence to date of the efficacy of psychotherapy [in the treatment of peptic ulcer disease] is that psychotherapy, even for brief periods of time, offers more lasting benefits in social adjustment and symptom reduction than symptomatic medical treatment alone, measured by recurrences and complications."

Essential Hypertension

The treatment of clients with hypertension is directed toward lowering blood pressure in an attempt to halt or reverse progressive organ damage. Some individuals can lower their blood pressure by altering their lifestyle. If the individual is unable or unwilling to do so, pharmacological therapy is recommended. Many individuals are treated with a combination of both approaches.

Dietary Modifications

Two effective nonpharmacological modalities for the reduction of elevated blood pressure are weight reduction and sodium restriction. It may also be necessary for the individual who is on diuretic therapy to ensure that there is a sufficient intake of potassium, either through diet or with supplements. It is also important for the individual with high blood pressure to decrease intake of caffeine, alcohol, and saturated fats.

Environmental Factors

Individuals with hypertension should not smoke.

Physical Exercise

Increased physical activity (e.g., aerobic-type exercise for 30 minutes two to three times a week) has been shown to lower blood pressure in some hypertensive individuals, and it is thought to be a good preventive measure for individuals at risk for cardiovascular disease because of hypertension (Porth, 1994). Caution with isotonic exercises, such as weight lifting, is advised for hypertensive individuals, as an acute rise in blood pressure can occur.

Pharmacotherapy

Physicians usually take a "stepped-care" approach to prescribing antihypertensive medications. If weight control, dietary restrictions, and physical exercise are not sufficient to maintain a lowered pressure, the first step of pharmacological intervention is usually with a low dose of a diuretic, beta blocker, calcium channel blocker, or angiotensin-converting enzyme inhibitor. If these medications are not successful in lowering the pressure, either the dosage is increased or a second drug of a different classification is substituted or added. This continues until the desired blood pressure is achieved, side effects become intolerable, or the maximum amount of each drug has been reached (Walsh, 1995).

Relaxation Techniques

Relaxation techniques, such as meditation, yoga, hypnosis, and biofeedback reduce blood pressure in some individuals. They are especially useful for individuals with higher initial pressures and as adjunctive therapy to pharmacological treatment. Supportive psychotherapy, during which the individual is encouraged to express honest feelings, particularly anger, may also be helpful.

Migraine Headache

Pharmacological intervention for migraine headache is directed toward prevention with drugs such as propranolol, amitriptyline, fluoxetine, verapamil, or divalproex sodium. Once a migraine attack has begun, some physicians administer injection of a narcotic, such as meperidine or codeine, which blocks the pain and allows the individual to sleep until the attack subsides. A relatively new class of drugs, the seratonin agonists (sumatriptan and zolmitriptan), which are available in oral, injectable, and inhalant forms, has been shown to be effective in interrupting migraine attacks.

Other treatments during a migraine attack that may provide some relief include cold compresses to the head and neck; bedrest in a quiet, darkened room; application of pressure to the temples; and perhaps heat to neck and shoulder muscles that have contracted in response to headache pain.

Some medications are prescribed to be taken at the first sign of onset of a migraine attack. If taken in the prodromal phase at the very first sign, ergotamine tartrate may prevent the vasodilation that creates the pain of migraine. It is ineffective once the attack has begun. Ergotamine is available in combination with other drugs, such as caffeine, sedatives, and antiemetics, and is marketed in various forms, including tablets, suppositories, inhalants, and sublinquals. Ergotamine can safely be taken only once or twice a week at the most, so it is not appropriate for individuals who have headaches more often than this. It can be very harmful because of its vasoconstrictive properties and potential for preventing adequate tissue perfusion.

Robbins and Lang (1995) suggest the following nonpharmacological interventions to help a client prevent migraine attacks:

1. Discontinue or avoid any circumstances, events, foods, over-the-counter medications, or beverages that could have precipitated an attack.
2. If headaches seem related to the use of oral contraceptives or other prescription medications, discuss this with the physician. No medication should be discontinued without first consulting with the physician.
3. Learn relaxation techniques. Ensure that at least half an hour is set aside for relaxation exercises to reduce stress. Use of these exercises may help prevent poststress headaches.
4. Regularly participate in enjoyable hobbies and relaxing activities.
5. Regular physical exercise is advisable, unless it has been known to provoke migraine attacks.
6. It is best to obtain the same amount of sleep each night. Do not oversleep or go without sleep.
7. Biofeedback, behavior modification, yoga, or meditation appear to be worthwhile in some cases of migraine.
8. Migraine may be related to repressed or suppressed anger, hostility, and guilt. Honest expression of these feelings may remove some of the emotional predisposition to the disorder. Psychotherapy may be necessary in some instances, both to help relieve unre-

solved anger and to help modify some of the characteristics associated with "migraine personality."

9. Some individuals report relief from migraines after they quit smoking. It is possible that the products of combustion may play a role in dilating arteries.

Rheumatoid Arthritis

The goals of therapy for rheumatoid arthritis are to relieve discomfort and achieve remission. Treatment depends on the extent of the disability, psychosocial variables, and the results of laboratory examinations.

Pharmacological Treatment

Aspirin is the cornerstone of drug therapy for the client with rheumatoid arthritis. In large doses, it has potent anti-inflammatory action, as well as analgesic and antipyretic actions. Up to 4 g/day is prescribed for the client with rheumatoid arthritis. (Kaplan & Sadock, 1998). Diazepam may also be prescribed as a muscle relaxant and for anxiety.

Nonsteroidal anti-inflammatory agents (e.g., ibuprofen, fenoprofen, naproxen, sulindac) are used with clients for whom salicylate therapy is ineffective or inappropriate. Persistent articular inflammation may be treated with antirheumatic agents (e.g., gold, penicillamine, hydroxychloroquine sulfate). Corticosteroids (e.g., prednisone, prednisolone, hydrocortisone) dramatically alleviate pain and inflammation but are not often used because of their numerous adverse side effects. Antineoplastic agents (e.g., azathioprine, cyclophosphamide, methotrexate, sulfasalazine) have afforded some relief to clients with particularly severe and resistant forms of the disease (Cicero, 1991).

Surgical Treatment

Various surgical treatments are available for clients with rheumatoid arthritis. Synovectomy is performed to relieve pain and maintain muscle and joint balance. Joint fusion may provide stability to a joint and decrease deformity. Spinal fusion may be necessary to treat subluxation. Total joint replacements are considered for clients with severe deformities, significant functional disabilities, or poorly controlled pain (Cicero, 1991).

Psychological Treatment

Psychotherapy and prompt recognition and treatment of psychiatric morbidity help clients cope and adapt to this condition (Ananth, 1989). A client's initial reaction to the diagnosis of rheumatoid arthritis depends on the degree of incapacity at the time and the immediate threat to his or her lifestyle. Denial of the illness is a common initial response. Over time, a number of adaptive processes, including resignation, episodic anger, sadness, and anxiety, may occur (Ananth, 1989). Clients may blame themselves or believe that the disease is the result of past behaviors. Depression may need to be treated separately. Clients should be encouraged to function as independently as possible. The focus on cure should be deflected to a focus on control of the disease and prevention of disability.

Ulcerative Colitis

The goals of care for the client with ulcerative colitis are to relieve discomfort and promote and maintain remission of the disease. This is accomplished through nutritional therapy, pharmacological treatment, surgical intervention if necessary, and psychological support.

Nutritional Therapy

There are no general restrictions on diet. Clients should avoid foods that they identify as irritating. Usually a low-residue diet is initiated and advanced as tolerated with one food added at a time. Milk may be a problem for some clients. When the disease is severe or extensive, and absorption problems have resulted in dehydration and cachexia, total parenteral nutrition may be necessary.

Pharmacological Treatment

Sulfasalazine is the most commonly prescribed medication for inflammatory bowel disease (Sands, 1995b). It appears to have both anti-inflammatory and antimicrobial properties. Severe forms of the disease are treated with corticosteroids (e.g., hydrocortisone, prednisone, prednisolone). Corticosteroids provide relief through suppression of inflammation but do not cure ulcerative colitis. To provide symptomatic relief, antidiarrheals (e.g., loperamide, diphenoxylate) and antispasmodics (e.g., propantheline) may be prescribed. Antibiotics (e.g., metronidazole) may be administered when infectious diarrhea in present (Sands, 1995b).

Surgical Treatment

Surgery is indicated for the client with ulcerative colitis intractable to medical management or when complications such as persistent hemorrhage, perforation or strictures of the colon, or toxic megacolon are present (Sands, 1995b). Types of surgery that may be performed include proctocolectomy with permanent or continent ileostomy, total colectomy with ileorectal anastomosis, or total colectomy with ileoanal reservoir. Surgery is considered curative, and recurrences are few (Sands, 1995b).

Psychological Support

Ulcerative colitis can be a lifetime illness with periods of exacerbation and remission that can disrupt the person's life situation. Because emotions and stress have been known to play a role in exacerbation of the illness, psychological support may help to decrease the frequency of these attacks by helping the individual to recognize the stressors that precipitate exacerbations and identify more adaptive ways of coping. The person with ulcerative colitis often feels a lack of control over his or her life. Psychological support may help the client cope with feelings of insecurity, dependency, and depression. It is extremely important that the individual express feelings of repressed or suppressed anger and hostility.

Fears and anxieties associated with possible sexual dysfunction need to be explored. The individual who has undergone surgical intervention for ulcerative colitis may be

---

TEST YOUR CRITICAL THINKING SKILLS

Melinda, age 32, describes herself to the nurse on the stress-management unit as "a high achiever who has always been success oriented." She is the only child of parents who are both attorneys, and who encouraged her to strive for whatever in life she wanted to be. As a child, she observed her parents typically working 60 to 70 hours per week. She decided early in life that she wanted to be the president of a big corporation. It was with this goal in mind that she entered college and, with top grades, was accepted to the Harvard MBA program. She was determined to graduate at the top of her class and, in pursuing this end, she developed a duodenal ulcer. She was treated by an internist in the local area during intermittent flare-ups and continued on to fulfill her goal. After graduation, she landed a prime position with a large corporation in New York City. She worked long hours, socialized very little (except for business purposes), and received regular promotions that moved her up the corporate ladder. After 6 years, the job of executive vice president became available. She was in the prime position to move into the position, and everyone she spoke with told her they were sure she would. However, when the position was filled, a young man 2 years her junior got the job. She was furious, and immediately engaged an attorney to take her case of sexual discrimination. The case has been going on for 8 months, and although she is continuing to work on her job while the lawsuit is being conducted, she is uncomfortable and feels rejected by her coworkers and by the administration. Her ulcer has been acting up for several months, and she complains of "constant pain." Her family physician suggested she enroll in the stress-management program.

Answer the following questions related to Melinda:

1. What would be the priority nursing diagnosis for Melinda?
2. Describe some primary nursing interventions for Melinda.
3. What would be the long-term goal for Melinda?

RESEARCH NOTE

Depression is a risk factor for coronary artery disease in men: The precursors study. *Archives of Internal Medicine* **(1998, July 13), 158, 1422–1426.**

Ford, D.E., Mead, L.A., Chang, P.P., Cooper-Patrick, L., Wang, N.Y., and Klag, M.J.

Description of the Study: This study was conducted to determine if clinical depression is an independent risk factor for coronary artery disease. The subjects included 1190 male Johns Hopkins medical students enrolled between 1948 and 1964. The subjects were followed through 1995 and assessed on family history, health behaviors, and clinical depression. At baseline, the subjects showed no significant differences in the prevalence of known cardiac risk factors. Follow-up studies for cardiovascular disease were assessed with reviews of annual questionnaires, National Death Index searches, medical records, death certificates, and autopsy reports.

Results of the Study: The cumulative incidence of clinical depression in the medical students at 40 years of follow-up (assessed by self-reported symptoms, diagnoses, and treatments) was 12 percent. Multivariate analyses indicated that the men who reported clinical depression were twice as likely to develop coronary heart disease or suffer a myocardial infarction (MI) than the nondepressed men. The increased risk for MI was shown to persist for up to 10 years after onset of the first depressive episode.

Comments: The authors state that several studies have found depression to be an important predictor of poor outcome after the onset of coronary artery disease. This study finds that clinical depression may be an independent risk factor for coronary artery disease. The actual mechanism by which this occurs is speculative. It has been suggested that changes in the autonomic nervous system and increased platelet reactivity that occurs in clinical depression may play a role. The results of this study provide justification for consideration of clinical depression in the prevention and treatment of coronary artery disease in men.

---

experiencing a body image disturbance that could interfere with sexual functioning. The person must be given the opportunity to discuss these sexual concerns. He or she may require assistance in communicating these concerns to the sexual partner. Alternate ways of meeting sexuality needs can be explored.

SUMMARY

Psychophysiological disorders are those in which psychological factors contribute to the initiation or exacerbation of the physical condition. There is evidence of either demonstrable organic pathology or a known pathophysiological process involved. The *DSM-IV* (APA, 1994) identifies this category as "psychological factors affecting medical condition." Types of psychological factors identified by the *DSM-IV* include mental disorders, psycho-

INTERNET REFERENCES

- Additional information about psychophysiological disorders discussed in this chapter may be located at the following websites:
  a. http://www.nci.nih.gov
  b. http://www.cancer.org
  c. http://www.amhrt.org/
  d. http://www.headaches.org/
  e. http://www.pslgroup.com/ASTHMA.HTM
  f. http://www.pharminfo.com/disease/immun/asthma/asthma_info.html
  g. http://www.gastro.org/adhf/ulcers.html
  h. http://www.pslgroup.com/HYPERTENSION.HTM
  i. http://www.pharminfo.com/disease/ra/ra-site.html
  j. http://www.mediconsult.com/ibd/shareware/colitis/contents.html

logical symptoms, personality traits or coping styles, maladaptive health behaviors, stress-related physiological responses, and others.

Virtually any organic disorder can be considered psychophysiological. The following disorders were discussed in this chapter:

- Asthma
- Cancer
- Coronary heart disease
- Peptic ulcer disease
- Essential hypertension
- Migraine headache
- Rheumatoid arthritis
- Ulcerative colitis

Psychophysiological disorders are thought to occur when the body remains in a prolonged state of moderate-to-severe anxiety. This prolonged period of arousal may contribute to the initiation or exacerbation of the physical symptoms in otherwise predisposed individuals.

Predisposing factors to the development of psychophysiological disorders include heredity, allergies, environmental conditions, viruses, elevated serum lipoproteins, cigarette smoking, alcohol abuse, specific foods, and dysfunctional immune system. The following personality characteristics have also been implicated in the predisposition to psychophysiological disorders:

- Asthma: unfulfilled dependency needs.
- Cancer: repressed anger and low self-esteem (type C personality).
- Coronary heart disease: competitive drive and continual sense of time urgency (type A personality).
- Peptic ulcer: unfulfilled dependency needs.
- Hypertension: repressed anger.
- Migraine headache: repressed anger, perfectionism.
- Rheumatoid arthritis: repressed anger, self-sacrificing traits.
- Ulcerative colitis: repressed anger, dependency.

Nursing care of the client with psychophysiological disorders is accomplished using the steps of the nursing process. Background assessment data were presented, along with nursing diagnoses common to each disorder and to the general psychophysiological condition. Interventions appropriate to each general nursing diagnosis and relevant outcome criteria for each were included. An overview of current medical treatment modalities for each disorder was discussed.

Nurses in all areas of clinical practice should be aware of client potential for psychophysiological responses and the possible psychosocial influences associated with these disorders. Nurses will most likely (at least initially) encounter these clients in areas other than psychiatry.

REVIEW QUESTIONS

SELF-EXAMINATION/LEARNING EXERCISE

Match the following psychophysiological disorders to the psychosocial profile with which it has been associated:

_____ 1. Asthma

_____ 2. Cancer

_____ 3. Coronary heart disease

_____ 4. Peptic ulcer disease

_____ 5. Essential hypertension

_____ 6. Migraine headache

_____ 7. Rheumatoid arthritis

_____ 8. Ulcerative colitis

a. Competitive; aggressive; ambitious; no time for leisure; never satisfied with accomplishments; easily aroused hostility.

b. Obsessive-compulsive by nature; anxious; rigid; excessively neat; repressed anger; depression is common.

c. Unfulfilled dependency needs; views separation from significant other as abandonment or rejection.

d. Self-sacrificing; inhibited; perfectionistic; repressed anger; depression is common.

e. Unfulfilled dependency needs; suppressed anxiety; resentment and frustration resulting in increased gastric secretion.

f. Perfectionistic; somewhat rigid; compulsive; sets unrealistic expectations; suppresses or represses anger.

g. "The nice guy"; suppresses anger; low self-esteem; depression is common; feelings of hopelessness.

h. Suppresses anger; longs for approval from others; stems from childhood fears of loss of love if showed anger toward parents.

9. Which of the following is the primary nursing diagnosis for clients in the general category of psychophysiological disorders?
   a. Pain, evidenced by classic pain behaviors.
   b. Ineffective individual coping, evidenced by exacerbation of physical symptoms.
   c. Altered role performance, evidenced by inability to perform usual responsibilities.
   d. Activity intolerance, evidenced by inability to participate in activities.

REFERENCES

Abraham, T. (1995). Management of persons with dysrhythmias and coronary artery disease. In W.J. Phipps, V.L. Cassmeyer, J.K. Sands, & M.K. Lehman (Eds.), *Medical-surgical nursing: Concepts and clinical practice.* St. Louis: Mosby.

American Heart Association. (1999). Blood pressure statistics. [On-line]. Available: http://www.amhrt.org

American Psychiatric Association. (1994). *Diagnostic and statistical manual of mental disorders* (4th ed.). Washington, DC: American Psychiatric Association.

Ananth, J. (1989). Rheumatoid arthritis. In H.I. Kaplan & B.J. Sadock (Eds.), *Comprehensive textbook of psychiatry* (5th ed.). Baltimore: Williams & Wilkins.

Anderson, K.L. (1991). Obstructive respiratory disorders. In M.L. Patrick et al. (Eds.), *Medical-surgical nursing* (2nd ed.). Philadelphia: J.B. Lippincott.

Cicero, T.F. (1991). Musculoskeletal inflammation and connective tissue disorders. In M.L. Patrick et al. (Eds.), *Medical-surgical nursing* (2nd ed.). Philadelphia: J.B. Lippincott.

Cunningham, S.L. (1991). Hypertension. In M.L. Patrick et al. (Eds.), *Medical-surgical nursing* (2nd ed.). Philadelphia: J.B. Lippincott.

Deters, G.E. (1995). Cancer. In W.J. Phipps, V.L. Cassmeyer, J.K. Sands, & M.K. Lehman (Eds.), *Medical-surgical nursing* (5th ed.). St. Louis: Mosby.

Engel, G.L. (1955). Studies in ulcerative colitis: The nature of the psychologic process. *American Journal of Medicine, 19,* 231.

Friedman, M., & Rosenman, R.H. (1974). *Type A behavior and your heart.* New York: Alfred A. Knopf.

Hackett, T.P., Rosenbaum, J.F., & Cassem, N.H. (1989). Cardiovascular disorders. In H.I. Kaplan & B.J. Sadock (Eds.), *Comprehensive textbook of psychiatry* (5th ed.). Baltimore: Williams & Wilkins.

Hafen, B.Q., Karren, K.J., Frandsen, K.J., & Smith, N.L. (1996). *Mind/body health: The effects of attitudes, emotions, and relationships.* Boston: Allyn & Bacon.

Heitkemper, M., & Martin, D.L. (1991). Infectious and inflammatory gastrointestinal disorders. In M.L. Patrick et al. (Eds.), *Medical-surgical nursing* (2nd ed.). Philadelphia: J.B. Lippincott.

Kaplan, H.I. (1989). History of psychosomatic medicine. In H.I. Kaplan & B.J. Sadock (Eds.), *Comprehensive textbook of psychiatry* (5th ed.). Baltimore: Williams & Wilkins.

Kaplan, H.I., & Sadock, B.J. (1985). *Modern synopsis of comprehensive textbook of psychiatry* (4th ed.). Baltimore: Williams & Wilkins.

Kaplan, H.I., & Sadock, B.J. (1998). *Synopsis of psychiatry: Behavioral sciences/clinical psychiatry* (8th ed.). Baltimore: Williams & Wilkins.

LeShan, L. (1977). *You can fight for your life.* New York: M. Evans.

LeShan, L. (1966). An emotional life-history pattern associated with neoplastic disease. *Annals of the New York Academy of Sciences, 3,* 780–793.

Lipsitt, D.R. (1989). Gastrointestinal disorders. In H.I. Kaplan & B.J. Sadock (Eds.), *Comprehensive textbook of psychiatry* (5th ed.). Baltimore: Williams & Wilkins.

Marek, J.F., Buergin, P.S., & Paskert, K.M. (1995). Management of persons with inflammatory and degenerative disorders of the musculoskeletal system. In W.J. Phipps, V.L. Cassmeyer, J.K. Sands, & M.K. Lehman (Eds.), *Medical-surgical nursing* (5th ed.). St. Louis: Mosby.

Massie, B.M. (1996). Heart. In L.M. Tierney Jr., S.J. McPhee, & M.A. Papadakis (Eds.), *Current medical diagnosis and treatment* (35th ed.). Stamford, CT: Appleton & Lange.

National Cancer Institute. (1999a). U.S. cancer death rate 1973–1995: All races, both sexes. [On-line]. Available: http://rex.nci.nih.gov/massmedia/pressreleases/GRAPHS3_12/graphs.html#anchor6498467.

National Cancer Institute. (1999b). What are some common symptoms of cancer? [On-line]. Available: http://cis.nci.nih.gov/contact/symptoms.html

Pelletier, K.R. (1992). *Mind as healer, mind as slayer*. New York: Dell.

Peplau, H. (1963). A working definition of anxiety. In S. Burd & M. Marshall (Eds.), *Some clinical approaches to psychiatric nursing*. New York: Macmillan.

Phipps, W.J., & Brucia, J.J. (1995). Management of persons with problems of the lower airway. In W.J. Phipps, V.L. Cassmeyer, J.K. Sands, & M.K. Lehman (Eds.), *Medical-surgical nursing: Concepts and clinical practice* (5th. ed.). St. Louis: Mosby.

Porth, C.M. (1994). *Pathophysiology: Concepts of altered health states* (4th ed.). Philadelphia: J.B. Lippincott.

Robbins L., & Lang, S.S. (1995). *Headache help*. Boston: Houghton Mifflin.

Roseman, R.H., et al. (1975). Coronary heart disease in the western collaborative group study: Final follow-up experience of eight-and-one-half years. *JAMA, 8*, 233.

Sands, J.K. (1995a). Management of persons with problems of the stomach and duodenum. In W.J. Phipps, V.L. Cassmeyer, J.K. Sands, & M.K. Lehman (Eds.), *Medical-surgical nursing* (5th ed.). St. Louis: Mosby.

Sands, J.K. (1995b). Management of persons with problems of the intestines. In W.J. Phipps, V.L. Cassmeyer, J.K. Sands, & M.K. Lehman (Eds.), *Medical-surgical nursing* (5th ed.). St. Louis: Mosby.

Schenk, E. (1995). Management of persons with problems of the brain. In W. J. Phipps, V.L. Cassmeyer, J.K. Sands, & M.K. Lehman (Eds.), *Medical-surgical nursing* (5th ed.). St. Louis: Mosby.

Selye, H. (1976). *The stress of life*. New York: McGraw-Hill.

Simmons, L.M., & Heitkemper, M. (1991). Ulcers of the gastrointestinal tract. In M.L. Patrick et al. (Eds.), *Medical-surgical nursing* (2nd ed.). Philadelphia: J.B. Lippincott.

Simonton, O.C., & Simonton, S. (1975). Belief systems and management of the emotional aspects of malignancy. *Journal of Transpersonal Psychology, 7*(1), 29–48.

Sobel, D.S., & Ornstein, R. (1996). *The healthy mind healthy body handbook*. New York: Patient Education Media.

Vachon, L. (1989). Respiratory disorders. In H.I. Kaplan & B.J. Sadock (Eds.), *Comprehensive textbook of psychiatry* (5th ed.). Baltimore: Williams & Wilkins.

Vaughn, L. (1987, August). Smile your way to a longer life. *Prevention*, 87–94.

Walsh, M.E. (1995). Management of persons with vascular problems. In W.J. Phipps, V.L. Cassmeyer, J.K. Sands, & M.K. Lehman (Eds.), *Medical-surgical nursing* (5th ed.). St. Louis: Mosby.

Wheeler, V. (1991). Cancer therapy and principles of nursing management. In M.L. Patrick et al. (Eds.), *Medical-surgical nursing* (2nd ed.). Philadelphia: J.B. Lippincott.

Woods, S.L., Underhill, S.L., & Cowan, M. (1991). Coronary heart disease: Myocardial ischemia and infarction. In M.L. Patrick et al. (Eds.), *Medical-surgical nursing* (2nd ed.). Philadelphia: J.B. Lippincott.

34
C H A P T E R

PERSONALITY DISORDERS

CHAPTER OUTLINE

OBJECTIVES

INTRODUCTION

HISTORICAL ASPECTS

TYPES OF PERSONALITY DISORDERS

APPLICATION OF THE NURSING PROCESS

TREATMENT MODALITIES

SUMMARY

REVIEW QUESTIONS

KEY TERMS

personality
schizoid
schizotypal

histrionic
narcissism
passive-aggressive

splitting
object constancy

OBJECTIVES

After reading this chapter, the student will be able to:

1. Define *personality.*
2. Compare stages of personality development according to Sullivan, Erikson, and Mahler.
3. Identify various types of personality disorders.
4. Discuss historical and epidemiological statistics related to various personality disorders.
5. Describe symptomatology associated with borderline personality disorder and antisocial personality disorder, and use these data in client assessment.
6. Identify predisposing factors to borderline personality disorder and antisocial personality disorder.

7. Formulate nursing diagnoses and goals of care for clients with borderline personality disorder and antisocial personality disorder.
8. Describe appropriate nursing interventions for behaviors associated with borderline personality disorder and antisocial personality disorder.
9. Evaluate nursing care of clients with borderline personality disorder and antisocial personality disorder.
10. Discuss various modalities relevant to treatment of personality disorder.

he word **"personality"** is derived from the Greek term *persona*. It was used originally to describe the theatrical mask worn by some dramatic actors at the time. Over the years, it lost its connotation of pretense and illusion and came to represent the person behind the mask—the "real" person. Kaplan and Sadock (1998) define personality as:

"a person's characteristic totality of emotional and behavioral traits apparent in ordinary life, a totality that is usually stable and predictable." (p. 775)

The *DSM-IV* (American Psychiatric Association [APA], 1994) defines personality *traits* as "enduring patterns of perceiving, relating to, and thinking about the environment and oneself that are exhibited in a wide range of social and personal contexts." Personality *disorders* occur when these traits become inflexible and maladaptive and cause either significant functional impairment or subjective distress. These disorders are coded on axis II of the multiaxial diagnostic system used by the APA (see Chapter 2 for an explanation of this system). Virtually all individuals exhibit some behaviors associated with the various personality disorders from time to time. It is only when significant functional impairment occurs in response to these personality characteristics that the individual is thought to have a personality disorder.

Personality development occurs in response to a number of biological and psychological influences. These variables include (but are not limited to) heredity, temperament, experiential learning, and social interaction. A number of theorists have attempted to provide information about personality development. Most suggest that it occurs in an orderly, step-wise fashion. These stages overlap, however, as maturation occurs at different rates in different individuals. The theories of Sullivan (1953), Erikson (1963), and Mahler (Mahler, Pine, & Bergman, 1975) were presented at length in Chapter 3. The stages of personality development according to these three theorists are compared in Table 34.1. The nurse should understand "normal" personality development before learning about what is considered dysfunctional.

Historical and epidemiological aspects of personality disorders are discussed in this chapter. Predisposing factors that have been implicated in the etiology of personality disorders are presented. Symptomatology is explained to provide background knowledge for assessing clients with personality disorders.

Individuals with personality disorders are not often treated in acute care settings for the personality disorder as their primary psychiatric diagnosis. However, many clients with other psychiatric and medical diagnoses manifest symptoms of personality disorders. Nurses are likely to encounter clients with these personality characteristics frequently in all health care settings.

Nurses working in psychiatric settings may often encounter clients with borderline and antisocial personality characteristics. The behavior of borderline clients is very unstable, and hospitalization is often required as a result of attempts at self-injury. The client with antisocial personality disorder may enter the psychiatric arena as a result of judicially ordered evaluation. Psychiatric intervention may be an alternative to imprisonment for antisocial behavior if it is deemed potentially helpful.

Nursing care of clients with borderline personality disorder or antisocial personality disorder is presented in this chapter in the context of the nursing process. Various medical treatment modalities for personality disorders are explored.

HISTORICAL ASPECTS

The concept of a personality disorder has been present throughout the history of medicine (Frances & Widiger, 1986; Millon, 1981). In the 4th century BC, Hippocrates concluded that all disease stemmed from an excess of or imbalance among four bodily humors: yellow bile, black bile, blood, and phlegm. Hippocrates identified four fundamental personality styles that he concluded stemmed from excesses in the four humors: the irritable and hostile choleric (yellow bile); the pessimistic melancholic (black bile); the overly optimistic and extraverted sanguine (blood); and the apathetic phlegmatic (phlegm).

Within the profession of medicine, the first recognition that personality disorders, apart from psychosis, were cause for their own special concern was in 1801, with the recognition that an individual can behave irrationally even when the powers of intellect are intact. Nineteenth-century psychiatrists embraced the term *moral insanity*, the concept of which defines what we know today as personality disorders (Perry & Vaillant, 1989).

A major difficulty for psychiatrists has been the establishment of a classification of personality disorders. The *DSM-IV* provides specific criteria for diagnosing these disorders. The *DSM-IV* groups the personality disorders into three clusters. These clusters, and the disorders classified under each, are described as follows:

1. Cluster A: behaviors described as odd or eccentric.
   a. Paranoid personality disorder
   b. Schizoid personality disorder
   c. Schizotypal personality disorder
2. Cluster B: behaviors described as dramatic, emotional, or erratic.
   a. Antisocial personality disorder
   b. Borderline personality disorder
   c. Histrionic personality disorder
   d. Narcissistic personality disorder
3. Cluster C: behaviors described as anxious or fearful.
   a. Avoidant personality disorder

TABLE 34.1 COMPARISON OF PERSONALITY DEVELOPMENT—SULLIVAN, ERIKSON, AND MAHLER

MAJOR DEVELOPMENTAL TASKS AND DESIGNATED AGES

SULLIVAN	ERIKSON	MAHLER
Birth to 18 months: Relief from anxiety through oral gratification of needs. 18 months to 6 years: Learning to experience a delay in personal gratification without undo anxiety. 6 to 9 years: Learning to form satisfactory peer relationships. 9 to 12 years: Learning to form satisfactory relationships with persons of the same sex; the initiation of feelings of affection for another person. 12 to 14 years: Learning to form satisfactory relationships with persons of the opposite sex; developing a sense of identity. 14 to 21 years: Establishing self-identity; experiences satisfying relationships; working to develop a lasting, intimate opposite-sex relationship.	Birth to 18 months: To develop a basic trust in the mothering figure and be able to generalize it to others. 18 months to 3 years: To gain some self-control and independence within the environment. 3 to 6 years: To develop a sense of purpose and the ability to initiate and direct own activities. 6 to 12 years: To achieve a sense of self-confidence by learning, competing, performing successfully, and receiving recognition from significant others, peers, and acquaintances. 12 to 20 years: To integrate the tasks mastered in the previous stages into a secure sense of self. 20 to 30 years: To form an intense, lasting relationship or a commitment to another person, a cause, an institution, or a creative effort. 30 to 65 years: To achieve the life goals established for oneself, while also considering the welfare of future generations. 65 years to death: To review one's life and derive meaning from both positive and negative events, while achieving a positive sense of self-worth.	Birth to 1 month: Fulfillment of basic needs for survival and comfort. 1 to 5 months: Developing awareness of external source of need fulfillment. 5 to 10 months: Commencement of a primary recognition of separateness from the mothering figure. 10 to 16 months: Increased independence through locomotor functioning; increased sense of separateness of self. 16 to 24 months: Acute awareness of separateness of self; learning to seek "emotional refueling" from mothering figure to maintain feeling of security. 24 to 36 months: Sense of separateness established; on the way to object constancy: able to internalize a sustained image of loved object/person when it is out of sight; resolution of separation anxiety.

b. Dependent personality disorder
c. Obsessive-compulsive personality disorder

NOTE: The *DSM-III-R* (APA, 1987) included passive-aggressive personality disorder in cluster C. In the *DSM-IV*, this disorder has been included in the section on *Criteria Provided for Further Study.* For purposes of this text, passive-aggressive personality disorder will be described with the cluster C disorders.

Historically, individuals with personality disorders have been labeled as "immoral" or "bad," as deviating from social norms, and as extremes on the continuum of normal personality dimensions (Perry & Vaillant, 1989). The events and sequences that result in pathology of the personality are complicated and difficult to unravel. Continued study is needed to facilitate understanding of this complex behavioral phenomenon.

TYPES OF PERSONALITY DISORDERS

Paranoid Personality Disorder

Definition and Epidemiological Statistics

The *DSM-IV* defines paranoid personality disorder as "a pattern of behavior, beginning by early adulthood and present in a variety of contexts, of pervasive distrust and suspiciousness of others such that their motives are interpreted as malevolent" (APA, 1994). Kaplan and Sadock (1998) identify the characteristic feature as a longstanding suspiciousness and mistrust of people in general. Prevalence is difficult to establish because individuals with the disorder seldom seek assistance for their problem or require hospitalization. When they present for treatment at the insistence of others, they may be able to pull themselves together sufficiently so that their behavior does not appear maladaptive. The disorder is more commonly diagnosed in men than in women.

Clinical Picture

Individuals with paranoid personality disorder are constantly on guard, hypervigilant, and ready for any real or imagined threat. They appear tense and irritable. They have developed a hard exterior and become immune or insensitive to the feelings of others. They avoid interactions with other people, lest they be forced to relinquish some of their own power. They always feel that others are there to take advantage of them.

They are extremely oversensitive and tend to misinterpret even minute cues within the environment, magnifying and distorting them into thoughts of trickery and deception. Because they trust no one, they are constantly "testing" the honesty of others. Their intimidating manner provokes almost everyone with whom they come in contact into exasperation and anger.

Paranoid persons maintain their self-esteem by attributing their shortcomings to others. Millon (1981) has stated:

> "Paranoids transform events to suit their self-image and aspirations. They do this by denial of any personal weakness and malevolence, the projection of these traits upon others, and the aggrandizement of self through grandiose and persecutory fantasies."

They are envious and hostile toward others who are highly successful and believe the only reason they are not as successful is because they have been treated unfairly. Paranoid persons are extremely vulnerable and are constantly on the defensive. Any real or imagined threat can release hostility and anger that is fueled by animosities from the past. The desire for reprisal and vindication is so intense that a possible loss of control can result in aggression and violence. These outbursts are usually brief, and the paranoid person soon regains the external control, rationalizes the behavior, and reconstructs the defenses central to his or her personality pattern.

The *DSM-IV* diagnostic criteria for paranoid personality disorder are presented in Table 34.2.

Predisposing Factors

Research has indicated a possible hereditary link in paranoid personality disorder. Studies have revealed a higher incidence of paranoid personality disorder among relatives of clients with schizophrenia than among control subjects (Kaplan & Sadock, 1998).

Psychosocially, paranoid persons may have been subjected to parental antagonism and harassment. They likely served as scapegoats for displaced parental aggression and gradually relinquished all hope of affection and approval. They learned to perceive the world as harsh and unkind, a place calling for protective vigilance and mistrust. They entered the world with a chip-on-the-shoulder attitude and were met with many rebuffs and rejections from others. Anticipating humiliation and betrayal by others, the paranoid person learned to attack first.

Schizoid Personality Disorder

Definition and Epidemiological Statistics

Schizoid personality disorder is characterized primarily by a profound defect in the ability to form personal relationships or to respond to others in any meaningful, emotional way (Phillips & Gunderson, 1994). These individuals display a lifelong pattern of social withdrawal, their discomfort with human interaction being very apparent. Prevalence of schizoid personality disorder within the general population has been estimated at between 3 and 7.5 percent. Significant numbers of people with the disorder are never observed in a clinical setting. Sex ratio of the disorder is unknown, although it is diagnosed more frequently in men.

TABLE 34.2 DIAGNOSTIC CRITERIA FOR PARANOID PERSONALITY DISORDER

A. A pervasive distrust and suspiciousness of others such that their motives are interpreted as malevolent, beginning by early adulthood and present in a variety of contexts, as indicated by four (or more) of the following:
  1. Suspects, without sufficient basis, that others are exploiting, harming, or deceiving him or her.
  2. Is preoccupied with unjustified doubts about the loyalty or trustworthiness of friends or associates.
  3. Is reluctant to confide in others because of unwarranted fear that the information will be used maliciously against him or her.
  4. Reads hidden demeaning or threatening meanings into benign remarks or events.
  5. Persistently bears grudges (i.e., is unforgiving of insults, injuries, or slights).
  6. Perceives attacks on his or her character or reputation that are not apparent to others and is quick to react angrily or to counterattack.
  7. Has recurrent suspicions, without justification, regarding fidelity of spouse or sexual partner.
B. Does not occur exclusively during the course of schizophrenia, a mood disorder with psychotic features, or another psychotic disorder, and is not due to the direct physiological effects of a general medical condition.

SOURCE: From APA (1994), with permission.

Clinical Picture

Persons with schizoid personality disorder appear cold, aloof, and indifferent to others. They prefer to work in isolation and are unsociable, with little need or desire for emotional ties (Kaplan & Sadock, 1998). They are able to invest enormous affective energy in intellectual pursuits.

In the presence of others they appear shy, anxious, or uneasy. They are inappropriately serious about everything and have difficulty acting in a lighthearted manner. Their behavior and conversation exhibit little or no spontaneity. Typically they are unable to experience pleasure, and their affect is commonly bland and constricted.

The *DSM-IV* diagnostic criteria for schizoid personality disorder are presented in Table 34.3.

Predisposing Factors

Although the role of heredity in the etiology of schizoid personality disorder is unclear, the feature of introversion appears to be a highly inheritable characteristic (Phillips & Gunderson, 1994). Further studies are required before definitive statements can be made.

Psychosocially, the development of schizoid personality is probably influenced by early patterns of object relations, familial interactive style, and culture (Perry & Vaillant, 1989). The childhoods of these individuals have often been characterized as bleak, cold, unempathic, and notably lacking in nurturing. A child brought up with this type of parenting may become a schizoid adult if that child possesses a temperamental disposition that is shy, anxious, and introverted. Phillips and Gunderson (1994) state:

> "Clinicians have noted that schizoid personality disorder occurs in adults who experienced cold, neglectful, and ungratifying relationships in early childhood, which leads these persons to assume that relationships are not valuable or worth pursuing." (p. 709)

Schizotypal Personality Disorder

Definition and Epidemiological Statistics

Individuals with **schizotypal** personality disorder were once described as "latent schizophrenics." Their behavior is odd and eccentric but does not decompensate to the level of schizophrenia. Schizotypal personality is a graver form of the pathologically less severe schizoid personality pattern. Recent studies indicate that approximately 3 percent of the population have this disorder (APA, 1994).

Clinical Picture

Individuals with schizotypal personality disorder are aloof and isolated and behave in a bland and apathetic manner. Magical thinking, ideas of reference, illusions, and depersonalization are part of their everyday world. Examples include superstitiousness; belief in clairvoyance, telepathy, or "sixth sense"; or beliefs that "others can feel my feelings" (APA, 1994).

The speech pattern is odd, sometimes bizarre. People with this disorder often cannot orient their thoughts logically and become lost in personal irrelevancies and in tangential asides that seem vague, digressive, and with no pertinence to the topic at hand. This feature of their personality only further alienates them from others.

Under stress, these individuals may decompensate and demonstrate psychotic symptoms, such as delusional thoughts, hallucinations, or bizarre behaviors, but they are usually of brief duration (Kaplan & Sadock, 1998). They often talk or gesture to themselves, as if "living in their own world." Affect is bland or inappropriate, such as expressing silly laughter when discussing their problems (Phillips & Gunderson, 1994).

The *DSM-IV* diagnostic criteria for schizotypal personality disorder are presented in Table 34.4.

TABLE 34.3   DIAGNOSTIC CRITERIA FOR SCHIZOID PERSONALITY DISORDER

A. A pervasive pattern of detachment from social relationships and a restricted range of expression of emotions in interpersonal settings, beginning by early adulthood and present in a variety of contexts, as indicated by four (or more) of the following:
   1. Neither desires nor enjoys close relationships, including being part of a family
   2. Almost always chooses solitary activities
   3. Has little if any interest in having sexual experiences with another person
   4. Takes pleasure in few, if any, activities
   5. Lacks close friends or confidants other than first-degree relatives
   6. Appears indifferent to the praise or criticism of others
   7. Shows emotional coldness, detachment, or flattened affectivity
B. Does not occur exclusively during the course of schizophrenia, a mood disorder with psychotic features, another psychotic disorder, or a pervasive developmental disorder and is not due to the direct physiological effects of a general medical condition.

SOURCE: From APA (1994), with permission.

TABLE 34.4 DIAGNOSTIC CRITERIA FOR SCHIZOTYPAL PERSONALITY DISORDER

A. A pervasive pattern of social and interpersonal deficits marked by acute discomfort with, and reduced capacity for, close relationships as well as by cognitive or perceptual distortions and eccentricities of behavior, beginning by early adulthood and present in a variety of contexts, as indicated by five (or more) of the following:
  1. Ideas of reference (excluding delusions of reference).
  2. Odd beliefs or magical thinking that influences behavior and is inconsistent with subcultural norms (e.g., superstitiousness, belief in clairvoyance, telepathy, or "sixth sense"; in children and adolescents, bizarre fantasies or preoccupations).
  3. Unusual perceptual experiences, including bodily illusions.
  4. Odd thinking and speech (e.g., vague, circumstantial, metaphorical, overly elaborate, or stereotyped).
  5. Suspiciousness or paranoid ideation.
  6. Inappropriate or constricted affect.
  7. Behavior or appearance that is odd, eccentric, or peculiar.
  8. Lack of close friends or confidants other than first-degree relatives.
  9. Excessive social anxiety that does not diminish with familiarity and that tends to be associated with paranoid fears rather than negative judgments about self.
B. Does not occur exclusively during the course of schizophrenia, a mood disorder with psychotic features, another psychotic disorder, or a pervasive developmental disorder.

SOURCE: From APA (1994), with permission.

Predisposing Factors

Some evidence suggests that schizotypal personality disorder is more common among the first-degree biological relatives of people with schizophrenia than among the general population, indicating a possible hereditary factor (APA, 1994). Other biogenic factors that, although speculative, may contribute to the development of this disorder include anatomical deficits or neurochemical dysfunctions resulting in diminished activation, minimal pleasure-pain sensibilities, and impaired cognitive functions. These possible biological etiological factors support the close link between schizotypal personality disorder and schizophrenia and are considered in classifying schizotypal personality disorder with schizophrenia rather than with the personality disorders in the *International Classification of Diseases (ICD-10)* (Phillips & Gunderson, 1994).

The early family dynamics of the individual with schizotypal personality disorder may have been characterized by indifference, impassivity, or formality, leading to a pattern of discomfort with personal affection and closeness. Early on, affective deficits made them unattractive and unrewarding social companions. They were likely shunned, overlooked, rejected and humiliated by others, resulting in feelings of low self-esteem and a marked distrust of interpersonal relations. Having failed repeatedly to cope with these adversities, they began to withdraw, "tune out" reality, and reduce contact with persons and events that evoked nothing but shame and agony (Millon, 1981). This new inner world would provide them with an existence that was more significant and potentially rewarding than the one experienced in reality.

Antisocial Personality Disorder

Definition and Epidemiological Statistics

Antisocial personality disorder is a pattern of socially irresponsible, exploitative, and guiltless behavior that reflects a disregard for the rights of others (Phillips & Gunderson, 1994). There is a tendency to fail to conform to the law or to sustain consistent employment, to exploit and manipulate others for personal gain, and to fail to develop stable relationships. It is one of the oldest and best researched of the personality disorders and has been included in all editions of the APA's *Diagnostic and Statistical Manual of Mental Disorders*. In the United States, prevalence estimates range from 3 percent in men to less than 1 percent in women (APA, 1994). The disorder is more common among the lower socioeconomic classes, and particularly so among highly mobile residents of impoverished urban areas (Perry & Vaillant, 1989). The *ICD-10* identifies this disorder as *dissocial personality disorder*.

NOTE: The clinical picture, predisposing factors, nursing diagnoses, and interventions for care of clients with antisocial personality disorder are presented later in this chapter.

Borderline Personality Disorder

Definition and Epidemiological Statistics

Borderline personality disorder is characterized by a pattern of intense and chaotic relationships, with affective instability and fluctuating attitudes toward other people. These individuals are impulsive, directly and indirectly self-destructive, and lack a clear sense of identity. Prevalence estimates of borderline personality range from 2 percent to 3 percent of the population. It is the most common form of personality disorder, occurring in every culture (Phillips & Gunderson, 1994). It is twice as common in women as in men (Kaplan & Sadock, 1998). The *ICD-10* identifies this disorder as *emotionally unstable personality disorder*.

> **NOTE:** The clinical picture, predisposing factors, nursing diagnoses, and interventions for care of clients with borderline personality disorder are presented later in this chapter.

Histrionic Personality Disorder

Definition and Epidemiological Statistics

This disorder is characterized by colorful, dramatic, and extroverted behavior in excitable, emotional persons (Perry & Vaillant, 1989). They have difficulty maintaining long-lasting relationships, although they require constant affirmation of approval and acceptance from others. Prevalence of the disorder is thought to be about 2 to 3 percent, and it is more common in women than in men.

Clinical Picture

Histrionic persons have a tendency to be self-dramatizing, attention-seeking, overly gregarious, and seductive. They use manipulative and exhibitionistic behaviors in their demands to be the center of attention. Persons with histrionic personality disorder often demonstrate, in mild pathological form, what our society tends to foster and admire in its members: to be well liked, successful, popular, extroverted, attractive, and sociable (Millon, 1981). Beneath these surface characteristics, however, is a driven quality, a consuming need for approval, a desperate striving to be conspicuous and to evoke affection or attract attention at all costs. Failure to evoke the attention and approval they seek often results in feelings of dejection and anxiety.

Individuals with this disorder are highly distractible and flighty by nature. They have difficulty paying attention to detail. They can portray themselves as carefree and sophisticated on the one hand and as inhibited and naive on the other. They tend to be highly suggestible, impressionable, and rather easily influenced by others. They are strongly dependent.

Interpersonal relationships are fleeting and superficial. The histrionic person, having failed throughout life to develop the richness of inner feelings and lacking resources on which to draw, lacks the ability to provide another with genuinely sustained affection. Somatic complaints are not uncommon in these individuals, and fleeting episodes of psychosis may occur during periods of extreme stress. The *DSM-IV* diagnostic criteria for histrionic personality disorder are presented in Table 34.5.

Predisposing Factors

Biological hypotheses have been proposed in the predisposition to histrionic personality disorder. These include ease of sympathetic arousal, adrenal hyperreactivity, and neurochemical imbalances (Millon, 1981). Heredity may be a factor, as the disorder is apparently more common among first-degree biological relatives of people with the disorder than in the general population (Pfohl, 1994).

Phillips and Gunderson (1994) report on research that suggests that the behavioral characteristics of histrionic personality disorder may be associated with a biogenetically determined temperament. From this perspective, histrionic personality disorder would arise out of "an extreme variation of temperamental disposition."

From a psychosocial perspective, learning experiences may contribute to the development of histrionic personality disorder. The child may have come to learn that positive reinforcement was contingent on the ability to perform parentally approved and admired behaviors. It is likely that the child rarely received either positive or negative feedback. Parental acceptance and approval came inconsistently and only when the behaviors met parental expectations. Millon (1981) stated:

▰ TABLE 34.5 DIAGNOSTIC CRITERIA FOR HISTRIONIC PERSONALITY DISORDER

A pervasive pattern of excessive emotionality and attention seeking, beginning by early adulthood and present in a variety of contexts, as indicated by five (or more) of the following:

1. Is uncomfortable in situations in which he or she is not the center of attention.
2. Interaction with others is often characterized by inappropriate sexually seductive or provocative behavior.
3. Displays rapidly shifting and shallow expression of emotions.
4. Consistently uses physical appearance to draw attention to self.
5. Has a style of speech that is excessively impressionistic and lacking in detail.
6. Shows self-dramatization, theatricality, and exaggerated expression of emotion.
7. Is suggestible (i.e., easily influenced by others or circumstances).
8. Considers relationships to be more intimate than they actually are.

SOURCE: From APA (1994), with permission.

"These types of experiences have several consequences in terms of personality. They appear to create behaviors that are designed primarily to evoke rewards, create a feeling of competence and acceptance only if others acknowledge and commend one's performances, and build a habit of seeking approval for its own sake. All three of these traits are characteristic of the histrionic personality."

Narcissistic Personality Disorder

Definition and Epidemiological Statistics

Persons with narcissistic personality disorder have an exaggerated sense of self-worth. They lack empathy and are hypersensitive to the evaluation of others. They believe that they have the inalienable right to receive special consideration and that their desire is justification for possessing whatever they seek. This diagnosis appeared for the first time in the *DSM-III* (APA, 1980). However, the concept of **narcissism** has its roots in the 19th century. It was viewed by early psychoanalysts as a normal phase of psychosexual development. Epidemiological patterns have not been fully investigated, but anecdotal reports suggest the disorder is more common in men than it is in women (Perry & Vaillant, 1989). The *DSM-IV* (APA, 1994) estimates the prevalence of the disorder as from 2 to 16 percent in the clinical population and less than 1 percent in the general population.

Clinical Picture

Individuals with narcissistic disorder appear to lack humility, being overly self-centered and exploiting others to fulfill their own desires. They often do not even conceive of their behavior as being inappropriate or objectionable. Because they view themselves as "superior" beings, they believe they are entitled to special rights and privileges.

Their mood, though often grounded in grandiose distortions of reality, is usually optimistic, relaxed, cheerful, and carefree. This mood can easily change, however, as a result of their very fragile self-esteem. If they do not meet self-expectations, do not receive the positive feedback they expect from others, or draw criticism from others, they may respond with rage, shame, humiliation, or dejection. They may turn inward and fantasize rationalizations that convince them of their continued stature and perfection.

The exploitation of others for self-gratification results in impaired interpersonal relationships. In selecting a mate, narcissistic individuals frequently choose a person who will be obedient, solicitous, and subservient, without expecting anything in return except strength and assurances of fidelity (Millon, 1981).

The *DSM-IV* diagnostic criteria for narcissistic personality disorder are presented in Table 34.6.

Predisposing Factors

Several psychodynamic theories exist regarding the predisposition to narcissistic personality disorder. Phillips and Gunderson (1994) suggest that, as children, these individuals have had their fears, failures, or dependency needs responded to with criticism, disdain, or neglect. They grow up with contempt for these behaviors in themselves and others, and are unable to view others as sources of comfort and support. They project an image of invulnerability and self-sufficiency that conceals their true sense of emptiness and contributes to their inability to feel deeply.

Millon (1981) suggests that the family dynamics of a person with narcissistic personality disorder are those that foster omnipotence and grandiosity in the child. The family world revolves around the child, and the parents acquiesce to and indulge their every whim. There is no give-and-take on the part of the child—only taking. Often adding to this predisposing influence is a minimal amount of parental guidance, discipline, and control.

TABLE 34.6 DIAGNOSTIC CRITERIA FOR NARCISSISTIC PERSONALITY DISORDER

A pervasive pattern of grandiosity (in fantasy or behavior), need for admiration, and lack of empathy, beginning by early adulthood and present in a variety of contexts, as indicated by five (or more) of the following:

1. Has a grandiose sense of self-importance (e.g., exaggerates achievements and talents, expects to be recognized as superior without commensurate achievements).
2. Is preoccupied with fantasies of unlimited success, power, brilliance, beauty, or ideal love.
3. Believes that he or she is "special" and unique and can only be understood by, or should associate with, other special or high-status people (or institutions).
4. Requires excessive admiration.
5. Has a sense of entitlement (i.e., unreasonable expectations of especially favorable treatment or automatic compliance with his or her expectations).
6. Is interpersonally exploitative (i.e., takes advantage of others to achieve his or her own ends).
7. Lacks empathy: is unwilling to recognize or identify with the feelings and needs of others.
8. Is often envious of others or believes that others are envious of him or her.
9. Shows arrogant, haughty behaviors or attitudes.

SOURCE: From APA (1994), with permission.

Narcissism may also develop from an environment in which parents attempt to live their lives vicariously through their child. They expect the child to achieve the things they did not achieve, possess that which they did not possess, and have life better and easier than they did. The child is not subjected to the requirements and restrictions that may have dominated the parents' lives, and thereby grows up believing he or she is above that which is required for everyone else. Horney (1939) wrote:

> "Parents who transfer their own ambitions to the child and regard the boy as an embryonic genius or the girl as a princess, thereby develop in the child the feeling that he is loved for imaginary qualities rather than for his true self."

Avoidant Personality Disorder

Definition and Epidemiological Statistics

The individual with avoidant personality disorder is extremely sensitive to rejection and because of this may lead a very socially withdrawn life. It is not that he or she is asocial; in fact, there may be a strong desire for companionship. The extreme shyness and fear of rejection, however, create needs for unusually strong guarantees of uncritical acceptance (Kaplan & Sadock, 1998). Prevalence of the disorder in the general population is between 0.5 percent and 1 percent, and it appears to be equally common in men and women (APA, 1994).

Clinical Picture

Individuals with this disorder are awkward and uncomfortable in social situations. They may be perceived by others from a distance as timid, withdrawn, or perhaps cold and strange. Those who have closer relationships with them, however, soon learn of their sensitivities, touchiness, evasiveness, and mistrustful qualities.

Their speech is usually slow and constrained, with frequent hesitations, fragmentary thought sequences, and occasional confused and irrelevant digressions. They are often lonely and express feelings of being unwanted. They view others as critical, betraying, and humiliating. They desire to have close relationships but avoid them because of their fear of being rejected. Depression, anxiety, and anger at oneself for failing to develop social relations are commonly experienced. The *DSM-IV* diagnostic criteria for avoidant personality disorder are presented in Table 34.7.

Predisposing Factors

Millon (1981) suggests that there may be a hereditary influence with avoidant personality disorder, as there appears to be a higher-than-chance correspondence rate among family members. Some infants who exhibit traits of hyperirritability, crankiness, tension, and withdrawal behaviors may possess a temperamental disposition toward an avoidant pattern.

The primary psychosocial predisposing influence to avoidant personality disorder is parental rejection and criticism (Phillips & Gunderson, 1994). These children are often reared in a family in which they are belittled, abandoned, and censured, such that any natural optimism is extinguished and replaced with feelings of low self-worth and social alienation. They learn to be suspicious and to view the world as hostile and dangerous.

Dependent Personality Disorder

Definition and Epidemiological Statistics

Dependent personality disorder is characterized by "a pervasive and excessive need to be taken care of that leads to submissive and clinging behavior and fears of separation" (APA, 1994). These characteristics are evident in the tendency to allow others to make decisions, to feel helpless when alone, to act submissively, to subordinate needs to others, to tolerate mistreatment by others, to demean oneself to gain acceptance, and to fail to function adequately in situations that require assertive or dominant behavior.

The disorder is relatively common. Kaplan and Sadock (1998) discuss the results of one study of personality disorders in which 2.5 percent of the sample were diagnosed

---

TABLE 34.7 DIAGNOSTIC CRITERIA FOR AVOIDANT PERSONALITY DISORDER

A pervasive pattern of social inhibition, feelings of inadequacy, and hypersensitivity to negative evaluation, beginning by early adulthood and present in a variety of contexts, as indicated by four (or more) of the following:

1. Avoids occupational activities that involve significant interpersonal contact, because of fears of criticism, disapproval, or rejection.
2. Is unwilling to get involved with people unless certain of being liked.
3. Shows restraint within intimate relationships because of the fear of being shamed or ridiculed.
4. Is preoccupied with being criticized or rejected in social situations.
5. Is inhibited in new interpersonal situations because of feelings of inadequacy.
6. Views self as socially inept, personally unappealing, or inferior to others.
7. Is unusually reluctant to take personal risks or to engage in any new activities because they may prove embarrassing.

SOURCE: From APA (1994), with permission.

with dependent personality disorder. It is more common in women than in men and more common in the youngest children of a family than the older ones.

Clinical Picture

Individuals with dependent personality disorder have a notable lack of self-confidence that is often apparent in their posture, voice, and mannerisms. They are typically passive and acquiescent to the desires of others. They are overly generous and thoughtful, while underplaying their own attractiveness and achievements. They may appear to others to "see the world through rose-colored glasses," but, once alone, they may feel pessimistic, discouraged, and dejected. Others are not made aware of these feelings; their "suffering" is done in silence.

Individuals with dependent personality disorder assume the passive and submissive role in relationships. They are willing to let others make their important decisions. Should the dependent relationship end, they feel helpless and fearful because they feel incapable of caring for themselves (Phillips & Gunderson, 1994). They may hastily and indiscriminately attempt to establish another relationship with someone they believe can provide them with the nurturance and guidance they need.

They avoid positions of responsibility and become anxious when forced into them. They have feelings of low self-worth and are easily hurt by criticism and disapproval. They will do almost anything, even if it is unpleasant or demeaning, in order to earn the acceptance of others.

The *DSM-IV* criteria for dependent personality disorder are presented in Table 34.8.

Predisposing Factors

An infant may be genetically predisposed to a dependent temperament. Twin studies measuring submissiveness have shown a higher correlation between identical twins than fraternal twins (Phillips & Gunderson, 1994).

Psychosocially, dependency is fostered in infancy when stimulation and nurturance are experienced exclusively from one source. The infant becomes attached to one source, to the exclusion of all others. If this exclusive attachment continues as the child grows, the dependency is nurtured. A problem may arise when parents become overprotective and discourage independent behaviors on the part of the child. Parents who make new experiences unnecessarily easy for the child and refuse to allow him or her to learn by experience encourage their children to give up their efforts at achieving autonomy. Dependent behaviors may be subtly rewarded in this environment, and the child may come to fear a loss of love or attachment from the parental figure if independent behaviors are attempted.

Obsessive-Compulsive Personality Disorder

Definition and Epidemiological Statistics

Individuals with obsessive-compulsive personality disorder are very serious and formal and have difficulty expressing emotions. They are overly disciplined, perfectionistic, and preoccupied with rules. They are inflexible about the way in which things must be done and have a devotion to productivity at the exclusion of personal pleasure. An intense fear of making mistakes leads to difficulty with decision making. The disorder is relatively common and occurs more often in men than in women. Within the family constellation, it appears to be most common in oldest children.

Clinical Picture

Individuals with obsessive-compulsive personality disorder are inflexible and lack spontaneity. They are very meticulous and work diligently and patiently at tasks that require

---

▰ **TABLE 34.8 DIAGNOSTIC CRITERIA FOR DEPENDENT PERSONALITY DISORDER**

A pervasive and excessive need to be taken care of that leads to submissive and clinging behavior and fears of separation, beginning by early adulthood and present in a variety of contexts, as indicated by five (or more) of the following:
1. Has difficulty making everyday decisions without an excessive amount of advice and reassurance from others.
2. Needs others to assume responsibility for most major areas of his or her life.
3. Has difficulty expressing disagreement with others because of fear of loss of support or approval. (**Note:** Do not include realistic fears of retribution.)
4. Has difficulty initiating projects or doing things on his or her own (because of a lack of self-confidence in judgment or abilities rather than a lack of motivation or energy).
5. Goes to excessive lengths to obtain nurturance and support from others, to the point of volunteering to do things that are unpleasant.
6. Feels uncomfortable or helpless when alone because of exaggerated fears of being unable to care for himself or herself.
7. Urgently seeks another relationship as a source of care and support when a close relationship ends.
8. Is unrealistically preoccupied with fears of being left to take care of himself or herself.

SOURCE: From APA (1994), with permission.

accuracy and discipline. They are especially concerned with matters of organization and efficiency and tend to be rigid and unbending about rules and procedures.

Social behavior tends to be polite and formal. They are very "rank conscious," a characteristic that is reflected in their contrasting behaviors with "superiors" as opposed to "inferiors." They can be very solicitous to and ingratiating with authority figures. However, with subordinates the compulsive person is quite autocratic and condemnatory, often appearing pompous and self-righteous.

People with obsessive-compulsive personality disorder typify the "bureaucratic personality," the so-called company man. They see themselves as conscientious, loyal, dependable and responsible and are contemptuous of people whose behavior they consider frivolous and impulsive. Emotional behavior is considered immature and irresponsible.

Although these individuals appear on the surface to be very calm and controlled, underneath this exterior lies a great deal of ambivalence, conflict, and hostility. Individuals with this disorder commonly use the defense mechanism of reaction formation. Not daring to expose their true feelings of defiance and anger, they withhold these feelings so strongly that the opposite feelings come forth. The defenses of isolation, intellectualization, displacement, and undoing are also commonly evident (Perry & Vaillant, 1989).

The *DSM-IV* diagnostic criteria for obsessive-compulsive personality disorder are presented in Table 34.9.

Predisposing Factors

In the psychoanalytical view, the parenting style in which the individual with obsessive-compulsive personality disorder was reared is one of overcontrol. These parents expect their children to live up to their imposed standards of conduct and condemn them if they do not. Praise for positive behaviors is bestowed on the child with much less frequency than punishment for undesirable behaviors. In this environment, individuals become experts in learning what they must *not* do, so as to avoid punishment and condemnation, rather than what they *can* do to achieve attention and praise. They learn to heed rigid restrictions and rules. Positive achievements are expected, taken for granted, and only occasionally acknowledged by their parents; comments and judgments are almost exclusively limited to pointing out infractions of rules and boundaries the child must never transgress (Millon, 1981).

Passive-Aggressive Personality Disorder

Definition and Epidemiological Statistics

The *DSM-IV* defines this disorder as a pervasive pattern of negativistic attitudes and passive resistance to demands for adequate performance in social and occupational situations that begins by early adulthood and occurs in a variety of contexts. The name of the disorder is based on the assumption that such people are passively expressing covert aggression (Kaplan & Sadock, 1998). **Passive-aggressive** disorder has been included in all editions of the *DSM* and, although no statistics exist that speak to its prevalence, it appears to be a relatively common syndrome.

Clinical Picture

Pfohl (1994) describes the passive-aggressive personality in the following manner:

> "Passive-aggressive personality disorder is characterized by passive resistance and general obstructiveness in response to the expectations of others. Such individuals would rarely be assertive enough to openly disagree with a treatment plan but may express disagreement indirectly by 'losing' a prescription or 'forgetting' the psychotherapy homework assignment."

TABLE 34.9 DIAGNOSTIC CRITERIA FOR OBSESSIVE-COMPULSIVE PERSONALITY DISORDER

A pervasive pattern of preoccupation with orderliness, perfectionism, and mental and interpersonal control, at the expense of flexibility, openness, and efficiency, beginning by early adulthood and present in a variety of contexts, as indicated by four (or more) of the following:

1. Is preoccupied with details, rules, lists, order, organization, or schedules to the extent that the major point of the activity is lost.
2. Shows perfectionism that interferes with task completion (e.g., is unable to complete a project because his or her own overly strict standards are not met).
3. Is excessively devoted to work and productivity to the exclusion of leisure activities and friendships (not accounted for by obvious economic necessity).
4. Is overconscientious, scrupulous, and inflexible about matters of morality, ethics, or values (not accounted for by cultural or religious identification).
5. Is unable to discard worn out or worthless objects even when they have no sentimental value.
6. Is reluctant to delegate tasks or to work with others unless they submit to exactly his or her way of doing things.
7. Adopts a miserly spending style toward both self and others; money is viewed as something to be hoarded for future catastrophes.
8. Shows rigidity and stubbornness.

SOURCE: From APA (1994), with permission.

Passive-aggressive individuals feel cheated and unappreciated. They believe that life has been unkind to them, and they express envy and resentment over the "easy life" that they perceive others having. When they feel they have been wronged by another, they may go to great lengths to seek retribution, or "get even," but always in a subtle and passive manner rather than discussing their feelings with the offending individual. As a tactic of interpersonal behavior, passive-aggressive individuals commonly switch among the roles of the martyr, the affronted, the aggrieved, the misunderstood, the contrite, the guilt-ridden, the sickly, and the overworked. In this way, they are able to vent their anger and resentment subtly, while gaining the attention, reassurance, and dependency they crave.

The *DSM-IV* research criteria for passive-aggressive personality disorder are presented in Table 34.10.

Predisposing Factors

The family dynamics of children who eventually develop a passive-aggressive personality involve contradictory parental attitudes and inconsistent training methods (Millon, 1981). At any moment, and without provocation, these children may receive either the kindness and support they crave or hostility and rejection. Parental responses are inconsistent and unpredictable, and these children internalize the conflicting attitudes toward themselves and others. For example, they do not know whether to think of themselves as competent or incompetent and are unsure as to whether they love or hate those on whom they depend. Double-bind communication may also be exhibited in these families. Expressions of concern and affection may be verbalized, only to be negated and undone through subtle and devious behavioral manifestations. This *approach-avoidance* pattern is modeled by the child, who then becomes equally equivocal and ambivalent in his or her own thinking and actions.

Through this type of environment, the child learns to control his or her anger for fear of provoking parental withdrawal and not receiving love and support—even on an inconsistent basis. Overtly the child appears polite and

undemanding; hostility and inefficiency are manifested only covertly and indirectly.

APPLICATION OF THE NURSING PROCESS

Borderline Personality Disorder

Background Assessment Data

Historically, there have been a group of clients who did not classically conform to the standard categories of neuroses or psychoses. Stern (1938) first used the designation "borderline" to identify these clients who seemed to fall on the border between the two categories. Other theorists who have attempted to identify this disorder have used terminology such as *ambulatory schizophrenia, pseudoneurotic schizophrenia,* and *emotionally unstable personality.* When the term *borderline* was first proposed for inclusion in the *DSM-III* (APA, 1980), some psychiatrists feared it may be used as a "wastebasket" diagnosis for difficult-to-treat clients. However, a specific set of criteria has been established for diagnosing what Schmideberg (1956) described as a consistent and "stable course of unstable behavior" (Table 34.11).

Clinical Picture

Individuals with borderline personality disorder always seem to be in a state of crisis. Their affect is one of extreme intensity and their behavior reflects frequent changeability. These changes can occur within a matter of days, hours, or even minutes. Often these individuals exhibit a single, dominant affective tone, such as depression, which may give way periodically to anxious agitation or inappropriate outbursts of anger.

Chronic Depression. Depression is so common in clients with this disorder that before the inclusion of borderline personality disorder in the *DSM-III* (APA, 1980) many of these clients were diagnosed as depressed. Depression occurs in response to feelings of abandonment by

---

TABLE 34.10   RESEARCH CRITERIA FOR PASSIVE-AGGRESSIVE PERSONALITY DISORDER

A. A pervasive pattern of negativistic attitudes and passive resistance to demands for adequate performance, beginning by early adulthood and present in a variety of contexts, as indicated by four (or more) of the following:
   1. Passively resists fulfilling routine social and occupational tasks.
   2. Complains of being misunderstood and unappreciated by others.
   3. Is sullen and argumentative.
   4. Unreasonably criticizes and scorns authority.
   5. Expresses envy and resentment toward those apparently more fortunate.
   6. Voices exaggerated and persistent complaints of personal misfortune.
   7. Alternates between hostile defiance and contrition.
B. Does not occur exclusively during major depressive episodes and is not better accounted for by dysthymic disorder.

SOURCE: From APA (1994), with permission.

TABLE 34.11   DIAGNOSTIC CRITERIA FOR BORDERLINE PERSONALITY DISORDER

A pervasive pattern of instability of interpersonal relationships, self-image, and affects, and marked impulsivity beginning by early adulthood and present in a variety of contexts, as indicated by five (or more) of the following:

1. Frantic efforts to avoid real or imagined abandonment.
   (**Note:** Do not include suicidal or self-mutilating behavior covered in criterion 5.)
2. A pattern of unstable and intense interpersonal relationships characterized by alternating between extremes of idealization and devaluation.
3. Identity disturbance: markedly and persistently unstable self-image or sense of self.
4. Impulsivity in at least two areas that are potentially self-damaging (e.g., spending, sex, substance abuse, reckless driving, binge eating). (**Note:** Do not include suicidal or self-mutilating behavior covered in criterion 5.)
5. Recurrent suicidal behavior, gestures, or threats, or self-mutilating behavior.
6. Affective instability due to marked reactivity of mood (e.g., intense episodic dysphoria, irritability, or anxiety, usually lasting a few hours and only rarely more than a few days).
7. Chronic feelings of emptiness.
8. Inappropriate, intense anger or difficulty controlling anger (e.g., frequent displays of temper, constant anger, recurrent physical fights).
9. Transient, stress-related paranoid ideation or severe dissociative symptoms.

SOURCE: From APA (1994), with permission.

---

the mother in early childhood (see "Predisposing Factors"). Underlying the depression is a sense of rage that is sporadically turned inward on the self and externally on the environment. Seldom is the individual aware of the true source of these feelings until well into long-term therapy.

Inability to Be Alone. Because of this chronic fear of abandonment, clients with borderline personality disorder have little tolerance for being alone. They prefer a frantic search for companionship, no matter how unsatisfactory, to sitting with feelings of loneliness, emptiness, and boredom (Kaplan & Sadock, 1998).

Patterns of Interaction

Clinging and Distancing. The client with borderline personality disorder commonly exhibits a pattern of interaction with others that is characterized by clinging and distancing behaviors. When clients are clinging to another individual, they may exhibit helpless, dependent, or even childlike behaviors. They overidealize a single individual with whom they want to spend all their time, with whom they express a frequent need to talk, or from whom they seek constant reassurance. Acting-out behaviors, even self-mutilation, may result when they cannot be with this chosen individual. Distancing behaviors are characterized by hostility, anger, and devaluation of others, arising from a feeling of discomfort with closeness. Devaluation, which often occurs in response to separations, limits, or confrontations, is the tendency to discredit or undermine the strengths and personal significance of important others (Gunderson, 1989).

Splitting. **Splitting** is a primitive ego defense mechanism that is common in persons with borderline personality disorder. It arises from their lack of achievement of object constancy and is manifested by an inability to integrate and accept both positive and negative feelings. In their view, people—including themselves—and life situations are either all good or all bad.

Manipulation. In their efforts to prevent the separation they so desperately fear, clients with this disorder become masters of manipulation. Virtually any behavior becomes an acceptable means of achieving the desired result: relief from separation anxiety. Playing one individual against another is a common ploy to allay these fears of abandonment.

Self-Destructive Behaviors. Repetitive, self-mutilative behaviors are classic manifestations of borderline personality disorder. Even though these acts can be potentially fatal, most commonly they are manipulative gestures designed to elicit a rescue response from significant others. Suicide attempts are not uncommon and result from feelings of abandonment following separation from a significant other. The endeavor is often attempted, however, in a relatively "safe" place (e.g., swallowing pills in an area where the person will surely be discovered by others; or swallowing pills and making a phone call to report the deed to someone).

Other types of destructive behaviors include cutting, scratching, and burning. Various theories abound regarding why these individuals are able to inflict pain on themselves. One hypothesis suggests they may have higher levels of endorphins in their bodies than most people, thereby increasing their threshold for pain. Another theory relates to the individual's personal identity disturbance. It proposes that since much of the self-mutilating behaviors take place when the individual is in a state of depersonalization and derealization, he or she does not initially feel the pain. They continue to mutilate until the pain is felt, in an effort to counteract the feelings of unreality. Some clients with borderline personality disorder have reported that ". . . to feel pain is better than to feel nothing." Pain validates their existence.

Impulsivity. Individuals with borderline personality disorder have poor impulse control based on primary process functioning. Impulsive behaviors associated with borderline personality disorder include substance abuse, gambling, promiscuity, reckless driving, and binging and purging (APA, 1994). Many times these acting-out behaviors occur in response to real or perceived feelings of abandonment.

Predisposing Factors

According to the theory of object relations (Mahler, Pine, & Bergman, 1975), the infant passes through six phases from birth to 36 months, when a sense of separateness from the parenting figure is finally established. These phases are discussed below.

Phase 1 (Birth to 1 Month), Autistic Phase. During this period, the baby spends most of his or her time in a half-waking, half-sleeping state. The main goal is fulfillment of needs for survival and comfort.

Phase 2 (1 to 5 Months), Symbiotic Phase. At this time, there is a type of psychic fusion of mother and child. The child views the self as an extension of the parenting figure, although there is a developing awareness of external sources of need fulfillment.

Phase 3 (5 to 10 Months), Differentiation Phase. The child is beginning to recognize that there is a separateness between the self and the parenting figure.

Phase 4 (10 to 16 Months), Practicing Phase. This phase is characterized by increased locomotor functioning and the ability to explore the environment independently. A sense of separateness of the self is increased.

Phase 5 (16 to 24 Months), Rapprochement Phase. Awareness of separateness of the self becomes acute. This is frightening to the child, who wants to regain some lost closeness but not return to symbiosis. The child wants the mother there as needed for "emotional refueling" and to maintain feelings of security.

Phase 6 (24 to 36 Months), On the Way to Object Constancy Phase. In this phase, the child completes the individuation process and learns to relate to objects in an effective, constant manner. A sense of separateness is established, and the child is able to internalize a sustained image of the loved object or person when out of sight. Separation anxiety is resolved.

The individual with borderline personality disorder becomes fixed in the rapprochement phase of development. This occurs when the child shows increasing separation and autonomy. The mother, who feels secure in the relationship as long as the child is dependent, begins to feel threatened by the child's increasing independence. The mother may indeed be experiencing her own fears of abandonment. In response to separation behaviors, the mother withdraws the emotional support or "refueling" that is so vitally needed during this phase in order for the child to feel secure. Instead, the mother rewards clinging, dependent behaviors, while punishing (withholding emo-

tional support) independent behaviors. With his or her sense of emotional survival at stake, the child learns to behave in a manner that satisfies the parental wishes. An internal conflict develops within the child, based on fear of abandonment. He or she wants to achieve independence common to this stage of development, but fears that the mother will withdraw emotional support as a result. This unresolved fear of abandonment remains with the child into adulthood. Unresolved grief for the nurturing they failed to receive results in internalized rage that manifests itself in the depression so common in those with borderline personality disorder.

Gunderson (1989) has stated:

"This pattern of a hostile and conflictual relationship with the mother is not counterbalanced by a positive relationship with the father: both parents usually have significant psychopathology. Mothers tend to be erratic and depressed, whereas fathers are often absent or characterologically disturbed. These families are frequently flawed by a variety of disruptive acts including incest, violence, and alcoholism."

Diagnosis/Outcome Identification

Nursing diagnoses are formulated from the data gathered during the assessment phase and with background knowledge regarding predisposing factors to the disorder. Some common nursing diagnoses for the client with borderline personality disorder include:

Risk for self-mutilation related to parental emotional deprivation (unresolved fears of abandonment).

Dysfunctional grieving related to maternal deprivation during rapprochement phase of development (internalized as a loss, with fixation in anger stage of grieving process), evidenced by depressed mood, acting-out behaviors.

Impaired social interaction related to extreme fears of abandonment and engulfment, evidenced by alternating clinging and distancing behaviors.

Personal identity disturbance related to underdeveloped ego, evidenced by feelings of depersonalization and derealization.

Anxiety (severe to panic) related to unconscious conflicts based on fear of abandonment, evidenced by transient psychotic symptoms (disorganized thinking, misinterpretation of the environment).

Self-esteem disturbance related to lack of positive feedback, evidenced by manipulation of others and inability to tolerate being alone.

The following criteria may be used for measurement of outcomes in the care of clients with borderline personality disorder.

THE CLIENT:

1. Has not harmed self.
2. Seeks out staff when desire for self-mutilation is strong.

3. Is able to identify true source of anger.
4. Expresses anger appropriately.
5. Relates to more than one staff member.
6. Completes activities of daily living independently.
7. Does not manipulate one staff member against the other in order to fulfill own desires.

Planning/Implementation

In Table 34.12, selected nursing diagnoses common to the client with borderline personality disorder are presented in a plan of care. Outcome criteria are included, along with appropriate nursing interventions and rationales.

Evaluation

Reassessment is conducted to determine if the nursing actions have been successful in achieving the objectives of care. Evaluation of the nursing actions for the client with borderline personality disorder may be facilitated by gathering information using the following types of questions:

1. Has the client been able to seek out staff when feeling the desire for self-harm?
2. Has the client avoided self-harm?
3. Can the client correlate times of desire for self-harm to times of elevation in level of anxiety?
4. Can the client discuss feelings with staff (particularly feelings of depression and anger)?
5. Can the client identify the true source toward whom the anger is directed?
6. Can the client verbalize understanding of basis for anger?
7. Can the client express anger appropriately?
8. Can the client function independently?
9. Can the client relate to more than one staff member?
10. Can the client verbalize the knowledge that the staff members will return and are not abandoning the client when leaving for the day?
11. Can the client separate from the staff in an appropriate manner?
12. Can the client delay gratification and refrain from manipulating others in order to fulfill own desires?
13. Can the client verbalize resources within the community from whom he or she may seek assistance in times of extreme stress?

Antisocial Personality Disorder

Background Assessment Data

In the *DSM-I*, antisocial behavior was categorized as a "sociopathic or psychopathic" reaction that was symptomatic of any of several underlying personality disorders. The *DSM-II* represented it as a distinct personality type, a distinction that has been retained in subsequent editions. The *DSM-IV* diagnostic criteria for antisocial personality disorder are presented in Table 34.13.

Individuals with antisocial personality disorder are not often seen in most clinical settings, and when they are, it is commonly a way to avoid legal consequences. Sometimes they are admitted to the health care system by court order for psychological evaluation. Most frequently, however, these individuals may be encountered in prisons, jails, and rehabilitation services.

Clinical Picture

Phillips and Gunderson (1994) describe antisocial personality disorder as a pattern of socially irresponsible, exploitative, and guiltless behavior that reflects a disregard for the rights of others. There is a tendency to fail to conform to the law or to sustain consistent employment, to exploit and manipulate others for personal gain, and to fail to develop stable relationships. These individuals appear cold and callous, often intimidating others with their brusque and belligerent manner. They tend to be argumentative and, at times, cruel and malicious. They lack warmth and compassion and are often suspicious of these qualities in others.

Individuals with antisocial personality have a very low tolerance for frustration, act impetuously, and are unable to delay gratification. They are restless and easily bored, often taking chances and seeking thrills, acting as if they were immune to danger.

When things go their way, individuals with this disorder act cheerful, even gracious and charming. Because of their low tolerance for frustration, this pleasant exterior can change very quickly. When what they desire at the moment is challenged, they are likely to become furious and vindictive. Easily provoked to attack, their first inclination is to demean and dominate. They believe that "good guys come in last," and show contempt for the weak and underprivileged. They exploit others to fulfill their own desires, showing no trace of shame or guilt for their behavior.

Individuals with antisocial personalities see themselves as victims, using projection as the primary ego defense mechanism. They do not accept responsibility for the consequences of their behavior. Gorman, Sultan, and Raines (1996) state:

"These individuals have come to suspect that any person or institution may try to control them, rendering them powerless and vulnerable to attack." (p. 228)

In their own minds, this perception justifies their malicious behavior, lest they be the recipient of unjust persecution and hostility from others.

Satisfying interpersonal relationships are not possible, for individuals with antisocial personalities have learned to place their trust only in themselves. Their basic philosophy of life allows that "everyone is out to 'help number one' and that one should stop at nothing to avoid being pushed around" (APA, 1994).

TABLE 34.12 CARE PLAN FOR THE CLIENT WITH BORDERLINE PERSONALITY DISORDER

NURSING DIAGNOSIS: RISK FOR SELF-MUTILATION

RELATED TO: Parental emotional deprivation (unresolved fears of abandonment)

OUTCOME CRITERIA	NURSING INTERVENTIONS	RATIONALE
Client will not harm self.	1. Observe client's behavior frequently. Do this through routine activities and interactions; avoid appearing watchful and suspicious. 2. Secure a verbal contract from client that he or she will seek out staff member when urge for self-mutilation is felt. 3. If self-mutilation occurs, care for client's wounds in a matter-of-fact manner. Do not give positive reinforcement to this behavior by offering sympathy or additional attention. 4. Encourage client to talk about feelings he or she was having just prior to this behavior. 5. Act as a role model for appropriate expression of angry feelings and give positive reinforcement to client when attempts to conform are made. 6. Remove all dangerous objects from client's environment. 7. If warranted by high acuity of the situation, staff may need to be assigned on a one-to-one basis.	1. Close observation is required so that intervention can occur if required to ensure client's (and others') safety. 2. Discussing feelings of self-harm with a trusted individual provides a degree of relief to the client. A contract gets the subject out in the open, and places some of the responsibility for his or her safety with the client. An attitude of acceptance of the client as a worthwhile individual is conveyed. 3. Lack of attention to the maladaptive behavior may decrease repetition of its use. 4. To problem solve the situation with the client, knowledge of the precipitating factors is important. 5. It is vital that the client express angry feelings, as suicide and other self-destructive behaviors are often viewed as a result of anger turned inward on the self. 6. Client safety is a nursing priority. 7. Because of their extreme fear of abandonment, leaving clients with this disorder alone at a stressful time may cause an acute rise in anxiety and agitation levels.

NURSING DIAGNOSIS: DYSFUNCTIONAL GRIEVING

RELATED TO: Maternal deprivation during rapprochement phase of development (internalized as a loss, with fixation in anger stage of grieving process)

EVIDENCED BY: Depressed mood, acting-out behaviors

OUTCOME CRITERIA	NURSING INTERVENTIONS	RATIONALE
Client will be able to identify true source of anger, accept ownership of the feelings, and express them in a socially acceptable manner in an effort to initiate progression through the grief process.	1. Convey an accepting attitude—one that creates a nonthreatening environment for the client to express feelings. Be honest and keep all promises. 2. Identify the function that anger, frustration, and rage serve for the client. Allow him or her to express these feelings within reason. 3. Encourage client to discharge pent-up anger through participation in large motor activities (e.g., brisk walks, jogging, physical exercises, volleyball, punching bag, exercise bike).	1. An accepting attitude conveys to the client that you believe he or she is a worthwhile person. Trust is enhanced. 2. Verbalization of feelings in a nonthreatening environment may help client come to terms with unresolved issues. 3. Physical exercise provides a safe and effective method for discharging pent-up tension.

4. Explore with client the true source of the anger. This is a painful therapy that often leads to regression as the client deals with the feelings of early abandonment.

5. As anger is displaced onto the nurse or therapist, caution must be taken to guard against the negative effects of countertransference. These are very difficult clients who have the capacity for eliciting a whole array of negative feelings from the therapist.

6. Explain the behaviors associated with the normal grieving process. Help the client recognize his or her position in this process.

7. Help client to understand appropriate ways to express anger. Give positive reinforcement for behaviors used to express anger appropriately. Act as a role model.

8. Set limits on acting-out behaviors and explain consequences of violation of those limits. Be supportive yet consistent and firm in caring for this client.

4. Reconciliation of the feelings associated with this stage is necessary before progression through the grieving process can continue.

5. The existence of negative feelings by the nurse or therapist must be acknowledged, but they must not be allowed to interfere with the therapeutic process.

6. Knowledge of the acceptability of the feelings associated with normal grieving may help to relieve some of the guilt that these responses generate.

7. Positive reinforcement enhances self-esteem and encourages repetition of desirable behaviors.

8. Client lacks sufficient self-control to limit maladaptive behaviors, so assistance is required from staff. Without consistency on the part of all staff members working with this client, however, a positive outcome will not be achieved.

NURSING DIAGNOSIS: IMPAIRED SOCIAL INTERACTION

RELATED TO: Extreme fears of abandonment and engulfment

EVIDENCED BY: Alternating clinging and distancing behaviors and staff splitting

OUTCOME CRITERIA	NURSING INTERVENTIONS	RATIONALE
Client will exhibit no evidence of splitting or clinging and distancing behaviors in relationships with staff and/or peers.	1. Encourage client to examine these behaviors (to recognize that they are occurring).	1. Client may be unaware of splitting or clinging and distancing pattern of interaction with others. Recognition must occur before change can occur.
	2. Help client realize that you will be available, without reinforcing dependent behaviors.	2. Knowledge of your availability may provide needed security for the client.
	3. Give positive reinforcement for independent behaviors.	3. Positive reinforcement enhances self-esteem and encourages repetition of desirable behaviors.
	4. Rotate staff who work with the client in order to avoid client's developing dependence on particular staff members.	4. Client must learn to relate to more than one staff member in an effort to decrease use of splitting and diminish fears of abandonment.
	5. Explore feelings that relate to fears of abandonment and engulfment with client. Help client understand that clinging and distancing behaviors are engendered by these fears.	5. Exploration of feelings with a trusted individual may help client come to terms with unresolved issues.
	6. Help client understand how these behaviors interfere with satisfactory relationships.	6. Client may be unaware of others' perception of him or her and why these behaviors are not acceptable to others.
	7. Assist client to work toward achievement of object constancy. Be available, without promoting dependency.	7. This may help client resolve fears of abandonment and develop the ability to establish satisfactory intimate relationships.

TABLE 34.13   DIAGNOSTIC CRITERIA FOR ANTISOCIAL PERSONALITY DISORDER

A. A pervasive pattern of disregard for and violation of the rights of others occurring since age 15 years, as indicated by three (or more) of the following:
   1. Failure to conform to social norms with respect to lawful behaviors as indicated by repeatedly performing acts that are grounds for arrest.
   2. Deceitfulness, as indicated by repeated lying, use of aliases, or conning others for personal profit or pleasure.
   3. Impulsivity or failure to plan ahead.
   4. Irritability and aggressiveness, as indicated by repeated physical fights or assaults.
   5. Reckless disregard for safety of self or others.
   6. Consistent irresponsibility, as indicated by repeated failure to sustain consistent work behavior or honor financial obligations.
   7. Lack of remorse, as indicated by being indifferent to or rationalizing having hurt, mistreated, or stolen from another.
B. Individual at least 18 years old.
C. Conduct disorder evident before age 15 years.
D. Antisocial behavior not occurring exclusively during the course of schizophrenia or a manic episode.

SOURCE: From APA (1994), with permission.

One of the most distinctive characteristics of antisocial personalities is their tendency to ignore conventional authority and rules. They act as though established social norms and guidelines for self-discipline and cooperative behavior do not apply to them. They are flagrant in their disrespect for the law and for the rights of others.

Predisposing Factors

Biological Influences. The *DSM-IV* reports that antisocial personality is more common among first-degree biological relatives of those with the disorder than among the general population (APA, 1994). Cadoret (1994) reports on studies that implicate the role of genetics in antisocial personality disorder. These studies of families of individuals with antisocial personality show higher numbers of relatives with antisocial personality or alcoholism than are found in the general population. Additional studies have shown that children of parents with antisocial behavior are more likely to be diagnosed as antisocial personality, even though separated at birth from biological parents.

Characteristics associated with temperament in the newborn may be significant in the predisposition to antisocial personality. Parents who bring their behavior-disordered children to clinics often report that the child displayed temper tantrums from infancy and would get furious when frustrated, either when awaiting the bottle or feeling uncomfortable in a wet diaper (Millon, 1981). As these children mature, they commonly develop a bullying attitude toward other children. Parents report that they are undaunted by punishment and generally quite unmanageable. They are daring and foolhardy in their willingness to chance physical harm and seem unaffected by pain.

Mannuzza and associates (1998) identified attention-deficit hyperactivity disorder and conduct disorder during prepuberty as predisposing factors to antisocial personality disorder.

While these biogenetic influences may describe some familial pattern to the development of antisocial personality disorder, no basic pathology process has yet been determined as an etiological factor. Cadoret (1994) states:

"While abnormalities of electroencephalography or autonomic nervous system reactivity have been described more frequently in antisocial populations, many antisocials still do not show such abnormalities. Any basic structural, biochemical, or functional abnormality eludes us at present." (p. 212)

Family Dynamics. Antisocial personality disorder frequently arises from a chaotic home environment (Cadoret, 1994). Parental deprivation during the first 5 years of life appears to be a critical predisposing factor in the development of antisocial personality disorder. Separation due to parental delinquency appears to be more highly correlated with the disorder than is parental loss from other causes. The presence or intermittent appearance of inconsistent impulsive parents, not the loss of a consistent parent, is environmentally *most* damaging.

A consistent finding in the histories of individuals with antisocial personality disorder is having been severely physically abused (Lewis, 1989). The abuse contributes to the development of antisocial behavior in several ways. First, it provides a model for behavior. Second, it may result in injury to the child's central nervous system, thereby impairing the child's ability to function appropriately. Finally, it engenders rage in the victimized child, which is then displaced onto others in the environment.

Townsend (1997) cites several sources that have implicated family functioning as an important factor in determining whether or not an individual develops antisocial personality. The following circumstances may influence the predisposition to antisocial personality disorder:

1. Absence of parental discipline.
2. Extreme poverty.

3. Removal from the home.
4. Growing up without parental figures of both sexes.
5. Erratic and inconsistent methods of discipline.
6. Being "rescued" each time they are in trouble (never having to suffer the consequences of their own behavior).
7. Maternal deprivation.

Diagnosis/Outcome Identification

Nursing diagnoses are formulated from the data gathered during the assessment phase and with background knowledge regarding predisposing factors to the disorder. Some common nursing diagnoses for the client with antisocial personality disorder include:

Risk for violence: directed at others related to rage reactions, negative role-modeling, inability to tolerate frustration.

Defensive coping related to dysfunctional family system, evidenced by disregard for societal norms and laws, absence of guilty feelings, or inability to delay gratification.

Self-esteem disturbance related to repeated negative feedback resulting in diminished self-worth, evidenced by manipulation of others to fulfill own desires or inability to form close, personal relationships.

Impaired social interaction related to negative role-modeling and low self-esteem, evidenced by inability to develop a satisfactory, enduring, intimate relationship with another.

Knowledge deficit (self-care activities to achieve and maintain optimal wellness) related to lack of interest in learning and denial of need for information, evidenced by demonstration of inability to take responsibility for meeting basic health practices.

The following criteria may be used to measure outcomes in the care of the client with antisocial personality disorder:

THE CLIENT:

1. Discusses angry feelings with staff and in group sessions.
2. Has not harmed self or others.
3. Can rechannel hostility into socially acceptable behaviors.
4. Follows rules and regulations of the milieu environment.
5. Can verbalize which of his or her behaviors are not acceptable.
6. Shows regard for the rights of others by delaying gratification of own desires when appropriate.
7. Does not manipulate others in an attempt to increase feelings of self-worth.

8. Verbalizes understanding of knowledge required to maintain basic health needs.

Planning/Implementation

Table 34.14 presents a care plan of selected nursing diagnoses common to the client with antisocial personality disorder. Outcome criteria are presented, along with appropriate nursing interventions and rationales.

Evaluation

Reassessment is conducted to determine if the nursing actions have been successful in achieving the objectives of care. Evaluation of the nursing actions for the client with antisocial personality disorder may be facilitated by gathering information using the following types of questions:

1. Does the client recognize when anger is getting out of control?
2. Can the client seek out staff instead of expressing anger in an appropriate manner?
3. Can the client use other sources for rechanneling anger (e.g., physical activities)?
4. Has harm to others been avoided?
5. Can the client follow rules and regulations of the milieu with little or no reminding?
6. Can the client verbalize which behaviors are appropriate and which are not?
7. Does the client express a *desire* to change?
8. Can the client delay gratifying own desires in deference to those of others when appropriate?
9. Does the client manipulate others in an attempt to have his or her own desires fulfilled?
10. Does the client fulfill activities of daily living willingly and independently?
11. Can the client verbalize methods of achieving and maintaining optimal wellness?
12. Can the client verbalize community resources from whom he or she can seek assistance with daily living and health care needs when required?

TREATMENT MODALITIES

Few would argue that treatment of individuals with personality disorders is difficult and, in some instances, may even seem impossible. Personality characteristics are learned very early in life and perhaps may even be genetic. It is not surprising, then, that these enduring patterns of behavior may take years to change, if change occurs. Widiger and Frances (1988) state, "In most cases it is unrealistic to set a goal of fundamental alteration of the personality style. A more practical goal would be to lessen the inflexibility of the maladaptive traits and to reduce their

TABLE 34.14 CARE PLAN FOR THE CLIENT WITH ANTISOCIAL PERSONALITY DISORDER

NURSING DIAGNOSIS: RISK FOR VIOLENCE: DIRECTED AT OTHERS
RELATED TO: Rage reactions, negative role-modeling, inability to tolerate frustration

OUTCOME CRITERIA	NURSING INTERVENTIONS	RATIONALE
Client will not harm self or others.	1. Convey an accepting attitude toward this client. Feelings of rejection are undoubtedly familiar to the client. Work on development of trust. Be honest, keep all promises, and convey the message that it is not him or her but the behavior that is unacceptable.	1. An attitude of acceptance promotes feelings of self-worth. Trust is the basis upon which a therapeutic relationship is established.
	2. Maintain low level of stimuli in client's environment (low lighting, few people, simple decor, low noise level).	2. A stimulating environment may increase agitation and promote aggressive behavior.
	3. Observe client's behavior frequently during routine activities and interactions, but avoid appearing watchful and suspicious.	3. Close observation is required so that intervention can occur if required to ensure client's (and others') safety.
	4. Remove all dangerous objects from client's environment.	4. Client safety is a nursing policy.
	5. Help client identify the true object of his or her hostility.	5. Because of weak ego development, client may be misusing the defense mechanism of displacement. Helping him or her recognize this in a nonthreatening manner may help reveal unresolved issues so that they may be confronted.
	6. Encourage client to gradually verbalize hostile feelings.	6. Verbalization of feelings in a nonthreatening environment may help client come to terms with unresolved issues.
	7. Explore with client alternative ways of handling frustration (e.g., large motor skills that channel hostile energy into socially acceptable behaviors).	7. Physically demanding activities help to relieve pent-up tension.
	8. Staff should maintain and convey a calm attitude.	8. Anxiety is contagious and can be transferred from staff to client. A calm attitude provides client with a feeling of safety and security.
	9. Have sufficient staff available to present a show of strength to client if necessary.	9. This conveys to client evidence of control over the situation and provides some physical security for the staff.
	10. Administer tranquilizing medications as ordered by physician or obtain an order if necessary. Monitor for effectiveness and for adverse side effects.	10. Antianxiety agents (e.g., diazepam, chlordiazepoxide, oxazepam) produce a calming effect and may help to allay hostile behaviors. (*Note:* Medications are not often prescribed for clients with this disorder because of these individuals' strong susceptibility to addictions.)
	11. If client is not calmed by "talking down" or by medication, use of mechanical restraints may be necessary. Be sure to have sufficient staff available to assist. Follow protocol established by the institution in executing this intervention. Most	11. Client safety is a nursing priority.

states require that the physician reevaluate and issue a new order for restraints every 3 hr, except between the hours of midnight and 8:00 AM. If client has refused medication, administer after restraints have been applied. Most states consider this intervention appropriate in emergency situations or in the event that a client would likely harm self or others. Never use restraints as a punitive measure but rather as a protective measure for a client who is out of control. Observe the client in restraints every 15 min (or according to institutional policy). Ensure that circulation to extremities is not compromised (check temperature, color, pulses). Assist client with needs related to nutrition, hydration, and elimination. Position client so that comfort is facilitated and aspiration can be prevented.

NURSING DIAGNOSIS: DEFENSIVE COPING

RELATED TO: Dysfunctional family system

EVIDENCED BY: Disregard for societal norms and laws, absence of guilty feelings, inability to delay gratification

OUTCOME CRITERIA	NURSING INTERVENTIONS	RATIONALE
Client will be able to follow rules and delay personal gratification.	1. From the onset, client should be made aware of which behaviors are acceptable and which are not. Explain consequences of violation of the limits. A consequence must involve something of value to the client. All staff must be consistent in enforcing these limits. Consequences should be administered in a matter-of-fact manner immediately following the infraction.	1. Because client cannot (or will not) impose own limits on maladaptive behaviors, they must be delineated and enforced by staff. Undesirable consequences may help to decrease repetition of these behaviors.
	2. Do not attempt to coax or convince client to do the "right thing." Do not use the words "You should (or shouldn't) . . . "; instead, use "You will be expected to . . . " The ideal would be for client to eventually internalize societal norms, beginning with this step-by-step, "either/or" approach (either you do [don't do] this, or this will occur).	2. Explanations must be concise, concrete, and clear, with little or no capacity for misinterpretation.
	3. Provide positive feedback or reward for acceptable behaviors.	3. Positive reinforcement enhances self-esteem and encourages repetition of desirable behaviors.
	4. Begin to increase the length of time requirement for acceptable behavior in order to achieve the reward. For example, 2 hr of acceptable behavior may be exchanged for a phone call, 4 hr for 2 hr of television; 1 day of acceptable behavior for a recreational therapy bowling activity, 5 days for a weekend pass.	4. This type of intervention may assist the client in learning to delay gratification.

Continued on following page

TABLE 34.14 *(Continued)*

5. A milieu unit provides the appropriate environment for the client with antisocial personality.	5. The democratic approach, with specific rules and regulations, community meetings, and group therapy sessions, emulates the type of societal situation in which the client must learn to live. Feedback from peers is often more effective than confrontation from an authority figure. The client learns to follow the rules of the group as a positive step in the progression toward internalizing the rules of society.
6. Help client to gain insight into his or her own behaviors. Often these individuals rationalize to such an extent that they deny that what they have done is wrong (e.g., "The owner of this store has so much money, he'll never miss the little bit I take. He has everything, and I have nothing. It's not fair! I deserve to have some of what he has.")	6. Client must come to understand that certain behaviors will not be tolerated within the society and that severe consequences will be imposed upon those individuals who refuse to comply. Client must *want* to become a productive member of society before he or she can be helped.
7. Talk about past behaviors with client. Discuss behaviors which are acceptable by society and those which are not. Help client identify ways in which he or she has exploited others. Encourage client to explore how he or she would feel if the circumstances were reversed.	7. An attempt may be made to enlighten the client to the sensitivity of others by promoting self-awareness in an effort to help the client gain insight into his or her own behavior.
8. Throughout relationship with client, maintain attitude of "It is not *you*, but your *behavior*, that is unacceptable."	8. An attitude of acceptance promotes feelings of dignity and self-worth.

interference with everyday functioning and meaningful relationships."

Little research exists to guide the decision of which therapy is most appropriate in the treatment of personality disorders. Selection of intervention is generally based on the area of greatest dysfunction, such as cognition, affect, behavior, or interpersonal relations. Following is a brief description of various types of therapies and the disorders to which they are customarily suited.

Interpersonal Psychotherapy

Depending on the therapeutic goals, interpersonal psychotherapy for personality disorders is either brief and time-limited or long-term exploratory psychotherapy. Interpersonal psychotherapy may be particularly appropriate because personality disorders largely reflect problems in interpersonal style. Widiger and Frances (1988) suggest the following approach:

"The strategy is to adopt an interpersonal style that encourages more flexible and adaptive functioning in the client to break the collusive pattern of mutually debilitating relationships. Oppositional and controlling clients may be directed toward more adaptive functioning by being explicitly encouraged to escalate their maladaptive personality traits."

Interpersonal psychotherapy is suggested for clients with paranoid, schizoid, schizotypal, borderline, dependent, narcissistic, and obsessive-compulsive personality disorders.

Psychoanalytical Psychotherapy

The treatment of choice for individuals with histrionic personality disorder has been psychoanalytical psychotherapy (Phillips & Gunderson, 1994). Treatment focuses on the unconscious motivation for seeking total satisfaction from others and for being unable to commit oneself to a stable, meaningful relationship.

Milieu or Group Therapy

This treatment is especially appropriate for individuals with antisocial personality disorder, who respond more adaptively to support and feedback from peers; in milieu or group therapy, feedback from peers is more effective than in one-to-one interaction with a therapist. Group therapy—particularly homogeneous supportive groups that emphasize the development of social skills—may be helpful in overcoming social anxiety and developing interpersonal trust and rapport in clients with avoidant personality disorder (Phillips & Gunderson, 1994). Feminist consciousness-raising groups can be useful in helping dependent clients struggling with social-role stereotypes.

Cognitive/Behavioral Therapy

Behavioral strategies offer reinforcement for positive change. Social skills training and assertiveness training teach alternative ways to deal with frustration. Cognitive strategies help the client recognize and correct inaccurate internal mental shemata (Phillips & Gunderson, 1994). This type of therapy may be useful for clients with obsessive-compulsive, passive-aggressive, antisocial, and avoidant personality disorders.

TEST YOUR CRITICAL THINKING SKILLS

Lana, age 32, had been diagnosed with borderline personality disorder when she was 26 years old. Her husband had taken her to the emergency department at that time when he walked into the bathroom and found her cutting her legs with a razor blade. At that time, assessment revealed that Lana had a long history of self-mutilation, which she had carefully hidden from her husband and others. Lana began long-term psychoanalytical psychotherapy on an outpatient basis. Therapy revealed that Lana had been physically and sexually abused as a child by both her mother and her father, both now deceased. She admitted to having chronic depression, and her husband related episodes of rage reactions. Lana has been hospitalized on the psychiatric unit for a week because of suicidal ideations. After making a no-suicide contract with the staff, she is allowed to leave the unit on pass to keep a dental appointment that she made a number of weeks ago. She has just returned to the unit and says to her nurse, "I just took 20 Desyrel while I was sitting in my car in the parking lot."

Answer the following questions related to Lana:

1. The nurse is well acquainted with Lana and believes this is a manipulative gesture. How should the nurse handle this situation?
2. What is the priority nursing diagnosis for Lana?
3. Lana likes to "split" the staff into "good guys" and "bad guys." What is the most important intervention for splitting by a person with borderline personality disorder?

RESEARCH NOTE

Reported pathological childhood experiences associated with the development of borderline personality disorder. *American Journal of Psychiatry* (1997, August), 154, 1101–1106.
Zanarini, M.C., Williams, A.A., Lewis, R.E., Reich, R.B., Vera, S.C., Marino, M.F., Levin, A., Yong, L., and Frankenburg, F.R.

Description of the Study: The purpose of this study was to assess a full range of pathological childhood experiences reported by clients with borderline personality disorder in comparison with clients with other personality disorders. The sample included 467 inpatients with personality disorders: 358 with borderline personality disorder and 109 with other personality disorders. Information was gathered by interviewers, who used a semistructured research interview tool and had no knowledge of clinical diagnosis.

Results of the Study: Of the 358 clients with borderline personality, 91 percent reported some type of abuse and 92 percent reported having been neglected before the age of 18. This compared with approximately 75 percent of the clients with other personality disorders. Clients with borderline personality disorder were significantly more likely to have been emotionally and physically abused by a caretaker, sexually abused by noncaretaker, and to have had a caretaker withdraw from them emotionally, treat them inconsistently, deny their thoughts and feelings, place them in the role of a parent, and fail to protect them. Over 60 percent of clients with borderline personality disorder reported having been sexually abused, and these clients were more likely than those without such a history to report having experienced all types of abuse and neglect studied.

Comments: When considering all significant risk factors together, four were found to be significant predictors of borderline personality disorder: female gender, sexual abuse by a male noncaretaker, emotional denial by a male caretaker, and inconsistent treatment by a female caretaker. The authors conclude that the results suggest that sexual abuse is neither necessary nor sufficient for the development of borderline personality disorder and that other childhood experiences, particularly neglect by caretakers of both genders, represent significant risk factors.

Psychopharmacology

Psychopharmacology may be helpful in some instances. Although these drugs have no direct effect in the treatment of the disorders themselves, some symptomatic relief can be achieved. Antipsychotic medications are helpful in the treatment of psychotic decompensations experienced by clients with paranoid and schizotypal personality disorders (Phillips & Gunderson, 1994).

A variety of pharmacological interventions have been used with borderline personality disorder. Carbamazepine and monoamine oxidase inhibitors have been successful in decreasing impulsivity and self-destructive acts in these clients (Phillips & Gunderson, 1994). Antipsychotics have resulted in improvement in illusions,

INTERNET REFERENCES

● Additional information about personality disorders may be located at the following websites:
  a. http://www.mental-health-matters.com/borderline.html
  b. http://www.cmhc.com/guide/person.htm
  c. http://www.usd.edu/~pwyss/person.dis.html
  d. http://www.dhearts.org/community/Mental_Health/Personality_Disorders/
  e. http://www.mentalhealth.com/dis/p20-pe04.html
  f. http://www.mentalhealth.com/dis/p20-pe08.html
  g. http://www.mentalhealth.com/dis/p20-pe05.html
  h. http://www.mentalhealth.com/dis/p20-pe09.html
  i. http://www.mentalhealth.com/dis/p20-pe06.html
  j. http://www.mentalhealth.com/dis/p20-pe07.html
  k. http://www.mentalhealth.com/dis/p20-pe10.html
  l. http://www.mentalhealth.com/dis/p20-pe01.html
  m. http://www.mentalhealth.com/dis/p20-pe02.html
  n. http://www.mentalhealth.com/dis/p20-pe03.html
  o. http://www.mentalhealth.com/p13.html#Per

ideas of reference, paranoid thinking, anxiety, and hostility in some clients. The selective serotonin reuptake inhibitors fluoxetine (Prozac), sertraline (Zoloft), and paroxetine (Paxil) have been very successful in clients with borderline personality in reducing anger, impulsiveness, and mood instability (Salzman, 1996).

Lithium carbonate and propranolol (Inderal) may be useful for the violent episodes observed in clients with antisocial personality disorder (Cadoret, 1994). Caution must be used in prescribing medications outside the structured setting because of the high risk for substance abuse by these individuals.

For the client with avoidant personality disorder, anxiolytics are sometimes helpful whenever previously avoided behavior is being attempted. The mere possession of the medication may be reassurance enough to help the client through the stressful period. Antidepressants, such as imipramine (Tofranil) or fluoxetine (Prozac) may be useful with these clients if panic disorder develops.

SUMMARY

Clients with personality disorders are undoubtedly some of the most difficult ones health care workers are likely to encounter. Personality characteristics are formed very early in life and are difficult, if not impossible, to change. In fact, some clinicians believe the therapeutic approach is not to try to change the characteristics but rather to decrease the inflexibility of the maladaptive traits and reduce their interference with everyday functioning and meaningful relationships.

This chapter presents a review of the development of personality according to Sullivan, Erikson, and Mahler. The stages identified by these theorists represent the "normal" progression and establish a foundation for studying dysfunctional patterns.

The concept of a personality disorder has been present throughout the history of medicine. Problems have arisen in the attempt to establish a classification system for three disorders. The *DSM-IV* groups them into these clusters. Cluster A (behaviors described as odd or eccentric) includes paranoid, schizoid, and schizotypal personality disorders. Cluster B (behaviors described as dramatic, emotional, or erratic) includes antisocial, borderline, histrionic, and narcissistic personality disorders. Cluster C (behaviors described as anxious or fearful) includes avoidant, dependent, obsessive-compulsive, and passive-aggressive personality disorders.

Nursing care of the client with a personality disorder is accomplished using the steps of the nursing process. Background assessment data were presented, along with information regarding possible etiological implications for each disorder. An overview of current medical treatment modalities for each disorder was presented.

Care of clients with borderline personality disorder and antisocial personality disorder was described at length. Individuals with borderline personality disorder may enter the health care system because of their instability and frequent attempts at self-destructive behavior. The individual with antisocial personality disorder may become part of the health care system to avoid legal consequences or because of a court order for psychological evaluation. Nursing diagnoses common to each disorder were presented, along with appropriate interventions and relevant outcome criteria for each.

Nurses who work in all types of clinical settings should be familiar with the characteristics associated with personality-disordered individuals. Nurses working in psychiatry must be knowledgeable about appropriate intervention with these clients, for it is unlikely that many of their other types of clients will match the challenge these clients present.

REVIEW QUESTIONS

SELF-EXAMINATION/LEARNING EXERCISE

Select the answer that is most appropriate for each of the following questions:

1. Kim has a diagnosis of borderline personality disorder. She often exhibits alternating clinging and distancing behaviors. The most appropriate nursing intervention with this type of behavior would be to:
   a. Encourage Kim to establish trust in one staff person, with whom all therapeutic interaction should take place.
   b. Secure a verbal contract from Kim that she will discontinue these behaviors.
   c. Withdraw attention if these behaviors continue.
   d. Rotate staff members who work with Kim so that she will learn to relate to more than one person.

2. Kim manipulates the staff in an effort to fulfill her own desires. All of the following may be examples of manipulative behaviors in the borderline client *except:*
   a. Refusal to stay in room alone, stating, "It's so lonely."
   b. Asking Nurse Jones for cigarettes after 30 minutes, knowing the assigned nurse has explained she must wait 1 hour.
   c. Stating to Nurse Jones, "I really like having you for my nurse. You're the best one around here."
   d. Cutting arms with razor blade after discussing dismissal plans with physician.

3. "Splitting" by the client with borderline personality disorder denotes:
   a. Evidence of precocious development.
   b. A primitive defense mechanism in which the client sees objects as all good or all bad.
   c. A brief psychotic episode in which the client loses contact with reality.
   d. Two distinct personalities within the borderline client.

4. According to Margaret Mahler, predisposition to borderline personality disorder occurs when developmental tasks go unfulfilled in which of the following phases?
   a. Autistic phase, during which the child's needs for security and comfort go unfulfilled.
   b. Symbiotic phase, during which the child fails to bond with the mother.
   c. Differentiation phase, during which the child fails to recognize a separateness between self and mother.
   d. Rapprochement phase, during which the mother withdraws emotional support in response to the child's increasing independence.

Jack was arrested for breaking into a jewelry store and stealing thousands of dollars worth of diamonds. At his arraignment, the judge ordered a psychological evaluation. He has just been admitted by court order to the locked unit. Based on a long history of maladaptive behavior, he has been given the diagnosis of antisocial personality disorder.

5. Which of the following characteristics would you expect to assess in Jack?
   a. Lack of guilt for wrongdoing.
   b. Insight into his own behavior.
   c. Ability to learn from past experiences.
   d. Compliance with authority.

6. Milieu therapy is a good choice for clients with antisocial personality disorder because it:
   a. Provides a system of punishment and rewards for behavior modification.
   b. Emulates a social community in which the client may learn to live harmoniously with others.
   c. Provides mostly one-to-one interaction between the client and therapist.
   d. Provides a very structured setting in which the clients have very little input into the planning of their care.

7. In evaluating Jack's progress, which of the following behaviors would be considered the most significant indication of positive change?

    a. Jack got angry only once in group this week.

    b. Jack was able to wait a whole hour for a cigarette without verbally abusing the staff.

    c. On his own initiative, Jack sent a note of apology to a man he had injured in a recent fight.

    d. Jack stated that he would no longer start any more fights.

8. Donna and Katie work in the secretarial pool of a large organization. It is 30 minutes until quitting time when a supervisor hands Katie a job that will take an hour and says he wants it before she leaves. She then says to Donna, "I can't stay over! I'm meeting Bill at 5:00 PM! Be a doll, Donna. Do this job for me!" Donna agrees, although silently she is furious at Katie since this is the third time this has happened in 2 weeks. Katie leaves and Donna says to herself, "This is crazy. I'm not finishing this job for her. Let's see how she likes getting in trouble for a change." Donna leaves without finishing the job. This is an example of which type of personality characteristic?

    a. Antisocial.

    b. Paranoid.

    c. Passive-aggressive.

    d. Obsessive-compulsive.

9. Carol is a new nursing graduate being oriented on a medical/surgical unit by the head nurse, Mrs. Carey. When Carol describes a new technique she has learned for positioning immobile clients, Mrs. Carey states, "What are you trying to do . . . tell me how to do my job? We have always done it this way on this unit, and we will continue to do it this way until I say differently!" This is an example of which type of personality characteristic?

    a. Antisocial.

    b. Paranoid.

    c. Passive-aggressive.

    d. Obsessive-compulsive.

10. Which of the following behavioral patterns is characteristic of individuals with histrionic personality disorder?

    a. They belittle themselves and their abilities.

    b. They inappropriately overreact to minor stimuli.

    c. They are suspicious and mistrustful of others.

    d. They have a lifelong pattern of social withdrawal.

REFERENCES

American Psychiatric Association. (1980). *Diagnostic and statistical manual of mental disorders* (3rd ed.). Washington, DC: American Psychiatric Association.

American Psychiatric Association. (1987). *Diagnostic and statistical manual of mental disorders* (3rd ed., rev.), Washington, DC: American Psychiatric Association.

American Psychiatric Association. (1994). *Diagnostic and statistical manual of mental disorders.* (4th ed.). Washington, DC: American Psychiatric Association.

Cadoret, R. (1994) Antisocial personality. In G. Winokur & P.J. Clayton (Eds.), *The medical basis of psychiatry.* Philadelphia: W.B. Saunders.

Erikson, E. (1963). *Childhood and society* (2nd ed.). New York: W.W. Norton.

Frances, A., & Widiger, T. (1986). A critical review of four *DSM-III* personality disorders: An overview of problems and solutions. In A. Frances & R. Hales (Eds.), *Psychiatry update: The American Psychiatric Association annual review* (Vol. 5.). Washington, DC: American Psychiatric Press.

Gorman, L., Sultan, D.F., & Raines, M.L. (1996). *Davis's manual of psychosocial nursing for general patient care.* Philadelphia: F.A. Davis.

Gunderson, J.G. (1989). Borderline personality disorder. In H.I. Kaplan & B.J. Sadock (Eds.), *Comprehensive textbook of psychiatry* (Vol. 2), (5th ed.). Baltimore: Williams & Wilkins.

Horney, K. (1939). *New ways in psychoanalysis.* New York: WW Norton.

International Classification of Diseases (10th ed.). (1992). *Classification of mental and behavioral disorders: Clinical descriptions and diagnostic guidelines.* Geneva: World Health Organization.

Kaplan, H.I., & Sadock, B.J. (1998). *Synopsis of psychiatry: Behavioral sciences/clinical psychiatry* (8th ed.). Baltimore: Williams & Wilkins.

Lewis, D.O. (1989). Adult antisocial behavior and criminality. In H.I. Kaplan & B.J. Sadock (Eds.), *Comprehensive textbook of psychiatry* (Vol. 2) (5th ed.). Baltimore: Williams & Wilkins.

Mahler, M., Pine, F., & Bergman, A. (1975). *The psychological birth of the human infant.* New York: Basic Books.

Mannuzza, S., et al. (1998, April). Adult psychiatric status of hyperactive boys grown up. *American Journal of Psychiatry, 155,* 493–498.

Millon, T. (1981). *Disorders of personality.* New York: John Wiley.

Perry, J.C., & Vaillant, G.E. (1989). Personality disorders. In H.I. Kaplan & B.J. Sadock (Eds.), *Comprehensive textbook of psychiatry* (Vol. 2) (5th ed.). Baltimore: Williams & Wilkins.

Phillips, K.A., & Gunderson, J.G. (1994). Personality disorders. In R.E. Hales, S.C. Yudofsky, & J.A. Talbott (Eds.), *The American Psychiatric Press textbook of psychiatry* (2nd ed.). Washington, DC: American Psychiatric Press.

Pfohl, B. (1994). Personality disorders. In G. Winokur & P.J. Clayton (Eds.), *The medical basis of psychiatry* (2nd ed.). Philadelphia: W.B. Saunders.

Salzman, C. (1996). What drug treatments are available for borderline personality disorder? *The Harvard Mental Health Letter, 13*(3), 8.

Schmideberg, M. (1956). The borderline patient. In S. Arieti (Ed.), *American handbook of psychiatry* (Vol. 1). New York: Basic Books.

Stern, A. (1938). Psychoanalytic investigation of and therapy in the borderline group of neuroses. *Psychoanalytic Quarterly, 7*, 467–489.

Sullivan, H.S. (1953). *The interpersonal theory of psychiatry.* New York: W.W. Norton & Co.

Townsend, M.C. (1997). *Nursing diagnoses in psychiatric nursing: A pocket guide for care plan construction* (4th ed.). Philadelphia: F.A. Davis.

Widiger, T.A., & Frances, A.J. (1988). Personality disorders. In J.A. Talbott et al. (Eds.), *The American Psychiatric Press textbook of psychiatry.* Washington, DC: American Psychiatric Press.

Bibliography

Atlas, J.A. (1995, December). Association between history of abuse and borderline personality disorder for hospitalized adolescent girls. *Psychological Reports, 77*, 1346.

Black, D.W., & Braun, D. (1998, June). Antisocial patients: A comparison of those with and those without childhood conduct disorder. *Annals of Clinical Psychiatry, 10*, 53–57.

Coccaro, E.F. (1998). Clinical outcome of psychopharmacologic treatment of borderline and schizotypal personality disordered subjects. *Journal of Clinical Psychiatry, 59* (Suppl. 1), 30–37.

Diaferia, G., et al. (1997, January–February). Relationship between obsessive-compulsive personality disorder and obsessive-compulsive disorder. *Comprehensive Psychiatry, 38*, 38–42.

Figueroa, E.F., & Silk, K.R. (1997, Spring). Biological implications of childhood sexual abuse in borderline personality disorder. *Journal of Personality Disorders, 11*, 71–92.

Figueroa, E.F., Silk, K.R., Huth, A., & Lohr, N.E. (1997, January–February). History of childhood sexual abuse and general psychopathology. *Comprehensive Psychiatry, 38*, 23–30.

Greene, H. (1995, December). The "stably unstable" borderline personality disorder: History, theory and nursing intervention. *Journal of Psychosocial Nursing and Mental Health Services, 33*(12), 26–30.

Langbehn, D.R., et al. (1998, September). Distinct contributions of conduct and oppositional defiant symptoms to adult antisocial behavior: Evidence from an adoption study. *Archives of General Psychiatry, 55*, 821–829.

Mckay, D., & Neziroglu, F. (1996, June). Social skills training in a case of obsessive-compulsive disorder with schizotypal personality disorder. *Journal of Behavior Therapy and Experimental Psychiatry, 27*, 189–194.

Miller, C.R. (1994, August). Creative coping: A cognitive-behavioral group for borderline personality disorder. *Archives of Psychiatric Nursing, 8*(4), 280–285.

Myers, M.G., Stewart, D.G., & Brown, S.A. (1998, April). Progression from conduct disorder to antisocial personality disorder following treatment for adolescent substance abuse. *American Journal of Psychiatry, 155*, 479–485.

Pajer, K.A. (1998, July). What happens to "bad" girls? A review of the adult outcomes of antisocial adolescent girls. *American Journal of Psychiatry, 155*, 862–870.

Robins, L.N. (1998, August). The intimate connection between antisocial personality and substance abuse. *Social Psychiatry and Psychiatric Epidemiology, 33*, 393–399.

Sansone, R.A., Sansone, L.A., & Wiederman, M. (1995, May). The prevalence of trauma and its relationship to borderline personality symptoms and self-destructive behaviors in a primary care setting. *Archives of Family Medicine, 4*, 439–442.

Silk, K.R., Lee, S., Hill, E.M., & Lohr, N.E. (1995, July). Borderline personality disorder symptoms and severity of sexual abuse. *American Journal of Psychiatry, 152*, 1059–1064.

Waller, G. (1994, January). Childhood sexual abuse and borderline personality disorder in the eating disorders. *Child Abuse and Neglect, 18*, 97–101.

Unit Four

Special Topics in Psychiatric/Mental Health Nursing

THE AGING INDIVIDUAL

KEY TERMS

gerontology	short-term memory	Medicare
geriatrics	long-term memory	Medicaid
geropsychiatry	bereavement overload	"granny-bashing"
menopause	attachment	"granny-dumping"
osteoporosis	disengagement	reminiscence therapy

OBJECTIVES

After reading this chapter, the student will be able to:

1. Discuss societal perspectives on aging.
2. Describe an epidemiological profile of aging in the United States.
3. Discuss various theories of aging.
4. Describe aspects of the normal aging process:
   a. Biological
   b. Psychological
   c. Sociocultural
   d. Sexual
5. Discuss retirement as a special concern to the aging individual.
6. Explain personal and sociological perspectives of long-term care of the aging individual.
7. Describe the problem of elder abuse as it exists in today's society.
8. Discuss the implications of the increasing number of suicides among the elderly population.
9. Apply the steps of the nursing process to the care of aging individuals.

hat is it like to grow old? It is not likely that many people in the American culture would state that it is something they want to do. Most would agree, however, that it is "better than the alternative."

Bowen (1944) tells the following often-told tale of Supreme Court Justice Oliver Wendell Holmes, Jr. In the year before he retired at age 91 as the oldest justice ever to sit on the Supreme Court of the United States, Holmes and his close friend Justice Louis Brandeis, then a mere 74 years old, were out for one of their frequent walks on Washington's Capitol Hill. On this particular day, the justices spotted a very attractive young woman approaching them. As she passed, Holmes paused, sighed, and said to Brandeis, "Oh, to be 70 again!" Obviously, being old is relative to the individual experiencing it.

Growing old has not been popular among the youth-oriented American culture. However, with 66 million "baby-boomers" reaching their 65th birthdays by the year 2030, greater emphasis is being placed on the needs of an aging population. The disciplines of **gerontology** (the study of the aging process), **geriatrics** (the branch of clinical medicine specializing in problems of the elderly), and **geropsychiatry** (the branch of clinical medicine specializing in psychopathology of the elderly) are expanding rapidly in response to this predictable demand.

Growing old in a society that has been obsessed with youth may have a critical impact on the mental health of many people. This situation has serious implications for psychiatric nursing.

What is it like to grow old? More and more people will be able to answer this question as the 21st century progresses. Perhaps they will also be asking the question that Roberts (1991) asks: "How did I get here so fast?"

This chapter focuses on physical and psychological changes associated with the aging process, as well as special concerns of the elderly, such as retirement, long-term care, elder abuse, and rising suicide rates. The nursing process is presented as the vehicle for delivery of nursing care to elderly individuals.

HOW OLD IS *OLD?*

The concept of "old" has changed drastically over the years. Our prehistoric ancestors probably had a life span of 40 years, with an average life span of around 18 years. As civilization developed, mortality rates remained high as a result of periodic famine and frequent malnutrition. An improvement in the standard of living was not truly evident until about the middle of the 17th century. Since that time, assured food supply, changes in food production, better housing conditions, and more progressive medical and sanitation facilities have contributed to population growth, declining mortality rates, and substantial increases in longevity.

In 1900, the average life expectancy in the United States was 47 years, and only 4 percent of the population was age 65 or over. By 1985, the average life expectancy at birth was 71.2 years for men and 78.2 years for women (Butler, 1989).

The U.S. Census Bureau has created a system for classification of older Americans:

Older	55 through 64 years
Elderly	65 through 74 years
Aged	75 through 84 years
Very old	85 years and older

Some gerontologists have elected to used a simpler classification system:

Young old	60 through 74 years
Middle old	75 through 84 years
Old old	85 years and older

So how old is *old?* Obviously the term cannot be defined by a number. Myths and stereotypes of aging have long obscured our understanding of the aged and the process of aging. Kermis (1986) identifies the following potentially damaging myths of old age:

1. Old people are all alike.
2. Old people are all poor.
3. Old people are all sick.
4. Old people are incapable of change.
5. Old people are all depressed.
6. Old people always think about death.
7. If we live long enough, we will all become senile.

Myths and stereotypes of this type affect the way elderly people are treated. They even shape the pattern of aging of the people who believe them. They can become self-fulfilling prophecies, in that persons believe they should behave in certain ways and therefore act according to those beliefs. Generalized assumptions can in fact be demeaning and interfere with the quality of life for older individuals.

Just as there are many differences in individual adaptation at earlier stages of development, so it is in the elderly person. Erikson (1963) has suggested that the mentally healthy older person possesses a sense of ego integrity and self-acceptance that will help in adapting to the ambiguities of the future with a sense of security and optimism.

Murray and Zentner (1997) state:

"Having accomplished the earlier [developmental] tasks, the person accepts life as his or her own and as the only life for the self. He or she would wish for none other and would defend the meaning and the dignity of the lifestyle. The person has further refined the characteristics of maturity described for the middle-aged adult, achieving both wisdom and an enriched perspective about life and people." (p. 739)

Everyone, particularly health care workers, should see aging persons as individuals, each with specific needs and abilities, rather than as a stereotypical group. Some individuals may seem "old" at 40, whereas others may not seem "old" at 70. Variables such as attitude, mental health, physical health, and degree of independence strongly influence how an individual perceives himself or herself. Surely, in the final analysis, whether or not one is considered "old" must be self-determined.

EPIDEMIOLOGICAL STATISTICS

The Population

In 1980, Americans 65 years of age or older numbered 25.5 million. By 1996, these numbers had increased to approximately 33.9 million, representing 12.8 percent of the population (Duncker & Greenberg, 1997). This trend is expected to continue, with a projection for 2030 at 70.2 million, or 20 percent of the population.

Marital Status

In 1995, of individuals age 65 and older, 76 percent of men and 43 percent of women were married (Duncker & Greenberg, 1997). Forty-seven percent of all women in this age group were widowed. There were five times as many widows as widowers because women live longer than men and tend to marry men older themselves.

Living Arrangements

The majority of individuals age 65 or older live alone, with a spouse, or with relatives (Duncker & Greenberg, 1997). At any one time, fewer than 5 percent of people in this age group live in institutions (Moody, 1994). See Figure 35.1 for a distribution of living arrangements.

Economic Status

Approximately 3.4 million persons age 65 or older were below the poverty level in 1996 (Duncker & Greenberg, 1997). Older women, and particularly older black women, had a higher poverty rate than older men. Poor people who have worked all their lives can expect to become poorer in old age, and others will become poor only *after* becoming old (Butler, 1989). However, there are still a substantial number of affluent and middle-income older persons who enjoy a high quality of life.

Seventy-eight percent of individuals in this age group owned their own homes in 1995 (Duncker & Greenberg, 1997). However, the housing of this population of Americans is usually older and less adequate than that of the younger population, so a higher percentage of income must be spent on maintenance and repairs.

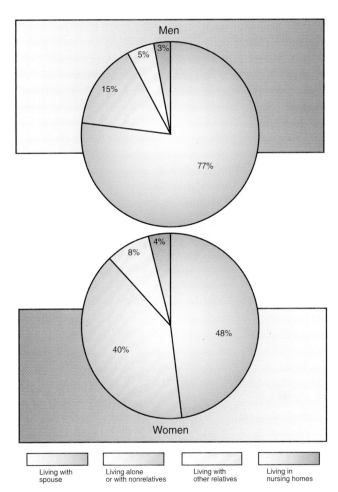

Figure 35.1 Living arrangement of persons aged 65 and over (1995).

Employment

With the passage of the Age Discrimination in Employment Act in 1967, forced retirement has been virtually eliminated in the workplace. Evidence suggests that involvement in purposive activity is vital to successful adaptation and even to survival (Butler, 1989). Individuals age 65 or older constituted 2.7 percent of the U.S. labor force in 1996 (Duncker & Greenberg, 1997).

Health Status

The number of days in which usual activities are restricted because of illness or injury increases with age. Persons 65 years of age or older averaged 35 such days in 1994 and accounted for 38 percent of all hospital stays (Duncker & Greenberg, 1997). Most older individuals have at least one chronic medical condition, and many have more than one. The most commonly occurring conditions for the elderly in 1994 (in descending order of frequency) were arthritis, hypertension, heart disease, hearing impairments, cataracts, orthopedic impairments, sinusitis, and diabetes (Duncker & Greenberg, 1997).

Emotional and mental illnesses increase over the life cycle. Depression is particularly prevalent and suicide is increasing among elderly Americans. Organic mental disease increases dramatically in old age (Butler, 1989).

THEORIES OF AGING

Biological Theories

Busse (1989) has identified the following eight biological theories regarding the aging process. Despite these propositions, a single, satisfactory biological theory has yet to be empirically demonstrated.

1. **The Exhaustion Theory.** This theory suggests that the body contains a finite amount of energy that is gradually used up over time. When the energy is gone, the body dies.
2. **The Accumulation Theory.** According to this theory, harmful material such as lipofuscin develops late in life and destroys cells.
3. **The Biological Programming Theory.** This theory says that cells are genetically programmed to live for a specific period, leading to inevitable death.
4. **The Error Theory.** This theory states that, in senescence, alterations occur in the structure of deoxyribonucleic acid (DNA). When the errors are transmitted to messenger ribonucleic acid (mRNA), there is a build-up of defective enzymes, leading ultimately to the death of the cell and organism.
5. **The Cross-Linkage or Eversion Theory.** This theory suggests that the linkages holding together the polypeptide strands of collagen change, rendering collagen less permeable and elastic and therefore less capable of sustaining normal life.
6. **The Immunological Theory.** This theory postulates that with time the protective mechanisms of the immune system weaken. Consequently, the system may become autoaggressive, leading to destruction of the body tissue.
7. **The "Aging Clock" Theory.** This "clock" is said to reside in the hypothalmus. The hypothalamus is central to a variety of brain and endocrine functions, and cell loss in this site has a particularly important role in decline of homeostatic mechanisms with age.
8. **The Free Radical Theory.** Free radicals are molecules with unpaired electrons that exist normally in the body, as well as being produced by ionizing radiation, ozone, and chemical toxins. According to this theory, these free radicals cause DNA damage, cross-linkage of collagen, and the accumulation of age pigments.

Psychosocial Theories

1. **The Activity Theory of Aging.** Kaplan and Sadock (1998) suggest that social integration is the prime factor in determining psychosocial adaptation in later life. Social integration refers to how the aging individual is included and takes part in the life and activities of his or her society. This theory holds that the maintenance of activities is important to most people as a basis for deriving and sustaining satisfaction, self-esteem, and health.
2. **Continuity Theory.** Atchley (1989) proposed that whereas the basic social structure of the individual remains intact over time, a variety of adaptive changes occur that require the aging person to make choices. Choices are made based on the preservation of inner psychological continuity and external continuity of social behaviors. Maintenance of internal continuity is motivated by the need for preservation of self-esteem, ego integrity, cognitive function, and social support. As they age, individuals maintain their self-concept by reinterpreting their current experiences so that old values can take on new meanings in keeping with present circumstances (Kaufman, 1986). Internal self-concepts and beliefs are not readily vulnerable to environmental change; and external continuity in skills, activities, roles, and relationships can remain remarkably stable into the 70s. Physical illness or death of friends and loved ones may preclude continued social interaction (Kaplan & Sadock, 1998).

Personality Theories

Personality theories of aging are influenced by the fact that, as they traverse life experiences, people become increasingly different (Sadavoy, Lazarus, & Jarvik, 1991). In extreme old age, however, people show greater similarity in certain characteristics, probably because of similar declines in biological functioning and societal opportunities.

Neugarten and associates (1964) found that when comparing 60-year-olds with 40-years-olds, the older individuals seem to see the environment as more complex and more dangerous. Their world becomes more internally oriented. In addition, older men seem to be more receptive than younger men to their nurturing and sensual capacities, whereas older women become more accepting of their own "aggressive and egocentric impulses."

In a study by Reichard, Livson, and Peterson (1962), the personalities of older men were classified into five major categories according to their patterns of adjustment to aging:

1. *Mature men* are well-balanced persons who maintain close personal relationships. They accept both the strengths and weaknesses of their age, finding little to regret about retirement and approaching

most problems in a relaxed or convivial manner without continually having to assess blame.

2. *"Rocking chair"* personalities are found in passive-dependent individuals who are content to lean on others for support, to disengage, and to let most of life's activities pass them by.

3. *Armored men* have well-integrated defense mechanisms, which serve as adequate protection. Rigid and stable, they present a strong silent front and often rely on activity as an expression of their continuing independence.

4. *Angry men* are bitter about life, themselves, and other people. Aggressiveness is common, as is suspicion of others, especially of minorities or women. With little tolerance for ambiguity or frustration, they have always shown some instability in work and their personal lives, and now feel extremely threatened by old age.

5. *Self-haters* are similar to angry men, except that most of their animosity is turned inward on themselves. Because they see themselves as dismal failures, being old only depresses them all the more.

The investigators identified the mature, "rocking chair," or armored categories as characteristic of healthy, adjusted individuals, and the angry and self-hater categories as less successful agers. In all cases, the evidence suggested that the personalities of the subjects, though distinguished by age-specific criteria, had not changed appreciably throughout most of adulthood.

THE NORMAL AGING PROCESS

Biological Aspects of Aging

Individuals are unique in their physical and psychological aging processes, as influenced by their predisposition or resistance to illness; the effects of their external environment and behaviors; their exposure to trauma, infections, and past diseases; and the health and illness practices they have adopted during their life span (Leventhal, 1991). As the individual ages, there is a quantitative loss of cells and changes in many of the enzymatic activities within cells, resulting in a diminished responsiveness to biological demands made on the body. Age-related changes occur at different rates for different individuals, even though in actuality, when growth stops aging begins; virtually all growth ceases with puberty (Leventhal, 1991). This section presents a brief overview of the normal biological changes that occur with the aging process.

Skin

One of the most dramatic changes that occurs in aging is the loss of elastin in the skin. This effect, as well as changes in collagen, causes aged skin to wrinkle and sag.

Excessive exposure to sunlight compounds these changes and increases the risk of developing skin cancer (Williams, 1995).

Fat redistribution results in a loss of the subcutaneous cushion of adipose tissue. Thus, older people lose "insulation" and are more sensitive to extremes of ambient temperature than are younger people (Kenney, 1989). Fewer blood vessels to the skin result in a slower rate of healing.

Cardiovascular System

The age-related decline in the cardiovascular system is thought to be the major determinant of decreased tolerance for exercise and loss of conditioning, and thus the major factor contributing to feelings of agedness and overall decline in energy reserve (Leventhal, 1991). The aging heart is characterized by modest hypertrophy with reduced ventricular compliance and diminished cardiac output (Kaplan & Sadock, 1998; Murray & Zentner, 1997). This results in a decrease in response to work demands and some diminishment of blood flow to the brain, kidneys, liver, and muscles. Heart rate also slows with time. If arteriosclerosis is present, cardiac function is further compromised.

Respiratory System

Thoracic expansion is diminished by an increase in fibrous tissue and loss of elastin. Pulmonary vital capacity decreases, and the amount of residual air increases. Scattered areas of fibrosis in the alveolar septae interfere with exchange of oxygen and carbon dioxide. These changes are accelerated by the use of cigarettes or other inhaled substances. Cough and laryngeal reflexes are reduced, causing decreased ability to defend the airway. Decreased pulmonary blood flow and diffusion ability result in reduced efficiency in responding to sudden respiratory demands.

Musculoskeletal System

Skeletal aging involving the bones, muscles, ligaments, and tendons probably generates the most frequent limitations on activities of daily living (ADLs) experienced by aging individuals (Leventhal, 1991). Loss of muscle mass is significant, although this occurs more slowly in men than in women. Demineralization of the bones occurs at a rate of about 1 percent per year throughout the life span in both men and women. However, this increases to approximately 10 percent in women around **menopause,** making them particularly vulnerable to **osteoporosis.**

Individual muscle fibers become thinner and less elastic with age. Muscles become less flexible following disuse. There is diminished storage of muscle glycogen, resulting in loss of energy reserve for increased activity. These changes are accelerated by nutritional deficiencies and inactivity.

Gastrointestinal System

In the oral cavity, the teeth show a reduction in dentine production, shrinkage and fibrosis of root pulp, gingival retraction, and loss of bone density in the alveolar ridges (Leventhal, 1991). There is some loss of peristalsis in the stomach and intestines, and gastric acid production decreases. Levels of intrinsic factor may also decrease, resulting in vitamin B_{12} malabsorption in some aging individuals. A significant decrease in absorptive surface area of the small intestine may be associated with some decline in nutrient absorption. Motility slowdown of the large intestine, combined with poor dietary habits, dehydration, lack of exercise, and some medications, may give rise to problems with constipation.

There is a modest decrease in size and weight of the liver, resulting in losses in enzyme activity that deactivate certain medications by the liver. These age-related changes can influence the metabolism and excretion of these medications. These changes, along with the pharmacokinetics of the drug, must be considered when giving medications to aging individuals.

Endocrine System

A decreased level of thyroid hormones causes a lowered basal metabolic rate. Decreased amounts of adrenocorticotropic hormone may result in less efficient stress response.

Impairments in glucose tolerance are evident in aging individuals (Leventhal, 1991). Studies of glucose challenges show that insulin levels are equivalent or slightly higher than those from younger challenged individuals, although peripheral insulin resistance appears to play a significant role in carbohydrate intolerance. The observed glucose clearance abnormalities and insulin resistance in older people may be related to many factors other than biological aging (e.g., obesity, family history of diabetes) and may be influenced substantially by diet or exercise.

Genitourinary System

Age-related declines in renal function occur because of a steady attrition caused by sclerosis of nephrons over time (Leventhal, 1991). The total renal blood flow declines at a steady rate of about 10 percent a year after age 20, so that glomerular filtration has decreased approximately 50 percent by age 80 (Pikna, 1994). Elderly persons are prone to develop the syndrome of inappropriate antidiuretic hormone secretion, and levels of blood urea nitrogen and creatinine may be elevated slightly. The overall decline in re-

nal functioning has serious implications for physicians in prescribing medications for elderly individuals.

In men, enlargement of the prostate gland is common as aging occurs. Prostatic hypertrophy is associated with an increased risk for urinary retention and may also be a cause of urinary incontinence (Williams, 1995). Loss of muscle and sphincter control, as well as the use of some medications, may cause urinary incontinence in women. Not only is this problem a cause of social stigma but also, left untreated, it increases the risk of urinary tract infection and local skin irritation.

Normal changes in the genitalia are discussed in the section of "Sexual Aspects of Aging."

Immune System

Aging results in changes in both cell-mediated and antibody-mediated immune responses (Larocco, 1994). The size of the thymus gland declines continuously from just beyond puberty to about 15 percent of its original size at age 50. The consequences of these changes include a greater susceptibility to infections and a diminished inflammatory response that results in delayed healing. There is also evidence of an increase in various autoantibodies (e.g., rheumatoid factor) as a person ages, increasing the risk of autoimmune disorders (Pikna, 1994).

Because of the overall decrease in efficiency of the immune system, the proliferation of abnormal cells is facilitated in the elderly individual. Cancer is the best example of aberrant cells allowed to proliferate due to the ineffectiveness of the immune system.

Nervous System

With aging, there is an absolute loss of neurons, which correlates with decreases in brain weight of about 10 percent by age 90 (Murray & Zentner, 1997). Gross morphological examination reveals gyral atrophy in the frontal, temporal, and parietal lobes; widening of the sulci; and ventricular enlargement. However, it must be remembered that these changes have been identified in careful study of adults with normal intellectual function.

The brain has enormous reserve, and little cerebral function is lost over time, although greater functional decline is noted in the periphery (Leventhal, 1991). There appears to be a disproportionately greater loss of cells in the cerebellum, the locus ceruleus, the substantia nigra, and olfactory bulbs, accounting for some of the more characteristic aging behaviors such as mild gait disturbances, sleep disruptions, and decreased smell and taste perception (Williams, 1995).

Some of the age-related changes within the nervous system may be due to alterations in neurotransmitter release, uptake, turnover, catabolism, or receptor functions (Shader & Kennedy, 1989). A great deal of attention is being given to brain biochemistry and in particular to the neurotransmitters acetylcholine, dopamine, norepinephrine, and epinephrine. These biochemical changes may be responsible for the altered responses of many older persons to stressful events and some biological treatments.

Sensory Systems

Vision. Visual acuity begins to decrease in mid-life. Presbyopia (blurred near vision) is the standard marker of aging of the eye. It is caused by a loss of elasticity of the crystalline lens, and results in compromised accommodation.

Cataract development is inevitable if the individual lives long enough for the changes to occur. Cataracts are formed when pigment is laid down in specific patterns in the lens over time and is coupled with increased rigidity of the lenticular proteins (Leventhal, 1991).

The color in the iris may fade, and the pupil may become irregular in shape. A decrease in production of secretions by the lacrimal glands may cause dryness and result in increased irritation and infection. The pupil may become constricted, requiring an increase in the amount of light needed for reading.

Hearing. Hearing changes significantly with the aging process. Gradually over time, the ear loses its sensitivity to discriminate sounds because of damage to the hair cells of the cochlea. The most dramatic decline appears to be in perception of high-frequency sounds.

Although hearing loss is significant in all aging individuals, the decline is more dramatic in men than in women. This may be related to deterioration from occupational exposure to noise (Leventhal, 1991).

Taste and Smell. Taste sensitivity decreases over the life span. Taste discrimination decreases, and bitter taste sensations predominate. Sensitivity to sweet and salty tastes is diminished.

The deterioration of the olfactory bulbs is accompanied by loss of smell acuity. The aromatic component of taste perception diminishes.

Touch and Pain. Organized sensory nerve receptors on the skin continue to decrease throughout the life span; thus, the touch threshold increases with age (Leventhal, 1991). The ability to feel pain also decreases in response to these changes, and the ability to perceive and interpret painful stimuli changes. These changes have critical implications for the elderly in their potential lack of ability to use sensory warnings for escaping serious injury.

PSYCHOLOGICAL ASPECTS OF AGING

Memory Functioning

Age-related memory deficiencies have been extensively reported in the literature. Although **short-term memory** seems to deteriorate with age, perhaps as a consequence of poorer sorting strategies, **long-term memory** does not show similar changes. However, in nearly every instance, well-educated, mentally active people do not exhibit the same decline in memory functioning as their age peers who lack similar opportunities to flex their minds. Nevertheless, with few exceptions, the time required for memory scanning is longer for both recent and remote recall among older people, perhaps more because of social and health factors than any irreversible effects of age (Williams, 1995).

Intellectual Functioning

There appears to be a high degree of regularity in intellectual functioning across the adult age span. Crystallized abilities, or knowledge acquired in the course of the socialization process, tend to remain stable over the adult life span. Fluid abilities, or abilities involved in solving novel problems, tend to decline gradually from young to old adulthood (Schaie, 1990). In other words, intellectual abilities of older people do not decline but do become obsolete. The age of their formal educational experiences is reflected in their intelligence scoring.

Learning Ability

The ability to learn is not diminished by age. Studies, however, have shown that some aspects of learning do change with age. The ordinary slowing of reaction time with age for nearly all tasks or the overarousal of the central nervous system may account for lower performance levels on tests requiring rapid responses. Under conditions that allow self-pacing by the participant, differences in accuracy of performance diminishes. Ability to learn continues throughout life, although strongly influenced by interests, activity, motivation, health, and income (Williams, 1995). Adjustments do need to be made in teaching methodology and time allowed for learning.

Adaptation to the Tasks of Aging

Loss and Grief. Individuals experience losses from the very beginning of life. By the time individuals reach their 60s and 70s, they have experienced numerous losses, and mourning has become a lifelong process. Those who are most successful at adapting earlier in life will similarly cope better with the losses and grief inherent in aging (Cath & Sadavoy, 1991). Unfortunately, with the aging process comes a convergence of losses, the timing of which makes it impossible for the aging individual to complete the grief process in response to one loss before another occurs. Because grief is cumulative, this can result in **bereavement overload,** which has been implicated in the predisposition to depression in the elderly.

Attachment and Disengagement. Many studies have confirmed the importance of interpersonal relationships at all stages in the life cycle. So important is the need for **attachment** that studies have shown that having a confidant, or the availability of a formal or informal caregiver, is the most critical factor discriminating between elderly persons who remain in the community and those who are institutionalized (Williams, 1995). These findings are consistent with the activity theory of aging that correlates the importance of social integration with successful adaptation in later life.

A contrasting theory, that of **disengagement**, suggests that (1) the process of mutual withdrawal of aging persons and society from each other is typical of most aging persons; (2) this process is biologically and psychologically intrinsic and inevitable; and (3) the disengagement process not only is correlated with successful aging but also is usually necessary for aging (Cumming & Henry, 1961). There have been many critics of this theory, and the attachment theory is currently more widely accepted than the disengagement theory.

Maintenance of Self-Identity. Several authors have asserted that self-concept and self-image remain stable and do not become impoverished or negative in old age (Cath & Sadavoy, 1991). A study by Vaillant and Vaillant (1990) found that the factors that favored good psychosocial adjustment in later life were sustained family relationships, maturity of ego defenses, absence of alcoholism, and absence of depressive disorder. Studies show that the elderly have a strong need for and remarkable capability of retaining a persistent self-concept in the face of the many changes that create the instability so evident in later life.

Dealing with Death. Death anxiety among the aging is apparently more of a myth than a reality. Studies have not supported the negative view of death as an overriding psychological factor in the aging process (Cath & Sadavoy, 1991). Various investigators who have worked with dying persons report that it is not death itself but rather abandonment, pain, and confusion that are feared. What many desire most is someone to talk with, to show them their life's meaning is not shattered merely because they are about to die (Kübler-Ross, 1969; Murray & Zentner, 1997).

Psychiatric Disorders in Later Life. The later years constitute a time of especially high risk for emotional distress. Kaplan, Sadock, and Grebb (1994) state:

"A number of psychosocial risk factors predispose the elderly to mental disorders. Those risk factors include loss of social roles, loss of autonomy, the deaths of friends and relatives, declining health, increased isolation, financial constraints, and decreased cognitive functioning."

Dementing disorders are the most common causes of psychopathology in elderly persons (Kaplan & Sadock, 1998). About half of these disorders are of the Alzheimer's type, which is characterized by an insidious onset and a gradually progressive course of cognitive impairment. No curative treatment is currently available. Symptomatic treatments, including pharmacological interventions, attention to the environment, and family support, can help to maximize the client's level of functioning.

Delirium is one of the most common and important forms of psychopathology in later life. A number of factors have been identified that predispose elderly people to delirium, including structural brain disease, reduced capacity for homeostatic regulation, impaired vision and hearing, a high prevalence of chronic disease, reduced resistance to acute stress, and age-related changes in the pharmacokinetic and pharmacodynamics of drugs. Delirium needs to be recognized and the underlying condition treated as soon as possible. A high mortality is associated with this condition (Williams, 1995).

Depressive disorders are the most common affective illnesses occurring after the middle years. The incidence of increased depression among the elderly population is influenced by the variables of physical illness, functional disability, cognitive impairment, and loss of spouse (Kaplan & Sadock, 1998; Williams, 1995). Hypochondriacal symptoms are common in the depressed elderly. Symptomatology often mimics that of dementia, a condition that is referred to as pseudodementia (see Table 23.2 for a comparison of the symptoms of dementia and pseudodementia.) Suicide is more prevalent in the elderly population, with economic status being considered an important influencing factor. Treatment of depression in elderly persons is with psychotropic medications or electroconvulsive therapy.

Schizophrenia and delusional disorders may continue into old age or may manifest themselves for the first time only during senescence (Blazer, 1994). In most instances, individuals who manifest psychotic disorders early in life show a decline in psychopathology as they age. Late-onset schizophrenia (after age 60) is not common, but when it does occur, it is often characterized by delusions or hallucinations of a persecutory nature. The course is chronic, and treatment is with neuroleptics and supportive psychotherapy.

Most anxiety disorders begin in early to middle adulthood, but some appear for the first time after age 60. Kaplan and Sadock (1998) state:

"The fragility of the autonomic nervous system in older people may account for the development of anxiety after a major stressor. Because of concurrent physical disability, older people react more severely to posttraumatic stress disorder than younger people." (p. 1297)

In older adults, symptoms of anxiety and depression tend to accompany each other, making it difficult to determine which disorder is dominant (Williams, 1995).

Personality disorders are also uncommon in the elderly population. The incidence peaks between 25 and 44 years and declines thereafter, with an incidence of less than 5 percent after age 65 (Guterman & Eisdorfer, 1989). These investigators suggest the following three explanations for this decline: (1) personality disorders improve with increasing age past middle age; (2) behavior patterns undergo deterioration to more severe states (e.g., psychoses); and (3) persons with such psychopathology do not survive to old age. Most elderly people with personality disorder have likely manifested the symptomatology for many years.

Sleep disorders are very common in the aging individual. Epidemiological surveys have reported as many as 35 percent of older persons suffer from and complain of chronic poor sleep quality (Blazer, 1994). Some common causes of sleep disturbances among elderly people include age-dependent decreases in the ability to sleep ("sleep decay"); increased prevalence of sleep apnea; depression; dementia; anxiety; pain; impaired mobility; medications; and psychosocial factors such as loneliness, inactivity, and boredom. Benzodiazepines are often used as sleep aids with elderly clients, along with nonpharmacological approaches. Changes in aging associated with metabolism and elimination must be considered when maintenance benzodiazepine therapy is administered for chronic insomnia in the aging client.

Sociocultural Aspects of Aging

Old age brings many important socially induced changes, some of which have the potential for negative effect on both the physical and mental well-being of older persons. In American society, old age is arbitrarily defined as being 65 or older because that is the age when most people can retire with full Social Security and other pension benefits.

Elderly people in virtually all cultures share some basic needs and interests. Palmore and Maddox (1977) have summarized these into the following five categories:

1. To live as long as possible or at least until life's satisfactions no longer compensate for its privations.
2. To get some release from the necessity of wearisome exertion at humdrum tasks and to have protection from too great exposure to physical hazards.
3. To safeguard or even strengthen any prerogatives acquired in midlife, such as skills, possessions, rights, authority, and prestige.
4. To remain active participants in the affairs of life in either operational or supervisory roles, any sharing in group interests being preferred to idleness and indifference.
5. To withdraw from life when necessity requires it, as timely, honorably, and comfortably as possible.

From the beginning of human culture, the aged have had a special status in society. Even today, in some cultures the aged are the most powerful, the most engaged, and the most respected members of the society. This has not been the case in the modern industrial societies, although trends in the status of the aged differ widely between one industrialized country and another. For example, the status and integration of the aged in Japan have remained relatively high when compared with the other industrialized nations. The aged are awarded a position of honor in cultures that place emphasis on family cohesiveness. In these cultures, the aged are revered for their knowledge and wisdom gained through their years of life experiences (Giger & Davidhizar, 1991).

Many negative stereotypes color the perspective on aging in the United States. Ideas that elderly individuals are always tired or sick, slow and forgetful, isolated and lonely, unproductive, and angry determine the way younger individuals relate to the elderly in this society. Increasing disregard for the elderly has resulted in a type of segregation, as aging individuals voluntarily seek out or are involuntarily placed in special residences for the aged. The growing segregation of the aged has been described by Breen (1960) as follows:

> "Homes for the aged, public housing projects, medical institutions, recreation centers, and communities which are devoted to the exclusive use of the retired have been increasing in number and size in recent years. Retirement "villages" have been sponsored by philanthropic organizations, unions, church groups, and others. Even established communities which are now known as 'retirement centers' have become inundated by older migrants seeking identification and spatial contiguity with 'the clan.'"

Since this description was written, the concept has blossomed. In 1996, about half (52 percent) of persons age 65 and older lived in nine states, with the majority in California, Florida, and New York (Duncker & Greenberg, 1997). It is important for elderly individuals to feel part of an integrated group, and they are migrating to these areas in an effort to achieve this integration. This phenomenon provides additional corroboration for the activity theory of aging and the importance of attachment to others.

Employment is another area in which the elderly experience discrimination. Even though compulsory retirement has been virtually eliminated, discrimination still exists in hiring and promotion practices. Many employers are not eager to retain or hire older workers. It is difficult to determine how much of the failure to hire and promote is due to discrimination based on age alone and how much of it is related to a realistic and fair appraisal of the aged employee's ability and efficiency. Undoubtedly, many elderly individuals are no longer capable of doing as good a job as a younger worker. However, surveys have shown that some employers accepted the negative stereotypes of the elderly and believe that older workers are hard to please, set in their ways, less productive, frequently absent, and involved in more accidents.

The status of the elderly population may improve with

time and as their numbers increase with the aging of the "baby-boomers." As older individuals gain political power, the benefits and privileges designed for the elderly will increase. There is power in numbers, and the 21st century promises power for individuals 65 and older.

Sexual Aspects of Aging

Sexuality and the sexual needs of elderly people are frequently misunderstood, condemned, stereotyped, ridiculed, repressed, and ignored (Neugarten, 1986). Americans have grown up in a society that has liberated sexual expression for all other age groups, but still retains certain Victorian standards regarding sexual expression by elderly individuals. Neugarten (1986) describes some stereotyped notions that younger individuals possess concerning sexual interest and activity of the elderly:

1. Old people do not have sexual desires or engage in sexual activity.
2. Older people could not engage in intercourse, even if they wanted to, because they are too fragile physically and might hurt themselves.
3. Elderly people are unattractive, which makes them sexually undesirable.
4. Sexuality among the aged is shameful and perverse.

These cultural stereotypes undoubtedly play a large part in the misperception many people hold regarding sexuality of the aged, and they may be reinforced by the common tendency of the young to deny the inevitability of aging. Masters and Johnson (1966) have stated that reasonable good health and an interesting and interested partner should ensure an active sexual life even into the 80s and beyond.

Physical Changes Associated with Sexuality

Many of the changes in sexuality that occur in later years are related to the physical changes that take place then.

Changes in the Female. Menopause may begin anytime during the 40s or early 50s (Kaplan, Sadock, & Grebb, 1994). At this time there is a gradual decline in the functioning of the ovaries and the subsequent production of estrogen, which results in a number of changes. The walls of the vagina become thin and inelastic, the vagina itself shrinks in both width and length, and the amount of vaginal lubrication decreases noticeably. Orgastic uterine contractions may become spastic. All of these changes can result in painful penetration, vaginal burning, pelvic aching, or irritation on urination. In some women, the discomfort may be severe enough to result in an avoidance of intercourse. Paradoxically, these symptoms are more likely to occur with infrequent intercourse of only one time a month or less. Regular and more frequent sexual

activity results in a greater capacity for sexual performance (Masters & Johnson, 1966). Other symptoms that are associated with menopause in some women include hot flashes, night sweats, sleeplessness, irritability, mood swings, short-term memory loss, migraine headaches, urinary incontinence, and weight gain (Beck et al., 1992).

About 15 percent of menopausal American women take hormone replacement therapy for relief of these changes and symptoms (Seligmann, Friday, & Wingert, 1992). With estrogen therapy, the symptoms of menopause are minimized or do not occur at all. However, some women chose not to take the hormone because of an increased risk of breast cancer and, when given alone, an increased risk of endometrial cancer. To combat this latter effect, most women also take a second hormone, progesterone. Taken for 7 to 10 days during the month, progesterone decreases the risk of estrogen-induced endometrial cancer. Some physicians are electing to prescribe a low dose of progesterone that is taken, along with estrogen, for the entire month.

Changes in the Male. Testosterone production declines gradually over the years, beginning between ages 40 and 60. A major change resulting from this hormone reduction is that erections occur more slowly and require more direct genital stimulation to achieve. There may also be a modest decrease in the firmness of the erection in men older than age 60. The refractory period lengthens with age, increasing the amount of time following orgasm before the man may achieve another erection. The volume of ejaculate gradually decreases, and the force of ejaculation lessens. The testes become somewhat smaller, but viable sperm are produced by some men well into their 90s (Hyde, 1986). Prolonged control over ejaculation in middle-aged and elderly men may bring increased sexual satisfaction for both partners.

Sexual Behavior in the Elderly

Masters and Johnson (1966) found that coital frequency in early marriage and the overall quantity of sexual activity between age 20 and 40 correlate significantly with frequency patterns of sexual activity during aging. Although sexual interest and behavior do appear to decline somewhat with age, studies show that significant numbers of elderly men and women have active and satisfying sex lives well into their 80s. A survey by Brecher and associates (1984) presented a revealing depiction of sexual behavior among the elderly population. Some statistics from the survey are summarized in Table 35.1.

The information from this survey clearly indicates that all forms of sexual activity can and do continue well past the 70s for healthy active individuals who have regular opportunities for sexual expression. Reinisch (1990) states:

"Some sexual patterns established early in life may continue as we age. Those who had lower frequencies of sexual activity in their youth may continue to have sex less frequently,

◢ TABLE 35.1   SEXUAL BEHAVIOR IN THE ELDERLY

SEX	AGES	PERCENTAGE OF RESPONDENTS (n = ~4200)
Women		
Women who have sex with their husbands (frequency):	50–59	88 (1.3 times/wk)
	60–69	76 (1.0 times/wk)
	70+	65 (0.7 times/wk)
Women who masturbate (frequency):	50–59	47 (0.7 times/wk)
	60–69	37 (0.6 times/wk)
	70+	33 (0.7 times/wk)
Engaged in extramarital sex after age 50:		8
Engaged in homosexual experience after age 50:		2
Men		
Men who have sex with their wives (frequency):	50–59	87 (1.3 times/wk)
	60–69	78 (1.0 times/wk)
	70+	59 (0.6 times/wk)
Men who masturbate (frequency):	50–59	66 (1.2 times/wk)
	60–69	50 (0.8 times/wk)
	70+	43 (0.7 times/wk)
Engaged in extramarital sex after age 50:		24
Engaged in homosexual experience after age 50:		4

SOURCE: Adapted from Brecher et al. (1984).

while whose who were more active are likely to continue being so in later years." (p. 228)

SPECIAL CONCERNS OF THE ELDERLY POPULATION

Retirement

Statistics reflect that a larger percentage of Americans of both sexes are living longer and that many of them are retiring earlier. Reasons often given for the increasing pattern of early retirement include health problems, Social Security and other pension benefits, attractive "early buyout" packages offered by companies, and long-held plans (e.g., turning a hobby into a money-making situation). Even eliminating the mandatory retirement age and the possibility of delaying the age of eligibility for Social Security benefits from 65 to 67 by the year 2027 is not expected to have a significant effect on the trend toward earlier retirement.

Kaplan, Sadock, and Grebb (1994) report that of those persons who voluntarily retire, a majority reenter the work force within 2 years. The reasons they give for doing this include negative reactions to being retired, feelings of being unproductive, economic hardship, and loneliness.

About 3.8 million older Americans were in the labor force (working or actively seeking work) in 1997. These included 2.2 million men and 1.5 million women, and constituted 2.7 percent of the U.S. labor force (Duncker & Greenberg, 1997).

Retirement has both social and economical implications for elderly individuals. The role is fraught with a great deal of ambiguity and is one that requires many adaptations on the part of those involved.

Social Implications

Retirement is often anticipated as an achievement in principle but met with a great deal of ambiguity when in actually occurs. Our society places a great deal of importance on productivity, making as much money as possible, and doing it at as young an age as possible. These types of values contribute to the ambiguity associated with retirement. Although leisure has been acknowledged as a legitimate reward for workers, leisure during retirement historically has lacked the same social value. Adjustment to this life-cycle event becomes more difficult in the face of societal values that are in direct conflict with the new lifestyle.

Historically, many women have derived a good deal of their self-esteem from their families—birthing them, rearing them, and being a "good mother." Likewise, many men have achieved self-esteem through work-related activities—creativity, productivity, and earning money. With the termination of these activities may come a loss of self-worth, resulting in depression in some individuals who are unable to adapt satisfactorily. Hendricks and Hendricks (1977) described a pattern that focuses on the continuity of environmental influences that *reinforce* appropriate adaptation to retirement. They have said:

"If the positive reinforcements present during early life and working adulthood are removed by retirement, the likelihood of adjustment is jeopardized. If a worker perceived money to be the most important reward for working, the significant decline in income after retirement will complicate the process of adjustment. If friends or feelings of autonomy were the reinforcing component of work, then retirement may pose markedly fewer problems." (p. 251)

American society often identifies an individual by his or her occupation. This is reflected in the conversation of people who are meeting each other for the first time. Undoubtedly, most everyone has either asked or been asked at some point in time, "What do you do?" or "Where do you work?" Occupation determines status, and retirement represents a significant change in status. The basic ambiguity of retirement occurs in an individual's or society's definition of this change. Is it undertaken voluntarily or involuntarily? Is it desirable or undesirable? Is one's status made better or worse by the change?

In looking at the trend of the past two decades, we may

presume that retirement is becoming, and will continue to become, more accepted by societal standards. With more and more individuals retiring earlier and living longer, the growing number of aging persons will spend a significantly longer time in retirement. At present, retirement has become more of an institutionalized expectation and there appears to be increasing acceptance of it as a social status.

Economic Implications

Because retirement is generally associated with a 20 to 40 percent reduction in personal income, the standard of living after retirement may be adversely affected (Petras & Petras, 1991). Most older adults derive retirement income from a combination of Social Security benefits, public and private pensions, and income from savings or investments.

In 1996, the median income in households headed by persons 65 or older was $28,983 and 3.4 million elderly persons were below the poverty level (Duncker & Greenberg, 1997). The rate of those living in poverty was higher among blacks and Hispanics than whites, and among women than men.

The Social Security Act of 1935 promised assistance with financial security for elderly Americans. Since then, the original legislation has been modified, yet the basic philosophy remains intact. Its effectiveness, however, is now being questioned. Faced with staggering deficits, the program is forced to pay benefits to those currently retired from both the reserve funds and moneys being collected at present. There is genuine concern about future generations, when undoubtedly there will be no reserve funds. Because many of the programs that benefit older adults depend on contributions from the younger population, the growing ratio of older Americans to younger persons may affect society's ability to supply the goods and services necessary to meet this expanding demand.

The **Medicare** and **Medicaid** systems were established by the government to provide medical care benefits for elderly and indigent Americans. Medicaid funds are matched by the states, and coverage varies significantly from state to state. Medicare covers only a percentage of health care costs, so to reduce risk related to out-of-pocket expenditures, many older adults purchase private "medigap" policies designed to cover charges in excess of those approved by Medicare.

The magnitude of retirement earnings depends almost entirely on preretirement income. The poor will remain poor and the wealthy are unlikely to lower their status during retirement; but for many in the middle classes, the relatively fixed income sources may be inadequate, possibly forcing them to face financial hardship for the first time in their lives.

Long-Term Care

Long-term care refers to a variety of formal and informal services needed for an extended period by people with limitations in function, as a result of one or more chronic illnesses or conditions, that interfere with daily living (Schechter & Butler, 1989). Long-term care facilities are defined by the level of care they provide. They may be skilled nursing facilities (SNFs), intermediate care facilities (ICFs), or a combination of the two. Some institutions provide convalescent care for individuals recovering from acute illness or injury, some provide long-term care for individuals with chronic illness or disabilities, and still others provide both types of assistance.

Most elderly individuals prefer to remain in their own homes or in the homes of family members for as long as this can meet their needs without deterioration of family or social patterns. Many elderly individuals are placed in institutions as a last resort only after heroic effects have been made to keep them in their own or a relative's home. The increasing emphasis on home health care has extended the period of independence for aging individuals.

In 1995, approximately 5 percent of the population aged 65 and older lived in nursing homes (Duncker & Greenberg, 1997). The percentage increased dramatically with age, ranging from 1 percent for persons aged 65 to 74 to 5 percent for persons aged 75 to 84, and 15 percent for persons aged 85 and older. A profile of the "typical" elderly nursing home resident is about 80 years of age, white, female, widowed, with multiple chronic health conditions (Duncker & Greenberg, 1997; Ignatavicius, 1998).

In determining who in our society will need long-term care, several factors have been identified that appear to place people at risk (Ignatavicius, 1998; Williams, 1995). The following risk factors are taken into consideration to predict potential need for services and to estimate future costs.

Age. Because people grow older in very different ways, and the range of differences becomes greater with the passage of time, age is becoming a less relevant characteristic than it was historically. However, because of the high prevalence of chronic health conditions and disabilities, as well as the greater chance of diminishing social supports associated with advancing age, the 65-and-older population is often viewed as an important long-term care target group.

Health. Level of functioning, as determined by ability to perform various behaviors or activities such as bathing, eating, mobility, meal preparation, handling finances, judgment, and memory, is a measurable risk factor. The need for ongoing assistance from another person is critical in determining the need for long-term care.

Mental Health Status. Mental health problems are risk factors in assessing need for long-term care. Many of the symptoms associated with certain mental disorders, (especially the dementias) such as memory loss, impaired judgment, impaired intellect, and disorientation, would render the individual incapable of meeting the demands of daily living independently.

Socioeconomic and Demographic Factors. Low income is generally associated with greater physical and mental health problems among the elderly. Because many elderly individuals have limited finances, they are less able to purchase care resources available outside of institutions (e.g., home health care), although Medicare and Medicaid now contribute a limited amount to this type of noninstitutionalized care. Women are at greater risk of being institutionalized than men, not because they are less healthy but because they tend to live longer and thus are usually older and more likely to be widowed. Whites have a higher rate of institutionalization than nonwhites. This may be related to cultural and financial influences.

Marital Status, Living Arrangement, and the Informal Support Network. Individuals who are married and live with a spouse are the least likely of all disabled people to be institutionalized. Those who live alone without resources for home care and few or no relatives living nearby to provide informal care are at higher risk for institutionalization.

Attitudinal Factors

Williams (1995) states:

> "The diversified highly regulated nursing home of today is a far cry from the nursing home of 30 years ago or the unsupervised, limited service, privately financed home for the poor that was common at the turn of the century." (p. 103)

State and national licensing boards perform periodic inspections to ensure that standards set forth by the federal governments are being met. These standards address quality of patient care as well as adequacy of the nursing home facility. Yet many elderly individuals and their families perceive nursing homes as a place to go to die, and the fact that many of these institutions are poorly equipped, understaffed, and disorganized keeps this societal perception alive. There are, however, many excellent nursing homes that strive to go beyond the minimum federal regulations for Medicaid and Medicare reimbursement. In addition to medical, nursing, rehabilitation, and dental services, social and recreational services are provided to increase the quality of life for the elderly living in nursing homes. These activities include playing cards, bingo, and other games; parties; church activities; books; television; movies; arts and crafts, and other classes. Some nursing homes provide occupational and professional counseling. These facilities strive to enhance opportunities for improving quality of life and for becoming "places to live," rather than "places to die."

Elder Abuse

Abuse of the elderly, which at times has been referred to in the media as **"granny-bashing,"** is a prevalent and serious form of family violence. Kaplan & Sadock (1998) estimate that 10 percent of individuals older than age 65 are the victims of abuse or neglect. The abuser is often a relative who lives with the elderly person and may be the assigned caregiver. Typical caregivers who are likely to be abusers of the elderly were described by Murray and Zentner (1997) as being under economic stress, substance abusers, themselves the victims of previous family violence, and exhausted and frustrated by the caregiver role. Identified risk factors for victims of abuse included being a white female 70 and older, mentally or physically impaired, unable to meet daily self-care needs, and having care needs that exceeded the caretaker's ability.

Adelman and Butler (1989) define three general categories of abuse of elderly persons—psychological, physical, and financial—and two categories of neglect—intentional and unintentional. Psychological abuse includes yelling, insulting, harsh commands, threats, silence, and social isolation. Physical abuse is described as striking, shoving, beating, or restraint. Financial abuse refers to misuse or theft of finances, property, or material possessions. Neglect implies failure to do the obviously necessary things that a person cannot do independently. Unintentional neglect is inadvert, whereas intentional neglect is deliberate. Additionally, elderly individuals may be the victims of sexual abuse, which is sexual intimacy between two persons that occurs without the consent of one of the persons involved. Another type of abuse, which has been called **"granny-dumping"** by the media, involves abandoning elderly individuals at emergency departments, nursing homes, or other facilities—literally leaving them in the hands of others when the strain of caregiving becomes intolerable. Types of elder abuse are summarized in Table 35.2.

Elder victims often minimize the abuse or deny that it has occurred (Kaplan, Sadock, & Grebb, 1994). The elderly person may be unwilling to disclose information because of fear of retaliation, embarrassment about the existence of abuse in the family, protectiveness toward a family member, or an unwillingness to institute legal action. Adding to this unwillingness to report is the fact that infirm elders are often isolated, so that their mistreatment is less likely to be noticed by those who might be alert to symptoms of abuse. For these reasons, detection of abuse in the elderly is difficult at best.

Factors that Contribute to Abuse

King (1984) describes a number of factors that contribute to abuse of elderly individuals.

Longer Life. The 65-and-older age group has become the fastest growing segment of the population, and within this segment, the number of elderly older than age 75 has increased most rapidly. This trend is expected to continue into the 21st century. The 75-and-older age group is the

TABLE 35.2 EXAMPLES OF ELDER ABUSE

Physical Abuse
Striking, hitting, beating
Shoving
Bruising
Cutting
Restraining

Psychological Abuse
Yelling
Insulting, name calling
Harsh commands
Threats
Ignoring, silence, social isolation

Neglect (intentional or unintentional)
Withholding food and water
Inadequate heating
Unclean clothes and bedding
Lack of needed medication
Lack of eyeglasses, hearing aids, false teeth

Financial Abuse or Exploitation
Misuse of the elderly person's income by the caregiver
Forcing the elderly person to sign over financial affairs
   to another person against his or her will or without
   sufficient knowledge about the transaction

Sexual Abuse
Sexual molestation; rape
Any type of sexual intimacy against the elderly person's will

SOURCE: Adapted from Kaplan & Sadock (1998) and Murray & Zenter (1997).

one most likely to be physically or mentally impaired, requiring assistance and care from family members. This group also is the most vulnerable to abuse from caregivers.

Dependency. Dependency is the most common precondition in domestic abuse. Changes associated with normal aging or induced by chronic illness often result in loss of self-sufficiency in the elderly, requiring that they become dependent on another for assistance with daily functioning. Long life may also consume finances to the point that the elderly individual becomes financially dependent on another as well. This dependence increases the elderly person's vulnerability to abuse.

Stress. The stress inherent in the caregiver role is a factor in most abuse cases. Some clinicians believe that elder abuse results from individual or family psychopathology. Others suggest that even psychologically healthy family members can become abusive as the result of the exhaustion and acute stress caused by overwhelming caregiving responsibilities. This is compounded in an age group that has been dubbed the "sandwich generation"—those individuals who elected to delay childbearing so that they are now at a point in their lives when they are "sandwiched" between providing care for their children and providing care for their aging parents.

Learned Violence. Children who have been abused or witnessed abusive and violent parents are more likely to evolve into abusive adults. Renvoise (1978) found that children who abuse their parents were most likely to have been abused by them as children. She also found that drinking alcohol was associated with violence in almost half the cases she studied.

Identifying Elder Abuse

Because so many elderly individuals are reluctant to report personal abuse, health care workers need to be able to detect signs of mistreatment when they are in a position to do so. Table 35.2 listed a number of *types* of elder abuse. Adelman and Butler (1989) have identified the following *manifestations* of the various categories of abuse:

* Indicators of psychological abuse include a broad range of behaviors such as the symptoms associated with pathological depression, excessive anxiety, and increased confusion or agitation.
* Indicators of physical abuse may include bruises, welts, lacerations, burns, punctures, evidence of hair pulling, and skeletal dislocations and fractures.
* Neglect may be manifested as inadequate warm clothing or heat in the home; lack of necessary supervision; substandard living conditions in relation to financial assets; failure to obtain eyeglasses, hearing aids, dentures, or prostheses; and failure to provide food and water, leading to malnutrition and dehydration.
* Possible sexual abuse may be suspected when the elderly person is presented with unexplained venereal disease or unusual genital infections.
* Financial abuse may be occurring when there is an obvious disparity between assets and satisfactory living conditions or when the elderly person complains of a sudden lack of sufficient funds for daily living expenses.

Health care workers often feel intimidated when confronted with cases of elder abuse. In these instances, referral to an individual experienced in management of victims of such abuse may be the most effective approach to evaluation and intervention. Intervention usually takes into consideration each individual case and ranges from counseling and court advocacy to supplying homemaker support or nursing home placement (Adelman & Butler, 1989). A family-oriented approach to intervention is favorable.

Increased efforts need to be made to provide health care providers with comprehensive training in the detection of and intervention in elder abuse. More research is needed to increase knowledge and understanding of the phenomenon of elder abuse and ultimately to effect more sophisticated strategies for prevention, intervention, and treatment.

Suicide

Although persons older than age 65 comprise only 12 percent of the population, they represent a disproportionately high percentage of individuals who commit suicide. Of all suicides, 17 percent are committed by this age group, and suicide is now one of the top 10 causes of death among the elderly population (Moody, 1994).

The group especially at risk appears to be white men. Predisposing factors include social isolation, loss of spouse, anxiety due to financial instability, and undertreated mood disorders (Ghosh & Victor, 1994).

Although the rate of suicide among the elderly population remains high, the number of suicides among this age group dropped steadily from 1930 to 1980. Investigators who study these trends surmise that this decline was due to increases in services for older people and an understanding of their problems in society. However, from 1980 to 1986 the number of suicides among those 65 and older increased by 25 percent, which suggests that other factors are contributing to the problem. Dr. Richard Sattin, a researcher at the Centers for Disease Control in Atlanta, suggests that increased social isolation may be a contributing factor to suicide among the elderly (Kaufman, 1991). The number of elderly individuals who are divorced, widowed, or otherwise living alone has increased. Divorce is a clear risk factor for elderly suicide, with the suicide rate for divorced men older than 65 three times that of married men older than 65 (Kaufman, 1991).

The American Association of Suicidology, however, suggests that isolation itself is not the key determinant, but the presence of a psychiatric disorder is the most important factor (Kaufman, 1991). A study conducted by the association revealed the presence of depression, alcoholism, or drug dependence (usually to prescription drugs) to be a factor in a majority of cases. Approximately one third suffered from a terminal illness or a severe and chronic medical condition.

Sadly, many elderly individuals express symptoms associated with depression that are never recognized as such. Any sign of helplessness or hopelessness should elicit a supportive intervening response. In assessing suicide intention, direct questions should be asked, but concern and compassion should be used:

- Have you ever had thoughts of suicide in the past?
- Have you ever attempted suicide?
- Are you currently experiencing thoughts of suicide?
- Do you have a plan for committing suicide?
- Do you have the means to carry out your plan? (Ghosh & Victor, 1994).

Components of intervention with a suicidal elderly person should include demonstrations of genuine concern, interest, and caring; indications of empathy for their fears and concerns; and help in identifying, clarifying, and formulating a plan of action to deal with the unresolved issue. If the elderly person's behavior seems particularly lethal, additional family or staff coverage and contact should be arranged to prevent isolation.

APPLICATION OF THE NURSING PROCESS

Assessment

Assessment of the elderly individual may follow the same framework used for all adults, but with consideration of the possible biological, psychological, sociocultural, and sexual changes that occur in the normal aging process described previously in this chapter. In no other area of nursing is it more important for nurses to practice holistic nursing than with the elderly. Older adults are likely to have multiple physical problems that contribute to problems in other areas of their lives. Obviously, these components cannot be addressed as separate entities. Nursing the elderly is a multifaceted, challenging process because of the multiple changes occurring at this time in the life cycle and the way in which each change affects every aspect of the individual.

Several considerations are unique to assessment of the elderly. Assessment of the older person's thought processes is a primary responsibility. Knowledge about the presence and extent of disorientation or confusion will influence the way in which the nurse approaches elder care.

Information about sensory capabilities is also extremely important. Because hearing loss is common, the nurse should lower the pitch and loudness of his or her voice when addressing the older person. Looking directly into the face of the older person when talking facilitates communication. Questions that require a declarative sentence in response should be asked; in this way, the nurse is able to assess the client's ability to use words correctly. Visual acuity can be determined by assessing adaptation to the dark, color matching, and the perception of color contrast. Knowledge about these aspects of sensory functioning is essential in the development of an effective care plan.

The nurse should be familiar with the normal physical changes associated with the aging process. Examples of some of these changes include:

- Less effective response to changes in environmental temperature, resulting in hypothermia.
- Decreases in oxygen use and the amount of blood pumped by the heart, resulting in cerebral anoxia or hypoxia.
- Skeletal muscle wasting and weakness, resulting in difficulty in physical mobility.
- Limited cough and laryngeal reflexes, resulting in risk of aspiration.
- Demineralization of bones, resulting in spontaneous fracturing.

- Decrease in gastrointestinal motility, resulting in constipation.
- Decrease in the ability to interpret painful stimuli, resulting in risk of injury.

Common psychosocial changes associated with aging include:

- Prolonged and exaggerated grief, resulting in depression.
- Physical changes, resulting in altered body image.
- Changes in status, resulting in loss of self-worth.

This list is by no means exhaustive. The nurse should consider many other alterations in his or her assessment of the client. Knowledge of the client's functional capabilities is essential for determining the physiological, psychological, and sociological needs of the elderly individual. Age alone does not preclude the occurrence of all these changes. The aging process progresses at a wide range of variance, and each client must be assessed as a unique individual.

Diagnosis/Outcome Identification

Virtually any nursing diagnosis may be applicable to the aging client, depending on individual needs for assistance. Based on normal changes that occur in the elderly, the following nursing diagnoses may be considered:

Physiologically Related Diagnoses

Risk for trauma related to confusion, disorientation, muscular weakness, spontaneous fractures, falls.

Hypothermia related to loss of adipose tissue under the skin, evidenced by increased sensitivity to cold and body temperature below 98.6 degrees.

Decreased cardiac output related to decreased myocardial efficiency secondary to age-related changes, evidenced by decreased tolerance for activity and decline in energy reserve.

Ineffective breathing pattern related to increase in fibrous tissue and loss of elasticity in lung tissue, evidenced by dyspnea and activity intolerance.

Risk for aspiration related to diminished cough and laryngeal reflexes.

Impaired physical mobility related to muscular wasting and weakness, evidenced by need for assistance in ambulation.

Altered nutrition, less than body requirements, related to inefficient absorption from gastrointestinal tract, difficulty chewing and swallowing, anorexia, difficulty in feeding self, evidenced by wasting syndrome, anemia, weight loss.

Constipation related to decreased motility; inadequate diet; insufficient activity or exercise, evidenced by decreased bowel sounds; hard, formed stools; or straining at stool.

Stress incontinence related to degenerative changes in pelvic muscles and structural supports associated with increased age, evidenced by reported or observed dribbling with increased abdominal pressure or urinary frequency.

Urinary retention related to prostatic enlargement, evidenced by bladder distention, frequent voiding of small amounts, dribbling, or overflow incontinence.

Sensory-perceptual alteration related to age-related alterations in sensory transmission, evidenced by decreased visual acuity, hearing loss, diminished sensitivity to taste and smell, or increased touch threshold.

Sleep pattern disturbance related to age-related decrease in ability to sleep ("sleep decay"), dementia, or medications, evidenced by interrupted sleep, early awakening, or falling asleep during the day.

Pain related to degenerative changes in joints, evidenced by verbalization of pain or hesitation to use weight-bearing joints.

Self-care deficit (specify) related to weakness, confusion, or disorientation, evidenced by inability to feed self, maintain hygiene, dress/groom self, or toilet self without assistance.

Risk for impaired skin integrity related to alterations in nutritional state, circulation, sensation, or mobility.

Psychosocially Related Diagnoses

Altered thought processes related to age-related changes that result in cerebral anoxia, evidenced by short-term memory loss, confusion, or disorientation.

Dysfunctional grieving related to bereavement overload, evidenced by symptoms of depression.

Risk for self-directed violence related to depressed mood and feelings of low self-worth.

Powerlessness related to lifestyle of helplessness and dependency on others, evidenced by depressed mood, apathy, or verbal expressions of having no control or influence over life situation.

Self-esteem disturbance related to loss of preretirement status, evidenced by verbalization of negative feelings about self and life.

Fear related to nursing home placement, evidenced by symptoms of severe anxiety and statements such as, "Nursing homes are places to go to die."

Body image disturbance related to age-related changes in skin, hair, fat distribution, evidenced by verbalization of negative feelings about body.

Altered sexuality patterns related to dyspareunia, evidenced by reported dissatisfaction with decrease in frequency of sexual intercourse.

Sexual dysfunction related to medications (e.g., antihypertensives) evidenced by inability to achieve an erection.

Social isolation related to total dependence on others, evidenced by expression of inadequacy in or absence of significant purpose in life.

Risk for trauma (elder abuse) related to caregiver role strain.

Caregiver role strain related to severity and duration of the care receiver's illness; lack of respite and recreation for the caregiver, evidenced by feelings of stress in relationship with care receiver; feelings of depression and anger; or family conflict around issues of providing care.

The following criteria may be used for measurement of outcomes in the care of the elderly client.

THE CLIENT:

1. Has not experienced injury.
2. Maintains reality orientation consistent with cognitive level of functioning.
3. Manages own self-care with assistance.
4. Expresses positive feelings about self, past accomplishments, and hope for the future.
5. Compensates adaptively for diminished sensory perception.

CAREGIVERS:

1. Can problem solve effectively regarding care of elderly client.
2. Demonstrate adaptive coping strategies for dealing with stress of caregiver role.
3. Openly express feelings.
4. Express desire to join support group of other caregivers.

Planning/Implementation

In Table 35.3, selected nursing diagnoses are presented for the elderly client. Outcome criteria are identified, along with appropriate nursing interventions and rationales.

Reminiscence therapy is especially helpful with elderly clients. This therapeutic intervention is highlighted in Table 35.4.

Evaluation

Reassessment is conducted in order to determine if the nursing actions have been successful in achieving the objectives of care. Evaluation of the nursing actions for the elderly client may be facilitated by gathering information using the following types of questions:

1. Has the client escaped injury from falls, burns, or other means to which he or she is vulnerable because of age?

2. Can caregivers verbalize means of providing a safe environment for the client?
3. Does the client maintain reality orientation at an optimum for his or her cognitive functioning?
4. Can the client distinguish between reality-based and non–reality-based thinking?
5. Can caregivers verbalize ways in which to orient client to reality, as needed?
6. Is the client able to accomplish self-care activities independently to his or her optimum level of functioning?
7. Does the client seek assistance for aspects of self-care that he or she is unable to perform independently?
8. Does the client express positive feelings about himself or herself?
9. Does the client reminisce about accomplishments that have occurred in his or her life?
10. Does the client express some hope for the future?
11. Does the client wear eyeglasses or a hearing aid, if needed, to compensate for sensory deficits?

TEST YOUR CRITICAL THINKING SKILLS

Mrs. M, age 76, is seeing her primary physician for her regular 6-month physical exam. Mrs. M's husband died 2 years ago, at which time she sold her home in Kansas and came to live in California with her only child, a daughter. The daughter is married and has three children (one in college and two teenagers at home). The daughter reports that her mother is becoming increasingly withdrawn, stays in her room, and eats very little. She has lost 13 lb since her last 6-month visit. The primary physician refers Mrs. M to a psychiatrist, who hospitalizes her for evaluation. He diagnoses Mrs. M with major depression.

Mrs. M tells the nurse, "I didn't want to leave my home, but my daughter insisted. I would have been all right. I miss my friends and my church. Back home I drove my car everywhere. But there's too much traffic out here. They sold my car, and I have to depend on my daughter or grandkids to take me places. I hate being so dependent! I miss my husband so much. I just sit and think about him and our past life all the time. I don't have any interest in meeting new people. I want to go home!!"

Mrs. M admits to having some thoughts of dying, although she denies feeling suicidal. She denies having a plan or means for taking her life. "I really don't want to die, but I just can't see much reason for living. My daughter and her family are so busy with their own lives. They don't need me—or even have time for me!"

Answer the following questions about Mrs. M:

1. What would be the *primary* nursing diagnosis for Mrs. M.?
2. Formulate a short-term goal for Mrs. M.
3. From the assessment data, identify the major problem that may be a long-term focus of care for Mrs. M.

12. Does the client consistently look at others in the face to facilitate hearing when they are talking to him or her?

13. Does the client use helpful aids, such as signs identifying various rooms, to help maintain orientation?

14. Can the caregivers work through problems and make decisions regarding care of the elderly client?

15. Do the caregivers include the elderly client in the decision-making process, if appropriate?

TABLE 35.3 CARE PLAN FOR THE ELDERLY CLIENT

NURSING DIAGNOSIS: RISK FOR TRAUMA

RELATED TO: Confusion, disorientation, muscular weakness, spontaneous fractures, falls

OUTCOME CRITERIA	NURSING INTERVENTIONS	RATIONALE
Client will not experience injury.	1. The following measures may be instituted: a. Arrange furniture and other items in the room to accommodate client's disabilities. b. Store frequently used items within easy access. c. Keep bed in unelevated position. Pad siderails and headboard if client has history of seizures. Keep bedrails up when client is in bed. d. Assign room near nurses' station; observe frequently. e. Assist client with ambulation. f. Keep a dim light on at night. g. If client is a smoker, cigarettes and lighter or matches should be kept at the nurses' station and dispensed only when someone is available to stay with client while he or she is smoking. h. Frequently orient client to place, time, and situation. i. Soft restraints may be required if client is very disoriented and hyperactive.	1. To ensure client safety.

NURSING DIAGNOSIS: ALTERED THOUGHT PROCESSES

RELATED TO: Age-related changes that result in cerebral anoxia

EVIDENCED BY: Short-term memory loss, confusion, or disorientation.

OUTCOME CRITERIA	NURSING INTERVENTIONS	RATIONALE
Client will interpret the environment accurately and maintain reality orientation to the best of his or her cognitive ability.	1. Frequently orient client to reality. Use clocks and calendars with large numbers that are easy to read. Notes and large, bold signs may be useful as reminders. Allow client to have personal belongings. 2. Keep explanations simple. Use face-to-face interaction. Speak slowly and do not shout. 3. Discourage rumination or delusional thinking. Talk about real events and real people. 4. Monitor for medication side effects.	1. To help maintain maintain orientation and aid in memory and recognition. 2. To facilitate comprehension. Shouting may create discomfort and in some instances may provoke anger. 3. Rumination promotes disorientation. Reality orientation increases sense of self-worth and personal dignity. 4. Physiological changes in the elderly can alter the body's response to certain medications. Toxic effects may intensify altered thought processes.

NURSING DIAGNOSIS: SELF-CARE DEFICIT (SPECIFY)
RELATED TO: Weakness, disorientation, confusion, or memory deficits
EVIDENCED BY: Inability to fulfill activities of daily living

OUTCOME CRITERIA	NURSING INTERVENTIONS	RATIONALE
Client will accomplish activities of daily living to the best of his or her ability. Unfulfilled needs will be met by caregivers.	1. Provide a simple, structured environment: a. Identify self-care deficits and provide assistance as required. Promote independent actions as able. b. Allow plenty of time for client to perform tasks. c. Provide guidance and support for independent actions by talking the client through the task one step at a time. d. Provide a structured schedule of activities that do not change from day to day. e. Activities of daily living should follow home routine as closely as possible. f. Allow consistency in assignment of daily caregivers.	1. To minimize confusion.

NURSING DIAGNOSIS: CAREGIVER ROLE STRAIN
RELATED TO: Severity and duration of the care receiver's illness; lack of respite and recreation for the caregiver
EVIDENCED BY: Feelings of stress in relationship with care receiver; feelings of depression and anger; family conflict around issues of providing care.

OUTCOME CRITERIA	NURSING INTERVENTIONS	RATIONALE
Caregivers will achieve effective problem-solving skills and develop adaptive coping mechanisms to regain equilibrium.	1. Assess prospective caregivers' ability to anticipate and fulfill client's unmet needs. Provide information to assist caregivers with this responsibility. Ensure that caregivers are aware of available community support systems from whom they can seek assistance when required. Examples include adult day-care centers, housekeeping and homemaker services, respite care services, or perhaps a local chapter of the Alzheimer's Disease and Related Disorders Association. This organization sponsors a nationwide 24-hour hot line to provide information and link families who need assistance with nearby chapters and affiliates. The hot-line number is 1-800-621-0379. 2. Encourage caregivers to express feelings, particularly anger. 3. Encourage participation in support groups composed of members with similar life situations.	1. Caregivers require relief from the pressures and strain of providing 24-hour care for their loved one. Studies have shown that elder abuse arises out of caregiving situations that place overwhelming stress on the caregivers. 2. Release of these emotions can serve to prevent psychopathology, such as depression or psychophysiological disorders, from occurring. 3. Hearing others who are experiencing the same problems discuss ways in which they have coped may help caregiver adopt more adaptive strategies. Individuals who are experiencing similar life situations provide empathy and support for each other.

Continued on following page

TABLE 35.3 *(Continued)*

NURSING DIAGNOSIS: SELF-ESTEEM DISTURBANCE
RELATED TO: Loss of preretirement status
EVIDENCED BY: Verbalization of negative feelings about self and life

OUTCOME CRITERIA	NURSING INTERVENTIONS	RATIONALE
Client will demonstrate increased feelings of self-worth by expressing positive aspects of self and past accomplishments.	1. Encourage client to express honest feelings in relation to loss of prior status. Acknowledge pain of loss. Support client through process of grieving. 2. If lapses in memory are occurring, devise methods for assisting client with memory deficit. Examples: 　a. Name sign on door identifying client's room 　b. Identifying sign on outside of dining room door. 　c. Identifying sign on outside of restroom door. 　d. Large clock with oversized numbers and hands, appropriately placed. 　e. Large calendar, indicating one day at a time, with month, day, and year in bold print. 　f. Printed, structured daily schedule, with one copy for client and one posted on unit wall. 　g. "News board" on unit wall where current news of national and local interest may be posted. 3. Encourage client's attempts to communicate. If verbalizations are not understandable, express to client what you think he or she intended to say. It may be necessary to reorient client frequently. 4. Encourage reminiscence and discussion of life review (see Table 35.4). Also discuss present-day events. Sharing picture albums, if possible, is especially good. 5. Encourage participation in group activities. May need to accompany client at first, until he or she feels secure that the group members will be accepting, regardless of limitations in verbal communication. 6. Encourage client to be as independent as possible in self-care activities. Provide written schedule of tasks to be performed. Intervene in areas where client requires assistance.	1. Client may be fixed in anger stage of grieving process, which is turned inward on the self, resulting in diminished self-esteem. 2. Memory aids may assist client to function more independently, thereby increasing self-esteem. 3. The ability to communicate effectively with others may enhance self-esteem. 4. Reminiscence and life review help client resume progression through the grief process associated with disappointing life events and increase self-esteem as successes are reviewed. 5. Positive feedback from group members will increase self-esteem. 6. The ability to perform independently preserves self-esteem.

NURSING DIAGNOSIS: SENSORY-PERCEPTUAL ALTERATION

RELATED TO: Age-related alterations in sensory transmission

EVIDENCED BY: Decreased visual acuity, hearing loss, diminished sensitivity to taste and smell, and increased touch threshold.

OUTCOME CRITERIA	NURSING INTERVENTIONS*	RATIONALE
Client will attain optimal level of sensory stimulation. Client will not experience injury due to diminished sensory perception.	1. The following nursing strategies are indicated: a. Provide meaningful sensory stimulation to all special senses through conversation, touch, music, or pleasant smells. b. Encourage wearing of glasses, hearing aids, prostheses, and other adaptive devices. c. Use bright, contrasting colors in the environment. d. Provide large-print reading materials, such as books, clocks, calendars, and educational materials. e. Maintain room lighting that distinguishes day from night and that is free of shadows and glare. f. Teach client to scan the environment to locate objects. g. Help client to locate food on a plate using "clock" system, and describe food if client is unable to visualize; assist with feeding as needed. h. Arrange physical environment to maximize functional vision. i. Place personal items, call button, and so forth, within client's field of vision. j. Teach client to watch the person who is speaking. k. Reinforce wearing of hearing aid; if client does not have an aid, use a communication device. l. Communicate clearly, distinctly, and slowly; use a low-pitched voice and face client; avoid overarticulation. m. Remove as much necessary background noise as possible. n. Do not use slang or extraneous words. o. As speaker, position self at eye level and no farther than 6 ft away. p. Get the client's attention before speaking. q. Avoid speaking directly into the client's ear. r. If the client does not understand what is being said, rephrase the statement rather than simply repeating it.	1. To assist client with diminished sensory perception and because client safety is a nursing priority.

Continued on following page

TABLE 35.3 *(Continued)*

	s. Help client select foods from the menus that will ensure a discrimination between various tastes and smells.
	t. Ensure that food has been properly cooled so that client with diminished pain threshold is not burned.
	u. Ensure that bath or shower water is appropriate temperature.
	v. Use backrubs and massage as therapeutic touch to stimulate sensory receptors.

*The interventions for this nursing diagnosis were adapted from Rogers-Seidl (1991), with permission.

TABLE 35.4   REMINISCENCE THERAPY WITH THE ELDERLY

Butler (1974) states:
> "The life review is characterized by a progressive return to consciousness of past experience, in particular the resurgence of unresolved conflicts which can now be surveyed and integrated. If unresolved conflicts and fears are successfully reintegrated they can give new significance and meaning to an individual's life."

Studies have indicated that *reminiscence*, or thinking about the past and reflecting on it, may promote better mental health in old age. An early study of reminiscence found that elderly individuals who spend time thinking about the past are less likely to suffer depression (McMahon & Rhudick, 1967). Some psychologists believe that life review may help some people adjust to memories of an unhappy past. Others view reminiscence and life review as ways to bolster self-esteem, particularly in older people who can no longer remain active (Haight, 1991).

Reminiscence therapy can take place on a one-to-one basis or in a group setting. In reminiscence groups, elderly individuals share significant past events with peers. The nurse leader facilitates the discussion of topics that deal with specific life transitions, such as childhood, adolescence, marriage, childbearing, grandparenthood, and retirement. Members share both positive and negative aspects, including personal feelings, about these life-cycle events.

Reminiscence on a one-to-one basis can provide a way for elderly individuals to work through unresolved issues from the past. Painful issues may be too difficult to discuss in the group setting. As the individual reviews his or her life process, the nurse can validate feelings and help the elderly client come to terms with painful issues that may have been long suppressed. This process is necessary if the elderly individual is to maintain (or attain) a sense of positive identity and self-esteem and ultimately achieve the goal of ego integrity as described by Erikson (1963).

A number of creative measures can be used to facilitate life review with the elderly individual. Having the client keep a journal for sharing may be a way to stimulate discussion (as well as providing a permanent record of past events for significant others). Pets, music, and special foods have a way of provoking memories from the client's past. Photographs of family members and past significant events are an excellent way of guiding the elderly client through his or her autobiographical review.

Kermis (1986) states,
> "Depending upon the person, the life review can be mild or extreme. In its mildest form, the person tells stories about the past and verbalizes successes and regrets. The life review can be more problematic in others, especially if they must conduct their review in isolation. Anxiety, guilt, depression, despair, and even suicide may result if the person cannot resolve problems or accept them. The life review can become tragic if the person decides that life was useless. However, positive results can also come of the life review. The person can take pride in past accomplishments and feel satisfied with his or her life. This can produce a sense of serenity and inner peace in the older client."

RESEARCH NOTE

Spousal interactions in Alzheimer's disease and stroke caregiving: Relationship to care recipients' functional abilities and physical and emotional health. *Journal of the American Psychiatric Nurses Association* **(1998, December), 4(6), 169–181.**
Wright, L.K., Hickey, J.V., Buckwalter, K.C., Kelechi, T., and Hendrix, S.A.

Description of the Study: The objective of this study was to examine spousal interactions along two illness trajectories, Alzheimer's disease (AD) and stroke, and to determine effect of spousal interaction on functional ability and physical and emotional health. The sample in this study included 42 couples equally divided among three groups. One group consisted of 14 persons afflicted with early-phase AD and their spousal caregivers. The second group consisted of 14 persons who had had a stroke and their 14 caregiver spouses. The third group was a control group of 14 healthy couples randomly selected from the community. Demographics were matched among the three groups according to age (mean, 65 years; range 49 to 85 years) and length of marriage (mean, 36 years; range 1 to 57 years). Data was collected in face-to-face interviews at baseline and 6-month follow-up, using various questionnaires to measure cognitive impairment, functional abilities, and physical and emotional health. Spousal interactions were measured by the Dyadic Adjustment Rating (DAR) Scale, with the subscale of "affection" being expanded to include the following items: kissing the spouse, touching the spouse lovingly, caressing, holding hands, putting an arm around the spouse, and sleeping in the same bed. Present interactions were considered during the time frame of the preceding 2 weeks. Past spousal interactions were referred to as "prior to illness onset" for the AD and stroke couples and "prior to retirement" for the well couples.

Results of the Study: At baseline assessment, functional ability in both the AD and stroke groups was similar. Quality and quantity of spousal interactions in the AD group were lower than for both the stroke and well group. Little change had occurred in the quality and quantity of spousal interactions after 6 months for all three groups, the one exception being increased quantity of interaction in the AD group. Both AD and stroke groups showed increases in depression at the 6-month follow-up. Spousal interaction was found to be positively correlated to functional ability, physical health, and lower depression in AD care recipients. No significant correlation was found between stroke couples' interactions and stroke care recipients' depression or physical health. Significant correlation was found only with increased functional ability at the 6-month follow-up.

Comments: This study revealed that positive spousal interactions are predominantly related to better physical and emotional health in AD care recipients and to increased functional ability in persons who have had a stroke. The authors suggest that these results provide a better understanding of changes in caregiver and care recipient interactions as well as knowledge of factors that could have an impact on the functioning and health of ill spouses. They further suggest the need for additional studies with larger sample sizes over longer periods.

---

16. Can the caregivers demonstrate adaptive coping strategies for dealing with the strain of long-term caregiving?
17. Are the caregivers open and honest in expression of feelings?
18. Can the caregivers verbalize community resources to whom they can go for assistance with their caregiving responsibilities?
19. Have the caregivers joined a support group?

SUMMARY

Care of the aging individual presents one of the greatest challenges for nursing. The growing population of individuals aged 65 and older suggests that the challenge will progress well into the 21st century.

America is a youth-oriented society. It is not desirable to be old; in fact, to some it is repugnant. Most, however, if faced with a choice, would choose growing old to the alternative, death. In some cultures, the elderly are revered and hold a special place of honor within the society, but in highly industrialized countries such as the United States, status declines with the decrease in productivity and participation in the mainstream of society.

Individuals experience many changes as they age. Physical changes occur in virtually every body system.

Psychologically, there may be age-related memory deficiencies, particularly for recent events. Intellectual functioning does not decline with age, but length of time required for learning increases.

INTERNET REFERENCES

- Additional sources related to aging may be located at the following websites:
  a. http://www.noah.cuny.edu/aging/ushc/menopause.html
  b. http://www.4woman.org/
  c. http://pr.aoa.dhhs.gov/aoa/stats/statpage.html
  d. http://www.interinc.com/NCEA
  e. http://www.aarp.org/
  f. http://www.oaktrees.org/elder/
  g. http://www.acjnet.org/docs/eldabpfv.html
  h. http://www.ssa.gov/
  i. http://www.nfcacares.org/home.html
  j. http://www.nih.gov/nia/
  k. http://www.medicare.gov/
  l. http://www.seniorlaw.com/
  m. http://www.growthhouse.org/cesp.html
  n. http://www.agenet.com/
  o. http://www.aoa.dhhs.gov/elderpage.html
  p. http://www.senior.com/
  q. http://www.nsclc.org/
  r. http://www.anti-age.com/

Aging individuals experience many losses, potentially leading to bereavement overload. They are vulnerable to depression and to feelings of low self-worth. The number of suicides increased 25 percent in the 65 and older age group from 1980 to 1986. Dementing disorders are the most frequent causes of psychopathology in the elderly. Sleep disorders are very common.

The need for sexual expression by the elderly is often misunderstood within our society. Although many physical changes occur at this time of life that alter an individual's sexuality, if he or she has reasonably good health and a willing partner, sexual activity can continue well past the 70s for most people.

Retirement has both social and economical implications for elderly individuals. Society often equates an individual's status with his or her occupation, and loss of employment may result in the need for adjustment in the standard of living, as retirement income may be reduced by 20 to 40 percent of preretirement earnings.

Less than 5 percent of the population aged 65 and older live in nursing homes. A profile of the typical elderly nursing home resident is a white woman about 78 years old, widowed, with multiple chronic health conditions. Much stigma is attached to what some still call "rest homes" or "old age homes," and many elderly people still equate them with a place "to go to die."

The strain of the caregiver role has become a major dilemma in our society. Elder abuse is sometimes inflicted by caregivers for whom the role has become overwhelming and intolerable. There is an intense need to find assistance for these people, who must provide care for their loved ones on a 24-hour basis. Home health care, respite care, support groups, and financial assistance are needed to ease the burden of this role strain.

Nursing of the elderly individual is accomplished through the six steps of the nursing process. Assessment requires that changes occurring in the normal aging process—biological, psychological, sociocultural, and sexual—be taken into consideration before an accurate plan of care can be formulated.

Nursing of elderly individuals requires a special kind of inner strength and compassion. The following poem, which has undoubtedly become very familiar over the years, is excellent in eliciting empathy for what the elderly must feel. I thank the anonymous author for sharing. It conveys a powerful message.

WHAT DO YOU SEE, NURSE?

What do you see, nurse, what do you see?
What are you thinking when you look at me?
A crabbed old woman, not very wise.
Uncertain of habit, with faraway eyes.
Who dribbles her food and makes not reply
When you say in a loud voice, "I do wish you'd try."
Who seems not to notice the things that you do
And forever is losing a stocking or shoe.
Who unresisting or not, lets you do as you will
With bathing and feeding, the long day to fill.
Is that what you're thinking, is that what you see?
Then open your eyes, you're not looking at me.
I'll tell you who I am as I sit there so still.
As I move at your bidding, as I eat at your will.
I'm a small child of ten with a father and mother,
Brothers and sisters who love one another.
A young girl at sixteen with wings on her feet
Dreaming that soon now a lover she'll meet.
A bride soon at twenty—my heart gives a leap
Remembering the vows that I promised to keep.
At twenty-five, now, I have young of my own
Who need me to build a secure happy home.
A woman of thirty, my young now grow fast
Bound to each other with ties that should last.
At forty my young now will soon be gone,
But my man stays beside me to see I don't mourn.
At fifty once more babies play round my knee.
Again we know children, my loved one and me.
Dark days are upon me, my husband is dead.
I look at the future, I shudder with dread.
For my young are all busy rearing young of their own.
And I think of the years and the love I have known.
I'm an old woman now and nature is cruel.
Tis her jest to make old age look like a fool.
The body it crumbles, grace and vigor depart.
There is now just a stone where I once had a heart.
But inside this old carcass a young girl still dwells.
And now and again my battered heart swells.
I remember the joys, I remember the pain.
And I'm loving and living life all over again.
I think of the years all too few—gone so fast.
And accept the stark fact that nothing can last.
So open your eyes, nurse, open and see.
Not a crabbed old woman—look closer—SEE ME.

Author unknown.

REVIEW QUESTIONS

SELF-EXAMINATION/LEARNING EXERCISE

Select the answer that is most appropriate for the questions that follow this situation.

Situation: Stanley, a 72-year-old widower, was brought to the hospital by his son, who reports that Stanley has become increasingly withdrawn. He has periods of confusion and forgetfulness, but most of the time his thought processes are intact. He eats very little and has lost some weight. His wife died 5 years ago and the son reports, "He did very well, didn't even cry." Stanley attended the funeral of his best friend 1 month ago, after which these symptoms began. Stanley has been admitted for testing and evaluation.

1. In her admission assessment, the nurse notices an open sore on Stanley's arm. When she questions him about it he says, "I scraped it on the fence 2 weeks ago. It's smaller than it was." How might the nurse analyze these data?

   a. Stanley was trying to commit suicide.
   b. The delay in healing may indicate that Stanley has developed cancer of the skin.
   c. A diminished inflammatory response in the elderly person increases healing time.
   d. Age-related skin changes and distribution of adipose tissue delay healing in the elderly.

2. Stanley is deaf on his right side. Which is the most appropriate nursing intervention for communicating with Stanley?

   a. Speak loudly into his left ear.
   b. Speak to him from a position on his left side.
   c. Speak face-to-face in a high-pitched voice.
   d. Speak face-to-face in a low-pitched voice.

3. Why is it important to have the nurse check the temperature of the water before Stanley takes a shower?

   a. Stanley may catch cold if the water temperature is too low.
   b. Stanley may burn himself because of a higher pain threshold.
   c. Stanley has difficulty discriminating between hot and cold.
   d. The water must be exactly 98.6°F.

4. From the information provided in the situation, which would be the priority nursing diagnosis for Stanley?

   a. Dysfunctional grieving.
   b. Altered nutrition: less than body requirements.
   c. Social isolation.
   d. High risk for injury.

5. The physician diagnoses Stanley with major depression. A suicide assessment is conducted. Why is Stanley at high risk for suicide?

   a. All depressed people are at high risk for suicide.
   b. Stanley is in the age group in which the highest percentage of suicides occur.
   c. Stanley is a white man, recently bereaved, living alone.
   d. His son reports that Stanley owns a gun.

6. Which of the following would be a priority nursing intervention with Stanley?

   a. Take blood pressure once each shift.
   b. Ensure that Stanley attends group activities.
   c. Encourage Stanley to eat all of the food on his food tray.
   d. Encourage Stanley to talk about his wife's death.

7. In group exercise, Stanley becomes tired and short of breath very quickly. This is most likely due to:

   a. Age-related changes in the cardiovascular system.
   b. Stanley's sedentary lifestyle.
   c. The effects of pathological depression.
   d. Medication the physician has prescribed for depression.

8. Stanley says to the nurse, "I'm all alone now. My wife is gone. My best friend is gone. My son is busy with his work and family. I might as well just go, too." Which is the best response by the nurse?

   a. "Are you thinking that you want to die, Stanley?"
   b. "You have lots to live for, Stanley."
   c. "Cheer up, Stanley. It's almost time for activity therapy."
   d. "Tell me about your family, Stanley."

9. Stanley says to the nurse, "I don't want to go to that crafts class. I'm too old to learn anything." Based on knowledge of the aging process, which of the following is a true statement?

   a. Memory functioning in the elderly most likely reflects loss of long-term memories of remote events.
   b. Intellectual functioning declines with advancing age.
   c. Learning ability remains intact, but time required for learning increases with age.
   d. Cognitive functioning is rarely affected in aging individuals.

10. According to the literature, which of the following is most important for Stanley to maintain a healthy, adaptive old age?

    a. To remain socially interactive.
    b. To disengage slowly in preparation of the last stage of life.
    c. To move in with his son and family.
    d. To maintain total independence and accept no help from anyone.

REFERENCES

Adelman, R.D., & Butler, R.N. (1989). Elder abuse and neglect. In H.I. Kaplan & B.J. Sadock (Eds.), *Comprehensive textbook of psychiatry* (Vol. 2) (5th ed.). Baltimore: Williams & Wilkins.

Atchley, R.C. (1989). A continuity theory of normal aging. *Gerontologist, 29,* 183–190.

Beck, M., et al. (1992, May 25). Menopause. *Newsweek, 119* (21), 38–42.

Blazer, D. (1994). Geriatric psychiatry. In R.E. Hales, S.C. Yudofsky, & J.A. Talbott (Eds.), *Textbook of psychiatry* (2nd ed.). Washington, DC: American Psychiatric Press.

Bowen, C.D. (1944). *Yankee from Olympus.* Boston: Little, Brown.

Brecher, E.M., et al. (1984). *Love, sex, and aging.* Mount Vernon, NY: Consumers Union.

Breen, L.A. (1960). The aging individual. In C. Tibbits (Ed.), *Handbook of social gerontology.* Chicago: University of Chicago Press.

Busse, E.W. (1989). The myth, history, and science of aging. In E.W. Busse & D.G. Blazer (Eds.), *Geriatric psychiatry.* Washington, DC: American Psychiatric Press.

Butler, R.N. (1974). Successful aging and the role of the life review. *Journal of the American Geriatrics Society, 22,* 529–535.

Butler, R.N. (1989). Psychosocial aspects of aging. In H.I. Kaplan & B.J. Sadock (Eds.), *Comprehensive textbook of psychiatry* (Vol. 2) (5th ed.). Baltimore: Williams & Wilkins.

Cath, S.H., & Sadavoy, J. (1991). Psychosocial aspects. In J. Sadavoy et al. (Eds.), *Comprehensive review of geriatric psychiatry.* Washington, DC: American Psychiatric Press.

Cumming, E., & Henry, W. E. (1961). *The process of disengagement.* New York: Basic Books.

Duncker, A.P., & Greenberg, S.R. (1997). *A profile of older Americans.* Washington, DC: Resource Services Group, American Association of Retired Persons and the Administration on Aging, U.S. Department of Health and Human Services.

Erikson, E.H. (1963). *Childhood and society* (2nd ed.). New York: W.W. Norton.

Ghosh, T.B., & Victor, B.S. (1994). Suicide. In R.E. Hales, S.C. Yudofsky, & J.S. Talbott (Eds.), *The American Psychiatric Press textbook of psychiatry* (2nd ed.). Washington, DC: American Psychiatric Press.

Giger, J.N., & Davidhizar, R.E. (1991). *Transcultural nursing: Assessment and intervention.* St. Louis: Mosby Year Book.

Guterman, A., & Eisdorfer, C. (1989). Other psychiatric conditions of the elderly. In H.I. Kaplan & B.J. Sadock (Eds.), *Comprehensive textbook of psychiatry* (Vol. 2) (5th ed.). Baltimore: Williams & Wilkins.

Haight, B.K. (1991). Reminiscing: The state of the art as a basis for practice. *International Journal of Aging and Human Development, 33*(1), 1–32.

Hendricks, J. & Hendricks, C.D. (1977). *Aging in mass society.* Cambridge, MA: Winthrop Publishers.

Hyde, J.S. (1986). *Understanding human sexuality* (3rd ed.). New York: McGraw-Hill.

Ignatavicius, D.D. (1998). *Introduction to long-term care nursing: Principles and practice.* Philadelphia: F.A. Davis.

Kaplan, H.I., & Sadock, B.J. (1998). *Synopsis of psychiatry: Behavioral sciences/clinical psychiatry* (8th ed.). Baltimore: Williams & Wilkins.

Kaplan, H.I., Sadock, B.J., & Grebb, J.A. (1994). *Synopsis of psychiatry* (7th ed.). Baltimore: Williams & Wilkins.

Kaufman, M. (1991, October 2). Elderly suicide increase baffling. *The Wichita Eagle,* 1a.

Kaufman, S.R. (1986). *The ageless self: Sources of meaning in late life.* Madison: University of Wisconsin Press.

Kenney, A.R. (1989). *Physiology of aging: A synopsis* (2nd ed.). Chicago: Year Book Medical Publishers.

Kermis, M.D. (1986). *Mental health in late life: The adaptive process.* Boston: Jones & Bartlett.

King, N.R. (1984). Exploitation and abuse of older family members: An overview of the problem. In J.J. Costa (Ed.), *Abuse of the elderly*. Lexington, MA: D.C. Health.

Kluger, J. (1996, November 25). Can we stay young? *Time, 148*(24), 89–99.

Kübler-Ross, E. (1969). *On death and dying*. New York: Macmillan.

Larocco, M. (1994). Inflammation and immunity. In C. M. Porth (Ed.), *Pathophysiology: Concepts of altered health states* (4th ed). Philadelphia: J.B. Lippincott.

Leventhal, E.A. (1991). Biological aspects. In J. Sadavoy et al. (Eds.), *Comprehensive review of geriatric psychiatry*. Washington, DC: American Psychiatric Press.

Masters, W. H., & Johnson, V.E. (1966). *Human sexual response*. Boston: Little, Brown.

McMahon, AW., & Rhudick, P.J. (1967). Reminiscing in the aged: An adaptational response. In S. Lvein & R.J. Kahana (Eds.), *Psychodynamic studies on aging: Creativity, reminiscing, and dying*. New York: International Universities Press.

Moody, H.R. (1994). *Aging: Concepts and controversies*. Thousand Oaks, CA: Pine Forge Press.

Murray, R.B., & Zentner, J.P. (1997). *Health assessment and promotion strategies through the life span* (6th ed.). Stamford, CT: Appleton & Lange.

Neugarten, B.L. (1986). Personality in late life. In M.D. Kermis (Ed.), *Mental health in late life: The adaptive process*. Boston: Jones & Bartlett.

Neugarten, B.L., et al. (1964) *Personality in middle and late life*. New York: Atherton.

Palmore, E., & Maddox, G.L. (1977). Sociological aspects of aging. In E.W. Busse & E. Pfeiffer (Eds.), *Behavior and adaptation in late life*. Boston: Little, Brown.

Petras, K., & Petras, R. (1991). *The only retirement guide you'll ever need*. New York: Poseidon Press.

Physician Payment Review Commission. (1989). *Annual report to Congress*. Washington, DC: U.S. Government Printing Office.

Pikna, J.K. (1994). Concepts of altered health in older adults. In C.M. Porth (Ed.), *Pathophysiology: Concepts of altered health states* (4th ed.). Philadelphia: J.B. Lippincott.

Reichard, S., Livson, F., & Peterson, P. G. (1962). *Aging and personality*. New York: John Wiley & Sons.

Reinisch, J.M. (1990). *The Kinsey Institute new report on sex*. New York: St. Martin's Press.

Renvoise, J. (1978). *Web of violence: A study of family violence*. London: Routledge & Kegan Paul.

Roberts, C.M. (1991). *How did I get here so fast?* New York: Warner Books.

Rogers-Seidl, F.F. (1991). *Geriatric nursing care plans*. St. Louis: Mosby Year Book.

Sadavoy, J., Lazarus, L.W., & Jarvik, L.F. (1991). *Comprehensive review of geriatric psychiatry*. Washington, DC: American Psychiatric Press.

Schaie, K.W. (1990). Intellectual development in adulthood. In J.E. Biffen & K.W. Schaie (Eds.), *Handbook of the psychology of aging* (3rd ed.). New York: Academic.

Schechter, M., & Butler, R.N. (1989). Long-term care. In H.I. Kaplan & B.J. Sadock (Eds.), *Comprehensive textbook of psychiatry* (Vol. 2) (5th ed.) Baltimore: Williams & Wilkins.

Seligmann, J., Friday, C., & Wingert, P. (1992, May 25). Every woman for herself. *Newsweek, 119*(21), 43–44.

Shader, R.I., & Kennedy, J.S. (1989). Biological treatments. In H.I. Kaplan & B.J. Sadock (Eds.), *Comprehensive textbook of psychiatry* (Vol. 2) (5th ed.). Baltimore: Williams & Wilkins.

Vaillant, G., & Vaillant, C.O. (1990). Natural history of male psychosocial health: A 45-year study of predictors of successful aging at age 65. *American Journal of Psychiatry, 147*, 31–37.

Williams, M.E. (1995). *The American Geriatrics Society's complete guide to aging and health*. New York: Harmony Books.

THE INDIVIDUAL WITH HIV DISEASE

CHAPTER OUTLINE

KEY TERMS

human immunodeficiency virus
acquired immunodeficiency syndrome
T4 lymphocytes
persistent generalized lymphadenopathy

seroconversion
opportunistic infection
HIV wasting syndrome
pneumocystis pneumonia
Kaposi's sarcoma

HIV-associated dementia
Standard Precautions
Transmission-Based Precautions
hospice

OBJECTIVES

After reading this chapter, the student will be able to:

1. Discuss the **human immunodeficiency virus** (HIV) as the causative agent in the development of **acquired immunodeficiency syndrome** (AIDS).
2. Describe the pathophysiology incurred by HIV.
3. Discuss historical perspectives associated with AIDS.
4. Relate epidemiological statistics associated with AIDS.
5. Identify predisposing factors to AIDS.
6. Describe symptomatology associated with HIV infection and AIDS and use this data in client assessment.
7. Formulate nursing diagnoses and goals of care for clients with AIDS.
8. Describe appropriate nursing interventions for clients with AIDS.
9. Identify topics for client and family teaching relevant to HIV disease.
10. Evaluate nursing care of clients with AIDS.
11. Discuss various modalities relevant to treatment of clients with AIDS.

IDS was first recognized as a lethal clinical syndrome in 1981 (Wolcott, Dilley, & Mitsuyasu, 1989). Since that time, it has grown in epidemic proportions and has been declared the number one health priority in the United States today. Much research is now focused on HIV infection as a possible means of altering the course of the epidemic.

The human immunodeficiency virus (HIV) is the etiological agent that produces the immunosuppression resulting in AIDS. Individuals are diagnosed as having HIV infection when the virus is directly identified in host tissues by virus isolation or indirectly identified by the presence of HIV antibodies in body fluid using laboratory immunoassay testing (Osmond, 1990a).

Many individuals with HIV infection remain asymptomatic for years, with a mean time of approximately 10 years between exposure and development of AIDS (Hollander & Katz, 1996).

Since 1993, HIV disease has been defined as "a specific group of diseases or conditions which are indicative of severe immunosuppression related to infection with the human immunodeficiency virus (HIV)" (CDC, 1995). HIV disease identifies a full spectrum of conditions caused by HIV infection, including asymptomatic HIV infection, symptomatic infection, and AIDS (Douglas & Pinsky, 1996). The individual with HIV infection is considered to have "CDC-defined AIDS" when the T4 lymphocyte count falls to less than 200/mm^3.

This chapter presents physical and psychological manifestations of AIDS. Delivery of nursing care is described in terms of the nursing process. Various medical treatment modalities are discussed.

PATHOPHYSIOLOGY INCURRED BY THE HIV VIRUS

Normal Immune Response

Cells responsible for nonspecific immune reactions include neutrophils, monocytes, and macrophages. They work to destroy the invasive organism and initiate and facilitate damaged tissue. If these cells are not effective in accomplishing a satisfactory healing response, specific immune mechanisms take over.

Specific immune mechanisms are divided into two major types: the cellular response and the humoral response. The controlling elements of the cellular response are the T lymphocytes (T cells), and those of the humoral response are called B lymphocytes (B cells). When the body is invaded by a specific antigen, the T cells—and particularly the **T4 lymphocytes** (also called *T helper cells*)—become sensitized to and specific for the foreign antigen. These antigen-specific T4 cells divide many times, producing antigen-specific T4 cells with other functions. One of these, the T killer cell, destroys viruses that re-

produce inside other cells by puncturing the cell membrane of the host cell and allowing the contents of the cell, including viruses, to spill out into the bloodstream, where they can be engulfed by macrophages (Perdew, 1990). Another cell produced through division of the T4 cells is the suppressor T cell, which serves to stop the immune response once the foreign antigen has been destroyed (Scanlon & Sanders, 1995).

The humoral response is activated when antigen-specific T4 cells communicate with B cells in the spleen and lymph nodes. These B cells in turn produce the antibodies specific to the foreign antigen. Antibodies attach themselves to foreign antigens so that they are unable to invade body cells. These invader cells are then destroyed without being able to multiply.

The Immune Response to HIV

The most conspicuous immunological abnormality associated with HIV infection is a striking depletion of T4 lymphocytes (Rosenberg & Fauci, 1989). The HIV infects the T4 lymphocyte, thereby destroying the very cell the body needs to direct an attack on the virus. T4 lymphocytes are called T4 cells, after the receptor they bear (Lisanti & Zwolski, 1997).

An individual with a healthy immune system may present with a T4 count between 600 and 1200 mm^3. The individual with HIV infection may experience a drop at the time of acute infection, with a subsequent increase when the acute stage subsides. Typically, the T-cell count is about 500 to 600 when the individual begins to develop chronic **persistent generalized lymphadenopathy** (PGL). Opportunistic infections are common when the T-cell count reaches 200 (Sweet, 1992). For someone with advanced HIV disease, it is not uncommon to find fewer than 10 T4 cells/mm3 (Grady, 1992).

When an individual is infected with HIV, T4 lymphocytes become the main target of attack by the virus. Rapid viral production within the cell causes destruction of the lymphocyte that has either direct or indirect control over virtually every other response of the human immune system (Roitt, Brostoff, & Male, 1989). The remaining T4 cells seem to lose the ability to function at full capacity and are therefore unable to initiate responses by various other components of the immune system. Because of this, the B cells demonstrate a decreased ability to mount an antibody response to a *new* antigen (Dietz, 1994).

The HIV continues to infiltrate new T4 cells, reproducing until they burst out of the cell membrane and begin to float freely in the blood, infecting other T4 cells, of which the body has a limited supply. B cells are stimulated by free-floating HIVs to start producing antibodies. Unfortunately, by the time enough antibodies to HIV are produced to mount an effective attack, the viruses have invaded other cells where they are safe from the attacking antibodies (Perdew, 1990). Protection by monocytes and macrophages is also compromised as a result of lack of stimulation by T4 cells and additionally because some monocytes and macrophages are directly infected by HIV.

Investigators and clinicians require a great deal more knowledge about the effects of HIV on the immune system. Currently, researchers are actively trying to develop a vaccine against HIV that could prevent infection or clinical progression. Until there is a greater understanding of what type of immunity will provide a protective response to HIV, development of a vaccine remains in the future.

HISTORICAL ASPECTS

The first description of what was later to be called AIDS appeared in the CDC's *Morbidity and Mortality Weekly Report* of June 5, 1981. The report described unusual outbreaks of PCP and KS among specific groups of young homosexual men in California and New York. Appearance of these syndromes was considered unusual because of the frequency with which they were occurring and the population being affected. Historically, these conditions were seen infrequently and generally only in severely immunosuppressed individuals (Essex, 1988).

Because these first cases were identified only in homosexual and bisexual men, investigators assumed that the immune deficiency was etiologically related to the gay lifestyle. The disease was even referred to at that time as gay-related immune deficiency (Flaskerud, 1992a).

Numbers of reported cases were mounting rapidly. Within a brief period, AIDS cases began appearing in other special populations: heterosexual intravenous (IV) drug users and hemophiliacs. Soon after, the first AIDS cases associated with blood transfusions were suspected. These individuals were found to have a history of receiving blood transfusions within the preceding 3 to 5 years (Essex, 1988).

Meanwhile, a number of researchers began to postulate that a mutant variant of the human T-lymphotropic retrovirus (HTLV) might be the etiological agent of AIDS (Essex et al., 1984; Gallo et al., 1983). Soon after, Gallo and associates (1984) confirmed the link to a T-lymphotropic retrovirus, which they called human T-lymphotropic virus type III (HTLV-III). Today the name has been standardized worldwide and is called HIV type 1 (HIV-1). Once the virus had been isolated, a test for identifying HIV antibodies in the blood was developed, making it possible to determine if individuals had been infected by HIV. Screening of blood and blood products also became possible, curbing transmission of the virus through blood transfusion.

The HTLV may have originated in Africa with a virus called simian T-cell leukemia virus (STLV) found in more than 30 species of monkeys and apes. Spread of the virus progressed from subprimate to African humans.

Early reports of its presence were cited in African persons living in southwestern Japan (Gallo et al., 1986). The virus then reportedly moved at elevated rates to the Caribbean and northern South America and at lower rates to North America and Europe. Recent cultural changes, such as gay liberation, relaxed heterosexual sexual mores, and post-1960 increases in IV drug use, may have amplified the spread of HIV in the United States (Osmond, 1990b).

In the early 1980s, Haitians were considered to be a distinct high-risk group for the development of AIDS. They did indeed constitute approximately 5 percent of all cases (Steis & Broder, 1985). However, they have been reclassified by the CDC into the "heterosexual contact" group and are no longer considered a separate group at risk for AIDS. According to Landesman, Ginzburg, and Weiss (1985), it does not appear that "being of Haitian extraction by itself, in isolation from other risk factors, increases the relative risk of being exposed to HTLV-III (HIV-1)."

The AIDS epidemic has assumed major proportions, with the numbers of cases continuing to grow internationally. Virtually every major country in the world is confronting what has become the major health crisis of modern times. If progression is not curtailed, it will undoubtedly come to be ranked among history's greatest killers.

EPIDEMIOLOGICAL STATISTICS

Estimates by the United Nations Joint Programme on HIV/AIDS (UNAIDS) and the World Health Organization (WHO), a cosponsor of the Joint Programme, indicate that by the beginning of 1998 more than 30 million people were infected with HIV, and that 11.7 million people around the world had already lost their lives to the disease (UNAIDS/WHO, 1998). The largest number of infections (approximately 89 percent) are concentrated in sub-Saharan Africa and South and in Southeast Asia.

Current estimates are that about 1 million Americans are infected with HIV (Hollander & Katz, 1996). As of December 1997, 619,690 cases of AIDS had been reported in the United States (CDC, 1997). AIDS is now the second leading cause of death (behind accidental injury) among individuals between 25 and 44 years of age (Aids Education & Research Trust [AVERT], 1999).

In the United States, HIV disease has now been reported in all 50 states and the District of Columbia. Geographical distribution shows the highest number of cases in New York, Florida, and California, and the lowest in North Dakota and South Dakota (AVERT, 1999).

Behavioral changes have resulted in a decline in the number of cases among homosexual men. However, the number of cases transmitted through heterosexual contact and IV drug use has increased (CDC, 1998).

Nursing care of AIDS clients is moving away from the acute care hospitals. Length of acute care hospital stays is decreasing, and a greater focus is being placed on alternative services, such as expanded outpatient clinics, day-care facilities, chronic-care facilities, and home care and hospice programs (Bartlett & Finkbeiner, 1996).

The epidemiology of HIV/AIDS changes rapidly, and current information becomes outdated almost before it is published. Nurses must maintain awareness of the latest available information about the disease and the issues that affect provision and outcome of nursing care of clients with HIV/AIDS.

PREDISPOSING FACTORS

The etiological agent associated with AIDS is HIV. It is currently known to have two subtypes which have been called type 1 and type 2 (HIV-1 and HIV-2). Most of the cases of AIDS worldwide are linked to HIV-1 with the exception of Africa, where HIV-2 is prevalent. HIV-1 and HIV-2 are clinically similar, except that HIV-2 appears to be less harmful to the cells of the immune system and reproduces more slowly than HIV-1 (Stine, 1993). There may be other subtypes of HIV, which are now classified as HIV type O (HIV-O) (Kaplan & Sadock, 1998).

The major routes for transmission of HIV are sexual, bloodborne, and perinatal transmission. There has been a shift in the identification of at-risk populations from that of merely belonging to a specific group to identifying characteristic behaviors that place individuals at risk. The risk for HIV infection is having sex with someone who is infected or being exposed to blood that is infected. The risk is not being a member of any particular group.

Sexual Transmission

It is now clear that both homosexual and heterosexual activity play major roles in the transmission of HIV infection worldwide. In the United States and Europe, most AIDS cases are homosexual men; in Africa, however, most cases result from heterosexual transmission of HIV (AVERT, 1999).

Heterosexual Transmission

The virus is found in greater concentration in semen than in vaginal secretions, which more readily facilitates transmission from men to women than from women to men (Bartlett & Finkbeiner, 1996). Male-to-female transmission has been reported in cases of HIV-positive female partners of hemophiliacs, bisexual men, and male IV drug users, and in women artificially inseminated by specimens from HIV-infected men.

HIV may be transmitted from an infected man to his female sexual partner by vaginal or anal intercourse. The possibility of oral transmission through sexual practices such as fellatio seems to be relatively low. Although data on female-to-male transmission in the United States have been limited, this mode of transmission is biologically plausible because HIV has been isolated in vaginal secretions (Bartlett & Finkbeiner, 1996) and cases of female-to-male transmission have been documented (Flaskerud, 1992b).

Homosexual Transmission

The most significant risk factors for homosexual transmission of HIV are receptive anal intercourse and the number of male sexual partners. Other behaviors that may injure rectal mucosa increase the risk of viral invasion. The lining of the anal canal is delicate and prone to tearing and bleeding, making anal intercourse an easy way for infections to be passed from one person to another (Bell, 1998). The presence of concomitant infections with other diseases such as hepatitis, herpes, and other sexually transmitted diseases increases the risk of infection with HIV because of antigenic overload in the host, resulting in acceleration of pathogenesis of immunodeficiency (Flaskerud, 1992b).

Bloodborne Transmission

Transfusion with Blood Products

Buehler, Petersen, and Jaffe (1995) state:

> "The only mode of HIV transmission that has been virtually eliminated in the United States is transmission related to transfusion of blood and blood products. Although cases of transfusion-acquired AIDS continue to be diagnosed and reported (692 cases reported in 1992), nearly all such cases resulted from transfusions that occurred before 1985, when routine screening of donated blood for antibodies to HIV was initiated." (p. 7)

Although laboratory tests are more than 99 percent sensitive, screening problems may occur when donations are received from recently HIV-1–infected individuals who have not yet developed antibody or from persistently antibody-negative HIV-1–infected donors (Donegan, 1990). In March, 1996, the American Red Cross (ARC) implemented the HIV-1 p24 antigen test. This test, when used in combination with the HIV antibody test, further improves the safety of the blood supply for transfusions. The ARC reports that the risk of HIV infection through transfusion is now 1 in 676,000 units. This new test also may shorten the period between infection and serum antigen detection to an average of 16 days (ARC, 1998).

Individuals at highest risk for HIV infection from blood transfusion are hemophiliacs, simply because of their massive requirements for blood products. Other individuals who require blood because of temporary illness or surgery also may be at risk.

Transmission by Needles Infected with HIV-1

The highest number of cases occurring via this route are among IV drug users who share needles and other equipment contaminated with HIV-1–infected blood. In some areas of the country, this is the most prevalent mode of transmission. IV drug abusers are also at higher risk because of the immunosuppressive factors associated with many of the drugs of abuse and the common underlying existence of malnutrition. Some regions (e.g., New York City) have established programs to provide drug users with clean needles in an effort to diminish the spread of HIV.

A second bloodborne mode of transmission of HIV with contaminated needles is through accidental needle sticks by health care workers, as well as by other means and with other contaminated equipment used for therapeutic purposes. Some examples include:

- Needle sticks caused by recapping needles and by improper disposal of syringes.
- Coming in contact with blood or other body fluids during treatments without wearing gloves and while having chapped hands or cuts on the hands.
- Having blood or other body fluids splashed on face during treatments, causing entry through ocular, nasal, or oral mucous membranes.
- Being cut with a sharp object that has been contaminated with the blood of an HIV-positive client.
- Dressing open wounds without wearing gloves.

Perinatal Transmission

Fifteen to forty percent of infants born to HIV-infected women are infected with the virus (Douglas & Pinsky, 1996). Modes of transmission include transplacental, through exposure to maternal blood and vaginal secretions during delivery, and through breast milk. The method of delivery (vaginal or cesarean) appears to play no significant role in HIV transmission; however, advanced stage of HIV infection with evidence of clinical illness may be influential (Nokes, 1992). Because breast milk has been implicated as a mode of transmission, women should be counseled to use other forms of infant feeding when possible.

The risk of perinatal transmission has been significantly reduced in recent years with the advent of free or low-cost prenatal care, provision of access to anti-HIV medication during pregnancy, and education about the dangers of breastfeeding. Kaplan and Sadock (1998) report that treating pregnant HIV-positive women with zidovudine and protease inhibitors has prevented perinatal transmission in more than 95 percent of cases.

Other Possible Modes of Transmission

To date, HIV has been isolated from blood, semen, vaginal secretions, saliva, tears, breast milk, cerebrospinal fluid, and amniotic fluid. However, only blood, semen, vaginal secretions, and breast milk have been epidemiologically linked to transmission of the virus (Douglas & Pinsky, 1996). Anecdotal accounts have described isolated cases of casual transmission. Some examples of these include:

- A mother who was infected by her infant son who had received contaminated blood at birth. Apparently the mother failed to follow recommended precautions when exposing herself to the child's secretions (CDC, 1986).
- A child who was infected by a sibling through a bite that did not break the skin (Allen & Curran, 1988).
- A woman who was infected by her HIV-positive husband through passionate kissing via small lesions in her oral mucous membranes. The man had been infected through blood transfusion and was known to be impotent (Haverkos & Edelman, 1988).

Bartlett and Finkbeiner (1996) state:

"HIV is found in low number in saliva, so deep kissing, mouth-to-mouth resuscitation, biting, being spat upon, and the like might potentially transmit the virus. It is noteworthy that HIV is actually found in saliva in only about 1 or 2 percent of people with HIV infection. Moreover, even in these people, the numbers of the virus are so low that researchers believe that transmission through saliva is biologically improbable and perhaps impossible. For this reason, the CDC has removed saliva as a potential source of infection for health care workers." (p. 33)

The risk of being infected with HIV through casual, nonsexual contact is so low as to be virtually nonexistent. Even in those isolated cases that have been reported, most consistently exhibit additional risk factors that may account for the infection (Gershon, Vlahov, & Nelson, 1990).

APPLICATION OF THE NURSING PROCESS

Background Assessment Data

The CDC now identifies HIV infection as a continuous and progressive process. Several authors have divided the diseases into stages according to signs and symptoms (Boswell & Hirsch, 1992; Stine, 1993; Volberding, 1992). These stages are summarized in Table 36.1.

■ TABLE 36.1 STAGES AND SYMPTOMS OF HIV DISEASE

STATE (T4 CELLS/MM^3)	CONDITION/SYMPTOMS
Early Stage (1000–500)	**Acute HIV Infection** Fever, malaise, sore throat, lymphadenopathy, anorexia, nausea and vomiting, headaches, skin rash, diarrhea **Seroconversion** HIV antibodies are detected in the blood (can occur any time from 1 week to 1 year after exposure) **Asymptomatic Infection** No manifestations of illness. Blood tests may reveal immunological and hematological abnormalities, such as leukopenia, anemia, or thrombocytopenia. This period may last 5 to 10 years or longer.
Middle Stage (500–200)	**Persistent Generalized Lymphadenopathy** Lymph notes of the neck, armpit, and groin swell and remain swollen for months. **Systemic Complaints** Fever, night sweats, chronic diarrhea, fatigue, minor oral infections, headaches, weight loss
Late Stage (≤200)	**HIV Wasting Syndrome** Severe weight loss; large-volume diarrhea; fever and weakness **Opportunistic Infections** *Pneumocystis carinii* pneumonia (fever, dyspnea, cough) Cryptosporidiosis (profuse watery diarrhea) Toxoplasmosis (neurological abnormalities) Candidiasis (lesions in oral cavity, esophagus, vagina) Cryptococcosis (meningitis) Cytomegalovirus (retinitis, enteritis, pneumonitis, cerebral disease, hepatitis, adrenal necrosis, and others) Herpes simplex (watery blisters orally and on genitals) Herpes zoster (painful, blistery lesions on skin along nerve track; disseminated disease may involve lungs and CNS) *Mycobacterium avium* (HIV wasting syndrome) *Mycobacterium tuberculosis* (tuberculosis) Others **AIDS-Related Malignancies** Kaposi's sarcoma (pigmented lesions that transform into tumors form on the body and in any organ system) Non-Hodgkin's lymphoma Hodgkin's disease Malignant melanoma Testicular cancers Primary hepatocellular carcinoma Invasive cervical cancer **Altered Mental States** Delirium (fluctuating consciousness, abnormal vital signs, and psychotic phenomena) Dementia (cognitive, motor, and behavioral changes)

Early-Stage HIV Disease (1000 to 500 T4 cells/mm3)

Acute HIV Infection. The acute HIV infection is identified by a characteristic syndrome of symptoms that occurs from 6 days to 6 weeks after exposure to the virus. The symptoms have an abrupt onset, are somewhat vague, and are similar to those sometimes seen in mononucleosis. Symptoms of acute HIV infection include fever, myalgia, malaise, lymphadenopathy, sore throat, anorexia, nausea and vomiting, headaches, skin rash, and diarrhea (Bartlett & Finkbeiner, 1996). Most symptoms resolve themselves in 1 to 3 weeks, with the exception of fever, myalgia, lymphadenopathy, and malaise, which may continue for several months.

Seroconversion, the detectability if HIV antibodies in the blood, most often is detected between 6 and 12 weeks (Kaplan & Sadock, 1998). Over 95 percent of people will show positive for HIV by 6 months after infection. In rare cases, seroconversion has taken up to 12 months. The time between infection and seroconversion is called the *window period.*

Asymptomatic Infection. The acute infection progresses to an asymptomatic stage. Probably the largest number of HIV-infected individuals fall within this group (Abrams, 1988). Individuals may remain in this asymptomatic stage for 10 or more years. The progression of the illness is much faster in infants and children than it is in adults.

These asymptomatic HIV-infected persons may develop immunological and hematological abnormalities of varying severity, including leukopenia, anemia, thrombocytopenia, hypergammaglobulinemia, decreased T4 lymphocytes, or any combination of these conditions.

Middle-Stage HIV Disease
(500 to 200 T4 cells/mm³)

Persistent Generalized Lymphadenopathy. Following the asymptomatic period, clients with HIV infection develop a generalized lymphadenopathy, in which lymph nodes in at least two different locations in the body swell and remain swollen for months, with no other signs of a related infectious disease (Bartlett & Finkbeiner, 1996). The swollen nodes may or may not be painful or visible externally. This syndrome often occurs within a few months of seroconversion for HIV antibody.

Other Symptoms of Middle-Stage HIV Disease

Fever. Fever is common during this stage, even in the absence of any specific **opportunistic infection.** Management is frequently through intermittent or long-term use of nonsteroidal anti-inflammatory drugs.

Night Sweats. The most common description of this symptom is severe drenching night sweats that occur repeatedly over at least a 2-week period (Volberding, 1992). They are often associated with the fever and may be controlled through the regular use of antipyretic agents.

Chronic Diarrhea. In middle-stage HIV disease, diarrhea can be induced by HIV infection of the cells of the gastrointestinal (GI) tract itself (Volberding, 1992). The diarrhea can be severe enough to result in dehydration and general debilitation. At this stage, it is treated symptomatically and effectively with common antidiarrheal medications. In late-stage HIV disease, diarrhea is usually associated with opportunistic GI pathogens.

Fatigue. This symptom can range from mild limitations in a usually active lifestyle to severe debilitation (Volberding, 1992). At this stage, the client should be evaluated for depression, of which fatigue is a common symptom and which is quite treatable in individuals with HIV disease. In late-stage HIV disease, fatigue may be associated with endocrine malfunction.

Minor Oral Infections. Oral infections with *Candida albicans* are common in early symptomatic HIV disease. Various topical and oral agents are successful in treating the symptom, although a high rate of recurrence is common (Volberding, 1992).

Headache. Headaches are a common symptom in all stages of the illness. These may be quite severe and are often identified as bifrontal or occipital. Treatment is symptomatic, and nonsteroidal anti-inflammatory agents are preferred over narcotics, owing to the chronicity of this complaint (Volberding, 1992).

Late-Stage HIV Disease
(200 or less T4 cells/mm³)

HIV Wasting Syndrome. **HIV wasting syndrome**, involving diarrhea and weight loss occurs in up to 80 percent of clients with AIDS (Volberding, 1992). Symptoms are associated with nutrient malabsorption, or enterocolitis or intestinal injury related to an opportunistic pathogen. Involuntary weight loss of more than 10 percent of baseline body weight is common. Large-volume diarrhea, fever, and weakness accompany the syndrome. A low-fat, lactose-free diet supplemented with medium-chain triglycerides may be beneficial. Parenteral nutrition may be used in refractory cases (Bartlett & Finkbeiner, 1996).

Opportunistic Infections. Opportunistic infections have long been a defining characteristic of AIDS. Common ones are defined here.

Pneumocystis carinii pneumonia. The most common, life-threatening opportunistic infection seen in clients with AIDS is **pneumocystis pneumonia** (Bartlett & Finkbeiner, 1996). Symptoms include fever, exertional dyspnea, and nonproductive cough.

Cryptosporidiosis. This parasitic infection may cause chronic profuse watery diarrhea in AIDS clients. Some clients may have up to 20 or more bowel movements a day.

Toxoplasmosis. This protozoan infection frequently causes central nervous system (CNS) disease in AIDS clients. Common presenting symptoms include impaired level of consciousness, fever, headache, seizures, and focal neurological signs, such as hemiparesis, cognitive deficits, ataxia, aphasia, and movement disorders (Bartlett & Finkbeiner, 1996).

Candidiasis. Most commonly caused by the fungus *Candida albicans*, this infection usually occurs in the oral cavity and esophagus of the HIV-infected individual. Vaginal and anal infections are seen less frequently. Oral candidiasis, commonly called thrush, is characterized by white plaques on the oral mucosa. Esophageal candidiasis presents with painful lesions in the esophagus, making swallowing difficult.

Cryptococcosis. This yeast infection, caused by *Cryptococcus neoformans*, most commonly causes meningitis in AIDS clients (Bartlett & Finkbeiner, 1996). Symptoms include fever, stiff neck, severe headache, and double vision.

Cytomegalovirus. Cytomegalovirus (CMV) is common in most human populations. In most instances, it is latent and asymptomatic. Immunosuppression by HIV reactivates the virus. In about 30 percent of AIDS clients CMV is recognized as a major contributor to death (Kovacs & Masur, 1988). CMV causes retinitis (and possible blindness), enteritis (manifested by profuse watery diarrhea), pneumonitis, cerebral disease, myelitis, pericarditis, endometritis, glomerulitis, epididymitis, hepatitis, and adrenal necrosis.

Herpes Simplex. This is a common virus, with up to 50 percent of the general population having had oral infections and 20 to 30 percent having had the infection on their genitals (Bartlett & Finkbeiner, 1996). Symptoms include watery blisters, pain, and fever. In people with HIV infection, the symptoms may last over a month. An antiviral medication may be prescribed continuously. Herpes simplex colitis is usually confined to the rectum and may result in itching, burning, pain, bloody stool, and fever (Kovacs & Masur, 1988).

Herpes Zoster. Herpes zoster has been found to cause both dermatomal (shingles) and disseminated disease in clients with HIV infection. It has been estimated that within 4 years of diagnosis of dermatomal zoster, nearly 50 percent of HIV-infected clients will have developed AIDS (Kovacs & Masur, 1988). After initial infection (usually in childhood), herpes zoster lies latent in the dorsal root ganglia of the peripheral nerves. Reactivation results in painful lesions on the skin area supplied by the affected nerve (Cohen, 1991). Dissemination to the lung or CNS can result in pneumonia or encephalitis. Ophthalmic nerve involvement can cause blindness.

Mycobacteria. Mycobacterium avium-intracellulare complex (MAC) and *M. tuberculosis* occur with great frequency among HIV-infected clients (Kovacs & Masur, 1988). MAC may contribute to the HIV wasting syndrome, with symptoms of diarrhea and malabsorption. Other symptoms include high, swinging fever; weight loss; malaise; anorexia; weakness; myalgia; night sweats; cough; and headache (Cohen, 1991). *M. tuberculosis* is associated with the development of tuberculosis in HIV-infected clients. The primary manifestation is pulmonary lesions. Extrapulmonary lesions involving bone, kidney, brain, lymph nodes, and virtually every other site have been reported (Kovacs & Masur, 1988).

AIDS-Related Malignancies

Kaposi's Sarcoma. Kaposi's sarcoma (KS) is caused by a newly discovered virus called Kaposi's sarcoma herpes virus (KSHV), or herpes virus 8 (because 7 prior herpes viruses have been named) (Bartlett & Finkbeiner 1996). Lesions associated with KS may appear on any body surface or in the viscera. KS lesions are usually painless, nonpruritic, and nonblanching (Heyer et al., 1990).

In light-skinned people, they appear reddish to purple in color, whereas in dark-skinned people, they are generally dark brown to black. Flat "patchy" lesions become elevated and develop into papules or plaques. Eventually the plaques enlarge, coalesce, and form tumor nodules. Skin lesions may form anywhere on the body, although characteristic sites include the tip of the nose, the eyelid, the hard palate and posterior pharynx, the glans penis, and the sole of the foot (Heyer et al., 1990). Virtually any organ system, including the heart and lungs, may be affected. GI involvement is common and may result in impaired swallowing, obstruction, or perforation. Clients with pulmonary KS may present with symptoms similar to those of pneumonia, thereby creating some difficulty with differential diagnosis. KS rarely involves the CNS. Lymphedema from lymphatic obstruction is common in the face, lower extremities, scrotum, and abdomen. In the lower extremities, the collecting fluid is usually very firm and nonpitting (Heyer et al., 1990). KS is not viewed as a metastatic disease, but rather one with multifocal origin. A poor prognosis is associated with visceral involvement (Heyer et al., 1990).

Bartlett & Finkbeiner (1996) state:

> "Some have argued that KS is a sexually transmitted disease because it is extremely common in gay men with HIV infection and is quite unusual in hemophiliacs, children, or those who became infected through transfusions. If KSHV (or herpes virus 8) is sexually transmitted, the safer sex practices that prevent transmission of HIV also seem to prevent transmission of KSHV; among gay men with HIV infection KS is disappearing." (p. 139)

Other Malignancies. HIV-positive individuals are at increased risk for developing non-Hodgkin's lymphoma (Wolcott, Dilley, & Mitsuyasu, 1989). Extranodal sites, including the CNS and bone marrow, are frequently involved. Major primary extranodal sites have been identified as the brain, anus, rectum, head, neck, lung, and liver (Biggar, 1990). Clinical features are consistent with regional involvement. Hodgkin's disease, squamous-cell carcinomas, malignant melanoma, testicular cancers, and primary hepatocellular carcinoma have been reported in association with AIDS; however, a direct correlation with HIV-induced immune deficiency has not been established (Volberding, 1990a).

Altered Mental States

Delirium. Delirium is one of the most common cognitive disorders seen in AIDS clients. Clinical manifestations may include a fluctuating level of consciousness, reversal of the sleep-wake cycle, abnormal vital signs, and psychotic phenomena (e.g., hallucinations). Contributing factors to the development of delirium include CNS infections, CNS neoplastic disease, side effects of various chemotherapeutic agents, hypoxemia from respiratory compromise, electrolyte imbalance, and sensory deprivation. In some clients, delirium may be superimposed on, or evolve into, dementia.

Depressive Syndromes. Anticipatory or actual grief, which may be acute or chronic, normal or pathological, is an important cause of depressive symptoms in AIDS clients (Wolcott, Dilley, & Mitsuyasu, 1989). Transient suicidal ideation on learning of HIV positivity is quite common, although the incidence of serious suicidal behavior is low. Depression in AIDS clients may be related to receiving a new diagnosis of HIV positivity or AIDS, perceiving rejection by loved ones, experiencing multiple losses of friends to the disease, having an inadequate social and financial support system, and presence of an early cognitive disorder.

HIV-Associated Dementia. Previously referred to as AIDS dementia complex, **HIV-associated dementia** (HAD) is a neuropathological syndrome experienced by 20 to 30 percent of people with HIV infection, usually in the late stages (Bartlett & Finkbeiner, 1996). Kaplan and Sadock (1998) suggest that possible etiologies of the dementia include "HIV encephalopathy, central nervous system (CNS) infections, CNS neoplasms, CNS abnormalities caused by systemic disorders and endocrinopathies, and adverse CNS responses to drugs." Early clinical manifestations include subtle cognitive, behavioral, and motor symptoms, which become more severe with progression of the disease (Table 36.2). HIV-associated dementia is the most frequent neurological complication of HIV infection (Wise & Gray, 1994).

Psychosocial Implications of HIV/AIDS. The psychosocial problems that confront a person with AIDS can be overwhelming. Health care workers still face a number of unknowns related to the disease, thereby setting AIDS clients apart from individuals with other life-threatening illnesses. Persons with AIDS (PWAs) are often the victims of discrimination because fear of contagion, prejudices, and stigmatization founded in societal attitudes toward groups most commonly afflicted. Dilley (1990) lists the following facts that contribute to the psychosocial problems experienced by PWAs:

1. AIDS is still a relatively new and complicated disease that is not well understood by the general population. Well-intentioned but uninformed individuals can have unfounded fears of contagion and be restrained toward people with AIDS.
2. AIDS is most frequently a sexually transmitted disease. In addition, it is commonly found among IV drug users, who spread it through sharing "dirty needles." Both of these issues, sexuality and illicit drug use, can raise moral issues, thereby making it easy for clients and nonclients alike to develop an attitude of blaming the victim for the illness.
3. Gay people have historically been stigmatized solely on the basis of their homosexuality. Similarly, individuals who use IV drugs share, at best, a public image of being troubled, difficult, or frightening.
4. At this time, AIDS is an incurable disease that in the United States predominantly strikes men in their early adult years.

The individual with newly diagnosed HIV seropositivity commonly responds with shock and disbelief, followed by guilt, anger, and depression. In some instances, a symptom complex similar to posttraumatic stress disorder is common in the first few weeks after a person receives notification of his or her HIV positivity. The person may become extremely anxious and hypervigilant about physical symptoms, exhibiting marked dependence on health care workers. Feelings of guilt prevail over previous life activities as well as self-blame for becoming infected. Depressive thoughts are common, and acute suicidal crises may occur. Other responses to initial diagnosis of HIV seropositivity have included transient or chronic sexual dysfunction and social withdrawal resulting from fear of infecting others or of social rejection (Wolcott, Dilley, & Mitsuyasu, 1989). Crisis intervention with newly diagnosed HIV-positive persons is aimed at restoring a positive psychological equilibrium and providing education for making the necessary lifestyle behavioral changes to protect self and others.

Denial is a common defense mechanism among individuals with high-risk behaviors. Denial prevents individuals from undergoing HIV testing; it delays some HIV-positive individuals from seeking early medical care; and

TABLE 36.2 SIGNS AND SYMPTOMS OF HIV-ASSOCIATED DEMENTIA

EARLY	LATE
Cognitive	**Cognitive**
Forgetfulness	Severe cognitive deficits
Loss of concentration	Mutism
Confusion	
Slowness of thought	
Motor	**Motor**
Loss of balance	Psychomotor retardation
Leg weakness	Ataxia
Deterioration in	Hypertonia
handwriting	Paraparesis
	Quadriparesis
	Hemiparesis
	Tremors
	Vegetative state
Behavioral	**Behavioral**
Apathy	Organic psychosis—persistent
Social withdrawal	Vacant staring
Dysphoric mood	Lethargy
Organic psychosis	Hypersomnolence
Regressed behavior	
Other	**Other**
Headache	Bowel and bladder
Seizures	incontinence
	Myoclonus
	Seizures

SOURCE: Adapted from Bartlett & Finkbeiner (1996); Navia, Jordon, & Price (1985); Navia & Price (1986); Price & Brew (1988).

it prevents some HIV-positive individuals from changing their behavior to prevent HIV transmission.

Significant others of clients with HIV disease face a great many stresses associated with the client's illness. Initially they may experience emotions typical of the grief response. The reality of the situation is felt when the person begins to accept the immense responsibility for the physical and emotional care of their loved one. They may experience financial concerns and lack of social support.

When the significant other is a gay lover, guilt over having infected the partner or fear of having been infected by the partner may be felt. The gay lover may be rejected by the client's family members, who themselves may be experiencing unique stresses associated with learning for the first time of their relative's lifestyle. Parents may blame themselves and their childrearing practices. The family may experience a lack of social support owing to the stigma attached to the illness. Grief responses by family members are common.

Psychiatric Disorders Common in Clients with HIV Infections. At least 50 percent of HIV-infected clients will experience a psychiatric disorder during the course of their illness (Holland, Jacobsen, & Brietbart, 1992). Adjustment disorder with depressed and/or anxious features accounts for about two thirds of the diagnoses. Other psychiatric disorders common to HIV-infected individuals include panic disorder, generalized anxiety disorder, major depression, mania, cognitive disorders (dementia and delirium), and substance-related disorders (Holland, Jacobsen, & Brietbart, et al., 1992).

Anxiety Disorders. The most common emotion in individuals with HIV infection is uncertainty about the future and fears of illness (Holland, Jacobsen, & Brietbart, 1992). Symptoms of intense anxiety may remit when a crisis can be temporarily resolved. However, persistence of anxiety symptoms for weeks to months can become a diagnosable anxiety disorder requiring evaluation and treatment. Holland, Jacobsen, & Brietbart (1992) state:

> "Supportive psychotherapy and counseling are central to helping patients cope with distress and anxiety. This means giving patients accurate information in a reassuring manner about HIV-related disease and treatment, and rehearsing what may occur during a feared anticipated procedure or event. Counseling should be built into medical management from the beginning." (p. 350)

Major Depression. Symptoms associated with the diagnosis of major depression in individuals with HIV disease include depressed mood, dysphoria, low self-esteem, hopelessness, worthlessness, guilt, helplessness, and suicidal ideation. Physical signs, such as fatigue, anorexia, insomnia, weakness, and diminished libido, which are often used to diagnose major depression in healthy individuals, may be related to the disease process in HIV-infected individuals and are not considered in making the diagnosis of major depression (Holland, Jacobsen, & Brietbart, 1992).

Other symptoms, such as apathy, withdrawal, mental slowing, and avoidance of complex tasks, which are considered common symptoms of major depression, may be related to early symptoms of cognitive impairment of HIV-associated dementia (Perry, 1990). Taking a careful history and making a clinical examination are required for a differential diagnosis. The management of major depression in HIV-infected individuals entails (1) supportive psychotherapy; (2) the control of distressing physical symptoms, especially pain; (3) adjunctive measures such as behavioral interventions; and (4) psychopharmacological measures (Holland, Jacobsen, & Brietbart, 1992).

AIDS is associated with an increased frequency of suicidal ideation, suicide attempts, and suicides. The risk of suicide is 10 to 20 times higher in HIV-infected individuals than in the general population (Holland, Jacobsen, & Brietbart, 1992). Feelings of hopelessness, guilt about past behavior, multiple bereavements, absent or inadequate social supports, and isolation from family and friends have been identified as common predisposing factors. Early and sustained counseling of high-risk individuals can avert suicide, and clients often reconsider the idea of suicide when the physician acknowledges the legitimacy of that option and the client's need to retain a sense of control over life and death (Holland, Jacobsen, & Brietbart, 1992).

Capaldini (1995) states:

> "Rational suicide and euthanasia are extremely controversial issues within the medical profession. Nonetheless, practitioners must realize that many HIV-positive patients have at least considered suicide as an option for themselves. Thus, it is important for practitioners to examine their feelings about this issue because they are likely to be approached about it by their patients. In some cases, a candid and empathic discussion about terminal and palliative care issues may help relieve the patient's concerns about intractable physical or emotional suffering." (p. 310)

Mania. AIDS-related mania often occurs late in the course of the disease. The manic symptoms may present as an adverse reaction to AIDS medications, as the first manifestation of an opportunistic or systemic illness, or as a complication of HIV-related cognitive disorder (Capaldini, 1995). Research shows that mania in AIDS carries a poor prognosis. In one study, more than one quarter of the clients died within 6 months of the onset of manic symptoms (El-Mallakh, 1991).

Dementia and Delirium. HAD was discussed previously in this chapter. It is not uncommon for delirium to be superimposed on HAD and to occur with greater frequency in advanced disease owing to organ system failure resulting in hypoxia, metabolic disturbances, septicemia, and bleeding (Holland, Jacobsen, & Brietbart, 1992). Delirium can also be an adverse reaction to medications, such as high-dose corticosteroids. Symptoms of delirium include fluctuating level of consciousness, misperceptions, delusions, sleep-wake cycle loss, and agitation or withdrawal. General treatment measures include maintaining orientation, restoring the sleep-wake cycle, and administering appropriate medications to treat agitation (Capaldini, 1995).

Diagnosis/Outcome Identification

Nursing diagnoses are formulated from the data gathered during the assessment phase and with background knowledge regarding predisposing factors to the disorder. The following nursing diagnoses may be used for the client with HIV disease:

Altered protection related to compromised immune status secondary to diagnosis of HIV disease, evidenced by laboratory values indicating decreased numbers of T4 cells and presence of opportunistic infections manifested by fever, night sweats, copious watery diarrhea, weight loss, fatigue, malaise, swollen lymph glands, cough, dyspnea, rash, skin lesions, white patches in mouth, headache, ataxia, anorexia, bleeding, bruising, and various neurological effects.

Altered family processes related to crisis associated with having a family member diagnosed with HIV disease, evidenced by difficulty making decisions that affect all family members; inability to meet physical, emotional, spiritual, and security needs of its members.

Knowledge deficit (prevention of transmission and protection of the client) related to lack of exposure to accurate information, evidenced by inaccurate statements by client and family.

Altered thought processes related to primary HIV infection, opportunistic infections that invade the CNS, and/or adverse effects of therapy, evidenced by confusion, disorientation, memory deficits, and inappropriate non–reality-based thinking. (Refer to Table 23.3, Care Plan for Client with a Cognitive Disorder.)

Risk for self-directed violence related to new diagnosis of HIV disease, evidenced by statements of wishing to take own life and rather dying than facing future with AIDS. (Refer to Table 26.7, Care Plan for Depressed Client.)

Impaired adjustment related to change in health status requiring modification in lifestyle, evidenced by elevated level of anxiety and fear of the future. (Refer to Table 32.2, Care Plan for the Client with Adjustment Disorder.)

The following criteria may be used for measurement of outcomes in the care of the client with HIV/AIDS.

THE CLIENT:

1. Shows no new signs or symptoms of infection.
2. Does not experience respiratory distress.
3. Maintains optimal nutrition and hydration.
4. Has experienced no further weight loss.
5. Maintains integrity of skin and mucous membranes.
6. Manifests evidence of wound healing.
7. Attains and maintains normal fluid and electrolyte balance.
8. Has fewer bowel movements, with increased stool consistency.
9. Explores feelings about self and illness.
10. Verbalizes understanding about disease process, modes of transmission, and prevention of infection.

THE FAMILY/SIGNIFICANT OTHERS:

1. Discuss feelings regarding client's diagnosis and prognosis.
2. Can make rational decisions regarding care of their loved one and the effect on family function.
3. Can verbalize precautions for preventing transmission of HIV to themselves and others and infection of the client.
4. Verbalize knowledge of resources within the community from whom they may seek support and assistance.

Planning/Implementation

Table 36.3 provides a plan of care for the client with HIV/AIDS. Nursing diagnoses are presented, along with outcome criteria, appropriate nursing interventions, and rationales.

Client/Family Education

The role of client teacher is important in the psychiatric area, as it is in all areas of nursing. A list of topics for client and family education relevant to HIV disease is presented in Table 36.4.

Evaluation

Reassessment is conducted in order to determine if the nursing actions have been successful in achieving the objectives of care. Evaluation of the nursing actions for the clients with HIV/AIDS may be facilitated by gathering information using the following types of questions:

1. Have precautions been successful in preventing new infection of the client?
2. Have fever and night sweats been controlled?
3. Has there been a decrease in frequency and increase in consistency of stools?
4. Have weight and nutritional status stabilized?
5. Are fluid and electrolyte values within normal limits?

TABLE 36.3 CARE PLAN FOR THE CLIENT WITH HIV/AIDS*

NURSING DIAGNOSIS: ALTERED PROTECTION

RELATED TO: Compromised immune status secondary to diagnosis of HIV disease

EVIDENCED BY: Laboratory values indicating decreased numbers of T4 cells and presence of opportunistic infections manifested by fever, night sweats, diarrhea, weight loss, fatigue, malaise, swollen lymph glands, cough, dyspnea, rash, skin lesions, white patches in mouth, headache, ataxia, anorexia, bleeding, bruising, and various neurological effects.

OUTCOME CRITERIA	NURSING INTERVENTIONS	RATIONALE
Client safety and comfort will be maximized.	1. Implement universal blood and body fluid precautions. 2. Wash hands with antibacterial soap before entering and on leaving client's room. 3. Monitor vital signs at regular intervals. 4. Monitor complete blood counts (CBCs) for leukopenia/neutropenia. 5. Monitor for signs and symptoms of specific opportunistic infections. 6. Protect client from individuals with infections. 7. Maintain meticulous sterile technique for dressing changes and any invasive procedure. 8. Administer antibiotics as ordered. 9. Provide low-residue, high-protein, high-calorie, soft, bland diet. Maintain hydration with adequate fluid intake. 10. Obtain daily weight and record intake/output. 11. Monitor serum electrolytes and CBCs. 12. If client is unable to eat, provide isotonic tube feedings as tolerated. Check for gastric residual frequently. 13. If client is unable to tolerate oral intake/tube feedings, consult physician regarding possibility of parenteral hyperalimentation. Observe hyperalimentation administration site for signs of infection. 14. Administer antidiarrheals and antiemetics as ordered. 15. Perform frequent oral care. Promote prevention and healing of lesions in the mouth. 16. Have the client eat small, frequent meals with high-calorie snacks rather than three large meals per day. 17. Monitor skin condition for signs of redness and breakdown. 18. Reposition client every 1 to 2 hours. 19. Encourage ambulation and chair activity as tolerated. 20. Use "egg crate" mattress or air mattress on bed.	1–8. To prevent infection in an immunocompromised individual. 9–16. To restore nutritional status and decrease nausea/vomiting and diarrhea. 17–26. To promote improvement of skin and mucous membrane integrity.

21. Wash skin daily with soap and rinse well with water.
22. Apply lotion to skin to maintain skin softness.
23. Provide wound care as ordered for existing pressure sores or lesions.
24. Cleanse skin exposed to diarrhea thoroughly and protect rectal area with ointment.
25. Apply artificial tears to eyes as appropriate.
26. Perform frequent oral care; apply ointment to lips.
27. Assess respiratory status frequently:
    a. Monitor depth, rate, and rhythm of respirations.
    b. Auscultate lung fields every 2 hr and p.r.n.
    c. Monitor arterial blood gases.
    d. Check color of skin, nail beds, and sclerae.
    e. Assess sputum for color, odor, and viscosity.
28. Encourage coughing and deep-breathing exercises.
29. Provide humidified oxygen as ordered.
30. Suction as needed using sterile technique.
31. Space nursing care to allow client adequate rest periods between procedures.
32. Administer analagesics or sedatives judiciously to prevent respiratory depression.
33. Administer bronchodilators and antibiotics as ordered.
34. Follow protocol for maintenance of skin integrity.
35. Provide safe environment to minimize falling or bumping into objects.
36. Provide soft toothbrush or "toothette" swabs for cleaning teeth and gums.
37. Ensure that client does not take aspirin or other medications that increase the potential for bleeding.
38. Clean up areas contaminated by client's blood with household bleach (5.25% sodium hypochlorite) diluted 1:10 with water (Bartlett & Finkbeiner, 1996).
39. Provide frequent tepid water sponge baths.
40. Provide antipyretic as ordered by physician (avoid aspirin).
41. Place client in cool room, with minimal clothing and bed covers.
42. Encourage intake of cool liquids (if not contraindicated).

27–33. To maximize oxygen consumption and minimize respiratory distress.

34–38. To minimize the potential for easy bleeding caused by HIV-induced thrombocytopenia.

39–42. To maintain near-normal body temperature.

Continued on following page

TABLE 36.3 *(Continued)*

NURSING DIAGNOSIS: ALTERED FAMILY PROCESSES

RELATED TO: Crisis associated with having a family member diagnosed with HIV disease

EVIDENCED BY: Difficulty making decisions that affect all family members; inability to meet physical, emotional, spiritual, and security needs of its members

OUTCOME CRITERIA	NURSING INTERVENTIONS	RATIONALE
Family will verbalize areas of dysfunction and demonstrate ability to cope more effectively. Family members will express feelings regarding loved one's diagnosis and prognosis.	1. Create an environment that is comfortable, supportive, private, and promotes trust. 2. Encourage each individual member to express feelings regarding loved one's diagnosis and prognosis. 3. If the client is homosexual, and this is family's first awareness, help them deal with guilt and shame they may experience. Help parents to understand they are not responsible, and their child is still the same individual they have always loved. 4. Serve as facilitator between client's family and homosexual lover. The family may have difficulty accepting the lover as a person who is as significant as a spouse. Clarify roles and responsibilities of family and lover. Do this by bringing both parties together to define and distribute the tasks involved in the client's care. 5. Encourage use of stress management techniques (e.g., relaxation exercises, guided imagery, attendance at support group meetings for significant others of AIDS clients). 6. Provide educational information about AIDS and opportunity to ask questions and express concerns. 7. Make family referrals to community organizations that provide supportive help or financial assistance to AIDS clients.	1. Basic needs of the family must be met before crisis resolution can be attempted. 2. Each individual is unique and must feel that his or her private needs can be met within the family constellation. 3. Resolving guilt and shame enables family members to respond adaptively to the crisis. Their response can affect the client's remaining future and the family's future as well (Christ, Siegel, & Moynihan, 1988). 4. By minimizing the lack of legally defined roles, and by focusing on the need for making realistic decisions about the client's care, communication and resolution of conflict are enhanced (Christ, Siegel, & Moynihan, 1988). 5. Reduction of stress and support from others who share similar experiences enable individuals to begin to think more clearly and develop new behaviors to cope with this situational crisis. 6. Many misconceptions about the disease abound within the public domain. Clarification may calm some of the family's fears and facilitate interaction with the client. 7. Extended care can place a financial burden on client and family members. Respite care may provide family members with occasional much-needed relief away from the stress of physical and emotional caregiving responsibilities.

NURSING DIAGNOSIS: KNOWLEDGE DEFICIT (PREVENTION OF TRANSMISSION AND PROTECTION OF THE CLIENT)

RELATED TO: Lack of exposure to accurate information

EVIDENCED BY: Inaccurate statements by client and family

OUTCOME CRITERIA	NURSING INTERVENTIONS	RATIONALE

Client and family will be able to verbalize accurate information regarding transmission of HIV, as well as protection of the immunodeficient client.	1. Teach that HIV cannot be contracted from:
	  a. Casual or household contact with an AIDS client.
	  b. Shaking hands, hugging, social (dry) kissing, holding hands, or other nonsexual physical contact.
		All of this information may be given to client and significant others in an effort to clarify misconceptions, calm fears, and support an environment of appropriate interventions for care of the client with AIDS.

    c. Touching unsoiled linens or clothing, money, furniture, or other inanimate objects.

    d. Being near someone who has AIDS at work, school, restaurants, elevators.

    e. Toilet seats, bathtubs, towels, showers, or swimming pools.

    f. Dishes, silverware, or food handled by a person with AIDS.

    g. Animals (pets may transmit opportunistic organisms).

    h. (Very unlikely spread by) coughing, sneezing, spitting, kissing, tears, saliva.

2. AIDS virus dies quickly outside the body because it requires living tissue to survive. It is readily killed by soap, cleansers, hot water, and disinfectants.

3. Teach client to protect self from infections by taking the following precautions:

    a. Avoid unpasteurized milk or milk products.

    b. Cook all raw vegetables and fruits before eating.   Raw or improperly washed foods may transmit microbes.

    c. Cook all meals well before eating.

    d. Avoid direct contact with persons with known contagious illnesses.

    e. Consult physician before getting a pet.   Pets require extra infection control precautions owing to the opportunistic organisms carried by animals.

    f. Avoid touching animal feces, urine, emesis, litter boxes, aquariums, or bird cages. Always wear mask and gloves when cleaning up after a pet.

    g. Avoid traveling in countries with poor sanitation.

    h. Avoid vaccines or vaccinations that contain live organisms.   Vaccination with live organisms may be fatal to severely immunosuppressed persons.

    i. Exercise regularly.

    j. Control stress factors. A counselor or support group may be helpful.

    k. Stop smoking.   Smoking predisposes to respiratory infections.

    l. Maintain good personal hygiene.

4. Teach client/significant others about prevention of transmission:

    a. Do not donate blood, plasma, body organs, tissues, or semen.

    b. Inform physician, dentist, and anyone providing care that you have AIDS.

    c. Do not share needles or syringes.

    d. Do not share personal items, such as toothbrushes, razors, or other implements that may be contaminated with blood or body fluids.

    e. Do not eat or drink from the same dinnerware and utensils without washing them between use.

    f. Avoid becoming pregnant if at risk for HIV infection.

Continued on following page

TABLE 36.3 (*Continued*)

g. Engage in only "safer" sexual practices (those *not* involving exchange of body fluids).

h. Avoid sexual practices medically classified as "unsafe," such as anal or vaginal intercourse and oral sex.

i. Avoid the use of recreational drugs because of their immunosuppressive effects.

5. Teach the home caregiver(s) to protect self from HIV infection by taking the following precautions:

a. Wash hands thoroughly with liquid antibiotic soap before and after each client contact. Use moisturizing lotion afterward to prevent dry, cracking skin.

b. Wear gloves when in contact with blood or body fluids (e.g., open wounds, suctioning, feces). Gown or aprons may be worn if soiling is likely.

c. Wear a mask:

(1) When client has a productive cough and tuberculosis has not been ruled out.

(2) To protect client if caregiver has a cold.

(3) During suctioning.

d. Bag disposable gloves and masks with client's trash.

e. Dispose of the following in the toilet:

(1) Organic material on clothes or linen before laundering.

(2) Blood or body fluids.

(3) Soiled tissue or toilet paper.

(4) Cleaners or disinfectants used to clean contaminated articles.

(5) Solutions contaminated with blood or body fluids.

f. Double-bag client's trash and soiled dressings in an impenetrable, plastic bag. *Tie* the bag shut and discard with household trash.

g. Do not recap needles, syringes, and other sharp items. Use puncture-proof covered containers for disposal (e.g., coffee cans, jars).

h. Place soiled linen and clothing in a plastic bag and tie shut until washed. Launder these separately from other laundry. Use bleach or other disinfectant in hot water.

i. When house cleaning, all equipment used in care of the client, as well as bathroom and kitchen surfaces, should be cleaned with a 1:10 dilute bleach solution.

j. Mops, sponges, and other items used for cleaning should be reserved specifically for that purpose.

---

*The nursing interventions for this care plan have been adapted from "Nursing Care Plan for the AIDS Patient," written by the nursing staff of Hospice, Inc., Wichita, KS, 1989, with permission.

TABLE 36.4   TOPICS FOR CLIENT/FAMILY EDUCATION RELATED TO HIV DISEASE

Nature of the Illness
1. What is HIV infection?
2. What is AIDS?
3. How can you find out if you have it?
4. Discuss usual progression of the illness:
   a. Time dimensions
   b. Symptoms associated with various stages
   c. Associated medical conditions

Management of the Illness
1. Discuss methods of transmission:
   a. Sexually
   b. Bloodborne
   c. Perinatal
   d. Ways to prevent transmission of the virus to others:
      (1) Safer sex
      (2) Don't share needles
      (3) Prevent pregnancy
      (4) Don't breastfeed
2. Dispel myths regarding transmission.
3. Provide guidelines to caregivers for preventing transmission of HIV during home care.
4. Discuss ways to prevent transmission of infections to the HIV-infected person.
5. Provide guidelines for when to seek medical assistance
6. Discuss opportunistic infections
7. Discuss treatment modalities and medication:
   a. Reverse transcriptase inhibitors
   b. Protease inhibitors
   c. Medications for opportunistic infections
   d. Antianxiety agents
   e. Antidepressants
   f. Antimanics
   g. Antipsychotics
8. Discuss legal issues
9. Discuss financial issues
10. Discuss psychological and social issues

Support Services
1. Support groups
2. Individual psychotherapy
3. AIDS hotline number: 1-800-342-AIDS
4. HIV-associated dementia hotline: Project Inform: 1-800-822-7422

---

6. Does the client experience respiratory distress?
7. Have bleeding and bruising been avoided?
8. Are skin and mucous membranes intact?
9. Do family members/significant others verbalize feelings (including anger) regarding the client's diagnosis and prognosis?
10. Can members identify areas of dysfunction within the family?
11. If the client has a homosexual lover, has any conflict been resolved?
12. Have caregiving responsibilities been defined and distributed in a manner acceptable to all?
13. Have the parents worked through feelings of guilt and shame?
14. Are the client and family/significant other(s) able to verbalize educational information presented regarding ways in which HIV can and cannot be transmitted, ways to protect the client from infec-

tions, and ways to prevent transmission to caregivers and others?
15. Can the client and family/significant other(s) identify resources within the community from whom they may seek support and assistance (e.g., AIDS support groups, home care, respite care, hospice, financial support)?

TREATMENT MODALITIES

Pharmacology

Antiretroviral Therapy

Yarchoan and Broder (1988) base the rationale for use of antiretroviral therapy in clients with HIV disease on the following premises that they consider to be true in *most* cases:

1. That active replication of HIV is important in the pathogenesis and maintenance of the disease state.
2. That at any one point in time, most helper T cells (or other relevant cells) are not infected with HIV.
3. That infected cells die in a relatively short time.
4. That it is possible to stop the replication of HIV and thus to block the spread of the virus.
5. That the damaged organs have at least some regenerative potential.

The first antiretroviral agent approved by the FDA in the treatment of HIV infection is zidovudine (azidothymidine [AZT]). Marketed under the trade name of Retrovir, it was initially prescribed for clients with severe symptomatic HIV disease (fewer than 200 T4 cells). More recent data, however, justify treating all clients who have fewer than 500 T4 cells (Hollander & Katz, 1996; Volberding, 1990b). Zidovudine belongs to the classification of drugs known as *nucleoside reverse transcriptase inhibitors* (NRTIs).

Since the approval of zidovudine by the FDA, a number of other NRTIs have been approved in the treatment of HIV infection. These include didanosine [ddI] (Videx), lamivudine [3TC] (Epivir), stavudine [d4T] (Zerit), and others. The latest is abacavir (Ziagen), which was approved in December 1998. A second classification of antiretroviral drugs is the *non-nucleoside reverse transcriptase inhibitors* (NNRTIs). Examples of NNRTIs include delavirdine (Rescriptor) and nevirapine (Viramune). Both the NRTIs and NNRTIs work (albeit in different ways) by disabling the HIV reproductive enzyme called *reverse transcriptase*. In doing so, viral replication inside the host cell is inhibited.

A different class of antiretrovirals, called *protease inhibitors*, are being used by some individuals who cannot tolerate or no longer benefit from the originally approved antiretrovirals. Protease inhibitors, which include saquinavir (Invirase), indinavir (Crixivan), nelfinavir (Viracept), and ritonavir (Norvir), prevent or slow down the action of an HIV enzyme called *protease*, which is needed by the HIV to break down proteins for replication. Protease inhibitors have been very effective in increasing T4 cell counts and decreasing viral load within the blood. However, in clinical trials with individuals who exhibited high levels of the virus, eventual resistance to the drug occurred (Douglas & Pinsky, 1996). Single-drug therapy is no longer the treatment of choice. Triple-drug therapy with two nucleosides and one protease inhibitor is the most potent antiretroviral treatment available (Kaplan & Sadock, 1998).

Other Chemotherapeutic Agents

Various other drugs are used in HIV-infected individuals to treat the opportunistic infections and malignancies associated with the disease. Some examples include antibiotics, antifungal agents, antiviral agents, and antineoplastic agents. Douglas & Pinsky (1996) state:

"When individuals with HIV disease develop minor infections, they should be treated quickly and thoroughly. Ongoing infection may put a strain on the immune system and worsen the course of HIV infection. HIV-infected people may need to be treated with longer courses of medication or higher dosages than patients not infected with HIV." (p. 63)

The U.S. Public Health Service has officially recommended that physicians offer primary preventive treatment for *Pneumocystis carinii* pneumonia (PCP) to all HIV-infected people with a T4 count below 200 (Douglas & Pinsky, 1996). The combination drug trimethoprim/sulfamethoxazole (Bactrim; Septra) is the prophylactic agent of choice (Hollander & Katz, 1996). Other drugs used to prevent opportunistic infections include dapsone (prophalaxis for PCP); rifabutin (prevention of disseminated *Mycobacterium avium*); fluconazole (prevention of fungal infections); and acyclovir (treatment and prophylaxis of herpes infections). Some studies have indicated that zidovudine may be helpful in slowing or preventing the symptoms of HIV-associated dementia (Bartlett & Finkbeiner, 1996; Kaplan & Sadock, 1998).

Psychotropic Medications

Antianxiety Agents. Benzodiazepines, such as oxazepam or lorazepam, are often prescribed for relief of anxiety in clients with HIV disease. Buspirone (BuSpar) may be useful in the management of chronic anxiety symptoms, although it takes from 2 to 3 weeks for it to become effective as an anxiolytic. Imipramine, clonazepam, and the selective serotonin reuptake inhibitors (SSRIs) (e.g., sertaline, fluoxetine, paroxetine) may be considered in the case of panic disorder.

Antidepressants. The tricyclic antidepressants are widely used for relief of depression in clients with HIV disease. In addition to relieving the symptoms of depression, some of the tricyclics (e.g., nortriptyline, amitriptyline, desipramine) also ameliorate peripheral neuropathy (Capaldini, 1995) and relieve chronic pain in some individuals with advanced HIV disease.

The SSRIs may be selected because of their minimal anticholinergic side effects, a benefit for HIV clients who suffer from excessive dryness of the mouth. They are also less sedating than the tricyclics. Their main disadvantages are that initially they may produce a stimulant effect that may aggravate anxiety in HIV clients and that they tend to cause sexual dysfunction.

Monoamine oxidase inhibitors (MAOIs), although highly effective antidepressants, may be a risky choice for HIV-infected clients with cognitive defects because of the diet and concomitant medication restrictions required with administration of these drugs. Stimulants, such as methylphenidate (Ritalin) and dextroamphetamine, have successfully treated depression in the medically ill (Capaldini, 1995). The effects are more rapid than with antidepressants, and they are especially effective for clients with despondency related to acute medical disease.

Antimanics. Lithium has been the drug of choice for manic symptoms. However, lithium therapy poses potential problems for clients with HIV disease. Lithium toxicity is particularly risky with these clients because of altered renal function, dehydration, vomiting, and diarrhea. If the manic behavior can be attributable to a medication being administered to the HIV-infected client, the medication should be decreased or stopped as soon as is medically feasible. Carbamazepine (Tegretol) and valproic acid (Depakote) have been used successfully to stabilize mood in clients with HIV-associated mania.

Antipsychotics. Psychotic symptoms are often seen in the HIV-infected client experiencing delirium. Certain medications administered for HIV-related problems may also result in psychosis. Capaldini (1995) states:

> "Because of the increased risk of both neuroleptic malignant syndrome and extrapyramidal syndromes with high-dose and high-potency neuroleptics, both dosage and duration of neuroleptic therapy should be minimized. Midpotency neuroleptics, such as perphenazine (Trilafon), represent a good compromise between avoiding the anticholinergic side effects of low-potency neuroleptics and avoiding the higher risk of extrapyramidal symptoms with high-potency agents, such as haloperidol." (p. 309.)

Universal Isolation Precautions*

In January 1996, the Centers for Disease Control and Prevention (CDC) issued new guidelines for isolation precautions in hospitals. The guidelines, based on the latest epidemiologic information on transmission of infection in hospitals, are intended primarily for use in acute-care hospitals, although some of the recommendations may be applicable to subacute-care or extended-care facilities. The recommendations are not intended for use in day care, well care, or domiciliary care programs.

The revised guidelines contain two tiers of precautions. In the first, and most important, tier are those precautions designed for the care of all patients in hospitals regardless of their diagnosis or presumed infection status. Implementation of these "Standard Precautions" is the primary strategy for successful nosocomial infection control. In the second tier are precautions designed only for the care of specified patients. These additional "Transmission-Based Precautions" are used for patients known or suspected to be infected or colonized with epidemiologically important pathogens that can be transmitted by airborne or droplet transmission or by contact with dry skin or contaminated surfaces.

Standard Precautions synthesize the major features

of Universal (Blood and Body Fluid) Precaution (designed to reduce the risk of transmission of pathogens from moist body substances). Standard Precautions apply to (1) blood; (2) all body fluids, secretions, and excretions *except sweat*, regardless of whether they contain visible blood; (3) nonintact skin; and (4) mucous membranes. Standard Precautions are designed to reduce the risk of transmission of both recognized and unrecognized sources of infection in hospitals.

Transmission-Based Precautions are designed for patients documented or suspected to be infected or colonized with highly transmissible or epidemiologically important pathogens for which additional precautions beyond Standard Precautions are needed to interrupt transmission in hospitals. There are three types of Transmission-Based Precautions: *Airborne Precautions, Droplet Precautions,* and *Contact Precautions.* They may be combined for diseases that have multiple routes of transmission. When used either singly or in combination, they are to be used in addition to Standard Precautions. [**Author's Note:** Knowledge of Transmission-Based Precautions is important in caring for clients with opportunistic infections associated with HIV disease.]

Standard Precautions

The following Standard Precautions, or the equivalent, should be used for the care of all patients.

- **Handwashing:**
  1. Wash hands after touching blood, body fluids, secretions, excretions, and contaminated items, whether or not gloves are worn. Wash hands immediately after gloves are removed, between patient contacts, and when otherwise indicated to avoid transfer of microorganisms to other patients or environments. It may be necessary to wash hands between tasks and procedures on the same patient to prevent cross-contamination of different body sites.
  2. Use a plain (nonantimicrobial) soap for routine handwashing.
  3. Use an antimicrobial agent or a waterless antiseptic agent for specific circumstances (e.g., control of outbreaks or hyperendemic infections), as defined by the infection control program.
- **Gloves:** Wear gloves (clean, nonsterile gloves are adequate) when touching blood, body fluids, secretions, excretions, and contaminated items. Put on clean gloves just before touching mucous membranes and nonintact skin. Change gloves between tasks and procedures on the same patient after contact with material that may contain a high concentration of microorganisms. Remove gloves promptly after use, before touching noncontaminated items and environmental surfaces, and before going to another patient,

---

*This section is from *Taber's Cyclopedic Medical Dictionary* (18th ed.) (1997). Philadelphia: F.A Davis. Reprinted with permission.

and wash hands immediately to avoid transfer of microorganisms to other patients or environments.

- **Mask, Eye Protection, Face Shield:** Wear a mask and eye protection or a face shield to protect mucous membranes of the eyes, nose, and mouth during procedures and patient-care activities that are likely to generate splashes or sprays of blood, body fluids, secretions, and excretions.
- **Gown:** Wear a gown (a clean, nonsterile gown is adequate) to protect skin and to prevent soiling of clothing during procedures and patient-care activities that are likely to generate splashes or sprays of blood, body fluids, secretions, or excretions. Select a gown that is appropriate for the activity and amount of fluid likely to be encountered. Remove a soiled gown as promptly as possible, and wash hands to avoid transfer of microorganisms to other patients or environments.
- **Patient-Care Equipment:** Handle used patient-care equipment soiled with blood, body fluids, secretions, and excretions in a manner that prevents skin and mucous membrane exposures, contamination of clothing, and transfer of microorganisms to other patients and environments. Ensure that reusable equipment is not used for the care of another patient until it has been cleaned and reprocessed appropriately. Ensure that single-use items are discarded properly.
- **Environmental Control:** Ensure that the hospital has adequate procedures for the routine care, cleaning, and disinfection of environmental surfaces, beds, bedrails, bedside equipment, and other frequently touched surfaces, and ensure that these procedures are being followed.
- **Linen:** Handle, transport, and process used linen soiled with blood, body fluids, secretions, and excretions in a manner that prevents skin and mucous membrane exposures and contamination of clothing, and that avoids transfer of microorganisms to other patients and environments.
- **Occupational Health and Bloodborne Pathogens:**
  1. Take care to prevent injuries when using needles, scalpels, and other sharp instruments or devices; when handling sharp instruments after procedures; when cleaning used instruments; and when disposing of used needles. Never recap used needles, or otherwise manipulate them using both hands, or use any other technique that involves directing the point of a needle toward any part of the body; rather, use either a one-handed "scoop" technique or a mechanical device designed for holding the needle sheath. Do not remove used needles from disposable syringes by hand, and do not bend, break, or otherwise manipulate used needles by hand. Place used disposable syringes and needles, scalpel

blades, and other sharp items in appropriate puncture-resistant containers, which are located as close as practical to the area in which the items were used, and place reusable syringes and needles in a puncture-resistant container for transport to the reprocessing area.
  2. Use mouthpieces, resuscitation bags, or other ventilation devices as an alternative to mouth-to-mouth resuscitation methods in areas where the need for resuscitation is predictable.
- **Patient Placement:** Place a patient who contaminates the environment or who does not (or cannot be expected to) assist in maintaining appropriate hygiene or environmental control in a private room. If a private room is not available, consult with infection control professionals regarding patient placement or other alternatives.

Hospice Care

Hospice is a program that provides palliative and supportive care to meet the special needs arising out of the physical, psychosocial, spiritual, social, and economical stresses that are experienced during the final stages of illness and during bereavement (Lemus, 1990). Various models of hospice exist, including freestanding institutions that provide both inpatient and home care; those affiliated with hospitals in which hospice services are provided within the hospital setting; and hospice organizations that provide home care only. Historically, the hospice movement in the United States has evolved mainly as a system of home-based care.

Candace and Walter (1988) state:

"The goal of hospice care is to enable persons who are dying to function optimally, in spite of the devastating effects of their physical condition, by preventing pain and other symptoms, anticipating and minimizing the side effects of drugs and fatigue, and allowing control and independent decision making by the patient and caregivers [significant others]."

The National Hospice Organization (1994) has published guidelines for standards of care that are directed at the hospice program concept. These standards of care are presented in Table 36.5.

Hospice follows an interdisciplinary team approach to provide care for the individual with AIDS in the familiar surroundings of the home environment. The interdisciplinary team consists of nurses, attendants (homemakers, home health aides), physicians, social workers, volunteers, and other health care workers from other disciplines as required for individual clients.

Candace and Walter (1988) identify seven components on which the hospice approach is based. They include the interdisciplinary team, pain and symptom management, emotional support to client and family, pastoral and spir-

◢ TABLE 36.5   NATIONAL HOSPICE ORGANIZATION—PRINCIPLES OF CARE

1. Hospice offers palliative care to all terminally ill people and their families regardless of age, gender, nationality, race, creed, sexual orientation, disability, diagnosis, availability of a primary caregiver, or ability to pay.
2. The unit of care in hospice is the patient and family.
3. A highly qualified, specially trained team of hospice professionals and volunteers work together to meet the physiological, psychological, social, spiritual, and economic needs of hospice patient/families facing terminal illness and bereavement.
4. The hospice interdisciplinary team collaborates continuously with the patient's attending physician to develop and maintain a patient-directed, individualized plan of care.
5. Hospice provides a safe, coordinated program of palliative and supportive care, in a variety of appropriate settings, from the time of admission through bereavement, with the focus on keeping terminally ill patients in their own home as long as possible.

   NOTE: Palliative care is defined by hospice as treatment which enhances comfort and improves the quality of a patient's life. The goals of intervention are pain control, symptom management, quality-of-life enhancement, and spiritual-emotional comfort for patients and the primary care support. Each patient's needs are continuously assessed, and all treatment options are explored and evaluated in the context of the patient's values and symptoms.
6. Hospice care is available 24 hours a day, 7 days a week, and services continue without interruption if the patient care setting changes.
7. Hospice is accountable for the appropriate allocation and utilization of its resources in order to provide optimal care consistent with patient and family needs.
8. Hospice maintains a comprehensive and accurate record of services provided in all care settings for each patient and family.
9. Hospice has an organized governing body that has complete and ultimate responsibility for the organization.
10. The hospice governing body entrusts the hospice administrator with overall management responsibility for operating the hospice including planning, organizing, staffing, and evaluating the organization and its services.
11. Hospice is committed to continuous assessment and improvement of the quality and efficiency of its services.

SOURCE: Adapted from NHO (1994), with permission.

---

itual care, bereavement counseling, 24-hour on-call nurse/counselor, and staff support. These are the ideal, and not all hospice programs may include all of these services.

Interdisciplinary Team

Nurses. A registered nurse usually acts as case manager for care of hospice clients. The nurse assesses the client and family's needs, establishes the goals of care, supervises and assists caregivers, evaluates care, serves as client advocate, and provides educational information as needed to client, family, and caregivers. He or she also provides physical care when needed, including IV therapy.

Attendants. These individuals are usually the members of the team who spend the most time with the client. They assist with personal care as well as all activities of daily living. Without these daily attendants, many AIDS clients would be unable to spend their remaining days in their home. Attendants may be noncertified and provide basic housekeeping services; they may be certified nursing assistants who assist with personal care; or they may be licensed vocational or practical nurses who provide more specialized care, such as dressing changes or tube feedings.

Physicians. The client's primary physician, as well as the hospice medical consultant, have input into the care of the AIDS hospice client. Orders may continue to come from the primary physician, while pain and symptom management may come from the hospice consultant. Ideally, these physicians attend weekly client care confer-

ences and provide inservice education for hospice staff as well as others in the medical community.

Social Workers. The social worker assists the client and family members with psychosocial issues, including those associated with the diagnosis of AIDS and its prognosis, financial issues, legal needs, and bereavement concerns. The social worker provides information on community resources from which client and family may receive support and assistance. Some of the functions of the nurse and social worker may overlap at times.

Trained Volunteers. Volunteers are vital to the hospice concept. They provide services that may otherwise be financially impossible. They are specially selected and extensively trained, and provide such services as transportation, companionship, respite care, recreational activities, light housekeeping, and in general are sensitive to the needs of families in stressful situations (Martin, 1990).

Rehabilitation Therapists. Physical therapists may assist hospice clients in an effort to minimize physical disability. They may assist with strengthening exercises and provide assistance with special equipment needs. Occupational therapists may help the debilitated client learn to accomplish activities of daily living as independently as possible. Other consultants, such as speech therapists, may be called upon for the client with special needs.

Dietitian. A nutritional consultant may be helpful to the AIDS client who is experiencing nausea and vomiting, diarrhea, anorexia, and weight loss. A nutritionist can ensure that the client is receiving the proper balance of calories and nutrients.

Counseling Services. The hospice client may require the services of a psychiatrist or psychologist if there is a history of mental illness, or if AIDS-related dementia or depressive syndrome has become evident. The AIDS client with a history of substance abuse may benefit from the services of a substance abuse counselor to provide assistance in dealing with these special needs.

Pain and Symptom Management

Improved quality of life at all times is a primary goal of hospice care. Thus, a major intervention for all caregivers is to ensure that the client is as comfortable as possible, whether experiencing pain or nausea, vomiting, or diarrhea, which are commonly associated with the AIDS client.

Emotional Support

Members of the hospice team encourage clients and families to discuss the eventual outcome of the disease process. Some individuals find discussing issues associated with death and dying uncomfortable, and if so, their decision is respected. However, honest discussion of these issues provides a sense of relief for some people, and they are more realistically prepared for the future. It may even draw some clients and families closer together during this stressful time.

Pastoral and Spiritual Care

Hospice philosophy supports the individual's right to seek guidance or comfort in the spiritual practices most suited to that person. Treatment team members must be aware and accepting of the fact that many AIDS clients seek spiritual support from various alternatives to traditional Western religions or spiritual practices. In the gay population, this may be partly due to the rejection they have experienced from some traditional religious organizations. The hospice team members help the client obtain the spiritual support and guidance for which he or she expresses a preference.

Bereavement Counseling

Hospice provides a service to surviving family members or significant others after the death of their loved one. This is usually provided by a bereavement counselor, but when one is not available, volunteers with special training in bereavement care may be of service. A grief support group may be helpful for the bereaved and provide a safe place for them to discuss their own fears and concerns about the death of a loved one.

Twenty-Four-Hour On-Call

The standards of care set forth by the National Hospice Organization state that care shall be available 24 hours a day, 7 days a week. A nurse or counselor is usually available either by phone or for home visits around the clock. The knowledge that emotional or physical support is available at any time, should it be required, provides considerable support and comfort to significant others or family caregivers.

Staff Support

Team members (all who work closely and frequently with the client) often experience emotions similar to those of

---

TEST YOUR CRITICAL THINKING SKILLS

George, a 37-year-old man, presents himself to his physician complaining of fever, sore throat, anorexia, and fatigue. These symptoms have persisted for about 3 weeks. George says, "I've had these flu symptoms, but they just don't seem to go away."

George is a professional writer and has had two of his novels published. He is gay and has been in a monogamous relationship for 9 years. He and his partner, Steve, both were found to be negative for HIV in tests they took 6 years ago. George confides to the physician that one night about 5 months ago after an argument with Steve, he left the apartment angry, went to a bar, and met a man with whom he had an unprotected sexual encounter. The next day, he and Steve resumed their relationship, and he never saw the man from the bar again.

A lab test reveals that George is HIV-positive. The acute symptoms disappear, and George has no further symptoms of the illness. However, George is devastated by the diagnosis and begins experiencing symptoms of anxiety and depression. He becomes preoccupied with dying. He cannot sleep without having nightmares about dying. He cannot eat, and he continues to lose weight. He cannot write, and he refuses to see anyone.

Steve tests negative for HIV at this time. George has moved out of their apartment and has rented a room for himself. Steve goes to see him every day. George is obsessed with reading everything he can find about AIDS but panics when he hears about people he knows dying of the disease. He has become nonfunctional and just sits and stares out his window. Steve talks him into seeing a psychiatrist who hospitalizes George with a diagnosis of adjustment disorder with mixed anxiety and depressed mood.

Answer the following questions related to George:

1. Describe priority information the nurse must gather during the intake assessment interview.
2. List the two priority nursing diagnoses for George.
3. Identify three important nursing interventions in working with George.

RESEARCH NOTE

College students' AIDS risk perception. *Journal of Psychosocial Nursing* (1998, September), 36(9), 25–30. Brown, E.J.

Description of the Study: This study was conducted to determine college students' AIDS risk perceptions (ARP) for themselves, their friends and peers, and to describe their AIDS-related risk behavior. The sample was self-selected, and consisted of 75 percent women and 25 percent men; 72 percent Caucasian, 18 percent African Americans, and 10 percent Latino Americans. The average age was 19.3 years. Information was gathered by survey and audiotaped in face-to-face semistructured interviews. Subjects were asked to rate their risk of acquiring AIDS given the following choices: nil, small, moderate, large, and great.

Results of the Study: The majority of the students in this study appraised their risk for AIDS as nil or small. They based this judgment on being in a monogamous relationship, feeling trust in their partner, and feeling secure in the relationship. Although most students rated their friends' behavior in a similar manner, most suggested that their friends (and especially their peers) were engaging in unprotected sex more often than themselves. In other words, ARP increased as distance from the student increased. In discussing what they considered risk factors for AIDS, sexual behavior (unprotected sex and multiple sex partners) and drug use were recurring themes. Most of the Latino-American students reported that they were virgins.

Comments: The conclusion of the author is that because college students tend to underestimate their AIDS risk, based on their monogamous status or by the trust or security they feel, educational forums for prevention strategies may not be sufficient to ensure behavior change or that ARP will be congruent with actual behavior. Situations in which ARP is challenged when not congruent with the riskiness of their behavior are suggested, such as: (1) encounter groups; (2) publication of HIV/AIDS prevalence and incidence data among college students in college papers; (3) periodic lectures that focus on the asymptomatic physical appearance of individuals with HIV disease; (4) employment of nonjudgmental health care workers to counsel, educate, and provide information that will enhance students' self-awareness of their risks for HIV disease.

the person with AIDS or their family and/or significant others. They may experience anger, frustration, or fears of contagion or of death and dying—all of which must be addressed through staff support groups, team conferences, time off, and adequate and effective supervision (Martin, 1990). Burnout is a common problem among hospice staff. Stress can be reduced, trust enhanced, and team functioning more effective if lines of communication are kept open among all members (medical director through volunteer), if information is readily accessible through staff conferences and inservice education, and if staff know they are appreciated and feel good about what they are doing (Candace & Walter, 1988).

SUMMARY

AIDS is likely to be one of this century's major killers. The disease is the terminal end of a continuum of syndromes identified by HIV infection. The continuum begins with the acute response that occurs when the individual is initially infected with the virus, and progresses to a period of asymptomatic infection that may last for as long as 10 years. Advanced stages of the disease present with lymphadenopathy, neurological involvement, opportunistic infections, HIV wasting syndrome, malignancies, and finally death.

The HIV invades the T4 cells (normal range 600/mm^3 to 1200/mm^3) until in the very advanced stage of the disease the individual may have fewer than 10/mm^3. Examples of opportunistic infections that attack the body of an individual with AIDS include *Pneumocystis carinii* pneumonia (PCP), candidiasis cytomegalovirus (CMV), herpes, *M. tuberculosis*, and toxoplasmosis. Many of these were rarely observed before the AIDS epidemic. Common malignancies associated with AIDS include KS and non-Hodgkin's lymphoma. Any infectious or other disease process can prove fatal to an individual with AIDS whose immune system is so severely depressed.

Approximately 70 percent to 95 percent of AIDS clients develop HAD, which is thought to be the most common CNS complication of HIV infection. Cognitive, motor, and behavioral processes are affected to a point when the individual may become totally vegetative. Psychiatric syndromes commonly associated with HIV infection include depression, anxiety, mania, and psychosis.

Transmission of HIV infection is via three major routes: sexual, bloodborne, and perinatal. Sexual transmission can occur through any activity in which there is an exchange of body fluids with an infected individual. Although most sexual transmission in the past has occurred within the homosexual population, increasing numbers of cases are occurring

INTERNET REFERENCES

● Additional information about HIV/AIDS may be located at the following websites:
   a. http://www.avert.org/
   b. http://www.kc-reach.org/
   c. http://www.infoweb.org/
   d. http://www.aegis.com/main/
   e. http://www.aidsnews/index.html
   f. http://www.critpath.org/
   g. http://www.healthcg.com/hiv/
   h. http://www.medscape.com/Home/Topics/
      AIDS/AIDS.htm
   i. http://www.HIVpositive.com/
   j. http://www.guides4living.com/links.html
   k. http://research.med.umkc.edu/teams/
      cml/AIDS.html
   l. http://www.alzheimer-europe.org/
      aids.html

from heterosexual contact. Bloodborne transmission can occur when an individual is transfused with blood or blood products that have been contaminated with HIV. Other modes of bloodborne transmission include the sharing of contaminated needles by IV drug users and accidental sticks with contaminated needles by health care workers. Perinatal transmission occurs in infants born to HIV-infected women through exposure to maternal blood and vaginal secretions during delivery. It can also occur transplacentally and through infant feeding with breast milk.

This chapter discussed delivery of care to the client with HIV disease via the steps of the nursing process. Background assessment data included a description of the predisposing factors as well as symptomatology associated with various aspects of the disease. Nursing diagnoses and a plan of care for the client with HIV disease were presented, along with outcome criteria and guidelines for evaluation of nursing care. Other treatment modalities including pharmacology, universal isolation precautions, and hospice care were discussed.

REVIEW QUESTIONS

SELF-EXAMINATION/LEARNING EXERCISE

Select the answer that is most appropriate for the questions that follow this situation:

Situation: Joe is a 34-year-old homosexual man. He and his partner were both tested and found to be HIV-positive 8 years ago. His partner died 2 years ago. Joe had taken care of him until his death. Joe has seen his primary physician, who is admitting him to the hospital with a loss of 15 lb in the past 2 weeks, fever, night sweats, persistent diarrhea, and enlarged cervical, axillary, and inguinal lymph nodes. His laboratory T4 count is 400/mm³. Oral candidiasis (thrush) is evident upon examination. This is his third hospitalization in 15 months. He previously had a diagnosis of persistent generalized lymphadenopathy.

1. During the initial nursing assessment, Joe says to the nurse, "I didn't mention it to my doctor, but I found this spot on my foot yesterday that I hadn't noticed before. It doesn't hurt or anything." Upon inspection, the nurse observes a small, bluish spot that is slightly raised on the sole of Joe's foot. Taking note of this symptom, of what might the nurse be concerned?

   a. Herpes simplex
   b. Candidiasis
   c. Herpes zoster
   d. Kaposi's sarcoma

2. Oral candidiasis presents with which of the following symptoms?

   a. Bleeding gums.
   b. Dry, cracking lips.
   c. White patches on the oral mucosa.
   d. Blisters on the tongue.

3. What type of organism is *Candida?*

   a. Fungus.
   b. Protozoan.
   c. Bacterium.
   d. Virus.

4. Joe's physician prescribed the antiretroviral agent zidovudine for him 5 years ago. What is the rationale behind administration of this medication?

   a. It cures HIV infection.
   b. It prevents the HIV-infected person from getting other viruses.
   c. It slows down the progression from HIV infection to full-blown AIDS.
   d. It prevents entry of HIV into the CNS.

5. In providing nursing care for Joe, which of the following interventions would be most appropriate for preventing transmission to the caregiver?

   a. Wear a gown to carry in Joe's food tray.
   b. Do not recap Joe's medication injection needles.
   c. Wear a mask when changing the linen on Joe's bed.
   d. Wear gloves to change the bag on Joe's continuous IV fluids.

6. Which of the following interventions would be most appropriate for prevention of infection to Joe?

   a. Allow only one staff person to provide care for Joe.
   b. Place Joe in protective isolation.
   c. Put a "no visitors" sign on Joe's door.
   d. Wash hands before entering Joe's room.

7. Joe is discharged from the hospital after 2 weeks. Which of the following would be appropriate to teach Joe and his caregivers?

   a. Joe should cook all vegetables and fruits before eating them.

   b. Joe should abstain from all sexual activities.

   c. Joe should refrain from exercising because of weakness and fatigue.

   d. Joe should not kiss anyone on the mouth.

8. Fourteen months later Joe is readmitted. He has lost a great deal more weight. He is unable to take nourishment by mouth and has apparent difficulty breathing. He has a dry, nonproductive cough, and a fever of 101.2°F. The physician diagnoses PCP. PCP is an example of:

   a. An opportunistic infection

   b. A hospital-acquired infection

   c. An infection acquired due to lack of immunization

   d. A hypersensitivity reaction to a medication Joe has been taking for his AIDS

9. Joe's condition continues to deteriorate and he is transferred to hospice care. The primary goal of hospice care is:

   a. To assist with legal and financial problems of long-term care and dying.

   b. To provide quality of life for the terminally ill person until death occurs.

   c. To assist family and significant others through their loved one's dying process.

   d. To fulfill the emotional and spiritual needs of the client and family and/or significant others.

10. Which of the following is *not* necessarily true about hospice care?

   a. Joe's family will be able to call someone from hospice on a 24-hour basis.

   b. Hospice services to Joe and his family will be discontinued upon Joe's death.

   c. Joe will be allowed to remain in his home during his terminal illness.

   d. Psychiatric services may be provided through the hospice program if deemed necessary.

REFERENCES

Abrams, D. (1998) The pre-AIDS syndromes. *Infectious Disease Clinics of North America, 2*(2), 343–351.

Aids Education & Research Trust (AVERT). (1999, February). Worldwide HIV & AIDS estimates. [On-line]. Available: http://www.avert.org/wwstatsg.htm.

Allen, J.R., & Curran, J.W. (1988). Prevention of AIDS and HIV-infection: Needs and priorities for epidemiologic research. *American Journal of Public Health, 78*, 381–386.

American Red Cross (ARC). (1998). HIV antigen test and risk of HIV transmission. [On-line]. Available: http://biomed.redcross.org/home/hiv-ant.htm

Bartlett, J.G., & Finkbeiner, A.K. (1996). *The guide to living with HIV infection* (3rd ed.). Baltimore: Johns Hopkins University Press.

Bell, R. (1998). *Changing bodies, changing lives* (3rd ed.). New York: Times Books.

Biggar, R.J. (1990). Cancer in acquired immunodeficiency syndrome: An epidemiological assessment. *Seminars in Oncology, 17*, 251–260.

Boswell, S.L., & Hirsch, M.S. (1992). Therapeutic approach to the HIV-seropositive patient. In V.T. DeVita, S. Hellman, & S.A. Rosenberg (Eds.), *AIDS: Etiology, diagnosis, treatment, and prevention* (3rd ed.). Philadelphia: J.B. Lippincott.

Buehler, J.W., Petersen, L.R., & Jaffe, H.W. (1995). Current trends in the epidemiology of HIV/AIDS. In M.A. Sande & P.A. Volberding (Eds.), *The medical management of AIDS* (4th ed.). Philadelphia: W.B. Saunders.

Candace, R., & Walter, M. (1988). The hospice approach to care. In A. Lewis (Ed.), *Nursing care of the person with AIDS/ARC.* Rockville, MD: Aspen Publishers.

Capaldini, L. (1995). HIV disease: Psychosocial issues and psychiatric complications. In M.A. Sande & P.A. Volberding (Eds.), *The medical management of AIDS* (4th ed.). Philadelphia: W.B. Saunders.

Centers for Disease Control (CDC). (1998, June). Twelfth World AIDS Conference, Geneva, Switzerland. Historical trends in AIDS incidence. [On-line]. Available: http://www.cdcnpin.org/geneva98/trends/trends_2.htm.

Centers for Disease Control (CDC). (1997). *HIV/AIDS surveillance report, 9*(2).

Centers for Disease Control. (1995). *HIV/AIDS surveillance report, 7*(1), 1–20.

Centers for Disease Control. (1986). Apparent transmission of human T-lymphotrophic virus type III/lymphadenopathy-associated virus from a child to a mother providing health care. *Morbidity and Mortality Weekly Report, 35*, 76–79.

Centers for Disease Control. (1981, June 5). Pneumocystic pneumonia. *Morbidity and Mortality Weekly Report, 30*, 205.

Christ, G.H., Siegel, K., & Moynihan, R.T. (1988). Psychosocial issues: Prevention and treatment. In V.T. DeVita, S. Hellman, & S.A. Rosenberg (Eds.), *AIDS: Etiology, diagnosis, treatment, and prevention* (2nd ed.). Philadelphia: J.B. Lippincott.

Cohen, F.L. (1991). The clinical spectrum of HIV infection and its treatment. In J.D. Durham & F.L. Cohen (Eds.), *The person with AIDS: Nursing perspectives.* New York: Springer.

Dietz, S.E. (1994). Acquired immunodeficiency syndrome (AIDS). In C.M. Porth (Ed.), *Pathophysiology: Concepts of altered health states* (4th ed.). Philadelphia: J.B. Lippincott.

Dilley, J. (1990). Psychosocial impact of AIDS: Overview. In P.T. Cohen, M.A. Sande, & P.A. Volberding (Eds.), *The AIDS knowledge base.* Waltham, MA: The Medical Publishing Group.

Donegan, E. (1990). Transmission of HIV in blood products. In P.T. Cohen, M.A. Sande, & P.A. Volberding (Eds.), *The AIDS knowledge base.* Waltham, MA: The Medical Publishing Group.

Douglas, P.H., & Pinsky, L. (1996). *The essential AIDS fact book.* New York: Simon & Schuster.

El-Mallakh, R. (1991). Mania in AIDS: Clinical significance and theoretical considerations. *International Journal of Psychiatry and Medicine, 21*, 383–391.

Essex, M. (1988). Origins of AIDS. In V.T. DeVita, S. Hellman, & S.A. Rosenberg (Eds.), *AIDS: Etiology, diagnosis, treatment, and prevention* (2nd ed.). Philadelphia: J.B. Lippincott.

Essex, M., et al. (1984). Seroepidemiology of HTLV in relation to immunosuppression and the acquired immunodeficiency syndrome. In R.C. Gallo et al. (Eds.), *Human T-cell leukemia viruses.* Cold Spring Harbor, NY: Cold Spring Harbor Press.

Flaskerud, J.H. (1992a). Overview: HIV disease and nursing. In J.H. Flaskerud & P.J. Ungvarski (Eds.), *HIV/AIDS: A guide to nursing care* (2nd ed.). Philadelphia: W.B. Saunders.

Flaskerud, J.H. (1992b). Cofactors in HIV and public health education. In J.H. Flaskerud & P.J. Ungvarski (Eds.), *HIV/AIDS: A guide to nursing care* (2nd ed.). Philadelphia: W.B. Saunders.

Gallo., R.C., et al. (1983). Isolation of human T-cell leukemia virus in acquired immune deficiency syndrome (AIDS). *Science, 220,* 865.

Gallo, R.C., et al. (1984). Frequent detection and isolation of cytopathic retroviruses (HTLV-III) from patients with AIDS and at risk for AIDS. *Science, 224,* 500–502.

Gallo, R.C., et al. (1986). Origins of human T-lymphotropic viruses. *Nature, 320,* 219.

Gershon, R.R.M., Vlahov, D., & Nelson, K.E. (1990). The risk of transmission of HIV-1 through non-percutaneous, non-sexual modes. A review. *AIDS, 4,* 645–650.

Grady, C. (1992). HIV disease: Pathogenesis and treatment. In J.H. Flaskerud & P.J. Ungvarski (Eds.), *HIV/AIDS: A guide to nursing care* (2nd ed.). Philadelphia: W.B. Saunders.

Haverkos, H.W., & Edelman, R. (1988). The epidemiology of acquired immunodeficiency syndrome among heterosexuals. *Journal of the American Medical Association, 260,* 1922–1929.

Heyer, D.M., et al. (1990). HIV-related Kaposi's sarcoma. In P.T. Cohen, M.A. Sande, & P.A. Volberding (Eds.), *The AIDS knowledge base.* Waltham, MA: The Medical Publishing Group.

Holland, J.C., Jacobsen, P., & Brietbart, W. (1992). Psychiatric and psychosocial aspects of HIV infection. In V.T. DeVita, S. Hellman, & S.A. Rosenberg (Eds.), *AIDS: Etiology, diagnosis, treatment, and prevention* (3rd ed.). Philadelphia: J.B. Lippincott.

Hollander, H., & Katz, M.H. (1996). HIV Infection. In L.M. Tierney, S.J. McPhee, & M.A. Papadakis (Eds.), *Current medical diagnosis and treatment* (35th ed.). Stamford, CT: Appleton & Lange.

Kaplan, H.I., & Sadock, B.J. (1998). *Synopsis of psychiatry: Behavioral sciences/clinical psychiatry* (8th ed.). Baltimore: Williams & Wilkins.

Kovacs, J.A., & Masur, H. (1988). Opportunistic infections. In V.T. DeVita, S. Hellman, & S.A. Rosenberg (Eds.), *AIDS: Etiology, diagnosis, treatment, and prevention* (2nd ed.). Philadelphia: J.B. Lippincott.

Landesman, S.H., Ginzburg, H.M., & Weiss, S.H. (1985). The AIDS epidemic. *New England Journal of Medicine, 312,* 521–525.

Lemus, E. (1990). Definition and standards of hospice care. In P.T. Cohen, M.A. Sande, & P.A. Volberding (Eds.), *The AIDS knowledge base.* Waltham, MA: The Medical Publishing Group.

Lisanti, P., & Zwolski, K. (1997). Understanding the devastation of AIDS. *American Journal of Nursing, 97*(7), 26–35.

Martin, J. (1990). Psychosocial and spiritual concerns. In P.T. Cohen, M.A. Sande, & P.A. Volberding (Eds.), *The AIDS knowledge base.* Waltham, MA: The Medical Publishing Group.

National Hospice Organization (NHO). (1994). Standards of a hospice program of care. *The Hospice Journal, 9*(4), 39–74.

Navia, B.A., Jordon, B.D., & Price, R.W. (1985). The AIDS dementia complex: I. Clinical features. *Annals of Neurology, 19*(6), 517.

Navia, B.A., & Price, R.W. (1986). Central and peripheral nervous system complications of AIDS. *Clinics in Immunology and Allergy, 6*(3), 543–558.

Nokes, K.M. (1992). HIV infection in women. In J.H. Flaskerud & P.J. Ungvarski (Eds.), *HIV/AIDS; A guide to nursing care* (2nd ed.). Philadelphia: W.B. Saunders.

Osmond, D. (1990a). Definitions and codes for HIV infection and AIDS. In P.T. Cohen, M.A. Sande, & P.A. Volberding (Eds.), *The AIDS knowledge base.* Waltham, MA: The Medical Publishing Group.

Osmond, D. (1990b). AIDS in Africa. In P.T. Cohen, M.A. Sande, & P.A. Volberding (Eds.), *The AIDS knowledge base.* Waltham, MA: The Medical Publishing Group.

Perdew, S. (1990). *Facts about AIDS: A guide for health care providers.* Philadelphia: J.B. Lippincott.

Perry, S.W. (1990). Organic mental disorders caused by HIV: Update on early diagnosis and treatment. *American Journal of Psychiatry, 147,* 696.

Price, R.W., & Brew, B. (1988). The AIDS dementia complex. *Journal of Infectious Diseases, 158,* 1079–1083.

Roitt, I., Brostoff, J., & Male, D. (1989). *Immunology* (2nd ed.). St. Louis: C.V. Mosby.

Rosenberg, Z., & Fauci, A. (1989). The immunopathogenesis of HIV infection. *Advances in immunology, 47,* 377–431.

Scanlon, V.C., & Sanders, T. (1995). *Essentials of anatomy and physiology* (2nd ed.). Philadelphia: F.A. Davis.

Steis, R., & Broder, S. (1985). AIDS: A general overview. In V.T. DeVita, S. Hellman, & S.A. Rosenberg (Eds.), *AIDS: Etiology, diagnosis, treatment, and prevention.* Philadelphia: J.B. Lippincott.

Stine, G.J. (1993). *Acquired immune deficiency syndrome: Biological, medical, social, and legal issues.* Englewood Cliffs, NJ: Prentice Hall.

Sweet, D. (1992, April 4). *AIDS information: Understanding the disease.* Paper presented at the continuing Education Conference on Psychosocial Aspects of HIV/AIDS. University of Kansas School of Medicine, Wichita.

United Nations Joint Programme on HIV/AIDS (UNAIDS) and World Health Organization (WHO). (1998, June). *Report on the global HIV/AIDS epidemic.* [On-line]. Available: http://www.unaids.org/unaids/document/epidemio/June98/global_report/index.html.

Volberding, P.A. (1992). Clinical spectrum of HIV disease. In V.T. DeVita, S. Hellman, & S.A. Rosenberg (Eds.), *AIDS: Etiology, diagnosis, treatment, and prevention* (3rd ed.). Philadelphia: J.B. Lippincott.

Volberding, P.A. (1990a). Other cancers in HIV-infected patients. In P.T. Cohen, M.A. Sande, & P.A. Volberding (Eds.), *The AIDS knowledge base.* Waltham, MA: The Medical Publishing Group.

Volberding, P.A. (1990b). Clinical applications of antiviral therapy: Use of zidovudine. In P.T. Cohen, M.A. Sande, & P.A. Volberding (Eds.), *The AIDS knowledge base.* Waltham, MA: The Medical Publishing Group.

Wise, M.G., & Gray, K.F. (1994). Delirium, dementia, and amnestic disorders. In R.E. Hales, S.C. Yudofsky, & J.A. Talbott (Eds.), *The American Psychiatric Press textbook of psychiatry* (2nd ed.). Washington, DC: American Psychiatric Press.

Wolcott, D.L., Dilley, J.W., & Mitsuyasu, R.T. (1989). Psychiatric aspects of acquired immune deficiency syndrome. In H.I. Kaplan & B.J. Sadock (Eds.), *Comprehensive textbook of psychiatry* (Vol. 2) (5th ed.). Baltimore: Williams & Wilkins.

Yarchoan, R., & Broder, S. (1988). Pharmacologic treatment of HIV infection. In V.T. DeVita, S. Hellman, & S.A. Rosenberg (Eds.), *AIDS: Etiology, diagnosis, treatment, and prevention* (2nd ed.) Philadelphia: J.B. Lippincott.

PROBLEMS RELATED TO ABUSE OR NEGLECT

CHAPTER OUTLINE

OBJECTIVES

INTRODUCTION

HISTORICAL PERSPECTIVES

PREDISPOSING FACTORS

APPLICATION OF THE NURSING PROCESS

TREATMENT MODALITIES

SUMMARY

REVIEW QUESTIONS

KEY TERMS

battering
cycle of battering
emotional injury
physical neglect
emotional neglect
sexual exploitation of a child

child sexual abuse
incest
rape
date rape
marital rape
statutory rape

expressed response pattern
controlled response pattern
compounded rape reaction
silent rape reaction
safe house
shelter

OBJECTIVES

After reading this chapter, the student will be able to:

1. Discuss historical perspectives associated with spouse abuse, child abuse, and sexual assault.
2. Describe epidemiological statistics associated with spouse abuse, child abuse, and sexual assault.
3. Discuss characteristics of victims and victimizers.
4. Identify predisposing factors to abusive behaviors.
5. Describe physical and psychological effects

on the victim of spouse abuse, child abuse, and sexual assault.
6. Identify nursing diagnoses, goals of care, and appropriate nursing interventions for care of victims of spouse abuse, child abuse, and sexual assault.
7. Evaluate nursing care of victims of spouse abuse, child abuse, and sexual assault.
8. Discuss various modalities relevant to treatment of victims of abuse.

buse—the maltreatment of one person by another—is on the rise in this society. Books, newspapers, movies, and television inundate their readers and viewers with stories of "man's inhumanity to man" (no gender bias intended).

It has been estimated that there are 1.8 million battered wives in the United States, excluding divorced women and women battered on dates (Kaplan & Sadock, 1998). More injuries are attributed to **battering** than to all rapes, muggings, and automobile accidents combined (Silver & Yudofsky, 1992). Rape is vastly underreported in the United States; however, West (1983) reported that in 1980 the rate of reported rape and attempted rape in the United States was 18 times higher than the corresponding rate for England and Wales.

An increase in the incidence of child abuse and related fatalities has also been documented. In 1994, about 1 million cases of child abuse and neglect were substantiated by the National Committee for the Prevention of Child Abuse (Kaplan & Sadock, 1998). Child abuse and neglect accounts for 2000 to 4000 deaths each year in the United States.

Abuse affects all populations equally. It occurs among all races, religions, economic classes, ages, and educational backgrounds (Meierhoffer, 1992). The phenomenon is cyclical in that many abusers were themselves victims of abuse as children.

This chapter discusses battering of partners, child abuse (including neglect), and sexual assault. Elder abuse is discussed in Chapter 35. Factors that predispose individuals to commit acts of abuse against others, as well as the physical and psychological effects on the victims, are examined.

Nursing of individuals who have experienced abusive behavior from others is presented within the context of the nursing process. Various treatment modalities are described.

HISTORICAL PERSPECTIVES

Family violence is not a new problem; in fact, it is probably as old as humankind and has been documented as far back as Biblical times (Dickstein & Nadelson, 1989). In the United States, spouse and child abuse arrived with the Puritans; however, it was not until 1973 that public outrage initiated an active movement against the practice. Child abuse became a mandatory reportable occurrence in the United States in 1968, and in 1985, elder abuse was added to federal statutes as H.R. 1674 (Dickstein & Nadelson, 1989). These events have made it possible for individuals who once felt powerless to stop the abuse against themselves to come forward and seek advice, support, and protection.

Historically, violence against female partners (whether in a married or an unmarried intimate relationship) has not been considered a social problem but rather a fact of life. Some individuals have been socialized within their cultural context to the acceptance of violence against women in their relationships (American Nurses Association [ANA], 1998).

From Roman times until the beginning of the 20th century, women were considered the personal property of men. Very early on in Roman times, women were purchased as brides, and their status, as well as that of their children, was closely akin to that of slaves. Violent beatings and even death occurred if women acted contrary to their husbands' wishes or to the social code of the time (Martin, 1988).

Women have historically been socialized to view themselves as sexual objects. Even in early Biblical times, women were expected to subjugate themselves to the will of men, and those who refused were seen as witches (Hays, 1964). Rape is largely a crime against women, although men and children also fall victim to this heinous act. Rape is the extreme manifestation of the domination of one individual over another. Rape is a ritual of power (Moynihan, 1988).

During the Puritan era, "spare the rod and spoil the child" was a theme supported by the Bible. Children were considered the property of their parents and could be treated accordingly. Harsh treatment by parents was justified by the belief that severe physical punishment was necessary to maintain discipline, transmit educational decisions, and expel evil spirits (Hamilton, 1988). Change began in the mid-19th and early 20th centuries with the child welfare movement and the passage of laws for the protection of children.

Historical examination reveals an inclination toward violence among human beings from very early in civilization. Little has changed, for violence permeates every aspect of today's society, the victims of which are inundating the health care system. Campbell (1992) states:

> "[Violence] is costing all of us, in terms of health care dollars, human potential squandered, and even in terms of our personal sense of security and well being."

PREDISPOSING FACTORS

What predisposes individuals to be abusive? Although no one really knows for sure, several theories have been espoused. A brief discussion of ideas associated with biological, psychological, and sociocultural views is presented here.

Biological Theories

Neurophysiological Influences

Various components of the neurological system in both humans and animals have been implicated in both the facilitation and inhibition of aggressive impulses. Areas of the brain that may be involved include the temporal lobe, the limbic system, and the amygdaloid nucleus (Tardiff, 1994).

Biochemical Influences

Studies show that various neurotransmitters, in particular norepinephrine, dopamine, and serotonin, may play a role in the facilitation and inhibition of aggressive impulses (Silver & Yudofsky, 1992). This theory is consistent with the "fight or flight" arousal described by Selye (1956) in his theory of the response to stress (see Chapter 1).

Genetic Influences

Various genetic components related to aggressive behavior have been investigated. Some studies have linked increased aggressiveness with selective inbreeding in mice, suggesting the possibility of a direct genetic link. Another genetic characteristic that was once thought to have some implication for aggressive behavior was the genetic karyotype XYY. The XYY syndrome has been found to contribute to aggressive behavior in a small percentage of cases (Kaplan, Sadock, & Grebb, 1994). The evidence linking this chromosomal aberration to aggressive and deviant behavior has not yet been firmly established.

Disorders of the Brain

Organic brain syndromes associated with various cerebral disorders have been implicated in the predisposition to aggressive and violent behavior (Silver & Yudofsky, 1992). Brain tumors, particularly in the areas of the limbic system and the temporal lobes; trauma to the brain, resulting in cerebral changes; and diseases, such as encephalitis (or medications that may effect this syndrome) and epilepsy, particularly temporal lobe epilepsy, have all been implicated.

Psychological Theories

Psychodynamic Theory

The psychodynamic theorists imply that unmet needs for satisfaction and security result in an underdeveloped ego and a weak superego. It is thought that when frustration occurs, aggression and violence supply this individual with a dose of power and prestige that boosts the self-image and validates a significance to his or her life that is lacking. The immature ego cannot prevent dominant id behaviors from occurring, and the weak superego is unable to produce feelings of guilt.

Learning Theory

Children learn to behave by imitating their role models, which are usually their parents. Models are more likely to be imitated when they are perceived as prestigious or influential, or when the behavior is followed by positive reinforcement (Berndt, 1992). Children may have an idealistic perception of their parents during the very early developmental stages but, as they mature, may begin to imitate the behavior patterns of their teachers, friends, and others. Individuals who were abused as children or whose parents disciplined with physical punishment are more likely to behave in an abusive manner as adults (Tardiff, 1994).

Adults and children alike model many of their behaviors after individuals they observe on television and in movies. Unfortunately, modeling can result in maladaptive as well as adaptive behavior, particularly when children view heroes triumphing over villains by using violence. Some theorists believe that those individuals who have a biological influence toward aggressive behavior are more likely to be affected by external models than those without this predisposition (Kaplan & Sadock, 1998).

Sociocultural Theories

Societal Influences

Although they agree that perhaps some biological and psychological aspects are influential, social scientists believe that aggressive behavior is primarily a product of one's culture and social structure (West, 1983).

American society was essentially founded on a general acceptance of violence as a means of solving problems. Wrightsman (1977) states:

> "One explanation for the origin of revolutions and other collective violence uses the concept of relative deprivation. When a group suffers an abrupt shift away from past increases in socioeconomic and political satisfaction, its members are more likely to revolt or express collective violence." (p. 241)

Indeed, the United States was populated by the violent actions of one group of people over another. Since that time, much has been said and written, and laws have been passed, regarding the civil rights of all people. However, to this day many people would agree that the statement "All men are created equal" is hypocritical in our society.

Societal influences may also contribute to violence when individuals realize that their needs and desires are not being met relative to other persons (Tardiff, 1994). When poor and oppressed people find that they have limited access through legitimate channels, they are more likely to resort to delinquent behaviors in an effort to obtain desired ends. This lack of opportunity and subsequent delinquency may even contribute to a subculture of violence within a society.

APPLICATION OF THE NURSING PROCESS

Background Assessment Data

Spouse Abuse

Definition. Several definitions have been set forth for the term *battering*. Martin (1988) offers the following:

"The infliction of physical pain or injury with the intent to cause harm which may include slaps, punches, biting, and hair pulling, but in frequency or occurrence generally involves more serious assaults including choking, kicking, breaking bones, stabbing, or shooting; or forcible restraint which may include locking in homes or closets, being tied or handcuffed."

Campbell and Humphreys (1993) define *battering* as:

" . . . repeated physical and/or sexual assault of an intimate partner within a context of coercive control."

Finally, a definition by Sadock (1989) states:

"Spouse abuse is the mistreatment or misuse of one spouse by the other. It can range from shoving and pushing to choking and severe battering, involving broken limbs, broken ribs, internal bleeding, and brain damage. The face and breasts are the most frequent sites of assault, and when the woman is pregnant, her husband often batters her abdomen."

Physical abuse between domestic partners may be known as spouse abuse, domestic or family violence, wife or husband battering, or partner or relationship abuse. Approximately 95 percent of the victims of domestic violence are women (*Domestic Violence: The Facts*, 1996). A woman is beaten every 15 seconds, and domestic violence is the leading cause of injury to women between ages 15 and 44 in the United States (Edwards, 1996). Female to male violence is increasing, according to statistics from the Thirteenth World Congress of Sociology (1994). The fact that percentages remain low may relate to the following: (1) fewer men than women report incidences of severe assault, (2) our society looks upon men as "wimps" if they can't stand up to women, and (3) because most men are larger and stronger than their female partners, serious injury is less likely to occur.

Profile of the Victim. Battered women represent all age, racial, religious, cultural, educational, and socioeconomic groups (Dickstein & Nadelson, 1989). They may be married or single, housewives or business executives. According to Walker (1979), many women who are battered have low self-esteem, commonly adhere to feminine sex-role stereotypes, and typically accept the blame for the batterer's actions. Feelings of guilt, anger, fear, and shame are common. They may be isolated from family and support systems.

Many women who are in such relationships grew up in abusive homes and may have left those homes, even married, at a very young age in order to escape the abuse. The battered woman views her relationship as male dominant, and as the battering continues, her ability to see the options available to her and to make decisions concerning her life (and possibly those of her children) decreases. The phenomenon of *learned helplessness* may be applied to the woman's progressing inability to act on her own behalf. Learned helplessness occurs when an individual comes to understand that regardless of his or her behavior, the outcome is unpredictable, and usually undesirable.

Profile of the Victimizer. Men who batter are usually characterized as persons with low self-esteem. Pathologically jealous, they present a "dual personality," exhibit limited coping ability, and have severe stress reactions (Project for Victims of Family Violence, 1999). The typical abuser is very possessive and perceives his spouse as a possession. He becomes very threatened when she shows any sign of independence or attempts to share herself and her time with others. Small children are often ignored by the abuser; however, they too become the targets of abuse as they grow older, particularly if they attempt to protect their mother from abuse. The abuser may also use threats of taking the children away as another tactic of emotional abuse.

The abusing man typically wages a continuous campaign of degradation against his female partner. He insults and humiliates her and everything she does at every opportunity. He strives to keep her isolated from others and totally dependent on him. He demands to know where she is at every moment, and when she tells him he challenges her honesty. He achieves power and control through intimidation.

Cycle of Battering. Walker (1979), in her work with battered women and analysis of their battering relationships, has identified a cycle of predictable behaviors that are repeated over time. The behaviors can be divided into three distinct phases that vary in time and intensity both within the same relationship and among different couples. Figure 37.1 shows the three phases of the **cycle of battering.**

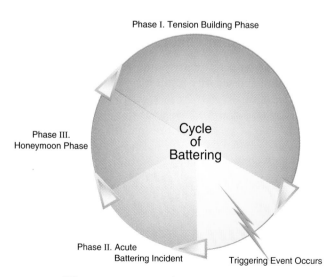

Figure 37.1   The cycle of battering.

Phase I. The Tension-Building Phase. During this phase, the woman senses that the man's tolerance for frustration is declining. He becomes angry with little provocation but, after lashing out at her, may be quick to apologize. The woman may become very nurturing and compliant, anticipating his every whim in an effort to prevent his anger from escalating. She may just try to stay out of his way.

Minor battering incidents may occur during this phase, and in a desperate effort to avoid more serious confrontations, the woman accepts the abuse as legitimately directed toward her. She denies her anger and rationalizes his behavior (e.g., "I need to do better;" "He's under so much stress at work;" "It's the alcohol. If only he didn't drink"). She assumes the guilt for the abuse, even reasoning that perhaps she *did* deserve the abuse, just as her aggressor suggests.

The minor battering incidents continue and the tension mounts, as the woman waits for the impending explosion. The abuser begins to fear that his partner will leave him. His jealousy and possessiveness increase, and he uses threats and brutality to keep her in his captivity. Battering incidents become more intense, after which the woman becomes less and less psychologically capable of restoring equilibrium. She withdraws from him, which he misinterprets as rejection, further escalating his anger toward her. Phase I may last from a few weeks to many months or even years.

Phase II. The Acute Battering Incident. This phase is the most violent and the shortest, usually lasting up to 24 hours. A triggering event occurs, and the violence most often begins with the batterer justifying his behavior to himself. By the end of the incident, however, he cannot understand what has happened, only that in his rage he has lost control over his behavior.

This incident may begin with the batterer wanting to "just teach her a lesson." In some instances, the woman may intentionally provoke the behavior. Having come to a point in phase I in which the tension is unbearable, long-term battered women know that once the acute phase is behind them, things will be better.

During phase II, women feel their only option is to find a safe place to hide from the batterer. The beating is severe, and many women can describe the violence in great detail, almost as if a dissociation from their bodies had occurred. The batterer generally minimizes the severity of the abuse. Help is usually sought only in the event of severe injury or if the woman fears for her life or those of her children.

Phase III. Calm, Loving, Respite ("Honeymoon") Phase. In this phase, the batterer becomes extremely loving, kind, and contrite. He promises that the abuse will never recur and begs her forgiveness. He is afraid she will leave him, and uses every bit of charm he can muster to ensure this does not happen. He believes he can now control his behavior, and besides, since he has now "taught her a lesson," he believes she will not "act up" again.

He plays on her feelings of guilt, and she desperately wants to believe him. She wants to believe that he *can* change, and that she will no longer have to suffer abuse. During this phase the woman relives her original dream of ideal love and chooses to believe that *this* is what her partner is *really* like.

This loving phase becomes the focus of the woman's perception of the relationship. She bases her reason for remaining in the relationship on this "magical" ideal phase and hopes against hope that the previous phases will not be repeated. This hope is evident even in those women who have lived through a number of horrendous cycles.

Although phase III usually lasts somewhere between the lengths of time associated with phases I and II, it can be so short as to almost pass undetected. In most instances, the cycle all too soon begins again with renewed tensions and minor battering incidents. In an effort to "steal" a few precious moments of the phase III kind of loving, the battered woman becomes a collaborator in her own abusive lifestyle. Victim and batterer become locked together in an intense, symbiotic relationship.

Why Does She Stay? Probably the most common response that battered women give for staying is that they fear for their life and/or the lives of their children. As the battering progresses, the man gains power and control through intimidation and instilling fear with threats such as, "I'll kill you and the kids if you don't do as I say" (Smith, 1987b). Challenged by these threats, and compounded by her low self-esteem and sense of powerlessness, the woman sees no way out. In fact, she may try to leave only to return when confronted by her partner and the psychological power he holds over her. Moss (1991) lists the following other reasons for the woman's staying in the marriage:

1. **Lack of a support network for leaving.** Our society glorifies the position of marriage and family, and some women report that family members encourage her to stay in the relationship and "try to work things out."
2. **Religious beliefs.** Many religious organizations denounce divorce and encourage the cohesion of the family. Some women have reported that their clergy told them this was "their cross to bear."
3. **Lack of financial independence to support herself and her children.**

Martin (1988) states:

"While some women have limited access to 'legitimate' resources, such as cash, a supportive network of family or friends, or strong assertive and communication skills, to assist them in leaving an abusive partner, almost all battered women seek help from traditional institutions or systems. The medical, mental health, and criminal justice/legal systems are the traditional formal sources of assistance sought by battered women. Yet each of these systems has reflected the pervasive cultural myths and stereotypes about battering and have generally been unresponsive to the needs of battered women."

Child Abuse

Erik Erikson (1963) stated, "The worst sin is the mutilation of a child's spirit." Children are vulnerable and relatively powerless, and the effects of maltreatment are infinitely deep and long-lasting. Child maltreatment typically includes physical or emotional injury, physical or emotional neglect, or sexual acts inflicted upon a child by a caregiver. The Child Abuse Prevention and Treatment Act (CAPTA), as amended and reauthorized in October 1996, identifies a minimum set of acts or behaviors that characterize maltreatment (National Clearinghouse on Child Abuse and Neglect [NCCAN], 1998). States may use these as foundations upon which to establish state legislation.

Physical Injury. Physical injury to a child includes any *nonaccidental physical* injury as a result of punching, beating, kicking, biting, burning, shaking, or otherwise harming a child (NCCAN, 1998). Maltreatment is considered whether the caretaker intended to cause harm or even if the injury resulted from overdiscipline or physical punishment. The most obvious way to detect it is by outward physical signs. However, behavioral indicators may also be evident.

Physical Signs. Indicators of physical abuse may include any of the following (ANA, 1998: Kansas Child Abuse Prevention Council [KCAPC], 1992, Tower, 1992).

1. Bruises, especially numerous bruises of different colors (indicating various stages of healing) over multiple parts of the body; bruises around the head and face.
2. Bite marks; skin welts.
3. Burns, such as:
   a. Glovelike burns that indicate the hand has been immersed in hot liquid.
   b. Cigarette burns.
   c. Burns in the shape of an object such as a poker or iron.
4. Fractures, scars, or serious internal injuries.
5. Lacerations, abrasions, or unusual bleeding.
6. Bald spots indicative of severe hair pulling.

Behavioral Signs. Following are common behavioral indicators of physical abuse (KCAPC, 1992; Tower, 1992). These behaviors alone do not necessarily indicate physical abuse.

1. Behavioral extremes, including very aggressive or demanding conduct.
2. Fear of the parent or caretaker.
3. Extreme rage, or passivity and withdrawal.
4. Apprehension when other children cry.

5. Verbal reporting of abuse.
6. Extreme hyperactivity, distractibility, or irritability.
7. Disorganized thinking; self-injurious or suicidal behavior.
8. Running away from home or engaging in illegal behavior such as drug abuse or stealing.
9. Displaying severe depression, flashbacks (including hallucinatory experiences), and dissociative disorders.
10. Cheating, lying, or low achievement in school.
11. Inability to form satisfactory peer relationships.
12. Wearing clothing that covers the body and that may be inappropriate for warm weather.
13. Regressiveness; demonstrating age-inappropriate behavior.

Emotional Injury. **Emotional injury** involves a pattern of behavior on the part of the parent or caretaker that results in serious impairment of the child's social, emotional, or intellectual functioning. Examples of emotional injury include belittling or rejecting the child, ignoring the child, blaming the child for things over which he or she has no control, isolating the child from normal social experiences, and using harsh and inconsistent discipline. Behavioral indicators of emotional injury may include (KCAPC, 1992; Tower, 1992):

1. Age-inappropriate behaviors.
2. Daytime anxiety and unrealistic fears.
3. Sleep problems; nightmares.
4. Behavioral extremes (e.g., overly happy or affectionate).
5. Social isolation.
6. Self-destructive behavior.
7. Inappropriate affect (e.g., laughing at something sad).
8. Vandalism, stealing, cheating, substance abuse.
9. Rocking, thumb sucking, enuresis, or other habitual problems.
10. Anorexia nervosa (especially in adolescents).

Physical Neglect. **Physical neglect** of a child includes refusal of or delay in seeking health care, abandonment, expulsion from the home or refusal to allow a runaway to return home, and inadequate supervision (NCCAN, 1998). The following physical and behavioral characteristics are associated with physical neglect of a child (ANA, 1998; Tower, 1992):

1. Clothing may be soiled and in need of repair; often fit is too small or too large; may be inappropriate for weather.
2. Child always seems hungry; steals and hoards food from others.
3. Child often appears listless and tired.
4. Child may demonstrate poor hygiene, with bad breath and body odor.
5. Medical problems, such as infected sores, and

dental problems, such as decayed or abscessed teeth, may be evident.

6. Delinquent behavior, such as stealing and vandalism, may be prevalent.
7. Poor school performance and attendance record may exist.
8. Poor peer relationships may be evident.
9. Child may be emaciated or have distended abdomen, indicative of malnutrition.

Emotional Neglect. **Emotional neglect** refers to a chronic failure by the parent or caretaker to provide the child with the hope, love, and support necessary for the development of a sound, healthy personality. The KCAPC (1992) identifies the following behavioral indicators of emotional neglect by the parent or caretaker of a child:

1. Ignoring the child's presence.
2. Rebuffing attempts by the child to establish meaningful interaction.
3. Ignoring the child's social, educational, recreational, and developmental needs.
4. Denying the child opportunities to receive positive reinforcement.

Sexual Abuse of a Child. Various definitions of child sexual abuse are available in the literature. CAPTA defines child sexual abuse as:

"Employment, use, persuasion, inducement, enticement, or coercion of any child to engage in, or assist any other person to engage in, any sexually explicit conduct or any simulation of such conduct for the purpose of producing any visual depiction of such conduct; or rape, and in cases of caretaker or interfamilial relationships, statutory rape, molestation, prostitution, or other form of sexual exploitation of children, or incest with children." (NCCAN, 1998.)

Included in the definition is **sexual exploitation of a child,** in which a child is induced or coerced into engaging in sexually explicit conduct for the purpose of promoting any performance, and **child sexual abuse,** in which a child is being used for the sexual pleasure of an adult (parent or caretaker) or any other person.

Incest is the occurrence of sexual contacts or interaction between, or sexual exploitation of, close relatives, or between participants who are related to each other by a kinship bond that is regarded as a prohibition to sexual relations (e.g., caretakers, stepparents, stepsiblings). (Kaplan & Sadock, 1998).

Indicators of Sexual Abuse. The following signs and symptoms may be indicators of child sexual abuse (Kaplan & Sadock, 1998; KCAPC, 1992; Tower, 1992):

PHYSICAL INDICATORS

1. Frequent urinary infections.
2. Any venereal disease or gonorrhea infection of the throat.
3. Difficulty or pain in walking or sitting.
4. Foreign matter in the bladder, rectum, urethra, or vagina.
5. Sleep problems (e.g., nightmares, insomnia).
6. Rashes or itching in the genital area; scratching the area a great deal or fidgeting when seated.
7. Bruising or pain in the genital area.
8. Genital or rectal bleeding; vaginal discharge.

BEHAVIORAL INDICATORS

1. Seductive behavior, advanced sexual knowledge for the child's age, promiscuity, prostitution.
2. Expressing fear of a particular person or place.
3. Compulsive masturbation, precocious sex play, excessive curiosity about sex.
4. Sexually abusing another child.
5. Appearance of an inordinate number of gifts or money from a questionable source.
6. Drop in school performance or sudden nonparticipation in school activities.
7. Sudden onset of enuresis.
8. Excessive anxiety.
9. Expression of low self-worth; verbalizations of being "damaged."
10. Excessive bathing.
11. Running away from home.
12. Suicide attempts.

Characteristics of the Abuser. A number of factors have been associated with adults who abuse or neglect their children. Kaplan and Sadock (1998) report that 90 percent of parents who abuse their children were severely physically abused by their own mothers or fathers. Murray and Zentner (1997) identify the following as additional characteristics that may be associated with abusive parents:

- Experiencing a stressful life situation (e.g., unemployment, poverty)
- Having few, if any, support systems; being commonly isolated from others
- Lacking understanding of child development or care needs
- Lacking in adaptive coping strategies; angers easily; has difficulty trusting others
- Expecting child to be perfect; may exaggerate any mild difference child manifests from the "usual"

The Incestual Relationship. A great deal of attention has been given to the study of father-daughter incest. In these cases there is usually an impaired sexual relationship between the parents. Communication between the parents is ineffective, which prevents them from correcting their problems. Typically, the father is domineering, impulsive, and physically abusing; whereas the mother is passive and submissive, and denigrates her role as wife and mother. She is often aware of, or at least strongly suspects, the incestual behavior between the father and daughter but may believe in or fear her husband's absolute authority over the family. She may deny that her daughter is being harmed and may actually be grateful that her husband's sexual demands are being met by someone other than herself.

Onset of the incestual relationship typically occurs when the daughter is 8 to 10 years of age and commonly begins with genital touching and fondling. In the beginning, the child may accept the sexual advances from her father as signs of affection. As the incestuous behavior continues and progresses, the daughter usually becomes more bewildered, confused, and frightened, never knowing whether her father will be paternal or sexual in his interactions with her (Kaplan & Sadock, 1998).

The relationship may become a love-hate situation on the part of the daughter. She continues to strive for the ideal father-daughter relationship but is fearful and hateful of the sexual demands he places on her. The mother may be alternately caring and competitive, as she witnesses her husband's possessiveness and affections directed toward her daughter. Out of fear that his daughter may expose their relationship, the father may attempt to interfere with her normal peer relationships (Kaplan & Sadock, 1998).

Mrazek (1981) suggests that some fathers who participate in incestuous relationships may have unconscious homosexual tendencies and have difficulty achieving a stable heterosexual orientation. On the other hand, some men have frequent sex with their wives and several of their own children but are unwilling to seek sexual partners outside the nuclear family because of a need to maintain the public facade of a stable and competent patriarch. Although the oldest daughter in a family is most vulnerable to becoming a participant in father-daughter incest, some fathers form sequential relationships with several daughters, each lasting for an extended period, often over many years (Sadock, 1989; Murray & Zentner, 1997).

The Adult Survivor of Incest. Several common characteristics have been identified in adults who have experienced incest as children. Basic to these characteristics is a fundamental lack of trust resulting from an unsatisfactory parent-child relationship, which causes low self-esteem and a poor sense of identity. Children of incest often feel trapped, for they have been admonished not to talk about the experience and may be afraid, or even fear for their lives, if they are exposed. If they do muster the courage to report the incest, particularly to the mother, they are frequently not believed. This is confusing to the child, who is then left with a sense of self-doubt and the inability to trust his or her own feelings. The child develops feelings of guilt with the realization over the years that the parents are using him or her in an attempt to solve their own problems.

Childhood sexual abuse is likely to distort the development of a normal association of pleasure with sexual activity (Bass & Davis, 1994). Peer relationships are often

delayed, altered, inhibited, or perverted. In some instances, individuals who were sexually abused as children completely retreat from sexual activity and avoid all close interpersonal relationships throughout life. Other adult manifestations of childhood sexual abuse in women include diminished libido, vaginismus, nymphomania, and promiscuity. In male survivors of childhood sexual abuse, impotence, premature ejaculation, exhibitionism, and compulsive sexual conquests may occur. Kreidler and Carlson (1991) report the results of various studies that suggest that adult survivors of incest are at risk for flashbacks, nightmares, drug and alcohol abuse, anxiety attacks, denial, avoidance, emotional numbing, prostitution, depression, suicide, feelings of powerlessness, guilt, victimization, eating and sleeping disorders, sexual dysfunction, and problems with trust and nonsexual intimacy and with being abusers themselves.

The conflicts experienced by sexually abused children associated with pain (either physical or emotional) and sexual pleasure are commonly manifested symbolically in adult relationships. Women who were abused as children commonly enter into relationships with men who abuse them physically, sexually, and/or emotionally (Bird et al., 1992).

Adult survivors of incest who decide to come forward with their stories are usually estranged from nuclear family members. They are blamed by family members for disclosing the "family secret" and often accused of overreacting to the incest. Frequently the estrangement becomes permanent when family members continue to deny the behavior, and the individual is accused of lying. In recent years, a number of celebrities have come forward with stories of their childhood sexual abuse. Some have chosen to make the disclosure only after the death of their parents. Revelation of these past activities can be one way of contributing to the healing process for which incest survivors so desperately strive.

Sexual Assault

Definition. Over the years, a number of definitions have emerged regarding the crime of **rape,** but one theme is common: rape is an act of aggression, not one of passion. Rape has been defined as the expression of power and dominance by means of sexual violence, most commonly by men over women, although men may also be rape victims. Sexual assault is viewed as any type of sexual act that an individual is threatened, coerced, or forced to submit to against his or her will. Rape, a type of sexual assault, occurs over a broad spectrum of experiences ranging from the surprise attack by a stranger to insistence on sexual intercourse by an acquaintance or spouse (Moynihan, 1988).

Date rape is a term applied to situations in which the rapist is known to the victim (Kaplan & Sadock, 1998).

They may be out on a first date, may have been dating for a number of months, or merely be acquaintances or schoolmates. College campuses are the location for a staggering number of these types of rapes, a great many of which go unreported. An increasing number of colleges and universities are establishing programs for rape prevention and counseling for victims of rape.

Marital rape, which has been recognized only in recent years as a legal category, is the case in which a spouse may be held liable for sexual abuse directed at a marital partner against that person's will. Historically, with societal acceptance of the concept of women as marital property, the legal definition of rape held an exemption within the marriage relationship. Mahoney (1998) states:

> "Today, under at least one section of the sexual offense codes (usually those regarding force), marital rape is a crime in all 50 states. However, since March 1996, 17 states and the District of Columbia have abolished the marital rape exemption completely."

Statutory rape is defined as unlawful intercourse between a man older than 16 years of age and a woman under the age of consent (Kaplan & Sadock, 1998). The age of consent varies from state to state, ranging from age 14 to 21. A man who has intercourse with a woman under the age of consent can be arrested for statutory rape, even though the interaction is likely to have occurred between consenting individuals. The charges, when they occur, are usually brought by the young woman's parents.

Profile of the Victimizer. One of the older profiles of the individual who rapes was described by Abrahamsen (1960), who identified the rapist's mother as "seductive but rejecting." Macdonald (1971) also supported the mother-dominated childhood as influential. The behavior of the mother toward the son is described as overbearing, with seductive undertones. Mother and son share little secrets, and she rescues him when his delinquent acts create problems with others. She is quick to withdraw her love and attention when he goes against her wishes, a rejection that can be powerful and unyielding. She is domineering and possessive of the son, a dominance that often continues into his adult life. Macdonald (1971) stated:

> "The seductive mother arouses overwhelming anxiety in her son with great anger which may be expressed directly toward her but more often is displaced onto other women. When this seductive behavior is combined with parental encouragement of assaultive behavior, the setting is provided for personality development in the child which may result in sadistic, homicidal sexual attacks on women in adolescence or adult life."

Many rapists report growing up in abusive homes (Scully, 1990). Even when the parental brutality is discharged by the father, the anger may be directed toward the mother who did not protect her child from physical assault (Macdonald, 1971). More recent feminist theories suggest that the rapist displaces this anger on the rape victim because he cannot directly express it toward other men (Kaplan & Sadock, 1998).

Statistics show that the greatest number of rapists are between the ages of 25 and 44. Fifty-one percent are white, 47 percent are black, and the remaining 2 percent come from all other races (Kaplan & Sadock, 1998). Many are either married or cohabiting at the time of their offenses (Scully, 1990). For those with previous criminal activity, the majority of their convictions are for crimes against property rather than against people. The majority of rapists do not have histories of mental illness.

The Victim. Rape can occur at virtually any age. Although victims have been reported as young as 15 months old and as old as 82 years, the high-risk age group appears to be 16 to 24 years (Kaplan & Sadock, 1998; Macdonald, 1971; Sadock, 1989). Seventy percent to 75 percent of rape victims are single women, and the attack frequently occurs in or close to the victim's own neighborhood.

Scully (1990), in a study of a prison sample of rapists, found that in "stranger rapes," victims were not chosen for any reason having to do with appearance or behavior, but simply because the individual happened to be in a certain place at a certain time. Scully states:

> "The most striking and consistent factor in all the stranger rapes, whether committed by a lone assailant or a group, is the unfortunate fact that the victim was 'just there' in a location unlikely to draw the attention of a passerby. Almost every one of these men said exactly the same thing, 'It could have been any woman,' and a few added that because it was dark, they could not even see what their victim looked like very well."

In her study, Scully found that 62 percent of the rapists used a weapon, most frequently a knife. The majority suggested that they used the weapon to terrorize and subdue the victim but not to inflict serious injury. The presence of a weapon (real or perceived) appears to be the principal measure of the degree to which a woman resists her attacker.

Rape victims who present themselves for care shortly after the crime has occurred may likely be experiencing an overwhelming sense of violation and helplessness that began with the powerlessness and intimidation experienced during the rape. Burgess (1984) identifies two emotional patterns of response that may occur within hours after a rape and with which health care workers may be confronted in the emergency department or rape crisis center. In the **expressed response pattern,** the victim expresses feelings of fear, anger, and anxiety through such behaviors as crying, sobbing, smiling, restlessness, and tension. In the **controlled response pattern,** the feelings are masked or hidden, and a calm, composed, or subdued affect is seen.

The following manifestations may be evident in the days and weeks after the attack (Burgess, 1984):

1. Contusions and abrasions about various parts of the body.

2. Headaches, fatigue, sleep pattern disturbances.
3. Stomach pains, nausea and vomiting.
4. Vaginal discharge and itching, burning upon urination, rectal bleeding and pain.
5. Rage, humiliation, embarrassment, desire for revenge, self-blame.
6. Fear of physical violence and death.

The long-term effects of sexual assault depend largely on the individual's ego strength, social support system, and the way he or she was treated as a victim (Burgess, 1984). Various long-term effects include increased restlessness, dreams and nightmares, and phobias (particularly those having to do with sexual interaction). Some women report that it takes years to get over the experience (Kaplan & Sadock, 1998); they describe a sense of vulnerability and a loss of control over their own lives during this period. They feel defiled and unable to wash themselves clean, and some women are unable to remain living alone in their home or apartment.

Some victims develop a **compounded rape reaction,** in which additional symptoms such as depression and suicide, substance abuse, and even psychotic behaviors may be noted (Burgess, 1984). Still another variation has been called the **silent rape reaction,** in which the victim tells no one about the assault. Anxiety is suppressed and the emotional burden may become overwhelming. The unresolved sexual trauma may not be revealed until the woman is forced to face another sexual crisis in her life that reactivates the previously unresolved feelings.

Diagnosis/Outcome Identification

Nursing diagnoses are formulated from the data gathered during the assessment phase and with background knowledge regarding predisposing factors to the situation. Some common nursing diagnoses for victims of abuse include:

Rape-trauma syndrome related to sexual assault, evidenced by verbalizations of the attack; bruises and lacerations over areas of body; severe anxiety.
Powerlessness related to cycle of battering, evidenced by verbalizations of abuse; bruises and lacerations over areas of body; fear for her safety and that of her children; verbalizations of no way to get out of relationship.
Altered growth and development related to abusive family situation, evidenced by sudden onset of enuresis, thumb sucking, nightmares, inability to perform self-care activities appropriate for age.

The following criteria may be used to measure outcomes in the care of abuse victims:

The Client Who Has Been Sexually Assaulted:

1. Is no longer experiencing panic anxiety.
2. Demonstrates a degree of trust in the primary nurse.

3. Has received immediate attention to physical injuries.
4. Has initiated behaviors consistent with the grief response.

The Client Who Has Been Physically Battered:

1. Has received immediate attention to physical injuries.
2. Verbalizes assurance of his or her immediate safety.
3. Discusses life situation with primary nurse.
4. Can verbalize choices from which he or she may receive assistance.

The Child Who Has Been Abused:

1. Has received immediate attention to physical injuries.
2. Demonstrates trust in primary nurse by discussing abuse through the use of play therapy.
3. Is demonstrating a decrease in regressive behaviors.

Planning/Implementation

Table 37.1 provides a plan of care for the client who has been a victim of abuse. Nursing diagnoses are presented, along with outcome criteria, appropriate nursing interventions, and rationales.

Evaluation

Evaluation of nursing actions to assist victims of abuse must be considered on both a short- and a long-term basis.

Short-term evaluation may be facilitated by gathering information using the following types of questions:

1. Has the individual been reassured of his or her safety?
2. Is this evidenced by a decrease in panic anxiety?
3. Have wounds been properly cared for and provision made for follow-up care?
4. Have emotional needs been attended to?
5. Has trust been established with at least one person to whom the client feels comfortable relating the abusive incident?
6. Have available support systems been identified and notified?
7. Have options for immediate circumstances been presented?

Long-term evaluation may be conducted by health care workers who have contact with the individual long after management of the immediate crisis.

1. Is the individual able to conduct activities of daily living satisfactorily?
2. Have physical wounds healed properly?
3. Is the client appropriately progressing through the behaviors of grieving?

TABLE 37.1 CARE PLAN FOR VICTIMS OF ABUSE

NURSING DIAGNOSIS: RAPE-TRAUMA SYNDROME

RELATED TO: Sexual assault

EVIDENCED BY: Verbalizations of the attack; bruises and lacerations over areas of bod

OUTCOME CRITERIA	NURSING INTERVENTIONS	
Client will begin a healthy grief resolution; initiating the process of healing (both physically and psychologically).	1. Smith (1987a) relates the importance of communicating the following four phases to the rape victim: • I am very sorry this happened to you. • You are safe here. • I am very glad you are alive. • You are not to blame. You are a victim. It was not your fault. Whatever decisions you made at the time of the assault were the right ones because you are alive.	1. The woman w… assaulted fears for h… be reassured of her safety. … also be overwhelmed with … doubt and self-blame, and these statements instill trust and validate self-worth.
	2. Explain every assessment procedure that will be conducted and why it is being conducted. Ensure that data collection is conducted in a caring, nonjudgmental manner.	2. This may serve to decrease fear/anxiety and increase trust.
	3. Ensure that the client has adequate privacy for all immediate postcrisis interventions. Try to have as few people as possible providing the immediate care or collecting immediate evidence.	3. The posttrauma client is extremely vulnerable. Additional people in the environment increase this feeling of vulnerability and serve to escalate anxiety.
	4. Encourage the client to give an account of the assault. Listen, but do not probe.	4. Nonjudgmental listening provides an avenue for catharsis that the client needs to begin healing. A detailed account may be required for legal follow-up, and a caring nurse, as client advocate, may help to lessen the trauma of evidence collection.
	5. Discuss with the client whom to call for support or assistance. Provide information about referrals for aftercare.	5. Because of severe anxiety and fear, the client may need assistance from others during this immediate post-crisis period. Provide referral information in writing for later reference (e.g., psychotherapist, mental health clinic, community advocacy group).

NURSING DIAGNOSIS: POWERLESSNESS

RELATED TO: Cycle of battering

EVIDENCED BY: Verbalizations of abuse; bruises and lacerations over areas of body; fear for own safety and that of children; verbalizations of no way to get out of relationship

OUTCOME CRITERIA	NURSING INTERVENTIONS	RATIONALE
Client will recognize and verbalize choices available, thereby perceiving some control over life situation.	1. In collaboration with physician, ensure that all physical wounds, fractures, and burns receive immediate attention. Take photographs if the victim will permit (Smith, 1987b; Burgess, 1990).	1. Client safety is a nursing priority. Photographs may be called in as evidence if charges are filed.
	2. Take the woman to a private area to do the interview.	2. If the client is accompanied by the man who did the battering, she is not likely to be truthful about her injuries.

Continued on following page

3. If she has come alone or with her children, assure her of her safety. Encourage her to discuss the battering incident. Ask questions about whether this has happened before, whether the abuser takes drugs, whether the woman has a safe place to go, and whether she is interested in pressing charges.

4. Ensure that "rescue" efforts are not attempted by the nurse. Offer support, but remember that the final decision must be made by the client.

5. Stress the importance of safety. Smith (1987b) suggests a statement such as, "Yes, it has happened. Now where do you want to go from here?" Burgess (1990) states, "The victim needs to be made aware of the variety of resources that are available to her. These may include crisis hot lines, community groups for women who have been abused, shelters, a variety of counseling opportunities (i.e., couples, individual, or group), and information regarding the victim's rights in the civil and criminal justice system." Following a discussion of these available resources, the woman may choose for herself. If her decision is to return to the marriage and home, this choice, too, must be respected.

3. Some women will attempt to keep secret how their injuries occurred in an effort to protect the partner or because they are fearful that the partner will kill them if they tell.

4. Making her own decision will give the client a sense of control over her life situation. Imposing judgments and giving advice are nontherapeutic.

5. Knowledge of available choices decreases the victim's sense of powerlessness, but true empowerment comes only when she chooses to use that knowledge for her own benefit.

NURSING DIAGNOSIS: ALTERED GROWTH AND DEVELOPMENT

RELATED TO: Abusive family situation

EVIDENCED BY: Sudden onset of enuresis, thumb sucking, nightmares, inability to perform self-care activities appropriate for age

OUTCOME CRITERIA	NURSING INTERVENTIONS	RATIONALE
Client will develop trusting relationship with nurse and report how evident injuries were sustained. Negative regressive behaviors (enuresis, thumb sucking, nightmares) will diminish.	1. Perform complete physical assessment of the child. Take particular note of bruises (in various stages of healing), lacerations, and client complaints of pain in specific areas. Do not overlook or discount the possibility of sexual abuse. Assess for nonverbal signs of abuse: aggressive conduct, excessive fears, extreme hyperactivity, apathy, withdrawal, age-inappropriate behaviors.	1. An accurate and thorough physical assessment is required to provide appropriate care for the client.
	2. Conduct an in-depth interview with the parent or adult who accompanies the child. Consider: If the injury is being reported as an accident, is the explanation reasonable? Is the injury consistent with the explanation? Is the injury consistent with the child's developmental capabilities?	2. Fear of imprisonment or loss of child custody may place the abusive parent on the defensive. Discrepancies may be evident in the description of the incident, and lying to cover up involvement is a common defense that may be detectable in an in-depth interview.

3. Use games or play therapy to gain child's trust. Use these techniques to assist in describing his or her side of the story.

4. Determine whether nature of the injuries warrants reporting to authorities. Specific state statutes must enter into the decision whether to report suspected child abuse.

3. Establishing a trusting relationship with an abused child is extremely difficult. They may not even want to be touched. These types of play activities can provide a nonthreatening environment that may enhance the child's attempt to discuss these painful issues (Celano, 1990).

4. A report is commonly made if there is reason to suspect that a child has been injured as a result of physical, mental, emotional, or sexual abuse. "Reason to suspect" exists when there is evidence of a discrepancy or inconsistency in explaining a child's injury. Most states require that the following individuals report cases of suspected child abuse: all health care workers, all metal health therapists, teachers, child-care providers, firefighters, emergency medical personnel, and law enforcement personnel. Reports are made to the Department of Health and Human Services or a law enforcement agency.

4. Is the client free of sleep disturbances (nightmares, insomnia); psychosomatic symptoms (headaches, stomach pains, nausea/vomiting); regressive behaviors (enuresis, thumb sucking, phobias); and psychosexual disturbances?

5. Is the individual free from problems with interpersonal relationships?

6. Has the individual considered the alternatives for change in his or her personal life?

7. Has a decision been made relative to the choices available?

8. Is he or she satisfied with the decision that has been made?

TREATMENT MODALITIES

Crisis Intervention

The focus of the initial interview and follow-up with the client who has been sexually assaulted is on the rape incident alone. Problems identified but unassociated with the rape are not dealt with at this time. The goal of crisis intervention is to aid victims to return to their previous lifestyle as quickly as possible (Burgess, 1990).

The client should be involved in the intervention from the beginning. This promotes a sense of competency, control, and decision making. Because an overwhelming sense of powerlessness accompanies the rape experience,

active involvement by the victim is both an affirmation of competency and the beginning of recovery (Moynihan, 1988). Crisis intervention is time limited—usually 6 to 8 weeks. If problems resurface beyond this time, the victim is referred for assistance from other agencies (e.g., long-term psychotherapy from a psychiatrist or mental health clinic).

During the crisis period, attention is given to coping strategies for dealing with the symptoms common to the posttrauma client. Initially the individual undergoes a period of disorganization during which there is difficulty making decisions, extreme or irrational fears, and general mistrust. Observable manifestations may range from stark hysteria to expression of anger and rage to silence and withdrawal. Guilt and feelings of responsibility for the rape, as well as numerous physical manifestations, are common. The crisis counselor will attempt to help the victim draw upon previous successful coping strategies in order to regain control over his or her life.

If the client is a victim of battering, the counselor ensures that various resources and options are made known to the victim so that she may make a personal decision regarding what she wishes to do with her life. Support groups provide a valuable forum for reducing isolation and learning new strategies for coping with the aftermath of physical or sexual abuse (Moynihan, 1988). Particularly for the rape victim, the peer support group provides a therapeutic forum for reducing the sense of isolation she may feel in the aftermath of predictable social and interpersonal responses to her experience.

Moynihan (1988) states:

> "Rape affects almost every aspect of the victim's life, emotional, physical and social, and influences her future level of functioning as well. The manner in which a victim is treated at the moment of disclosure has a profound effect on recovery. Thus, the victim whose request for help is responded to by skepticism and doubt may respond by withdrawing, and closing communications. Feelings of guilt and self-blame may be exaggerated, and significant long-term effects will almost predictably occur."

The Safe House or Shelter

Most major cities in the United States now have **safe houses** or **shelters** where women can go to be assured of protection for themselves and their children. These shelters provide a variety of services, and the women receive emotional support from staff and each other. Most shelters provide individual and group counseling; help with bureaucratic institutions such as the police, legal representation, and social services; child care and children's programming; and aid for the woman in making future plans, such as employment counseling and linkages with housing authorities (Campbell, 1984a).

The shelters are usually run by a combination of professional and volunteer staff, including nurses, psychologists, lawyers, and others. Women who have been previously abused themselves are often among the volunteer staff members.

Group work is an important part of the service of shelters. Women in residence range from those in the immediate crisis phase to those who have progressed through a variety of phases of the grief process. Those newer members can learn a great deal from the women who have successfully resolved similar problems. Length of stay varies a great deal from individual to individual, depending on a number of factors, such as outside support network, financial situation, and personal resources.

The shelter not only provides a haven of physical safety for the battered woman, but also promotes expression of the intense emotions she may be experiencing regarding her situation. A woman will commonly exhibit depression, extreme fear, or even violent expressions of anger and rage. In the shelter, she learns that these feelings are normal and that others have also experienced these same emotions in similar situations. She is allowed to grieve for what has been lost and for what was expected but not achieved. Help is provided in overcoming the tremendous guilt associated with self-blame. This is a difficult step for someone who has accepted responsibility for another's behavior over a long period.

New arrivals at the shelter are given time to experience the relief from the safety and security provided. Making decisions is discouraged during the period of immediate crisis and disorganization. Once the woman's emotions have become more stable, planning for the future begins. Through information from staff and peers, she learns what resources are available to her within the community. Feedback is provided, but the woman makes her own decision about "where she wants to go from here." She is accepted and supported in whatever she chooses to do.

Family Therapy

Campbell (1984b) states, "Any family that uses physical punishment or any form of physical aggression can be considered at risk to become violent, because violence tends to escalate under stress." The focus of therapy with families who use violence is to help them develop democratic ways of solving problems. Studies show that the more a family uses the democratic means of conflict resolution, the less likely they are to engage in physical violence. Families need to learn to deal with problems in ways that can produce mutual benefits for all concerned, rather than engaging in power struggles among family members.

Parents also need to learn more effective methods of disciplining children, aside from physical punishment. Methods that emphasize the importance of positive rein-

Question from Hell

TEST YOUR CRITICAL THINKING SKILLS

Sandy is a psychiatric RN who works at a safe house for battered women. Lisa has just been admitted with her two small children, after being treated in the emergency department. She was severely beaten by her husband while he was intoxicated last night. She escaped with her children after he had passed out in their bedroom.

In her initial assessment, Sandy learns from Lisa that she has been battered by her husband for 5 years, beginning shortly after their marriage. She explained that she "knew he drank quite a lot before they were married, but thought he would stop after we had kids." Instead, the drinking has increased. Sometimes he doesn't even get home from work until 11 PM or midnight, after stopping to drink at the bar with his buddies.

Lately, he has begun to express jealousy and a lack of trust in Lisa, accusing her of numerous infidelities and indiscretions, none of which is true. Lisa says, "If only he wasn't under so much stress on his job, then maybe he wouldn't drink so much. Maybe if I tried harder to make everything perfect for him at home . . . I don't know. What do you think I should do to keep him from acting this way?"

Answer the following questions related to Lisa:

1. What is an appropriate response to Lisa's question?
2. Identify the priority psychosocial nursing diagnosis for Lisa.
3. What must the nurse ensure that Lisa learns from this experience?

R E S E A R C H   N O T E

Potential for abusive parenting by rural mothers with low-birth-weight children. *Image: Journal of Nursing Scholarship* (1999), 31(1), 21–25
Sachs, B., Hall, L.A., Lutenbacher, M., and Rayens, M.K.

Description of the Study: The purpose of this study was to describe factors influencing the potential for abusive parenting by rural mothers of low-birth-weight (LBW) children. The convenience sample in this study included 48 mothers of LBW children, ranging in age from 18 to 39 years, all living in a rural area of the state, and all living with their LBW infant at the time of the study. The average length of the children's hospitalization after birth was 6 weeks, and the average age at time of the study was 9 months. In-home interviews were conducted using structured questionnaires to assess the mothers' everyday stressors, depressive symptoms, functional social support, quality of family relationships, and child abuse potential.

Results of the Study: According to the questionnaires used for measurement, 54 percent of the mothers indicated a high level of depressive symptoms and 63 percent indicated a high potential for physical child abuse. No significant differences were noted in depressive symptoms and potential for child abuse by birth weight, health status of the child, or time since hospital discharge. Mothers with high child abuse potential reported more everyday stressors and depressive symptoms, less functional social support, and poorer family functioning. Because in this study everyday stressors and the two social support systems (functional social support and quality of family relationships) were examined as predictors of depressive symptoms, it is suggested that everyday stressors exert both a direct and an indirect effect on mothers' potential for child abuse. The strongest predictor of child abuse potential was mothers' depressive symptoms.

Comments: The researchers conclude that rural mothers of LBW children are at risk for abusive parenting. This study demonstrated the adverse effects of everyday stressors, minimal social resources, and depressive symptoms on mothers' potential for abusive parenting. Attention should be given to the mental health of mothers living in isolated, rural areas, including in particular those community resources offering social support, child care, and help for these mothers to improve parenting skills and promote more positive child health outcomes.

forcement for acceptable behavior can be very effective. Family members must be committed to consistent use of this behavior modification technique for it to be successful.

Teaching parents about expectations for various developmental levels may alleviate some of the stress that accompanies these changes. Knowing what to expect from individuals at various stages of development may provide needed anticipatory guidance to deal with the crises commonly associated with these stages.

Therapy sessions with all family members together may focus on problems with family communications. Members are encouraged to express honest feelings in a manner that is nonthreatening to other family members.

Active listening, assertiveness techniques, and respecting the rights of others are taught and encouraged. Barriers to effective communication are identified and resolved.

Referrals to agencies that promote effective parenting skills (e.g., Parent Effectiveness Training) may be made. Alternative agencies that may relieve the stress of parenting (e.g., "Mom's Day Out" programs, sitter-sharing organizations, and day-care institutions) may also be considered. Support groups for abusive parents may also be helpful, and assistance in locating or initiating such a group may be provided.

SUMMARY

This chapter provided a discussion of abuse—the maltreatment of one person by another. Spouse abuse, child abuse, and sexual assault are all on the rise in this country, and all populations are equally affected.

Abuse of women and children began early in the development of this country, when these individuals were considered the property of their husbands and fathers; this physical abuse was considered acceptable. Women came to believe that they deserved any physical or sexual abuse they encountered.

Various factors have been theorized as influential in the predisposition to violent behavior. Physiological and biochemical influences within the brain have been suggested, as has the possibility of a direct genetic link. Organic brain syndromes associated with various cerebral disorders have been implicated in the predisposition to aggressive and violent behavior.

INTERNET REFERENCES

- Additional information related to child abuse may be located at the following websites:
  a. http://www.endabuse.com/index.htm
  b. http://www.childabuse.org/
  c. http://www.cmhcsys.com/factsfam/sexabuse.htm
- Additional information related to sexual assault may be located at the following websites:
  a. http://www.cs.utk.edu/~bartley/saInfoPage.html
  b. http://www.ncweb.com/org/rapecrisis
- Additional information related to domestic violence may be located at the following websites:
  a. http://www.ndvh.org/
  b. http://www.cpsdv.org/
  c. http://home.cybergrrl.com/dv/book/toc.html
  d. http://software2.bu.edu/cohis/violence/helpvctm.htm
  e. http://www.domestic-violence.org/

Psychodynamic theorists relate the predisposition to violent behavior to an underdeveloped ego and a poor self-concept. Learning theorists suggest that children imitate the abusive behavior of their parents. This theory has been substantiated by studies that show that individuals who were abused as children or whose parents disciplined them with physical punishment are more likely to be abusive as adults. Societal influences, such as general acceptance of violence as a means of solving problems, have also been implicated.

Battered women usually take blame for their situation. They were often reared in abusive families and have come to expect this type of behavior. Battered women often see no way out of their present situation and may be encouraged by their social support network (family, friends, clergy) to remain in the abusive relationship.

Child abuse includes physical and emotional injury, physical and emotional neglect, and sexual abuse of a child. A child may experience many years of abuse without reporting it, out of fear of retaliation by the abuser. Some children report incest experiences to their mothers, only to be rebuffed by her and told to remain secretive about the abuse. Adult survivors of incest often experience a number of physical and emotional manifestations relating back to the incestual relationship.

Sexual assault is identified as an act of aggression, not passion. Many rapists report growing up in abusive homes, and some theorists relate the predisposition to rape to a "seductive, but rejecting, mother." Rape is a crisis situation; many women experience flashbacks, nightmares, rage, physical symptoms, depression, and thoughts of suicide for many years after the occurrence.

Nursing implementation with victims of abuse was discussed in the context of the nursing process. Assessment data, nursing diagnoses, outcome criteria, appropriate nursing interventions with rationale, and standards for evaluation were presented. Additional treatment modalities were described, including crisis intervention with the sexual assault victim, safe shelter for battered women, and therapy for families who use violence.

Problems related to abuse and neglect are becoming a national crisis in this country. Nurses are in a unique position to intervene at the primary, secondary, and tertiary levels of prevention with the victims of these problematic behaviors.

REVIEW QUESTIONS

SELF-EXAMINATION/LEARNING EXERCISE

Select the answer that is most appropriate for the questions that follow each situation.

Situation: Sharon is a 32-year-old woman who arrives at the emergency department with her three small children. She has multiple bruises around her face and neck. Her right eye is swollen shut.

1. Sharon says to the nurse, "I didn't want to come. I'm really okay. He only does this when he has too much to drink. I just shouldn't have yelled at him. " The best response by the nurse would be:

   a. "How often does he drink too much?"
   b. "It is not your fault. You did the right thing by coming here."
   c. "How many times has he done this to you?"
   d. "He is not a good husband. You have to leave him before he kills you."

2. In the interview, Sharon tells the nurse, "He's been getting more and more violent lately. He's been under a lot of stress at work the last few weeks, and so he drinks a lot when he gets home. He always gets mean when he drinks. I was getting scared. So I just finally told him I was going to take the kids and leave. He got furious when I said that and began beating me with his fists." With knowledge about the cycle of battering, what does this situation represent?

   a. Phase I. Sharon was desperately trying to stay out of his way and keep everything calm.
   b. Phase I. A minor battering incident for which Sharon assumes all the blame.
   c. Phase II. The acute battering incident that Sharon provoked with her threat to leave.
   d. Phase III. The honeymoon phase where the husband believes that he has "taught her a lesson and she won't act up again."

3. The *priority* nursing intervention for Sharon in the emergency department is:

   a. tending to the immediate care of her wounds.
   b. providing her with information about a safe place to stay.
   c. administering the p.r.n. tranquilizer ordered by the physician.
   d. explaining how she may go about bringing charges against her husband.

4. Sharon goes with her children to stay at a women's shelter. She participates in group therapy and receives emotional support from staff and peers. She is made aware of the alternatives open to her. Nevertheless, she decides to return to her home and marriage. The best response by the nurse upon Sharon's departure is:

   a. "I just can't believe you have decided to go back to that horrible man."
   b. "I'm just afraid he will kill you or the children when you go back."
   c. "What makes you think things have changed with him?"
   d. "I hope you have made the right decision. Call this number if you need help."

Situation: Carol is a school nurse. Five-year-old Jana has been sent to her office complaining of nausea. She lies down on the office cot, but eventually vomits and soils her blouse. When Carol removes Jana's blouse to clean it, she notices that Jana has a number of bruises on her arms and torso. Some are bluish in color; others are various shades of green and yellow. She also notices some small scars. Jana's abdomen protrudes on her small, thin frame.

5. From the objective physical assessment, the nurse suspects that:

   a. Jana is experiencing physical and sexual abuse.
   b. Jana is experiencing physical abuse and neglect.
   c. Jana is experiencing emotional neglect.
   d. Jana is experiencing sexual and emotional abuse.

6. Carol tries to talk to Jana about her bruises and scars, but Jana refuses to say how she received them. Another way in which Carol can get information from Jana is to:

   a. Have her evaluated by the school psychologist.
   b. Tell her she may select a "treat" from the treat box (e.g., sucker, balloon, junk jewelry) if she answers the nurse's questions.
   c. Explain to her that if she answers the questions, she may stay in the nurse's office and not have to go back to class.
   d. Use a "family" of dolls to role play Jana's family with her.

7. Carol strongly suspects that Jana is being abused. What would be the best way for Carol to proceed with this information?

   a. As a health care worker, report the suspicion to the Department of Health and Human Services.
   b. Check Jana again in a week and see if there are any new bruises.
   c. Meet with Jana's parents and ask them how Jana got the bruises.
   d. Initiate paperwork to have Jana placed in foster care.

Situation: Lana is an 18-year-old freshman at the state university. She was extremely flattered when Don, a senior star football player, invited her to a party. On the way home, he parked the car in a secluded area by the lake. He became angry when she refused his sexual advances. He began to beat her and finally raped her. She tried to fight him, but his physical strength overpowered her. He dumped her in the dorm parking lot and left. The dorm supervisor rushed Lana to the emergency department.

8. Lana says to the nurse, "It's all my fault. I shouldn't have allowed him to stop at the lake." The nurse's best response is:

   a. "Yes, you're right. You put yourself in a very vulnerable position when you allowed him to stop at the lake."
   b. "You are not to blame for his behavior. You obviously made some right decisions, because you survived the attack."
   c. "There's no sense looking back now. Just look forward, and make sure you don't put yourself in the same situation again."
   d. "You'll just have to see that he is arrested so he won't do this to anyone else."

9. The priority nursing intervention with Lana would be:

   a. Help her to bathe and clean herself up.
   b. Provide physical and emotional support during evidence collection.
   c. Provide her with a written list of community resources for rape victims.
   d. Discuss the importance of a follow-up visit to evaluate for sexually transmitted diseases.

10. Lana is referred to a support group for rape victims. She has been attending regularly for 6 months. From this group, she has learned that the most likely reason Don raped her was:

    a. He had had too much to drink at the party and was not in control of his actions.
    b. He had not had sexual relations with a girl in many months.
    c. He was predisposed to become a rapist by virtue of the poverty conditions under which he was reared.
    d. He was expressing power and dominance by means of sexual aggression and violence.

REFERENCES

Abrahamsen D. (1960). *The psychology of crime.* New York: John Wiley & Sons.

American Nurses Association (ANA). (1998). *Culturally competent assessment for family violence.* Washington, DC: American Nurses Publishing.

Bass, E,. & Davis, L. (1994). *The courage to heal: A guide for women survivors of child sexual abuse* (3rd ed.). New York: HarperCollins Publishers.

Berndt, T.J. (1992). *Child development.* Ft. Worth, TX: Harcourt Brace Jovanovich, Publishers.

Bird, H.R., et al. (1992). Stresses and traumas of childhood. In F.I. Kass,

J.M. Oldham, & H. Pardes (Eds.), *The Columbia University College of Physicians and Surgeons complete home guide to mental health.* New York: Henry Holt and Company.

Burgess, A. (1984). Intra-familial sexual abuse. In J. Campbell & J. Humphreys (Eds.), *Nursing care of victims of family violence.* Reston, VA: Reston Publishing.

Burgess, A. (1990). Victims of family violence: Incest and battering. In A.W. Burgess (Ed.), *Psychiatric nursing in the hospital and the community* (5th ed.). Norwalk, CT: Appleton & Lange.

Campbell, J. (1984a). Nursing care of abused women. In J. Campbell & J. Humphreys (Eds.), *Nursing care of victims of family violence.* Reston, VA: Reston Publishing.

Campbell, J. (1984b). Nursing care of families using violence. In J. Campbell & J. Humphreys (Eds.), *Nursing care of victims of family violence.* Reston, VA: Reston Publishing.

Campbell, J. (1992). Violence demands nursing solutions. *The American Nurse, 24*(4), 4.

Campbell, J., & Humphreys, J. (1993). *Nursing care of survivors of family violence.* St. Louis: Mosby.

Celano, M.P. (1990). Activities and games for group psychotherapy with sexually abused children. *International Journal of Group Psychotherapy, 40*(4), 419–428.

Dickstein, L.J., & Nadelson, C.C. (Eds.). (1989). *Family violence: Emerging issues of a national crisis.* Washington, DC: American Psychiatric Press.

Domestic violence: The facts. (1996). Boston: Peace At Home (formerly Battered Women Fighting Back).

Edwards, R.E. (1996). *The courage of a woman* [On-line]. Available: http://www.biz.arkansas.net/lordandedw/book.htm

Erikson, E.H. (1963). *Childhood and society* (2nd ed.). New York: W.W. Norton & Co.

Hamilton, J. (1988). Child abuse and family violence. In N. Hutchings (Ed.), *The violent family: Victimization of women, children, and elders.* New York: Human Sciences Press.

Hays, H.R. (1964). *The dangerous sex: The myth of feminine evil.* New York: Putnam.

Kansas Child Abuse Prevention Council (KCAPC). (1992). *A guide about child abuse and neglect.* Wichita, KS: National Committee for Prevention of Child Abuse and Parents Anonymous.

Kaplan, H.I., & Sadock, B.J. (1998). *Synopsis of psychiatry: Behavioral sciences/clinical psychiatry* (8th ed.). Baltimore: Williams & Wilkins.

Kaplan, H.I., Sadock, B.J., & Grebb, J.A. (1994). *Kaplan and Sadock's synopsis of psychiatry* (7th ed.). Baltimore: Williams & Wilkins.

Kreidler, M.C., & Carlson, R.E. (1991). Breaking the incest cycle: The group as a surrogate family. *Journal of Psychosocial Nursing, 29*(4), 28–32.

Macdonald, J.M. (1971). *Rape: Offenders and their victims.* Springfield, IL: Charles C. Thomas.

Mahoney, P. (1998). The wife rape information page. [Online]. Available: http://www.wellesley.edu/WCW/projects/mrape.html.

Martin, M. (1988). Battered women. In N. Hutchings (Ed.), *The violent family: Victimization of women, children, and elders.* New York: Human Sciences Press.

Meierhoffer, L.L. (1992, April). Nurses battle family violence. *The American Nurse, 24*(4), 1, 7–8.

Moss, V.A. (1991). Battered women and the myth of masochism. *Journal of Psychosocial Nursing, 29*(7), 18–23.

Moynihan, B. (1988). The rape victim. In N. Hutchings (Ed.), *The violent family: Victimization of women, children, and elders.* New York: Human Sciences Press.

Mrazek, P.B. (1981). The nature of incest: A review of contributing factors. In P.B. Mrazek & C.H. Kempe (Eds.), *Sexually abused children and their families.* Oxford: Pergamon Press.

Murray, R.B., & Zentner, J.P. (1997). *Health assessment and promotion strategies through the life span* (6th ed.). Stamford, CT: Appleton & Lange.

National Clearinghouse on Child Abuse and Neglect (NCCAN). (1998). *What is child maltreatment?* [On-line]. Available: http://www.calib.com/nccanch/pubs/.

Person, E.S. (1992). Women's issues at a time of social change. In F.I. Kass, J.M. Oldham, & H. Pardes (Eds.), *The Columbia University College of Physicians and Surgeons complete home guide to mental health.* New York: Henry Holt and Company.

Project for Victims of Family Violence. (1999). *How to help someone you know who is being abused.* [On-line]. Available: http://www.biz.arkansas.net/lordandedw/warning.htm.

Sadock, V.A. (1989). Rape, spouse abuse, and incest. In H.I. Kaplan & B.J. Sadock (Eds.), *Comprehensive textbook of psychiatry,* Vol. I (5th ed.). Baltimore: Williams & Wilkins.

Scully, D. (1990). *Understanding sexual violence: A study of convicted rapists.* Boston: Unwin Hyman.

Selye, H. (1956). *The stress of life.* New York: McGraw-Hill.

Silver, J.M., & Yudofsky, S. (1992). In F.I. Kass, J.M. Oldham, & H. Pardes (Eds.), *The Columbia University College of Physicians and Surgeons complete home guide to mental health.* New York: Henry Holt and Company.

Smith, L.S. (1987a). Sexual assault: The nurse's role. *AD Nurse, 2*(2), 24–28.

Smith, L.S. (1987b). Battered women: The nurse's role. *AD Nurse, 2*(5), 21–24.

Tardiff, K. (1994). Violence. In R.E. Hales, S.C. Yudofsky, & J.A. Talbott (Eds.), *Textbook of psychiatry* (2nd ed.) Washington, DC: The American Psychiatric Press.

Thirteenth World Congress of Sociology (1994, July 19). *Men and domestic violence.* [On-line]. Available: http://www.vix.com/pub/men/battery/trends.html.

Tower, C.C. (1992). *The role of educators in the prevention and treatment of child abuse and neglect.* [On-line]. Available: http://www.calib.com/nccanch/pubs/educator/section3.htm

Walker, L.E. (1979). *The battered woman.* New York: Harper & Row.

West, D.J. (1983). Sex offenses and offending. In M. Tonry & N. Morris (Eds.), *Crime and justice: An annual review of research.* Chicago: University of Chicago Press.

Wrightsman, L.B. (1977). *Social psychology* (2nd ed.). Monterey, CA: Brooks/Cole.

Bibliography

Brookoff, D., et al. (1997, August 20). Characteristics of participants in domestic violence. Assessment at the scene of domestic assault. *Journal of the American Medical Association, 278*(7) 547–548.

DiVitto, S. (1998). Empowerment through self-regulation; Group approach for survivors of incest. *Journal of the American Psychiatric Nurses Association, 4*(3), 77–89.

Gallop, R., et al. (1998). A survey of psychiatric nurses regarding working with clients who have a history of sexual abuse. *Journal of the American Psychiatric Nurses Association,4*(1), 9–17.

Garber, A., Grindel, C.G., & Mitchell, D. (1997). Assessing for sexual abuse. *Journal of Psychosocial Nursing, 35*(3), 26–30.

Holmes, M.M., Resnick, H.S., & Frampton, D. (1998, August). Follow-up of sexual assault victims. *American Journal of Obstetrics and Gynecology, 179,* 336–342.

McCauley, J., et al. (1997, May 7). Clinical characteristics of women with a history of childhood abuse: Unhealed wounds. *Journal of the American Medical Association, 277*(17), 1400–1401.

Putz, M., Thomas, B.K., & Cowles, K.V. (1996, December). Sexual assault victims' compliance with follow-up care at one sexual assault treatment center. *Journal of Emergency Nursing, 22,* 560–565.

Rynerson, B.C., & Fishel, A. H. (1998). Expressions of men who batter: Implications for nursing. *Journal of the American Psychiatric Nurses Association, 4*(2), 41–47.

COMMUNITY MENTAL HEALTH NURSING

CHAPTER OUTLINE

KEY TERMS

deinstitutionalization
prospective payment
diagnostically related
    groups (DRGs)
primary prevention

secondary prevention
tertiary prevention
case management
managed care
case manager

community
shelters
store-front clinics
mobile outreach units

OBJECTIVES

After reading this chapter, the student will be able to:

1. Discuss the changing focus of care in the field of mental health.
2. Define the concepts of care associated with the model of public health:
   a. Primary prevention.
   b. Secondary prevention.
   c. Tertiary prevention.
3. Differentiate between the roles of basic level and advanced practice psychiatric/mental health registered nurses.
4. Define the concepts of case management and identify the role of case management in community mental health nursing.
5. Discuss primary prevention of mental illness within the community.
6. Identify populations at risk for mental illness within the community.
7. Discuss nursing intervention in primary prevention of mental illness within the community.
8. Discuss secondary prevention of mental illness within the community.
9. Describe treatment alternatives related to secondary prevention within the community.
10. Discuss tertiary prevention of mental illness within the community as it relates to the chronically and homeless mentally ill.
11. Relate historical and epidemiological factors associated with caring for the chronically and homeless mentally ill within the community.

12. Identify treatment alternatives for care of the chronically and homeless mentally ill within the community.
13. Apply steps of the nursing process to care of the

chronically and homeless mentally ill within the community.
14. Describe principal aspects of the role of the mental health nurse in rural settings.

his chapter explores the concepts of primary and secondary prevention of mental illness within communities. Additional focus is placed on tertiary prevention of mental illness: treatment with community resources of the chronically mentally ill and the homeless mentally ill. Emphasis is given to the role of the psychiatric nurse in the various treatment alternatives within the community setting.

THE CHANGING FOCUS OF CARE

Before 1840, there was no known treatment for individuals who were mentally ill. Because mental illness was perceived as incurable, the only "reasonable" intervention was thought to be removing these ill persons from the community to a place where they would do no harm to themselves or others.

In 1841, Dorothea Dix, a former school teacher, began a personal crusade across the land on behalf of institutionalized mentally ill clients. The efforts of this self-appointed "inspector" resulted in more humane treatment of the mentally ill, as well as the establishment of a number of hospitals for the mentally ill.

After the movement initiated by Dix, the number of hospitals for the mentally ill increased, although unfortunately not as rapidly as did the mentally ill population. The demand soon outgrew the supply, and hospitals became overcrowded and understaffed, with conditions that would have sorely distressed Dorothea Dix.

The community mental health movement had its impetus in the 1940s. With establishment of the National Mental Health Act of 1946, the U.S. government awarded grants to the states to develop mental health programs outside of state hospitals. Outpatient clinics and psychiatric units in general hospitals were inaugurated. Then, in 1949, as an outgrowth of the National Mental Health Act, the National Institute of Mental Health (NIMH) was established. The U.S. government has charged this agency with the responsibility for mental health in the United States.

In 1955, the Joint Commission on Mental Health and Illness was established by Congress "for the purpose of surveying the nation's mental health needs and to recommend new approaches to improve mental health care" (Chamberlain, 1983). In 1961, the Joint Commission published the report, *Action for Mental Health*, in which recommendations were made for treatment of the men-

tally ill, training for caregivers, and improvements in education and research of mental illness. With consideration given to these recommendations, Congress passed the Mental Retardation Facilities and Community Mental Health Centers Construction Act (often called the Community Mental Health Centers Act) of 1963. This act called for the construction of comprehensive community health centers, the cost of which would be shared by federal and state governments. The **deinstitutionalization** movement (the closing of state mental hospitals and discharging of mentally ill individuals) had begun.

Unfortunately, many state governments did not have the capability to match the federal funds required for the establishment of these mental health centers. Some communities found it difficult to follow the rigid requirements for services required by the legislation that provided the grant.

In 1980 the Community Mental Health Systems Act, which was to have played a major role in renovation of mental health care, was established. Funding was authorized for community mental health centers, services to high-risk populations, ambulatory mental health care centers, a prevention unit and associate director for minority concerns at NIMH, and rape research and services (Wilson & Kneisl, 1992). However, before this plan could be enacted, the newly inaugurated administration set forth its intention to diminish federal involvement. Budget cuts reduced the number of mandated services, and federal funding for community mental health centers was terminated in 1984.

Meanwhile, costs of care for hospitalized psychiatric clients continued to rise. The problem of the "revolving door" began to intensify. The chronically mentally ill had no place to go than back to the hospital when their illness exacerbated. Individuals without support systems remained in the hospital for extended periods because of lack of appropriate community services. Hospital services were paid for by cost-based, retrospective reimbursement: Medicaid, Medicare, and private health insurance. Retrospective reimbursement encouraged hospital expenditure; the more services provided, the more payment received.

This system of delivery of health care was interrupted in 1983 with the advent of **prospective payment,** the Reagan administration's proposal of cost containment. It was directed at control of Medicare costs by setting forth pre-established amounts that would be reimbursed for specific diagnoses, or **diagnostically related groups (DRGs).** Since that time, prospective payment has also been integrated by the states (Medicaid) and by some private insurance companies, drastically affecting the amount of reimbursement for health care services.

Mental health services have been influenced by prospective payment. General hospital services to psychiatric clients have been severely restricted. Clients who present with acute symptoms, such as acute psychosis, suicidal ideations or attempts, or manic exacerbations, constitute the largest segment of the psychiatric hospital census. Clients with less serious illnesses (e.g., moderate depression, adjustment disorders) may be hospitalized, but length of stay has been shortened considerably by the reimbursement guidelines. Clients are being discharged from the hospital with a greater need for aftercare than in the past, when hospital stays were longer.

Deinstitutionalization continues to be the changing focus of mental health care in the United States. Care for the client in the hospital has become cost prohibitive whereas care for the client in the community is cost effective. Shirley Smoyak (1991) has stated,

> ". . . how and what health care is provided is more of a political and funding issue than one driven by scientific knowledge. That is not to say that science is not important, or that it is not needed, but to emphasize the reality that it is not the number-one factor in how decisions get made to either seek or provide services." (p. 7)

Provision of outpatient mental health services not only is the wave of the future but also has become a necessity today. We must serve the consumer by providing the essential services to assist with health promotion or prevention, to initiate early intervention, and to ensure rehabilitation or prevention of long-term disability.

THE PUBLIC HEALTH MODEL

The premise of the model of public health is based largely on the concepts set forth by Gerald Caplan (1964) during the initial community mental health movement, which include **primary prevention, secondary prevention,** and **tertiary prevention.** These concepts no longer have relevance only to mental health nursing but have been widely adapted as guiding principles in many clinical and community settings over a range of nursing specialties.

Primary prevention is defined as reducing the incidence of mental disorders within the population. It targets both individuals and the environment. Emphasis is twofold:

1. Assisting individuals to increase their ability to cope effectively with stress.
2. Targeting and diminishing harmful forces (stressors) within the environment.

Nursing in primary prevention is focused on the targeting of groups at risk and the provision of educational programs. Examples include:

1. Teaching parenting skills and child development to prospective new parents.
2. Teaching physical and psychosocial effects of alcohol/drugs to elementary school students.
3. Teaching techniques of stress management to virtually anyone who desires to learn.
4. Teaching groups of individuals ways to cope with the changes associated with various maturational stages.
5. Teaching concepts of mental health to various groups within the community.
6. Providing education and support to unemployed or homeless individuals.
7. Providing education and support to other individuals in various transitional periods (e.g., widows and widowers, new retirees, and women entering the work force in middle life).

These are only a few examples of the types of services nurses provide in primary prevention. These services can be offered in a variety of settings that are convenient for the public: churches, schools, colleges, community centers, YM/YWCAs, workplace of employee organizations, meetings of women's groups, or civic or social organizations such as PTAs, health fairs, and community shelters, to name only a few.

Secondary prevention is reducing the prevalence of psychiatric illness by shortening the course (duration) of the illness (Kaplan & Sadock, 1998). This is accomplished through early identification of problems and prompt initiation of effective treatment.

Nursing in secondary prevention focuses on recognition of symptoms and provision of, or referral for, treatment. Examples include:

1. Ongoing assessment of individuals at high risk for illness exacerbation (e.g., during home visits, day care, community health centers, or in any setting where screening of high-risk individuals might occur).
2. Provision of care for individuals in whom illness symptoms have been assessed (e.g., individual or group counseling, medication administration, education and support during period of increased stress [crisis intervention], staffing rape crisis centers, suicide hotlines, homeless shelters, shelters for abused women, or mobile mental health units).
3. Referral for treatment of individuals in whom illness symptoms have been assessed. Referrals may come from support groups, community mental health centers, emergency services, psychiatrists or psychologists, and day or partial hospitalization. Inpatient therapy on a psychiatric unit of a general hospital or in a private psychiatric hospital may be necessary. Chemotherapy and various adjunct therapies may be initiated as part of the treatment.

Secondary prevention has been addressed extensively in Unit Three of this text. Nursing assessment, diagnosis/

outcome identification, plan/implementation, and evaluation were discussed for the majority of mental illnesses identified in the *DSM-IV* (APA, 1994). These concepts may be applied in any setting where nursing is practiced.

Tertiary prevention is reducing the residual defects that are associated with severe or chronic mental illness. This is accomplished in two ways:

1. Preventing complications of the illness.
2. Promoting rehabilitation that is directed toward achievement of each individual's maximum level of functioning.

Kaplan, Sadock, and Grebb (1994) suggest that the term *chronic mental illness*, which has historically been associated with long hospitalizations that resulted in loss of social skills and increased dependency, now may also refer to clients from the deinstitutionalized generation. These individuals may never have experienced hospitalization, but they still do not possess adequate skills to live productive lives within the community.

Nursing in tertiary prevention focuses on helping clients learn or relearn socially appropriate behaviors so that they may achieve a satisfying role within the community. Examples include:

1. Consideration of the rehabilitation process at the time of initial diagnosis and treatment planning.
2. Teaching the client daily living skills and encouraging independence to his or her maximum ability.
3. Referring clients for various aftercare services (e.g., support groups, day treatment programs, partial hospitalization programs, psychosocial rehabilitation programs, group home or other transitional housing).
4. Monitoring effectiveness of aftercare services (e.g., through home health visits or follow-up appointments in community mental health centers).
5. Making referrals for support services when required (e.g., some communities have programs linking individuals with chronic mental disorders to volunteers who serve to develop friendships with the individuals and who may assist with household chores, shopping, and other activities of daily living with which the individual is having difficulty, in addition to participating in social activities with the individual).

Nursing care at the tertiary level of prevention can be administered on an individual or group basis and in a variety of settings, such as inpatient hospitalization, day or partial hospitalization, group home or halfway house, shelters, home health care, nursing homes, and community mental health centers.

THE ROLE OF THE NURSE

One emphasis of the National Mental Health Act of 1946 was to increase the supply of mental health professionals. This Act named four major mental health disciplines: psy-

chiatry, clinical psychology, social work, and nursing. To increase the numbers of trained mental health professionals, grants were provided to institutions, and stipends and fellowships were awarded to individuals.

Nurses who work in the field of psychiatry may practice at one of two levels: the psychiatric/mental health registered nurse or the psychiatric/mental health advanced practice registered nurse. These two levels have been differentiated through the efforts of the Coalition of Psychiatric Nursing Organizations, under the leadership of the Executive Committee of the American Nurses Association's (ANA) Council on Psychiatric and Mental Health Nursing.

The Psychiatric/Mental Health Registered Nurse

Definition:	A registered nurse (RN) who is educationally prepared in nursing and licensed to practice in his or her individual state (ANA, 1994).
Education:	Baccalaureate degree in nursing (BSN) and demonstrated clinical skills, within the specialty, exceeding those of a beginning RN or novice in the specialty (ANA, 1994).
Additional credentialing:	In addition to professional licensure by the state, psychiatric/mental health RNs may apply to sit for ANA examinations that certify them as basic level psychiatric/mental health nurses (ANA, 1994).
Employment settings:	Inpatient psychiatric hospital unit, day treatment and partial hospitalization programs, community health centers, home health care, long-term care centers.
Professional responsibilities:	Health promotion and health maintenance, intake screening and evaluation, case management, provision of a therapeutic environment (e.g., milieu therapy), tracking clients and assisting them with self-care activities, administering and monitoring psychobiological treatment regimens (including prescribed psychopharmacological agents and their effects), health teaching, crisis intervention and counseling, and outreach activities such as home visits and community action (ANA, 1994).

The Psychiatric/Mental Health Advanced Practice Registered Nurse

Definition: A licensed RN who is educationally prepared at the graduate level and nationally certified as a clinical specialist in psychiatric/mental health nursing (ANA, 1994).

Education: Minimum of a master's degree in psychiatric and mental health nursing. This preparation is distinguished by a depth of knowledge of theory and practice, supervised clinical practice, and competence in advanced clinical nursing skills (ANA, 1994).

Additional credentialing: Master's- or doctorate-prepared nurses may sit for ANA examinations that certify them as psychiatric/mental health clinical specialists. In addition, some states have special licensure that may be granted to nurses with advanced education that permits them to practice at a more independent level (Advanced Practice Registered Nurse [APRN]) and that makes them eligible for prescriptive authority, admission privileges, and third-party reimbursement (ANA, 1994).

Employment settings: Inpatient psychiatric hospital units; day treatment and partial hospitalization programs; community mental health centers; private mental health facilities; individual private practice; crisis intervention services; or in the capacity of mental health consultant, supervisor, educator, administrator, or researcher.

Professional responsibilities: In addition to those required at the basic RN level, the RN in advanced psychiatric/mental health nursing practice must demonstrate expertise in psychotherapy modalities associated with various client systems (individual, couple, group, family, and community). Additional knowledge of psychobiological interventions involved in the diagnosis and treatment of mental disorders is required. These include the prescription of psychoactive medications and the ordering of appropriate diagnostic and laboratory tests, according to state nursing regulations. Advanced practice RNs provide clinical supervision to assist others in further developing their clinical practice skills. They may also practice consultation-liaison nursing to provide consultation and direct care services in nonpsychiatric settings (ANA, 1994).

CASE MANAGEMENT

Because of the rising costs of hospitalization and in keeping with the concept of deinstitutionalization, there has become a need for managing the care of clients (particularly the chronically ill) in an outpatient setting. **Case management** for a selected group of clients at the secondary level of prevention (acute care center) was presented in Unit Three of this text. Case management in the acute care setting strives to organize client care through an episode of illness so that specific clinical and financial outcomes are achieved within an allotted time frame (Zander, 1988). Commonly, this time frame is determined by the established protocols for length of stay as defined by the DRGs.

Ideally, case management incorporates concepts of care at the primary, secondary, and tertiary levels of prevention. Various definitions have emerged and should be clarified:

Managed care is a concept purposefully designed to control the balance between cost and quality of care (Zander, 1988). In a managed-care program, individuals receive health care based on need, as assessed by coordinators of the providership. Managed care exists in many settings, including (but not limited to):

● Insurance-based programs.
● Employer-based medical providerships.
● Social service programs.
● The public health sector.

Managed care may exist in virtually any setting in which medical providership is a part of the service; that is, in any setting in which an organization (whether it be private or government-based) is responsible for payment of health care services for a group of people. Examples of managed care are health maintenance organizations (HMOs) and preferred provider organizations (PPOs).

Case management is the method used to achieve managed care. It is the actual coordination of services required to meet the needs of the client. Goals of case management are to "facilitate access to needed services and coordinate care for clients within the fragmented health care delivery system, prevent avoidable episodes of illness among at-risk clients, and control or reduce the cost of care borne by the client or third-party payers" (Bower, 1992). Types of clients who benefit from case management include (but are not limited to):

- The frail elderly.
- The developmentally disabled.
- The physically handicapped.
- The mentally handicapped.
- Individuals with long-term medically complex problems that require multifaceted, costly care (e.g., high-risk infants, persons with human immunodeficiency virus or AIDS, transplant patients).
- Individuals who are severely compromised by an acute episode of illness or an acute exacerbation of a chronic illness (e.g., schizophrenia).

The **case manager** is responsible for negotiating with multiple health care providers to obtain a variety of services for the client. Bower (1992) states: "Nurses are particularly suited to provide case management for clients with multiple health problems that have a health-related component." The very nature of nursing that incorporates knowledge about the biological, psychological, and sociocultural aspects related to human functioning makes nurses highly appropriate as case managers. The ANA recommends that the minimum preparation for a nurse case manager is a baccalaureate in nursing with 3 years of appropriate clinical experience (Bower, 1992). Some case management programs prefer master's-prepared clinical nurse specialists who have experience working with the specific populations for whom the case management service will be rendered.

Case management is becoming a recommended method of treatment for individuals with a chronic mental illness. This type of care enhances functioning by increasing the individual's ability to solve problems, improving work and socialization skills, promoting leisure time activities, and endeavoring to diminish dependency on others.

THE COMMUNITY AS CLIENT

Primary Prevention

Lancaster (1980) defines community as:

" . . . a group of people living in close proximity and having some dependency on each other. Community encompasses the place where people live, work, raise children, and in general carry on the activities necessary for daily living. A given community is composed of individuals who are engaged in some degree of social interaction within a defined geographic area and who have one or more common ties. The community is the social environment in which hazards are experienced and supports are provided."

Primary prevention within communities encompasses the twofold emphasis defined earlier in this chapter. These include:

1. Identifying stressful life events that precipitate crises and targeting the relevant populations at high risk.
2. Intervening with these high-risk populations to prevent or minimize harmful consequences.

Populations at Risk

One way to view populations at risk is to focus on types of crises that individuals experience in their lives. Two broad categories are maturational crises and situational crises.

Maturational Crises. Maturational crises are crucial experiences that are associated with various stages of growth and development. Erikson (1963) described eight stages of the life cycle during which individuals struggle with developmental "tasks." Crises can occur during any of the developmental stages, although several periods or events have been commonly identified as having increased crisis potential: adolescence, marriage, parenthood, midlife, and retirement (Pasquali, Arnold, & DeBasio, 1989).

Adolescence. The task for adolescence according to Erikson (1963) is *identity versus role confusion*. This is the time in life when individuals ask questions such as "Who am I?" "Where am I going?" and "What is life all about?"

Adolescence is a transition into young adulthood. It is a very volatile time in most families. Commonly, there is conflict over issues of control. Parents sometimes have difficulty relinquishing even a minimal amount of the control they have had throughout their adolescent's infancy, toddlerhood, and school-age years, while the adolescent seeks to be independent. It may seem that the adolescent is 25 years old one day and 5 years old the next. An often-quoted definition of an adolescent, by an anonymous author, is: "A toddler with hormones and wheels."

At this time, adolescents are "trying out their wings," although they possess an essential need to know that the parents (or surrogate parents) are available if support is required. Mahler, Pine, and Bergman (1975) have termed this vital concept "emotional refueling," and although they were referring to toddlers when they coined the term, it is highly applicable to adolescents as well. In fact, it is believed that the most frequent immediate precipitant to adolescent suicide is loss, or threat of loss, or abandonment by parents or closest peer relationship.

Adolescents have many issues to deal with and many choices to make. Some of these include issues that relate to self-esteem and body image (in a body that is undergoing rapid changes), peer relationships (with both genders), education and career selection, establishing a set of values and ideals, sexuality and sexual experimentation (including issues of birth control and prevention of sexually transmitted diseases), drug and alcohol abuse, and physical appearance.

Nursing interventions with adolescents at the primary level of prevention focuses on providing adolescents with support and accurate information to ease the difficult transition they are undergoing. Educational offerings can be presented in schools, churches, youth centers, or any location in which groups of teenagers gather. Types of programs may include (but are not limited to):

1. Alateen groups for adolescents with alcoholic parent(s).
2. Other support groups for teenagers who are in need of assistance to cope with stressful situations (e.g., children dealing with divorce of their parents, pregnant teenagers, teenagers coping with abortion, adolescents coping with the death of a parent).
3. Educational programs that inform about and validate bodily changes and emotional feelings about which there may be some concerns.
4. Educational programs that inform about nutritional needs specific for this age group.
5. Educational programs that inform about sexuality, pregnancy, contraception, and sexually transmitted diseases.
6. Educational programs that inform about the use and abuse of alcohol and other drugs.

Marriage. The "American Dream" of the 1950s—especially that of the American woman—was to marry, have 2.5 children, buy a house in the suburbs, and drive a station wagon. To not be at least betrothed by the mid-20s caused many women to fear becoming an "old maid." Living together without the benefit of marriage was not only unacceptable but rarely even considered an option.

Times have changed considerably in 40 years. Today's young women are choosing to pursue careers before entering into marriage, to continue their careers after marriage, or to not get married at all. Many couples are deciding to live together without being married, and as with most trends, the practice now receives more widespread societal acceptance than it once did.

Why is marriage considered one of the most common maturational crises? Sheehy (1976) wrote:

"No two people can possibly coordinate all their developmental crises. The timing of outside opportunities will almost never be the same. But more importantly, each one has an inner life structure with its own idiosyncrasies. Depending on what has gone before, each one will alternate differently between times of feeling full of certainty, hope, and heightened potential and times of feeling vulnerable, unfocused, and scared." (p.138)

Additional conflicts sometimes also arise when the marriage is influenced by crossovers in religion, ethnicity, social status, or race, although these types of differences have become more individually and societally acceptable than they once were.

Nursing interventions at the primary level of prevention with individuals in this stage of development involve education regarding what to expect at various stages in the marriage. Many high schools now offer courses in marriage and family living in which students role play through anticipatory marriage and family situations. Nurses could offer these kinds of classes within the community to individuals considering marriage. Too many people enter marriage with the notion that, as sure as the depth of their love, their soon-to-be husband or wife will discontinue his or her "undesirable" traits and change into the perceived ideal spouse. Primary prevention with these individuals involves:

● Encouraging honest communication.
● Determining what each person expects from the relationship.
● Ascertaining whether or not each individual can accept compromise.

This type of intervention can be effective in individual or couple therapy or in support/educational groups of couples experiencing similar circumstances.

Parenthood. Lancaster (1980) states:

"The developmental crisis precipitated by the birth of a child necessitates an alteration in the family system. With the introduction of a third person, the initial dyadic relationship is altered. Each additional child similarly affects the existing family constellation."

There is probably no developmental stage that creates the upheaval in life equal to that of the arrival of a child. Even when the child is desperately wanted and pleasurably anticipated, his or her arrival usually results in some degree of chaos within the family system.

Because the family operates as a system, the addition of a new member influences all parts of the system as a whole. If it is a first child, the relationship between the spouses is likely to be affected by the demands of caring for the infant on a 24-hour basis. If there are older children, they may resent the attention showered on the new arrival and show their resentment in a variety of creative ways.

The concept of having a child (particularly the first one) is often romanticized, with little or no consideration given to the realities and responsibilities that accompany this "bundle of joy." Many young parents are shocked to realize that such a tiny human can create so many changes in so many lives. It is unfortunate that parenting is one of the most important positions an individual will hold in life and one for which he or she is often least prepared.

Nursing intervention at the primary level of prevention with the developmental stage of parenthood must begin long before the child is even born. How do we prepare individuals for parenthood? *Anticipatory guidance* is the term used to describe the interventions used to help new parents know what they might expect. Volumes have been written on the subject, but it is also important for expectant parents to have a support person or network with whom they can talk, express feelings, excitement, and fears. Nurses can provide the following type of information to help ease the transition into parenthood (McCabe, 1979; Murray & Zentner, 1997).

1. Prepared childbirth classes: what most likely will happen but with additional information about possible variations from that which is expected.
2. Information about what to expect after the baby arrives:
   a. **Parent-Infant Bonding.** Expectant parents should know that it is not unusual for parent-infant bonding not to occur immediately. The strong attachment will occur as parent and infant get to know each other.
   b. **Changing Husband-Wife Relationships.** The couple should be encouraged to engage in open honest communication and role-playing of typical situations that are likely to arise after the baby becomes a part of the family.
   c. **Clothing and Equipment.** Expectant parents need to know what is required to care for a newborn child. Family economics, space available, and lifestyle should be considered.
   d. **Feeding.** Advantages and disadvantages of both breastfeeding and formula-feeding should be presented. The couple should be supported in whatever method it chooses. Anticipatory guidance related to technique should be provided for one or both methods, as the expectant parents request.
   e. **Other Expectations.** It is important for expectant parents to receive anticipatory guidance about the infant's sleeping and crying patterns, bathing the infant, care of the circumcision and cord, toys that provide stimulation of the newborn's senses, aspects of providing a safe environment, and when to call the physician.
3. Stages of Growth and Development. It is very important for parents to understand what behaviors should be expected at what stage of development. It is also important to know that their child may not necessarily follow the age guidelines associated with these stages. However, a substantial deviation from these guidelines should be reported to their physician.

Midlife. What is middle age? A colleague once remarked that upon turning 50 years of age she stated, "Now I can say I am officially middle aged . . . until I began thinking about how few individuals I really knew who were 100!"

The occurrence of midlife crises is not defined by a specific number. Various sources in the literature identify these conflicts as occurring anytime between age 35 and 65.

What is a midlife crisis? This, too, is very individual, but a number of patterns have been identified within three broad categories:

1. **An Alteration in Perception of the Self.** One's perception of self may occur slowly. One may suddenly become aware of being "old" or "middle aged." The individual looks in the mirror and sees changes that others may have noticed for some time. Gray thinning hair and wrinkles, coarsening features, decreased muscular tone, weight gain, varicosities, and capillary breakage may suddenly become frighteningly apparent to the individual (Murray & Zentner, 1997).

Other biological changes that occur naturally with the aging process may also impact on the crises that occur at this time. In women, a gradual decrease in the production of estrogen initiates the menopause, which results in a variety of physical and emotional symptoms. Some physical symptoms include "hot flashes," vaginal dryness, cessation of menstruation, loss of reproductive ability, night sweats, insomnia, headaches, and minor memory disturbances. Emotional symptoms include anxiety, depression, crying for no reason, and temper outbursts.

Although the menopausal period in men is not as evident as it is in women, most clinicians subscribe to the belief that men undergo a climacteric experience related to the gradual decrease in production of testosterone. Sperm production decreases, although viable sperm may still be produced at age 90 (Hyde, 1986). Some men experience hot flashes, sweating, chills, dizziness, and heart palpitations (Murray & Zentner, 1997), whereas others may experience severe depression and an overall decline in physical vigor (Kaplan & Sadock, 1998). An alteration in sexual functioning is not uncommon (see Chapter 35).

2. **An Alteration in Perception of Others.** A change in relationship with adult children requires a sensitive shift in caring. Ebersole and Gustin (1979) state:

> "An adult parent must care enough to allow the child to struggle through decisions, mistakes, indecision—providing support when needed and willingly staying in the background rather than inflicting one's own values or experience."

These experiences are particularly difficult when parents' values conflict with the relationships and types of lifestyles their children choose.

An alteration in perception of one's parents also begins to occur during this time. Having always looked to parents for support and comfort, the middle-aged individual may suddenly find that the roles are beginning to reverse. Aging parents may look to their children for assistance with making decisions regarding their everyday lives and for assistance with chores that they have previously accomplished independently. When parents die, middle-aged individuals must come to terms with their own mortality. The process of recognition and resolution of one's own finitude begins in earnest at this time.

3. **An Alteration in Perception of Time.** Middle age

has been defined as the end of youth and the beginning of old age. Individuals often experience a sense that time is running out: "I haven't done all I want to do or accomplished all I intended to accomplish!" Depression and a sense of loss may occur as individuals realize that some of the goals established in their youth may indeed go unmet.

"The empty nest" syndrome has been identified as the adjustment period parents experience when the last child leaves home to establish an independent residence. The crisis is often more profound for the mother who has devoted her life to nurturing her family. As the last child leaves, she may perceive her future as uncertain and meaningless.

Some women who have devoted their lives to rearing their children decide to develop personal interests and pursue personal goals once the children are grown. This occurs at a time when many husbands have begun to decrease what may have been a compulsive drive for occupational security during the earlier years of their lives. This disparity in common goals may create conflict between husband and wife. At a time when she is experiencing more value in herself and her own life, he may begin to feel less valued. This may also relate to a decrease in the amount of time and support from the wife to which the husband has become accustomed. This type of role change will require numerous adaptations on the part of both spouses.

Finally, an alteration in one's perception of time may be related to the societal striving for eternal youth. Murray and Zentner (1997) state:

"Whether a man or a woman, the person who lacks self-confidence and who cannot accept the changing body, has a compulsion to try cosmetics, clothes, hair styles, and the other trappings of youth in the hope that the physical attributes of youth will be attained. The person tries to regain a youthful figure and face, perhaps through surgery; tints the hair to cover signs of gray; and turns to hormone creams to restore the skin." (p. 677)

This yearning for youth may take the form of sexual promiscuity or extramarital affairs with much younger individuals, in an effort to prove that one "still has what it takes." Some individuals reach for the trappings of youth with regressive-type behaviors, such as the middle-aged man who buys a motorcycle and joins a motorcycle gang and the 50-year-old woman who wears mini skirts and flirts with her daughter's boyfriends. These individuals may be denying their own past and experience. With a negative view of self, they strongly desire to relive their youth.

Nursing intervention at the primary level of prevention with the developmental stage of midlife involves providing accurate information regarding changes that occur during this time of life and support for adapting to these changes effectively. These interventions might include:

1. Nutrition classes to inform individuals in this age group about the essentials of diet and exercise. Educational materials on how to avoid obesity or reduce weight can be included, along with the importance of good nutrition.
2. Assistance with ways to improve health (e.g., quit smoking, cease or reduce alcohol consumption, reduce fat intake).
3. Discussions of the importance of having regular physical examinations, including Pap and breast examinations for women and prostate examinations for men. Monthly breast self-examinations should be taught and yearly mammograms encouraged.
4. Classes on menopause should be given. Provide information about what to expect. Myths that abound regarding this topic should be expelled. Support groups for women (and men) undergoing the menopausal experience should be formed.
5. Support and information related to physical changes occurring in the body during this time of life. Assist with the grief response that some individuals will experience in relation to loss of youth, "empty nest," and sense of identity.
6. Support and information related to care of aging parents should be given. Individuals should be referred to community resources for respite and assistance before strain of the caregiver role threatens to disrupt the family system.

Retirement. Retirement, which is often anticipated as an achievement in principle, may be met with a great deal of ambiguity when it actually occurs. Our society places a great deal of importance on productivity and on earning as much money as possible at as young an age as possible. These types of values contribute to the ambiguity associated with retirement. Although leisure has been acknowledged as a legitimate reward for workers, leisure during retirement is generally not accorded the same social value. Adjustment to this life-cycle event becomes more difficult in the face of societal values that are in direct conflict with the new lifestyle.

Historically many women have derived much of their self-esteem from having children, rearing children, and being a "good mother." Likewise, many men have achieved self-esteem through work-related activities—creativity, productivity, and earning money. With the termination of these activities may come a loss of self-worth. Depression may be the result for some individuals who are unable to adapt satisfactorily.

Hendricks and Hendricks (1977) described a pattern that focuses on the continuity of environmental influences that *reinforce* appropriate adaptation to retirement. They have said:

"If the positive reinforcements present during early life and working adulthood are removed by retirement, the likelihood of adjustment is jeopardized. If a worker perceived money to be the most important reward for working, the significant decline in income after retirement will complicate the process of adjustment. If friends or feelings of autonomy were the reinforcing component of work, then retirement may pose markedly fewer problems." (p. 251)

In an early study by Reichard, Livson, and Peterson (1962), men nearing retirement appeared to be especially vulnerable psychologically. They showed increased feelings of inadequacy and tended to be resentful, depressed, and pessimistic. In addition, they were apathetic or contemptuous of themselves. The investigators interpreted these results as indicating that the time shortly before retirement is a critical adjustment period for men.

A later study by Lazarus and DeLongis (1983) did not support this conclusion. It would appear that retirement is becoming, and will continue to become, more accepted by societal standards. With more and more individuals retiring earlier and living longer, the growing number of aging persons will spend a significantly longer time in retirement. At present, retirement has become more of an institutionalized expectation, and there appears to be increasing acceptance of it as a social status.

Nursing intervention at the primary level of prevention with the developmental task of retirement involves providing information and support to individuals who have retired or are considering retirement.

Support can be on a one-to-one basis to assist these individuals to sort out their feelings regarding retirement. Murray and Zentner (1997) state:

"The retiree may be faced with these questions: Can I face loss of job satisfaction? Will I feel the separation from people close to me at work? If I need continued employment on a part-time basis to supplement Social Security payments, will the old organization provide it, or must I adjust to a new job? Shall I remain in my present home or seek a different one because of easier maintenance or reduced cost of upkeep? Might a different climate be better, and if so, will I miss my relatives and neighbors?" (p. 750)

Support can also be provided in a group environment. Support groups of individuals undergoing the same types of experiences can be extremely helpful. Nurses can form and lead these types of groups to assist retiring individuals through this critical period. These groups can also serve to provide information about available resources that offer assistance to individuals in or nearing retirement, such as information concerning Medicare, Social Security, and Medicaid; information related to organizations that specialize in hiring retirees; and information regarding ways to use newly acquired free time constructively.

Situational Crises. Situational crises are acute responses that occur as a result of an external circumstantial stressor. The number and types of situational stressors are limitless and may be real or exist only in the perception of the individual. Some types of situational crises that put individuals at risk for mental illness include the following.

Poverty. A number of studies have identified poverty as a direct correlation to emotional illness. This may have to do with the direct consequences of poverty, such as inadequate and crowded living conditions, nutritional deficiencies, medical neglect, unemployment, and the newest at-risk population, the homeless.

High Rate of Life Change Events. Holmes and Rahe (1967) found that frequent changes in life patterns due to a large number of significant events occurring in close proximity tend to decrease a person's ability to deal with stress, and physical or emotional illness may be the result. These include life change events such as death of a loved one, divorce, fired from job, change in living conditions, change in place of employment or residence, physical illness, or change in body image due to loss of a body part or function.

Environmental Conditions. These can create situational crises. Tornados, floods, hurricanes, and earthquakes have wreaked devastation on thousands of individuals and families in recent years.

Trauma. Individuals who have encountered traumatic experiences must be considered at risk for emotional illness. These include traumatic experiences usually considered outside the range of usual human experience, such as military combat, violent personal assault, torture, being taken hostage or kidnapped, or being the victim of a natural or manmade disaster (APA, 1994).

Nursing intervention at the primary level of prevention with individuals experiencing situational crises is aimed at maintaining the highest possible level of functioning while offering support and assistance with problem solving during the crisis period. Interventions for nursing of clients in crisis include the following:

1. Use a reality-oriented approach. The focus of the problem is on the here and now.
2. Remain with the individual who is experiencing panic anxiety.
3. Establish a rapid working relationship by showing unconditional acceptance, by active listening, and by attending to immediate needs.
4. Discourage lengthy explanations or rationalizations of the situation; promote an atmosphere for verbalization of true feelings.
5. Set firm limits on aggressive, destructive behaviors. At high levels of anxiety, behavior is likely to be impulsive and regressive. Establish at the outset what is acceptable and what is not, and maintain consistency.
6. Clarify the problem that the individual is facing. The nurse does this by describing his or her perception of the problem and comparing it with the individual's perception of the problem.
7. Help the individual determine what he or she believes precipitated the crisis.

8. Acknowledge feelings of anger, guilt, helplessness, and powerlessness, while taking care not to provide positive feedback for these feelings.
9. Guide the individual through a problem-solving process by which he or she may move in the direction of positive life change:
    a. Help the individual confront the source of the problem that is creating the crisis response.
    b. Encourage the individual to discuss changes he or she would like to make. Jointly determine whether or not desired changes are realistic.
    c. Encourage exploration of feelings about aspects that cannot be changed, and explore alternative ways of coping more adaptively in these situations.
    d. Discuss alternative strategies for creating changes that are realistically possible.
    e. Weigh benefits and consequences of each alternative.
    f. Assist the individual to select alternative coping strategies that will help alleviate future crisis situations.
10. Identify external support systems and new social networks from whom the individual may seek assistance in times of stress.

Nursing at the level of primary prevention focuses largely on education of the consumer to prevent initiation or exacerbation of mental illness. An example of just one type of teaching plan for use in primary prevention situations is presented in Table 38.1.

Secondary Prevention

Populations At Risk

Secondary prevention within communities relates to using early detection and prompt intervention with individuals experiencing mental illness symptoms. The same maturational and situational crises that were presented in the previous section on primary prevention are used to discuss intervention at the secondary level of prevention.

Maturational Crises

Adolescence. The need for intervention at the secondary level of prevention in adolescence occurs when disruptive and age-inappropriate behaviors become the norm, and the family can no longer cope adaptively with the situation. All levels of dysfunction are considered, from dysfunctional family coping to the need for hospitalization of the adolescent.

Nursing intervention with the adolescent at the secondary level of prevention may occur in the community setting at community mental health centers, physician's offices, schools, public health departments, and crisis intervention centers. They may work with families to prob-lem solve and improve coping and communication skills, or they may work on a one-to-one basis with the adolescent in an attempt to modify behavior patterns.

Adolescents may be hospitalized for a variety of reasons. The *DSM-IV* (APA, 1994) identifies a number of problems, the severity of which would determine whether or not the adolescent required inpatient care. Conduct disorders, adjustment disorders, eating disorders, substance-related disorders, depression, and anxiety disorders are the most common diagnoses for which adolescents are hospitalized. Nursing care of adolescents in the hospital setting focuses on problem identification and stabilizing a crisis situation. Once stability has been achieved, clients are commonly discharged to outpatient care. If an adolescent's home situation has been deemed unsatisfactory, the state may take custody and the child is then discharged to a group or foster home. Care plans for intervention with the adolescent at the secondary level of prevention can be found in Chapter 22.

Marriage. Problems in a marriage are as far-reaching as the individuals who experience them. Problems that are not uncommon to the disruption of a marriage relationship include substance abuse on the part of one or both partners and disagreements on issues of sex, money, children, gender roles, and infidelity, among others. Murray and Zentner (1997) state:

> "Staying married to one person and living with the frustrations, conflicts, and boredom that any close and lengthy relationship imposes requires constant work by both parties." (p. 566)

Nursing intervention at the secondary level of prevention with individuals encountering marriage problems may include one or more of the following:

1. Counseling with the couple or with one of the spouses on a one-to-one basis.
2. Referral to a couples' support group.
3. Identification of the problem and possible solutions. Support and guidance as changes are undertaken.
4. Referral to a sex therapist.
5. Referral to a financial advisor.
6. Referral to parent effectiveness training.

Murray and Zentner (1997) state:

> "When marriage fails and bonds are broken, aloneness, anger, mistrust, hostility, guilt, shame, a sense of betrayal, fear, disappointment, loss of identity, anxiety, and depression, alone or in combination, can appear both in the divorcee and the one initiating the divorce." (p. 625)

In Holmes and Rahe's (1967) life stress inventory, divorce was second only to death of a spouse in severity of stress experienced. This is indeed an area in which nurses can intervene to help ease the transition and prevent emotional breakdown. In community health settings, nurses can lead support groups for newly divorced individuals.

TABLE 38.1 CLIENT EDUCATION FOR PRIMARY PREVENTION: DRUGS OF ABUSE

CLASS OF DRUGS	EFFECTS	SYMPTOMS OF OVERDOSE	TRADE NAMES	COMMON NAMES	EFFECTS ON THE BODY (CHRONIC OR HIGH-DOSE USE)
CNS Depressants					
Alcohol	Relaxation, loss of inhibitions, lack of concentration, drowsiness, slurred speech, sleep.	Nausea, vomiting; shallow respirations; cold, clammy skin; weak, rapid pulse; coma; possible death.	Ethyl alcohol, beer, gin, rum, vodka, bourbon, whiskey, liqueurs, wine, brandy, sherry, champagne.	Booze, alcohol, liquor, drinks, cocktails, highballs, nightcaps, moonshine, white lightning, firewater.	Peripheral nerve damage, skeletal muscle wasting, encephalopathy, psychosis, cardiomyopathy, gastritis, esophagitis, pancreatitis, hepatitis, cirrhosis of the liver, leukopenia, thrombocytopenia, sexual dysfunction.
Other (barbiturates and non-barbiturates)	Same as alcohol.	Anxiety, fever, agitation, hallucinations, disorientation, tremors, delirium, convulsions, possible death.	Seconal, Nembutal, Amytal, Valium, Librium Chloral hydrate Equanil, Miltown	Red birds, yellow birds, blue birds Blues/yellows Green and whites Mickies Downers	Decreased REM sleep, respiratory depression, hypotension, possible kidney or liver damage, sexual dysfunction.
CNS Stimulants					
Amphetamines and related drugs	Hyperactivity, agitation, euphoria, insomnia, loss of appetite.	Cardiac arrhythmias, headache, convulsions, hypertension, rapid heart rate, coma, possible death.	Dexedrine, Didrex, Tenuate, Preludin, Ritalin, Plegine, Cylert, Ionamin, Sanorex	Uppers, pep pills, wakeups, bennies, eye-openers, speed, black beauties, sweet A's	Aggressive, compulsive behavior; paranoia; hallucinations; hypertension.
Cocaine	Euphoria, hyperactivity, restlessness, talkativeness, increased pulse, dilated pupils.	Hallucinations, convulsions, pulmonary edema, respiratory failure, coma, cardiac arrest, possible death.	Cocaine hydrochloride	Coke, flake, snow, dust, happy dust, gold dust, girl, cecil, C, toot, blow, crack	Pulmonary hemorrhage; myocardial infarction; ventricular fibrillation.
Opioids					
	Euphoria, lethargy, drowsiness, lack of motivation.	Shallow breathing, slowed pulse, clammy skin, pulmonary edema, respiratory arrest, convulsions, coma, possible death.	Heroin Morphine Codeine Dilaudid Demerol Methadone Percodan Talwin Opium	Snow, stuff, H, Harry, horse M, morph, Miss Emma Schoolboy Lords Doctors Dollies Perkies T's Big O, black stuff	Respiratory depression, constipation, fecal impaction, hypotension, decreased libido, retarded ejaculation, impotence, orgasm failure.

TABLE 38.1 CLIENT EDUCATION FOR PRIMARY PREVENTION: DRUGS OF ABUSE

CLASS OF DRUGS	EFFECTS	SYMPTOMS OF OVERDOSE	TRADE NAMES	COMMON NAMES	EFFECTS ON THE BODY (CHRONIC OR HIGH-DOSE USE)
Hallucinogens	Visual hallucinations, disorientation, confusion, paranoid delusions, euphoria, anxiety, panic, increased pulse.	Agitation, extreme hyperactivity, violence, hallucinations, psychosis, convulsions, possible death.	LSD PCP Mescaline DMT STP	Acid, cube, big D Angel dust, Hog crystal Mesc Businessman's trip Serenity and peace	Panic reaction, acute psychosis, flashbacks.
Cannabinols	Relaxation, talkativeness, lowered inhibitions, euphoria, mood swings.	Fatigue, paranoia, delusions, hallucinations, possible psychosis.	Cannabis Hashish	Marijuana, pot, grass, joint, Mary Jane, MJ Hash, rope, Sweet Lucy	Tachycardia, orthostatic hypotension, chronic bronchitis, problems with infertility, amotivational syndrome.

REM = rapid eye movement.

They can also provide one-to-one counseling for individuals experiencing the emotional chaos engendered by the dissolution of a marriage relationship.

Divorce also has an impact on the children involved. Nurses can intervene with the children of divorce in an effort to prevent dysfunctional behaviors associated with the break-up of a marriage.

Parenthood. Intervention at the secondary level of prevention with parents can be required for a number of reasons. Only a few of these include:

1. Physical, emotional, or sexual abuse of a child.
2. Physical or emotional neglect of a child.
3. Birth of an imperfect child.
4. Diagnosis of a terminal illness in a child.
5. Death of a child.

Nursing intervention at the secondary level of prevention includes being able to recognize the physical and behavioral signs that indicate possible abuse of a child. The child may be cared for in the emergency room or as an inpatient on the pediatric unit or child psychiatric unit of a general hospital.

Nursing intervention with parents may include teaching effective methods of disciplining children, aside from physical punishment. Methods that emphasize the importance of positive reinforcement for acceptable behavior can be very effective. Family members must be committed to consistent use of this behavior modification technique for it to be successful.

Parents should also be informed about behavioral expectations at the various levels of development. Knowledge of what to expect from children at various stages of development may provide needed anticipatory guidance to deal with the crises commonly associated with these various stages.

Therapy sessions with all family members together may focus on problems with family communications. Members are encouraged to express honest feelings in a manner that is nonthreatening to other family members. Active listening, assertiveness techniques, and respect for the rights of others are taught and encouraged. Barriers to effective communication are identified and resolved.

Referrals to agencies that promote effective parenting skills may be made (e.g., parent effectiveness training). Alternative agencies that may provide relief from the stress of parenting may also be considered (e.g., "Mom's Day Out" programs, sitter-sharing organizations, and daycare institutions). Support groups for abusive parents may also be helpful, and assistance in locating or initiating such a group may be provided.

The nurse can assist parents who are grieving the loss of a child or the birth of an imperfect child by helping them to express their true feelings associated with the loss. Feelings such as shock, denial, anger, guilt, powerlessness, and hopelessness need to be expressed in order for the parents to progress through the grief response.

Home health care assistance can be provided for the family with an imperfect child. This can be done by making referrals to other professionals, such as speech, physical, and occupational therapists, medical social workers, psychologists, and nutritionists. If the child with special needs is hospitalized, the home health nurse can provide specific information to hospital staff that may be helpful in providing continuity of care for the client and help in the transition for the family.

Nursing intervention also includes providing assistance in the location of and referral to support groups that deal with loss of a child or birth of a child with special needs. Some nurses may serve as leaders of these types of groups in the community.

Midlife. Nursing care at the secondary level of prevention during midlife becomes necessary when the individual is unable to integrate all of the changes that are occurring during this period. An inability to accept the physical and biological changes, the changes in relationships between themselves and their adult children and aging parents, and the loss of the perception of youth may result in depression for which the individual may require help to resolve.

Retirement. Retirement can also result in depression for individuals who are unable to satisfactorily grieve for the loss of this aspect of their lives. This is more likely to occur if the individuals have not planned for retirement and if they have derived most of their self-esteem from their employment.

Nursing intervention at the secondary level of prevention with depressed individuals takes place in both inpatient and outpatient settings. Severely depressed clients with suicidal ideations will need close observation in the hospital setting, whereas those with mild to moderate depression may be treated in the community. Nursing care plans for the client with depression are found in Chapter 26 of this text. These concepts apply to the secondary level of prevention and may be used in all nursing care settings.

The physician may elect to use pharmacotherapy with antidepressants. Nurses may intervene by providing information to the client about what to expect from the medication, possible side effects, adverse effects, and how to self-administer the medication.

Situational Crises. Nursing care at the secondary level of prevention with clients undergoing situational crises occurs only if crisis intervention at the primary level failed and the individual is unable to function socially or occupationally. Exacerbation of mental illness symptoms requires intervention at the secondary level of prevention. These disorders were addressed extensively in Unit Three of this text. Nursing assessment, diagnosis and outcome identification, plan and implementation, and evaluation were discussed for the majority of mental illnesses identified in the *DSM-IV* (APA, 1994). These skills may be applied in any setting where nursing is practiced.

A case study situation of nursing care at the secondary level of prevention in a community setting is presented in Table 38.2.

Tertiary Prevention

The Chronically Mentally Ill

Historical and Epidemiological Aspects. In 1955, more than half a million individuals resided in public mental hospitals. More recent statistics indicate that approximately 120,000 mentally ill persons inhabit these institutions on a long-term basis (Talley & Coleman, 1992).

Deinstitutionalization of chronically mentally ill persons began in the 1960s as national policy changed in response to a strong belief in the individual's right to freedom. Other considerations included the deplorable conditions of some of the state asylums, the introduction of neuroleptic medications, and the cost-effectiveness of caring for these individuals in the community setting.

Deinstitutionalization began to occur rapidly and without sufficient planning for the needs of these individuals as they reentered the **community.** Those who were fortunate enough to have support systems to provide assistance with living arrangements and sheltered employment experiences most often received the outpatient treatment they required. However, those without adequate support either managed to survive on a meager existence or were forced to join the ranks of the homeless. Some ended up in nursing homes meant to provide care for individuals with physical disabilities.

Large segments of our population with chronic mental illness problems are left untreated: the elderly, the "working poor," the homeless, and those individuals previously covered by funds that have been cut by various social reforms (Talley & Coleman, 1992). These circumstances have promoted in the chronically mentally ill a greater number of crisis-oriented emergency department visits and hospital admissions, as well as repeated confrontations with law enforcement officials.

The community-based mental health system is not working for the chronically mentally ill. The Coalition of Psychiatric Nursing Organizations (COPNO) has developed a position paper in which barriers to care have been described and essential services delineated (Krauss, 1993). The Coalition identified the following five barriers:

1. **Public Attitudes.** A social stigma still exists regarding attitudes toward mental illness, even in light of the fact that in 1990, 41 million adults had some form of mental disorder. In fact, a study by the NIMH revealed that one in three adult Americans meets the criteria for a mental disorder at some point during his or her lifetime (Krauss, 1993). The unfortunate fact is that having cancer is considered more "socially appropriate" than having a mental disorder.

2. **Fragmented Systems.** Our nation's health policy ignores the biopsychosocial aspects of illness. Body and mind cannot be separated, yet our system is not properly prepared to meet the general health care

TABLE 38.2   SECONDARY PREVENTION CASE STUDY: PARENTHOOD

The identified patient was a petite, doll-like 4-year-old girl named Tanya. She was the oldest of two children in a Latino American family. The other child was a boy named Joseph, aged 2. The mother was 5 months pregnant with their third child. The family had been referred to the nurse after Tanya was placed in foster care following a report to Department of Human Services (DHS) by her nursery school teacher that the child had marks on her body suspicious of child abuse.

The parents, Paulo and Annette, were in their mid-20s. Paulo had lost his job at an aircraft plant 3 months ago and had been unable to find work since. Annette brought in a few dollars from cleaning houses for other people, but the family was struggling to survive.

Paulo and Annette were angry at having to see the nurse. After all, "Parents have the right to discipline their children." The nurse did not focus on the *intent* of the behavior, but instead looked at factors in the family's life that could be viewed as stressors. This family had multiple stressors: poverty, the father's unemployment, the age and spacing of the children, the mother's chronic fatigue from work at home as well as in other people's homes, and finally, having a child removed from the home against the parents' wishes.

During therapy with this family, the nurse discussed the behaviors associated with various developmental levels. She also discussed possible deviations from these norms and when they should be reported to the physician. The nurse and the family discussed Tanya's behavior, and how it compared with the norms.

The parents also discussed their own childhoods. They were able to relate some of the same types of behaviors that they observed in Tanya. But they both admitted that they came from families whose main method of discipline was physical punishment. Annette had been the oldest child in her large family, and had been expected to "keep the younger ones in line." When she had not done so, she was punished with her father's belt. She expressed anger toward her father, although she had never been allowed to express it at the time.

Paulo's father had died when he was a small boy, and Paulo had been expected to be the "man of the family." He had worked at odd jobs from the time he was very young to bring money into the home. Because of this, he had had little time for the usual activities of childhood and adolescence. He held much resentment toward the young men who "had everything and never had to work for it."

Paulo and Annette had high expectations for Tanya. In effect, they expected her to behave in a manner well beyond her developmental level. These expectations were based on the reflections of their own childhoods. They were uncomfortable with the spontaneity and playfulness of childhood, for they had had little personal experience with these behaviors. When Tanya balked and expressed the verbal assertions common to early childhood, Paulo and Annette interpreted these behaviors as defiance toward them, and retaliated with anger in the manner in which they had been parented.

With the parents, the nurse explored feelings and behaviors from their past so that they were able to understand the correlation to their current behaviors. They learned to negotiate ways to deal with Tanya's age-appropriate behaviors. In combined therapy with Tanya, they learned how to relate to her childishness, and even how to enjoy playing with both of their children.

The parents ceased blaming each other for the family's problems. Annette had spent a good deal of her time deprecating Paulo for his lack of support of his family, and Paulo blamed Annette for being "unable to control her daughter." Communication patterns were clarified, and life in the family became more peaceful.

Without a need to "prove himself" to his wife, Paulo's efforts to find employment met with success, as he no longer felt the need to turn down jobs that he knew his wife would perceive to be beneath his capabilities. Annette no longer works outside the home, and both she and Paulo participate in the parenting chores. Tanya and her siblings continue to demonstrate age-appropriate developmental progression.

---

needs on a holistic level. Because of fragmented and diminished services, many consumers cannot achieve the level of care required to maintain a satisfactory community existence.

3. **Poverty and Race.** Poor people have limited access to mental health services because of economics and cultural implications, yet studies show that poverty increases one's risk of psychiatric illness by twofold. Children born into poverty are two to three times more likely to develop emotional or behavioral problems (Krauss, 1993).

4. **Private Insurance.** Coverage for mental health services by private insurance companies is and always has been far less comprehensive than for physical illness. Benefits and reimbursements are lower and deductibles and copayments higher. Some individuals who have insurance coverage refuse to file claims for mental health care for fear that they may suffer repercussions from disclosure of such information.

5. **Public Funding.** Public funding of mental health services comes from various state and federal sources. Most is apportioned to pay for costly inpatient treatment of individuals who require acute care because of decompensation of their illness (which may have been prevented if less costly outpatient care had been available).

The Coalition outlined the following essential services for mental health reform:

1. **Primary Care Mental Health Services.** Krauss (1993) states:

> "Community-based primary care settings should serve as an essential consumer pathway to mental health services. Such settings must be prepared to provide mental

health promotion and education programs, case finding, diagnostic assessments, routine treatment, and referral."

2. **Universal Access to a Basic Mental Health Package.** The Coalition advocates a universal minimum-benefit package that ensures access to mental health services (both inpatient and outpatient) to all individuals across the life span.

3. **Long-Term Care.** The Coalition recommends assurance of long-term or rehabilitative services for clients with mental impairment. The Coalition proposes that "Such care should be financed by public funds and sliding-scale service fees, and authorized by a care coordinator or case manager."

4. **Managed Care.** The Coalition views the "concept of managed care as a cost-effective monitoring system for the delivery of mental health services," as well as a way to "ensure that maximum value is received from the resources used in the production and delivery of health care services."

If these proposals became reality, it would surely mean improvement in the care of chronically mentally ill individuals. Many nurse leaders see this period of health care reform as an opportunity for nurses to expand their roles and assume key positions in education, prevention, assessment, and referral. Nurses are, and will continue to be, in key positions to assist chronically mentally ill clients to remain as independent as possible, to manage their illness within the community setting, and to strive to minimize the number of hospitalizations required.

Treatment Alternatives

Community Mental Health Centers. The goal of community mental health centers in caring for the chronically mentally ill is to improve coping ability and prevent exacerbation of acute symptoms. A major obstacle in meeting this goal has been the lack of advocacy or sponsorship for clients who require services from a variety of sources. This has placed responsibility for health care on a mentally ill individual who is often barely able to cope with everyday life (Pittman, 1989). Case management is becoming a recommended method of treatment for individuals with a chronic mental illness.

The ANA (1988) has endorsed case management as an effective method of providing care for clients in the community who require long-term assistance:

"Nurses—with their theoretical background in the biological and social sciences, and the humanities; their knowledge of health maintenance, disease processes, and medications; and their experience in collaboration—are uniquely equipped to become case managers."

Bower (1992) has identified five core components and nursing role functions that blend with the steps of the nursing process to form a framework for nursing case management. The core components include:

Interaction. The nurse must develop a trusting relationship with the client, family members, and other service providers. During an initial screening process the nurse determines if the client is eligible for case management according to preestablished guidelines and, if not, refers the client for appropriate assistance elsewhere.

Assessment: Establishment of a Database. The nurse conducts a comprehensive assessment of the client's physical health status, functional capability, mental status, personal and community support systems, financial resources, and environmental conditions. The data are then analyzed and appropriate nursing diagnoses formulated.

Planning. A service care plan is devised with client participation. The plan should include mutually agreed-on goals, specific actions directed toward goal achievement, and selection of essential resources and services through collaboration among health care professionals, the client, and the family or significant others.

Implementation. In this phase, the client receives the needed services from the appropriate providers. In some instances the nursing case manager is also a provider of care, whereas in others, he or she is only the coordinator of care.

Evaluation. The case manager continuously monitors and evaluates the client's responses to interventions and progress toward preestablished goals. Regular contact is maintained with client, family or significant others, and direct service providers. Ongoing care coordination continues until outcomes have been achieved. The client may then be discharged or assigned to inactive status, as appropriate.

A case study of nursing case management within a community mental health center is presented in Table 38.3.

Day-Evening Treatment/Partial Hospitalization Programs. Day or evening treatment programs (also called partial hospitalization) are designed to ease the transition from hospital to community living, as well as to prevent institutionalization (Pittman, Parson, & Peterson, 1990). Various types of treatment are offered. Most include therapeutic community (milieu) activities; individual, group, and family therapies; therapeutic recreational activities; and occupational therapy. Many programs offer medication administration and monitoring as part of their care.

Day treatment programs generally offer a comprehensive treatment plan formulated by an interdisciplinary team of psychiatrists, psychologists, nurses, occupational and recreational therapists, and social workers. Swearingen (1987) described eight broad categories of goals used in day treatment:

1. Stabilization of psychiatric symptoms.
2. Medication trial or adjustment.
3. Stabilization of living environment.
4. Improvement in activities of daily living.
5. Learning to structure time.

TABLE 38.3 NURSING CASE MANAGEMENT IN THE COMMUNITY MENTAL HEALTH CENTER: A CASE STUDY

Michael, 73 years old with a history of multiple psychiatric admissions, has lived in various adult foster homes and boarding houses for the past 10 years. He was originally diagnosed as having schizophrenia, but he was recently rediagnosed as having bipolar disorder, mania. His symptoms are well controlled with lithium 300 mg three times a day, which is prescribed by the outpatient psychiatrist.

The nurse practitioner/case manager in the outpatient clinic coordinates Michael's care, advocates for his needs, and counsels him regarding his health problems. She orders routine blood tests to assess his lithium levels. When Michael experienced visual disturbances, she referred him for an emergency eye evaluation. He was found to have a retinal detachment and was sent to a local VA hospital for emergency surgery. After his eye surgery, the nurse practitioner arranged transportation to his follow-up visits with the eye doctor and instructed him about his eye care and instillation of his eyedrops. Michael did not like putting eyedrops in his eye and tended to neglect doing it. Because he also had glaucoma and required ongoing treatment with pilocarpine and timolol maleate eyedrops twice daily, he needed a great deal of education and reassurance to continue using the eyedrops.

In addition to routine quarterly visits for ongoing case management, the nurse practitioner also performs his annual health assessment consisting of history, review of systems, mental status exam, and physical assessment. During Michael's last physical exam, the nurse practitioner detected a thyroid mass and referred him for a complete evaluation including thyroid function tests, a thyroid scan, and evaluation by a surgeon and an endocrinologist. She discussed his thyroid problem with the surgeon and the endocrinologist, and they determined that Michael would best benefit from thyroid replacement therapy (i.e., levothyroxine sodium 0.1 mg daily).

Because Michael eats all of his meals in restaurants, the nurse was concerned about his diet. A brief diet review revealed that his diet was low in vitamin C. He was then instructed in which foods and juices he should include in his daily menu. The nurse practitioner discussed ways that Michael could get the best nutrition for the least cost.

Michael is currently living in a boarding house and is totally responsible for taking his own medication, attending to his activities of daily living, and managing his own money. He has very limited income and depends on donations for many of his clothing needs.

Despite his age, he is quite active and alert. He attends many VA-sponsored social activities and does daily volunteer work at the VA, such as pushing wheelchairs, running errands, and escorting other veterans to clinic appointments. His nurse case manager arranged for him to receive free lunches as a reward for some of his volunteer activities.

Nursing case management has helped this elderly gentleman with chronic psychiatric illness and many years of hospitalization to live independently within the community setting.

SOURCE: From Pittman (1989), with permission.

---

6. Development of social skills.
7. Acquisition of a volunteer or paid employment position.
8. Follow-up on medical and dental concerns.

Individualized weekly goals were used to measure progression toward achievement of these eventual outcomes.

Wilkinson (1991) describes a specialty program within the framework of a day treatment program. Because chronically mentally ill individuals are frequently noncompliant with psychotropic medications, Wilkinson and colleagues established a medication clinic and medication group, each of which met on a weekly basis to provide education and support of individuals on long-term psychopharmacological therapy. During medication clinic appointments, clients are evaluated in relation to effectiveness of and side effects or adverse reactions associated with their medication. Medication groups are assembled according to type of drug being used (e.g., individuals taking antipsychotics compose one group, those taking antidepressants another). The groups are time limited and led by the psychiatric clinical nurse specialist, who provides education and support as needed. As a result of these efforts, Wilkinson reports a 96 percent success rate with medication compliance and subsequent client adjustment to community living.

Nurses take a leading role in the administration of day and evening treatment programs. They lead groups, provide crisis intervention, conduct individual counseling, act as role models, and make necessary referrals for specialized treatment. Use of the nursing process provides continual evaluation of the program, and modifications can be made as necessary.

Pittman, Parson, and Peterson (1990) state:

"Day programs for the chronically mentally ill have been shown to be effective in preventing hospitalization. They help to facilitate the transition from the hospital back into the mainstream of the community. They can improve the quality of life of the deinstitutionalized person by providing social skills training, adding structure and support to the person's daily life, and providing opportunities for socialization."

Community Residential Facilities. Community residential facilities for the chronically mentally ill are known by many names: group homes, halfway houses, foster homes, boarding homes, sheltered care facilities, transitional housing, independent living programs, social-rehabilitation residences, and others. These facilities differ by the purpose for which they exist and the activities that they offer.

Some of these facilities provide basically food, shelter, housekeeping, and minimal supervision and assistance with activities of daily living. Others offer a variety of therapies and serve as a transition between hospital and independent living. In addition to the basics, services might include individual and group counseling, medical care, job training or employment assistance, and leisure-time activities.

A wide variety of personnel staff these facilities. Some facilities have live-in professionals who are available at all times, some have professional staff who are on call for intervention during crisis situations, and some are staffed by volunteers and individuals with little knowledge or background for understanding and treating the chronically mentally ill.

The concept of transitional housing for chronically mentally ill clients is sound and has proved in many instances to be a successful means of therapeutic support and intervention for maintaining these individuals within the community. However, without guidance and planning, transition to the community can be futile. These individuals may be ridiculed and rejected by the community. They may be targets of unscrupulous individuals who take advantage of their inability to care for themselves satisfactorily. These behaviors may increase maladaptive responses to the demands of community living and exacerbate the mental illness. A period of structured reorientation to the community in a living situation that is supervised and monitored by professionals is more likely to result in a successful transition for the chronically mentally ill individual.

The Homeless Population

Historical and Epidemiological Aspects. Dr. Richard Lamb (1992) has stated:

"Alec Guinness, in his memorable role as a British Army colonel in *Bridge on the River Kwai*, exclaims at the end of the film when he finally realizes he has been working to help the enemy, 'What have I done?' As a vocal advocate and spokesman for deinstitutionalization and community treatment of severely mentally ill patients for well over two decades, I often find myself asking that same question."

The number of homeless in the United States has been estimated at somewhere between 250,000 and 4 million. It is difficult to determine the true scope of the problem, for even the statisticians who collect the data have difficulty defining the homeless. Criteria have included: "those people who sleep in shelters or public spaces" (Susser, Conover, & Struening, 1990). This approach results in underestimates because available shelter services are insufficient to meet the numbers of homeless people (U.S. Conference of Mayors, 1998).

Two methods of counting the homeless are commonly used (National Coalition for the Homeless ([NCH], 1999). The point-in-time method attempts to count all the people who are literally homeless on a given day or during a given week. The second method (called *period prevalence counts*) examines the number of people who are homeless over a given period of time. This second method may result in a more accurate count because the extended time period would allow for including the people who are homeless one day (or week) but find employment and affordable housing later, removing them from the homeless count. At the same time during this extended period, others would lose housing and become homeless.

Who Are the Homeless?

The numbers of homeless continues to increase at about 17 percent a year (Blau, 1992). They are increasingly a heterogeneous group. The NCH (1999) provides the following demographics:

Age. Studies have produced a variety of statistics related to the age of the homeless: 25 percent are younger than 18 years of age; individuals between 31 and 50 comprise 51 percent; and the range of persons aged 55 to 60 has been estimated at 2.5 to 19.4 percent.

Gender. More men than women are homeless. The U.S. Conference of Mayors (1998) study found that single men comprised 45 percent of the urban homeless population and single women 14 percent.

Families. Families with children are among the fastest growing segments of the homeless population. Families comprise 38 percent of the urban homeless population, but research indicates that this number is likely higher in rural areas, where families, single mothers, and children make up the largest group of homeless people.

Ethnicity. The study by the U.S. Conference of Mayors (1998) found that the homeless population was 53 percent African American, 35 percent Caucasian, 12 percent Hispanic, 4 percent Native American, and 3 percent Asian. The ethnic makeup of homeless populations varies according to geographic location.

Mental Illness and Homelessness

It is thought that approximately 20 to 25 percent of the single adult homeless population suffers from some form of severe and persistent mental illness (Koegel, Burnam, & Baumohl, 1996). Who are these individuals, and why are they homeless? Some blame the deinstitutionalization movement. Between 1955 and 1981, the population of state and county mental hospitals dropped nationally from 559,000 to 125,000 clients (Dato & Rafferty, 1985). Those without families to return to sought residence in board and care homes of varying quality. Halfway houses and supportive group living arrangements were helpful, but scarce. Many of those with families returned to their homes, but because families received little if any instruction or support, the consequences of their mentally ill loved one returning to live at home were often turbulent, resulting in the individual frequently leaving home.

Types of Mental Illness Among the Homeless. A number of studies have been conducted, primarily in large, urban areas, that have addressed the most common types of mental illness identified among the homeless. Frequently described as the most common diagnosis is schizophrenia. Other prevalent disorders include bipolar affective disorder, substance abuse and dependence, depression, personality disorders, and organic mental disorders. Many exhibit psychotic symptoms, many are former residents of long-term care institutions for the mentally ill, and many have such a strong desire for independence that they isolate themselves in an effort to avoid being identified as a part of the mental health system. Many of them are clearly a danger to themselves or others, yet they do not see themselves as ill (Torrey, 1997).

Contributing Factors to Homelessness Among the Mentally Ill

Deinstitutionalization. As previously stated, deinstitutionalization is frequently implicated as a contributing factor to homelessness among the mentally ill. Deinstitutionalization began out of expressed concern by mental health professionals and others who described the "deplorable conditions" under which mentally ill individuals were housed.

The advent of psychotropic medications and the community mental health movement began a growing philosophical view that mentally ill individuals receive better and more humanitarian treatment in the community than in state hospitals far removed from their homes. It was believed that commitment and institutionalization in many ways deprived these individuals of their civil rights (Lamb, 1992). Not the least of the motivating factors for deinstitutionalization was the financial burden these clients placed on state governments.

In fact, deinstitutionalization has not failed completely. About 50 percent of the mentally ill population—those who have insight into their illness and need for medication—have done reasonably well since leaving the hospital (Torrey, 1997). It is the other 50 percent who lack such insight and often stop taking their medication who end up on the streets.

However, because the vast increases in homelessness did not occur until the 1980s, the release of severely mentally ill people from institutions cannot be solely to blame. A number of other factors have been implicated.

Poverty. Cuts in various government entitlement programs have depleted the allotments available for chronically mentally ill individuals living in the community. The job market is prohibitive for individuals whose behavior is incomprehensible or even frightening to many. The stigma and discrimination associated with mental illness may be diminishing slowly, but it is highly visible to those who suffer from its effects.

A Scarcity of Affordable Housing. Wallsten (1992) states:

> "Economic policies and issues have contributed to the growing numbers and different profiles of the homeless. Urban redevelopment projects eliminated a considerable amount of low-cost housing options for poor people. A growing number of impoverished families have been doubling and tripling up in single housing units as affordable housing becomes more scarce. A sizable proportion of residents in these renewal areas were poor elderly renting rooms in houses, residential hotels, and missions."

In addition, the number of single-room-occupancy (SRO) hotels has diminished drastically. These SRO hotels provided a means of relatively inexpensive housing for chronic psychiatric clients. Although some people believe that these facilities nurtured isolation, they provided adequate shelter from the elements for their occupants. So many individuals currently frequent the shelters of our cities that there is concern that the shelters are becoming mini-institutions for the chronically mentally ill.

Other Factors. The NCH (1999) identified several other factors that may contribute to homelessness. They include:

- **Lack of Affordable Health Care.** For families barely able to scrape together enough money to pay for day-to-day living, a catastrophic illness can create the level of poverty that starts the downward spiral to homelessness.
- **Domestic Violence.** The study by the U.S. Conference of Mayors (1998) revealed that 46 percent identified domestic violence as a primary cause of homelessness. Battered women are often forced to choose between an abusive relationship and homelessness.
- **Addiction Disorders.** For individuals with alcohol or drug addictions, in the absence of appropriate treatment, the chances increase for being forced into life on the street. The NCH (1999) cites the following as obstacles to addiction treatment for homeless persons: lack of health insurance; lack of documentation; waiting lists; scheduling difficulties; daily contact requirements; lack of transportation; ineffective treatment methods; lack of supportive services; and cultural insensitivity.

Community Resources for the Homeless

Interfering Factors. Among the many issues that complicate service planning for the homeless mentally ill is this population's penchant for mobility. This frequent relocation confounds service delivery and interferes with providers' efforts to ensure appropriate care (Bachrach, 1987). Bachrach identifies three types of mobility reflected in the geographic movements of homeless mentally ill individuals:

1. **Residential Instability.** Some chronically mentally ill individuals may be affected by homelessness only

temporarily or intermittently. These individuals are sometimes called the *episodically homeless.*

2. **Seasonal Mobility.** Some of the homeless mentally ill move around within neighborhoods or cities as needs change and based on whether or not they can obtain needed services.

3. **Migration.** Some members of the homeless mentally ill population exhibit continuous unbounded movement over wide geographical areas.

Not all of the homeless mentally ill population are mobile. Some studies have indicated that a large percentage remain in the same location over a number of years. Health care workers must identify movement patterns of the homeless in their area in order to at least try to bring the best care possible to this unique population. This may indeed mean delivering services to those individuals who do not seek out services on their own.

Health Issues. Life as a homeless person can have severe consequences in terms of health. Exposure to the elements, poor diet, sleep deprivation, risk of violence, injuries, and little or no health care lead to a precarious state of health and exacerbate any preexisting illnesses (Glasser, 1994). One of the major afflictions is alcoholism. Currently, alcohol abuse affects an estimated two fifths of the U.S. homeless population, with the majority being men (Glasser, 1994). In a privately funded program of health care for the homeless, researchers found that the alcohol abuser was at greater risk for neurological impairment, heart disease and hypertension, chronic lung disease, gastrointestinal (GI) disorders, hepatic dysfunction, and trauma, in comparison to the rest of the homeless individuals in the program (Wright & Weber, 1987).

Thermoregulation is a health problem for all homeless individuals because of their exposure to all kinds of weather. It is a compounded problem for the homeless alcoholic who spends much time in an altered level of consciousness.

It is difficult to determine whether mental illness is a cause or an effect of homelessness. Wright and Weber (1987) state that behaviors such as rummaging through the garbage for food or urinating in public may seem deviant to some but that in actuality may be adaptations to life on the street. It has been suggested that some homeless individuals may even seek hospitalization in psychiatric institutions in an attempt to get off the streets for a while.

A recent increase in the incidence of tuberculosis, especially the drug-resistant form, has been noted (Glasser, 1994). A number of factors have been implicated in the increase of this disease, including the growth of the number of people living in congregate living situations and an increase of poverty and homelessness (Gostin, 1993).

Dietary deficiencies are a continuing problem for homeless individuals. Not only is the homeless person commonly in a poor nutritional state but the condition itself exacerbates a number of other health problems. Wright and Weber (1987) found that homeless people are significantly more ill than their generational counterparts in the general population, suffering from higher mortality rates and a greater number of serious disorders.

Sexually transmitted diseases are a serious problem for the homeless. In one sample of homeless single adults, almost 8 percent of the men and 11 percent of the women had gonorrhea or syphilis, and one third reported previous infection (Breakey et al., 1989). One of the most serious sexually transmitted diseases prevalent among the homeless is HIV infection. Street life is precarious for individuals whose systems are immunosuppressed by the AIDS virus. Rummaged food scraps are often spoiled, and exposure to the elements is a continuous threat. HIV-infected individuals who stay in **shelters** are often exposed to the infectious diseases of others, which can be life-threatening in their vulnerable condition.

HIV disease is increasing among the homeless population. The NCH (1997) reports that one study revealed a seropositive rate of 2.3 percent for homeless persons under the age of 25. Another suggested that up to 50 percent of persons living with HIV/AIDS are expected to need housing assistance of some kind during their lifetimes.

Homeless children have special health needs. Studies have indicated an increased rate of respiratory infections, minor skin ailments, ear disorders, GI disorders, infestational ailments, developmental delays, and psychological problems among homeless children, when compared with control samples (Rafferty & Shinn, 1991; Wright & Weber, 1987).

Types of Resources Available

Homeless Shelters. The system of shelters for the homeless in the United States varies widely, from converted warehouses that provide cots or floor space on which to sleep overnight, to significant operations that provide a multitude of social and health care services. They are run by volunteers and paid professionals and are sponsored by churches, community governments, and a variety of social agencies.

It is impossible, then, to describe a "typical" shelter. One profile may be described as the provision of lodging, food, and clothing to individuals who are in need of these services. Some shelters also provide medical and psychiatric evaluations, first aid and other health care services, and even referral for case management services by nurses or social workers.

Individuals who seek services from the shelter are generally assigned a bed or cot, issued a set of clean linen, provided a place to shower, shown laundry facilities, and offered a meal in the shelter kitchen or dining hall. Most shelters attempt to separate dormitory areas for men and women, with various consequences for those who violate the rules.

Shelters cover expenses through private and corporate donations, church sponsorships, and government grants. From the outset, shelters were conceptualized as "temporary" accommodations for individuals who needed a place to spend the night. Realistically, they have become permanent lodging for homeless individuals with little hope for improving their situation. Some individuals use shelters for their mailing address.

In the early 1980s, New York City instituted the Work Experience Program (WEP), which required all employable residents to work 20 hours a week for a $12.50 stipend. Evaluation of the program suggested that WEP kept the residents busy and enhanced their self-esteem, while preventing idleness and depression (Human Resources Administration [HRA], 1983). Today, under a comprehensive program of welfare reform, more than 250,000 people have moved through the WEP (HRA, 1998).

Shelters provide a safe and supportive environment for homeless individuals who have no other place to go. Some homeless people who inhabit shelters use the resources offered to improve their lot in life, whereas others become hopelessly dependent on the shelter's provisions. To a few, the availability of a shelter may even mean the difference between life and death.

Health Care Centers and Store-Front Clinics. Some communities have established "street clinics" to serve the homeless population. Many of these clinics are operated by nurse practitioners who work in consultation with physicians in the area. In recent years, some of these **store-front clinics** have provided clinical rotation sites for nursing students in their community health rotation. Some have been staffed by faculties of nursing schools who have established group practices in the community setting.

A wide variety of services are offered at these clinics, including administering medications, assessing vital signs, screening for tuberculosis and other communicable diseases, giving immunizations and flu shots, changing dressings, and administering first aid (Brunner & Suddarth, 1992). Physical and psychosocial assessments, health education, and supportive counseling are also frequent interventions.

Mayo (1992), reporting on the Nurse Clinic for the Homeless at Charleston's Interfaith Crisis Ministry, related that the most frequent health problems for which homeless individuals presented themselves at the clinic were foot injuries and infections; ingrown toenails; respiratory infections; problems with eyes, ears, nose, and throat; skin conditions such as rashes and lice infestation; GI problems including ulcers, flu, vomiting, and diarrhea; and accidental injuries involving musculoskeletal damage from trauma or work-related injuries. Referrals are made

to local hospitals and physicians who provide pro bono services when necessary.

Nursing in store-front clinics for the homeless provides many special challenges, not the least of which is poor working conditions. These clinics often operate under severe budgetary constraints with inadequate staffing, supplies, and equipment, in high-crime neighborhoods in rundown facilities that provide inadequate heat in the winter, poor to no air-conditioning in the summer, broken plumbing, vermin infestation, and a scarcity of secure parking facilities (Brunner & Suddarth, 1992).

Frustration is often high among nurses who work in these clinics, as they are seldom able to see measurable progress in their homeless clients. Maintenance of health management is virtually impossible for many individuals who have no resources outside the health care setting. When return appointments for preventive care are made, the lack of follow-through is high.

Mobile Outreach Units. Outreach programs literally reach out to the homeless in their own environment in an effort to provide health care. Volunteers and paid professionals form teams to drive or walk around and seek out homeless individuals who are in need of assistance. They offer coffee, sandwiches, and blankets in an effort to show concern and establish trust. If assistance can be provided at the site, it is done so. If not, every effort is made to ensure that the individual is linked with a source that can provide the necessary services.

Mobile outreach units provide assistance to homeless individuals who are in need of physical or psychological care. Blau (1992) presents the following report about the Center City Project, established in 1984 by the Philadelphia Office of Mental Health and Mental Retardation to address the special needs of the homeless mentally ill:

> "The project consisted of a network of twenty-one service sites that provided aggressive outreach to the homeless. Careful planning linked services, so that an outreach team could bring someone they engaged on the street to an intake center. From there, the homeless could be referred to a "low-demand" facility to ease their way into the system, and then, as their capacity to tolerate rules increased, to a facility offering specialized care." (p.129)

The emphasis of outreach programs is to accommodate the homeless who refuse to seek treatment elsewhere. Most target the mentally ill segment of the population. When trust has been established, and the individual agrees to come to the team's office, medical and psychiatric treatment is initiated. Involuntary hospitalization is initiated when an individual is deemed harmful to self or others or otherwise meets the criteria for being considered "gravely disabled."

The Homeless Client and the Nursing Process. Nursing process with the homeless client is demonstrated by the following case study:

CASE STUDY

ASSESSMENT

Joe, age 46, is brought to the Community Health Clinic by two of his peers, who report: "He just had a fit. He needs a drink bad!" Joe is dirty, unkempt, has visible tremors of the upper extremities, and is weak enough to require assistance when ambulating. He is cooperative as the nurse completes the intake assessment. He is coherent, although thought processes are slow. He is disoriented to time and place. He appears somewhat frightened as he scans the unfamiliar surroundings. He is unable to tell the nurse when he had his last drink. He reports no physical injury, and none is observable.

Joe carries a small bag with a few personal items inside, among which is a VA Benefit Card, identifying him as a veteran of the Vietnam War. The nurse finds a cot for Joe to lie down, ensures that his vital signs are stable, and telephones the number on the VA card.

The clinic nurse discovers that Joe is well known to the admissions personnel at the VA. He has a 24-year history of schizophrenia, with numerous hospitalizations. At the time of his last discharge, he was taking fluphenazine (Prolixin) 10 mg twice a day. He told the clinic nurse that he took the medication for a few months after he got out of the hospital but then did not have the prescription refilled. He could not remember when he had last taken fluphenazine.

Joe also has a long history of alcohol-related disorders and has been through the VA substance rehabilitation program three times. He has no home address and receives his VA disability benefit checks at a shelter address. He reports that he has no family. The nurse makes arrangements for VA personnel to drive Joe from the clinic to the VA hospital, where he is admitted for detoxification. She sets up a case management file for Joe and arranges with the hospital to have Joe return to the clinic after discharge.

DIAGNOSIS/OUTCOME IDENTIFICATION

The following nursing diagnosis was formulated for Joe:

Altered health maintenance related to ineffective coping skills, evidenced by abuse of alcohol, lack of follow-through with neuroleptic medication, and lack of personal hygiene.

Ongoing criteria were selected as outcomes for Joe. They include:

1. Follows the rules of the group home and maintains his residency status.
2. Attends weekly sessions of group therapy at the VA day treatment program.
3. Attends weekly sessions of Alcoholics Anonymous and maintains sobriety.
4. Reports regularly to the health clinic for injections of fluphenazine.
5. Volunteers at the VA hospital 3 days a week.
6. Secures and retains permanent employment.

PLAN/IMPLEMENTATION

During Joe's hospitalization, the clinic nurse remained in contact with his case. Joe received complete physical and dental examinations and treatment during his hospital stay. The clinic nurse attended the treatment team meeting for Joe as his outpatient case manager. It was decided at the meeting to try giving Joe injections of fluphenazine decanoate because of his history of noncompliance with his daily oral medications. The clinic nurse would administer the injection every 4 weeks.

At Joe's follow-up clinic visit the nurse explains to Joe that she has found a group home where he may live with others who have personal circumstances similar to his. At the group home, meals will be provided and the group home manager will ensure that Joe's basic needs are fulfilled. A criterion for remaining at the residence is for Joe to remain alcohol free. Joe is agreeable to these living arrangements.

With Joe's concurrence, the clinic nurse also performs the following interventions:

1. Goes shopping with Joe to purchase some new clothing, allowing Joe to make decisions as independently as possible.
2. Helps Joe move into the group home and introduces him to the manager and residents.
3. Helps Joe change his address from the shelter to the group home so that he may continue to receive his VA benefits.
4. Enrolls Joe in the weekly group therapy sessions of the day treatment facility connected with the VA hospital.
5. Helps Joe locate the nearest Alcoholics Anonymous group and identifies a sponsor who will ensure that Joe gets to the meetings.
6. Sets up a clinic appointment for Joe to return in 4 weeks for his fluphenazine injection; telephones Joe 1 day in advance to remind him of his appointment.
7. Instructs Joe to return to or call the clinic if any of the following symptoms occur: sore throat, fever, nausea and vomiting, severe headache, difficulty urinating, tremors, skin rash, or yellow skin or eyes.
8. Assists Joe in securing transportation to and from appointments.
9. Encourages Joe to set realistic goals for his life and offers recognition for follow-through.
10. When Joe is ready, discusses employment alternatives with him; suggests the possibility of starting with a volunteer job (perhaps as a VA hospital volunteer).

EVALUATION

Evaluation of the nursing process with the homeless mentally ill must be highly individualized. Statistics show that chances for relapse with this population are high. Therefore, it is extremely important that outcome criteria be realistic so as not to set the client up for failure.

RURAL MENTAL HEALTH NURSING

Approximately 25 percent of the U.S. population reside in rural areas. These rural communities make up a type of subculture with their own set of beliefs, attitudes, and values that differ comparatively with the urban population. These differences affect the way in which individuals in the rural areas view mental health and mental illness and the care of mentally ill individuals.

Mental health assistance is much less readily available to rural residents than it is to individuals who reside in urban areas. Not only do fewer general hospitals exist in rural America, but psychiatric services are seldom provided within these institutions. Because of this, rural residents often must travel long distances to procure mental health services. In reality, only about half of rural residents with emotional problems ever seek treatment (Hendrix, 1990), and most commonly, the mental health services are provided by a general practitioner, public health nurse, or social service worker. Knowledge of crisis intervention techniques is essential for the rural mental health nurse, as the denial of emotional illness and delay in treatment often necessitates emergency services.

A number of characteristics have been identified in describing the rural population. In comparison to the population in general, rural residents are commonly more religious, conservative, traditional, family-centered, clannish, inflexible, and work-oriented (Flax et al., 1979). These particular values influence not only the way in which rural residents interpret psychopathological behaviors but also the initiative to seek treatment and the type of treatment sought.

The rural mental health nurse must by necessity serve as a generalist. That is, he or she must be able to assess the physical and emotional needs of individuals and make referrals when needed. He or she should also possess the ability to intervene with a variety of skills in a diversity of situations. As a practitioner, the rural mental health nurse may staff a community health center, make home visits, or even serve as primary therapist in crisis intervention, and short- and long-term individual counseling.

Trust may be difficult to establish in the rural community. Because of the stigma attached to mental illness and the ideology that "one takes care of one's own problems," it is less likely that individuals would seek treatment for emotional problems but more likely that they would seek assistance for related physical complaints, as these would be more socially acceptable. Personal disclosure is difficult among individuals who "know everyone and everyone's business." Suspicions surrounding confidentiality may interfere with treatment in group situations.

The role of educator is most significant to the rural mental health nurse. Because many individuals who live in rural settings have had little or no health education, the choice of topics is vast. Examples range from basic nutrition and hygiene to information about numerous physical illnesses, how to prevent them, identify symptoms, and treat them. The rural mental health nurse also has an opportunity to decrease stigma surrounding mental illness by increasing knowledge about pathological behaviors and how to prevent and treat them. Information can be dispensed in a variety of ways, including during community health fairs and club meetings, in schools and churches, and in the home or community health clinic.

Change is difficult under the best of circumstances. Because of the characteristic of inflexibility identified as common among rural residents, change presents an even greater challenge for the rural mental health nurse. But the opportunity for change is bountiful, and with enough patience and fortitude the rural mental health nurse can serve as change agent on many levels, including individual, community, state, and even national. Expansion of mental health services in rural areas is sorely needed, and the legislative arena is the most probable source for assistance in generating the resources required to provide these services. A keen opportunity exists for rural mental health nurses to become active in the political process, particularly at this time of volatile health care reform.

Outreach programs have been shown to be effective in providing care to underserved areas, and mental health nurses are important members of the team that provides these services (Santos et al., 1993). Nurses in outreach programs provide ongoing assessment and intervention to rural residents within their own homes. For some chronically mentally ill individuals, this home treatment may be the only alternative to institutionalization. Not only are these outreach services the "least restrictive" alternative, but they have also been shown to be very efficient and cost-effective without diminishing quality of care.

In 1989, the ANA's Councils on Community Health and Gerontological Nursing issued a statement on rural nursing. This ANA statement is presented in Table 38.4.

SUMMARY

The trend in psychiatric care is shifting from that of inpatient hospitalization to a focus of outpatient care within the community. This trend is largely due to the need for greater cost-effectiveness in the provision of medical care to the masses. The community mental health movement began in the 1960s with the closing of state hospitals and the deinstitutionalization of many chronically mentally ill individuals.

Mental health care within the community targets primary prevention (reducing the incidence of mental disorders within the population), secondary prevention (reducing the prevalence of psychiatric illness by shortening the course of the illness), and tertiary prevention (reducing

TABLE 38.4   AMERICAN NURSES' ASSOCIATION STATEMENT ON RURAL NURSING

Rural Americans are now more than ever experiencing significant obstacles to attaining the nation's goal of a healthy America. The rural health care system is fragile and often unable to provide accessible, high-quality, comprehensive, coordinated health care services. Frequently rural communities have a maldistribution and a shortage in numbers and types of qualified health providers.

The crisis in rural health. Compared with urban residents, rural Americans have higher infant and maternal morbidity and mortality rates, a higher incidence of occupational injuries, considerable exposure to pollution, and a greater prevalence of serious health conditions. Individuals who live in rural areas give less positive self-reports of health status, compared with their nonrural counterparts. The rural economic crisis is reflected among rural residents in an increasing incidence of stress-related behaviors and illness. Disease prevention and health promotion programs are hampered in rural America by economic barriers such as inadequate or unavailable health insurance coverage. Available and affordable transportation is often nonexistent, rendering even less accessible those services that might be available, particularly for children, the poor, and the elderly.

Rural nurse supply and demand. Data and further research are needed to explore more fully the issues of supply and demand for rural nurses. Compensation for rural nurses lags behind that for urban nurses, despite rural similarities to the work conditions that have led to recent increases in urban nurse compensation: increased patient acuity, an older client population with special needs, and increasingly complex health-care needs in institutional and community settings. The complexity and diversity of their client/patient mix challenge rural nurses to be generalists in an era of specialization, requiring proficiency in a wide range of nursing practice areas. Other allied personnel are absent or in short supply in rural settings, to the extent that rural nurses often perform physical therapy, respiratory therapy, and many other skills as part of their duties. In addition, rural nurses have limited opportunities for career development, professional continuing education, advanced education in nursing, and professional networking. Despite these stressors, rural staff nurses and nurse leaders are performing at an outstanding level. Rural public health nurses may be the only health professionals in some counties. Without nurse anesthetists, rural hospitals would certainly have to significantly curtail or close surgical suites.

Nursing's approaches to problems in rural health. The American Nurses' Association is concerned about the validity and quality of health services for rural residents. The Association is also concerned about the image and low visibility of rural nursing. Activities are underway, however, to address the problems affecting rural nursing. A number of innovative programs have developed across the nation that not only attract potential rural residents into nursing but may also provide rural nurses more accessible routes to baccalaureate and higher degrees. The nation's nursing schools have been preparing an increasing number of nurse practitioners, nurse midwives, and nurses with other advanced preparation at the graduate level who form the cadre of those prepared for leadership in rural nursing. A body of knowledge is growing that describes the concerns and proposed solutions to problems of recruitment, retention, and other factors affecting rural nursing.

ANA's recommendations on access, education, and payment. Programs and incentives are needed to ensure that rural residents have access to nurses. Other programs are needed to develop and demonstrate how nursing knowledge can be used in service to rural citizens. Providing student nurses with rural clinical placements has helped address image and recruitment problems for rural nurses. Support for nursing education programs is needed to develop similar plans that might consider preceptorships as a cost-effective method of providing rural clinical placements. To help meet the networking needs of rural nurse leadership, graduate nurse clinical experiences and consultation experiences with nursing colleagues in rural settings should be facilitated. These clinical experiences would be for postbasic nurses completing their baccalaureate, as well as master's degree nursing students. Loans and/or scholarships need to be provided to rural residents willing to pursue a career, or a second career, in nursing. Accessible, affordable continuing professional education is essential if rural nurses are to define the practice of rural nursing and achieve the proficiency and career development characteristic of professional nursing practice.

Access to nursing is a necessity if rural health delivery systems are to be responsive to needs, family centered, and prevention focused. It is essential to obtain direct reimbursement for the services provided by all rural nurses, particularly by nurse practitioners, nurse midwives, and nurses with other advanced preparation, to ensure that nursing can continue to demonstrate the unique contributions nurses can make in primary care, in nursing care management, in disease prevention, and in health promotion. All nurses are cost-effective providers of high-quality care, but in this era of cost containment they may not be hired by employers if direct reimbursement is not available for their services.

The American Nurses' Association urges continued enthusiastic support for these and other efforts directed toward the well-being of rural Americans.

---

the residual defects that are associated with severe or chronic mental illness). Primary prevention focuses on identification of populations at risk for mental illness, increasing their ability to cope with stress, and targeting and diminishing harmful forces within the environment. The focus of secondary prevention is accomplished through early identification of problems and prompt initiation of effective treatment. Tertiary prevention focuses on pre-venting complications of the illness and promoting rehabilitation that is directed toward achievement of the individual's maximum level of functioning.

Registered nurses serve as providers of psychiatric/mental health care in the community setting. Nurses may practice at the basic level or at the advanced practice level, depending on their education, experience, and credentialing. Many nurses serve as case managers for chronically

R E S E A R C H   N O T E

Managing health problems among homeless women with children in a transitional shelter. *Image: Journal of Nursing Scholarship* **(1997, Spring), 29(1), 33–37.** Hatton, D.C.

Description of the Study: This study was conducted to examine the health concerns of homeless women with children, to analyze how they managed various ailments, and when and how they sought assistance from health care providers. The study was conducted at a shelter for homeless women which serves 600 to 700 women a year. The convenience sample included 13 Latina, 11 white, and 6 African-American women ranging in age from 20 to 30. All but two of the women had children, and the two without children were pregnant. Data were gathered through in-depth, semistructured interviews. Subjects were asked to evaluate their health, express any concerns they had about particular diseases, discuss the last time they saw a health care provider, describe various symptoms they experienced and how they managed them, and report how they decided on various treatments.

Results of the Study: Typically, the respondents reported that they dealt with health problems prior to entering the shelter by "overcoming it alone." They ignored signs and symptoms of illness and hoped they would go away. As for lack of management of health care problems, four patterns of consequence emerged: shame (too embarrassed to seek help for a specific problem); fear (afraid that if they admit to having some kind of problem they may lose their children); lack of information (limited information about their children's and their own health needs and where to seek it); and lack of eligibility (unable to seek care or medication because could not afford it and were ineligible for government assistance). Most of the women, when asked to describe their health, tended to describe their mental health concerns and minimize physical concerns. They reported alcohol/drug abuse, bipolar disorders, depression, suicidal behaviors, self-mutilation, and anxiety, while giving little consideration to conditions such as cystitis, otitis media, and sexually transmitted disease.

Comments: The author concluded that, even when the homeless women with children received supportive services from their transitional living situation, they continued to have difficulty knowing when health problems needed professional attention, and they generally attempted to deal with the problems by overcoming them alone. Clinical nursing interventions that address shame, fear, lack of information, and eligibility for services could improve health outcomes among women and children living in transitional shelters.

mentally ill persons, to ensure that a wide range of services are made available as needed. Case management has been shown to enhance the client's functioning by increasing ability to solve problems, improving work and socialization skills, promoting leisure-time activities, and endeavoring to diminish dependency on others.

Nurses provide outpatient care for chronically mentally ill individuals in community mental health centers, in day and evening treatment programs, in partial hospitalization programs, in community residential facilities, and with psychiatric home health care (addressed in Chapter 41).

The homeless mentally ill provide a special challenge for the community mental health nurse. Care is provided within homeless shelters, at health care centers or storefront clinics, and through mobile outreach programs.

The mental health needs of individuals who live in rural areas are largely underserved. Nurses who choose to work in these areas encounter enormous challenge as well as abundant opportunities for creating positive change. The rural mental health nurse can be a compelling force for providing quality care at all three levels of prevention to residents of rural areas of our country.

REVIEW QUESTIONS

SELF-EXAMINATION/LEARNING EXERCISE

Select the answer that is most appropriate for each of the following questions.

1. Which of the following represents a nursing intervention at the primary level of prevention?
   a. Teaching a class in parent effectiveness training.
   b. Leading a group of adolescents in drug rehabilitation.
   c. Referring a married couple for sex therapy.
   d. Leading a support group for battered women.

2. Which of the following represents a nursing intervention at the secondary level of prevention?
   a. Teaching a class about menopause to middle-aged women.
   b. Providing support in the emergency room to a rape victim.
   c. Leading a support group for women in transition.
   d. Making monthly visits to the home of a client with schizophrenia to ensure medication compliance.

3. Which of the following represents a nursing intervention at the tertiary level of prevention?
   a. Serving as case manager for a mentally ill homeless client.
   b. Leading a support group for newly retired men.
   c. Teaching prepared childbirth classes.
   d. Caring for a depressed widow in the hospital.

4. John, a homeless person, has just come to live in the shelter. The shelter nurse is assigned to his care. Which of the following is a *priority* intervention on the part of the nurse?
   a. Referring John to a social worker.
   b. Developing a plan of care for John.
   c. Conducting a behavioral and needs assessment on John.
   d. Helping John apply for Social Security benefits.

5. John has a history of paranoid schizophrenia and noncompliance with medications. Which of the following medications might be the best choice of neuroleptic for John?
   a. Haldol.
   b. Navane.
   c. Lithium carbonate.
   d. Prolixin decanoate.

6. Ann is a rural mental health nurse. She has just received an order to begin regular visits to Mrs. W, a 78-year-old widow who lives alone. Mrs. W's primary care physician has diagnosed her as depressed. Based on knowledge of rural residents, which of the following statements would most likely apply to Mrs. W?
   a. She will most likely have little difficulty establishing trust with the nurse.
   b. She will probably resist therapy for emotional illness.
   c. She will most likely welcome the nurse without question.
   d. She would most likely do better in a group situation than one-to-one with the nurse.

7. Based on a needs assessment, which of the following problems would Ann address during her first visit?
   a. Dysfunctional grieving.
   b. Social isolation.
   c. Risk for injury.
   d. Sleep pattern disturbance.

8. Mrs. W says to Ann, "What's the use? I don't have anything to live for anymore." Which is the best response on the part of the nurse?

    a. "Of course you do, Mrs. W. Why would you say such a thing?"

    b. "You seem so sad. I'm going to do my best to cheer you up."

    c. "Let's talk about why you are feeling this way."

    d. "Have you been thinking about harming yourself in any way?"

9. The physician orders trazadone (Desyrel) for Mrs. W, 150 mg to take at bedtime. Which of the following statements about this medication would be appropriate for Ann to make in teaching Mrs. W about trazadone?

    a. "You may feel dizzy when you stand up, so go slowly when you get up from sitting or lying down."

    b. "You must be sure and not eat any chocolate while you are taking this medicine."

    c. "We will need to draw a sample of blood to send to the lab every month while you are on this medication."

    d. "If you don't feel better right away with this medicine, the doctor can order a different kind for you."

10. Which of the following statements is true about rural mental health services?

    a. Services are generally adequate to meet the demands.

    b. Rural mental health nurses must be generalists in an era of specialization.

    c. Rural residents are compliant and eager to accept opportunities for change.

    d. Direct reimbursement for services by rural nurses historically has not been a problem.

REFERENCES

American Nurses' Association (ANA). (1988). *Nursing case management.* Kansas City, MO: American Nurses' Association.

American Nurses' Association (ANA). (1989). *A statement on rural nursing.* Kansas City, MO: American Nurses' Association.

American Nurses' Association (ANA). (1994). *A statement on psychiatric-mental health clinical nursing practice and standards of psychiatric-mental health clinical nursing practice.* Washington, DC: American Nurses Publishing.

American Psychiatric Association (APA). (1994). *Diagnostic and statistical manual of mental disorders* (4th ed.). Washington, DC: American Psychiatric Association.

Bachrach, L.L. (1987). Geographic mobility and the homeless mentally ill. *Hospital and Community Psychiatry, 38*(1), 27–28.

Blau, J. (1992). *The visible poor: Homelessness in the United States.* New York: Oxford University Press.

Bower, K.A. (1992). *Case management by nurses.* Washington, DC: American Nurses Publishing.

Breakey, W.R., et al. (1989). Health and mental health problems of homeless men and women in Baltimore. *Journal of the American Medical Association, 262*(10), 1352–1357.

Brunner, L.S., & Suddarth, D.S. (1992). *Textbook of medical-surgical nursing* (7th ed.). Philadelphia: J.B. Lippincott.

Caplan, G. (1964). *Principles of preventive psychiatry.* New York: Basic Books.

Chamberlain, J.G. (1983). The role of the federal government in development of psychiatric nursing. *Journal of Psychosocial Nursing and Mental Health Services, 21*(4), 11–18.

Dato, C., & Rafferty, M. (1985). The homeless mentally ill. *International Nursing Review, 32*(6), 170–173.

Ebersole, P., & Gustin, K. (1979). The middle-aged family. In D.P. Hymovich & M.U. Barnard (Eds.), *Family health care* (2nd ed.). New York: McGraw-Hill.

Erikson, E. (1963). *Childhood and society* (2nd ed.). New York: W.W. Norton.

Flax, J.W., et al. (1979). *Mental health and rural America: An overview and annotated bibliography.* Washington, DC: National Institute of Mental Health.

Glasser, I. (1994). *Homelessness in global perspective.* New York: G.K. Hall.

Gostin, L.O. (1993). Controlling the resurgent tuberculosis epidemic. *Journal of the American Medical Association, 262*(2), 255–261.

Hendricks, J., & Hendricks, C.D. (1977). *Aging in mass society.* Cambridge, MA: Winthrop Publishers.

Hendrix, M.J. (1990). The rural community mental health nurse. In A.W. Burgess (Ed.), *Psychiatric nursing in the hospital and the community* (5th ed.). Norwalk, CT: Appleton & Lange.

Holmes, T., & Rahe, R. (1967). The social readjustment rating scale. *Journal of Psychosomatic Research, 11*, 213–218.

Human Resources Administration (HRA). (1983). *Harlem shelter work experience program.* New York: HRA.

Human Resources Administration (HRA). (1998). *Inhouse report, Winter 1998.* New York: HRA.

Hyde, J.S. (1986). *Understanding human sexuality* (3rd ed.). New York: McGraw-Hill.

Kaplan, H.I., & Sadock, B.J. (1998). *Synopsis of psychiatry: Behavioral sciences/clinical psychiatry* (8th ed.). Baltimore: Williams & Wilkins.

Kaplan, H.I., Sadock, B.J., & Grebb, J.A. (1994). *Synopsis of psychiatry: Behavioral sciences/clinical psychiatry* (7th ed.). Baltimore: Williams & Wilkins.

Koegel, P., Burnam, M.A., & Baumohl, J. (1996). The causes of homelessness. In J. Baumohl (Ed.). *Homelessness in America.* Phoenix, AZ: Oryx Press.

Krauss, J.B. (1993). *Health care reform: Essential mental health services.* Waldorf, MD: American Nurses Publishing Distribution Center.

Lamb, H.R. (1992). Perspectives on effective advocacy for homeless mentally ill persons. *Hospital and Community Psychiatry, 43*(12), 1209–1212.

Lancaster, J. (1980). *Community mental health nursing: An ecological perspective.* St. Louis: C.V. Mosby.

Lazarus, R.S., & DeLongis, A. (1983). Psychological stress and coping in aging. *American Psychologist, 38*, 245–254.

Mahler, M., Pine, F., & Bergman, A. (1975). *The psychological birth of the human infant.* New York: Basic Books.

Mayo, K. (1992, November–December). Homelessness in the South: Excerpts from student journals. *Imprint*, 64–67.

McCabe, S.N. (1979). Anticipatory guidance for families with infants. In D.P. Hymovich & M.U. Barnard (Eds.), *Family health care: Developmental and situational crises* (2nd ed.). New York: McGraw-Hill.

Murray, R., & Zentner, J. (1997). *Health assessment and promotion strategies through the life span* (6th ed.). Stamford, CT: Appleton & Lange.

National Coalition for the Homeless (NCH). (1997). *HIV/AIDS and homelessness.* [On-line]. Available: http://www.ari.net/nch/hivaids. html.

National Coalition for the Homeless (NCH). (1999). *How many people experience homelessness?* [On-line]. Available: http://nch.ari.net/numbers.html.

Pasquali, E.A., Arnold, H.M., & DeBasio, N. (1989). *Mental health nursing: A holistic approach* (3rd ed.). St. Louis: C.V. Mosby.

Pittman, D.C. (1989). Nursing case management: Holistic care for the deinstitutionalized chronically mentally ill. *Journal of Psychosocial Nursing, 27*(11), 23–27.

Pittman, D.C., Parson, R., & Peterson, R.W. (1990). Easing the way: A multifaceted approach to day treatment. *Journal of Psychosocial Nursing, 28*(11), 6–11.

Rafferty, Y., & Shinn, M. (1991). The impact of homelessness on children. *American Psychologist, 46*(11), 1170–1179.

Reichard, S., Livson, F., & Peterson, P.G. (1962). *Aging and personality: A study of 87 older men.* New York: John Wiley.

Richie, F., & Lusky, K. (1987). Psychiatric home health nursing: A new role in community mental health. *Community Mental Health Journal, 23*(3), 229–235.

Santos, A.B., et al. (1993). Providing assertive community treatment for severely mentally ill patients in a rural area. *Hospital and Community Psychiatry, 44*(1), 34–39.

Sheehy, G. (1976). *Passages: Predictable crises of adult life.* New York: Bantam Books.

Smoyak, S.A. (1991). Psychosocial nursing in public versus private sectors: An introduction. *Journal of Psychosocial Nursing, 29*(8), 6–12.

Susser, E., Conover, S., & Struening, E.L. (1990). Mental illness in the homeless: Problems of epidemiologic method in surveys of the 1980s. *Community Mental Health Journal, 26*(5), 391–414.

Swearingen, L. (1987). Transitional day treatment: An individualized goal-oriented approach. *Archives of Psychiatric Nursing, 1*(2), 104–110.

Talley, B.S., & Coleman, M.A. (1992). The chronically mentally ill: Issues of individual freedom versus societal neglect. *Journal of Community Health Nursing, 9*(1), 33–41.

Torrey, E.F. (1997). *Madness in the streets.* [On-line]. Available: http://www.nami-nyc-metro.org/Torrey/deinst.html.

U.S. Conference of Mayors (USCM). (1998). *A status report on hunger and homelessness in America's cities: 1998.* Washington, DC: U.S. Conference of Mayors.

Wallsten, S.M. (1992). Geriatric mental health: A portrait of homelessness. *Journal of Psychosocial Nursing, 30*(9), 20–24.

Wilkinson, L. (1991). A collaborative model: Ambulatory pharmacotherapy for chronic psychiatric patients. *Journal of Psychosocial Nursing, 29*(12), 26–29.

Wilson, H.S., & Kneisl, C.R. (1992). *Psychiatric nursing* (4th ed.). Menlo Park, CA: Addison-Wesley Health Sciences Division.

Wright, J.D., & Weber, E. (1987). *Homelessness and health.* Washington, DC: McGraw-Hill's Healthcare Information Center.

Zander, K. (1988). Managed care within acute care settings: Design and implementation via nursing case management. *Health Care Supervisor, 6*(2), 27–43.

Bibliography

Bachrach, L.L., Santiago, J.M., & Berren, M.R. (1990). Homeless mentally ill patients in the community: Results of a general hospital emergency room study. *Community Mental Health Journal, 26*(5), 415–423.

Bassuk, E.L. (1990). Who are the homeless families? Characteristics of sheltered mothers and children. *Community Mental Health Journal, 26*(5), 425–434.

Bryson, K.K., et al. (1990). Brief admission program: An alliance of inpatient care and outpatient case management. *Journal of Psychosocial Nursing, 28*(12), 19–23.

Carr, S., Murray R., Harrington, Z., & Oge, J. (1998). Discharged residents' satisfaction with transitional housing for the homeless. *Journal of Psychosocial Nursing, 36*(7), 27–33.

Chafetz, L. (1990). Withdrawal from the homeless mentally ill. *Community Mental Health Journal, 26*(5), 449–461.

Connolly, P.M. (1991). Services for the underserved: A nurse-managed center for the chronically mentally ill. *Journal of Psychosocial Nursing, 29*(1), 15–20.

Drew, N. (1991). Combating the social isolation of chronic mental illness. *Journal of Psychosocial Nursing, 29*(6), 14–17.

Goering, P., et al. (1992). Gender differences among clients of a case management program for the homeless. *Hospital and Community Psychiatry, 43*(2), 160–165.

Goldfinger, S.M. (1990). Introduction: Perspectives on the homeless mentally ill. *Community Mental Health Journal, 26*(5), 387–390.

Harvey, S., & Seelman, M. (1991, March). Development of a mental health home care program. *Caring,* 20–22.

Henry, J.K. (1997, March–April). Community nursing centers: Models of nurse managed care. *Journal of Obstetric, Gynecologic, and Neonatal Nursing, 26,* 224–228.

Hochberger, J.M., & Fisher-James, L. (1992). A discharge group for chronically mentally ill: Easing the way. *Journal of Psychosocial Nursing, 30*(4), 25–28.

Hunter, J.K. (1992, December). Making a difference for homeless patients. *RN,* 48–53.

Jeffers, J.M., & Okeson, D.L. (1992, November–December). Homelessness in the Midwest. *Imprint,* 70–72.

Kline, E.N., & Saperstein, A.B. (1992). Homeless women: The context of an urban shelter. *Nursing Clinics of North America, 27*(4), 885–899.

Kozlak, J., & Thobaben, M. (1992). Treating the elderly mentally ill at home. *Perspectives in Psychiatric Care, 28*(2), 31–35.

Leifer, C., & Young, E.W. (1997, October). Homeless lesbians: Psychology of the hidden, the disenfranchised, and the forgotten. *Journal of Psychosocial Nursing and Mental Health Services, 35,* 28–33.

Lehman, L., & Kelly, J.H. (1993). Nursing interventions for anxiety, depression, and suspiciousness in the home care setting. *Home Healthcare Nurse, 11*(3), 35–40.

Lenehan, G.P. (1998, February). Free clinics and parish nursing offer unique rewards. *Journal of Emergency Nursing, 24,* 3–4.

Lindsey, A.M., & Gottesman, M.M. (1992, November–December). Overview: Homelessness in America. *Imprint,* 60–62.

Lindy, D.C., et al. (1991, March). The mobile crisis service. *Caring,* 29–31.

Martin, M.A. (1990). The homeless mentally ill and community-based care: Changing a mindset. *Community Mental Health Journal, 26*(5), 435–447.

Maurin, J.T. (1990). Case management: Caring for psychiatric clients. *Journal of Psychosocial Nursing, 28*(7), 6–14.

McDaniel, C. (1990). Reorganization of community psychiatric services by professional nurses. *Issues in Mental Health Nursing, 11,* 397–405.

Minick, P., et al. (1998, June). Nurses' perceptions of people who are homeless. *Western Journal of Nursing Research, 20,* 356–369.

Mound, B., et al. (1991). The expanded role of nurse case managers. *Journal of Psychosocial Nursing, 29*(6), 18–22.

Murray, R.B., & Baier, M. (1993). Use of therapeutic milieu in a community setting. *Journal of Psychosocial Nursing, 31*(10), 11–16.

Pessin, N., et al. (1991, March). Bringing the mental health clinic to the home. *Caring,* 24–28.

Power, J. (1991, May). Expanding the role of community mental health nurses. *The Canadian Nurse,* 20–21.

Shea, C.A. (1993). Mental health care reform: A historic town meeting of psychiatric nurses. *Journal of Psychosocial Nursing, 31*(8), 30–33.

Sheehy, G. (1993). *Menopause: The silent passage.* New York: Simon & Schuster.

Susser, E., Goldfinger, S.M., & White, A. (1990). Some clinical approaches to the homeless mentally ill. *Community Mental Health Journal, 26*(5), 463–479.

Testani-Dufour, L., Green, L., Green, R., & Carter, K.F. (1996). Establishing outreach health services for homeless persons: An emerging role for nurse managers. *Journal of Community Health Nursing, 13,* 221–235.

VanDongen, C.J., & Jambunathan, J. (1992). Pilot study results: The psychiatric RN case manager. *Journal of Psychosocial Nursing, 30*(11), 11–14.

CULTURAL CONCEPTS RELEVANT TO PSYCHIATRIC/MENTAL HEALTH NURSING

CHAPTER OUTLINE

OBJECTIVES

INTRODUCTION

HOW DO CULTURES DIFFER?

APPLICATION OF THE NURSING PROCESS

SUMMARY

REVIEW QUESTIONS

KEY TERMS

culture
ethnicity
stereotyping
territoriality

density
distance
folk medicine
shaman

yin and yang
curandero
curandera

OBJECTIVES

After reading this chapter, the student will be able to:

1. Define and differentiate between *culture* and *ethnicity*.
2. Describe six phenomena on which to identify cultural differences.
3. Identify cultural variances, based on the six phenomena, for
   a. Northern European Americans.
   b. African Americans.
   c. Native Americans.
   d. Asian Americans.
   e. Latino Americans.
   f. Western European Americans.
4. Apply the nursing process in the care of individuals from various cultural groups.

hat is **culture?** How does it differ from **ethnicity?** Why are these questions important? The answers lie in the changing face of America. Immigration is not new in the United States. Indeed, most U.S. citizens are either immigrants or descendents of immigrants. This pattern continues because of the many individuals who want to take advantage of the technological growth and upward mobility that exists in this country. Gordon (1995) states:

> "Although immigration is not new in the United States, its complexion has changed. The fact that the new immigrants are people of color has had a decided impact on many industries, health care included. The Bureau of Labor Statistics estimates that by the year 2005 there will be a total of 151 million people either in the work force or looking for work, an increase of 26 million from 1990. The bureau predicts a 32 percent increase in African Americans, a 75 percent increase in Hispanics, and a 74 percent increase in Asians, Native Americans, Pacific Islanders, Alaskan Natives, and others."

Culture describes a particular society's entire way of living, encompassing shared patterns of belief, feeling, and knowledge that guide people's conduct and are passed down from generation to generation. Ethnicity is a somewhat narrower term, and relates to people who identify with each other because of a shared heritage (Griffith & Gonzalez, 1994).

Why is this important? Cultural influences affect human behavior, the interpretation of human behavior, and the response to human behavior. It is therefore essential for nurses to understand the effects of these cultural influences if they are to work effectively with this diverse population. Caution must be taken, however, not to assume that all individuals who share a culture or ethnic group are clones. This constitutes **stereotyping,** and must be avoided. Geissler (1994) states, "The different values found within one culture may be as numerous as the variations found when comparing two different cultures." Every individual must be appreciated for his or her uniqueness.

This chapter explores the ways in which various cultures differ. The nursing process is applied to the delivery of psychiatric/mental health nursing care for individuals from the following cultural groups: Northern European Americans, African Americans, Native Americans, Asian Americans, Latino Americans, and Western European Americans.

HOW DO CULTURES DIFFER?

Giger and Davidhizar (1995) suggest six cultural phenomena that vary with application and use but yet are evidenced among all cultural groups: (1) communication, (2) space, (3) social organization, (4) time, (5) environmental control, and (6) biological variations.

Communication

All verbal and nonverbal behavior in the presence of another individual is communication. Therapeutic communication has always been considered an essential part of the nursing process and represents a critical element in the curricula of most schools of nursing. Communication has its roots in culture. Cultural mores, norms, ideas, and customs provide the basis for our way of thinking. Cultural values are learned and differ from society to society. Communication is expressed through language (the spoken vocabulary), paralanguage (the voice quality, intonation, rhythm, and speed of the spoken word), and gestures (touch, facial expression, eye movements, body posture, and physical appearance). The nurse who is planning care must have an understanding of the client's needs and expectations as they are being communicated. Being a third party, an interpreter often complicates matters, but one may be necessary when the client does not speak the same language as the nurse. However, interpreting is a very complex process that requires a keen sensitivity to cultural nuances, and not just the translating of words into another language.

Space

Spatial determinants relate to the place where the communication occurs and encompass the concepts of **territoriality, density,** and **distance.** Territoriality refers to the innate tendency to own space. The need for territoriality is met only if the individual has control of a space, can establish rules for that space, and is able to defend the space against invasion or misuse by others (Giger & Davidhizar, 1995). Density refers to the number of people within a given environmental space and has been shown to influence interpersonal interaction. Distance is the means by which various cultures use space to communicate. Hall (1966) identified three primary dimensions of space in interpersonal interactions in the Western culture: the intimate zone (0 to 18 inches), the personal zone (18 inches to 3 feet), and the social zone (3 to 6 feet).

Social Organization

Cultural behavior is socially acquired through a process called acculturation, which involves acquiring knowledge and internalizing values (Giger & Davidhizar, 1995). Children are acculturated by observing adults within their social organizations. Social organizations include families, religious groups, and ethnic groups.

Time

An awareness of the concept of time is a gradual learning process. Some cultures place great importance on values that are measured by clock time. Punctuality and efficiency are highly valued in the United States. Other cultures are actually scornful of clock time. For example, peasants in Algeria live with a total indifference to the passage of clock time and despise haste in human affairs (Giger & Davidhizar, 1995). Other cultural implications regarding time have to do with perception of time orientation. Whether individuals are present-oriented or future-oriented in their perception of time influences many aspects of their lives.

Environmental Control

This variable has to do with the degree to which individuals perceive that they have control over their environment. Cultural beliefs and practices influence how an individual responds to the environment during periods of wellness and illness. To provide culturally appropriate care, the nurse should not only respect the individual's unique beliefs but should also have an understanding of how these beliefs can be used to promote optimal health in the client's environment (Giger & Davidhizar, 1995).

Biological Variations

Biological differences exist among people in various racial groups (Giger & Davidhizar, 1995). These differences include body structure (both size and shape), skin color, physiological responses to medication, electrocardiographic patterns, susceptibility to disease, and nutritional preferences and deficiencies.

It is difficult to generalize about any one specific group in a country that is known for its heterogeneity. Within our American "melting pot" any or all of the characteristics described could apply to individuals within any or all of the cultural groups represented. As these stated differences continue to be integrated, one American culture will eventually emerge. This is already in evidence in certain regions of the country today. However, some differences still do exist, and it is important for nurses to be aware of certain cultural influences that may affect individuals' behaviors and beliefs, particularly as they apply to health care.

APPLICATION OF THE NURSING PROCESS

Background Assessment Data

Table 39.1 presents a format for cultural assessment that may be used to gather information related to culture and ethnicity that is important for planning client care.

Northern European Americans

The language of the Northern European Americans has its roots in the language of the first English settlers to the United States, with the influence of immigrants from around the world. The descendants of these immigrants now make up what is considered to be the dominant cultural group in the United States today. Specific dialects and rate of speech are common to various regions of the country. Northern European Americans value territory. Personal space is about 18 inches to 3 feet.

With the advent of technology and widespread mobility, less emphasis has been placed on the cohesiveness of the family. In 1996, the divorce rate was 4.3 divorces per 1000 population (American Association for Marriage and Family Therapy, 1999). The value that was once placed on religion also seems to be diminishing in the American culture, with an overall decline reported in church membership since 1970. According to a research study by the Barna Research Group of Glendale, California, church attendance in 1996 had sunk to its lowest level in two decades (Personal Pastor Program, 1998). Punctuality and efficiency are highly valued in the culture that promoted the work ethic, and most within this cultural group tend to be future-oriented (Murray & Zentner, 1997).

Northern European Americans, particularly those who achieve middle-class socioeconomic status, value preventive medicine and primary health care. This value follows along with the socioeconomic group's educational level, successful achievement, and financial capability to maintain a healthy lifestyle. Most recognize the importance of regular physical exercise. Northern European Americans have medium body structure and fair skin, the latter of which is thought to be an evolutionary result of living in cold, cloudy Northern Europe (Giger & Davidhizar, 1995).

Beef and certain seafoods, such as lobster, are regarded as high-status foods among people in this culture (Giger & Davidhizar, 1995). However, changing food habits may bring both good news and bad news. The good news is that people are learning about eating healthier by decreasing the amount of fat and increasing the nutrients in their diets. The bad news is that Americans still enjoy fast food, and it conforms to their fast-paced lifestyles.

African Americans

The language dialect of many African Americans is different from what is considered to be standard English. The origin of the black dialect is not clearly understood but is thought to be a combination of various African languages and the languages of other cultural groups (e.g., Dutch, French, English, and Spanish) present in the United States at the time of its settlement. Personal space tends to be smaller than that of the dominant culture.

Patterns of discrimination date back to the days of slavery, and evidence of segregation still exists. This can be observed in some cities with the existence of predominantly black neighborhoods, churches, and schools. Some

TABLE 39.1   CULTURAL ASSESSMENT TOOL

Client's name _____ Ethnic origin _____

Address _____ Birthdate_____

Name of significant other _____ Relationship _____

Primary language spoken _____ Second language spoken _____

How does client usually communicate with people who speak a different language?_____

Is an interpreter required? _____ Available? _____

Highest level of education achieved: _____ Occupation _____

Presenting problem: _____

Has this problem ever occurred before? _____

   If so, in what manner was it handled previously? _____

What is the client's usual manner of coping with stress?_____

Who is (are) the client's main support system(s)? _____

Describe the family living arrangements: _____

Who is the major decision maker in the family? _____

Describe client's/family members' roles within the family:_____

_____

Describe religious beliefs and practices: _____

   Are there any religious requirements or restrictions that place limitations on the client's care?_____

   If so, describe: _____

Who in the family takes responsibility for health concerns?_____

Describe any special health beliefs and practices:_____

From whom does family usually seek medical assistance in time of need?_____

Describe client's usual emotional/behavioral response to: _____

   Anxiety:_____

   Anger: _____

   Loss/change/failure: _____

   Pain: _____

   Fear: _____

Describe any topics that are particularly sensitive or that the client is unwilling to discuss (because of cultural taboos):_____

_____

Describe any activities in which the client is unwilling to participate (because of cultural customs or taboos)._____

_____

What are the client's personal feelings regarding touch? _____

What are the client's personal feelings regarding eye contact?_____

What is the client's personal orientation to time? (past, present, future)_____

Describe any particular illnesses to which the client may be bioculturally susceptible: _____

   (e.g., hypertension and sickle cell anemia in African Americans)

Describe any nutritional deficiencies to which the client may be bioculturally susceptible: _____

   (e.g., lactose intolerance in Native and Asian Americans)

Describe client's favorite foods: _____

Are there any foods the client requests or refuses because of cultural beliefs related to this illness? _____

   (e.g., "hot" and "cold" foods for Latino Americans and Asian Americans). If so, please describe: _____

_____

Describe client's perception of the problem and expectations of health care: _____

_____

_____

African Americans find it too difficult to try to assimilate into the mainstream culture and choose to remain within their own social organization.

In 1994, about one third of African-American households were headed by a woman (Bennett, 1997). Social support systems may be large and include sisters, brothers, aunts, uncles, cousins, boyfriends, girlfriends, neighbors, and friends. Many African Americans have a strong religious orientation, and most belong to the Protestant faith (Giger & Davidhizar, 1995).

African Americans who have assimilated into the dominant culture are likely to be well educated, professional, and future-oriented. Some who have not become assimilated believe that planning for the future is hopeless, a belief based on their previous experiences and encounters with racism and discrimination (Giger & Davidhizar, 1995). They are usually unemployed or have low-paying jobs, with little expectation for improvement. They are unlikely to value time or punctuality to the same degree as the dominant cultural group, which often causes them to be labeled as irresponsible.

Some African Americans, particularly those from the rural South, may reach adulthood never having encountered a physician. They receive their medical care from the local folk practitioner known as "granny," or "the old lady," or a "spiritualist." Incorporated into the system of **folk medicine** is the belief that health is a gift from God, whereas illness is a punishment from God or a retribution for sin and evil. Historically, African Americans have turned to folk medicine either because they could not afford the cost of medical treatment or because of the insensitive treatment by caregivers in the health care delivery system.

Height of African Americans varies little from their Northern European American counterparts. Skin color varies from white to very dark brown or black, which offered the ancestors of African Americans protection from the sun and tropical heat.

Hypertension occurs more frequently, and sickle cell anemia occurs predominantly in African Americans. Hypertension carries a strong hereditary risk factor, while sickle cell anemia is genetically derived. Alcoholism is a serious problem among the black community, leading to a high incidence of alcohol-related illness and death (Campinha-Bacote, 1998).

The diet of most African Americans differs little from the mainstream culture. However, some African Americans follow their heritage and still enjoy what has come to be known as "soul" food. Some of these foods include poke salad, collard greens, beans, corn, fried chicken, black-eyed peas, grits, okra, and cornbread. These foods are now considered typical Southern fare and are regularly consumed and enjoyed by most individuals who inhabit the southern region of the United States.

Native Americans

The Bureau of Indian Affairs (BIA) recognizes more than 554 Indian tribes and Alaskan native groups that speak more than 250 languages (BIA, 1998). Less than half of these still live on reservations, but most return home often to participate in family and tribal life and sometimes to retire. Touch is an aspect of communication that differs in Native Americans from the dominant American culture. Some Native Americans view the traditional handshake as somewhat aggressive. Instead, if a hand is offered to another, it may be accepted with a light touch or just a passing of hands. Some Native Americans will not touch a dead person (Giger & Davidhizar, 1995).

Native Americans may appear silent and reserved. They may be uncomfortable expressing emotions, as the culture encourages private thoughts to be kept to oneself.

The concept of space is very concrete to Native Americans. Living space is often crowded with members of both nuclear and extended families. A large network of kin is very important to Native Americans. However, a need for extended space exists, as demonstrated by a distance of many miles between individual homes or camps.

The primary social organizations of Native Americans are the family and the tribe. From infancy Native American children are taught the importance of these units. Traditions are passed down by the elderly, and children are taught to respect tradition and to honor wisdom.

Native Americans are very present-time oriented. The time sequences of importance for Native Americans are present, past, and future, with little emphasis on the future (Still & Hodgins, 1998). Not only are Native Americans not ruled by the clock, some do not even own clocks. The concept of time is very casual, and tasks are accomplished not with the notion of a particular time in mind but merely in a present-oriented time frame.

Religion and health practices are intertwined in the Native American culture. The medicine man (or woman) is called the **shaman,** and may use a variety of methods in his or her practice. Some depend on "crystal gazing" to diagnose illness, some sing and perform elaborate healing ceremonies, and some use herbs and other plants or roots to concoct remedies with healing properties. The Native American healers and U.S. Indian Health Service have worked together with mutual respect for many years. Giger and Davidhizar (1995) relate that a medicine man or medicine woman may confer with a physician regarding the care of a client in the hospital. Clients may sometimes receive hospital passes to participate in a healing ceremony held outside the hospital.

Research studies have continued to show the importance of each of these health care systems in the overall wellness of Native American people.

Native Americans are typically of average height with reddish-tinted skin that may be light to medium brown. Their cheek bones are usually high and their noses have high bridges, probably an evolutionary result of living in very dry climates.

The risks of illness and premature death from alcoholism, diabetes, tuberculosis, heart disease, accidents, homicide, suicide, pneumonia, and influenza are greater for Native Americans than for the U.S. population as a whole (Indian Health Service [IHS], 1998). Alcoholism is a widespread problem among Native Americans. It is thought to be a symptom of depression in many cases and to contribute to a number of other serious problems such as automobile accidents, homicides, spouse and child abuse, and suicides.

Nutritional deficiencies are not uncommon among tribal Native Americans. Fruits and green vegetables are often scarce in many of the federally defined Indian geographical regions. Meat and corn products are identified as preferred foods. Fiber intake is relatively low, while fat intake is often of the saturated variety. A large percentage of Native Americans receive commodity foods supplied by the U.S. Department of Agriculture's food distribution program (Giger & Davidhizar, 1995).

Asian/Pacific Islander Americans

Asian Americans comprise one of the largest ethnic groups in the United States today, totaling approximately 11 million people (Spector, 1996). The Asian American culture includes peoples (and their descendants) from Japan, China, Vietnam, the Philippines, Thailand, Cambodia, Korea, Laos, and the Pacific Islands. Although this discussion relates to these peoples as a single culture, it is important to keep in mind that a multiplicity of differences regarding attitudes, beliefs, values, religious practices, and language exist among these subcultures.

Many Asian Americans, particularly Japanese, are third- and even fourth-generation Americans. These individuals are likely to be very acculturated into the American culture. Sue (1981) describes three patterns common to Asian Americans in their attempt to adjust to the American culture:

1. The Traditionalists. These individuals tend to be the older-generation Asians who hold on to the traditional values and practices of their native culture.
2. The Marginal People. These individuals reject the traditional values and totally embrace Western culture. They tend to be members of the younger generations.
3. Asian Americans. These individuals incorporate traditional values and beliefs with Western values and beliefs. They become integrated into the American culture, while maintaining a connection with their ancestral culture.

The languages and dialects of Asian Americans are very diverse. In general, they do share a similar belief in harmonious interaction. To raise one's voice is likely to be interpreted as a sign of loss of control. The English language is

very difficult to master, and even bilingual Asian Americans may encounter communication problems because of the differences in meaning assigned to nonverbal cues, such as facial gestures, verbal intonation and speed, and body movements. Touching during communication has historically been considered unacceptable. However, with the advent of Western acculturation, younger generations of Asian Americans accept touching as more appropriate than did their ancestors. Eye contact is often avoided as it connotes rudeness and lack of respect in some Asian cultures. Acceptable personal and social spaces are larger than in the dominant American culture. Some Asian Americans have a great deal of difficulty expressing emotions. Because of their reserved public demeanor, Asian Americans may be perceived as shy, cold, or uninterested.

The family is the ultimate social organization in the Asian American culture, and loyalty to family is emphasized above all else. Children are expected to obey and honor their parents. Misbehavior is perceived as bringing dishonor to the entire family. Filial piety (one's social obligation or duty to one's parents) is highly regarded. Failure to fulfill these obligations can create a great deal of guilt and shame in an individual. A chronological hierarchy exists, with the elderly maintaining positions of authority. Several generations, or even extended families, may share a single household.

Although education is highly valued among Asian Americans, many remain undereducated. Religious beliefs and practices are very diverse and exhibit influences of Taoism, Buddhism, Islam, and Christianity (Giger & Davidhizar, 1995).

Many Asian Americans are both past- and present-oriented. Emphasis is placed on the wishes of one's ancestors, while adjusting to demands of the present. Little value is given to prompt adherence to schedules or rigid standards of activities.

Restoring the balance of **yin and yang** is the fundamental concept of Asian health practices (Giger & Davidhizar, 1995). Yin and yang represent opposite forces of energy, such as negative/positive, dark/light, cold/hot, hard/soft, and feminine/masculine. When there is a disruption in the balance of these forces of energy, illness can occur. In medicine, the opposites are expressed as "hot" and "cold," and health is the result of a balance between hot and cold elements (Giger & Davidhizar, 1995). Food, medicines, and herbs are classified according to their hot and cold properties, and are used to restore balance between yin and yang (cold and hot), thereby restoring health.

Asian Americans are generally small of frame and build. Obesity is very uncommon in this culture. Skin color ranges from white to medium brown, with yellow tones. Other physical characteristics include almond-shaped eyes with a slight droop to eyelids and sparse body hair, particularly in men, in whom chest hair is often absent. Hair on the head is commonly coarse, thick, straight, and black in color.

Rice, vegetables, and fish are the main staple foods of

Asian Americans. Milk is seldom used, as a large majority of Asian Americans experience lactose intolerance. With Western acculturation, the diet is changing, and unfortunately, with more meat being consumed, the percentage of fat in the diet is increasing.

Many Asian Americans believe that psychiatric illness is merely behavior that is out of control. They view this as a great shame to the individual and the family. They often attempt to manage the ill person on their own until they can no longer handle the situation. It is not uncommon for Asian Americans to somaticize. Expressing mental distress through various physical ailments may be viewed as more acceptable than expressing true emotions (Giger & Davidhizar, 1995).

The incidence of alcohol dependence is low among Asians. This may be a result of a possible genetic intolerance of the substance. Some Asians develop unpleasant symptoms, such as flushing, headaches, and palpitations, upon drinking of alcohol. Research indicates that this is due to an isoenzyme variant that quickly converts alcohol to acetaldehyde, as well as the absence of an isoenzyme that is needed to oxidize acetaldehyde. This results in a rapid accumulation of acetaldehyde that produces the unpleasant symptoms (Madden, 1984).

Latino Americans

Latino Americans trace their ancestry to countries such as Mexico, Spain, Puerto Rico, Cuba, and other countries of Central and South America. The common language is Spanish, spoken with a number of dialects by the various peoples. Touch is a common form of communication among Latinos; however, they are very modest and are likely to withdraw from any infringement on their modesty (Murray & Zentner, 1997). Latinos tend to be very tactful and diplomatic and will often appear agreeable on the surface out of courtesy for the person with whom they are communicating. It is only after the fact when agreements remain unfulfilled that the true context of the interaction becomes clear.

Latino Americans are very group-oriented. It is important for them to interact with large groups of relatives, where a great deal of touching and embracing occur. The family is the primary social organization and includes nuclear family members as well as numerous extended family members. The nuclear family is male dominated, and the father possesses ultimate authority.

Latino Americans tend to be present-oriented. The concept of being punctual and giving attention to activities that relate to concern about the future are perceived as less important than present-oriented activities which cannot again be retrieved beyond the present time.

Roman Catholicism is the predominant religion among Latino Americans. Most Latinos identify with the Roman Catholic church, even if they do not attend. Religious beliefs and practices are likely to be strong influences in their lives. Especially in times of crisis, such as with illness and hospitalization, Latino-Americans will rely on priest and family to carry out important religious rituals, such as promise making, offering candles, visiting shrines, and offering prayers (Spector, 1996).

Folk beliefs regarding health are a combination of elements incorporating views of Roman Catholicism and Indian and Spanish ancestries. The folk healer is called a **curandero** (male) or **curandera** (female). Among traditional Latino-Americans, the curandero is believed to have a gift from God for healing the sick and is often the first contact made when illness is encountered. Treatments used include massage, diet, rest, suggestions, practical advice, indigenous herbs, prayers, magic, and supernatural rituals (Giger & Davidhizar, 1995). Many Latino Americans still subscribe to the "hot and cold theory" of disease. This concept is similar to the Asian perception of yin and yang discussed earlier in this chapter. Diseases and the foods and medicines used to treat them are classified as "hot" or "cold," and the intention is to restore the body to a balanced state.

Latino Americans are usually shorter than the average member of the dominant American culture. Skin color can vary from light tan to dark brown. Research indicates that there is less mental illness among Latino Americans than the general population. This may have to do with the strong cohesiveness of the family and the support that is given during times of stress. Latino Americans also have clearly defined rules of conduct, which creates fewer role conflicts within the family.

Western European Americans

Western European Americans have their origin in France, Italy, and Greece. Each of these cultures possesses its own unique language with a number of dialects noticeable within each language. Western Europeans are known to be very warm and affectionate people. They tend to be very physically expressive, using a lot of body language, including hugging and kissing.

Like Latino Americans, Western European Americans are very family-oriented. They interact in large groups, and it is not uncommon for several generations to live together or in close proximity of each other. A strong allegiance to the cultural heritage exists, and it is not uncommon, particularly among Italians, to find settlements of immigrants clustering together.

Roles within the family are clearly defined, with the man as the head of the household. Western European women view their role as mother and homemaker, and children are prized and cherished. The elderly are held in positions of respect and often are cared for in the home rather than placed in nursing homes (Giger & Davidhizar, 1995).

Roman Catholicism is the predominant religion for the French and Italians; Greek Orthodox for the Greeks. A number of religious traditions are observed surrounding rites of passage. Masses and rituals are observed for births, first communions, marriages, anniversaries, and deaths.

Western Europeans tend to be present-oriented with a somewhat fatalistic view of the future. A priority is placed on the here and now, and whatever happens in the future is perceived as God's will.

Most Western European Americans follow health beliefs and practices of the dominant American culture, but some folk beliefs and superstitions still endure. Spector (1996) reports the following superstitions and practices of Italians as they relate to health and illness:

1. A woman can "mark" her unborn baby if she looks at an object or situation that is frightening to her.
2. Miscarriage or birth defect can occur if a pregnant woman is denied access to a food that she desires or smells.
3. A cold can be cured with warm camphor rubbed on the chest.
4. Individuals should attempt to stay warm and dry and out of drafts.
5. Women should avoid washing their hair during the menstrual period.

The author recalls her own Italian immigrant grandmother warming large collard greens in oil and placing them on swollen parotid glands during a bout with the mumps. The greens undoubtedly did nothing for the mumps, but they (along with the tender loving care) felt wonderful!

Western Europeans are typically of average stature. Skin color ranges from fair to medium brown. Hair and eyes are commonly dark, but some Italians have blue eyes and blond hair. Food is very important in the Western European American culture. Italian, Greek, and French cuisine is world famous, and food is used in a social manner, as well as for nutritional purposes. Wine is consumed by all (even the children) and is the beverage of choice with meals. However, among Greek Americans, drunkenness engenders social disgrace on the individual and the family (Tripp-Reimer & Sorofman, 1998).

Table 39.2 summarizes information related to the six cultural phenomena as they apply to the cultural groups discussed here.

Diagnosis/Outcome Identification

Nursing diagnoses are selected based on the information gathered during the assessment process. With background knowledge of various cultural variables and information uniquely related to the individual, the following nursing diagnoses may be appropriate:

Impaired verbal communication related to cultural differences, evidenced by inability to speak the dominant language.

Anxiety (moderate to severe) related to entry into unfamiliar health care system and separation from support systems, evidenced by apprehension and suspicion, restlessness, and trembling.

Alteration in nutrition, less than body requirements, related to refusal to eat unfamiliar foods provided in the health care setting, evidenced by loss of weight.

Spiritual distress related to inability to participate in usual religious practices because of hospitalization, evidenced by alterations in mood (e.g., anger, crying, withdrawal, preoccupation, anxiety, hostility, apathy, and so forth)

Outcome criteria related to these nursing diagnoses may include:

THE CLIENT:

1. Has had all basic needs fulfilled.
2. Has communicated with staff through an interpreter.
3. Has maintained anxiety at a manageable level by having family members stay with him or her during hospitalization.
4. Has maintained weight by eating foods that he or she likes brought to the hospital by family members.
5. Has restored spiritual strength through use of cultural rituals and beliefs and visits from spiritual leader.

Planning/Implementation

The following interventions have special cultural implications for nursing:

1. Use an interpreter if necessary to ensure that there are no barriers to communication. Be careful with nonverbal communication, as it is interpreted differently by different cultures (e.g., Asians and Native Americans may be uncomfortable with touch and direct eye contact, whereas Latinos and Western Europeans perceive touch as a sign of caring).
2. Make allowances for individuals from other cultures to have family members around them and even participate in their care. Large numbers of extended family members are very important to African Americans, Native Americans, Asian Americans, Latino Americans, and Western European Americans. To deny access to these family support systems could interfere with the healing process.
3. Ensure that the individual's spiritual needs are being met. Religion is an important source of support for many individuals, and the nurse must be tolerant of various rituals that may be connected with different cultural beliefs about health and illness.
4. Be aware of the differences in concept of time among the various cultures. Most members of the dominant American culture are future-oriented and

TABLE 39.2 SUMMARY OF SIX CULTURAL PHENOMENA IN COMPARISON OF VARIOUS CULTURAL GROUPS

CULTURAL GROUP AND COUNTRIES OF ORIGIN	COMMUNICATION	SPACE	SOCIAL ORGANIZATION	TIME	ENVIRONMENTAL CONTROL	BIOLOGICAL VARIATIONS
Northern European Americans (England, Ireland, Germany, others)	National languages (although many learn English very quickly) Dialects (often regional) English More verbal than nonverbal	Territory valued Personal space: 18 inches to 3 feet Uncomfortable with personal contact and touch	Families: nuclear and extended Religions: Jewish and Christian Organizations: social and community	Future-oriented	Most value preventive medicine and primary health care through traditional health care delivery system Alternative methods on the increase	Health concerns: Cardiovascular disease Cancer Diabetes mellitus
African Americans (Africa, West Indian islands, Dominican Republic, Haiti, Jamaica)	National languages Dialects (pidgin, Creole, Gullah, French, Spanish) Highly verbal and nonverbal	Close personal space Comfortable with touch	Large, extended families Many female-headed households Strong religious orientation, mostly Protestant Community social organizations	Present-oriented	Traditional health care delivery system Some individuals prefer to use folk practitioner ("granny" or voodoo healer) Home remedies	Health concerns: Cardiovascular disease Hypertension Sickle cell disease Diabetes mellitus Lactose intolerance
Native Americans (North America, Alaska, Aleutian Islands)	250 tribal languages recognized Comfortable with silence Direct eye contact considered rude	Large, extended space important Uncomfortable with touch	Families: nuclear and extended Children taught importance of tradition Social organizations: tribe and family most important	Present-oriented	Religion and health practices intertwined Medicine man or woman (shaman) uses folk practices to heal Shaman may work with modern medical practitioner	Health concerns: Alcoholism Tuberculosis Accidents Diabetes mellitus Heart disease
Asian/Pacific Islander Americans (Japan, China, Korea, Vietnam, Philippines, Thailand, Cambodia, Laos, Pacific Islands)	More than 30 different languages spoken Comfortable with silence Uncomfortable with eye-to-eye contact Nonverbal connotations may be misunderstood	Large personal space Uncomfortable with touch	Families: nuclear and extended Children taught importance of family loyalty and tradition Many religions: Taoism, Buddhism, Islam, and Christianity Community social organizations	Present-oriented Past important and valued	Traditional health care delivery system Some prefer to use folk practices (e.g., yin and yang; herbal medicine; and moxibustion)	Health concerns: Hypertension Cancer Diabetes mellitus Thalassemia Lactose intolerance

Continued on following page

TABLE 39.2   SUMMARY OF SIX CULTURAL PHENOMENA IN COMPARISON OF VARIOUS CULTURAL GROUPS *(Continued)*

CULTURAL GROUP AND COUNTRIES OF ORIGIN	COMMUNICATION	SPACE	SOCIAL ORGANIZATION	TIME	ENVIRONMENTAL CONTROL	BIOLOGICAL VARIATIONS
Latino Americans (Mexico, Spain, Cuba, Puerto Rico, other countries of Central and South America)	Spanish, with many dialects	Close personal space Lots of touching and embracing Very group oriented	Families: nuclear and large extended families Strong ties to Roman Catholicism Community social organizations	Present-oriented	Traditional health care delivery system Some prefer to use folk practitioner, called curandero or curandera Folk practices include "hot and cold" herbal remedies	Health concerns: Heart disease Cancer Diabetes mellitus Accidents Lactose intolerance
Western European Americans (France, Italy, Greece)	National languages Dialects	Close personal space Lots of touching and embracing Very group oriented	Families: nuclear and large extended families France and Italy: Roman Catholic religion Greece: Greek Orthodox	Present-oriented	Traditional health care delivery system Lots of home remedies and practices based on superstition	Health concerns: Heart disease Cancer Diabetes mellitus Thalassemia

SOURCES: Spector (1996); Purnell & Paulanka (1998); Murray & Zentner (1997); Geissler (1994); and Giger & Davidhizar (1995).

place a high value on punctuality and efficiency. Other cultures such as African Americans, Native Americans, Asian Americans, Latino Americans, and Western European Americans are more present-oriented. Nurses must be aware that such individuals may not share the value of punctuality. They may be late to appointments and appear to be indifferent to some aspects of their therapy. Nurses must be accepting of these differences and refrain from allowing existing attitudes to interfere with delivery of care.

5. Be aware of different beliefs about health care among the various cultures and recognize the importance of these beliefs to the healing process. If an individual from another culture has been receiving health care from a "spiritualist," or a "medicine man," or "granny," or "curandero," it is important for the nurse to listen to what has been done in the past and even to consult with these cultural healers about the care being given to the client.

6. Follow the health care practices that the client views as essential, provided they do no harm or interfere with the healing process of the client. For example, the concepts of yin and yang and the "hot and cold" theory of disease are very important to the well-being of some Asians and Latinos, respectively. Try to ensure that a balance of these foods are included in the diet as an important reinforcement for traditional medical care.

7. Be aware of favorite foods of individuals from different cultures. The health care setting may seem strange and somewhat isolated, and for some individuals it feels good to have anything around them that is familiar. They may even refuse to eat foods that are unfamiliar to them. If it does not interfere with his or her care, allow family members to provide favorite foods for the client.

8. The nurse working in psychiatry must realize that psychiatric illness is unacceptable in some cultures. Individuals who believe that expressing emotions is unacceptable (e.g., Asian Americans and Native Americans) will present unique problems when they are clients in a psychiatric setting. Nurses must have patience and work slowly to establish trust in order to provide these individuals with the assistance they require.

Evaluation

Evaluation of nursing actions is directed at achievement of the established outcomes. Part of the evaluation process is continuous reassessment to ensure that the selected actions are appropriate and the goals and outcomes are realistic. Including the family and extended support systems in the evaluation process is essential if cultural implications of nursing care are to be measured. Modifications to the plan of care are made as the need is determined.

SUMMARY

Culture encompasses shared patterns of belief, feeling, and knowledge that guide people's conduct and are passed down from generation to generation. Ethnic groups are tied together by shared heritage. Nurses must understand concepts as they relate to various cultural groups, with caution regarding the risk of stereotyping. Each person, regardless of cultural ties, must be considered unique.

Cultural groups differ in terms of communication, space, social organization, time, environmental control, and biological variations. Northern European Americans are the descendants of the first immigrants to the United States and make up the current dominant cultural group. They value punctuality, work responsibility, and a healthy lifestyle. The divorce rate is high within this cultural group and the structure of the family is changing. Religious ties have loosened.

African Americans trace their roots in the United States to the days of slavery. Many African Americans have assimilated into the dominant culture, but some remain tied to their own social organization by choice or by necessity. Approximately one third of all African American households are headed by women. The social support systems are large and many African Americans have strong religious ties, particularly to the Protestant faith. Some African Americans, particularly in the rural South, may still use folk medicine as a means of health care. Hypertension, sickle cell anemia, and alcoholism are serious health problems.

Many Native Americans still live on reservations. They speak many different languages and dialects. Native Americans appear silent and reserved and many are uncomfortable with touch and expressing emotions. A large network of family is important to Native Americans. They are very present-oriented and not ruled by a clock. Religion and health practices are intertwined, and the *shaman* (medicine man or woman) is the deliverer of care. Health problems include tuberculosis, diabetes, and alcoholism. Nutritional deficiencies are not uncommon.

Asian American language is very diverse. Touching during communication has historically been considered unacceptable. Asian Americans have difficulty expressing emotions, and may appear cold and aloof. Family loyalty is emphasized above all else, and extended family are very important. Health practices are based on the restoration of balance of yin and yang. Many Asian Americans believe that psychiatric illness is merely behavior that is out of control, and to behave in such a manner is to bring shame on the family.

The common language of Latino Americans is Spanish.

Large family groups are important to Latinos, and touch is a common form of communication. The predominant religion is Roman Catholicism, and the church is a source of strength in times of crisis. Health care may be delivered by a folk healer called a curandero, who uses various forms of treatment to restore the body to a balanced state.

Western European Americans have their origin in Italy, France, and Greece. They are warm and expressive, and use touch as a common form of communication. Western European Americans are very family-oriented, and most have a strong allegiance to the cultural heritage. The dominant religion is Roman Catholicism for the Italians and French, and Greek Orthodoxy for the Greeks. Most Western European Americans follow the health practices of the dominant culture, but some folk beliefs and superstitions still endure.

The nursing process was presented as the vehicle for delivery of care. A cultural assessment tool was included to assist in gathering information needed to plan appropriate care for individuals from various cultural groups.

REVIEW QUESTIONS

SELF-EXAMINATION/LEARNING EXERCISE

Select the answer that is most appropriate for each of the following questions.

1. Miss Lee is an Asian American on the psychiatric unit. She tells the nurse, "I must have the hot ginger root for my headache. It is the only thing that will help." What meaning does the nurse attach to this statement by Miss Lee?

    a. She is being obstinate and wants control over her care.
    b. She believes that ginger root has magical qualities.
    c. She subscribes to the restoration of health through the balance of yin and yang.
    d. Asian Americans refuse to take traditional medicine for pain.

2. Miss Lee (the same client from previous question) says she is afraid that no one from her family will visit her. On what belief does Miss Lee base her statement?

    a. Asian Americans do not believe in hospitals.
    b. Asian Americans do not have close family support systems.
    c. Asian Americans believe the body will heal itself if left alone.
    d. Asian Americans view psychiatric problems as bringing shame to the family.

3. Joe, a Native American, appears at the community health clinic with an oozing stasis ulcer on his lower right leg. It is obviously infected, and he tells the nurse that the shaman has been treating it with herbs. The nurse determines that Joe needs emergency care, but Joe states he will not go to the emergency department (ED) unless the shaman is allowed to help treat him. How should the nurse handle this situation?

    a. Contact the shaman and have him meet them at the ED to consult with the attending physician.
    b. Tell Joe that the shaman is not allowed in the ED.
    c. Explain to Joe that the shaman is at fault for his leg being in the condition it is in now.
    d. Have the shaman try to talk Joe into going to the ED without him.

4. When the shaman arrives at the hospital, Joe's physician extends his hand for a handshake. The shaman lightly touches the physician's hand, then quickly moves away. How should the physician interpret this gesture?

    a. The shaman is snubbing the physician.
    b. The shaman is angry that he was called away from his supper.
    c. The shaman does not believe in traditional medicine.
    d. The shaman does not feel comfortable with touch.

5. Sarah is an African American woman who receives a visit from the psychiatric home health nurse. A referral for a mental health assessment was made by the public health nurse, who noticed that Sarah was becoming exceedingly withdrawn. When the psychiatric nurse arrives, Sarah says to her, "No one can help me. I was an evil person in my youth, and now I must pay." How might the nurse assess this statement?

    a. Sarah is having delusions of persecution.
    b. Some African Americans believe illness is God's punishment for their sins.
    c. Sarah is depressed and just wants to be left alone.
    d. African Americans do not believe in psychiatric help.

6. Sarah says to the nurse, "Granny told me to eat a lot of poke greens and I would feel better." How should the nurse interpret this statement?

    a. Sarah's grandmother believes in the healing power of poke greens.
    b. Sarah believes everything her grandmother tells her.
    c. Sarah has been receiving health care from a "folk practitioner."
    d. Sarah is trying to determine if the nurse agrees with her grandmother.

7. Frank is a Latino American who has an appointment at the community health center for 1:00 PM. The nurse is angry when Frank shows up at 3:30 PM stating, "I was visiting with my brother." How must the nurse interpret this behavior?

   a. Frank is being passive-aggressive by showing up late.
   b. This is Frank's way of defying authority.
   c. Frank is a member of a cultural group that is present-oriented.
   d. Frank is a member of a cultural group that rejects traditional medicine.

8. The nurse must give Frank (Latino American) a physical examination. She tells him to remove his clothing and put on an examination gown. Frank refuses. How should the nurse interpret this behavior?

   a. Frank does not believe in taking orders from a woman.
   b. Frank is modest and embarrassed to remove his clothes.
   c. Frank doesn't understand why he must remove his clothes.
   d. Frank does not think he needs a physical examination.

9. Maria is an Italian American who is in the hospital after having suffered a miscarriage at 5 months' gestation. Her room is filled with relatives, who have brought a variety of foods and gifts for Maria. They are all talking, seemingly at the same time, and some, including Maria, are crying. They repeatedly touch and hug Maria and each other. How should the nurse handle this situation?

   a. Explain to the family that Maria needs her rest and they must all leave.
   b. Allow the family to remain and continue their activity as described, as long as they do not disturb other clients.
   c. Explain that Maria will not get over her loss if they keep bringing it up and causing her to cry so much.
   d. Call the family priest to come and take charge of this family situation.

10. Maria's mother says to the nurse, "If only Maria had told me she wanted the *biscotti*. I would have made them for her." What is the meaning behind Maria's mother's statement?

    a. Some Italian Americans believe a miscarriage can occur if a woman does not eat a food she craves.
    b. Some Italian Americans think *biscotti* can prevent miscarriage.
    c. Maria's mother is taking the blame for Maria's miscarriage.
    d. Maria's mother believes the physician should have told Maria to eat *biscotti*.

REFERENCES

American Association for Marriage and Family Therapy. (1999). *Divorce and marriage statistics*. [On-line]. Available: http://www.aamft.org/families/stats.htm.

Bennett, C.E. (1997). *Selected characteristics of black households, by type of householder: March 1994*. U.S. Department of Commerce. [On-line]. Available: http://www.thuban.com/census/tables/hh1_b94.html.

Bureau of Indian Affairs (BIA). (1998). *American Indian Today*. [On-line]. Available: http://www.doi.gov/bia/aitoday/aitoday.html.

Campinha-Bacote, J. (1998). African-Americans. In L.D. Purnell and B.J. Paulanka (Eds.). *Transcultural health care: A culturally competent approach*. Philadelphia: F.A. Davis.

Geissler, E.M. (1994). *Pocket guide to cultural assessment*. St. Louis: Mosby Year Book.

Giger, J.N., & Davidhizar, R.E. (1995). *Transcultural nursing: Assessment and intervention* (2nd ed.) St. Louis: Mosby Year Book.

Gordon, B.N. (1995). Cultural diversity: You make a difference. *The Oklahoma Nurse, 40*(3), 14–15.

Griffith, E.E.H., & Gonzalez, C.A. (1994). Essentials of cultural psychiatry. In R.E. Hales, S.C. Yudofsky, & J.A. Talbott (Eds.), *Textbook of psychiatry* (2nd ed.). Washington, DC: American Psychiatric Press.

Hall, E.T. (1966). *The hidden dimension*. Garden City, NY: Doubleday.

Indian Health Service (IHS). (1998). *Important strides in Indian health*. [On-line.] Available: http://www.tucson.his.gov/MedicalPrograms/Nursing/impstrih.asp.

Madden, J.S. (1984). *A guide to alcohol and drug dependence* (2nd ed.). Bristol, England: John Wright & Sons.

Murray, R.B., & Zentner, J.P. (1997). *Health assessment and promotion strategies through the life span* (6th ed.). Stamford, CT: Appleton & Lange.

Purnell, L.D., & Paulanka, B.J. (1998). *Transcultural health care: A culturally competent approach*. Philadelphia: F.A. Davis.

Personal Pastor Program. (1998). Church attendance reported at lowest level in two decades. *Presbyterian Outlook*, September 30, 1996. [On-line]. Available: http://www.personalpastor.org/pp03018.htm.

Spector, R.E. (1996). *Cultural diversity in health and illness* (4th ed.). Stamford, CT: Appleton & Lange.

Still, O., & Hodgins, D. (1998). Navajo Indians. In L.D. Purnell & B.J. Paulanka (Eds.), *Transcultural health care: A culturally competent approach*. Philadelphia: F.A. Davis.

Sue, D. (1981). *Counseling the culturally different: Theory and practice.* New York: John Wiley.

Tripp-Reimer, T., & Sorofman, B. (1998). Greek-Americans. In L.D. Purnell & B.J. Paulanka (Eds.), *Transcultural health care: A culturally competent approach.* Philadelphia: F.A. Davis.

Bibliography

Beeber, L.S., et al. (1993). The challenge of diversity. *Journal of Psychosocial Nursing, 31*(8), 23–29.

Delgado, M. (1983). Hispanic natural support systems: Implications for mental health services. *Journal of Psychosocial Nursing, 21*(4). 19–24.

Mohr, W.K. (1998). Cross-ethnic variations in the care of psychiatric patients: A review of contributing factors and practice considerations. *Journal of Psychosocial Nursing, 36*(5), 16–21.

Nurse-to-nurse: Social equity and diversity. (1998, Second Quarter). *Reflections* [Special issue]. Indianapolis, IN: Sigma Theta Tau International.

Nursing among diverse cultures. (1996, Fourth Quarter). *Reflections* [Special issue]. Indianapolis, IN: Sigma Theta Tau International.

Warren, B.J. (1994). Depression in African-American women. *Journal of Psychosocial Nursing, 32*(3), 29–33.

ETHICAL AND LEGAL ISSUES IN PSYCHIATRIC/MENTAL HEALTH NURSING

CHAPTER OUTLINE

OBJECTIVES

INTRODUCTION

DEFINITIONS

ETHICAL CONSIDERATIONS

LEGAL CONSIDERATIONS

SUMMARY

REVIEW QUESTIONS

KEY TERMS

ethics
bioethics
moral behavior
values
values clarification
right
utilitarianism
Kantianism
Christian ethics
natural law
ethical egoism

ethical dilemma
autonomy
beneficence
nonmaleficence
justice
veracity
statutory law
common law
civil law
tort

privileged
    communication
informed consent
false imprisonment
malpractice
negligence
defamation of character
slander
libel
assault
battery

OBJECTIVES

After reading this chapter, the student will be able to:

1. Differentiate among ethics, morals, values, and rights.
2. Discuss ethical theories including utilitarianism, Kantianism, Christian ethics, natural law theories, and ethical egoism.
3. Define *ethical dilemma*.
4. Discuss the ethical principles of autonomy, beneficence, nonmaleficence, and justice.
5. Use an ethical decision-making model to make an ethical decision.

6. Describe ethical issues relevant to psychiatric/mental health nursing.
7. Define *statutory law* and *common law*.
8. Differentiate between civil and criminal law.
9. Discuss legal issues relevant to psychiatric/mental health nursing.
10. Differentiate between *malpractice* and *negligence*.
11. Identify behaviors relevant to the psychiatric/mental health setting for which specific malpractice action could be taken.

*I*n the education of mental health care professionals, the teaching of ethical issues is inadequate (McGovern, 1991). This chapter provides a reference for the student and practicing nurse of the basic ethical and legal concepts and their relationship to psychiatric/mental health nursing.

Nurses are constantly faced with the challenge of making difficult decisions regarding good and evil or life and death. A discussion of ethical theory is presented as a foundation upon which ethical decisions may be made. The American Nurses' Association (ANA) (1985) has established a code of ethics for nurses to use as a framework within which to make ethical choices and decisions (Table 40.1).

Because legislation determines what is *right* or *good* within a society, legal issues pertaining to psychiatric/mental health nursing are also discussed. Definitions are presented, along with rights of psychiatric clients of which nurses must be aware. Nursing competency and client care accountability are compromised when the nurse has inadequate knowledge about the laws that regulate the practice of nursing.

TABLE 40.1 AMERICAN NURSES' ASSOCIATION CODE OF ETHICS FOR NURSES

1. The nurse provides services with respect for human dignity and the uniqueness of the client unrestricted by considerations of social or economic status, personal attributes, or the nature of health problems.
2. The nurse safeguards the client's right to privacy by judiciously protecting information of a confidential nature.
3. The nurse acts to safeguard the client and the public when health care and safety are affected by the incompetent, unethical, or illegal practice of any person.
4. The nurse assumes responsibility and accountability for individual nursing judgments and actions.
5. The nurse maintains competence in nursing.
6. The nurse exercises informed judgment and uses individual competence and qualifications as criteria in seeking consultations, accepting responsibilities, and delegating nursing activities to others.
7. The nurse participates in activities that contribute to the ongoing development of the profession's body of knowledge.
8. The nurse participates in the profession's efforts to implement and improve standards of nursing.
9. The nurse participates in the profession's efforts to establish and maintain conditions of employment conducive to high-quality nursing care.
10. The nurse participates in the profession's effort to protect the public from misinformation and misrepresentation and to maintain the integrity of nursing.
11. The nurse collaborates with members of the health profession and other citizens in promoting community and national efforts to meet the health needs of the public.

SOURCE: ANA (1985).

Knowledge of the legal and ethical concepts presented in this chapter will enhance the quality of care the nurse provides in his or her psychiatric/mental health nursing practice, while also protecting the nurse within the parameters of legal accountability. Indeed, the very right to practice nursing carries with it the responsibility to maintain a specific level of competency and to practice in accordance with certain ethical and legal standards of care.

DEFINITIONS

King (1984) defines **ethics** as "a branch of philosophy dealing with values related to human conduct, to the rightness and wrongness of certain actions, and to the goodness and badness of the motives and ends of such actions." **Bioethics** is the term applied to these principles when they refer to concepts within the scope of medicine, nursing, and allied health.

Moral behavior is defined as conduct that results from serious critical thinking about how individuals ought to treat others. Moral behavior reflects the way a person interprets basic respect for other persons, such as the respect for autonomy, freedom, justice, honesty, and confidentiality (Pappas, 1994).

Values are personal beliefs about the truth, beauty, or worth of a thought, object, or behavior (Leach, 1987). **Values clarification** is a process of self-discovery by which people identify their personal values and their value rankings (King, 1984). This process increases awareness about why individuals behave in certain ways. Values clarification is important in nursing to increase understanding about why certain choices and decisions are made over others, and how values affect nursing outcomes.

A **right** is that which an individual is entitled (by ethical or moral standards) to have, or to do, or to receive from others within the limits of the law (Goldstein, Perdew, & Pruitt 1989). A right is *absolute* when there is no restriction whatsoever upon the individual's entitlement. A *legal right* is one upon which the society has agreed and formalized into law. Both the National League for Nursing (NLN) and the American Hospital Association (AHA) have established guidelines of patients' rights. Although these are not considered legal documents, nurses and hospitals are considered responsible for upholding these rights of patients. In certain instances, courts have held this bill of rights to be part of a legal contract between hospital and patient, and therefore legally binding (Goldstein, Perdew, & Pruitt, 1989). The AHA Patient's Bill of Rights is presented in Table 40.2.

ETHICAL CONSIDERATIONS

Theoretical Perspectives

An *ethical theory* is a moral principle or a set of moral principles that can be used in assessing what is morally right

TABLE 40.2 AMERICAN HOSPITAL ASSOCIATION PATIENT'S BILL OF RIGHTS

1. The patient has the right to considerate and respectful care.

2. The patient has the right to obtain from his physician complete current information concerning his diagnosis, treatment, and prognosis in terms the patient can be reasonably expected to understand. When it is not medically advisable to give such information to the patient, the information should be made available to an appropriate person in his behalf. He has the right to know by name the physician responsible for coordinating his care.

3. The patient has the right to receive from his physician information necessary to give informed consent prior to the start of any procedure and/or treatment. Except in emergencies, such information for informed consent should include but not necessarily be limited to the specific procedure and/or treatment, the medically significant risks involved, and the probable duration of incapacitation. Where medically significant alternatives for care or treatment exist, or when the patient requests information concerning medical alternatives, the patient has the right to such information. The patient also has the right to know the name of the person responsible for the procedures and/or treatment.

4. The patient has the right to refuse treatment to the extent permitted by law and to be informed of the medical consequences of his action.

5. The patient has the right to every consideration of his privacy concerning his own medical care program. Case discussion, consultation, examination, and treatment are confidential and should be conducted discreetly. Those not directly involved in his care must have the permission of the patient to be present.

6. The patient has the right to expect that all communications and records pertaining to his care should be treated as confidential.

7. The patient has the right to expect that within its capacity a hospital must make reasonable response to the request of a patient for services. The hospital must provide evaluation, service, and/or referral as indicated by the urgency of the case. When medically permissible, a patient may be transferred to another facility only after he has received complete information and explanation concerning the needs for and alternatives to such a transfer. The institution to which the patient is to be transferred must first have accepted the patient for transfer.

8. The patient has the right to obtain information as to any relationship of his hospital to other health care and educational institutions insofar as his care is concerned. The patient has the right to obtain information as to the existence of any professional relationships among individuals, by name, who are treating him.

9. The patient has the right to be advised if the hospital proposes to engage in or perform human experimentation affecting his care or treatment. The patient has the right to refuse to participate in such research projects.

10. The patient has the right to expect reasonable continuity of care. He has the right to know in advance what appointment times and physicians are available and where. The patient has the right to expect that the hospital will provide a mechanism whereby he is informed by his physician or a delegate of the physician of the patient's continuing health care requirements following discharge.

11. The patient has the right to examine and receive an explanation of his bill regardless of source of payment.

12. The patient has the right to know what hospital rules and regulations apply to his conduct as a patient.

SOURCE: AHA (1992), with permission.

or morally wrong (Ellis & Hartley, 1995). These principles provide guidelines for ethical decision making.

Utilitarianism

The basis of **utilitarianism** is "the greatest-happiness principle." This principle holds that actions are right in proportion as they tend to promote happiness; wrong as they tend to produce the reverse of happiness. Thus, the good is happiness and the right is that which promotes the good. Conversely, the wrongness of an action is determined by its tendency to bring about unhappiness. An ethical decision based on the utilitarian view would look at the end results of the decision. Action would be taken based on the end results that produced the most good (happiness) for the most people.

Kantianism

Named for philosopher Immanuel Kant, this theory is in direct opposition to that of utilitarianism. Kant argued that it is not the consequences or end results that make an action right or wrong, but rather it is the principle or motivation on which the action is based that is the morally decisive factor. **Kantianism** suggests that our actions are bound by a sense of duty. This theory is often called *deontology* (from the Greek word *deon*, which means "that which is binding; duty"). Kantian-directed ethical decisions are made out of respect for moral law. For example, "I make this choice because it is morally right and my duty to do so" (not because of consideration for a possible outcome).

Christian Ethics

A basic principle that might be called a Christian philosophy is that which is known as the golden rule: "Do unto others as you would have them do unto you" and, alternatively, "Do not do unto others what you would not have them do unto you." The imperative demand of **Christian ethics** is to treat others as moral equals and to recognize the equality of other persons by permitting them to act as we do when they occupy a position similar to ours.

Natural-Law Theories

The most general moral precept of the **natural law** theory is "do good and avoid evil." Based on the writings of St. Thomas Aquinas, natural-law theorists contend that ethics must be grounded in a concern for the human good. Although the nature of this "human good" is not expounded upon, Catholic theologians view natural law as the law inscribed by God into the nature of things—as a species of divine law. According to this conception, the Creator endows all things with certain potentialities or tendencies that serve to define their natural end. The fulfillment of a thing's natural tendencies constitutes the specific good of that thing. For example, the natural tendency of an acorn is to become an oak. What then is the natural potential, or tendency, of human beings? Natural-law theorists focus on an attribute that is regarded as distinctively human, as separating human beings from the rest of worldly creatures—that is, the ability to live according to the dictates of reason. It is with this ability to reason that humans are able to choose "good" over "evil." In natural law, evil acts are never condoned, even if they are intended to advance the noblest of ends.

Ethical Egoism

Ethical egoism espouses that what is right and good is what is best for the individual making the decision. An individual's actions are determined by what is to his or her own advantage. The action may not be best for anyone else involved, but consideration is only for the individual making the decision.

Ethical Dilemmas

Ethical dilemmas arise when no explicit reasons exist that govern an action. Ethical dilemmas generally create a great deal of emotion. Often the reasons supporting each side of the argument for action are logical and appropriate. The actions associated with both sides are desirable in some respects and undesirable in others.

Phipps, Long, and Woods (1987) offer the following steps leading to an ethical dilemma:

1. Some evidence indicates that act X is morally right and some evidence indicates that act X is morally wrong.
2. Evidence on both sides is inconclusive.
3. The individual perceives that he or she ought and ought not perform the act.
4. Some action must be taken.
5. An ethical dilemma exists.

In most situations *taking no action is considered an action taken.*

Ethical Principles

Ethical principles are fundamental guidelines that influence decision making. The ethical principles of autonomy, beneficence, nonmaleficence, veracity, and justice are helpful and used frequently by health care workers to assist with ethical decision making.

Autonomy

The principle of **autonomy** arises from the Kantian duty of respect for persons as rational agents. This viewpoint emphasizes the status of persons as autonomous moral agents whose right to determine their destinies should always be respected. This presumes that individuals are always capable of making independent choices for themselves. Health care workers know this is not always the case. Children, comatose patients, and the seriously mentally ill are examples of clients who are incapable of making informed choices. In these instances, a representative of the individual is usually asked to intervene with consent. However, health care workers must ensure that respect for an individual's autonomy is not disregarded in favor of what another person may view as best for the client.

Beneficence

Beneficence refers to one's duty to benefit or promote the good of others. Health care workers who act in their clients' interests are beneficent, provided their actions really do serve the client's best interest. In fact, some duties do seem to take preference over other duties. For example, the duty to respect the autonomy of an individual may be overridden when that individual has been deemed harmful to self or others. Aiken (1994) states, "The difficulty that sometimes arises in implementing the principle of beneficence lies in determining what exactly is good for another and who can best make the decision about this good."

Nonmaleficence

Nonmaleficence is the requirement that health care providers do no harm to their clients, either intentionally or unintentionally (Aiken, 1994). Some philosophers suggest that this principle is more important than beneficence; that is, they support the notion that it is more important to avoid doing harm than it is to do good. In any event, ethical dilemmas often arise when a conflict exists between an individual's rights (the duty to promote good) and what is thought to best represent the welfare of the individual (the duty to do no harm). An example of this conflict might occur when administering chemotherapy to a cancer patient, knowing it will prolong his or her life, but creating "harm" (side effects) in the short term.

Justice

This principle has been referred to as the "justice as fairness" principle. It is sometimes referred to as *distributive justice*, and its basic premise lies with the right of individuals to be treated equally regardless of race, sex, marital status, medical diagnosis, social standing, economic level, or religious belief (Aiken, 1994). The concept of **justice** reflects a duty to treat all individuals equally and fairly. When applied to health care, this principle suggests that all resources within the society (including health care services) ought to be distributed evenly without respect to socioeconomic status. Thus, according to this principle, view the vast disparity in the quality of care dispensed to the various classes within our society would be considered unjust. A more equitable distribution of care for all individuals would be favored.

Veracity

The principle of **veracity** refers to one's duty to always be truthful. Aiken (1994) states, "Veracity requires that the health care provider tell the truth and not intentionally deceive or mislead clients." There are times when limitations must be placed on this principle, such as when the truth would knowingly produce harm or interfere with the recovery process. Being honest is not always easy. But rarely is lying justified. Clients have the right to know about their diagnosis, treatment, and prognosis.

A Model for Making Ethical Decisions

The following is a set of steps that may be employed in making an ethical decision. These steps closely resemble the steps of the nursing process, and are adapted from a model suggested by Shelly (1980).

1. **Assessment.** Gather the subjective and objective data about a situation.
2. **Problem Identification.** Identify the conflict between two or more alternative actions.
3. **Plan.**
   a. Explore the benefits and consequences of each alternative.
   b. Consider principles of ethical theories.
   c. Select an alternative.
4. **Implementation.** Act on the decision made and communicate the decision to others.
5. **Evaluation.** Evaluate outcomes.

A schematic of this model is presented in Figure 40.1. A case study using this decision-making model is presented

in Table 40.3. If the outcome is acceptable, action continues in the manner selected. If the outcome is unacceptable, benefits and consequences of the remaining alternatives are reexamined, and steps 3 through 7 in Table 40.3 are repeated.

Ethical Issues in Psychiatric/Mental Health Nursing

The Right to Refuse Medication

The AHA's (1992) Patient's Bill of Rights states: "The patient has the right to refuse treatment to the extent permitted by law and to be informed of the medical consequences of his action." In psychiatry, refusal of treatment primarily concerns the administration of psychotropic medications. "To the extent permitted by law" may be defined within the U.S. Constitution and several of its amendments (e.g., the First Amendment, which addresses the rights of speech, thought, and expression; the Eighth Amendment, which grants the right to freedom from cruel and unusual punishment; and the Fifth and Fourteenth Amendments, which grant due process of law and equal protection for all). In psychiatry, "the medical consequences of his action" may include such steps as involuntary commitment, legal competency hearing, or client discharge from the hospital.

Although many courts are supporting a client's right to refuse medications in the psychiatric area, some limitations do exist. In one case (*Davis v. Hubbard, Ohio*, 1980), a federal district court concluded that no state interest could provide justification for the administration of psychotropic drugs without the consent of a competent client, *unless the client presents a danger to self or to others in the institution* (Beis, 1984). In these types of emergency situations, then, it is considered appropriate to medicate forcibly. However, the client has the right to a hearing as soon as possible.

The Right to the Least-Restrictive Treatment Alternative

Health care personnel must attempt to provide treatment in a manner that least restricts the freedom of clients. The "restrictiveness" of psychiatric therapy can be described in the context of a continuum, based on severity of illness. Clients may be treated on an outpatient basis, in day hospitals, or in voluntary or involuntary hospitalization. Symptoms may be treated with verbal rehabilitative techniques and move successively to behavioral techniques, chemical interventions, mechanical restraints, or electroconvulsive therapy.

Psychiatric nurses frequently must make decisions about selection of treatment for clients in emergency situations when there is danger to the client or others. While attempting to adhere to the principle of least-restrictive

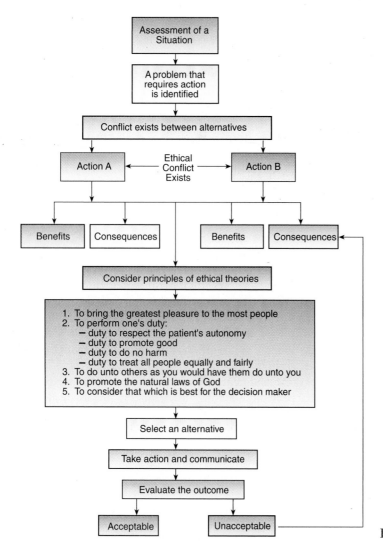

Figure 40.1 Ethical decision-making model.

alternative, harm must be avoided. Although physical restraints are the most restrictive form of treatment available to the nurse, this option is sometimes necessary to provide the needed controls, particularly if less-restrictive measures have not been effective. Because most institutions have their own policies and procedures associated with the use of restraints, the nurse should be familiar with those of his or her facility.

LEGAL CONSIDERATIONS

In 1980, the 96th Congress of the United States passed the Mental Health Systems Act, which includes a Patient's Bill of Rights, for recommendation to the states. An adaptation of these rights is presented in Table 40.4.

Nurse Practice Acts

The legal parameters of professional and practical nursing are defined within each state by the state nurse practice act. These documents are passed by the state legislature and in general are concerned with such provisions as:

1. The definition of important terms, including the definition of nursing and the various types of nurses recognized.
2. A statement of the education and other training or requirements for licensure and reciprocity.
3. A statement as to permitted nursing practices or acts (e.g., medical diagnosis) that may *not* be performed by a nurse.
4. Conditions under which a nurse's license may be suspended or revoked.
5. The general authority and powers of the state licensing agency having jurisdiction over nurses (Goldstein, Perdew, & Pruitt, 1989).

Most nurse practice acts are very general in their terminology and do not provide specific guidelines for practice. Nurses must understand the scope of practice that is protected by their license and should therefore seek assistance from legal counsel if unsure about the proper interpretation of a nurse practice act.

TABLE 40.3 ETHICAL DECISION MAKING—A CASE STUDY

Step 1. Assessment

Tonja is a 17-year-old girl who is currently on the psychiatric unit with a diagnosis of conduct disorder. Tonja reports that she has been sexually active since she was 14. She had an abortion when she was 15, and a second one just 6 weeks ago. She states that her mother told her she has "had her last abortion," and that she has to start taking birth control pills. She asks her nurse, Kimberly, to give her some information about the pills and tell her how to go about getting some. Kimberly believes Tonja desperately needs information about birth control pills, as well as other types of contraceptives, but the psychiatric unit is part of a Catholic hospital, and hospital policy prohibits distributing this type of information.

Step 2. Problem Identification

A conflict exists between the client's need for information, the nurse's desire to provide that information, and the institution's policy prohibiting the provision of that information.

Step 3. Alternatives—Benefits and Consequences

1. Alternative 1. Give the client information and risk losing job.
2. Alternative 2. Do not give client information and compromise own values of holistic nursing.
3. Alternative 3. Refer client to another source outside the hospital and risk reprimand from supervisor.

Step 4. Consider Principles of Ethical Theories

1. Alternative 1. Giving the client information would certainly respect the client's autonomy and would benefit the client by decreasing her chances of becoming pregnant again. It would not be to the best advantage of Kimberly, in that she would likely lose her job. And according to the beliefs of the Catholic hospital, the natural laws of God would be violated.
2. Alternative 2. Withholding information restricts the client's autonomy. It has the potential for doing harm, in that without the use of contraceptives, the client may become pregnant again (and she implies that this is not what she wants). Kimberly's Christian ethic is violated in that this action is not what she would want "done unto her."

3. Alternative 3. A referral would respect the client's autonomy, would promote good, would do no harm (except perhaps to Kimberly's ego from the possible reprimand), and this decision would comply with Kimberly's Christian ethic.

Step 5. Select an Alternative

Alternative 3 is selected based on the ethical theories of utilitarianism (does the most good for the greatest number), Christian ethics (Kimberly's belief of "Do unto others as you would have others do unto you"), Kantianism (to perform one's duty), and the ethical principles of autonomy, beneficence, and nonmaleficence. The success of this decision depends upon the client's follow-through with the referral and compliance with use of the con-traceptives.

Step 6. Take Action and Communicate

Taking action involves providing information in writing for Tonja, perhaps making a phone call and setting up an appointment for her with Planned Parenthood. Communicating suggests sharing the information with Tonja's mother. Communication also includes documentation of the referral in the client's chart.

Step 7. Evaluate the Outcome

An acceptable outcome might indicate that Tonja did indeed keep her appointment at Planned Parenthood and is complying with the prescribed contraceptive regimen. It might also include Kimberly's input into the change process in her institution to implement these types of referrals to other clients who request them.

An unacceptable outcome might be indicated by Tonja's lack of follow-through with the appointment at Planned Parenthood or lack of compliance in using the contraceptives, resulting in another pregnancy. Kimberly may also view a reprimand from her supervisor as an unacceptable outcome, particularly if she is told that she must select other alternatives should this situation arise in the future. This may motivate Kimberly to make another decision—that of seeking employment in an institution that supports a philosophy more consistent with her own.

Types of Law

There are two general categories or types of law that are of most concern to nurses: statutory law and common law. These laws are identified by their source or origin.

Statutory Law

Statutory laws are those that have been enacted by legislative bodies, such as a county or city council, state legislature, or the Congress of the United States. An example of statutory law would be the nurse practice acts.

Common Law

Common laws are derived from decisions made in previous cases. These laws apply to a body of principles that evolve from court decisions resolving various controver-sies. Because common law in the United States has been developed on a state basis, the law on specific subjects may differ from state to state. An example of a common law might be how different states deal with a nurse's refusal to provide care for a specific client.

Classifications Within Statutory and Common Law

Broadly speaking, there are two kinds of unlawful acts: civil and criminal. Both statutory law and common law have civil and criminal components.

Civil Law

Civil law protects the private and property rights of individuals and businesses. Private individuals or groups may bring a legal action to court for breach of civil

TABLE 40.4 BILL OF RIGHTS FOR PSYCHIATRIC PATIENTS

1. The right to appropriate treatment and related services in the setting that is most supportive and least restrictive to personal freedom.
2. The right to an individualized, written treatment or service plan; the right to treatment based on such plan; and the right to periodic review and revision of the plan based on treatment needs.
3. The right, consistent with one's capabilities, to participate in and receive a reasonable explanation of the care and treatment process.
4. The right to refuse treatment except in an emergency situation or as permitted by law.
5. The right not to participate in experimentation in the absence of informed, voluntary, written consent.
6. The right to freedom from restraint or seclusion except in an emergency situation.
7. The right to a humane treatment environment that affords reasonable protection from harm and appropriate privacy.
8. The right to confidentiality of medical records (also applicable following patient's discharge).
9. The right of access to medical records except information received from third parties under promise of confidentiality, and when access would be detrimental to the patient's health (also applicable following patient's discharge).
10. The right of access to use of the telephone, personal mail, and visitors, unless deemed inappropriate for treatment purposes.
11. The right to be informed of these rights in comprehensible language.
12. The right to assert grievances if rights are infringed.
13. The right to referral as appropriate to other providers of mental health services upon discharge.

SOURCE: Adapted from Mental Health Systems Act (1980).

law. These legal actions are of two basic types: torts and contracts.

Torts. A **tort** is a violation of a civil law in which an individual has been wronged. In a tort action, one party asserts that wrongful conduct on the part of the other has caused harm, and compensation for harm suffered is sought. A tort may be *intentional* or *unintentional*. Examples of unintentional torts are malpractice and negligence actions. An example of an intentional tort is the touching of another person without consent. Intentional touching (e.g., a medical treatment) without the client's consent can result in a charge of battery, an intentional tort.

Contracts. In a contract action, one party asserts that the other party has, in failing to fulfill an obligation, breached the contract, and either compensation or performance of the obligation is sought as remedy. An example might be an action by a mental health professional whose clinical privileges have been reduced or terminated in violation of an implied contract between the professional and a hospital (Beis, 1984).

Criminal Law

Criminal law provides protection from conduct deemed injurious to the public welfare. It provides for punishment of those found to have engaged in such conduct. This commonly includes imprisonment, parole conditions, a loss of privilege (such as a license), a fine, or any combination of these (Ellis & Hartley, 1995). An example of a violation of criminal law is the theft by a hospital employee of supplies or drugs.

Legal Issues in Psychiatric/Mental Health Nursing

Confidentiality and Right to Privacy

An individual's privacy is protected by the Fourth, Fifth, and Fourteenth Amendments to the Constitution of the United States. Most states have statutes protecting the confidentiality of client records and communications. The only individuals who have a right to observe a client or have access to medical information are those involved in his or her medical care.

Pertinent medical information may be released in a life-threatening situation without consent. If information is released in an emergency, the following information must be recorded in the client's record: date of disclosure, person to whom information was disclosed, reason for disclosure, reason written consent could not be obtained, and the specific information disclosed.

Most states have statutes that pertain to the doctrine of **privileged communication.** Although the codes differ markedly from state to state, most grant certain professionals privileges under which they may refuse to reveal information about and communications with clients. In most states, the doctrine of privileged communication applies to psychiatrists and attorneys; in some instances, psychologists, clergy, and nurses are also included.

In certain instances nurses may be called on to testify in cases in which the medical record is used as evidence. In most states, the right to privacy of these records is exempted in civil or criminal proceedings. It is therefore very important that nurses document with these possibilities in mind. Strict record keeping, using statements that are objective and nonjudgmental; care plans that are specific in their prescriptive interventions; and documentation that describes those interventions and their subsequent evaluation all serve the best interests of the client, the nurse, and the institution should questions regarding care arise. Documentation very often weighs heavily in malpractice case decisions.

The right to confidentiality is a basic one, and especially so in psychiatry. Even though societal attitudes are improving, individuals have been discriminated against in the past for no other reason than having a history of emotional illness. Nurses working in psychiatry must guard the privacy of their clients with great diligence.

Informed Consent

According to law, all persons have the right to decide whether to accept or reject treatment (Guido, 1997). A health care provider can be charged with assault and battery for providing life-sustaining treatment to a client when the client has not agreed to it. The rationale for the doctrine of **informed consent** is the preservation and protection of individual autonomy in determining what will and will not happen to the person's body (Guido, 1997).

Informed consent is a client's permission granted to a physician to perform a therapeutic procedure, prior to which information about the procedure has been presented to the client with adequate time given for consideration about the pros and cons. The client should receive information such as what treatment alternatives are available; why the physician believes this treatment is most appropriate; the possible outcomes, risks, and adverse effects; the possible outcome should the client select another treatment alternative; and the possible outcome should the client choose to have no treatment.

Goldstein, Perdew, and Pruitt (1989) state that informed consent should be obtained:

"… any time there is an inherent risk of death or serious bodily injury that the patient might not know about, or when the probability of success in a medical procedure is low. The rule applies equally to administration of investigational drugs, the performance of diagnostic tests, and the performance of major or minor surgical procedures." (p.113)

An example of a treatment in the psychiatric area that requires informed consent is electroconvulsive therapy.

There are some conditions under which treatment may be performed without obtaining informed consent. A client's refusal to accept treatment may be challenged under the following circumstances (Cournos & Petrila, 1992; Beis, 1984; Goldstein, Perdew, & Pruitt, 1989; Guido, 1997):

1. When a client is mentally incompetent to make a decision and treatment is necessary to preserve life or avoid serious harm.
2. When refusing treatment endangers the life or health of another.
3. An emergency in which a client is in no condition to exercise judgment.
4. When the client is a child (consent is obtained from parent or surrogate).
5. In the case of therapeutic privilege. In therapeutic privilege, information about a treatment may be withheld if the physician can show that full disclosure would

   a. Hinder or complicate necessary treatment
   b. Cause severe psychological harm
   c. Be so upsetting as to render a rational decision by the client impossible

Although most clients in psychiatric/mental health facilities are competent and capable of giving informed consent, those with severe psychiatric illness will not possess the cognitive ability to do so. If an individual has been legally determined as mentally incompetent, consent is obtained from the legal guardian. Difficulty arises when there has been no legal determination made, but the individual's current mental state prohibits informed decision making (e.g., the psychotic person, the unconscious person, the inebriated person). In these instances, informed consent is usually obtained from the individual's nearest relative, or if none exist and time permits, the physician may ask the court to appoint a conservator or guardian. When time does not permit court intervention, permission may even be sought from the hospital administrator.

A client or guardian always has the right to withdraw consent after it has been given. When this occurs, the physician should inform (or reinform) the client about the consequences of refusing treatment. If treatment has already been initiated, the physician should terminate treatment in a way least likely to cause injury to the client and inform the client or guardian of the risks associated with interrupted treatment (Guido, 1997).

The nurse's role in obtaining informed consent is usually defined by agency policy. A nurse may sign the consent form as witness for the client's signature. However, legal liability for informed consent lies with the physician. The nurse acts as client advocate to ensure that the three major elements of informed consent have been addressed:

1. **Knowledge**—that the client has received adequate information on which to base his or her decision.
2. **Competency**—that the individual's cognition is not impaired to an extent that would interfere with decision making or, if so, that the individual has a legal representative.
3. **Free Will**—that the individual has given consent voluntarily without pressure or coercion from others.

Restraints and Seclusion

An individual's privacy and personal security are protected by the U.S. Constitution and supported by the Mental Health Systems Act of 1980, out of which was conceived a Bill of Rights for psychiatric patients. These include "the right to freedom from restraint or seclusion except in an emergency situation."

In psychiatry, the term *restraints* generally refers to a set of leather straps that are used to restrain the extremities of an individual whose behavior is out of control and who poses a threat of harm to self or others. They are never to be used as punishment or for the convenience of staff. Less-restrictive measures to decrease agitation, such as "talking down" (verbal intervention) and chemical restraints (tranquilizing medication) are usually tried initially. When these interventions are ineffective, mechanical restraints may be instituted. *Seclusion* is another type of physical restraint in which the client is confined alone in a room from which he or she is unable to leave. The room is usually minimally furnished with items to promote the client's comfort and safety.

In an emergency, when a client threatens harm to self or others, restraint or seclusion may be implemented without a physician's written order. However, the written order of the physician who is responsible for the client's medical care should be obtained no more than eight hours after initial employment of the restraint or seclusion. An "as-needed" order is never permitted. Orders are time limited, and vary from state to state. This limited time period allows for periodic review and assessment by the physician before orders are renewed.

Clients in restraints or seclusion must be observed and assessed every 10 to 15 minutes with regard to circulation, respiration, nutrition, hydration, and elimination. Such attention should be documented in the client's record. Periodic (usually every 2 hours) release from restraints or seclusion is recommended (Goldstein, Perdew, & Pruitt, 1989).

False imprisonment is the deliberate and unauthorized confinement of a person within fixed limits by the use of verbal or physical means (Ellis & Hartley, 1995). Health care workers may be charged with false imprisonment for restraining or secluding against their wishes those clients who have sought hospital admission voluntarily. Should a voluntarily admitted client decompensate to a point that required restraint or seclusion for protection of self or others, court intervention to determine competency and involuntary commitment would be required to preserve the client's rights to privacy and freedom.

Commitment Issues

Voluntary Commitment

Each year, more than 1 million persons are committed to hospitals for psychiatric treatment. Approximately two thirds of these admissions are officially identified as voluntary commitments, while the remaining one third are involuntary (Durham, 1996). To be admitted voluntarily, an individual makes direct application to the institution for services and may stay as long as treatment is deemed necessary. He or she may sign out of the hospital at any time, unless following a mental status examination the health care professional determines that the client may be harmful to self or others and recommends that the admission status be changed form voluntary to involuntary. Durham (1996) states:

"Even though these hospital admissions are considered 'voluntary,' they are regulated by statute to ensure that (1) persons with mental disorders are sufficiently competent to make decisions of this kind, (2) inappropriate pressure or outright coercion has not been exerted on a person already in custody to admit themselves, and (3) the person is truly 'willing' to seek treatment, thereby improving the prospects for success." (p. 17)

Involuntary Commitment

Because involuntary hospitalization results in substantial restrictions of the rights of an individual, the admission process is subject to the guarantee of the Fourteenth Amendment to the U.S. Constitution that no state may "deprive any person of life, liberty, or property, without due process of law; nor deny to any person within its jurisdiction the equal protection of the laws" (Beis, 1984). Involuntary commitments are made for various reasons. Most states commonly cite the following criteria:

1. In an emergency situation (for the client who is dangerous to self or others).
2. For observation and treatment of mentally ill persons.
3. When an individual is unable to take care of basic personal needs (the "gravely disabled").

Under the Fourth Amendment, individuals are protected from unlawful searches and seizures without probable cause. Therefore, the individual seeking the involuntary commitment must show probable cause why the client should be hospitalized against his or her wishes—that is, to show that there is cause to believe that the person would be dangerous to self or others, is mentally ill and in need of treatment, or is gravely disabled.

Emergency Commitments. Emergency commitments are sought when an individual manifests behavior that is clearly and imminently dangerous to self or others. These admissions are usually instigated by relatives or friends of the individual, police officers, the court, or health care professional. Emergency commitments are time-limited, and a court hearing for the individual will be scheduled, usually within a 72-hour period. At that time the court may decide that the client may be discharged; or, if deemed necessary, and voluntary admission is refused by the client, an additional period of involuntary commitment may be ordered. In most instances, another hearing will be scheduled for a specified time (usually 7 to 21 days).

The Mentally Ill Person in Need of Treatment. A second type of involuntary commitment is for the observation and treatment of mentally ill persons in need of treatment. Most states have established definitions of what constitutes "mentally ill," for purposes of state involuntary admission statutes. Some examples include (Beis, 1984):

1. In Colorado: "Mentally ill person" means a person who is of such mental condition that he is in need of medical supervision, treatment, care, or restraint.
2. In Kansas: "Mentally ill person" is any person who:
   a. Is suffering from a severe mental disorder to the extent that such a person is in need of treatment.
   b. Lacks capacity to make an informed decision concerning treatment.
   c. Is likely to cause harm to self or others.
3. In Oregon: "Mentally ill person" means a person who, because of a mental disorder, is either:
   a. Dangerous to himself or others, or
   b. Unable to provide for his basic personal needs and is not receiving such care as is necessary for his health and safety.

In determining whether or not commitment is required, the court will look for substantial evidence of abnormal conduct—evidence that cannot be explained as the result of a physical cause. There must be "clear and convincing evidence" as well as "probable cause" to substantiate the need for involuntary commitment to ensure that an individual's rights under the Constitution are protected. The U.S. Supreme Court in *O'Connor v. Donaldson* held that the existence of mental illness alone does not justify involuntary hospitalization. State standards require a specific impact or consequence to flow from the mental illness that involves dangerousness or an inability to care for one's own needs (Beis, 1984). These clients are entitled to court hearings with representation, at which time determination of commitment and length of stay are considered. Legislative statutes governing involuntary commitments vary from state to state.

Involuntary Outpatient Commitment. Involuntary outpatient commitment (IOC) is a court-ordered mechanism used to compel a person with mental illness to submit to treatment on an outpatient basis. Maloy (1996) cites three determinants for commitment to outpatient treatment. These include:

1. Conditional release from inpatient hospitalization.
2. Commitment to an outpatient program as a less-restrictive alternative to hospitalization for persons who meet the inpatient commitment standard but would benefit from community treatment
3. Commitment to outpatient treatment (sometimes called preventive commitment) based on less stringent criteria than are required for inpatient commitment.

Twenty-five states enacted IOC legislation during the 1980s, and at least a dozen more currently have resolutions that speak to this topic on their agendas (Maloy, 1996). Most commonly, clients who are committed into the IOC programs are those with severe and persistent mental illness, such as schizophrenia. The rationale behind the legislation is to reduce the numbers of readmissions and lengths of hospital stays of these clients. Concern lies in the possibility of violating the individual rights of psychiatric clients without significant improvement in treatment outcomes. Maloy (1996) states, "IOC laws do not necessarily lead to improvements in services or enhancements of community mental health programs. Nonetheless, the ongoing attention given to outpatient commitment laws by state legislators suggests that state policymakers view IOC as a useful and appropriate response to the challenges and crises posed by severe and persistent mental illness." Ongoing research shows that IOC may indeed reduce hospital readmissions and lengths of stays. Continuing research is required to determine if IOC will improve treatment compliance and enhance quality of life in the community for individuals with severe and persistent mental illness.

The Gravely Disabled Client. A number of states have statutes that specifically define the "gravely disabled" client. For those that do not use this label, the description of the individual who, because of mental illness, is unable to take care of basic personal needs is very similar.

Gravely disabled is generally defined as a condition in which an individual, as a result of mental illness, is in danger of serious physical harm resulting from inability to provide for basic needs such as food, clothing, shelter, medical care, and personal safety. Inability to care for oneself cannot be established by showing that an individual lacks the resources to provide the necessities of life. Rather, it is the inability to make use of available resources (Beis, 1984).

Should it be determined that an individual is gravely disabled, a guardian, conservator, or committee will be appointed by the court to ensure the management of the person and his or her estate. To legally restore competency would then require another court hearing to reverse the previous ruling. The individual whose competency is being determined has the right to be represented by an attorney.

Nursing Liability

Mental health practitioners—psychiatrists, psychologists, psychiatric nurses, and social workers—have a duty to provide appropriate care based on the standards of their professions and the standards set by law. The standards of care for psychiatric/mental health nursing are presented in Chapter 7 of this text.

Malpractice and Negligence

The terms **malpractice** and **negligence** are often used interchangeably. *Negligence* (Black & Nolan, 1990) has been defined as:

"... the omission (of a person) to do something which a reasonable person, guided by those ordinary considerations which ordinarily regulate human affairs, would do, or the doing of something which a prudent and reasonable person would not do."

Any person may be negligent. In contrast, malpractice is a specialized form of negligence applicable only to professionals. In *Matthews v. Walker* in Ohio, 1973, malpractice was defined as:

"The failure of one rendering professional services to exercise that degree of skill and learning commonly applied under all the circumstances in the community by the average prudent reputable member of the profession with the result of injury, loss, or damage to the recipient of those services or to those entitled to rely upon them" (Black & Nolan, 1990).

In the absence of any state statutes, common law is the basis of liability for injuries to clients caused by acts of malpractice and negligence of individual practitioners. In other words, most decisions of negligence in the professional setting are based on legal precedent (decisions that have previously been made about similar cases) rather than any specific action taken by the legislature.

To summarize, then, when the breach of duty is characterized as malpractice, the action is weighed against the professional standard. When it is brought forth as negligence, action is contrasted with what a reasonably prudent professional would have done in the same or similar circumstances.

Goldstein, Perdew, and Pruitt (1989) state that every nursing malpractice suit must include the following basic elements:

1. A claim that the nurse owed the client a special duty of care.
2. A claim that the nurse was required to meet a specific standard of care in carrying out the nursing act or function in question.
3. A claim that the nurse failed to meet the required standard of care.
4. A claim that harm or injury resulted, for which compensation is sought.

For the client to prevail in a malpractice claim, each of these elements must be proved. Juries' decisions are generally based on the testimony of expert witnesses, since members of the jury are laypeople and cannot be expected to know what nursing interventions should have been carried out. Without the testimony of expert witnesses, a favorable verdict usually goes to the defendent nurse.

Types of Lawsuits That Occur in Psychiatric Nursing

Most malpractice suits against nurses are civil actions—that is, they are considered breach of conduct actions on the part of the professional, for which compensation is being sought. The nurse in the psychiatric setting should be aware of the types of behaviors that may result in charges of malpractice.

Basic to the psychiatric client's hospitalization is his or her right to confidentiality and privacy. A nurse may be charged with *breach of confidentiality* for revealing aspects about a client's case, or even for revealing that an individual has been hospitalized, if that person can show that making this information known resulted in harm.

When shared information is detrimental to the client's reputation, the person sharing the information may be liable for **defamation of character.** When the information is in writing, the action is called libel. Oral defamation is called **slander.** Defamation of character involves communication that is malicious and false (Ellis & Hartley, 1995). Occasionally, **libel** arises out of critical, judgmental statements written in the client's medical record. Nurses need to be very objective in their charting, backing up all statements with factual evidence.

Invasion of privacy is a charge that may result when a client is searched without probable cause. Many institutions conduct body searches on mental clients as a routine intervention. In these cases, there should be a physician's order and written rationale should show probable cause for the intervention. Many institutions are reexamining their policies regarding this procedure.

Assault is an act that results in a person's genuine fear and apprehension that he or she will be touched without consent. **Battery** is the unconsented touching of another person. These charges can result when a treatment is administered to a client against his or her wishes and outside of an emergency situation. Harm or injury need not have occurred for these charges to be legitimate.

For confining a client against his or her wishes, and outside of an emergency situation, the nurse may be charged with false imprisonment. Examples of actions that may invoke these charges include locking an individual in a room; taking a client's clothes for purposes of detainment against his or her will; and retaining in mechanical restraints a competent voluntary client who demands to be released.

Avoiding Liability

Goldstein, Perdew, and Pruitt (1989) suggest the following guidelines for avoiding liability:

1. Practice within the scope of the nurse practice act.
2. Observe the hospital's and department's policy manuals.
3. Measure up to established practice standards.
4. Always put the client's rights and welfare first.
5. Develop and maintain a good interpersonal relationship with each client and his or her family.

This final item is an extremely important guideline to follow. Some clients appear to be more *suit prone* than others. Suit-prone clients are often very critical, complaining, uncooperative, and even hostile. A natural response by the staff to these clients is to become defensive or withdrawn. Either of these behaviors increases the likelihood of a lawsuit should an unfavorable event occur (Ellis & Hartley, 1995). No matter how high a degree of technical competence and skill a nurse has, his or her insensitivity to a client's complaints and failure to meet the client's emotional needs often influence whether or not a lawsuit is generated. A great deal depends on the psychosocial skills of the health care professional.

SUMMARY

This chapter examined some of the ethical and legal issues relevant to psychiatric/mental health nursing in an effort to promote enhancement of quality of client care, as well as provide protection to the nurse within the parameters of legal accountability. Ethics is a branch of philosophy that deals with values related to human conduct, to the rightness and wrongness of certain actions, and to the goodness and badness of the motives and ends of such actions.

Clients have certain rights that are afforded them under the Constitution of the United States. Clients' rights have also been set forth by the AHA, the NLN, the American Civil Liberties Union, and the Mental Health Systems Act. Nurse practice acts and standards of professional practice guide the scope within which a nurse may legally practice. The ANA has established a Code for Nurses under which guidelines the professional nurse is expected to practice ethical nursing.

Ethical theories and principles are foundational guidelines that influence decision making. Ethical theories include utilitarianism, Kantianism, Christian ethics, natural-law theories, and ethical egoism. Ethical principles include autonomy, beneficence, nonmaleficence, veracity, and justice. An individual's ethical philosophy affects his or her decision-making and ultimately the outcomes of those decisions.

Ethical issues in psychiatric/mental health nursing include the right to refuse medication and the right to the least-restrictive treatment alternative. An ethical decision-making model was presented along with a case study for application of the process.

Statutory laws are those that have been enacted by legislative bodies, and common laws are derived from decisions made in previous cases. Civil law protects the private and property rights of individuals and businesses, and criminal law provides protection from conduct deemed injurious to the public welfare. Both statutory law and common law have civil and criminal components.

Legal issues in psychiatric/mental health nursing center around confidentiality and the right to privacy, informed consent, restraints and seclusion, and commitment issues. Nurses are accountable for their own actions in relation to these issues, and violation can result in malpractice lawsuits against the physician, the hospital, and the nurse. Nurses must be aware of the kinds of behaviors that place them at risk for malpractice action. Developing and maintaining a good interpersonal relationship with the client and his or her family appears to be a positive factor when the question of malpractice is being considered.

REVIEW QUESTIONS

SELF-EXAMINATION/LEARNING EXERCISE

Match the following decision-making examples with the appropriate ethical theory:

_____ 1. Carol decides to go against family wishes and tell the client of his terminal status because that is what she would want if she were the client.

_____ 2. Carol decides to respect family wishes and not tell the client of his terminal status because that would bring the most happiness to the most people.

_____ 3. Carol decides not to tell the client about his terminal status because it would be too uncomfortable for her to do so.

_____ 4. Carol decides to tell the client of his terminal status because her reasoning tells her that to do otherwise would be an evil act.

_____ 5. Carol decides to tell the client of his terminal status because she believes it is her duty to do so.

a. Utilitarianism

b. Kantianism

c. Christian ethics

d. Natural-law theories

e. Ethical egoism

Match the following nursing actions with the possible legal action with which the nurse may be charged:

_____ 6. The nurse assists the physician with electroconvulsive therapy on his client, who has refused to give consent.

_____ 7. When the local newspaper calls to inquire why the mayor has been admitted to the hospital, the nurse replies, "He's here because he is an alcoholic."

_____ 8. A competent, voluntary client has stated he wants to leave the hospital. The nurse hides his clothes in an effort to keep him from leaving.

_____ 9. Jack recently lost his wife and is very depressed. He is running for reelection to the Senate and asks the staff to keep his hospitalization confidential. The nurse is excited about having a senator on the unit and tells her boyfriend about the admission, which soon becomes common knowledge. Jack loses the election.

_____ 10. Joe is very restless and is pacing a lot. The nurse says to Joe, "If you don't sit down in the chair and be still, I'm going to put you in restraints!"

a. Breach of confidentiality

b. Defamation of character

c. Assault

d. Battery

e. False imprisonment

REFERENCES

Aiken, T.D. (1994). *Legal, ethical, and political issues in nursing.* Philadelphia: F.A. Davis.

American Hospital Association (AHA). (1992). *A Patient's Bill of Rights.* Chicago: American Hospital Association.

American Nurses' Association (ANA). (1985). *Code of ethics with interpretive statements.* Kansas City, MO: ANA.

Beis, E.B. (1984). *Mental health and the law.* Rockville, MD: Aspen Systems.

Black, H., & Nolan, J.R. (1990). *Black's law dictionary* (6th ed.). St. Paul, MN: West Publishing.

Cournos, F., & Petrila, J. (1992). Legal and ethical issues. In F.I. Kass, J.M. Oldham, & H. Pardes (Eds.), *The Columbia University College of Physicians and Surgeons complete guide to mental health.* New York: Henry Holt.

Durham, M.L. (1996). Civil commitment of the mentally ill: Research, policy and practice. In B.D. Sales & S.A Shaw (Eds.), *Mental health and law: Research, policy and services.* Durham, NC: Carolina Academic Press.

Ellis, J.R., & Hartley, C.L. (1995). *Nursing in today's world: Challenges, issues, and trends* (5th ed.). Philadelphia: J.B. Lippincott.

Goldstein, A.S., Perdew, S., & Pruitt S.S. (1989). *The nurse's legal advisor: Your guide to legally safe practice.* Philadelphia: J.B. Lippincott.

Guido, G.W. (1997). *Legal issues in nursing* (2nd ed.). Stamford, CT: Appleton & Lange.

King, E.C. (1984). *Affective education in nursing: A guide to teaching and assessment.* Rockville, MD: Aspen Systems.

Leach, A.M. (1987). Legal and ethical issues. In J. Haber, A.M. Leach, S.M. Schudy, & B.F. Sidelaw (Eds.), *Comprehensive psychiatric nursing* (3rd ed.). New York: McGraw-Hill.

Maloy, K.A. (1996). Does involuntary outpatient commitment work? In B.D. Sales & S.A. Shah (Eds.), *Mental health and law: Research, policy and services.* Durham, NC: Carolina Academic Press.

McGovern, T.F. (1991). Foreword. In P.J. Barker & S. Baldwin (Eds.), *Ethical issues in mental health.* London: Chapman & Hall.

Mental Health Systems Act. P.L. 96-398, Title V, Sect. 501.94 Stat. 1598, October 7, 1980.

Pappas, A. (1994). Ethical issues. In J. Zerwekh & J.C. Claborn (Eds.), *Nursing today: Transition and trends.* Philadelphia: W.B. Saunders.

Phipps, W.J., Long, B.C., & Woods, N.F. (1987). *Medical-surgical nursing: Concepts and clinical practice* (3rd ed.). St. Louis: C. V. Mosby.

Shelly, J.A. (1980). *Dilemma: A nurses' guide for making ethical decisions.* Downers Grove, IL: Inter-Varsity.

PSYCHIATRIC HOME NURSING CARE

KEY TERMS

home care
psychiatric home care
Medicare

Health Care Financing
    Administration
    (HCFA)

informed consent
abandonment

OBJECTIVES

After reading this chapter, the student will be able to:

1. Define *home care* and *psychiatric home care*.
2. Discuss historical aspects related to the growth in the home health care movement.
3. Identify agencies that provide, and sources of reimbursement for, psychiatric home nursing care.
4. Identify client populations that benefit most from psychiatric home nursing care.
5. Describe advantages and disadvantages associated with psychiatric home nursing care.
6. Discuss cultural and boundary issues associated with psychiatric home nursing care.
7. Describe the role of the nurse in psychiatric home nursing care.
8. Apply steps of the nursing process to psychiatric home nursing care.
9. Discuss legal and ethical issues that relate to psychiatric home nursing care.

ramatic changes in the health care delivery system and skyrocketing costs have created a need to find a way to provide cost-effective quality care to psychiatric clients. **Home care** has become one of the fastest-growing areas in the health care system, and it is now recognized by many reimbursement agencies as a preferred method of community-based service. Just what is home health care? The National Association for Home Care (NAHC) (1996) contributes the following definition:

> "Home care is a simple phrase that encompasses a wide range of health and social services. These services are delivered at home to recovering, disabled, chronically or terminally ill persons in need of medical, nursing, social, or therapeutic treatment and/or assistance with essential activities of daily living."

Duffey and Miller (1996) expound on the role of **psychiatric home care** in the delivery of mental health services to clients in their home setting:

> "Psychiatric home care nurses must have physical and psychosocial nursing skills to meet the demands of the patient population they serve. Inpatient psychiatric nurses are likely to have some familiarity with physical nursing skills. Psychiatric nurses in home care must adapt their skills to fit within the home care nursing arena." (p. 104)

This chapter examines some of the issues related to psychiatric home nursing care. Historical aspects and present-day statistics are presented. Strengths and limitations of the concept and role of the nurse are described. Nursing care of the psychiatric home care client is presented in the context of the nursing process. Pertinent legal and ethical issues related to psychiatric home nursing care are examined.

HISTORICAL ASPECTS

The root of home care is found in the practice of visiting nursing, which had its beginnings in the United States in the late 1800s (Humphrey & Milone-Nuzzo, 1996). When physicians began to limit their home visits to clients after World War II, much of this care was relegated to nurses. Visiting nurses associations were established throughout the first half of the 20th century, with much of their service directed toward the poor who could not afford hospital care. In 1965, with the passage of **Medicare** legislation, home nursing care increased dramatically, because it was one of the benefits that Medicare provided for elderly clients who were eligible for the service.

Psychiatric home nursing care did not enjoy the popularity of other types of home care nursing, largely because psychiatric home nursing care was not recognized by the **Health Care Financing Administration (HCFA)** as a reimbursable service until 1979. Growth through the 1980s was slow, with home care agencies employing psychiatric nurses mainly as consultants to their staff nurses

(Humphrey & Milone-Nuzzo, 1996). In recent years this has changed, and currently psychiatric home nursing care is experiencing the same rapid growth as general medical home nursing care.

GENERAL INFORMATION RELATED TO PSYCHIATRIC HOME NURSING CARE

In 1996, 3.4 percent of all clients receiving home care services had a primary psychiatric diagnosis (NAHC, 1999). Richie and Lusky (1987) cite the following reasons for a continuing need for psychiatric home care:

1. Earlier hospital discharges
2. Increased demand for home care as an alternative to institutional care
3. Broader third-party payment coverage
4. Greater physician acceptance of home care

Psychiatric home nursing care is provided through private home health agencies; private hospitals; public hospitals; government institutions, such as the Veterans Administration; and community mental health centers. Most often, home care is viewed as follow-up care to inpatient, partial, or outpatient hospitalization.

Payment for Home Care

The majority of home health care is paid for by Medicare. Other sources include Medicaid, private insurance, self-pay, and others. The statistics related to sources of payment are presented in Table 41.1. Medicare requires that the following criteria be met to qualify for psychiatric home care:

1. Certification by a physician that the client is homebound
2. Diagnosis of an acute psychiatric illness or an acute exacerbation of such an illness
3. Requirement by the client of the specialized knowledge, skills, and abilities of a psychiatric registered nurse (Pelletier, 1988)

Case (1993) reports:

> "Medicare's interpretation of 'homebound' status for psychiatric clients diverges from the medical application

TABLE 41.1 SOURCES OF PAYMENT FOR HOME CARE 1996

SOURCE OF PAYMENT	PERCENT
Medicare	38.7
Medicaid	27.2
Private insurance	12.2
Self-pay	20.5
Other	1.3

with which most have been familiar in the past. Patients don't have to be physically homebound; they can be mentally homebound. In other words, they can be patients physically able to leave their homes but mentally unwilling. It deals more with not wanting to leave the home because of factors such as anxiety, cognitive impairment, and vegetative depression. Agency nurses must be able to document that patients truly are homebound by such factors." (p. 61)

Although Medicare and Medicaid are the largest reimbursement providers, a growing number of health maintenance organizations (HMOs) and preferred provider organizations (PPOs) are beginning to recognize the cost-effectiveness of psychiatric home nursing care and are including it as part of their benefit packages. Most managed care agencies require that treatment, or even a specific number of visits, be preauthorized for psychiatric home nursing care. The plan of treatment and subsequent charting must explain why the client's psychiatric disorder keeps him or her at home as well as justify the need for services.

Types of Diagnoses

Homebound clients most often have diagnoses of schizophrenia, major depression, bipolar disorder, substance abuse, agoraphobia, paranoia, or generalized anxiety (Hellwig, 1993). Many elderly clients are homebound owing to medical conditions that impair mobility and necessitate home care.

Finkelman (1997) states:

"Psychiatric home care is provided to patients with psychiatric diagnoses who may or may not have been hospitalized in the past, to medical patients who do not have a formal psychiatric diagnosis but do have major psychiatric symptoms, and to medical patients with psychological responses to their medical illnesses."

Richie and Lusky (1987) identify three predominant client populations that benefit from psychiatric home health nursing:

1. **The Elderly.** These individuals are without a history of chronic mental illness but are experiencing acute psychosocial and developmental problems that have arisen from medical and sociocultural factors. Depression and social isolation are common.
2. **The Chronically Mentally Ill.** These individuals have a history of three or more psychiatric hospitalizations and require long-term medications and supportive care. Common diagnoses include depression, schizoaffective disorders, schizophrenia, and borderline personality disorder.
3. **Those With Acute Mental Health Problems.** These individuals are experiencing crisis situations and are in need of crisis intervention and/or short-term psychotherapy.

Advantages and Disadvantages of Home Care

Ongoing studies continue to support the cost-effectiveness of psychiatric home nursing care, but there are certain other aspects related to nursing the psychiatric client in his or her home that must be taken into consideration. Being able to observe the client within the context of family and home environment allows for the most comprehensive biopsychosocial assessment. Humphrey and Milone-Nuzzo (1996) state, "Psychiatric care provided in the home is often perceived as less threatening, especially to the elderly and the chronically mentally ill."

Harris (1987) suggests, however, that caring for a client in a home environment without the additional services of other professionals may be a disadvantage. If the client has never participated in home care before, he or she, and perhaps the family also, may be distrustful or somewhat confused about what this new form of treatment entails. Peplau (1995) asserts that, because the client's home is the domain of the family, the authority and autonomy of the nurse are constrained. She also suggests that the safety of the nurse may be an issue, citing a study reporting that persons with serious mental illness lived in unsafe, poorer neighborhoods than the overall population. She believes that nurses who plan to practice in psychiatric home care programs will need retraining in terms of safety issues.

Cultural and Boundary Issues

Duffey and Miller (1996) propose that there are several cultural and boundary issues in psychiatric home nursing care that differ from nursing in the institutional setting. Nurses have always learned that it is never appropriate to accept a gift from a client in the hospital. But what about in the home? Is it appropriate to accept a cup of coffee on a cold day? What about a small token of their appreciation for the care they see the nurse providing? Culturally, would it be an insult if the gift were refused by the nurse? It is important for the nurse to be aware of cultural influences that affect boundary issues when he or she enters the private domain of the client. These issues are not completely resolved and warrant further discussion and study.

ROLE OF THE NURSE

The American Nurses' Association (ANA) (1992) defines home health nursing as

" . . . the practice of nursing applied to a patient with a health deficit in the patient's place of residence. Patients and their designated caregivers are the focus of home health nursing practice. The goal of care is to initiate, manage, and evaluate the resources needed to promote the patient's optimal level of well-being." (p. 5)

Medicare requires that psychiatric home nursing care be provided by "psychiatrically trained nurses," which they define as, " . . . nurses who have special training and/or experience beyond the standard curriculum required for a registered nurse" (HCFA, 1999). Finkelman (1997) suggests that the ideal candidate for a psychiatric home health nurse has a minimum of 1 year of medical-surgical nursing experience, as well as several years of psychiatric inpatient treatment experience. Further training and experience in psychotherapy is viewed as an asset. However, psychotherapy is not the primary focus of psychiatric home nursing care. In fact, most reimbursement sources say they will not pay for exclusively insight-oriented "therapy" (Duffey & Miller, 1996). Peplau (1995) states, "Hands-on care, health teaching, coordination of care, and supervision of home health aides are all nursing functions in psychiatric home care." Crisis intervention is common in psychiatric home nursing care.

Table 41.2 presents several examples of education and experience accepted by Medicare for reimbursement purposes in psychiatric home nursing care.

Nurses who provide psychiatric home care must have an in-depth knowledge of psychopathology, psychopharmacology, and how medical and physical problems can be influenced by psychiatric impairments (Hellwig, 1993). These nurses must be highly adept at performing biopsychosocial assessments. They must be sensitive to changes in behavior that signal that the client is decompensating either psychiatrically or medically so that early intervention may be implemented.

Another important job of the psychiatric home health nurse is monitoring the client's compliance with the regimen of psychotropic medications. Some clients who are receiving injectable medications remain on home health care only until they can be placed on oral medications. Those clients receiving oral medications require close monitoring for compliance and assistance with the uncomfortable side effects of some of these drugs. Medication noncompliance is responsible for approximately two thirds of psychiatric hospital readmissions (Hellwig, 1993). Home health nurses can assist clients with this problem by helping them to see the relationship between control of their psychiatric symptoms and compliance with their medication regimen.

Richie and Lusky (1987) describe the scope of the nurse in psychiatric home health care as follows:

● **Comprehensive Care.** The psychiatric home health nurse provides comprehensive nursing care, incorporating interventions for physical and psychosocial problems into the treatment plan. The interventions are based on the client's mental and physical health status, sociocultural factors, and available resources.

● **Accountability.** The authors state:

> "Accountability to the client is initiated when the nurse contracts with the client for specific services, and the scope and nature of the therapeutic relationship are defined. It is maintained as the nurse uses professional standards as the basis for practice, and documented through accurate and comprehensive recording of each home visit. Accountability to the larger system or community in which the client resides is essential as the nurse seeks to promote adaptive functioning of the client within his or her social system." (p. 233)

● **Interdisciplinary Collaboration.** Collaboration with other members of the health team is essential in the nursing scope of home health practice. The team may include a psychiatrist who is overseeing medication therapy, a social worker who is doing therapy with the family, a psychologist who may be administering psychological testing, and others, such as occupational therapists and physical therapists.

The ANA standards of home health nursing practice are presented in Table 41.3.

APPLICATION OF THE NURSING PROCESS

Wheeler (1998) identifies the following components of the comprehensive assessment that must be completed during an initial visit or two with the client:

1. Client's perception of the problem and need for assistance
2. Information regarding client's strengths and personal habits
3. Health history

TABLE 41.2 EDUCATION AND EXPERIENTIAL REQUIREMENTS FOR REGISTERED NURSE MEDICARE REIMBURSEMENT IN PSYCHIATRIC HOME NURSING CARE

1. Registered nurses must have a master's degree in psychiatric or mental health nursing.
2. Registered nurses with diplomas or associate degrees must have at least 2 years' experience as a staff member in an active treatment unit of an inpatient psychiatric hospital or outpatient mental health clinic or department of a hospital.
3. Registered nurses with a bachelor's degree in nursing must have at least 1 year of experience in a setting detailed above.
4. On an individual basis, other combinations of education and experience will be considered.

SOURCE: Harper (1989) from HCFA *Intermediary Manual* (Pub. 13.3, 1979).

4. Recent changes
5. Support systems
6. Vital signs
7. Current medications
8. Client's understanding and compliance with medications
9. Nutritional and elimination assessment
10. Activities of daily living (ADLs) assessment
11. Substance-use assessment
12. Neurological assessment
13. Mental status examination (see Appendix B)
14. Comprehension of proverbs
15. Global Assessment of Functioning (GAF) scale rating

Other important assessments include information about acute or chronic medical conditions, patterns of sleep and rest, solitude and social interaction, use of leisure time, education and work history, issues related to religion or spirituality, and adequacy of the home environment.

A case study of psychiatric home health care and the nursing process is presented in Table 41.4. A plan of care for Mrs. C (the client in the case study) is presented in Table 41.5. Nursing diagnoses are presented along with outcome criteria, appropriate nursing interventions, and rationales.

Care for the Caregivers. Another aspect of psychiatric home health care is to provide support and assistance to primary caregivers. When family are the providers of care on a 7-day-a-week, 24-hour-a-day schedule for a loved one with a chronic mental disorder, it can be very exhausting and very frustrating. A care plan for primary caregivers is presented in Table 41.6.

■ TABLE 41.3 AMERICAN NURSES' ASSOCIATION STANDARDS OF HOME HEALTH NURSING PRACTICE

Standard I. Organization of home health services
   All home health services are planned, organized, and directed by a master's prepared professional nurse with experience in community health and administration.

Standard II. Theory
   The nurse applies theoretical concepts as a basis for decisions in practice.

Standard III. Data collection
   The nurse continuously collects and records data that are comprehensive, accurate, and systematic.

Standard IV. Diagnosis
   The nurse uses health assessment data to determine nursing diagnoses.

Standard V. Planning
   The nurse develops care plans that establish goals. The care plan is based on nursing diagnoses and the medical treatment plan, and it incorporates therapeutic, preventive, and rehabilitative nursing actions. The client and family participate in the planning process.

Standard VI. Intervention
   The nurse, guided by the care plan, intervenes to provide comfort; to restore, improve, and promote health; to prevent complications and sequelae of illness; and to effect rehabilitation.

Standard VII. Evaluation
   The nurse continually evaluates the client's and family's responses to interventions in order to determine progress toward goal attainment and to revise the database, nursing diagnosis, and plan of care.

Standard VIII. Continuity of care
   The nurse is responsible for the client's appropriate and uninterrupted care along the health care continuum, and therefore, uses discharge planning, case management, and coordination of community resources.

Standard IX. Interdisciplinary collaboration
   The nurse initiates and maintains a liaison relationship with all appropriate health care providers to ensure that all efforts effectively complement one another.

Standard X. Professional development
   The nurse participates in research activities that contribute to the profession's continuing development of knowledge of home health care.

Standard XI. Research
   The nurse participates in research activities that contribute to the profession's continuing development of knowledge of home health care.

Standard XII. Ethics
   The nurse uses the code for nurses established by the American Nurses' Association as a guide for ethical decision making in practice.

SOURCE: ANA (1986), with permission.

TABLE 41.4 PSYCHIATRIC HOME HEALTH CARE AND THE NURSING PROCESS: A CASE STUDY

ASSESSMENT

Mrs. C, aged 76, has been living alone in her small apartment for 6 months since the death of her husband, to whom she had been married for 51 years. Mrs. C had been an elementary school teacher for 40 years, retiring at age 65 with an adequate pension. She and her husband had no children. A niece looks in on Mrs. C regularly. It was she who contacted Mrs. C's physician when she observed that Mrs. C was not eating properly, was losing weight, and seemed to be isolating herself more and more. She had not left her apartment in weeks. Her physician referred her to psychiatric home health care.

On her initial visit, Carol, the psychiatric home health nurse, conducted a preliminary assessment revealing the following information about Mrs. C:

1. Blood pressure 90/60 mm Hg.
2. Height 5'5"; weight 102 lb.
3. Poor skin turgor; dehydration.
4. Subjective report of occasional dizziness.
5. Subjective report of loss of 20 lb since death of husband.
6. Oriented to time, place, person, and situation.
7. Memory (remote and recent) intact.
8. Flat affect.
9. Mood is dysphoric and tearful at times, but client is cooperative.
10. Denies thoughts to harm self, but states, "I feel so alone, so useless."
11. Subjective report of difficulty sleeping.
12. Subjective report of constipation.

DIAGNOSIS/OUTCOME IDENTIFICATION

The following nursing diagnoses were formulated for Mrs. C:

1. Dysfunctional grieving related to death of husband, evidenced by symptoms of depression such as withdrawal, anorexia, weight loss, difficulty sleeping, dysphoric/tearful mood.
2. Risk for injury related to dizziness and weakness from lack of activity, low blood pressure, and poor nutritional status.
3. Social isolation related to depressed mood and feelings of worthlessness, evidenced by staying home alone, refusing to leave her apartment.

Outcome Criteria. The following criteria were selected as measurement of outcomes in the care of Mrs. C:

1. Experiences no physical harm/injury.
2. Is able to discuss feelings about husband's death with nurse.
3. Sets realistic goals for self.
4. Is able to participate in problem solving regarding her future.
5. Eats a well-balanced diet with snacks to restore nutritional status and gain weight.
6. Drinks adequate fluid daily.
7. Sleeps at least 6 hr per night and verbalizes feeling well rested.
8. Shows interest in personal appearance and hygiene. Is able to accomplish self-care independently.
9. Seeks to renew contact with previous friends and acquaintances.
10. Verbalizes interest in participating in social activities.

PLAN/IMPLEMENTATION

A plan of care for Mrs. C is presented in Table 41.5.

EVALUATION

Mrs. C was started the second week on trazodone (Desyrel) 150 mg at bedtime. Her sleep was enhanced and within 2 weeks she showed a noticeable improvement in mood. She began to discuss how angry she felt about being all alone in the world. She admitted that she had felt anger toward her husband but experienced guilt and tried to suppress that anger. As she was assured that these feelings were normal, they became easier for her to express.

The nurse arranged for a local teenager to do some weekly grocery shopping for Mrs. C and contacted the local Meals on Wheels program, which delivered her noon meal to her every day. Mrs. C began to eat more and slowly to gain a few pounds. She still has an occasional problem with constipation but verbalizes improvement with the addition of vegetables, fruit, and a daily stool softener prescribed by her physician.

Mrs. C used her walker until she felt she was able to ambulate without assistance. She reports that she no longer experiences dizziness, and her blood pressure has stabilized at around 100/70 mm Hg.

Mrs. C has joined a senior citizens group and attends activities weekly. She has renewed previous friendships and formed new acquaintances. She sees her physician monthly for medication management and visits a local adult day health center for regular blood pressure and weight checks. Her niece still visits regularly, but her favorite relationship is the one she has formed with her constant canine companion, Molly, whom Mrs. C rescued from the local animal shelter and who continually demonstrates her unconditional love and gratitude.

TABLE 41.5   CARE PLAN FOR PSYCHIATRIC HOME HEALTH CARE OF DEPRESSED ELDERLY PERSON

NURSING DIAGNOSIS: DYSFUNCTIONAL GRIEVING
RELATED TO: Death of husband
EVIDENCED BY: Symptoms of depression such as withdrawal, anorexia, weight loss, difficulty sleeping, and dysphoric/tearful mood

OUTCOME CRITERIA	NURSING INTERVENTIONS	RATIONALE
Mrs. C will demonstrate adaptive grieving behaviors and evidence of progression toward resolution.	1. Assess Mrs. C's position in the grief process. 2. Develop a trusting relationship by showing empathy and caring. Be honest and keep all promises. Show genuine positive regard. 3. Explore feelings of anger and help Mrs. C direct them toward the source. Help her understand it is appropriate and acceptable to have feelings of anger and guilt about her husband's death. 4. Encourage Mrs. C to review honestly the relationship she had with her husband. With support and sensitivity, point out reality of the situation in areas where misrepresentations may be expressed. 5. Determine if Mrs. C has spiritual needs that are going unfulfilled. If so, contact spiritual leader for intervention with Mrs. C. 6. Refer Mrs. C to physician for medication evaluation.	1. Accurate baseline data are required to plan accurate care for Mrs. C. 2. These interventions provide the basis for a therapeutic relationship 3. Knowledge of acceptability of the feelings associated with normal grieving may help to relieve some of the guilt that these responses generate. 4. Mrs. C must give up an idealized perception of her husband. Only when she is able to see both positive and negative aspects about the relationship will the grieving process be complete. 5. Recovery may be blocked if spiritual distress is present and care is not provided. 6. Antidepressant therapy may help Mrs. C to function while confronting the dynamics of her depression.

NURSING DIAGNOSIS: RISK FOR INJURY
RELATED TO: Dizziness and weakness from lack of activity, low blood pressure, and poor nutritional status

OUTCOME CRITERIA	NURSING INTERVENTIONS	RATIONALE
Mrs. C will not experience physical harm or injury.	1. Assess vital signs at every visit. Report to physician should they fall below baseline. 2. Encourage Mrs. C to use walker until strength has returned. 3. Visit Mrs. C during mealtimes and sit with her while she eats. Encourage her niece to do the same. Ensure that easy-to-prepare, nutritious foods for meals and snacks are available in the house and that they are items that Mrs. C likes. 4. Contact local meal delivery service (e.g., Meals on Wheels) to deliver some of Mrs. C's meals. 5. Weigh Mrs. C each week. 6. Ensure that diet contains sufficient fluid and fiber.	1. Client safety is a nursing priority. 2. The walker will keep Mrs. C from falling. 3. She is more likely to eat what is convenient and what she enjoys. 4. This would ensure that she receives at least one complete and nutritious meal each day. 5. Weight gain is a measurable, objective means of assessing whether Mrs. C is eating. 6. Adequate dietary fluid and fiber will help to alleviate constipation. She may also benefit from a daily stool softener.

Continued on following page

TABLE 41.5 *(Continued)*

NURSING DIAGNOSIS: SOCIAL ISOLATION
RELATED TO: Depressed mood and feelings of worthlessness
EVIDENCED BY: Staying home alone, refusing to leave apartment

OUTCOME CRITERIA	NURSING INTERVENTIONS	RATIONALE
Mrs. C will renew contact with friends and participate in social activities.	1. As nutritional status is improving and strength is gained, encourage Mrs. C to become more active. Take walks with her; help her perform simple tasks around her house.	1. Increased activity enhances both physical and mental status.
	2. Assess lifelong patterns of relationships.	2. Basic personality characteristics will not change. Mrs. C will very likely keep the same style of relationship development that she had in the past.
	3. Help her identify present relationships that are satisfying and activities that she considers interesting.	3. She is the person who truly knows what she likes, and these personal preferences will facilitate success in reversing social isolation.
	4. Consider the feasibility of a pet.	4. There are many documented studies of the benefits to elderly individuals of companion pets.
	5. Suggest possible alternatives that Mrs. C may consider as she seeks to participate in social activities. These may include foster grandparent programs, senior citizens centers, church activities, craft groups, and volunteer activities. Help her to locate individuals with whom she may attend some of these activities.	5. She is more likely to attend and participate if she does not have to do so alone.

LEGAL AND ETHICAL ISSUES

Legal Issues

Basic legal concepts for psychiatric nursing in general are discussed in this section as they relate to home psychiatric nursing care. Both national and state laws influence a number of issues that may arise within a home care setting. The psychiatric home health nurse must be familiar with these laws for the protection of both the client and the nurse.

Confidentiality

Client confidentiality is protected by both federal and state statutes. Confidentiality affects all aspects of information that become known as a direct result of the agency-client relationship. The only other individuals who should have access to the client's records should be other professionals directly involved in the client's care. It is advisable that the agency nurse obtain written permission during the initial contact to share client medical information with these other staff professionals. Guido (1997) suggests that if this initial permission is not ob-

tained, a release form authorizing release of information should be obtained before medical records are shared with other staff professionals.

Third-party payers also require medical information for making payment for services. A release of information form for this purpose should be signed during the initial visit.

Clients may also request copies of their medical record, and indeed they have a legal right to the information contained therein. Generally, the original medical record becomes the property of the home health agency, but copies may be provided to the client. Finkelman (1997) presents an issue that may have legal implications for confidentiality. In home health care, does the sharing of medical information with family or significant other (SO) breach the confidentiality of the client? Finkelman (1997) states:

"Most psychiatric nurses have confronted this dilemma, and many have crossed the line and shared confidential information without the patient's consent. How often does a nurse obtain an adult patient's permission prior to talking with the patient's family/SO? How does a nurse encourage family/SO participation in the home without sharing information? How does a nurse plan for discharge from home care without the family/SO?" (p. 110)

TABLE 41.6   CARE PLAN FOR PRIMARY CAREGIVER OF CLIENT WITH CHRONIC MENTAL ILLNESS

NURSING DIAGNOSIS: CAREGIVER ROLE STRAIN

RELATED TO: Severity and duration of the care receiver's illness and lack of respite and recreation for the caregiver

EVIDENCED BY: Feelings of stress in relationship with care receiver, feelings of depression and anger, family conflict around issues of providing care

OUTCOME CRITERIA	NURSING INTERVENTIONS	RATIONALE
Caregivers will achieve effective problem-solving skills and develop adaptive coping mechanisms to regain equilibrium.	1. Assess prospective caregivers' abilities to anticipate and fulfill client's unmet needs. Provide information to assist caregivers with this responsibility. Ensure that caregivers encourage client to be as independent as possible.	1. Caregivers may be unaware of what the client can realistically accomplish. They may be unaware of the nature of the illness.
	2. Ensure that caregivers are aware of available community support systems from whom they can seek assistance when required. Examples include respite care services, day treatment centers, and adult day-care centers.	2. Caregivers require relief from the pressures and strain of providing 24-hour care for their loved one. Studies have shown that abuse arises out of caregiving situations that place overwhelming stress on the caregivers.
	3. Encourage caregivers to express feelings, particularly anger.	3. Release of these emotions can serve to prevent psychopathology, such as depression or psychophysiological disorders, from occurring.
	4. Encourage participation in support groups composed of members with similar life situations. Provide information about support groups that may be helpful: a. National Alliance for the Mentally Ill—(800)950-NAMI b. National Clearinghouse on Family Support—(800)628-1696 c. Association on Mental Retardation—(800)424-3688 d. Association for Retarded Citizens—(817)261-6003 e. Alzheimer's Disease and Related Disorders Association—(800)621-0379	4. Hearing others who are experiencing the same problems discuss ways in which they have coped may help the caregiver adopt more adaptive strategies. Individuals who are experiencing similar life situations provide empathy and support for each other.

This is an area in which a great deal more discussion is required. An initial consent from the client to share information with family or SO would be in the best interest of all concerned, and the home health nurse should know the policies established by his or her agency.

Another issue concerning confidentiality relates to the HIV and AIDS status of clients. Legal implications must be taken into account if the documentation will be made accessible to third-party payers. Humphrey and Milone-Nuzzo (1996) state:

> "Strict confidentiality of this information is the general rule, and release of this information without consent of the client (even to family members) could subject the nurse to legal actions by the client. Release of the information to others can

have serious legal, social, employment, housing, and financial consequences." (p. 176)

Home health care agencies should have policies concerning this type of documentation, and nurses should be aware of these guidelines. In some instances, the agency's policy may be affected by state laws concerning testing for HIV and AIDS (Humphrey & Milone-Nuzzo, 1996).

Finkelman (1997) lists some other instances in which states may have statutes that require reporting, regardless of confidentiality. These include:

● Child abuse
● Adult abuse
● Possession of illegal substances

- Specific communicable diseases
- Injuries that appear to have been caused by a dangerous weapon
- Deaths of uncertain nature
- Animal bites

It is important for nurses to be knowledgeable about state law, so that required information is reported without breaching client confidentiality.

Informed Consent

Informed consent is an educational process and interpersonal exchange between a client and his or her physician in which information from the physician assists the client to make decisions about health care or treatment. In psychiatry, there has long been conflict about whether or not clients have the competence to make informed decisions about their health care. As discussed in Chapter 40, there are exceptional instances when procedures may be instituted without client consent. These include situations in which treatment is required to prevent harm to the client or others and emergency situations in which the client is in no condition to exercise judgment. In regard to psychiatric clients, it must not be assumed that mental illness implies lack of capacity to make independent decisions about treatment. Trudeau (1993) defines lack of capacity as "the inability, due to mental impairment, to make reasoned decisions regarding treatment by evaluating information about the likelihood of therapeutic benefit, the risk of side effects, and the availability of alternative treatments." Information about the procedure must be given to the client in language that he or she can understand. Initially it is presented by the physician but later can be reinforced by the nurse, who may provide additional information or further explanation. Finkelman (1997) suggests that the client's level of competence can be assessed by asking the client to paraphrase the information or by questioning the client specifically about the information. Careful documentation of information presented and level of client comprehension is critical for reasons of legal consequence.

Ethical Issues

Right to Refuse Treatment

The right to refuse treatment is closely tied to informed consent. Treatment without consent is allowed in most states only under emergency conditions and circumstances of potential harm to self or others. Clients have the right to make reasoned decisions regarding their treatment. They also have the right to withdraw consent after it has been given. Verbal withdrawal of consent is adequate (Guido, 1997). It should be noted that refusal of treatment should also be based on informed consent. Clients should have sufficient information about the consequences of refusing treatment in order to make a reasoned decision. Careful documentation by the psychiatric home health nurse of the client's decision to refuse treatment is imperative.

Abandonment

Humphrey and Milone-Nuzzo (1996) define **abandonment** as:

RESEARCH NOTE

Long-term effects of nurse home visitation on children's criminal and antisocial behavior: Fifteen-year follow-up of a randomized controlled trial. *Journal of the American Medical Association* **(1998, October 14), 280, 1238–1244.** Olds, D., Henderson, C.R., Cole, R., Eckenrode, J., Kitzman, H., Luckey, D., Pettitt, L., Sidora, K., Morris, P., and Powers, J.

Description of the Study: Between April 1978 and September 1980, 400 pregnant women with no previous live births took part in this study in a semirural community in New York. The group was randomized into a control group that received standard prenatal and well-child care in a clinic, and a study group that received the standard prenatal care plus home nursing visits during the prenatal period as well as home nursing visits during the first 2 years of the child's life. The prenatal visits focused on positive health-related behaviors and counseling related to diet and reducing the stress of pregnancy. The visits following birth of the child emphasized competent care of the child and maternal personal development. Fifteen years later, interviews were conducted with the adolescents and their biological mothers or custodial parents. Main outcome measures included the adolescents' self-reports of running away, arrests, convictions, being sentenced to youth corrections, initiation of sexual intercourse, number of sex partners, and use of illegal substances; school records of suspensions; teachers' reports of the adolescents' disruptive behavior in school; and parents' reports of the adolescents' arrests and behavioral problems related to the children's use of alcohol and other drugs.

Results of the Study: Adolescents born to women who received nurse visits during pregnancy and in early childhood and who were unmarried and from households of low socioeconomic status (risk factors for antisocial behavior) reported fewer incidences of running away, fewer arrests, fewer convictions and violation of probation, fewer lifetime sex partners, fewer cigarettes smoked per day, and fewer days having consumed alcohol in the last 6 months than those in the control group. Parents of nurse-visited children reported that their children had fewer behavioral problems related to use of alcohol and other drugs.

Comments: The authors concluded that this program of prenatal and early childhood home visitation by nurses can reduce reported serious antisocial behavior and emergent abuse of substances on the part of adolescents born into high-risk families.

"A unilateral severance of the professional relationship between a health care provider and a client without reasonable notice at a time when there is still a need for continuing health care." (p. 180)

Abandonment may occur in home health care when the home health care agency decides it must terminate care while a client may still be in need of service. Humphrey and Milone-Nuzzo (1996) cite the following reasons why an agency may discontinue client care:

- The client refuses to cooperate in the provision of home care.
- Reimbursement for services has been denied, the agency has ceased to be a Medicaid or Medicare provider, and the client will not or cannot pay for the service.
- The client is unruly, obnoxious, or difficult to treat to the point that it is in the best interests of all concerned that the agency discontinue service.
- Certain environmental factors exist that endanger agency staff, such as physical threats, a dangerous dog, or sexual harassment.

To prevent client abandonment, it is important that a reasonable amount of notice be given to the client that discontinuation of services will be occurring. The amount of time considered reasonable depends on considerations such as the client's condition, the availability of alternative care, and urgency of need to terminate (e.g., danger to staff). Agency policies should address issues of abandonment. Ongoing communication with the physician and detailed documentation in the agency record are critical.

Least-Restrictive Alternative

Clients have the right to the least-restrictive alternative in treatment or care in the least restrictive setting. Psychiatric home nursing provides the client with a great deal of control and the least amount of restriction in his or her care. It is important for the nurse to understand this concept of least-restrictive alternative, for indeed there may be times when the client requires more intensive care. The psychiatric home care nurse has first-line access to the client in a crisis situation. Careful assessment and documentation are important to help determine the appropriate level of care for the client and make recommendations to the physician with the best interests of the client in mind.

SUMMARY

Psychiatric home nursing care has shown to be a cost-effective way to provide quality care to clients outside the hospital setting. The concept began with the visiting nurses associations that were established in the early 1900s. When Medicare legislation was passed in 1965,

---

TEST YOUR CRITICAL THINKING SKILLS

Sarah is a 71-year-old widow whose husband died 6 years ago. Until recently, Sarah has been very independent and lived in a small apartment in the same town with her daughter and her family. Sarah was active in church and club activities and had many friends and acquaintances.

Six months ago, Sarah began having chest pain and was admitted to the hospital for diagnostic testing. A cardiac catheterization revealed major blockage in three coronary arteries, and Sarah underwent triple coronary artery bypass graft surgery. The surgery was successful and Sarah's physical recovery has been unremarkable. She returned to her apartment and was referred by her cardiologist for home health care by a staff nurse and home health aide who made regular visits to assist Sarah with her postoperative care. She qualified for homebound status because of physical weakness, need for wound care, postoperative pain, and need for assistance with ADLs. Her follow-up medications include digoxin (Lanoxin) and propranolol (Inderal).

As Sarah's physical condition stabilized, the home health staff nurse began to notice Sarah's progressive withdrawal and depressed mood. Instead of increasing her level of activity as her physical strength returned, she became less active and refused to participate in her daily care. She showed no interest in resuming any of the activities in which she had participated prior to her surgery. She began to lose weight. She needed to be reminded to take her medication. She moved in with her daughter, son-in-law, and granddaughter, so that she would not have to be alone at night. The home health staff nurse reported these symptoms to the cardiologist, who referred Sarah's case to a psychiatrist. A computed tomography (CT) scan was ordered to rule out possible neurological disorder, and the results were negative. A psychiatric home nursing care service was enlisted to assess Sarah's condition. Home health aides continued to visit Sarah daily to assist with ADLs and hygiene needs.

During the nurse's first visit, she found Sarah to be very withdrawn. Her daughter reported that Sarah hardly leaves her room, and eats very little. Sarah was diagnosed with major depression.

Answer the following questions related to Sarah:

1. Describe initial assessments the psychiatric home care nurse would make in visiting with Sarah.
2. Identify two priority nursing diagnoses for Sarah.
3. What would be the goals of treatment for Sarah?
4. What medical treatment might the psychiatrist prescribe for Sarah based on the psychiatric home health nurse's assessment?

---

home health care was recognized as a benefit, and services escalated. It was not until 1979, however, that psychiatric home nursing care came to be recognized as a reimbursable service.

The majority of home health care is paid for by Medicare. Other sources include Medicaid, private insurance, self-pay, and others. Homebound clients most often have diagnoses of schizophrenia, major depression, bipolar disorder, substance abuse, agoraphobia, paranoia, and generalized anxiety.

Besides being cost-effective, home care offers the advantage of observation of the client within the context of family and environment, which allows for the most comprehensive biopsychosocial assessment. Treatment in the home may also be perceived by the client as less threatening than treatment in an institutional environment. Disadvantages to home nursing include lack of professional assistance for the nurse, constraints on the nurse within the client's home environment, and issues related to nursing in potentially unsafe neighborhoods.

Psychiatric home care nurses must have special training in psychiatric mental health nursing. Several years of psychiatric inpatient treatment experience plus 1 year of medical-surgical nursing is preferred. Psychiatric nurses are expected to perform hands-on, holistic nursing, not just insight-oriented psychotherapy.

The nursing process is the tool for delivery of nursing care for the psychiatric client in the home care setting. This chapter presented a case study of and care plan for a depressed elderly client receiving psychiatric home nursing care. A care plan for the primary caregiver of a client with a chronic mental illness was also presented.

Legal issues pertaining to home health, such as confidentiality and informed consent, were discussed along with ethical issues, including right to refuse treatment, abandonment, and least-restrictive alternative.

REVIEW QUESTIONS

SELF-EXAMINATION/LEARNING EXERCISE

Select the answer that is most appropriate for each of the following questions:

1. The primary reason that psychiatric nursing care in the home has experienced slower growth than general home nursing care is that:
   a. Studies have shown that psychiatric home nursing care is not cost-effective.
   b. HCFA did not recognize psychiatric home nursing care as reimbursable until much later than general staff home nursing care.
   c. Most psychiatric clients refuse to accept psychiatric nursing treatment in their homes.
   d. Psychiatric clients must also have a primary medical diagnosis before they can qualify for payment for home psychiatric services.

2. Psychiatric home nursing care has experienced a rapid growth in recent years because of all of the following reasons *except:*
   a. Broader third-party payment coverage
   b. Greater physician acceptance of home care
   c. Increased demand as an alternative to institutional care
   d. Lengthier hospital stays for severe and persistently mentally ill clients

3. The majority of home health care is paid for by:
   a. Medicare
   b. Medicaid
   c. Private insurance
   d. Self-pay

4. Medicare requires that all the following criteria be met in order to qualify for psychiatric home care *except:*
   a. Certification by a physician that the client is homebound.
   b. A physical reason for inability to leave the home.
   c. An acute psychiatric diagnosis or exacerbation of one.
   d. The need for the specialized skills of a psychiatric nurse.

5. Which of the following is considered a disadvantage of psychiatric home nursing care?
   a. Family involvement diminishes the nurse-client relationship.
   b. Studies have shown it is not cost-effective.
   c. The nurse's authority and autonomy are constrained in the home setting.
   d. The presence of family interferes with comprehensive biopsychosocial assessment.

6. Maria and Tony are part of an Italian family of three generations who live together in one large home. Twyla, a psychiatric home health nurse, was enlisted to make home visits when Maria started to have panic attacks and refused to leave her home. Twyla has been visiting Maria once a week for 6 weeks now, and Maria has improved and with support and medication is able to leave her home and carry out her activities as required. Two more visits are preauthorized, and Maria and Twyla have been discussing termination. When Twyla arrives for her visit this week, Maria has baked an Italian Easter bread for Twyla. She is very obviously excited to present the gift to Twyla. What is the most appropriate response on Twyla's part?
   a. She explains to Maria that her agency has a policy against accepting gifts from clients.
   b. She refuses the gift, knowing that if she accepts, it will interfere with the therapeutic relationship.
   c. She places a call to her supervisor at the home health agency to ask permission to accept the gift.
   d. She accepts the Easter bread knowing that in the Italian culture a refusal would be taken as an insult by Maria.

7. Referrals are an important part of psychiatric home nursing care, and often psychiatric home care nurses refer clients to support groups of individuals with similar types of problems. In the case of Maria, Twyla decides this is not an appropriate intervention. On what might Twyla have based her decision?

   a. Italians are very family-oriented and would prefer to care for Maria within the privacy of the family constellation.
   b. There are very few support groups for individuals with panic disorder because treatment of anxiety has been shown to be less than successful in a group situation.
   c. Twyla believes that Maria would be uncomfortable within a group setting, because Italians generally have a large personal distance.
   d. Twyla has decided that Maria is completely well and it is unlikely that she will ever need care or support in the future.

8. Maria asks Twyla what she writes about their visits together. She says to Twyla, "My friend told me that the medical record really belongs to me." What is the most appropriate response by Twyla?

   a. "I'm sorry, but I can't share this information with you."
   b. "I'll have to ask my supervisor if I can show you the record."
   c. "The actual record belongs to the agency, but I can get a copy for you."
   a. "I will be happy to tell you what I have written, but I can't show you the record."

9. Following a routine visit to Maria, which of the following situations would Twyla be required to report to the appropriate authority, regardless of confidentiality?

   a. Maria has a small bruise on her arm. She states, "Oh, Tony grabbed me a little too hard. He does that sometimes when he drinks too much."
   b. Maria has a small, open wound on her lower leg. She states, "I accidentally stepped on my neighbor's dog's tail and he bit me."
   c. Maria has itchy blisters on both arms. She states, "I got into the patch of poison ivy behind our house yesterday."
   d. Maria is upset. She is crying. "Tony didn't come home last night. He's done it before."

10. In the instance when a contract for treatment has been made between a client and a psychiatric home care nurse, if the client decides to withdraw from treatment before the contract expires or before discharge, what must be done?

    a. The client needs only to withdraw consent verbally.
    b. The client must present a written refusal of treatment.
    c. The client must have cosignature of family or significant other to withdraw treatment.
    d. The client does not have the right to refuse treatment until the nurse determines the appropriate time for discharge.

REFERENCES

American Nurses' Association (ANA). (1986). *Standards of home health nursing practice*. Washington, DC: American Nurses Association.

American Nurses' Association (ANA). (1992). *A statement on the scope of home health nursing practice*. Washington, DC: American Nurses Publishing.

Case, J. (Ed.). (1993, May). Special Focus: Psychiatric services. *Hospital Home Health, 10*(5), 61–68.

Duffey, J.M., & Miller, M.P. (1996, June). Toward resolving the issue: In-home psychiatric nursing. *Journal of the American Psychiatric Nurses Association, 2*(3), 104–106.

Finkelman, A.W. (1997). *Psychiatric home care*. Gaithersburg, MD: Aspen Publications.

Guido, G.W. (1997). *Legal issues in nursing* (2nd ed.). Stamford, CT: Appleton & Lange.

Harper, M.S. (1989, June). Providing mental health services in the homes of the elderly: A public policy perspective. *Caring, 5–9, 52–53.*

Harris, P. (1987). Psychiatric assessments in the home. *Quality Review Bulletin, 13*(4).

Health Care Financing Administration (HCFA). (1999). Coverage of services. In *Home health agency manual*. [On-line]. Available: http://www.hcfa.gov/

Hellwig, K. (1993). Psychiatric home care nursing: Managing patients in the community setting. *Journal of Psychosocial Nursing 31*(12), 21–24.

Humphrey, C.J., & Milone-Nuzzo, P. (1996). *Orientation to home care nursing*. Gaithersburg, MD: Aspen Publishers.

National Association for Home Care (NAHC). (1996). *How to choose a home care provider*. [On-line]. Available: http://www.nahc.org/Consumer/ wihc.html

National Association for Home Care (NAHC). (1999). *Basic statistics about home care.* [On-line]. Available: http://www.nahc.org/Consumer/hc-stats. html

Pelletier, L.R. (1988). Psychiatric home care. *Journal of Psychosocial Nursing, 26*(3), 22–27.

Peplau, H. E. (1995). Some unresolved issues in the era of biopsychosocial nursing. *Journal of the American Psychiatric Nurses Association, 1*(3), 92–96.

Richie, F., & Lusky, K. (1987). Psychiatric home health nursing: A new role in community mental health. *Community Mental Health Journal, 23*(3), 229–235.

Trudeau, M.E. (1993). Informed consent: The patient's right to decide. *Journal of Psychosocial Nursing, 31*(6), 9–12.

Wheeler, K. (1998). Psychiatric clinical pathways in home care. In P.C. Dykes (Ed.), *Psychiatric clinical pathways: An interdisciplinary approach.* Gaithersburg, MD: Aspen Publishers.

FORENSIC NURSING

KEY TERMS

forensic nursing
forensic

sexual assault nurse
examiner (SANE)

colposcope

OBJECTIVES

After reading this chapter, the student will be able to:

1. Define the terms *forensic* and *forensic nursing.*
2. Discuss historical perspectives of forensic nursing.
3. Identify areas of nursing within which forensic nurses may practice.
4. Describe forensic nursing specialties.
5. Apply the nursing process within the role of clinical forensic nursing in trauma care.
6. Apply the nursing process within the role of forensic psychiatric nursing in correctional facilities.

he many roles of nurses continue to increase with the ever-expanding health service delivery system. **Forensic nursing** is an example of a new concept of the nursing role that is rapidly increasing in its scope of practice. Nurses practicing in this unique specialty may apply their skills to the care of both victims and perpetrators of crime and in a variety of settings, including primary care facilities, hospitals, and correctional institutions. This chapter focuses on defining forensic nursing within varied aspects of the role. A discussion of historical perspectives is included, and care of the client is presented within the context of the nursing process.

WHAT IS FORENSIC NURSING?

The word **forensic** is defined by *Taber's Cyclopedic Medical Dictionary* (1997) as, "pertaining to the law; legal." How then is this terminology applied to nursing? Several definitions have emerged.

The International Association of Forensic Nurses (IAFN) and the American Nurses' Association (ANA) (1997) define forensic nursing as:

> "The application of forensic science combined with the bio-psychological education of the registered nurse, in the scientific investigation, evidence collection and preservation, analysis, prevention and treatment of trauma and/or death related medical-legal issues." (p. v)

Hufft and Peternelj-Taylor (1999) present the following definition:

> "A nursing specialty that integrates nursing and forensic science to bridge the gap between the health care system and the criminal justice system." (p. 1)

Lynch (1993) suggests that:

> "Forensic nursing is defined as the application of the medicolegal aspects of health care in the scientific investigation of trauma and/or death related issues." (p. 5)

Because this area of nursing is a continuing pioneering effort, roles, definitions, and educational programs are still being formulated.

HISTORICAL PERSPECTIVES

Forensic nursing has its roots in Alberta, Canada, around 1975, where nurses served as medical examiners' investigators in the field of death investigation (Lynch, 1993). They were valued for their biomedical education, their sensitivity in dealing with family members, and their ability to substitute in the role of the medical examiner when required. These are qualities that were often found

to be lacking in medically untrained criminal investigative personnel.

The discipline has made great advances since that time. The role of forensic nursing has expanded from concerns solely with death investigation to include the living—the survivors of violent crime—as well as the perpetrators of criminal acts. In 1992, seventy-four nurses, primarily sexual assault nurse examiners, met to form the International Association of Forensic Nurses (Bell, 1999). By 1997, this organization had grown to more than a thousand members.

Violence has reached epidemic proportions in the United States and has been identified as a major public health problem. It is with this in mind that the health care system and the legal system have joined in an attempt to respond to the increasing needs of crime victims. Lynch (1993) cites the following as goals for forensic nursing: "the empowerment of victims of all races and cultures, the treatment of perpetrators in preventive studies, and the protection of their human rights" (p. 6).

THE CONTEXT OF FORENSIC NURSING PRACTICE

The Forensic Nursing Service (FNS) (1999) has identified a variety of assignments within which the forensic nurse may intervene. They include the following.

1. Interpersonal violence
   - Domestic violence/sexual assault
   - Child and elder abuse/neglect
   - Physiological/psychological abuse
   - Drug/alcohol abuse
2. Public health and safety
   - Environmental hazards
   - Food and drug tampering
   - Holistic health investigation
   - Medically unsupervised abortion practices
   - Epidemiological issues
   - Anatomical gifts (tissue/organ donation)
3. Emergency/trauma nursing
   - Automobile and pedestrian accidents
   - Traumatic injuries
   - Suicide attempts
   - Work-related injuries
   - Fatal/near-fatal injuries
4. Patient care facilities
   - Accidents/injuries/neglect
   - Inappropriate treatment/medication administration
5. Police and corrections
   - Custody
   - Abuse

FORENSIC NURSING SPECIALTIES*

Clinical Forensic Nursing Specialty

Clinical forensic nursing is the management of crime victims from trauma to trial. Nurses working in clinical forensics collect evidence through assessment of living victims, survivors of traumatic injury, or those whose death is pronounced in the clinical environment (Lynch, 1995). Clinical forensic nursing involves making judgments related to patient treatment associated with court-related issues. The clinical forensic nurse assesses victims of child and elder abuse and domestic violence. Forensic nurses are asked to make distinctions between injuries that appear accidental and those that appear purposely inflicted. An essential skill required by the forensic nurse is the ability to assess patterned injury by differentiating such marks as defense wounds, grab marks, and fingernail marks. Clinical forensic nurses will focus on observation of the communication and interaction patterns of possible abuse victims and perpetrators. Many nurses come to forensic nursing from acute-care settings of emergency room nursing, critical care nursing, and perioperative nursing.

In the coroner's office, death notification entails stabilization of the family situation and grief support, skills basic to nursing. Expert skills in physical assessment, clinical history taking and interviewing, and the use of technology have helped to advance this nursing role.

Because of their awareness of the effects of violence in society and their ability to assess situations in which the potential for violence exists, clinical forensic nurses are often called upon for consultation. By identifying risk factors and cues for violence in health care and workplace settings, these nurses can assist in the development of strategies, policies, and protocols to manage risk and reduce violence and injury. They also assist in the debriefing or resolution of violent events in a workplace or community.

The Sexual Assault Nurse Examiner (SANE)

The **sexual assault nurse examiner (SANE)** is a clinical forensic registered nurse who has received specialized training to provide care to the sexual assault victim. The SANE is involved with physical and psychosocial examination and addresses collection of physical evidence, therapeutic interactions to minimize the trauma and initiate healing, coordination of referral and collaboration with community-based agencies involved in the rehabilitation of victims, and the judicial processing of sexual assault.

The first programs training SANEs were developed in the United States in the late 1970s. It is expected that national certification will be mandated in the near future.

Forensic Psychiatric Nursing Specialty

Forensic psychiatric nurses integrate psychiatric/mental health nursing philosophy and practice with knowledge of the criminal justice system and assessment of the sociocultural influences on the individual clients, their families, and the community, to provide comprehensive psychiatric and mental health nursing (Peternelj-Taylor & Hufft, 1997). Forensic psychiatric nurses work with mentally ill offenders and with victims of crime, helping victims cope with their emotional wounds, and in the assessment and care of perpetrators (Scales, Mitchell, & Smith, 1993). They focus on identification and change of behaviors that link criminal offenses and/or reactions to them. They help perpetrators and victims of crime to deal with the courts and other aspects of the criminal justice system, minimizing further victimization and promoting functional abilities.

Functional applications of forensic psychiatric nursing include assessment of inmates for fitness, criminal responsibility, disposition, and early release. Forensic psychiatric nurses also provide mental health treatment for convicted offenders and those who are not found criminally responsible. In the criminal justice system, forensic psychiatric nurses deal with destructive, aggressive, and socially unacceptable behavior, providing nursing interventions; this encourages individuals to exercise self control, foster individual change in behavior, and, in the process, protect property and other members of society.

Recently there has been an increase in the involvement of forensic psychiatric nurses—especially those prepared for advanced practice—in assessment and treatment of forensic psychiatric patients. These practitioners are involved in the development and refinement of clinical roles in forensic psychiatric nursing and are in a position to promote intervention strategies, which increases the likelihood of rehabilitation and reintegration of the forensic client into society.

Correctional/Institutional Nursing Specialty

Correctional/institutional nurses work in secure settings, providing treatment, rehabilitation, and health promotion to clients who have been charged with or convicted of crimes. Settings include jails, state and federal prisons, and halfway houses. Prior to the 1960s, most nurses gave little thought to working in the correctional system, even though jails and correctional facilities have always been a part of the community at large. There is a growing awareness of the potential for the correctional population as a

---

*This section was written by A. Hufft and C. Peternelj-Taylor. Reprinted with permission from *1999 Contemporary Professional Nursing Update*, J.T. Catalano (Ed.). Philadelphia: F.A. Davis.

target of successful health interventions. Some nurses have created private practices or consultation services in which they identify the health needs of people in custody and arrange for their care. These services are provided separately from acute care, which is located in a secured hospital or infirmary section of the institution. Such services are just emerging as health care alternatives and will serve as the model from which community-based care, aimed at decreasing recidivism among the incarcerated, will develop. To guide professional nursing practice, the ANA first published *Standards for Nursing Practice in Correctional Facilities* in 1985; this was revised and updated in 1995 (ANA, 1995). In addition to the specialties of forensic nursing previously discussed, nurses are continuing to develop roles based on the integration of forensic knowledge and nursing practice.

Nurses in General Practice

Nurses in general practice find forensic nursing knowledge of growing importance, as do nurses in specialty practice. Forensic applications in the acute care setting emphasize the use of forensic knowledge and awareness of criminal justice implications for assessment, documentation of care, and reporting of information to police or other law enforcement agencies. Nurses working in emergency rooms and in critical care units are often in a position to preserve evidence of what might be a criminal offense. A victim of a car accident or an apparent accidental overdose does not always show signs of what actually has happened, but knowledge of what to look for and how to collect evidence, in addition to whom to call and when, can be valuable in finding out the truth. Patients often come into acute care settings with what are first thought to be injuries that are the result of an accident. However, preservation of evidence such as stomach contents, clothing residue, or marks on the skin surface can provide a very different picture: one of a self-inflicted wound or violence perpetrated by another.

This chapter will focus on two specialties in forensic nursing: the clinical forensic nurse specialist in trauma care settings and the psychiatric forensic nurse in correctional facilities. The IAFN and ANA (1997) Standards of Care and Standards of Professional Performance for forensic nursing are presented in Table 42.1.

APPLICATION OF THE NURSING PROCESS IN CLINICAL FORENSIC NURSING IN TRAUMA CARE

Assessment

Lynch (1995) states that forensic nurses who work in trauma care settings may "become the designated clinicians who will evaluate and assess surviving victims of rape, drug and alcohol addiction, domestic violence (including abuse of spouse, children, elderly), assaults, automobile/pedestrian accidents, suicide attempts, occupationally related injuries, incest, medical malpractice and the injuries sustained therefrom, and food and drug tampering." All traumatic injuries in which liability is suspected are considered within the scope of forensic nursing. Reports to legal agencies are required to ensure follow-up investigation; however, the protection of clients' rights remains a nursing priority.

With the rise of violence in our society reaching epidemic proportions, the role of the clinical forensic nurse in the care of trauma clients in the emergency department is expanding. The forensic clinical nurse specialist may be the ideal liaison between legal and medical agencies.

Lynch (1995) identifies several areas of assessment in which the clinical forensic nurse specialist may become involved. They include the preservation of evidence, investigation of wound characteristics, and deaths in the emergency department.

Preservation of Evidence

Intentional traumas in the emergency department may be crime related or self-inflicted. Crime-related evidence is essential and must be safeguarded in a manner consistent with the investigation. Lynch (1995) identifies the most common types of evidence as clothing, bullets, blood stains, hairs, fibers, and small pieces of material such as fragments of metal, glass, paint, and wood. Often this type of evidence is destroyed in the clinical setting when health care personnel are unaware of its potential value in an investigation. It is important that this type of evidence be saved and documented in all medical or accident instances that have legal implications.

Investigation of Wound Characteristics

When clients present to the emergency department with wounds from undiagnosed trauma, it is important for the clinical forensic nurse specialist to make a detailed documentation of the injuries. Failure to do so may interfere with the administration of justice should legal implications later arise. Lynch (1995) identifies the following categories of medicolegal injuries:

1. Sharp injuries: sharp force injuries including stab wounds and other wounds resulting from penetration with a sharp object.
2. Blunt-force injuries: includes cuts and bruises resulting from the impact of a blunt object against the body.
3. Dicing injuries: multiple, minute cuts and abrasions caused by contact with shattered glass (e.g., injuries that often occur in motor vehicle accidents).

![] **Table 42.1 STANDARDS OF CARE AND STANDARDS OF PROFESSIONAL PERFORMANCE FOR FORENSIC NURSING**

STANDARDS OF CARE

Standard I. Assessment
The forensic nurse shall provide an accurate assessment, based upon data collected, of the physical and/or psychological issues of the client as related to forensic nursing and/or forensic pathology.

Standard II. Diagnosis
The forensic nurse shall analyze the assessment data to determine a diagnosis pertaining to forensic issues in nursing.

Standard III. Outcome identification
The forensic nurse will identify expected individual outcomes based on the forensic diagnoses of the client.

Standard IV. Planning
The forensic nurse develops a comprehensive plan of action for the forensic client appropriate to forensic interventions to attain expected outcomes.

Standard V. Implementation
The forensic nurse implements a plan of action based on forensic issues derived from assessment data, nursing diagnoses, and medical diagnoses, when applicable, and scientific knowledge.

Standard VI. Evaluation
The forensic nurse evaluates and modifies the plan of action to achieve expected outcomes.

STANDARDS OF PROFESSIONAL PERFORMANCE

Standard I. Quality of care
The forensic nurse systematically evaluates the quality and effectiveness of forensic nursing practice.

Standard II. Performance appraisal
The forensic nurse evaluates his/her own forensic nursing practice in relation to professional practice standards and relevant statutes and regulations.

Standard III. Education
The forensic nurse acquires and maintains current knowledge in forensic nursing practice.

Standard IV. Collegiality
The forensic nurse contributes to the professional development of peers, colleagues, and others.

Standard V. Ethics
The forensic nurse's decisions and actions are determined in an ethical manner.

Standard VI. Collaboration
The forensic nurse collaborates with the forensic client, family members, significant others, and multidisciplinary team members.

Standard VII. Research
The forensic nurse recognizes, values, and utilizes research as a method to further forensic nursing practice.

Standard VIII. Resource utilization
The forensic nurse considers factors related to safety, effectiveness, and cost in planning and delivering forensic services.

SOURCE: IAFN & ANA (1997).

4. Patterned injuries: specific injuries that reflect the pattern of the weapon used to inflict the injury.
5. Bite mark injuries: a type of patterned injury inflicted by human or animal.
6. Defense wounds: injuries that reflect the victim's attempt to defend himself or herself from attack.
7. Hesitation wounds: usually superficial, sharp-force wounds; often found perpendicular to the lower part of the body and may reflect self-inflicted wounds.
8. Fast-force injuries: usually gunshot wounds; may reflect various patterns of injury.

Nurses managing the client's care in the emergency department must be able to make assessments about the type of wound, the weapon involved, and an estimate of the length of time between the injury and presentation for treatment.

Deaths in the Emergency Department

When deaths occur in the emergency department as a result of abuse or accident, evidence must be retained, the death must be reported to legal authorities, and an investigation is conducted (Lynch, 1995). It is therefore essential that the nurse carefully document the appearance, condition, and behavior of the victim upon arrival at the hospital. The information gathered from the client and family (or others accompanying the client) may serve to facilitate the postmortem investigation and may be used during criminal justice proceedings.

The critical factor is to be able to determine if the cause of death is natural or unnatural. In the emergency department, most deaths are sudden and unexpected. Those that are considered natural most commonly involve the cardiovascular, respiratory, and central nervous systems (Lynch, 1995). Deaths that are considered unnatural include those from trauma, from self-inflicted acts, or from injuries inflicted by another. Legal authorities must be notified of all deaths related to unnatural circumstances.

Nursing Diagnosis

Clinical forensic nurse specialists in the trauma care setting analyze the information gathered during assessment of the client to formulate nursing diagnoses. Common nursing diagnoses relevant to forensic clients in the emergency department include:

1. Risk for posttrauma syndrome
2. Fear
3. Anxiety
4. Risk for self-mutilation
5. Risk for self-directed violence
6. Risk for dysfunctional grieving

Planning/Implementatation

Preservation of Evidence

When a trauma victim is admitted to the emergency department, the most obvious priority intervention is medical stabilization. This priority must be balanced against the need to protect rapidly deteriorating physical evidence that can be used to determine if a crime has occurred.

Wounds must be examined to speculate about the type of weapon used and to estimate age of the wound. Clothing must be checked for blood, semen, gunshot residue, or trace materials such as hair or fibers, or even paint chips, in the case of an automobile/pedestrian hit-and-run accident (Lynch, 1995). Clothing that is removed from a victim should not be shaken, so that any evidence that may be adhering to it is not lost. Each separate item of clothing should be placed carefully in a paper bag, sealed, dated, timed, and signed. Plastic bags should never be used because of the tendency for condensation to occur, the accumulation of which can cause deterioration of the evidence (Lynch, 1995).

When the trauma is sexual assault, a SANE may be called to the emergency department. SANEs usually work on-call, and because most sexual assault victims are women, female nurses are employed as SANEs. Male victims of sexual assault also most often prefer to work with a female SANE, because the perpetrators are usually men

and because of the subsequent mistrust of men following the attack.

Ledray and Arndt (1994) suggest the following five essential components of a forensic examination of the sexual assault survivor in the emergency department:

1. Treatment and Documentation of Injuries. Ledray and Arndt (1994) state:

"Unless the injuries are life threatening, proper forensic documentation should occur first. This documentation involves photographs, a written description of the injuries, and documentation on body drawings included as part of the sexual assault examination report. Documentation of physical injuries that show that force was used is important to demonstrate that the sexual contact was against the woman's will." (p. 9)

It is often expected that a sexual assault survivor must exhibit cuts and bruises in the genital or nongenital area. It has been estimated that there are no visible physical injuries in 40 percent to 60 percent of sexual assaults (American Medical Association [AMA], 1999). Absence of physical trauma does not necessarily mean that no force was used and that consent was given. This, however, is the case often used by defense attorneys in court. The AMA (1999) suggests the use of a traumagram—a diagram of a nude figure on which the locations of visible injuries are made. A written description of the color, size, and location of each wound, abrasion, and laceration is then documented. With the client's permission, photographs of the wounds should be taken for accurate documentation.

The nurse may use a **colposcope** to examine for tears and abrasions inside the vaginal area. A colposcope is an instrument that contains a magnifying lens and to which a 35-mm camera can be attached.

Some states have legally mandated procedures, and some acute care settings also have established protocols, for gathering evidence in cases of sexual assault. In some instances, "rape kits" are available for collecting specimens and lab samples in a competent manner that is consistent with legal requirements and that will not interfere with the victim's option to pursue criminal charges. In addition to the vaginal examination, oral and rectal examinations may be conducted. Fingernail scrapings and body, head, and pubic hair samples should also be collected. Client hair samples are important to be able to differentiate from those of the assailant. As previously stated, all evidence should be sealed in paper, *not* plastic, bags to prevent the possible growth of mildew from accumulation of moisture inside the plastic container, and the subsequent contamination of the evidence.

Some states may require a urine specimen to test for pregnancy or screen for drugs. It is best, if possible, to wait until the initial internal examination is complete before collecting the urine sample. However, the AMA (1999) states, "Patients needing to urinate before the internal examination should be allowed to do so, with a notation being made in the medical record."

2. Maintaining the Proper Chain of Evidence. Ledray and Arndt (1994) state that "improper documentation and handling of evidence of sexual assault is typically the greatest problem that occurs in institutions without nurse examiners." Unless the proper chain of evidence has been maintained, it cannot be used successfully in a court of law to convict an assailant. The AMA (1999) states:

> "To preserve the chain of evidence and the freshness of the samples, check to ensure that they are properly labeled, sealed, refrigerated when necessary, and kept under observation or properly locked until rendered to the proper legal authority."

3. Treatment and Evaluation of Sexually Transmitted Diseases (STDs). The AMA (1999) recommends counseling about, and prophylaxis for, STDs to sexual assault victims. Conducted within 72 hours of the attack, several tests and interventions are available. Prophylactic antibiotics may be given to prevent chlamydia, gonorrhea, trichomoniasis, and bacterial vaginosis according to guidelines from the Centers for Disease Control (CDC) (AMA, 1999). They also recommend postexposure prophylaxis using hepatitis B immunoglobulin. Information also should be provided describing symptoms of STDs for which there are no preventive measures. Because incubation periods vary, the importance of follow-up testing must be emphasized.

There is no proven prophylactic intervention for HIV infection, and this is a growing concern of sexual assault victims. Even though the CDC reports that the risk for acquiring HIV infection through sexual assault is low in most cases, some states mandate testing for HIV as part of the sexual assault protocol. The AMA (1999) states, "Baseline testing can diagnose or rule out preexisting HIV infection, but repeated testing after 6 months and again in 1 year is recommended, particularly when the assailant is known to be HIV positive or the serostatus is unknown."

4. Pregnancy Risk Evaluation and Prevention. It is important that sexual assault victims receive information related to risks and interventions for prevention of conception as a result of the assault. Evaluation of pregnancy risk is based on the client's ability to relay accurate information about the occurrence of her last menses so that an estimate can be made of time of ovulation. Prophylactic regimens are 97 percent to 98 percent effective if started within 24 hours of the sexual attack and are generally only recommended within 72 hours (AMA, 1999). If the client chooses, a regimen of ethinyl estradiol and norgestrel (Ovral) can be administered. Two tablets are taken at the time of treatment and two tablets are taken 12 hours later. An antiemetic, such as trimethobenzamide (Tigan), is usually given to prevent nausea and vomiting, the most common side effects of the medication.

5. Crisis Intervention and Arrangements for Follow-Up Counseling. In the hours immediately following the sexual assault, the rape victim experiences an over-whelming sense of violation and helplessness that began with the powerlessness and intimidation experienced during the rape (Hutchings, 1988). Burgess (1984) identifies two emotional response patterns that may occur within hours after a rape and that health care workers may encounter in the emergency department or rape crisis center. In the *expressed response pattern*, the victim expresses feelings of fear, anger, and anxiety through such behaviors as crying, sobbing, smiling, restlessness, and tension. In the *controlled response pattern*, the feelings are masked or hidden, and a calm, composed, or subdued affect is seen. Ledray and Arndt (1994) suggest that helping the victim to regain a sense of control—that is, helping her to make decisions about what she wants to do—can be an effective method of enhancing recovery. They state:

> "During this time of crisis, the survivor is more open and accessible to outside intervention that will promote effective coping and prevent the development of ineffective or maladaptive coping strategies. She needs an empathetic, supportive listener who will allow her to talk about the assault—without pressure—as she is ready to do so." (p. 11)

This is also an important time to ensure that the victim understands that she is not to blame for what has happened. She may be blaming herself and feeling guilty for certain behaviors, such as drinking or walking alone late at night, that may have placed her in a vulnerable position. Smith (1987) suggests the following four statements be made to the sexual assault survivor:

- I am very sorry this happened to you.
- You are safe here.
- I am very glad you are alive.
- You are not to blame. You are a victim. It was not your fault. Whatever decisions you made at the time of the assault were the right ones because you are alive.

Before she leaves the emergency department, the individual should be advised about the importance of returning for follow-up counseling. She should be given the names of individuals to call for support. Often a survivor will not follow up with aftercare because she is too ashamed or is fearful of having to relive the nightmare of the attack by sharing the information in group or individual counseling. For this reason, it may be important for the nurse to get permission from the individual to allow a counselor to call her to make a follow-up appointment.

Deaths in the Emergency Department

The emergency department becomes the scene of legal investigation when death occurs in the trauma care setting. Evidence is preserved and the body is protected until the investigation has been completed. Hufft and Peter-nelj-Taylor (1999) state:

"When investigating a death scene, the clinical forensic nurse interviews witnesses; takes charge of, examines, and photographs the body; secures physical evidence; arranges body transport; and gathers records. The coroner is usually in charge of death investigation. Nurses working in this capacity initiate or assist with death investigation under selected circumstances of homicide, violence, suicide, and suspicious circumstances that indicate a violation of criminal law (e.g., presence of illegal drugs, a body found in water, a fire or explosion)."

Anatomical Gifts. When a sudden and unexpected death occurs in the trauma care setting, the clinical forensic nurse may become involved in organ/tissue donation. Some states now require that a request for organ/tissue donation be made of the family when a death occurs under certain circumstances. This is a very painful period for family members, and nurses may feel it is an inappropriate time to present the information associated with an anatomical request. However, most nurses employed in trauma care recognize that organ/tissue recovery for transplantation is a requisite component of their work. Lynch (1995) states:

"As an expert in legal issues and with sensitivity to the deceased's family, a forensic nurse can be used (1) to provide consultation as necessary, (2) to foster staff education, and (3) to perform immediate interventions in the emergency department setting. As a nurse manager, the forensic nurse position can provide an opportunity to create or to advance existing protocol with greater emphasis on the coordination and cooperation between organ/tissue procurement and the medical examiner/coroner system."

Evaluation

Evaluation of the clinical forensic nursing process in the trauma care setting involves ongoing measurement of the diagnostic criteria aimed at resolution of identified real or potential problems. The following types of questions may provide assistance in the evaluation process:

1. Have the physical and psychological needs of the survivors who present themselves to the emergency department been met?
2. Has the evidence in potential criminal investigations been handled such that it can be used in a credible manner?
3. Has the sexual assault survivor received information related to choices pertaining to STDs, pregnancy, and follow-up counseling?
4. In the instance of sudden and unexpected death in the emergency department, have the needs of the grieving family been met?
5. Have the importance of anatomical donations been communicated?

The role of the clinical forensic nurse in trauma care continues to expand. With the level of societal violence at epidemic proportions, clinical forensic nurses potentially may intervene in the examination of victims of all types of abuse situations. The clinical forensic nurse specialist must also strive to be proactive, beginning with educating emergency department staff in the philosophy and interventions of clinical forensic nursing practice (Lynch, 1995). Within the community, proactive responsibilities may include providing information about environmental hazards and issues that may affect public health and safety. Effectiveness of these changes provides measurement for ongoing evaluation.

APPLICATION OF THE NURSING PROCESS IN FORENSIC PSYCHIATRIC NURSING IN CORRECTIONAL FACILITIES

Assessment

Deinstitutionalization as a concept has not been successful. Doyle (1998) states:

"The apparent failure of deinstitutionalization throughout the developed world, along with an international trend toward longer periods of incarceration as a sentencing option for violent or drug and alcohol-related crime has resulted in a rapid expansion of its incarcerated inpatient populations." (p. 25)

It was believed that deinstitutionalization increased the freedom of mentally ill individuals in accordance with the principle of "least-restrictive alternative." However, because of inadequate community-based services, many of these individuals drifted into poverty and homelessness, increasing their vulnerability to criminalization (Freeman & Roesch, 1989). Because the bizarre behavior of mentally ill individuals living on the street is sometimes offensive to community standards, law enforcement officials have the authority to protect the welfare of the public, as well as the safety of the individual, by initiating emergency hospitalization. However, legal criteria for commitment are so stringent in most cases that arrest becomes an easier way of getting the mentally ill person off the street if a criminal statute has been violated (Teplin & Voit, 1996). It is estimated that between 10 and 35 percent of all inmates have some form of psychological disorder or mental disability (Wark, 1998). Some of these individuals are incarcerated as a result of the increasingly popular "guilty but mentally ill" verdict. It is unfortunate that "prisons are becoming the 1990s' 'state psychiatric hospitals'" (Lego, 1995).

The U.S. Department of Justice recently reported that U.S. prisons and jails held a record 1.8 million inmates in 1998 (Fox News, 1999). The report stated that 41 percent of the national jail population were white, 41 percent were African American, 16 percent were Hispanic, and 2 percent were of other backgrounds, such as Asians Americans,

Native Americans, and Alaskan natives. Men accounted for 89 percent of the total.

Care of the mentally ill offender population is a highly specialized area of nursing practice. Reeder and Meldman (1991) identify four aims of imprisonment for criminal behavior:

● Retribution to society
● Deterrence of future crimes
● Reformation and repentance
● Protection of society

If an institution bases its orientation on retribution and deterrence of criminal activity, the prison will reflect a punishment-oriented atmosphere. If reformation and repentance are accepted as a basis for change, mental health programs that encourage reflection and insight may be a part of the correctional setting. Because at times these basic aims may seem incompatible with each other, nurses who work in correctional facilities may struggle with a cognitive dissonance founded in their basic nursing value system.

Assessing Mental Health Needs of the Incarcerated

Is the provision of mental health care within the custodial environment possible? Or are clinical care concerns incompatible with security issues? What special knowledge and skills must a psychiatric nurse possess to be successful in caring for the mentally ill offender?

Peternelj-Taylor (1998) suggests that three groups of psychiatric clients may be identified in the forensic population: (1) those who are mentally ill at the time of incarceration, (2) those who become mentally ill while incarcerated, and (3) those with antisocial personality disorder. Psychiatric diagnoses commonly identified at the time of incarceration include schizophrenia, affective psychoses, personality disorders, and substance disorders (Rice, Harris, & Quinsey, 1996). Common psychiatric behaviors include hallucinations, suspiciousness, thought disorders, anger/agitation, impulsivity, and denial of problems. In a study by Rice, Harris, & Quinsey (1996), the behavior, "denial of problems," ranked as most significant among this population. Use of substances and medication noncompliance are common obstacles to rehabilitation. Substance abuse has been shown to have a strong correlation with recidivism among the prison population (Rice, Harris, & Quinsey, 1996). Many individuals report that they were under the influence of illegal substances at the time of their criminal actions, and dual diagnoses are common. Detoxification frequency occurs in jails and prisons, and some inmates have died from the withdrawal syndrome because of lack of adequate treatment during this process (Bernier, 1991).

Reeder and Meldman (1991) point out that there is a fundamental difference between prisons and jails and that the U.S. Department of Justice (1980) defines a jail as "a locally administered confinement facility authorized to hold persons awaiting adjudication and/or those committed after adjudication to serve sentences of one year or less" (p. 42). A large portion of mentally ill offenders, particularly the acutely psychotic, never reach the prison system. Frequent arrests for minor offenses may lead to numerous jail incarcerations, a sense of loss of control, and a continual state of crisis, resulting in psychosocial consequences such as anger, anxiety, depression, despair, and learned helplessness (Reeder & Meldman, 1991). Tuskan and Thase (1983) report that inmates in U.S. prisons and jails manifest a rate of suicide at least three times greater than the population at large.

Special Concerns

Overcrowding and Violence. Numerous studies have shown that crowding affects the level of violence in prisons. More than half of all infractions committed by prisoners are violent in nature (Wark, 1998). The prison system is not capable of handling the burden of the large numbers of prisoners for which it has become responsible. These growing numbers are thought to be related to the increasing war on drugs, longer mandatory sentencing, and the "three strikes and you're out" laws. As this population continues to grow, the solution seems to be to continue to construct larger and larger complexes to house the growing numbers of inmates. In these crowded conditions, "the desired result of violent behavior is to gain a reputation or acquire material resources through force" (Wark, 1998).

Inmate violence directed toward prison staff is a common occurrence. Light (1991) reported the most frequently cited motives as: inmate resistance to officer's commands, protest of unjust treatment, resistance to searches and attempt to remove contraband, and staff intervention in fights between inmates. Peternelj-Taylor and Johnson (1995) state: "Violence also may be actual or implied verbal threats, or the constant barrage of swearing, which is the common everyday language of most offender clients" (p. 13).

Nurses who work in correctional facilities must be able to adjust to the commonality of physical and verbal aggression if they are to prevail in this chosen area of specialization.

Sexual Assault. The number of victims of sexual assault in American prisons is unknown. Studies have suggested that 9 to 20 percent of federal inmates have been victims of sexual assault (Kantor, 1998). Wark (1998) reports that it is likely that upwards of 75 percent of sexual assaults in prisons go unreported. The consequences of "ratting" on fellow prisoners is often far more serious than the rape itself.

Rape in prison is viewed as an act of dominance and power, rather than one which is sexually motivated, and the majority of both victims and victimizers are heterosexuals (Bernier, 1991). Wark (1998) describes the typical victim as "young, white, nonviolent, generally tall and slender with long hair." In other instances, sexual assault is used as a means of punishment and social control when the victim is believed to have violated certain unwritten prison codes. Gang rape is not uncommon, and severe physical injury is often the result if the victim attempts to defend himself.

HIV Infection in the Prison Population. The AIDS rate is seven times higher in state and federal prisons than in the general U.S. population (Kantor, 1998). In addition to sexual conduct, other means of HIV transmission among inmates include fights that result in lacerations, bites, or bleeding. Body piercing and tattooing are becoming more popular in prison, and clean instruments for these activities are not available. Intravenous drug use results in sharing of unsterilized injection equipment.

HIV has placed an enormous financial burden on a prison system that was already financially distressed. Some terminally ill prisoners with advanced AIDS are being granted early compassionate release to family or hospice care, with access to community health services (Kantor, 1998).

The most recent approach to prevention of HIV transmission has shifted from segregation to education. Education of the prison population about HIV is difficult because as many as 50 percent of American prisoners are functionally illiterate, and many do not speak English (Kantor, 1998). Educational programs to meet the communication needs of this special population would be required.

Female Offenders. Women comprise 6.3 percent of the total prison population (Wark, 1998). As a minority group, they appear to be discriminated against within the prison system. Their facilities are usually more isolated, making it more difficult for family visits. In some instances, separate institutions do not exist, making it necessary to house male and female offenders in co-correctional facilities. Men are given a greater number of opportunities regarding education and vocational training services.

Many women are single mothers who are unable to make adequate provision for their children while they serve their time in prison and who often lose custody of their children to the state. Prison health care is mostly inadequate, and the unique health needs of women often go unmet. Many of these women had very little before they were incarcerated, and have come to expect that little is what they deserve. Many report long histories of sexual and emotional abuse throughout their lives. Depression and acting-out behaviors are not uncommon in women's prisons. Desmond (1991) reported that women who made friends within the institution were less lonely than those

who did not and were better able to cope with the stress of incarceration.

Nursing Diagnosis

Forensic psychiatric nurse specialists in correctional facilities analyze the information gathered during assessment of the client to formulate nursing diagnoses. Common nursing diagnoses relevant to forensic clients in correctional facilities include:

1. Defensive coping
2. Dysfunctional grieving
3. Anxiety/fear
4. Altered thought processes
5. Powerlessness
6. Self-esteem disturbance
7. Risk for self-mutilation
8. Risk for violence, directed at self or others
9. Ineffective individual coping
10. Altered sexuality patterns
11. Risk for infection

Planning/Implementation

Psychiatric nurses who work in correctional facilities must be armed with extraordinary psychosocial skills and the knowledge to apply them in the most appropriate manner.

Development of a Therapeutic Relationship

Incarcerated individuals have difficulty trusting anyone associated with authority, including nurses. For most of these individuals, this likely relates back to very early stages of development and lack of nurturing.

Aside from the added difficulty of dealing with this special population, development of a therapeutic relationship in the correctional facility encompasses the same phases of interaction as it does with other clients. Chapter 5 of this text discusses the dynamics of this process at length.

Preinteraction Phase. During this phase the nurse must examine his or her feelings, fears, and anxieties about working with prisoners—violent offenders—perhaps murderers, rapists, or pedophiles. This is the phase in which the nurse must determine whether he or she is able to separate the *person* from the *behavior* and provide the unconditional positive regard that Rogers (1951) believed identified each individual as a worthwhile and unique human being.

Orientation (Introductory) Phase. This is the phase in which the nurse works to establish trust with the client. This is a lengthy and intense process with the prisoner population. The characteristics that have been identified as significant to the development of a therapeutic nurse-client relationship—rapport, trust, genuineness—are commonly met with suspicion on the part of the offender. Empathy may be used as a tool for manipulating the nurse. It is therefore imperative that limits be established and enforced by all of the nursing staff. Testing of limits will be commonplace, so consequences for violation must be consistently administered. Splitting nurse against other treatment team members ("You're the only one who understands me.") is a common ploy among inmates (Peternelj-Taylor & Johnson, 1995).

Touch and self-disclosure, two elements used in the establishment of trust with clients, are most commonly unacceptable with the prisoner population. A handshake may be appropriate, but any other form of touch between nurse and inmate of the opposite gender is usually restricted in most settings. Self-disclosure is commonly used to convey empathy and to promote trust by helping the client view the nurse as an ordinary human being. With the prisoner population, the client may seek personal information about the nurse in an effort to maintain control of the relationship. Nurses must maintain awareness of the situation and ensure that personal boundaries are not being violated.

Communication within the correctional facility may prove to be a challenge for the nurse. Slang terminology is commonplace and changes rapidly. Some of these terms are presented in Table 42.2.

Working Phase. This is the phase of the relationship during which the nursing skills are implemented. Promoting behavioral change is the primary goal of the working phase. This is extremely difficult with offenders, who commonly deny problems and resist change. Transference and countertransference issues are more common in working with this population than with other psychiatric clients. Issues are discussed in the treatment team meetings, and ongoing modifications are made as required. Following are some of the interventions associated with psychiatric forensic nursing in correctional institutions.

1. Counseling and Supportive Psychotherapy. Nurses may work with inmates who are experiencing feelings of powerlessness and grief. Women who have left children behind may fear the permanent loss of custody or of never seeing them again. Helping these individuals work through a period of mourning is an important nursing intervention.

Nurses may also counsel victims of sexual assault. Bernier (1991) states:

> "Psychologically, the victim experiences feelings of humiliation, depression, shame, anger, violent mood swings, flashbacks, nightmares, and an inability to concentrate. Since 'real men' do not discuss their emotions, assistance in resolution of these problems often does not occur." (p. 696)

These individuals often become withdrawn and isolated, and at a high risk for suicide. The nurse can recognize these symptoms and intervene as required. All unusual behavior should be shared with the treatment team.

2. Crisis Intervention. Behaviors such as aggression, self-mutilation, and suicide attempts, as well as acute psychotic episodes and posttrauma responses, require that the nurse be proficient in crisis intervention. Reeder and Meldman (1991) state:

> "Once people become inmates of a jail, they experience a loss of control and a sense of loss, which creates a continual state of crisis. A chaotic, overburdened criminal justice system often is unable to provide the inmates with much sense of what will happen to them or what, if any, control they have over their own situation. A strong, solid foundation in crisis intervention theory and techniques is an absolute prerequisite [for the nurse]." (p. 43)

Threatening behaviors must be reported immediately to all members of the treatment team. Techniques of crisis intervention are discussed in Chapter 11 of this text.

3. Education. Opportunities for teaching abound in the correctional facility. However, as was mentioned previously, because of the level of education of many incarcerated individuals, and because many of them speak little English, the teaching plan must be highly individualized. Many have no desire or motivation to learn and resist cooperating with these efforts. Important educational endeavors with these clients include:

- **Health Teaching.** Most criminals are not in good physical condition when they reach prison. They have lived rough lives of smoking, poor diets, substance abuse, and minimal health care. This is an opportunity for nurses to provide information about ways to achieve optimum wellness.
- **HIV/AIDS Education.** Kantor (1998) states:

> "All persons entering prison must be informed in clear, simple terms, *and in their own language*, about how to avoid transmission of HIV and other communicable diseases. Educational programs have reduced fears about HIV and its transmission among the majority of staff and inmates. Individual counseling, peer counseling, support groups, and special programs for women, designed for and by prisoners, have been successful in a number of institutions and seem to be the best educational tools."

Some correctional institutions now provide condoms to inmates, but this remains a point of controversy between legal and public health officials.

- **Stress Management.** Nurses can present information and demonstration of stress management techniques. They can help individuals practice reduction of anxiety without resorting to medications or substances.
- **Substance Abuse.** The National Commission on Correctional Health Care (NCCHC) (1999) states:

> "Substance abuse treatment is often a mandatory part of some offenders' sentences, and in many institutions, Alcoholics Anonymous (AA) is the only substance abuse group available. In recent months, however, the

TABLE 42.2 GLOSSARY OF PRISON SLANG

Ad-seg. Administrative segregation. A prisoner placed on ad-seg is being investigated and will go into isolation (the "hole") until the investigation is complete.

Beef. Criminal charges. As, "I caught a burglary beef this time around." Also used to mean a problem "I have a beef with that guy."

Big yard. The main recreation yard.

Bit. Prison sentence, usually relatively short. "I got a three-year bit." (opposite of *jolt*)

Bitch, bitched (v). To be sentenced as a "habitual offender."

Blocks. Cellhouses.

Books. Administratively controlled account ledger that lists each prisoner's account balance.

Bone yard. The visiting trailers, used for overnight visits of wives and/or families.

Bum beef. A false accusation. Also, a wrongful conviction.

Catch a ride. To ask a friend with drugs to get you high. "Hey, man, can I catch a ride?"

The chain. The bus transports that bring prisoners to prison. One is shackled and chained when transported. As, "I've been riding the chain," or "I just got in on the chain," or "Is there anyone we know on the chain?"

Check-in. Someone who has submitted to pressure, intimidation, debts, etc., and no longer feels secure in population and "checks in" to a protective custody (PC) unit.

Chi-mo. Child molester, "chester," "baby-raper," "short-eyes," (as "he has short-eyes," meaning he goes after young kids). The worst of the *rapo* class in the eyes of *convicts*.

Convict. Guys who count in prison; loyal to the code; aren't stool pigeons; their word is good (Opposite of *inmate*)

C.U.S. Custody unit supervisor/cellhouse supervisor.

De-seg. Disciplinary segregation. When a person is on de-seg, he is in isolation (the "hole") for an infraction.

Ding. A disrespectful term for a mentally ill prisoner.

Dry snitching. To inform on someone indirectly by talking loud or performing suspicious actions when officers are in the area.

Dummy up; get on the dummy. To shut up, to pipe down, to be quiet, especially about one's knowledge of a crime.

E.P.R.D. Earliest possible release date.

Fish. A new arrival, a first-timer, a bumpkin, not wise to prison life.

Gate money. Money the state gives a prisoner upon release.

Gate time. At most prisons they yell "gate time," meaning one can get in or out of the cell. See *lock-up*.

Hacks/hogs/pigs/snouts/screws/cops/bulls. The guards; called "corrections officers" by themselves and *inmates*.

Heat wave. Being under constant suspicion, thereby bringing attention to those around you.

Hit it. Go away, leave, get lost

Hold your mud. Not tell, even under pressure of punishment.

The hole. An isolation ("segregation") cell, used as punishment for offenses.

House. Cell.

Hustle. A professional criminal's avocation. Also refers to any scheme to obtain money or drugs while in prison.

I.K. Inmate kitchen.

I.M.U. Intensive management unit. Administration's name for "segregation" or "the hole."

Inmate. Derogatory term for prisoners. Used by guards, administrators, other inmates, or new arrivals who don't know the language yet. Opposite of *convict*.

Jacket. Prison file containing all information on a prisoner. "He's a child molester; it's in his jacket." Also reputation. Prisoners can put false jackets on other prisoners to discredit them.

Jolt. A long sentence. ("I got a life jolt.") Opposite of *bit*.

Jumping-out. Turning to crime. "I've been jumping out since I was a kid."

Keister. To hide something in the anal cavity.

Lag. A *convict*, as in, "He's an old lag, been at it all his life."

Lifer or **"all day."** Anyone doing a life sentence. A life *jolt*.

Lock-down. When prisoners are confined to their cells.

Lock-up. Free movement period for prisoners. See also *gate time*.

Lop. Same as *inmate*.

Mule. A person who smuggles drugs into the institution.

On the leg. A prisoner who is always chatting with and befriending guards.

Paper. A small quantity of drugs packaged for selling.

TABLE 42.2 GLOSSARY OF PRISON SLANG

P.C. Protective custody. Also as in "He's a PC case," meaning weak or untrustworthy.

Point/outfit. Syringe.

Pruno. Homemade wine.

Punk. Derogatory term meaning homosexual or weak individual.

Rapo. Anyone convicted of a sex crime—generally looked down on by *convicts*.

Rat/snitch/stool pigeon. n., informant. v., to inform.

Stand point. Watch for "the man" (guard)

Tag/write-up. Infraction of institution rules.

The bag/sack. Dope.

Tom or **George.** Meaning "no good" (Tom) or "okay"(George).Used in conversation to indicate if someone or something is okay or not.

Turned out. To be forced into homosexual acts, or to turn someone out to do things for you; to use someone for your own needs.

White money. Currency within the institution.

Yard-in/yard-out. Closing of the recreation yard (yard-in). Recreation yard opens (yard-out).

SOURCE: From Tenenbaum (1999), with permimssion.

---

courts have heard cases regarding mandatory attendance at AA and have begun to challenge prison officials' ability to force participation in AA due to the spiritual component of the program."

Nurses can provide information about the effects of substances on the body, the consequences of sharing needles, and form support groups for substance abusers if one does not exist in the institution.

Termination Phase. Ideally, the termination phase of the nurse-client relationship ensures therapeutic closure. This is not always possible in the correctional environment. Prisoners are transferred from one institution to another, and from one part of an institution to another, for a variety of reasons, not the least of which are safety and security of self or others. When possible, it is important for nurses to initiate termination with clients so that at least some semblance of closure can be achieved and a review of goal attainment can be accomplished. Community facilities for mentally ill ex-offenders are few, and recidivism is rampant. Bernier (1991) states:

"When inmates are nearing the time for parole, there is an excellent opportunity for the nurse to hold group meetings specifically focused on reentry into the community. Some ex-offenders have organized support groups in the community to assist those first coming out of prison."(p. 697)

Evaluation

Evaluation of the psychiatric forensic nursing process in the correctional environment involves ongoing

---

TEST YOUR CRITICAL THINKING SKILLS

Kim is a 27-year-old woman who recently moved from a small town in Texas to work in the city of Dallas as a reporter for one of the major newspapers. She is 5′6″ tall and weighs 115 lb. To keep in shape she likes to jog, which she did regularly in her home town. She doesn't know anyone in Dallas and has been lonely for her family since arriving. But she has moved into a small apartment in a quiet neighborhood and hopes to meet young people soon though her work and church.

On the first Saturday morning after she moved into her new apartment, Kim decided to get up early and go jogging. It was still dark out, but Kim was not afraid. She had been jogging alone in the dark many times in her home town. She donned her jogging clothes and headed down the quiet street toward a nearby park. As she entered the park, an individual came out from a dense clump of bushes, put a knife to her throat, and ordered her to the ground. She was raped and beaten unconscious. She remained in that condition until sunrise when she was found by another jogger who called emergency services, and Kim was taken to the closest emergency department. Upon regaining consciousness, Kim was hysterical, but a sexual assault nurse examiner (SANE) was called to the scene, and Kim was assigned to a quiet area of the hospital, where the post-rape examination was initiated.

Answer the following questions related to Kim.

1. What are the initial nursing interventions for Kim?
2. What treatments must the nurse ensure that Kim is aware are available for her?
3. What nursing diagnosis would the nurse expect to focus on with Kim in follow-up care?

measurement of the diagnostic criteria aimed at resolution of identified real or potential problems. The following types of questions may provide assistance in the evaluation process.

1. Has a degree of trust been established in the nurse-client relationship?
2. Has violence by the offender to self or others been prevented?
3. If victimization has occurred, has appropriate care and support been provided to the survivor?
4. Have limits been set on inappropriate behaviors and has consistency of consequences for violation of the limits been administered by all staff?
5. Have educational programs been established to provide information about health and wellness, HIV/AIDS, stress management, and substance abuse?

Evaluation is an ongoing process and must be assumed by the entire treatment team. Modification of the treatment plan as required is part of the ongoing evaluation process, and positive change within the system is the ultimate outcome. Nurses who work in correctional facilities are "pioneers" within the nursing profession. To share the knowledge gleaned from this specialty area is an important part of the nursing process.

SUMMARY

Forensic nursing, which is a growing area within the profession, is composed of a variety of areas of expertise. Forensic nurses take care of both victims and perpetrators of crime in a variety of settings, including primary care facilities, hospitals, and correctional institutions. The International Association of Forensic Nurses, founded in 1992, now has more than a thousand members.

Forensic nursing specialties include clinical forensic nursing, the sexual assault nurse examiner, forensic psychiatric nursing, and correctional/institutional nursing. Nurses in general practice also find forensic nursing knowledge of importance in their practices, particularly in emergency department and intensive care units.

This chapter presented discussions of two specialty areas of forensic nursing: clinical forensic nursing in trauma care and forensic psychiatric nursing in correctional facilities. Nursing care of these special populations was presented in the context of the nursing process.

The number of educational offerings pertaining to forensic nursing is growing. Some content is taught in traditional nursing courses, whereas some colleges and universities are establishing forensic nursing courses as electives. Forensic nursing is fertile ground for nursing research, and the complex nature of the specialty lends itself well to those nurses who seek a challenge within the profession.

REVIEW QUESTIONS

SELF-EXAMINATION/LEARNING EXERCISE

Indicate with a checkmark whether the following statements are true or false.

1. All traumatic injuries in which liability is suspected are considered within the scope of forensic nursing.

    a. _____ true   b. _____ false

2. Clinical forensic nursing in the trauma department encompasses preservation of evidence, investigation of wound characteristics, and sudden deaths in the emergency department (ED).

    a. _____ true   b. _____ false

3. Legal authorities must be notified of all deaths, natural or unnatural, that occur in the ED.

    a. _____ true   b. _____ false

4. When a trauma victim is admitted to the ED, the most obvious priority intervention is preservation of evidence.

    a. _____ true   b. _____ false

5. When clothing is removed, it should be shaken to remove any possible evidence that may be adhering to it.

    a. _____ true   b. _____ false

6. Rape victims can be treated prophylacticly for sexually transmitted diseases.

    a. _____ true   b. _____ false

7. The most common psychiatric behavior that has been identified among mentally ill offenders is thought disorder.

    a. _____ true   b. _____ false

8. The AIDS rate is higher in state and federal prisons than in the general population.

    a. _____ true   b. _____ false

9. Male offenders receive more educational opportunities in prison than female offenders.

    a. _____ true   b. _____ false

10. Correctional institutions are federally mandated to provide condoms to inmates to prevent the transmission of HIV.

    a. _____ true   b. _____ false

REFERENCES

American Medical Association (AMA). (1999). *Strategies for the treatment and prevention of sexual assault.* [On-line]. Available: http://www.ama-assn.org/public/releases/assault/sa-guide.htm

American Nurses' Association (ANA). (1995). *Standards of nursing practice in correctional facilities.* Washington, DC: American Nurses Association.

Bell, K. (1999, March). Forensic nursing. Paper presented at the meeting of the Oklahoma Association of Clinical Nurse Specialists, Stroud, Oklahoma.

Bernier, S.L. (1991). Mental health issues and nursing in corrections. In G.K. McFarland & M.D. Thomas (Eds.), *Psychiatric mental health nursing: Application of the nursing process.* Philadelphia: J.B. Lippincott.

Burgess, A. W. (1984). Intra-familial sexual abuse. In J. Campbell & J. Humphreys (Eds.), *Nursing care of victims of family violence.* Reston, VA: Reston Publishing.

Desmond, A.M. (1991). The relationship between loneliness and social interaction in women prisoners. *Journal of Psychosocial Nursing, 29*(3), 4–10.

Doyle, J. (1998). Prisoners as patients: The experience of delivering mental health nursing care in an Australian prison. *Journal of Psychosocial Nursing, 36*(12), 25–29.

Forensic Nursing Service (FNS). (1999). *About forensic nursing.* [On-line]. Available: http://www.forensicnursing.com/html/about.html/

Fox News. (1999). *News America Digital Publishing* [On-line]. Available: http://www.foxnews.com/nav/ js_stage.sml/

Freeman, R.J., & Roesch, R. (1989). Mental disorder and the criminal justice system: A review. *International Journal of Law and Psychiatry, 12*, 105–115.

Hufft, A., & Peternelj-Taylor, C. (1999). Forensic nursing: An emerging specialty. In J.T. Catalano (Ed.). *1999 contemporary professional nursing update.* Philadelphia: F.A. Davis.

Hutchings, N. (1998). *The violent family: Victimization of women, children, and elders.* New York: Human Sciences Press.

International Association of Forensic Nurses (IAFN) and American Nurses' Association (ANA). (1997). *Scope and standards of forensic nursing practice.* Washington, DC: American Nurses Publishing.

Kantor, E. (1998). AIDS and HIV infection in prisoners. *The AIDS knowledge base.* [On-line]. Available: http://hivinsite.ucsf.edu/akb/1997/01pris/

Ledray, L.E., & Arndt, S. (1994). Examining the sexual assault victim: A new model for nursing care. *Journal of Psychosocial Nursing, 32*(2), 7–12.

Lego, S. (1995). Book review: "Live from death row." *Journal of the American Psychiatric Nurses Association, 1*(5), 171–174.

Light, S. (1991). Assaults on prison officers: Interactional themes. *Justice Quarterly, 8*, 243–261.

Lynch, V.A. (1993). Forensic nursing: Diversity in education and practice. *Journal of Psychosocial Nursing, 31*(11), 7–14.

Lynch, V.A. (1995, September). Clinical forensic nursing: A new perspective in the management of crime victims from trauma to trial. *Critical Care Nursing Clinics of North America, 7*(3), 489–507.

National Commission on Correctional Health Care (NCCHC). (1999). *Secular groups help inmates battle substance abuse.* [On-line.] Available: http://www.corrections.com/ncchc/care.html/

Peternelj-Taylor, C.A. (1998). Forbidden love: Sexual exploitation in the forensic milieu. *Journal of Psychosocial Nursing, 36*(6), 17–23.

Peternelj-Taylor, C.A., & Hufft, A.G. (1997). Forensic psychiatric nursing. In B.S. Johnson (Ed.). *Psychiatric-mental health nursing: Adaptation and growth.* Philadelphia: Lippincott.

Peternelj-Taylor, C.A., & Johnson, R.L. (1995). Serving time: Psychiatric mental health nursing in corrections. *Journal of Psychosocial Nursing, 33*(8), 12–19.

Reeder, D., & Meldman, L. (1991). Conceptualizing psychosocial nursing in the jail setting. *Journal of Psychosocial Nursing, 29*(8), 40–44.

Rice, M.E., Harris, G.T., & Quinsey, V.L. (1996). Treatment for forensic patients. In B.D. Sales & S.A. Shah (Eds.), *Mental health and law: Research, policy and services.* Durham, NC: Carolina Academic Press.

Rogers, C.R. (1951). *Client centered therapy.* Boston: Houghton Mifflin.

Scales, C.J., Mitchell, J.L., & Smith, R.D. (1993). Survey report on forensic nursing. *Journal of Psychosocial Nursing, 31*(11), 39–44.

Smith, L. S. (1987). Sexual assault: The nurse's role. *AD Nurse, 2*(2), 24–28.

Taber's Cyclopedic Medical Dictionary (18th ed.). (1997). Philadelphia: F.A. Davis.

Tenenbaum, D. (1999). *Glossary of prison slang.* [On-line.] Available: http://www.halcyon.com/scripts/dante/cgi-pvt/pe/dpp/glossary.html/

Teplin, L.A., & Voit, E.S. (1996). Criminalizing the seriously mentally ill: Putting the problem in perspective. In B.D. Sales & S.A. Shah (Eds.), *Mental health and law: Research, policy, and services.* Durham, NC: Carolina Academic Press.

Tuskan, J.J., & Thase, M.E. (1983). Suicides in jails and prisons. *Journal of Psychosocial Nursing, 21*(5), 29–33.

U.S. Department of Justice. (1980). *Federal standards for prisons and jails.* Washington, DC: U.S. Government Printing Office.

Wark, D. (1998). *Prison violence: Homicide, assault, and rape.* [On-line]. Available: http://oak.cats.ohiou.edu/~dw101094/esp/soc4661.html/

Answers to Chapter Review Questions

CHAPTER 1

Introduction to Stress

1. b
2. d
3. a
4. b
5. 1. c
   2. d
   3. b
   4. a
6. 1. d
   2. a
   3. e
   4. b
   5. c

CHAPTER 2

Mental Health/Mental Illness

1. c
2. d
3. b
4. a
5. b
6. d
7. c
8. d
9. c
10. b
11. b
12. h
13. a
14. m
15. n
16. c
17. k
18. e
19. i
20. f
21. d
22. o

23. g
24. j
25. l

CHAPTER 3

Theories of Personality Development

1. b
2. c
3. d
4. b
5. b
6. b
7. a
8. c
9. a
10. b

CHAPTER 4

Concepts of Psychobiology

1. c
2. e
3. f
4. b
5. d
6. g
7. a
8. c
9. b
10. a
11. a
12. b
13. d

CHAPTER 5

Relationship Development

1. a. The mother-surrogate.
   b. The technician.

c. The manager.

d. The socializing agent.

e. The health teacher.

f. The counselor.

2. The counselor.

3. It is through establishment of a satisfactory nurse-client relationship that individuals learn to generalize the ability to achieve satisfactory interpersonal relationships to other aspects of their lives.

4. Most often the goal is directed at learning and growth promotion, in an effort to bring about some type of change in the client's life. This is accomplished through use of the problem-solving model.

5. The therapeutic use of self.

6. 1. d
   2. a
   3. e
   4. b
   5. c

7. 1. c
   2. a
   3. d
   4. b

CHAPTER 6

Therapeutic Communication

1. In the transactional model of communication, both persons are participating simultaneously. They are mutually perceiving each other, simultaneously listening to each other, and mutually and simultaneously engaged in the process of creating meaning in a relationship.

2. a. One's value system.
   b. Internalized attitudes and beliefs.
   c. Culture and/or religion.
   d. Social status.
   e. Gender.
   f. Background knowledge and experience.
   g. Age or developmental level.
   h. Type of environment in which the communication takes place.

3. Territoriality is the innate tendency to own space. People "mark" space as their own and feel more comfortable in these spaces. Territoriality affects communication in that an interaction can be more successful if it takes place on "neutral" ground rather than in a space "owned" by one or the other of the communicants.

4. Density refers to the number of people within a given environmental space. It may affect communication in that some studies indicate that a correlation exists between prolonged high-density situations and certain behaviors, such as aggression, stress, criminal activity, hostility toward others, and a deterioration of mental and physical health.

5. a. Intimate distance (0–18 inches)—kissing or hugging someone.
   b. Personal distance (18–40 inches)—close conversations with friends or colleagues.
   c. Social distance (4–12 feet)—conversations with strangers or acquaintances (e.g., at a cocktail party).
   d. Public distance (>12 feet)—speaking in public.

6. a. Physical appearance and dress (e.g., young men who have hair down past their shoulders may convey a message of rebellion against the establishment).
   b. Body movement and posture (e.g., a person with hands on hips standing straight and tall in front of someone seated who must look up to them is conveying a message of power over the seated individual).
   c. Touch (e.g., laying one's hand on the shoulder of another may convey a message of friendship and caring).
   d. Facial expressions (e.g., wrinkling up of the nose, raising the upper lip, or raising one side of the upper lip conveys a message of disgust for a situation).
   e. Eye behavior (e.g., direct eye contact, accompanied by a smile and nodding of the head, conveys interest in what the other person is saying).
   f. Vocal cues or paralanguage (e.g., a normally soft-spoken individual whose pitch and rate of speaking increases may be perceived as being anxious or tense).

7. S—Sit squarely facing the client.
   O—Observe an open posture.
   L—Lean forward toward the client.
   E—Establish eye contact.
   R—Relax.

8. a. Nontherapeutic technique: Disagreeing.
   b. The correct answer. Therapeutic technique: Voicing doubt.

9. a. The correct answer. Therapeutic technique: Giving recognition.
   b. Nontherapeutic technique: Complimenting—a judgment on the part of the nurse.

10. a. Nontherapeutic: Giving reassurance.
    b. Nontherapeutic: Giving disapproval.
    c. Nontherapeutic: Introducing an unrelated topic.
    d. Nontherapeutic: Indicating an external source of power.
    e. The correct answer. Therapeutic technique: Exploring.

11. a. Nontherapeutic: Requesting an explanation.
    b. Nontherapeutic: Belittling feelings expressed.
    c. Nontherapeutic: Rejecting.
    d. The correct answer. Therapeutic technique: Formulating a plan of action.
12. Therapeutic response: "Do you think you should tell him?" Technique: Reflecting.
    Nontherapeutic response: "Yes, you must tell your husband about your affair with your boss." Technique: Giving advice.
13. a. The correct answer. Therapeutic technique: Reflecting.
    b. Nontherapeutic: Requesting an explanation.
    c. Nontherapeutic: Indicating an external source of power.
    d. Nontherapeutic: Giving advice.
    e. Nontherapeutic: Defending.
    f. Nontherapeutic: Making stereotyped comments.

CHAPTER 7

The Nursing Process in Psychiatric/Mental Health Nursing

1. Assessment, diagnosis, outcome identification, planning, implementation, evaluation.
2. a. Implementation.
   b. Diagnosis.
   c. Evaluation.
   d. Assessment.
   e. Planning.
   f. Outcome identification.
3. Nursing diagnoses:
   a. Altered nutrition, less than body requirements.
   b. Social isolation.
   c. Self-esteem disturbance.
   Outcomes:
   a. Client will gain 2 lb/wk in next 3 weeks.
   b. Client will voluntarily spend time with peers and staff in group activities on the unit within 7 days.
   c. Client will verbalize positive aspects about herself (excluding any references to eating or body image) within 2 weeks.
4. Problem-oriented recording (SOAPIE); Focus Charting; PIE charting.

CHAPTER 8

Therapeutic Groups

1. A group is a collection of individuals whose association is founded upon shared commonalities of interest, values, norms, and/or purpose.

2. a. Teaching group.
      Laissez-faire leader.
   b. Supportive/therapeutic group.
      Democratic leader.
   c. Task group.
      Autocratic leader.
3. 1. b
   2. i
   3. k
   4. h
   5. e
   6. j
   7. a
   8. d
   9. f
   10. g
   11. c
4. 1. e
   2. h
   3. f
   4. d
   5. a
   6. c
   7. g
   8. b

CHAPTER 9

Intervention With Families

1. e
2. a
3. f
4. c
5. b
6. d
7. b
8. c
9. a
10. b

CHAPTER 10

Milieu Therapy—The Therapeutic Community

1. A scientific structuring of the environment in order to effect behavioral changes and to improve the psychological health and functioning of the individual.
2. The goal of milieu therapy/therapeutic community is for the client to learn adaptive coping, interaction, and relationship skills that can be generalized to other aspects of his or her life.

3. c
4. b
5. a
6. d
7. 1. f   8. e
   2. h   9. c
   3. b   10. k
   4. i   11. m
   5. g   12. l
   6. j   13. d
   7. a

CHAPTER 11

Crisis Intervention

1. c
2. d
3. a
4. b
5. c
6. a
7. d
8. b
9. b
10. d

CHAPTER 12

Relaxation Therapy

3a. (1) Anxiety (moderate to severe) related to lack of self-confidence and fear of making errors
   (2) Pain (migraine headaches) related to repressed severe anxiety
   (3) Sleep pattern disturbance related to anxiety
3b. Some outcome criteria for Linda might be:
   (1) Client will be able to perform duties on the job while maintaining anxiety at a manageable level by practicing deep-breathing exercises.
   (2) Client will verbalize a reduction in headache pain following progressive relaxation techniques.
   (3) Client is able to fall asleep within 30 minutes of retiring by listening to soft music and performing mental imagery exercises.
3c. The deep-breathing exercises would be especially good for Linda because she could perform them as many times as she needed to during the working day to relieve her anxiety. With practice, progressive relaxation techniques and mental imagery could also provide relief from anxiety attacks for Linda. Any of these relaxation techniques may be beneficial at bedtime to help induce relaxation and sleep. Biofeedback may provide assistance for relief from migraine headaches. Physical exercise, either in the early morning or late afternoon after work, may provide Linda with renewed energy and combat chronic fatigue. It also relieves pent-up tension.

CHAPTER 13

Assertiveness Training

1. a. AS
   b. PA
   c. NA
   d. AG
2. a. AG
   b. NA
   c. PA
   d. AS
3. a. NA
   b. AS
   c. PA
   d. AG
4. a. PA
   b. AG
   c. AS
   d. NA
5. a. AS
   b. NA
   c. PA
   d. AG
6. a. NA
   b. AS
   c. AG
   d. PA
7. a. AS
   b. PA
   c. AG
   d. NA
8. a. PA
   b. NA
   c. AG
   d. AS
9. a. AG
   b. NA
   c. AS
   d. PA
10. a. AS
    b. NA
    c. AG
    d. PA

CHAPTER 14

Promoting Self-Esteem

1. b
2. a

3. d
4. c
5. a
6. b
7. c
8. e
9. d
10. a

CHAPTER 15

Anger/Aggression Management

1. Past history of violence; diagnosis of alcohol abuse/intoxication; current behaviors: abusive and threatening.
2. b
3. c
4. c
5. a
6. Observe at least every 15 minutes; check circulation (temperature, color, pulses); assist with needs related to nutrition, hydration, and elimination; position for comfort and to prevent aspiration.
7. c
8. a, b, c
9. c
10. b

CHAPTER 16

The Suicidal Client

1. b
2. a
3. c
4. a
5. d
6. c
7. c
8. b
9. d
10. b

CHAPTER 17

Behavior Therapy

1. a
2. a
3. b
4. c
5. a
6. b
7. d

8. f, b, d, a, e, c

CHAPTER 18

Cognitive Therapy

1. b
2. d
3. a
4. c
5. c
6. a
7. d
8. a
9. b
10. c

CHAPTER 19

Psychopharmacology

1. a
2. c
3. d
4. b
5. c
6. b
7. a
8. b
9. c
10. c

CHAPTER 20

Electroconvulsive Therapy

1. c.
2. b
3. a
4. c
5. d
6. a
7. c
8. d
9. b
10. c

CHAPTER 21

Complementary Therapies

1. c
2. e
3. f

4. b
5. g
6. a
7. d
8. c
9. d
10. a

CHAPTER 22

Disorders of Infancy/Childhood/Adolescence

1. b
2. c
3. a
4. b
5. d
6. b
7. c
8. d
9. a
10. b

CHAPTER 23

Delirium, Dementia, and Amnestic Disorders

1. c
2. d
3. b
4. a
5. b
6. c
7. d
8. a
9. b
10. d

CHAPTER 24

Substance-Related Disorders

1. a
2. c
3. b
4. b
5. a
6. c
7. a
8. b
9. d
10. a

CHAPTER 25

Schizophrenia and Other Psychotic Disorders

1. b
2. b
3. c
4. d
5. d
6. a
7. c
8. b
9. c
10. d

CHAPTER 26

Mood Disorders

1. c
2. b
3. a
4. d
5. c
6. b
7. c
8. a
9. c
10. b

CHAPTER 27

Anxiety Disorders

1. d
2. c
3. d
4. a
5. b
6. c
7. b
8. c
9. a
10. d

CHAPTER 28

Somatoform and Sleep Disorders

1. b
2. d
3. a
4. d
5. c
6. a

7. b
8. d
9. b
10. c

CHAPTER 29

Dissociative Disorders

1. d
2. b
3. a
4. b
5. d
6. c
7. a
8. c
9. a
10. b

CHAPTER 30

Sexual and Gender Identity Disorders

1. b
2. c
3. d
4. a
5. b
6. b
7. d
8. a
9. e
10. c

CHAPTER 31

Eating Disorders

1. c
2. a
3. b
4. b
5. c
6. b
7. c
8. b
9. c
10. a

CHAPTER 32

Adjustment and Impulse Control Disorders

1. c

2. b
3. a
4. c
5. d
6. b
7. c
8. c
9. a
10. d

CHAPTER 33

Psychological Factors Affecting Medical Condition

1. c
2. g
3. a
4. e
5. h
6. f
7. d
8. b
9. b

CHAPTER 34

Personality Disorders

1. d
2. a
3. b
4. d
5. a
6. b
7. c
8. c
9. d
10. b

CHAPTER 35

The Aging Individual

1. c
2. d
3. b
4. a
5. c
6. d
7. a
8. a
9. c
10. a

CHAPTER 36

The Individual with HIV Disease

1. d
2. c
3. a
4. c
5. b
6. d
7. a
8. a
9. b
10. b

CHAPTER 37

Problems Related to Abuse or Neglect

1. b
2. c
3. a
4. d
5. b
6. d
7. a
8. b
9. b
10. d

CHAPTER 38

Community Mental Health Nursing

1. a
2. b
3. a
4. c
5. d
6. b
7. c
8. d
9. a
10. b

CHAPTER 39

Cultural Concepts Relevant to Psychiatric/Mental Health Nursing

1. c
2. d
3. a
4. d
5. b

6. c
7. c
8. b
9. b
10. a

CHAPTER 40

Ethical and Legal Issues in Psychiatric/Mental Health Nursing

1. c
2. a
3. e
4. d
5. b
6. d
7. b
8. e
9. a
10. c

CHAPTER 41

Psychiatric Home Nursing Care

1. b
2. d
3. a
4. b
5. c
6. d
7. a
8. c
9. b
10. a

CHAPTER 42

Forensic Nursing

1. a
2. a
3. b
4. b
5. b
6. a
7. b
8. a
9. a
10. b

Mental Status Assessment

Gathering the correct information about the client's mental status is essential to the development of an appropriate plan of care. The mental status examination is a description of all the areas of the client's mental functioning (Scheiber, 1994). The following are the components that are considered critical in the assessment of a client's mental status.

Identifying Data

1. Name.
2. Sex.
3. Age.
4. Race/culture.
5. Occupational/financial status.
6. Educational level.
7. Significant other.
8. Living arrangements.
9. Religious preference.
10. Allergies.
11. Special diet considerations.
12. Chief complaint.
13. Medical diagnosis.

General Description

Appearance

1. Grooming and dress.
2. Hygiene.
3. Posture.
4. Height and weight.
5. Level of eye contact.
6. Hair color and texture.
7. Evidence of scars, tattoos, or other distinguishing skin marks.
8. Evaluation of client's appearance compared with chronological age.

Motor Activity

1. Tremors.
2. Tics or other stereotypical movements.
3. Mannerisms and gestures.
4. Hyperactivity.
5. Restlessness or agitation.
6. Aggressiveness.
7. Rigidity.
8. Gait patterns.
9. Echopraxia.
10. Psychomotor retardation.
11. Freedom of movement (range of motion).

Speech Patterns

1. Slowness or rapidity of speech.
2. Pressure of speech.
3. Intonation.
4. Volume.
5. Stuttering or other speech impairments.
6. Aphasia.

General Attitude

1. Cooperative/uncooperative.
2. Friendly/hostile/defensive.
3. Uninterested/apathetic.
4. Attentive/interested.
5. Guarded/suspicious.

Emotions

Mood

1. Sad
2. Depressed
3. Despairing
4. Irritable
5. Anxious
6. Elated
7. Euphoric
8. Fearful
9. Guilty
10. Labile

Affect

1. Congruence with mood.
2. Constricted or blunted (diminished amount/range and intensity of emotional expression).
3. Flat (absence of emotional expression).
4. Appropriate or inappropriate (defines congruence of affect with the situation or with the client's behavior).

Thought Processes

Form of Thought

1. Flight of ideas.
2. Associative looseness.
3. Circumstantiality.
4. Tangentiality.
5. Neologisms.
6. Concrete thinking.
7. Clang associations.
8. Word salad.
9. Perseveration.
10. Echolalia.
11. Mutism.
12. Poverty of speech (restriction in the amount of speech).
13. Ability to concentrate.
14. Attention span.

Content of Thought

1. Delusions.
   a. Persecutory
   b. Grandiose
   c. Reference
   d. Control or influence
   e. Somatic
   f. Nihilistic
2. Suicidal or homicidal ideas.
3. Obsessions.
4. Paranoia/suspiciousness.
5. Magical thinking.
6. Religiosity.
7. Phobias.
8. Poverty of content (vague, meaningless responses).

Perceptual Disturbances

1. Hallucinations.
   a. Auditory
   b. Visual
   c. Tactile
   d. Olfactory
   e. Gustatory
2. Illusions.

3. Depersonalization (altered perception of the self).
4. Derealization (altered perception of the environment).

Sensorium and Cognitive Ability

1. Level of alertness/consciousness.
2. Orientation.
   a. Time
   b. Place
   c. Person
   d. Circumstances
3. Memory.
   a. Recent
   b. Remote
   c. Confabulation
4. Capacity for abstract thought.

Impulse Control

1. Ability to control impulses related to:
   a. Aggression
   b. Hostility
   c. Fear
   d. Guilt
   e. Affection
   f. Sexual feelings

Judgment and Insight

1. Ability to solve problems.
2. Ability to make decisions.
3. Knowledge about self.
   a. Awareness of limitations.
   b. Awareness of consequences of actions.
   c. Awareness of illness.
4. Adaptive/maladaptive use of coping strategies and ego defense mechanisms.

REFERENCES

Schieber, S.C. (1994). The psychiatric interview, psychiatric history, and mental status examination. In R.E. Hales, S.C. Yudofsky, & J.A. Talbott (Eds.), *Textbook of psychiatry* (2nd ed.). Washington, DC: American Psychiatric Press.

Bibliography

Farley-Toombs, C., & Hamilton, D.B. (1996). Psychiatric nursing: Content review and tests. In P.G. Beare (Ed.), *Davis's NCLEX-RN review* (2nd ed.). Philadelphia: F.A. Davis.

Kaplan, H.I., Sadock, B.J., & Grebb, J.A. (1994). *Kaplan and Sadock's synopsis of psychiatry* (7th ed.). Baltimore: Williams & Wilkins.

Reynolds, J.I., & Logsdon, J.B. (1979). Assessing your patient's mental status. *Nursing 79, 9*(8), 26–33.

DSM-IV
Classification

◼ AXES I AND II CATEGORIES AND CODES

DISORDERS USUALLY FIRST DIAGNOSED IN INFANCY, CHILDHOOD, OR ADOLESCENCE

Mental Retardation

317	Mild Mental Retardation
318.0	Moderate Retardation
318.1	Severe Retardation
318.2	Profound Mental Retardation
319	Mental Retardation, Severity Unspecified

Learning Disorders

315.00	Reading Disorder
315.1	Mathematics Disorder
315.2	Disorder of Written Expression
315.9	Learning Disorder Not Otherwise Specified (NOS)

Motor Skills Disorder

315.4	Developmental Coordination Disorder

Communication Disorders

315.31	Expressive Language Disorder
315.31	Mixed Receptive/Expressive Language Disorder
315.39	Phonological Disorder
307.0	Stuttering
315.39	Communication Disorder NOS

Pervasive Developmental Disorders

299.00	Autistic Disorder
299.80	Rett's Disorder
299.10	Childhood Disintegrative Disorder
299.80	Asperger's Disorder
299.80	Pervasive Developmental Disorder NOS

Attention-Deficit and Disruptive Behavior Disorders

314.xx	Attention-Deficit/Hyperactivity Disorder
314.01	Combined type
314.00	Predominantly inattentive type
314.01	Predominantly hyperactive-impulsive type
314.9	Attention-Deficit/Hyperactivity Disorder NOS
312.8	Conduct Disorder
	Specify Childhood- or Adolescent-Onset Type
313.81	Oppositional Defiant Disorder
312.9	Disruptive Behavior Disorder NOS

Feeding and Eating Disorders of Infancy or Early Childhood

307.52	Pica
307.53	Rumination Disorder
307.59	Feeding Disorder of Infancy or Early Childhood

Tic Disorders

307.23	Tourette's Disorder
307.22	Chronic Motor or Vocal Tic Disorder
307.21	Transient Tic Disorder
307.20	Tic Disorder NOS

Elimination Disorders

	Encopresis
787.6	With constipation and overflow incontinence
307.7	Without constipation and overflow incontinence
307.6	Enuresis (Not Due to a General Medical Condition)

Other Disorders of Infancy, Childhood, or Adolescence

309.21	Separation Anxiety Disorder
313.23	Selective Mutism
313.89	Reactive Attachment Disorder of Infancy or Early Childhood
307.3	Stereotypic Movement Disorder
313.9	Disorder of Infancy, Childhood, or Adolescence NOS

DELIRIUM, DEMENTIA, AMNESTIC, AND OTHER COGNITIVE DISORDERS

Delirium

293.0	Delirium Due to (indicate the general medical condition)
—	Substance Intoxication Delirium (refer to Substance Related Disorders for substance-specific codes)
—	Substance Withdrawal Delirium (refer to Substance Related Disorders for substance-specific codes)
—	Delirium Due to Multiple Etiologies (code each of the specific etiologies)
780.09	Delirium NOS

Dementia

290.xx	Dementia of the Alzheimer's Type With Early Onset: if onset at age 65 or below
290.10	Uncomplicated
290.11	With delirium
290.12	With delusions
290.13	With depressed mood
290.xx	Dementia of the Alzheimer's Type With Late Onset: if onset after age 65
290.00	Uncomplicated
290.3	With delirium

Continued on following page

AXES I AND II CATEGORIES AND CODES *(Continued)*

DELIRIUM, DEMENTIA, AMNESTIC, AND OTHER COGNITIVE DISORDERS *(continued)*

Dementia *(continued)*

290.20	With delusions
290.21	With depressed mood
290.xx	Vascular Dementia
290.40	Uncomplicated
290.41	With delirium
290.42	With delusions
290.43	With depressed mood
294.9	Dementia Due to Human Immunodeficiency Virus (HIV) Disease
294.1	Dementia Due to Head Trauma
294.1	Dementia Due to Parkinson's Disease
294.1	Dementia Due to Huntington's Disease
290.10	Dementia Due to Pick's Disease
290.10	Dementia Due to Creutzfeldt-Jakob Disease
294.1	Dementia Due to (indicate the general medical condition not listed above)

—	Substance-Induced Persisting Dementia (refer to Substance Related Disorders for substance-specified codes)
—	Dementia Due to Multiple Etiologies (code each of the specific etiologies)
294.8	Dementia NOS

Amnestic Disorders

294.0	Amnestic Disorder Due to (indicate the general medical condition)
—	Substance-induced Persisting Amnestic Disorder (refer to specific substance for code)
294.8	Amnestic Disorder NOS

Other Cognitive Disorders

294.9	Cognitive Disorder NOS

MENTAL DISORDERS DUE TO A GENERAL MEDICAL CONDITION NOT ELSEWHERE CLASSIFIED

293.89	Catatonic Disorder Due to (indicate the general medical condition)
310.1	Personality Change Due to (indicate the general medical condition)

293.9	Mental Disorder NOS Due to (indicate the general medical condition)

SUBSTANCE-RELATED DISORDERS

Alcohol-Related Disorders

Alcohol Use Disorders

303.90	Alcohol Dependence
305.00	Alcohol Abuse

Alcohol-Induced Disorders

303.00	Alcohol Intoxication
291.8	Alcohol Withdrawal
291.0	Alcohol Intoxication Delirium
291.0	Alcohol Withdrawal Delirium
291.2	Alcohol-Induced Persisting Dementia
291.1	Alcohol-Induced Persisting Amnestic Disorder
291.x	Alcohol-Induced Psychotic Disorder
291.5	With Delusions
291.3	With Hallucinations
291.8	Alcohol-Induced Mood Disorder
291.8	Alcohol-Induced Anxiety Disorder
292.8	Alcohol-Induced Sexual Dysfunction
292.89	Alcohol-Induced Sleep Disorder
291.9	Alcohol-Related Disorder NOS

Amphetamine (or Amphetamine-Like) Related Disorders

Amphetamine Use Disorders

304.40	Amphetamine Dependence
305.70	Amphetamine Abuse

Amphetamine-Induced Disorders

292.89	Amphetamine Intoxication
292.0	Amphetamine Withdrawal
292.81	Amphetamine Intoxication Delirium
292.xx	Amphetamine-Induced Psychotic Disorder
292.11	With Delusions
292.12	With Hallucinations
292.84	Amphetamine-Induced Mood Disorder
292.89	Amphetamine-Induced Anxiety Disorder
292.89	Amphetamine-Induced Sexual Dysfunction

292.89	Amphetamine-Induced Sleep Disorder
292.9	Amphetamine-Related Disorder NOS

Caffeine-Related Disorder

Caffeine-Induced Disorders

305.90	Caffeine Intoxication
292.89	Caffeine-Induced Anxiety Disorder
292.89	Caffeine-Induced Sleep Disorder
292.9	Caffeine-Related Disorder NOS

Cannabis-Related Disorders

Cannabis Use Disorders

304.30	Cannabis Dependence
305.20	Cannabis Abuse

Cannabis-Induced Disorders

292.89	Cannabis Intoxication
292.81	Cannabis Intoxication Delirium
292.xx	Cannabis-Induced Psychotic Disorder
292.11	With Delusions
292.12	With Hallucinations
292.89	Cannabis-Induced Anxiety Disorder
292.9	Cannabis-Related Disorder NOS

Cocaine-Related Disorders

Cocaine Use Disorders

304.20	Cocaine Dependence
305.60	Cocaine Abuse

Cocaine-Induced Disorders

292.89	Cocaine Intoxication
292.0	Cocaine Withdrawal
292.81	Cocaine Intoxication Delirium
292.xx	Cocaine-Induced Psychotic Disorder
292.11	With Delusions
292.12	With Hallucinations
292.84	Cocaine-Induced Mood Disorder
292.89	Cocaine-Induced Anxiety Disorder

SUBSTANCE-RELATED DISORDERS (*continued*)

292.89	Cocaine-Induced Sexual Dysfunction
292.89	Cocaine-Induced Sleep Disorder
292.9	Cocaine-Related Disorder NOS

Hallucinogen-Related Disorders

Hallucinogen Use Disorders

304.50	Hallucinogen Dependence
305.30	Hallucinogen Abuse

Hallucinogen-Induced Disorders

292.89	Hallucinogen Intoxication
292.89	Hallucinogen Persisting Perception Disorder (Flashbacks)
292.81	Hallucinogen Intoxication Delirium
292.xx	Hallucinogen-Induced Psychotic Disorder
292.11	With Delusions
292.12	With Hallucinations
292.84	Hallucinogen-Induced Mood Disorder
292.89	Hallucinogen-Induced Anxiety Disorder
292.9	Hallucinogen-Related Disorder NOS

Inhalant-Related Disorders

Inhalant Use Disorders

304.60	Inhalant Dependence
305.90	Inhalant Abuse

Inhalant-Induced Disorders

292.89	Inhalant Intoxication
292.81	Inhalant Intoxication Delirium
292.82	Inhalant-Induced Persisting Dementia
292.xx	Inhalant-Induced Psychotic Disorder
292.11	With Delusions
292.12	With Hallucinations
292.84	Inhalant-Induced Mood Disorder
292.89	Inhalant-Induced Anxiety Disorder
292.9	Inhalant-Related Disorder NOS

Nicotine-Related Disorders

Nicotine Use Disorders

305.10	Nicotine Dependence

Nicotine-Induced Disorders

292.0	Nicotine Withdrawal
292.9	Nicotine-Related Disorder NOS

Opioid-Related Disorders

Opioid Use Disorders

304.00	Opioid Dependence
305.50	Opioid Abuse

Opioid-Induced Disorders

292.89	Opioid Intoxication
292.0	Opioid Withdrawal
292.81	Opioid Intoxication Delirium
292.xx	Opioid-Induced Psychotic Disorder
292.11	With Delusions
292.12	With Hallucinations
292.84	Opioid-Induced Mood Disorder
292.89	Opioid-Induced Sexual Dysfunction
292.89	Opioid-Induced Sleep Disorder
292.9	Opioid-Related Disorder NOS

Phencyclidine (or Phencyclidine-like)–Related Disorders

Phencyclidine Use Disorders

304.90	Phencyclidine Dependence
305.90	Phencyclidine Abuse

Phencyclidine-Induced Disorders

292.89	Phencyclidine Intoxication
292.81	Phencyclidine Intoxication Delirium
292.xx	Phencyclidine-Induced Psychotic Disorder
292.11	With Delusions
292.12	With Hallucinations
292.84	Phencyclidine-Induced Mood Disorder
292.89	Phencyclidine-Induced Anxiety Disorder
292.9	Phencyclidine-Related Disorder NOS

Sedative-, Hypnotic-, or Anxiolytic-Related Disorders

Sedative, Hypnotic, or Anxiolytic Substance Use Disorders

304.10	Sedative, Hypnotic, or Anxiolytic Dependence
305.40	Sedative, Hypnotic, or Anxiolytic Abuse

Sedative-, Hypnotic-, or Anxiolytic-Induced Disorders

292.89	Sedative, Hypnotic, or Anxiolytic Intoxication
292.0	Sedative, Hypnotic, or Anxiolytic Withdrawal
292.81	Sedative, Hypnotic, or Anxiolytic Intoxication Delirium
292.81	Sedative, Hypnotic, or Anxiolytic Withdrawal Delirium
292.82	Sedative-, Hypnotic-, or Anxiolytic-Induced Persisting Dementia
292.83	Sedative-, Hypnotic-, or Anxiolytic-Induced Persisting Amnestic Disorder
292.xx	Sedative-, Hypnotic-, or Anxiolytic-Induced Psychotic Disorder
292.11	With Delusions
292.12	With Hallucinations
292.84	Sedative-, Hypnotic-, or Anxiolytic-Induced Mood Disorder
292.89	Sedative-, Hypnotic-, or Anxiolytic-Induced Anxiety Disorder
292.89	Sedative-, Hypnotic-, or Anxiolytic-Induced Sexual Dysfunction
292.89	Sedative-, Hypnotic-, or Anxiolytic-Induced Sleep Disorder
292.9	Sedative-, Hypnotic-, or Anxiolytic-Related Disorder NOS

Polysubstance-Related Disorder

304.80	Polysubstance Dependence

Other (or Unknown) Substance Use Disorders

304.90	Other (or Unknown) Substance Dependence
305.90	Other (or Unknown) Substance Abuse

Other (or Unknown) Substance-Induced Disorders

292.89	Other (or Unknown) Substance Intoxication
292.0	Other (or Unknown) Substance Withdrawal
292.81	Other (or Unknown) Substance-Induced Delirium
292.82	Other (or Unknown) Substance-Induced Persisting Dementia
292.83	Other (or Unknown) Substance-Induced Persisting Amnestic Disorder
292.xx	Other (or Unknown) Substance-Induced Psychotic Disorder
292.11	With Delusions
292.12	With Hallucinations
292.84	Other (or Unknown) Substance-Induced Mood Disorder
292.89	Other (or Unknown) Substance-Induced Anxiety Disorder
292.89	Other (or Unknown) Substance-Induced Sexual Dysfunction

Continued on following page

■ AXES I AND II CATEGORIES AND CODES (*Continued*)

SUBSTANCE-RELATED DISORDERS (*continued*)

Other (or Unknown) Substance-Induced Disorders (*Continued*)

292.89	Other (or Unknown) Substance-Induced Sleep Disorder	292.9	Other (or Unknown) Substance-Induced Disorder NOS

SCHIZOPHRENIA AND OTHER PSYCHOTIC DISORDERS

295.xx	Schizophrenia	297.3	Shared Psychotic Disorder (Folie à Deux)
295.30	Paranoid type	293.xx	Psychotic Disorder Due to a General Medical Condition
295.10	Disorganized type		
295.20	Catatonic type	293.81	With Delusions
295.90	Undifferentiated type	293.82	With Hallucinations
295.60	Residual type	—	Substance-Induced Psychotic Disorder (refer to Substance-Related Disorders for substance-specific codes)
295.40	Schizophreniform Disorder		
295.70	Schizoaffective Disorder		
297.1	Delusional Disorder		
298.8	Brief Psychotic Disorder	298.9	Psychotic Disorder NOS

MOOD DISORDERS

(Code current state of Major Depressive Disorder or Bipolar Disorder in Fifth digit: 0 = unspecified; 1 = mild; 2 = moderate; 3 = severe, without psychotic features; 4 = severe, with psychotic features; 5 = in partial remission; 6 = in full remission.)

Depressive Disorders

296.xx	Major Depressive Disorder	296.5x	most recent episode depressed
296.2x	Single episode	296.7	most recent episode unspecified
296.3x	Recurrent	296.89	Bipolar II Disorder (Specify current or most recent episode: Hypomanic or Depressed)
300.4	Dysthymic Disorder		
311	Depressive Disorder NOS	301.13	Cyclothymic Disorder
		296.80	Bipolar Disorder NOS

Bipolar Disorders

		293.83	Mood Disorder Due to (indicate the general medical condition)
296.xx	Bipolar I Disorder		
296.0x	single manic episode	—	Substance-Induced Mood Disorder (refer to Substance-Related Disorders for substance-specific codes)
296.40	most recent episode hypomanic		
296.4x	most recent episode manic		
296.6x	most recent episode mixed	296.90	Mood Disorder NOS

ANXIETY DISORDERS

300.01	Panic Disorder Without Agoraphobia	300.02	Generalized Anxiety Disorder
300.21	Panic Disorder with Agoraphobia	293.89	Anxiety Disorder Due to (indicate the general medical condition)
300.22	Agoraphobia Without History of Panic Disorder		
300.29	Specific Phobia	—	Substance-Induced Anxiety Disorder (refer to Substance-Related Disorders for substance-specific codes)
300.23	Social Phobia		
300.3	Obsessive-Compulsive Disorder		
309.81	Posttraumatic Stress Disorder	300.00	Anxiety Disorder NOS
308.3	Acute Stress Disorder		

SOMATOFORM DISORDERS

300.81	Somatization Disorder	307.89	Associated with Both Psychological Factors and a General Medical Condition
300.11	Conversion Disorder		
300.7	Hypochondriasis	300.82	Undifferentiated Somatoform Disorder
300.71	Body Dysmorphic Disorder Pain Disorder	300.89	Somatoform Disorder NOS
307.80	Associated with Psychological Factors		

FACTITIOUS DISORDERS

300.xx	Factitious Disorder	300.19	With combined psychological and physical signs and symptoms
300.16	With predominantly psychological signs and symptoms		
300.19	With predominantly physical signs and symptoms	300.19	Factitious Disorder NOS

DISSOCIATIVE DISORDERS

300.12	Dissociative Amnesia	300.6	Depersonalization Disorder
300.13	Dissociative Fugue	300.15	Dissociative Disorder NOS
300.14	Dissociative Identity Disorder		

SEXUAL AND GENDER IDENTITY DISORDERS

Sexual Dysfunctions

Sexual Desire Disorders
302.71 Hypoactive Sexual Desire Disorder
302.79 Sexual Aversion Disorder

Sexual Arousal Disorders
302.72 Female Sexual Arousal Disorder
302.72 Male Erectile Disorder

Orgasmic Disorders
302.73 Female Orgasmic Disorder
302.74 Male Orgasmic Disorder
302.75 Premature Ejaculation

Sexual Pain Disorders
302.76 Dyspareunia (Not Due to a General Medical Condition)
306.51 Vaginismus (Not Due to a General Medical Condition)

Sexual Dysfunctions Due to a General Medical Condition
625.8 Female Hypoactive Sexual Desire Disorder Due to (indicate the general medical condition)
608.89 Male Hypoactive Sexual Desire Disorder Due to (indicate the general medical condition)
607.84 Male Erectile Disorder Due to (indicate the general medical condition)
625.0 Female Dyspareunia Due to (indicate the general medical condition)

608.89 Male Dyspareunia Due to (indicate the general medical condition)
625.8 Other Female Sexual Dysfunction Due to (indicate the general medical condition)
608.89 Other Male Sexual Dysfunction Due to (indicate the general medical condition)
— Substance-Induced Sexual Dysfunction (refer to Substance-Related Disorders for substance-specific codes)
302.70 Sexual Dysfunction NOS

Paraphilias
302.4 Exhibitionism
302.81 Fetishism
302.89 Frotteurism
302.2 Pedophilia
302.83 Sexual Masochism
302.84 Sexual Sadism
302.3 Transvestic Fetishism
302.82 Voyeurism
302.9 Paraphilia NOS

Gender Identity Disorders
302.xx Gender Identity Disorder
302.6   In Children
302.85   In Adolescents or Adults
302.6 Gender Identity Disorder NOS
302.9 Sexual Disorder NOS

EATING DISORDERS

307.1 Anorexia Nervosa
307.51 Bulimia Nervosa

307.50 Eating Disorder NOS

SLEEP DISORDERS

Primary Sleep Disorders

Dyssomnias
307.42 Primary Insomnia
307.44 Primary Hypersomnia
347 Narcolepsy
780.59 Breathing-Related Sleep Disorder
307.45 Circadian Rhythm Sleep Disorder
307.47 Dyssomnia NOS

Parasomnias
307.47 Nightmare Disorder
307.46 Sleep Terror Disorder
307.46 Sleepwalking Disorder
307.47 Parasomnia NOS

Sleep Disorders Related to Another Mental Disorder
307.42 Insomnia Related to (indicate the Axis-I or Axis-II disorder)
307.44 Hypersomnia Related to (indicate the Axis-I or Axis-II disorder)

Other Sleep Disorders
780.xx Sleep Disorder due to (indicate the general medical condition)
780.52 Insomnia type
780.54 Hypersomnia type
780.59 Parasomnia type
780.59 Mixed type
— Substance-Induced Sleep Disorder (refer to Substance-Related Disorders for substance-specific codes)

IMPULSE CONTROL DISORDERS NOT ELSEWHERE CLASSIFIED

312.34 Intermittent Explosive Disorder
312.32 Kleptomania
312.33 Pyromania

312.31 Pathological Gambling
312.39 Trichotillomania
312.30 Impulse Control Disorder NOS

ADJUSTMENT DISORDERS

309.xx Adjustment Disorder
309.0   With Depressed Mood
309.24   With Anxiety
309.28   With Mixed Anxiety and Depressed Mood

309.3   With Disturbance of Conduct
309.4   With Mixed Disturbance of Emotions and Conduct
309.9   Unspecified

Continued on following page

AXES I AND II CATEGORIES AND CODES *(Continued)*

PERSONALITY DISORDERS

Note: These are coded on Axis II.

301.0	Paranoid Personality Disorder
301.20	Schizoid Personality Disorder
301.22	Schizotypal Personality Disorder
301.7	Antisocial Personality Disorder
301.83	Borderline Personality Disorder

301.50	Histrionic Personality Disorder
301.81	Narcissistic Personality Disorder
301.82	Avoidant Personality Disorder
301.6	Dependent Personality Disorder
301.4	Obsessive-Compulsive Personality Disorder
301.9	Personality Disorder NOS

OTHER CONDITIONS THAT MAY BE A FOCUS OF CLINICAL ATTENTION

(Psychological Factors) Affecting Medical Condition

316   *Choose name based on nature of factors:*
- Mental Disorder Affecting Medical Condition
- Psychological Symptoms Affecting Medical Condition
- Personality Traits or Coping Style Affecting Medical Condition
- Maladaptive Health Behaviors Affecting Medical Condition
- Stress-Related Physiological Response Affecting Medical Condition
- Other or Unspecified Psychological Factors Affecting Medical Condition

Medication-Induced Movement Disorders

332.1	Neuroleptic-Induced Parkinsonism
333.92	Neuroleptic Malignant Syndrome
333.7	Neuroleptic-Induced Acute Dystonia
333.99	Neuroleptic-Induced Acute Akathisia
333.82	Neuroleptic-Induced Tardive Dyskinesia
333.1	Medication-Induced Postural Tremor
333.90	Medication-Induced Movement Disorder NOS

Other Medication-Induced Disorder

995.2	Adverse Effects of Medication NOS

Relational Problems

V61.9	Relational Problem Related to a Mental Disorder or General Medical Condition

V61.20	Parent-Child Relational Problem
V61.1	Partner Relational Problem
V61.8	Sibling Relational Problem
V62.81	Relational Problem NOS

Problems Related to Abuse or Neglect

V61.21	Physical Abuse of Child
V61.21	Sexual Abuse of Child
V61.21	Neglect of Child
V61.1	Physical Abuse of Adult
V51.1	Sexual Abuse of Adult

Additional Conditions That May Be a Focus of Clinical Attention

V15.81	Noncompliance with Treatment
V65.2	Malingering
V71.01	Adult Antisocial Behavior
V71.02	Childhood or Adolescent Antisocial Behavior
V62.89	Borderline Intellectual Functioning (coded on Axis II)
780.9	Age-Related Cognitive Decline
V62.82	Bereavement
V62.3	Academic Problem
V62.2	Occupational Problem
313.82	Identity Problem
V62.61	Religious or Spiritual Problem
V62.4	Acculturation Problem
V62.89	Phase of Life Problem

ADDITIONAL CODES

300.9	Unspecified Mental Disorder (nonpsychotic)
V71.09	No Diagnosis or Condition on Axis I
799.9	Diagnosis or Condition Deferred on Axis I

V71.09	No Diagnosis on Axis II
799.9	Diagnosis Deferred on Axis II

DSM-IV CRITERIA SETS AND AXES PROVIDED FOR FURTHER STUDY

Text and criteria for these disorders will be provided to facilitate systematic clinical research:
- Postconcussional disorder
- Mild neurocognitive disorder
- Caffeine withdrawal
- Alternative dimensional descriptors for schizophrenia
- Postpsychotic depression of schizophrenia
- Simple schizophrenia
- Minor depressive disorder
- Alternative criteria B for dysthymic disorder
- Recurrent brief depressive disorder
- Premenstrual dysphoric disorder
- Mixed anxiety-depressive disorder
- Factitious disorder by proxy
- Dissociative trance disorder
- Binge eating disorder
- Depressive personality disorder
- Passive aggressive personality disorder (negativistic personality disorder)
- Medication-induced movement disorders
- Defensive Functioning Scale
- Global Assessment of Relational Functioning (GARF) Scale
- Social and Occupational Functioning Assessment Scale (SOFAS)

SOURCE: Adapted from APA (1994), pp 13–24, with permission.

Nursing Diagnoses Approved by NANDA (for Use and Testing)

Activity intolerance
Activity intolerance, risk for
Adaptive capacity, intracranial, decreased
Adjustment, impaired
Airway clearance, ineffective
Anxiety (specify level)
Anxiety, death
Aspiration, risk for

Body image disturbance
Body temperature, altered, risk for
Breastfeeding, effective
Breastfeeding, ineffective
Breastfeeding, interrupted
Breathing pattern, ineffective

Cardiac output, decreased
Caregiver role strain
Caregiver role strain, risk for
Communication, verbal, impaired
Confusion, acute
Confusion, chronic
Constipation
Constipation, colonic
Constipation, perceived
Constipation, risk of
Coping, defensive
Coping, community, ineffective
Coping, community, potential for enhanced
Coping, family, ineffective
Coping, family, compromised
Coping, family, disabling
Coping, family, potential for growth
Coping, individual, ineffective

Decisional conflict (specify)
Denial, ineffective
Dentition, altered
Development, risk for altered
Diarrhea
Disuse syndrome, risk for
Diversional activity deficit
Dysreflexia
Dysreflexia, risk for autonomic

Elimination, urinary, altered
Energy field, disturbance
Environmental interpretation syndrome, impaired

Failure to thrive, adult
Family processes, altered
Family processes, altered, alcoholism

Fatigue
Fear
Fluid volume deficit
Fluid volume deficit, risk for
Fluid volume excess
Fluid volume imbalance, risk for

Gas exchange, impaired
Grieving, anticipatory
Grieving, dysfunctional
Growth, risk for altered
Growth and development, altered

Health maintenance, altered
Health-seeking behaviors (specify)
Home maintenance management, impaired
Hopelessness
Hyperthermia
Hypothermia

Incontinence, bowel
Incontinence, urinary, functional
Incontinence, urinary, reflex
Incontinence, urinary, stress
Incontinence, urinary, total
Incontinence, urinary, urge
Infant behavior, disorganized
Infant behavior, disorganized, risk for
Infant behavior, organized, potential for enhancement
Infant feeding pattern, ineffective
Infection, risk for
Injury, risk for
Injury, risk for, perioperative positioning

Knowledge deficit (specify)

Latex allergy response
Latex allergy response, risk for
Loneliness, risk for

Management of therapeutic regimen, community, ineffective
Management of therapeutic regimen, families, ineffective
Management of therapeutic regimen, individual, ineffective
Memory, impaired
Mobility, bed, impaired
Mobility, physical, impaired
Mobility, wheelchair, impaired

Nausea
Noncompliance (specify)
Nutrition, altered: less than body requirements

Nutrition, altered: more than body requirements
Nutrition, altered: risk for more than body requirements

Oral mucous membrane, altered

Pain
Pain, chronic
Parent/infant, child attachment, altered, risk for
Parental role conflict
Parenting, altered
Parenting, altered, risk for
Peripheral neurovascular dysfunction, risk for
Personal identity disturbance
Poisoning, risk for
Post-trauma syndrome
Post-trauma syndrome, risk for
Powerlessness
Protection, altered

Rape-trauma syndrome
Rape-trauma syndrome: compound reaction
Rape-trauma syndrome: silent reaction
Relocation stress syndrome
Retention, urinary
Role conflict, parental
Role performance, altered

Self-care deficit (specify): feeding, bathing/hygiene, dressing/ grooming, toileting
Self-esteem, chronic low
Self-esteem disturbance
Self-esteem, situational low
Self-mutilation, risk for
Sensory/perceptual alteration (specify): visual, auditory, kines- thetic, gustatory, tactile, olfactory

Sexual dysfunction
Sexuality patterns, altered
Skin integrity, impaired
Skin integrity, impaired, risk for
Sleep deprivation
Sleep pattern disturbance
Social interaction, impaired
Social isolation
Sorrow, chronic
Spiritual distress
Spiritual distress, risk for
Spiritual well-being, potential for enhancement
Suffocation, risk for
Surgical recovery, delayed
Swallowing, impaired

Thermoregulation, ineffective
Thought processes, altered
Tissue integrity, impaired
Tissue perfusion, altered (specify): cerebral, cardiopulmonary, gastrointestinal, peripheral, renal
Transfer ability, impaired
Trauma, risk for

Unilateral neglect

Ventilation, inability to sustain spontaneous
Ventilatory weaning response, dysfunctional
Violence, risk for: directed at others
Violence, risk for: self-directed

Walking, impaired

SOURCE: Adapted from NANDA (1999).

Assigning Nursing Diagnoses to Client Behaviors

Following is a list of client behaviors and the NANDA nursing diagnoses which correspond to the behaviors and which may be used in planning care for the client exhibiting the specific behavorial symptoms.

BEHAVIORS	NANDA NURSING DIAGNOSES
Aggression; hostility	Risk for injury; risk for violence, directed at others
Anorexia or refusal to eat	Altered nutrition: less than body requirements
Anxious behavior	Anxiety (specify level)
Confusion; memory loss	Confusion, acute/chronic; altered thought processes
Delusions	Altered thought processes
Denial of problems	Ineffective denial
Depressed mood or anger turned inward	Dysfunctional grieving
Detoxification; withdrawal from substances	Risk for injury
Difficulty making important life decision	Decisional conflict (specify)
Difficulty with interpersonal relationships	Impaired social interaction
Disruption in capability to perform usual responsibilities	Altered role performance
Dissociative behaviors (depersonalization; derealization)	Sensory/perceptual alteration (kinesthetic)
Expresses feelings of disgust about body or body part	Body image disturbance
Expresses lack of control over personal situation	Powerlessness
Flashbacks, nightmares, obsession with traumatic experience	Posttrauma response
Hallucinations	Sensory/perceptual alteration (auditory; visual)
Highly critical of self or others	Self-esteem disturbance
HIV positive; altered immunity	Altered protection
Inability to meet basic needs	Self-care deficit (specify)
Insomnia or hypersomnia	Sleep pattern disturbance
Loose associations or flight of ideas	Impaired verbal communication
Manic hyperactivity	Risk for injury
Manipulative behavior	Ineffective individual coping
Multiple personalities; gender identity disturbance	Personal identity disturbance
Orgasm, problems with; lack of sexual desire	Sexual dysfunction
Overeating, compulsive	Altered nutrition: (risk for) more than body requirements
Phobias	Fear
Physical symptoms as coping behavior	Ineffective individual coping
Projection of blame; rationalization of failures; denial of personal responsibility	Defensive coping
Ritualistic behaviors	Anxiety (severe); ineffective individual coping
Seductive remarks; inappropriate sexual behaviors	Impaired social interaction

Continued on following page

(Continued)

BEHAVIORS	NANDA NURSING DIAGNOSES
Self-mutilative behaviors	Risk for self-mutilation
Sexual behaviors (difficulty, limitations, or changes in; reported dissatisfaction)	Altered sexuality patterns
Stress from caring for chronically ill person	Caregiver role strain
Stress from locating to new environment	Relocation stress syndrome
Substance use as a coping behavior	Ineffective individual coping
Substance use (denies use is a problem)	Ineffective denial
Suicidal	Risk for violence, directed at self
Suspiciousness	Altered thought processes; ineffective individual coping
Vomiting, excessive, self-induced	Risk for fluid volume deficit
Withdrawn behavior	Social isolation

Glossary

A

abandonment. A unilateral severance of the professional relationship between a health care provider and a client without reasonable notice at a time when there is still a need for continuing health care.

abreaction. "Remembering with feeling"; bringing into conscious awareness painful events that have been repressed, and reexperiencing the emotions that were associated with the events.

acquired immunodeficiency syndrome (AIDS). A condition in which the immune system becomes deficient in its efforts to prevent opportunistic infections, malignancies, and neurological disease. It is caused by the human immunodeficiency virus (HIV), which is passed from one individual to another through body fluids.

acupoints. In Chinese medicine, acupoints represent areas along the body that link pathways of healing energy.

acupressure. A technique in which the fingers, thumbs, palms, or elbows are used to apply pressure to certain points along the body. This pressure is thought to dissolve any obstructions in the flow of healing energy and to restore the body to a healthier functioning.

acupuncture. A technique in which hair-thin, sterile, disposable, stainless-steel needles are inserted into points along the body to dissolve obstructions in the flow of healing energy and restore the body to a healthier functioning.

adaptation. Restoration of the body to homeostasis following a physiological and/or psychological response to stress.

adjustment disorder. A maladaptive reaction to an identifiable psychosocial stressor that occurs within 3 months after onset of the stressor. The individual shows impairment in social and occupational functioning, or exhibits symptoms that are in excess of a normal and expectable reaction to the stressor.

affect. The behavioral expression of emotion; may be *appropriate* (congruent with the situation); *inappropriate* (incongruent with the situation); *constricted* or *blunted* (diminished range and intensity); or *flat* (absence of emotional expression).

aggression. Harsh physical or verbal actions intended (either consciously or unconsciously) to harm or injure another.

aggressiveness. Behavior that defends an individual's own basic rights by violating the basic rights of others (as contrasted with **assertiveness**).

agoraphobia. The fear of being in places or situations from which escape might be difficult (or embarrassing) or in which help might not be available in the event of a panic attack.

agranulocytosis. Extremely low levels of white blood cells. Symptoms include sore throat, fever, and malaise. This may be a side effect of long-term therapy with some antipsychotic medications.

AIDS. See **acquired immunodeficiency syndrome (AIDS)**.

akathesia. Restlessness; an urgent need for movement. A type of extrapyramidal side effect associated with some antipsychotic medications.

akinesia. Muscular weakness, or a loss or partial loss of muscle movement; a type of extrapyramidal side effect associated with some antipsychotic medications.

Alcoholics Anonymous (AA). A major self-help organization for the treatment of alcoholism. It is based on a 12-step program to help members attain and maintain sobriety. Once individuals have achieved sobriety, they in turn are expected to help other alcoholic persons.

allopathic medicine. Traditional medicine. The type traditionally, and currently, practiced in the United States and taught in U.S. medical schools.

alternative medicine. Practices that differ from usual traditional (allopathic) medicine.

altruism. One curative factor of group therapy (identified by Yalom) in which individuals gain self-esteem through mutual sharing and concern. Providing assistance and support to others creates a positive self-image and promotes self-growth.

altruistic suicide. Suicide based on behavior of a group to which an individual is excessively integrated.

amenorrhea. Cessation of the menses; may be a side effect of some antipsychotic medications.

amnesia. An inability to recall important personal information that is too extensive to be explained by ordinary forgetfulness.

amnesia, continuous. The inability to recall events occurring after a specific time up to and including the present.

amnesia, generalized. The inability to recall anything that has happened during the individual's entire lifetime.

amnesia, localized. The inability to recall all incidents associated with a traumatic event for a specific time period following the event (usually a few hours to a few days).

amnesia, selective. The inability to recall only certain incidents associated with a traumatic event for a specific time period following the event.

amnesia, systematized. The inability to remember events that relate to a specific category of information, such as one's family, a particular person, or an event.

anger. An emotional response to one's perception of a situation. Anger has both positive and negative functions.

anhedonia. The inability to experience or even imagine any pleasant emotion.

anomic suicide. Suicide that occurs in response to changes that occur in an individual's life that disrupt cohesiveness from a group and cause that person to feel without support from the formerly cohesive group.

anorexia. Loss of appetite.

anorexigenics. Drugs that suppress appetite.

anorgasmia. Inability to achieve orgasm.

anosmia. Inability to smell.

anticipatory grief. A subjective state of emotional, physical, and social responses to an anticipated loss of a valued entity. The grief response is repeated once the loss actually occurs, but it may not be as intense as it might have been if anticipatory grieving has not occurred.

antisocial personality disorder. A pattern of socially irresponsible, exploitative, and guiltless behavior, evident in the tendency to fail to conform to the law, develop stable relationships, or sustain consistent employment; exploitation and manipulation of others for personal gain is common.

anxiety. Vague diffuse apprehension that is associated with feelings of uncertainty and helplessness.

aphasia. Inability to communicate through speech, writing, or signs, caused by dysfunction of brain centers.

aphonia. Inability to speak.

apraxia. Inability to carry out motor activities despite intact motor function.

arbitrary inference. A type of thinking error in which the individual automatically comes to a conclusion about an incident without the facts to support it, or even sometimes despite contradictory evidence to support it.

ascites. Excessive accumulation of serous fluid in the abdominal cavity, occurring in response to portal hypertension caused by cirrhosis of the liver.

assault. An act that results in a person's genuine fear and apprehension that he or she will be touched without consent. Nurses may be guilty of assault for threatening to place an individual in restraints against his or her will.

assertiveness. Behavior that enables individuals to act in their own best interests, to stand up for themselves without undue anxiety, to express their honest feelings comfortably, or to exercise their own rights without denying those of others.

associative looseness. Sometimes called *loose associations*, a thinking process characterized by speech in which ideas shift from one unrelated subject to another. The individual is unaware that the topics are unconnected.

ataxia. Muscular incoordination.

attachment theory. The hypothesis that individuals who maintain close relationships with others into old age are more likely to remain independent and less likely to be institutionalized than those who do not.

attitude. A frame of reference around which an individual organizes knowledge about his or her world. It includes an emotional element and can have a positive or negative connotation.

autism. A focus inward on a fantasy world, while distorting or excluding the external environment; common in schizophrenia.

autistic disorder. The withdrawal of an infant or child into the self and into a fantasy world of his or her own creation. There is marked impairment in interpersonal functioning and communication and in imaginative play. Activities and interests are restricted and may be considered somewhat bizarre.

autocratic. A leadership style in which the leader makes all decisions for the group. Productivity is very high with this type of leadership, but morale is often low because of the lack of member input and creativity.

autoimmunity. A condition in which the body produces a disordered immunological response against itself. In this situation, the body fails to differentiate between what is normal and what is a foreign substance. When this occurs, the body produces antibodies against normal parts of the body to such an extent as to cause tissue injury.

automatic thoughts. Thoughts that occur rapidly in response to a situation, and without rational analysis. They are often negative and based on erroneous logic.

autonomy. Independence; self-governance. An ethical principle that emphasizes the status of persons as autonomous moral agents whose right to determine their destinies should always be respected.

aversive stimulus. A stimulus that follows a behavioral response and decreases the probability that the behavior will recur; also called punishment.

axon. The cellular process of a neuron that carries impulses away from the cell body.

B

battering. A pattern of repeated physical assault, usually of a woman by her spouse or intimate partner. Men are also battered, although this occurs much less frequently.

battery. The unconsented touching of another person. Nurses may be charged with battery should they participate in the treatment of a client without his or her consent and outside of an emergency situation.

behavior modification. A treatment modality aimed at changing undesirable behaviors, using a system of reinforcement to bring about the modifications desired.

belief. A belief is an idea that one holds to be true. It can be rational, irrational, taken on faith, or a stereotypical idea.

beneficence. An ethical principle that refers to one's duty to benefit or promote the good of others.

bereavement overload. An accumulation of grief that occurs when an individual experiences many losses over a short period of time and is unable to resolve one before another is experienced. This phenomenon is common among the elderly.

binge and purge. A syndrome associated with eating disorders, especially bulimia, in which an individual consumes thousands of calories of food at one sitting, and then purges through the use of laxatives or self-induced vomiting.

bioethics. The term used with ethical principles that refer to concepts within the scope of medicine, nursing, and allied health.

biofeedback. The use of instrumentation to become aware of processes in the body that usually go unnoticed and to bring them under voluntary control (e.g., the blood pressure or pulse); used as a method of stress reduction.

bipolar disorder. Characterized by mood swings from profound depression to extreme euphoria (mania), with intervening periods of normalcy. Psychotic symptoms may or may not be present.

body image. One's perception of his or her own body. It may also be how one believes *others* perceive his or her body. (See also **physical self.**)

borderline personality disorder. A disorder characterized by a pattern of intense and chaotic relationships, with affective instability, fluctuating and extreme attitudes regarding other people, impulsivity, direct and indirect self-destructive behavior, and lack of a clear or certain sense of identity, life plan, or values.

boundaries. The level of participation and interaction between individuals and between subsystems. Boundaries denote physical and psychological space individuals identify as their own. They are sometimes referred to as limits. Boundaries are appropriate when they permit appropriate contact with others while preventing excessive interference. Boundaries may be clearly defined (healthy) or rigid or diffuse (unhealthy).

C

cachexia. A state of ill health, malnutrition, and wasting; extreme emaciation.

cannabis. The dried flowering tops of the hemp plant. It produces euphoric effects when ingested or smoked and is commonly used in the form of marijuana or hashish.

carcinogen. Any substance or agent that produces or increases the risk of developing cancer in humans or lower animals.

case management. A health care delivery process, the goals of which are to provide quality health care, decrease fragmentation, enhance the client's quality of life, and contain costs. A case manager coordinates the client's care from admission to discharge and sometimes following discharge. Critical pathways of care are the tools used for the provision of care in a case management system.

case manager. The individual responsible for negotiating with multiple health care providers to obtain a variety of services for a client.

catastrophic thinking. Always thinking that the worst will occur without considering the possibility of more likely, positive outcomes.

catatonia. A type of schizophrenia that is typified by stupor or excitement, stupor characterized by extreme psychomotor retardation, mutism, negativism, and posturing; excitement characterized by psychomotor agitation, in which the movements are frenzied and purposeless.

catharsis. One curative factor of group therapy (identified by Yalom), in which members in a group can express both positive and negative feelings in a nonthreatening atmosphere.

cell body. The part of the neuron that contains the nucleus and is essential for the continued life of the neuron.

chi. In Chinese medicine, the healing energy that flows through pathways in the body called meridians.

child sexual abuse. Any sexual act, such as indecent exposure or improper touching to penetration (sexual intercourse), that is carried out with a child.

chiropractic. A system of alternative medicine based on the premise that the relationship between structure and function in the human body is a significant health factor and that such relationships between the spinal column and the nervous system are important because the normal transmission and expression of nerve energy are essential to the restoration and maintenance of health.

Christian ethics. The ethical philosophy that states one should treat others as moral equals, and recognize the equality of other persons by permitting them to act as we do when they occupy a position similar to ours; sometimes referred to as "the ethic of the golden rule."

circadian rhythm. A 24-hour biological rhythm controlled by a "pacemaker" in the brain that sends messages to other systems in the body. Circadian rhythm influences various regulatory functions, including the sleep-wake cycle, body temperature regulation, patterns of activity such as eating and drinking, and hormonal and neurotransmitter secretion.

circumstantiality. In speaking, the delay of an individual to reach the point of a communication, owing to unnecessary and tedious details.

civil law. Law that protects the private and property rights of individuals and businesses.

clang associations. A pattern of speech in which the choice of words is governed by sounds. Clang associations often take the form of rhyming.

classical conditioning. A type of learning that occurs when an unconditioned stimulus (UCS) that produces an unconditioned response (UCR) is paired with a conditioned stimulus (CS), until the CS alone produces the same response, which is then called a conditioned response (CR). Pavlov's example: food (i.e., UCS) causes salivation (i.e., UCR); ringing bell (i.e., CS) with food (i.e., UCS) causes salivation (i.e., UCR), ringing bell alone (i.e., CS) causes salivation (i.e., CR).

codependency. An exaggerated dependent pattern of learned behaviors, beliefs, and feelings that make life painful. It is a dependence on people and things outside the self, along with neglect of the self to the point of having little self-identity.

cognition. Mental operations that relate to logic, awareness, intellect, memory, language, and reasoning powers.

cognitive development. A series of stages described by Piaget through which individuals progress, demonstrating at each successive stage a higher level of logical organization than at each previous stage.

cognitive maturity. The capability to perform all mental operations needed for adulthood.

cognitive therapy. A type of therapy in which the individual is taught to control thought distortions that are considered to be a factor in the development and maintenance of emotional disorders.

colposcope. An instrument that contains a magnifying lens and to which a 35-mm camera can be attached. A colposcope is used to examine for tears and abrasions inside the vaginal area of a sexual assault victim.

common law. Laws that are derived from decisions made in previous cases.

community. A group of people living close to and depending to some extent on each other.

compensation. Covering up a real or perceived weakness by emphasizing a trait one considers more desirable.

complementary medicine. Practices that differ from usual traditional (allopathic) medicine, but may in fact supplement it in a positive way.

compounded rape reaction. Symptoms that are in addition to the typical rape response of physical complaints, rage, humiliation, fear, and sleep disturbances. They include depression and suicide, substance abuse, and even psychotic behaviors.

concrete thinking. Thought processes that are focused on specifics rather than on generalities and immediate issues rather than on eventual outcomes. Individuals who are experiencing concrete thinking are unable to comprehend abstract terminology.

confidentiality. The right of an individual to the assurance that his or her case will not be discussed outside the boundaries of the health care team.

contextual stimulus. Conditions present in the environment that support a focal stimulus and influence a threat to self-esteem.

contingency contracting. A written contract between individuals used to modify behavior. Benefits and consequences for fulfilling the terms of the contract are delineated.

controlled response pattern. The response to rape in which feelings are masked or hidden, and a calm, composed, or subdued affect is seen.

counselor. One who listens as the client reviews feelings related to difficulties he or she is experiencing in any aspect of life; one of the nursing roles identified by H. Peplau.

covert sensitization. An aversion technique used to modify behavior that relies on the individual's imagination to produce unpleasant symptoms. When the individual is about to succumb to undesirable behavior, he or she visualizes something that is offensive or even nauseating in an effort to block the behavior.

criminal law. Law that provides protection from conduct deemed injurious to the public welfare. It provides for punishment of those found to have engaged in such conduct.

crisis. Psychological disequilibrium in a person who confronts a hazardous circumstance that constitutes an important problem which for the time he or she can neither escape nor solve with usual problem-solving resources.

crisis intervention. An emergency type of assistance in which the intervener becomes a part of the individual's life situation. The focus is to provide guidance and support to help mobilize the resources needed to resolve the crisis and restore or generate an improvement in previous level of functioning. Usually lasts no longer than 6 to 8 weeks.

critical pathways of care. An abbreviated plan of care that provides outcome-based guidelines for goal achievement within a designated length of time.

culture. A particular society's entire way of living, encompassing shared patterns of belief, feeling, and knowledge that guide people's conduct and are passed down from generation to generation.

curandera. A female folk healer in the Latino culture.

curandero. A male folk healer in the Latino culture.

cycle of battering. Three phases of predictable behaviors that are repeated over time in a relationship between a batterer and a victim: tension-building phase; the acute battering incident; and the calm, loving, respite (honeymoon) phase.

cyclothymia. A chronic mood disturbance involving numerous episodes of hypomania and depressed mood, of insufficient severity or duration to meet the criteria for bipolar disorder.

D

date rape. A situation in which the rapist is known to the victim. This may occur during dating or with acquaintances or school mates.

decatastrophizing. In cognitive therapy, with this technique the therapist assists the client to examine the validity of a negative automatic thought. Even if some validity exists, the client is then encouraged to review ways to cope adaptively, moving beyond the current crisis situation.

defamation of character. An individual may be liable for defamation of character by sharing with others information about a person that is detrimental to his or her reputation.

deinstitutionalization. The removal of mentally ill individuals from institutions and the subsequent plan to provide care for these individuals in the community setting.

delirium. A state of mental confusion and excitement characterized by disorientation for time and place, often with hallucinations, incoherent speech, and a continual state of aimless physical activity.

delusions. False personal beliefs, not consistent with a person's intelligence or cultural background. The individual continues to have the belief in spite of obvious proof that it is false and/or irrational.

dementia. Global impairment of cognitive functioning that is progressive and interferes with social and occupational abilities.

dendrites. The cellular processes of a neuron that carry impulses toward the cell body.

denial. Refusal to acknowledge the existence of a real situation and/or the feelings associated with it.

density. The number of people in a given environmental space, influencing interpersonal interaction.

depersonalization. An alteration in the perception or experience of the self so that the feeling of one's own reality is temporarily lost.

derealization. An alteration in the perception or experience of the external world so that it seems strange or unreal.

detoxification. The process of withdrawal from a substance to which one has become dependent.

diagnostically related groups (DRGs). A system used to determine prospective payment rates for reimbursement of hospital care based on the client's diagnosis.

***Diagnostic and Statistical Manual of Mental Disorders*, 4th ed**

(*DSM-IV*). Standard nomenclature of emotional illness published by the American Psychiatric Association (APA) and used by all health care practitioners. It classifies mental illness and presents guidelines and diagnostic criteria for various mental disorders.

dichotomous thinking. In this type of thinking, situations are viewed in all-or-nothing, black-or-white, good-or-bad terms.

directed association. A technique used to help clients bring into consciousness events that have been repressed. Specific thoughts are guided and directed by the psychoanalyst.

discriminative stimulus. A stimulus that precedes a behavioral response and predicts that a particular reinforcement will occur. Individuals learn to discriminate between various stimuli that will produce the responses they desire.

disengagement. In family theory, disengagement refers to extreme separateness among family members. It is promoted by rigid boundaries or lack of communication among family members.

disengagement theory. The hypothesis that there is a process of mutual withdrawal of aging persons and society from each other that is correlated with successful aging. This theory has been challenged by many investigators.

displacement. Feelings are transferred from one target to another that is considered less threatening or neutral.

distraction. In cognitive therapy, when dysfunctional cognitions have been recognized, activities are identified that can be used to distract the client and divert him or her from the intrusive thoughts or depressive ruminations that are contributing to the client's maladaptive responses.

disulfiram. A drug that is administered to individuals who abuse alcohol as a deterrent to drinking. Ingestion of alcohol while disulfiram is in the body results in a syndrome of symptoms that can produce a great deal of discomfort, and can even result in death if the blood alcohol level is high.

double-bind communication. Communication described as contradictory that places an individual in a "double bind." It occurs when a statement is made and succeeded by a contradictory statement or when a statement is made accompanied by nonverbal expression that is inconsistent with the verbal communication.

dyspareunia. Pain during sexual intercourse.

dysthymic disorder. A depressive neurosis. The symptoms are similar to, if somewhat milder than, those ascribed to major depression. There is no loss of contact with reality.

dystonia. Involuntary muscular movements (spasms) of the face, arms, legs, and neck; may occur as an extrapyramidal side effect of some antipsychotic medications.

E

echolalia. The parrot-like repetition, by an individual with loose ego boundaries, of the words spoken by another.

echopraxia. An individual with loose ego boundaries attempting to identify with another person by imitating movements that the other person makes.

ego. One of the three elements of the personality, identified by Freud as the rational self or "reality principle." The ego seeks to maintain harmony between the external world, the id, and the superego.

ego defense mechanisms. Strategies employed by the ego for protection in the face of threat to biological or psychological integrity. (See individual defense mechanisms.)

egoistic suicide. The response of an individual who feels separate and apart from the mainstream of society.

electroconvulsive therapy (ECT). A type of somatic treatment in which electric current is applied to the brain through electrodes placed on the temples. A grand mal seizure produces the desired effect. This is used with severely depressed patients refractory to antidepressant medications.

emaciated. The state of being excessively thin or physically wasted.

emotional injury of a child. A pattern of behavior on the part of the parent or caretaker that results in serious impairment of the child's social, emotional, or intellectual functioning.

emotional neglect of a child. A chronic failure by the parent or caretaker to provide the child with the hope, love, and support necessary for the development of a sound, healthy personality.

empathy. The ability to see beyond outward behavior and sense accurately another's inner experiencing. With empathy, one can accurately perceive and understand the meaning and relevance in the thoughts and feelings of another.

enmeshment. Exaggerated connectedness among family members. It occurs in response to diffuse boundaries in which there is overinvestment, overinvolvement, and lack of differentiation between individuals or subsystems.

esophageal varices. Veins in the esophagus become distended because of excessive pressure from defective blood flow through a cirrhotic liver.

essential hypertension. Persistent elevation of blood pressure for which there is no apparent cause or associated underlying disease.

ethical dilemma. A situation that arises when on the basis of moral considerations an appeal can be made for taking each of two opposing courses of action.

ethical egoism. An ethical theory espousing that what is "right" and "good" is what is best for the individual making the decision.

ethics. A branch of philosophy dealing with values related to human conduct, to the rightness and wrongness of certain actions, and to the goodness and badness of the motives and ends of such actions.

ethnicity. The concept of people identifying with each other because of a shared heritage.

exhibitionism. A paraphilic disorder characterized by a recurrent urge to expose one's genitals to a stranger.

expressed response pattern. Pattern of behavior in which the victim of rape expresses feelings of fear, anger, and anxiety through such behavior as crying, sobbing, smiling, restlessness, and tenseness; in contrast to the rape victim who withholds feelings in the controlled response pattern.

extinction. The gradual decrease in frequency or disappearance of a response when the positive reinforcement is withheld.

extrapyramidal symptoms (EPS). A variety of responses that originate outside the pyramidal tracts and in the basal ganglion of the brain. Symptoms may include tremors, chorea, dystonia, akinesia, akathisia, and others; may occur as a side effect of some antipsychotic medications.

F

false imprisonment. The deliberate and unauthorized confinement of a person within fixed limits by the use of threat or force. A nurse may be charged with false imprisonment by placing a patient in restraints against his or her will in a non-emergency situation.

family structure. A family system in which the structure is founded on a set of invisible principles that influence the interaction among family members. These principles are established over time and become the "laws" that govern the conduct of various family members.

family system. A system in which the parts of the whole may be the marital dyad, parent-child dyad, or sibling groups. Each

of these subsystems is further divided into subsystems of individuals.

family therapy. A type of therapy in which the focus is on relationships within the family. The family is viewed as a system in which the members are interdependent, and a change in one creates change in all.

fetishism. A paraphilic disorder characterized by recurrent sexual urges and sexually arousing fantasies involving the use of nonliving objects.

fight or flight. A syndrome of physical symptoms that result from an individual's real or perceived perception that harm or danger is imminent.

flexible boundary. A personal boundary is flexible when, because of unusual circumstances, individuals can alter limits that they have set for themselves. Flexible boundaries are healthy boundaries.

flooding. Sometimes called implosion therapy, this technique is used to desensitize individuals to phobic stimuli. The individual is "flooded" with a continuous presentation (usually through mental imagery) of the phobic stimulus until it no longer elicits anxiety.

focal stimulus. A situation of immediate concern that results in a threat to self-esteem.

focus charting.® A type of documentation that follows a data, action, and response (DAR) format. The main perspective is a client "focus," which can be a nursing diagnosis, a client's concern, change in status, or significant event in the client's therapy. The focus cannot be a medical diagnosis.

folk medicine. A system of health care within various cultures that is provided by a local practitioner, not professionally trained, but who uses techniques specific to that culture in the art of healing.

forensic. Pertaining to the law; legal.

forensic nursing. The application of forensic science combined with the biopsychological education of the registered nurse in the scientific investigation, evidence collection, and preservation, analysis, prevention and treatment of trauma and/or death-related medical-legal issues.

free association. A technique used to help individuals bring to consciousness material that has been repressed. The individual is encouraged to verbalize whatever comes into his or her mind, drifting naturally from one thought to another.

frotteurism. A paraphilic disorder characterized by the recurrent preoccupation with intense sexual urges or fantasies involving touching or rubbing against a nonconsenting person.

fugue. A sudden unexpected travel away from home or customary work locale with the assumption of a new identity and an inability to recall one's previous identity; usually occurring in response to severe psychosocial stress.

G

gains. The reinforcements an individual receives for somaticizing.

gains, primary. The receipt of positive reinforcement for somaticizing through added attention, sympathy, and nurturing.

gains, secondary. The receipt of positive reinforcement for somaticizing by being able to avoid difficult situations because of physical complaint.

gains, tertiary. The receipt of positive reinforcement for somaticizing by causing the focus of the family to switch to him or her and away from conflict that may be occurring within the family.

Gamblers Anonymous (GA). An organization of inspirational group therapy, modeled after Alcoholics Anonymous (AA), for individuals who desire to, but cannot, stop gambling.

gender identity disorder. A sense of discomfort associated with an incongruence between biologically assigned gender and subjectively experienced gender.

generalized anxiety disorder. A disorder characterized by chronic (at least 6 months), unrealistic, and excessive anxiety and worry.

genogram. A graphic representation of a family system. It may cover several generations. Emphasis is on family roles and emotional relatedness among members. Genograms facilitate recognition of areas requiring change.

genotype. The total set of genes present in an individual at the time of conception, and coded in the DNA.

genuineness. The ability to be open, honest, and "real" in interactions with others; the awareness of what one is experiencing internally and the ability to project the quality of this inner experiencing in a relationship.

geriatrics. The branch of clinical medicine specializing in the care of the elderly and concerned with the problems of aging.

gerontology. The study of normal aging.

geropsychiatry. The branch of clinical medicine specializing in psychopathology of the elderly.

gonorrhea. A sexually transmitted disease caused by the bacterium *N. gonorrhoeae* and resulting in inflammation of the genital mucosa. Treatment is through the use of antibiotics, particularly penicillin. Serious complications occur if the disease is left untreated.

"granny-bashing." Media-generated term for abuse of the elderly.

"granny-dumping." Media-generated term for abandoning elderly individuals at emergency departments, nursing homes, or other facilities—literally, leaving them in the hands of others when the strain of caregiving becomes intolerable.

grief. A subjective state of emotional, physical, and social responses to the real or perceived loss of a valued entity. Change and failure can also be perceived as losses. The grief response consists of a set of relatively predictable behaviors that describe the subjective state that accompanies mourning.

grief, exaggerated. A reaction in which all of the symptoms associated with normal grieving are exaggerated out of proportion. Pathological depression is a type of exaggerated grief.

grief, inhibited. The absence of evidence of grief when it ordinarily would be expected.

grief, prolonged. Grief characterized by lack of resumption of normal activities of daily living within 4 to 8 weeks of a loss.

group therapy. A therapy group, founded in a specific theoretical framework, led by a person with an advanced degree in psychology, social work, nursing, or medicine. The goal is to encourage improvement in interpersonal functioning.

gynecomastia. Enlargement of the breasts in men; may be a side effect of some antipsychotic medications.

H

hallucinations. False sensory perceptions not associated with real external stimuli. Hallucinations may involve any of the five senses.

Health Care Financing Administration (HCFA). The division of the U.S. Department of Health and Human Services responsible for Medicare funding.

hepatic encephalopathy. A brain disorder resulting from the inability of the cirrhotic liver to convert ammonia to urea for excretion. The continued rise in serum ammonia results in progressively impaired mental functioning, apathy, euphoria or depression, sleep disturbances, increasing confusion, and progression to coma and eventual death.

histrionic personality disorder. Conscious or unconscious overly dramatic behavior for the purpose of drawing attention to oneself.

HIV: associated dementia (HAD). A neuropathological syndrome, possibly caused by chronic HIV encephalitis and myelitis and manifested by cognitive, behavioral, and motor symptoms that become more severe with progression of the disease.

HIV wasting syndrome. An absence of concurrent illness other than HIV infection, and presence of the following: fever, weakness, weight loss, and chronic diarrhea.

home care. A wide range of health and social services that are delivered at home to recovering, disabled, chronically or terminally ill persons in need of medical, nursing, social, or therapeutic treatment and/or assistance with essential activities of daily living.

homosexuality. A sexual preference for persons of the same gender.

hospice. A program that provides palliative and supportive care to meet the special needs arising out of the physical, psychosocial, spiritual, social, and economic stresses that are experienced during the final stages of illness and during bereavement.

human immunodeficiency virus (HIV). The virus that is the etiological agent that produces the immunosuppression resulting in AIDS.

humors. The four body fluids described by Hippocrates: blood, black bile, yellow bile, and phlegm. Hippocrates associated insanity and mental illness with these four fluids.

hypersomnia. Excessive sleepiness or seeking excessive amounts of sleep.

hypertensive crisis. A potentially life-threatening syndrome that results when an individual taking monoamine oxidase inhibitors eats a product high in tyramine. Symptoms include severe occipital headache, palpitations, nausea and vomiting, nuchal rigidity, fever, sweating, marked increase in blood pressure, chest pain, and coma. Foods with tyramine include aged cheeses or other aged, overripe, and fermented foods; broad beans; pickled herring; beef or chicken liver; preserved meats; beer and wine; yeast products; chocolate; caffeinated drinks; canned figs; sour cream; yogurt; soy sauce; and some over-the-counter cold medications and diet pills.

hypnosis. A treatment for disorders brought on by repressed anxiety. The individual is directed into a state of subconsciousness and assisted, through suggestions, to recall certain events that he or she cannot recall while conscious.

hypochondriasis. The unrealistic preoccupation with fear of having a serious illness.

hypomania. A mild form of mania. Symptoms are excessive hyperactivity, but not severe enough to cause marked impairment in social or occupational functioning or to require hospitalization.

hysteria. A polysymptomatic disorder characterized by recurrent, multiple somatic complaints often described dramatically.

I

id. One of the three components of the personality, identified by Freud as the "pleasure principle." The id is the locus of instinctual drives, is present at birth, and compels the infant to satisfy needs and seek immediate gratification.

identification. An attempt to increase self-worth by acquiring certain attributes and characteristics of an individual one admires.

illusion. A misperception of a real external stimulus.

implosion therapy. See **flooding**.

incest. Sexual exploitation of a child under 18 years of age by a relative or nonrelative who holds a position of trust in the family.

informed consent. Permission granted to a physician by a client to perform a therapeutic procedure, prior to which information about the procedure has been presented to the client with adequate time given for consideration about the pros and cons.

insomnia. Difficulty initiating or maintaining sleep.

insulin coma therapy. The induction of a hypoglycemic coma aimed at alleviating psychotic symptoms; a dangerous procedure, questionably effective, no longer used in psychiatry.

integration. The process used with individuals with dissociative identity disorder in an effort to bring all the personalities together into one; usually achieved through hypnosis.

intellectualization. An attempt to avoid expressing actual emotions associated with a stressful situation by using the intellectual processes of logic, reasoning, and analysis.

interdisciplinary care. A concept of providing care for a client in which members of various disciplines work together with common goals and shared responsibilities for meeting those goals.

intimate distance. The closest distance that individuals will allow between themselves and others. In the United States, this distance is 0 to 18 inches.

introjection. The beliefs and values of another individual are internalized and symbolically become a part of the self, to the extent that the feeling of separateness or distinctness is lost.

isolation. The separation of a thought or a memory from the feeling tone or emotions associated with it (sometimes called *emotional isolation*).

J

justice. An ethical principle reflecting that all individuals should be treated equally and fairly.

K

Kantianism. The ethical principle espousing that decisions should be made and actions taken out of a sense of duty.

Kaposi's sarcoma. Malignant areas of cell proliferation initially in the skin and eventually in other body sites; thought to be related to the immunocompromised state that accompanies AIDS.

kleptomania. A recurrent failure to resist impulses to steal objects not needed for personal use or monetary value.

Korsakoff's psychosis. A syndrome of confusion, loss of recent memory, and confabulation in alcoholics, caused by a deficiency of thiamine. It often occurs together with Wernicke's encephalopathy and may be termed Wernicke-Korsakoff's syndrome.

L

la belle indifference. A symptom of conversion disorder in which there is a relative lack of concern that is out of keeping with the severity of the impairment.

laissez-faire. A leadership type in which the leader lets group members do as they please. There is no direction from the leader. Member productivity and morale may be low, owing to frustration from lack of direction.

lesbian. A female homosexual.

libel. An action with which an individual may be charged for sharing with another individual, *in writing*, information that is detrimental to someone's reputation.

libido. Freud's term for the psychic energy used to fulfill basic physiological needs or instinctual drives such as hunger, thirst, and sexuality.

limbic system. The part of the brain that is sometimes called the "emotional brain." It is associated with feelings of fear and anxiety; anger and aggression; love, joy, and hope; and with sexuality and social behavior.

long-term memory. Memory for remote events, or those that occurred many years ago. The type of memory that is preserved in the elderly individual.

M

magical thinking. A primitive form of thinking in which an individual believes that thinking about a possible occurrence can make it happen.

magnification. A type of thinking in which the negative significance of an event is exaggerated.

maladaptation. A failure of the body to return to homeostasis following a physiological and/or psychological response to stress, disrupting the individual's integrity.

malpractice. The failure of one rendering professional services to exercise that degree of skill and learning commonly applied under all the circumstances in the community by the average prudent reputable member of the profession with the result of injury, loss, or damage to the recipient of those services or to those entitled to rely upon them.

managed care. A concept purposefully designed to control the balance between cost and quality of care. Examples of managed care are health maintenance organizations (HMOs) and preferred provider organizations (PPOs). The amount and type of health care that the individual receives are determined by the organization providing the managed care.

mania. A type of bipolar disorder in which the predominant mood is elevated, expansive, or irritable. Motor activity is frenzied and excessive. Psychotic features may or may not be present.

mania, delirious. A grave form of mania characterized by severe clouding of consciousness and representing an intensification of the symptoms associated with mania. The symptoms of delirious mania have become relatively rare since the availability of antipsychotic medications.

marital rape. Sexual violence directed at a marital partner against that person's will.

marital schism. A state of severe chronic disequilibrium and discord within the marital dyad, with recurrent threats of separation.

marital skew. A marital relationship in which there is lack of equal partnership. One partner dominates the relationship and the other partner.

masochism. Sexual stimulation derived from being humiliated, beaten, bound, or otherwise made to suffer.

Medicaid. A system established by the federal government to provide medical care benefits for indigent Americans. Medicaid funds are matched by the states, and coverage varies significantly from state to state.

Medicare. A system established by the federal government to provide medical care benefits for elderly Americans.

meditation. A method of relaxation in which an individual sits in a quiet place and focuses total concentration on an object, word, or thought.

melancholia. A severe form of major depressive episode. Symptoms are exaggerated, and interest or pleasure in virtually all activities is lost.

menopause. The period marking the permanent cessation of menstrual activity; usually occurs at approximately 48 to 51 years of age.

mental health. The successful adaptation to stressors from the internal or external environment, evidenced by thoughts, feelings, and behaviors that are age-appropriate and congruent with local and cultural norms.

mental illness. Maladaptive responses to stressors from the internal or external environment, evidenced by thoughts, feelings, and behaviors that are incongruent with the local and cultural norms, and interfere with the individual's social, occupational, and/or physical functioning.

mental imagery. A method of stress reduction that employs the imagination. The individual focuses imagination on a scenario that is particularly relaxing to him or her (e.g., a scene on a quiet seashore, a mountain atmosphere, or floating through the air on a fluffy white cloud).

meridians. In Chinese medicine, pathways along the body, linking acupoints, in which the healing energy (chi) flows.

migraine personality. Personality characteristics that have been attributed to the migraine-prone person. The characteristics include perfectionistic, overly conscientious, somewhat inflexible, neat and tidy, compulsive, hard worker, intelligent, exacting, and places a very high premium on success, setting high (sometimes unrealistic) expectations on self and others.

milieu. French for "middle"; the English translation connotes "surroundings, or environment."

milieu therapy. Also called therapeutic community, or therapeutic environment, this type of therapy consists of a scientific structuring of the environment in order to effect behavioral changes and to improve the individual's psychological health and functioning.

minimization. A type of thinking in which the positive significance of an event is minimized or undervalued.

mobile outreach units. Programs in which volunteers and paid professionals drive or walk around and seek out homeless individuals who need assistance with physical or psychological care.

modeling. Learning new behaviors by imitating the behaviors of others.

mood. An individual's sustained emotional tone, which significantly influences behavior, personality, and perception.

moral behavior. Conduct that results from serious critical thinking about how individuals ought to treat others; reflects respect for human life, freedom, justice, or confidentiality.

moral-ethical self. That aspect of the personal identity that functions as observer, standard setter, dreamer, comparer, and most of all evaluator of who the individual says he or she is. This component of the personal identity makes judgments that influence an individual's self-evaluation.

mourning. The psychological process (or stages) through which the individual passes on the way to successful adaptation to the loss of a valued object.

multidisciplinary care. A concept of providing care for a client in which individual disciplines provide specific services for the client without formal arrangement for interaction between the disciplines.

N

narcissistic personality disorder. A disorder characterized by an exaggerated sense of self-worth. These individuals lack empathy and are hypersensitive to the evaluation of others.

narcolepsy. A disorder in which the characteristic manifestation is sleep attacks. The individual cannot prevent falling asleep, even in the middle of a sentence or performing a task.

natural-law theory. The ethical theory that has as its moral precept to "do good and avoid evil" at all costs. Natural-law ethics are grounded in a concern for the human good that is based on man's ability to live according to the dictates of reason.

negative reinforcement. Increasing the probability that a behavior will recur by removal of an undesirable reinforcing stimulus.

negativism. Strong resistance to suggestions or directions; exhibiting behaviors contrary to what is expected.

negligence. The failure to do something which a reasonable person, guided by those considerations which ordinarily regulate human affairs, would do, or doing something which a prudent and reasonable person would not do.

neologism. New words that an individual invents that are meaningless to others but have symbolic meaning to the psychotic person.

neuroendocrinology. The study of hormones functioning within the neurological system.

neuroleptic. Antipsychotic medication used to prevent or control psychotic symptoms.

neuroleptic malignant syndrome (NMS). A rare but potentially fatal complication of treatment with neuroleptic drugs. Symptoms include severe muscle rigidity, high fever, tachycardia, fluctuations in blood pressure, diaphoresis, and rapid deterioration of mental status to stupor and coma.

neuron. A nerve cell; consists of a cell body, an axon, and dendrites.

neurotic disorder. A psychiatric disturbance, characterized by excessive anxiety and/or depression, disrupted bodily functions, unsatisfying interpersonal relationships, and behaviors that interfere with routine functioning. There is no loss of contact with reality.

neurotransmitter. A chemical that is stored in the axon terminals of the presynaptic neuron. An electrical impulse through the neuron stimulates the release of the neurotransmitter into the synaptic cleft, which in turn determines whether or not another electrical impulse is generated.

nonassertiveness. Individuals who are nonassertive (sometimes called passive) seek to please others at the expense of denying their own basic human rights.

nonmaleficence. The ethical principle that espouses abstaining from negative acts toward another, including acting carefully to avoid harm.

nursing diagnosis. A clinical judgment about individual, family, or community responses to actual and potential health problems/life processes. Nursing diagnoses provide the basis for selection of nursing interventions to achieve outcomes for which the nurse is accountable.

nursing process. A dynamic, systematic process by which nurses assess, diagnose, identify outcomes, plan, implement, and evaluate nursing care. It has been called "nursing's scientific methodology." Nursing process gives order and consistency to nursing intervention.

O

obesity. The state of having a body mass index of 30 or above.

object constancy. The phase in the separation/individuation process when the child learns to relate to objects in an effective, constant manner. A sense of separateness is established, and the child is able to internalize a sustained image of the loved object or person when out of sight.

obsessive-compulsive disorder. Recurrent thoughts or ideas (obsessions) that an individual is unable to put out of his or her mind, and actions that an individual is unable to refrain from performing (compulsions). The obsessions and compulsions are severe enough to interfere with social and occupational functioning.

oculogyric crisis. An attack of involuntary deviation and fixation of the eyeballs, usually in the upward position. It may last for several minutes or hours and may occur as an extrapyramidal side effect of some antipsychotic medications.

operant conditioning. The learning of a particular action or type of behavior that is followed by a reinforcement.

opportunistic infection. Infections with any organism, but especially fungi and bacteria, that occur due to the opportunity afforded by the altered physiological state of the host. Opportunistic infections have long been a defining characteristic of AIDS.

orgasm. A peaking of sexual pleasure, with release of sexual tension and rhythmic contraction of the perineal muscles and pelvic reproductive organs.

osteoporosis. A reduction in the mass of bone per unit of volume which interferes with the mechanical support function of bone. This process occurs because of demineralization of the bones and is escalated in women about the time of menopause.

overgeneralization. Also called *absolutistic thinking*. With overgeneralization, sweeping conclusions are made based on one incident—a type of all-or-nothing thinking.

overt sensitization. A type of aversion therapy that produces unpleasant consequences for undesirable behavior. An example is the use of disulfiram therapy with alcoholics, which induces an undesirable physical response if the individual has consumed any alcohol.

P

palilalia. Repeating one's own sounds or words (a type of vocal tic associated with Tourette's disorder).

panic disorder. A disorder characterized by recurrent panic attacks, the onset of which are unpredictable, and manifested by intense apprehension, fear, or terror, often associated with feelings of impending doom, and accompanied by intense physical discomfort.

paradoxical intervention. In family therapy, "prescribing the symptom." The therapist requests that the family continue to engage in the behavior that they are trying to change. Tension is relieved, and the family is able to view more clearly the possible solutions to their problem.

paralanguage. The gestural component of the spoken word. It consists of pitch, tone, and loudness of spoken messages, the rate of speaking, expressively placed pauses, and emphasis assigned to certain words.

paranoia. A term that implies extreme suspiciousness. Paranoid schizophrenia is characterized by persecutory delusions and hallucinations of a threatening nature.

paraphilias. Repetitive behaviors or fantasies that involve non-human objects, real or simulated suffering or humiliation, or nonconsenting partners.

parasomnia. Unusual or undesirable behaviors that occur during sleep (e.g., nightmares, sleep terrors, and sleepwalking).

passive-aggressive behavior. Behavior that defends an individual's own basic rights by expressing resistance to social and occupational demands. Sometimes called *indirect aggression*, this behavior takes the form of sly, devious, and undermining actions that express the opposite of what they are really feeling.

pathological gambling. A failure to resist impulses to gamble, and gambling behavior that compromises, disrupts, or damages personal, family, or vocational pursuits.

pedophilia. Recurrent urges and sexually arousing fantasies involving sexual activity with a prepubescent child.

peer assistance programs. A program established by the American Nurses' Association to assist impaired nurses. The individuals who administer these efforts are nurse members of the state associations, as well as nurses who are in recovery themselves.

perseveration. Persistent repetition of the same word or idea in response to different questions.

persistent generalized lymphadenopathy (PGL). A condition common in HIV-infected individuals in which there are lymph nodes greater than 1 cm in diameter at two extrainguinal sites persisting for 3 months or longer, not attributed to other causes, and not associated with other substantial constitutional symptoms.

personal distance. The distance between individuals who are having interactions of a personal nature, such as a close conversation. In the U.S. culture, personal distance is approximately 18 to 40 inches.

personal identity. An individual's self-perception that defines one's functions as observer, standard setter, and self-evaluator. It strives to maintain a stable self-image and relates to what the individual strives to become.

personal self. See **personal identity.**

personality. Deeply ingrained patterns of behavior, which include the way one relates to, perceives, and thinks about the environment and oneself.

personalization. Taking complete responsibility for situations without considering that other circumstances may have contributed to the outcome.

pharmacoconvulsive therapy. The chemical induction of a convulsion used in the past for the reduction of psychotic symptoms, a type of therapy no longer used in psychiatry.

phencyclidine HCl. An anesthetic used in veterinary medicine; used illegally as a hallucinogen, referred to as PCP or angel dust.

phenotype. Characteristics of physical manifestations that identify a particular genotype. Examples of phenotypes include eye color, height, blood type, language, and hair texture. Phenotypes may be genetic or acquired.

phobia. An irrational fear.

phobia, specific. A persistent fear of a specific object or situation, other than the fear of being unable to escape from a situation (agoraphobia) or the fear of being humiliated in social situations (social phobia).

phobia, social. The fear of being humiliated in social situations.

physical neglect of a child. The failure on the part of the parent or caregiver to provide for a child's basic needs, such as food, clothing, shelter, medical-dental care, and supervision.

physical self. A personal appraisal by an individual of his or her physical being; includes physical attributes, functioning, sexuality, wellness-illness state, and appearance.

PIE charting. More specifically called "APIE," this method of documentation has an assessment, problem, intervention, and evaluation (APIE) format and is a problem-oriented system used to document nursing process.

***Pneumocystis carinii* pneumonia (PCP).** The most common life-threatening opportunistic infection seen in patients with AIDS. Symptoms include fever, exertional dyspnea, and nonproductive cough.

positive reinforcement. A reinforcement stimulus that increases the probability that the behavior will recur.

postpartum depression. Depression that occurs during the postpartum period. It may be related to hormonal changes, tryptophan metabolism, or alterations in membrane transport during the early postpartum period. Other predisposing factors may also be influential.

posttraumatic stress disorder (PTSD). A syndrome of symptoms that develop following a psychologically distressing event that is outside the range of usual human experience (e.g., rape, war). The individual is unable to put the experience out of his or her mind, has nightmares, flashbacks, and panic attacks.

posturing. The voluntary assumption of inappropriate or bizarre postures.

preassaultive tension state. Behaviors predictive of potential violence. They include excessive motor activity, tense posture, defiant affect, clenched teeth and fists, and other arguing, demanding, and threatening behaviors.

precipitating event. A stimulus arising from the internal or external environment that is perceived by an individual as taxing or exceeding his or her resources and endangering his or her well-being.

predisposing factors. A variety of elements that influence how an individual perceives and responds to a stressful event. Types of predisposing factors include genetic influences, past experiences, and existing conditions.

Premack principle. This principle states that a frequently occurring response (R_1) can serve as a positive reinforcement for a response (R_2) that occurs less frequently. For example, a girl may talk to friends on phone (R_2) only if she does her homework (R_1).

premature ejaculation. Ejaculation that occurs with minimal sexual stimulation or before, upon, or shortly after penetration and before the person wishes it.

premenstrual dysphoric disorder. A disorder that is characterized by depressed mood, anxiety, mood swings, and decreased interest in activities during the week prior to menses and subsiding shortly after the onset of menstruation (*DSM-IV*, APA, 1994).

presenile. Pertaining to premature old age as judged by mental or physical condition. In presenile-onset dementia initial symptoms appear at age 65 or younger.

priapism. Prolonged painful penile erection; may occur as an adverse effect of some antidepressant medications, particularly trazodone.

primary dementia. Dementia, such as Alzheimer's disease, in which the dementia itself is the major sign of some organic brain disease not directly related to any other organic illness.

primary prevention. Reduction of the incidence of mental disorders within the population by helping individuals to cope more effectively with stress and by trying to diminish stressors within the environment.

privileged communication. A doctrine common to most states that grants certain privileges under which they may refuse to reveal information about and communications with clients.

problem-oriented recording (POR). A system of documentation that follows a subjective, objective, assessment, plan, implementation, and evaluation (SOAPIE) format. It is based on a list of identified patient problems to which each entry is directed.

progressive relaxation. A method of deep muscle relaxation in which each muscle group is alternately tensed and relaxed in a systematic order, with the person concentrating on the contrast of sensations experienced from tensing and relaxing.

projection. Attributing to another person feelings or impulses unacceptable to oneself.

prospective payment. The program of cost containment within the health care profession directed at setting forth preestablished amounts that would be reimbursed for specific diagnoses.

pseudocyesis. A condition in which an individual has nearly all the signs and symptoms of pregnancy but is not pregnant; a conversion reaction.

pseudodementia. Symptoms of depression that mimic those of dementia.

pseudohostility. A family interaction pattern characterized by a state of chronic conflict and alienation among family members. This relationship pattern allows family members to deny underlying fears of tenderness and intimacy.

pseudomutuality. A family interaction pattern characterized by a facade of mutual regard with the purpose of denying underlying fears of separation and hostility.

psychiatric home care. Care provided by psychiatric nurses in the client's home. Psychiatric home care nurses must have physical and psychosocial nursing skills to meet the demands of the client population they serve.

psychodrama. A specialized type of group therapy that employs a dramatic approach in which patients become "actors" in life situation scenarios. The goal is to resolve interpersonal conflicts in a less-threatening atmosphere than the real-life situation would present.

psychodynamic nursing. Being able to understand one's own behavior, to help others identify felt difficulties, and to apply principles of human relations to the problems that arise at all levels of experience.

psychoimmunology. The study of the implications of the immune system in psychiatry.

psychomotor retardation. Extreme slowdown of physical movements. Posture slumps; speech is slowed; digestion becomes sluggish. Common in severe depression.

psychophysiological. Referring to psychological factors contributing to the initiation or exacerbation of a physical condition. Either a demonstrable organic pathology or a known pathophysiological process is involved.

psychosomatic. See **psychophysiological.**

psychotic disorder. A serious psychiatric disorder in which there is a gross disorganization of the personality, a marked disturbance in reality testing, and the impairment of interpersonal functioning and relationship to the external world.

public distance. Appropriate interactional distance for speaking in public or yelling to someone some distance away. U.S. culture defines this distance as 12 feet or more.

pyromania. An inability to resist the impulse to set fires.

R

rape. The expression of power and dominance by means of sexual violence, most commonly by men over women, although men may also be rape victims. Rape is considered an act of aggression, not of passion.

rapport. The development between two people in a relationship of special feelings based on mutual acceptance, warmth, friendliness, common interest, a sense of trust, and a nonjudgmental attitude.

rationalization. Attempting to make excuses or formulate logical reasons to justify unacceptable feelings or behaviors.

reaction formation. Preventing unacceptable or undesirable thoughts or behaviors from being expressed by exaggerating opposite thoughts or types of behaviors.

receptor sites. Molecules situated on the cell membrane of the postsynaptic neuron that will accept only molecules with a complementary shape. These complementary molecules are specific to certain neurotransmitters that determine whether an electrical impulse will be excited or inhibited.

reciprocal inhibition. Also called counterconditioning, this technique serves to decrease or eliminate a behavior by introducing a more adaptive behavior, but one that is incompatible with the unacceptable behavior (e.g., introducing relaxation techniques to an anxious person; relaxation and anxiety are incompatible behaviors).

reframing. Changing the conceptual or emotional setting or viewpoint in relation to which a situation is experienced and placing it in another frame that fits the "facts" of the same concrete situation equally well or even better, and thereby changing its entire meaning. The *behavior* may not actually change, but the *consequences* of the behavior may change because of a change in the meaning attached to the behavior.

regression. A retreat to an earlier level of development and the comfort measures associated with that level of functioning.

religiosity. Excessive demonstration of or obsession with religious ideas and behavior; common in schizophrenia.

reminiscence therapy. A process of life review by elderly individuals that promotes self-esteem and provides assistance in working through unresolved conflicts from the past.

repression. The involuntary blocking of unpleasant feelings and experiences from one's awareness.

residual stimuli. Certain beliefs, attitudes, experiences, or traits that may contribute to an individual's low self-esteem.

retarded ejaculation. Delayed or absent ejaculation, even though the man has a firm erection and has had more than adequate stimulation.

retrograde ejaculation. Ejaculation of the seminal fluid backwards into the bladder; may occur as a side effect of antipsychotic medications.

right. That which an individual is entitled (by ethical or moral standards) to have, or to do, or to receive from others within the limits of the law.

rigid boundaries. A person with rigid boundaries is "closed" and difficult to bond with. Such a person has a narrow perspective on life, sees things one way, and cannot discuss matters that lie outside his or her perspective.

ritualistic behavior. Purposeless activities that an individual performs repeatedly in an effort to decrease anxiety (e.g., handwashing); common in obsessive-compulsive disorder.

S

sadism. Recurrent urges and sexually arousing fantasies involving acts (real, not simulated) in which the psychological or physical suffering (including humiliation) of the victim is sexually exciting.

safe house or **shelter.** An establishment set up by many cities to provide protection for battered women and their children.

scapegoating. Occurs when hostility exists in a marriage dyad and an innocent third person (usually a child) becomes the target of blame for the problem.

schemas (core beliefs). Cognitive structures that consist of the individual's fundamental beliefs and assumptions, which develop early in life from personal experiences and identification with significant others. These concepts are reinforced by further learning experiences and, in turn, influence the formation of other beliefs, values, and attitudes.

schizoid personality disorder. A profound defect in the ability to form personal relationships or to respond to others in any meaningful, emotional way.

schizotypal personality disorder. A disorder characterized by odd and eccentric behavior, not decompensating to the level of schizophrenia.

secondary dementia. Dementia which is caused by or related to another disease or condition, such as HIV disease or a cerebral trauma.

secondary prevention. Health care that is directed at reduction of the prevalence of psychiatric illness by shortening the course (duration) of the illness. This is accomplished through early identification of problems and prompt initiation of treatment.

selective abstraction (sometimes referred to as *mental filter*). A type of thinking in which a conclusion is drawn based on only a selected portion of the evidence.

self-concept. The composite of beliefs and feelings that one holds about oneself at a given time, formed from perceptions of others' reactions. The self-concept consists of the physical self, or body image; the personal self or identity; and the self-esteem.

self-consistency. The component of the personal identity that strives to maintain a stable self-image.

self-esteem. The degree of regard or respect that individuals have for themselves. It is a measure of worth that they place on their abilities and judgments.

self-expectancy. The component of the personal identity that is the individual's perception of what he or she wants to be, to do, or to become.

self-ideal. See **self-expectancy**.

senile. Pertaining to old age and the mental or physical weakness with which it is sometimes associated. In senile-onset dementia, the first symptoms appear after age 65.

sensate focus. A therapeutic technique used to treat individuals and couples with sexual dysfunction. The technique involves touching and being touched by another and focusing attention on the physical sensations encountered thereby. Clients gradually move through various levels of sensate focus that progress from nongenital touching to touching that includes the breasts and genitals; touching done in a simultaneous, mutual format rather than by one person at a time; and touching that extends to and allows eventually for the possibility of intercourse.

seroconversion. The development of evidence of antibody response to a disease or vaccine. The time at which antibodies may be detected in the blood.

sexual assault nurse examiner (SANE). A clinical forensic registered nurse who has received specialized training to provide care to the sexual assault victim.

sexual exploitation of a child. The inducement or coercion of a child into engaging in sexually explicit conduct for the purpose of promoting any performance (e.g., child pornography).

shaman. The Native American "medicine man" or folk healer.

shaping. In learning, one shapes the behavior of another by giving reinforcements for increasingly closer approximations to the desired behavior.

shelters. A variety of places designed to help the homeless, ranging from converted warehouses that provide cots or floor space on which to sleep overnight to significant operations that provide a multitude of social and health care services.

"ship of fools." The term given during the Middle Ages to sailing boats filled with severely mentally ill people that were sent out to sea with little guidance and in search of their lost rationality.

short-term memory. The ability to remember events that occurred very recently. This ability deteriorates with age.

silent rape reaction. The response of a rape victim in which he or she tells no one about the assault.

slander. An action with which an individual may be charged for *orally* sharing information that is detrimental to a person's reputation.

social distance. The distance considered acceptable in interactions with strangers or acquaintances, such as at a cocktail party or in a public building. U.S. culture defines this distance as 4 to 12 feet.

social skills training. Educational opportunities through role play for the person with schizophrenia to learn appropriate social interaction skills and functional skills that are relevant to daily living.

Socratic questioning (also called *guided discovery*). When the therapist questions the client with Socratic questioning, the client is asked to describe feelings associated with specific situations. Questions are stated in a way that may stimulate in the client a recognition of possible dysfunctional thinking and produce a dissonance about the validity of the thoughts.

somatization. A method of coping with psychosocial stress by developing physical symptoms.

splitting. A primitive ego defense mechanism in which the person is unable to integrate and accept both positive and negative feelings. In their view, people—including themselves—and life situations are either all good or all bad. This trait is common in borderline personality disorder.

standard precautions. Guidelines established by the Centers for Disease Control (CDC) designed to reduce the risk of transmission of pathogens from moist body substances. Standard precautions apply to blood; all body fluids, secretions, and excretions *except sweat;* nonintact skin; and mucous membranes.

statutory law. A law that has been enacted by legislative bodies, such as a county or city council, state legislature, or the U.S. Congress.

statutory rape. Unlawful intercourse between a man over age 16 and a female under the age of consent. The man can be arrested for statutory rape even when the interaction has occurred between consenting individuals.

stereotyping. The process of classifying all individuals from the same culture or ethnic group as identical.

stimulus generalization. The process by which a conditioned response is elicited from all stimuli *similar* to the one from which the response was learned.

store-front clinic. Establishments that have been converted into clinics that serve the homeless population.

stress. A state of disequilibrium that occurs when there is a disharmony between demands occurring within an individual's internal or external environment and his or her ability to cope with those demands.

stress management. Various methods used by individuals to reduce tension and other maladaptive responses to stress in their lives; includes relaxation exercises, physical exercise, music, mental imagery, or any other technique that is successful for a person.

stressor. A demand from within an individual's internal or external environment that elicits a physiological and/or psychological response.

sublimation. The rechanneling of personally and/or socially unacceptable drives or impulses into activities that are more tolerable and constructive.

subluxation. The term used in chiropractic medicine to describe vertebrae in the spinal column that have become displaced, possibly pressing on nerves and interfering with normal nerve transmission.

substance abuse. Use of psychoactive drugs that poses significant hazards to health and interferes with social, occupational, psychological, or physical functioning.

substance dependence. *Physical* dependence is identified by the inability to stop using a substance despite attempts to do so; a continual use of the substance despite adverse consequences; a developing tolerance; and the development of withdrawal symptoms upon cessation or decreased intake. *Psychological* dependence is said to exist when a substance is perceived by the user to be necessary to maintain an optimal state of personal well-being, interpersonal relations, or skill performance.

substitution therapy. The use of various medications to decrease the intensity of symptoms in an individual who is withdrawing from, or experiencing the effects of excessive use of, substances.

subsystems. The smaller units of which a system is composed. In family systems theory, the subsystems are composed of husband-wife, parent-child(ren), or sibling-sibling.

sundowning. A phenomenon in dementia in which the symptoms seem to worsen in the late afternoon and evening.

superego. One of the three elements of the personality identified by Freud that represents the conscience and the culturally determined restrictions that are placed on an individual.

suppression. The voluntary blocking from one's awareness of unpleasant feelings and experiences.

surrogate. One who serves as a substitute figure for another.

symbiotic relationship. A type of "psychic fusion" that occurs between two people; it is unhealthy in that severe anxiety is generated in either or both if separation is indicated. A symbiotic relationship is normal between infant and mother.

sympathy. The actual sharing of another's thoughts and behaviors. Differs from empathy, in that with empathy one experiences an objective understanding of what another is feeling, rather than actually sharing those feelings.

synapse. The junction between two neurons. The small space between the axon terminals of one neuron and the cell body or dendrites of another is called the synaptic cleft.

syphilis. A sexually transmitted disorder caused by the spirochete *T. pallidum* and resulting in a chancre on the skin or mucous membranes of the sexual organs. If left untreated, may go systemic. End-stage disease can have profound effects, such as blindness or insanity.

systematic desensitization. A treatment for phobias in which the individual is taught to relax and then asked to imagine various components of the phobic stimulus on a graded hierarchy, moving from that which produces the least fear to that which produces the most.

T

T-4 lymphocyte. The white blood cell that is the primary target of HIV. These cells are destroyed by the virus, causing the striking depletion of T4 cells associated with HIV infection.

tangentiality. The inability to get to the point of a story. The speaker introduces many unrelated topics, until the original topic of discussion is lost.

tardive dyskinesia. Syndrome of symptoms characterized by bizarre facial and tongue movements, a stiff neck, and difficulty swallowing. It may occur as an adverse effect of long-term therapy with some antipsychotic medications.

technical expert. Peplau's term for one who understands various professional devices and possesses the clinical skills necessary to perform the interventions that are in the best interest of the client.

temperament. A set of inborn personality characteristics that influence an individual's manner of reacting to the environment and ultimately influence his or her developmental progression.

territoriality. The innate tendency of individuals to own space. Individuals lay claim to areas around them as their own. This phenomenon can have an influence on interpersonal communication.

tertiary prevention. Health care that is directed toward reduction of the residual effects associated with severe or chronic physical or mental illness.

therapeutic group. Differs from group therapy in that there is a lesser degree of theoretical foundation. Focus is on group relations, interactions between group members, and the consideration of a selected issue. Leaders of therapeutic groups do not require the degree of educational preparation required of group therapy leaders.

thought-stopping technique. A self-taught technique that an individual uses each time he or she wishes to eliminate intrusive or negative, unwanted thoughts from awareness.

time out. An aversive stimulus or punishment during which the individual is removed from the environment where the unacceptable behavior is being exhibited.

token economy. In behavior modification, a type of contracting in which the reinforcers for desired behaviors are presented in the form of tokens, which may then be exchanged for designated privileges.

tort. The violation of a civil law in which an individual has been wronged. In a tort action, one party asserts that wrongful conduct on the part of the other has caused harm, and compensation for harm suffered is sought.

Transmission-Based Precautions. Guidelines established by the Centers for Disease Control (CDC) designed for a patient documented or suspected to be infected or colonized with highly transmissible or epidemiologically important pathogens for which additional precautions beyond standard precautions are needed to interrupt transmission in hospitals. There are three types of Transmission-Based Precautions: airborne precautions, droplet precautions, and contact precautions.

transsexualism. A disorder of gender identity or gender dysphoria (unhappiness or dissatisfaction with one's gender) of the most extreme variety. The individual, despite having the anatomical characteristics of a given gender, has the self-perception of being of the opposite gender, and may seek to have gender changed through surgical intervention.

transvestic fetishism. Recurrent urges and sexually arousing fantasies involving dressing in the clothes of the opposite gender.

triangles. A three-person emotional configuration which is considered the basic building block of the family system. When anxiety becomes too great between two family members, a third person is brought in to form a triangle. Triangles are dysfunctional in that they offer relief from anxiety through diversion rather than through resolution of the issue.

trichotillomania. The recurrent failure to resist impulses to pull out one's own hair.

type A personality. The personality characteristics attributed to individuals prone to coronary heart disease, including excessive competitive drive, chronic sense of time urgency, easy anger, aggressiveness, excessive ambition, and inability to enjoy leisure time.

type B personality. The personality characteristics attributed to individuals who are *not* prone to coronary heart disease; includes characteristics such as ability to perform even under pressure but without the competitive drive and constant sense of time urgency experienced by the type A personality. Type Bs can enjoy their leisure time without feeling guilty, and they are much less impulsive than type A individuals; that is, they think things through before making decisions.

type C personality. The personality characteristics attributed to the cancer-prone individual. Includes characteristics such as suppression of anger, calm, passive, puts the needs of others before their own, but holds resentment toward others for perceived "wrongs."

tyramine. An amino acid found in aged cheeses or other aged, overripe, and fermented foods; broad beans; pickled herring; beef or chicken liver; preserved meats; beer and wine; yeast products; chocolate; caffeinated drinks; canned figs; sour cream; yogurt; soy sauce; and some over-the-counter cold medications and diet pills. If foods high in tyramine content are consumed while an individual is taking monoamine oxidase inhibitors, a potentially life-threatening syndrome called hypertensive crisis can result.

U

unconditional positive regard. Carl Rogers' term for the respect and dignity of an individual regardless of his or her unacceptable behavior.

undoing. A mechanism used to symbolically negate or cancel out a previous action or experience that one finds intolerable.

universality. One curative factor of groups (identified by Yalom) in which individuals realize that they are not alone in a problem and in the thoughts and feelings they are experiencing. Anxiety is relieved by the support and understanding of others in the group who share similar experiences.

utilitarianism. The ethical theory that espouses "the greatest happiness for the greatest number." Under this theory, action would be taken based on the end results that will produce the most good (happiness) for the most people.

V

vaginismus. Involuntary constriction of the outer one third of the vagina that prevents penile insertion and intercourse.

values. Personal beliefs about the truth, beauty, or worth of a thought, object, or behavior that influence an individual's actions.

values clarification. A process of self-discovery by which people identify their personal values and their value rankings. This process increases awareness about why individuals behave in certain ways.

voyeurism. Recurrent urges and sexually arousing fantasies involving the act of observing unsuspecting people, usually strangers, who are either naked, in the process of disrobing, or engaging in sexual activity.

W

waxy flexibility. A condition by which the individual with schizophrenia passively yields all movable parts of the body to any efforts made at placing them in certain positions.

Wernicke's encephalopathy. A brain disorder caused by thiamine deficiency and characterized by visual disturbances, ataxia, somnolence, stupor, and, without thiamine replacement, death.

word salad. A group of words that are put together in a random fashion without any logical connection.

Y

yin and yang. The fundamental concept of Asian health practices. Yin and yang are opposite forces of energy such as negative/positive, dark/light, cold/hot, hard/soft, and feminine/masculine. Food, medicines, and herbs are classified according to their yin and yang properties and are used to restore a balance, thereby restoring health.

yoga. A system of beliefs and practices, the ultimate goal of which is to unite the human soul with the universal spirit. In Western countries, yoga uses body postures, along with meditation and breathing exercises, to achieve a balanced, disciplined workout that releases muscle tension, tones the internal organs, and energizes the mind, body, and spirit, so that natural healing can occur.

splitting. A primitive ego defense mechanism in which the person is unable to integrate and accept both positive and negative feelings. In their view, people—including themselves—and life situations are either all good or all bad. This trait is common in borderline personality disorder.

standard precautions. Guidelines established by the Centers for Disease Control (CDC) designed to reduce the risk of transmission of pathogens from moist body substances. Standard precautions apply to blood; all body fluids, secretions, and excretions *except sweat;* nonintact skin; and mucous membranes.

statutory law. A law that has been enacted by legislative bodies, such as a county or city council, state legislature, or the U.S. Congress.

statutory rape. Unlawful intercourse between a man over age 16 and a female under the age of consent. The man can be arrested for statutory rape even when the interaction has occurred between consenting individuals.

stereotyping. The process of classifying all individuals from the same culture or ethnic group as identical.

stimulus generalization. The process by which a conditioned response is elicited from all stimuli *similar* to the one from which the response was learned.

store-front clinic. Establishments that have been converted into clinics that serve the homeless population.

stress. A state of disequilibrium that occurs when there is a disharmony between demands occurring within an individual's internal or external environment and his or her ability to cope with those demands.

stress management. Various methods used by individuals to reduce tension and other maladaptive responses to stress in their lives; includes relaxation exercises, physical exercise, music, mental imagery, or any other technique that is successful for a person.

stressor. A demand from within an individual's internal or external environment that elicits a physiological and/or psychological response.

sublimation. The rechanneling of personally and/or socially unacceptable drives or impulses into activities that are more tolerable and constructive.

subluxation. The term used in chiropractic medicine to describe vertebrae in the spinal column that have become displaced, possibly pressing on nerves and interfering with normal nerve transmission.

substance abuse. Use of psychoactive drugs that poses significant hazards to health and interferes with social, occupational, psychological, or physical functioning.

substance dependence. *Physical* dependence is identified by the inability to stop using a substance despite attempts to do so; a continual use of the substance despite adverse consequences; a developing tolerance; and the development of withdrawal symptoms upon cessation or decreased intake. *Psychological* dependence is said to exist when a substance is perceived by the user to be necessary to maintain an optimal state of personal well-being, interpersonal relations, or skill performance.

substitution therapy. The use of various medications to decrease the intensity of symptoms in an individual who is withdrawing from, or experiencing the effects of excessive use of, substances.

subsystems. The smaller units of which a system is composed. In family systems theory, the subsystems are composed of husband-wife, parent-child(ren), or sibling-sibling.

sundowning. A phenomenon in dementia in which the symptoms seem to worsen in the late afternoon and evening.

superego. One of the three elements of the personality identified by Freud that represents the conscience and the culturally determined restrictions that are placed on an individual.

suppression. The voluntary blocking from one's awareness of unpleasant feelings and experiences.

surrogate. One who serves as a substitute figure for another.

symbiotic relationship. A type of "psychic fusion" that occurs between two people; it is unhealthy in that severe anxiety is generated in either or both if separation is indicated. A symbiotic relationship is normal between infant and mother.

sympathy. The actual sharing of another's thoughts and behaviors. Differs from empathy, in that with empathy one experiences an objective understanding of what another is feeling, rather than actually sharing those feelings.

synapse. The junction between two neurons. The small space between the axon terminals of one neuron and the cell body or dendrites of another is called the synaptic cleft.

syphilis. A sexually transmitted disorder caused by the spirochete *T. pallidum* and resulting in a chancre on the skin or mucous membranes of the sexual organs. If left untreated, may go systemic. End-stage disease can have profound effects, such as blindness or insanity.

systematic desensitization. A treatment for phobias in which the individual is taught to relax and then asked to imagine various components of the phobic stimulus on a graded hierarchy, moving from that which produces the least fear to that which produces the most.

T

T-4 lymphocyte. The white blood cell that is the primary target of HIV. These cells are destroyed by the virus, causing the striking depletion of T4 cells associated with HIV infection.

tangentiality. The inability to get to the point of a story. The speaker introduces many unrelated topics, until the original topic of discussion is lost.

tardive dyskinesia. Syndrome of symptoms characterized by bizarre facial and tongue movements, a stiff neck, and difficulty swallowing. It may occur as an adverse effect of long-term therapy with some antipsychotic medications.

technical expert. Peplau's term for one who understands various professional devices and possesses the clinical skills necessary to perform the interventions that are in the best interest of the client.

temperament. A set of inborn personality characteristics that influence an individual's manner of reacting to the environment and ultimately influence his or her developmental progression.

territoriality. The innate tendency of individuals to own space. Individuals lay claim to areas around them as their own. This phenomenon can have an influence on interpersonal communication.

tertiary prevention. Health care that is directed toward reduction of the residual effects associated with severe or chronic physical or mental illness.

therapeutic group. Differs from group therapy in that there is a lesser degree of theoretical foundation. Focus is on group relations, interactions between group members, and the consideration of a selected issue. Leaders of therapeutic groups do not require the degree of educational preparation required of group therapy leaders.

thought-stopping technique. A self-taught technique that an individual uses each time he or she wishes to eliminate intrusive or negative, unwanted thoughts from awareness.

time out. An aversive stimulus or punishment during which the individual is removed from the environment where the unacceptable behavior is being exhibited.

token economy. In behavior modification, a type of contracting in which the reinforcers for desired behaviors are presented in the form of tokens, which may then be exchanged for designated privileges.

tort. The violation of a civil law in which an individual has been wronged. In a tort action, one party asserts that wrongful conduct on the part of the other has caused harm, and compensation for harm suffered is sought.

Transmission-Based Precautions. Guidelines established by the Centers for Disease Control (CDC) designed for a patient documented or suspected to be infected or colonized with highly transmissible or epidemiologically important pathogens for which additional precautions beyond standard precautions are needed to interrupt transmission in hospitals. There are three types of Transmission-Based Precautions: airborne precautions, droplet precautions, and contact precautions.

transsexualism. A disorder of gender identity or gender dysphoria (unhappiness or dissatisfaction with one's gender) of the most extreme variety. The individual, despite having the anatomical characteristics of a given gender, has the self-perception of being of the opposite gender, and may seek to have gender changed through surgical intervention.

transvestic fetishism. Recurrent urges and sexually arousing fantasies involving dressing in the clothes of the opposite gender.

triangles. A three-person emotional configuration which is considered the basic building block of the family system. When anxiety becomes too great between two family members, a third person is brought in to form a triangle. Triangles are dysfunctional in that they offer relief from anxiety through diversion rather than through resolution of the issue.

trichotillomania. The recurrent failure to resist impulses to pull out one's own hair.

type A personality. The personality characteristics attributed to individuals prone to coronary heart disease, including excessive competitive drive, chronic sense of time urgency, easy anger, aggressiveness, excessive ambition, and inability to enjoy leisure time.

type B personality. The personality characteristics attributed to individuals who are *not* prone to coronary heart disease; includes characteristics such as ability to perform even under pressure but without the competitive drive and constant sense of time urgency experienced by the type A personality. Type Bs can enjoy their leisure time without feeling guilty, and they are much less impulsive than type A individuals; that is, they think things through before making decisions.

type C personality. The personality characteristics attributed to the cancer-prone individual. Includes characteristics such as suppression of anger, calm, passive, puts the needs of others before their own, but holds resentment toward others for perceived "wrongs."

tyramine. An amino acid found in aged cheeses or other aged, overripe, and fermented foods; broad beans; pickled herring; beef or chicken liver; preserved meats; beer and wine; yeast products; chocolate; caffeinated drinks; canned figs; sour cream; yogurt; soy sauce; and some over-the-counter cold medications and diet pills. If foods high in tyramine content are consumed while an individual is taking monoamine oxidase inhibitors, a potentially life-threatening syndrome called hypertensive crisis can result.

U

unconditional positive regard. Carl Rogers' term for the respect and dignity of an individual regardless of his or her unacceptable behavior.

undoing. A mechanism used to symbolically negate or cancel out a previous action or experience that one finds intolerable.

universality. One curative factor of groups (identified by Yalom) in which individuals realize that they are not alone in a problem and in the thoughts and feelings they are experiencing. Anxiety is relieved by the support and understanding of others in the group who share similar experiences.

utilitarianism. The ethical theory that espouses "the greatest happiness for the greatest number." Under this theory, action would be taken based on the end results that will produce the most good (happiness) for the most people.

V

vaginismus. Involuntary constriction of the outer one third of the vagina that prevents penile insertion and intercourse.

values. Personal beliefs about the truth, beauty, or worth of a thought, object, or behavior that influence an individual's actions.

values clarification. A process of self-discovery by which people identify their personal values and their value rankings. This process increases awareness about why individuals behave in certain ways.

voyeurism. Recurrent urges and sexually arousing fantasies involving the act of observing unsuspecting people, usually strangers, who are either naked, in the process of disrobing, or engaging in sexual activity.

W

waxy flexibility. A condition by which the individual with schizophrenia passively yields all movable parts of the body to any efforts made at placing them in certain positions.

Wernicke's encephalopathy. A brain disorder caused by thiamine deficiency and characterized by visual disturbances, ataxia, somnolence, stupor, and, without thiamine replacement, death.

word salad. A group of words that are put together in a random fashion without any logical connection.

Y

yin and yang. The fundamental concept of Asian health practices. Yin and yang are opposite forces of energy such as negative/positive, dark/light, cold/hot, hard/soft, and feminine/masculine. Food, medicines, and herbs are classified according to their yin and yang properties and are used to restore a balance, thereby restoring health.

yoga. A system of beliefs and practices, the ultimate goal of which is to unite the human soul with the universal spirit. In Western countries, yoga uses body postures, along with meditation and breathing exercises, to achieve a balanced, disciplined workout that releases muscle tension, tones the internal organs, and energizes the mind, body, and spirit, so that natural healing can occur.

An *f* following a page number indicates a figure; a *t* indicates a table.